Davis's
NCLEX-RN® Success

Money
Back Guarantee

If you are a graduate of a nursing program accredited in the United States, take the NCLEX-RN® for the first time, and do not pass after using *Davis's NCLEX-RN® Success,* return the book to **F. A. Davis Company, Customer Service, 404-420 N. 2nd Street, Philadelphia, PA 19123.** Enclose your original receipt for purchase of the book and copies of your official test results notification and your certification of graduation. We will refund the price you paid for the book. If you have any questions, please call 800-323-3555.

NCLEX-RN® is a registered trademark of National Council of State Boards of Nursing, Inc. (NCSBN).

Davis's
NCLEX-RN® Success

Second Edition

Edited by
Sally Lambert Lagerquist, RN, MS

Written by
Sally Lambert Lagerquist, RN, MS
Former Instructor of Undergraduate, Graduate, and Continuing Education in Nursing,
School of Nursing,
University of California, San Francisco,
President, Review for Nurses, Inc., and RN Tapes Company,
San Francisco, California

Janice Lloyd McMillin, RN, MSN, EdD
Lecturer in Perinatal Nursing, Division of Nursing, California State University, Sacramento
Staff Nurse, Labor and Delivery, Methodist Hospital, Sacramento

Robyn Marchal Nelson, DNSc, RN
Chair and Professor, Division of Nursing, California State University, Sacramento

Kathleen E. Snider, RN, MSN, CNS
Professor of Nursing, Los Angeles Valley College,
Valley Glen, California

 F.A. Davis Company • Philadelphia

F. A. Davis Company
1915 Arch Street
Philadelphia, PA 19103
www.fadavis.com

Printed in the United States of America

Last digit indicates print number: 10 9 8 7 6 5 4 3 2 1

Acquisitions Editor: Robert G. Martone
Developmental Editor: Alan Sorkowitz
Manager of Art & Design: Carolyn O'Brien

As new scientific information becomes available through basic and clinical research, recommended treatments and drug therapies undergo changes. The author(s) and publisher have done everything possible to make this book accurate, up to date, and in accord with accepted standards at the time of publication. The author(s), editors, and publisher are not responsible for errors or omissions or for consequences from application of the book, and make no warranty, expressed or implied, in regard to the contents of the book. Any practice described in this book should be applied by the reader in accordance with professional standards of care used in regard to the unique circumstances that may apply in each situation. The reader is advised always to check product information (package inserts) for changes and new information regarding dose and contraindications before administering any drug. Caution is especially urged when using new or infrequently ordered drugs.

Library of Congress Cataloging-in-Publication Data

Davis's NCLEX-RN success / edited by Sally Lambert Lagerquist ;
  written by Sally Lambert Lagerquist ... [et al.]. — 2nd ed.
    p. ; cm.
  Includes bibliographical references and index.
  ISBN 0-8036-1242-7 (pbk. : alk. paper)
  1. Nursing—Examinations, questions, etc. 2. National Council
Licensure Examination for Registered Nurses—Study guides.
I. Lagerquist, Sally L. II. Title: NCLEX-RN® success.
  [DNLM] 1. Nursing—Examination Questions. 2. Nursing—Outlines.
WY 18.2 D2651 2006:
RT55.D386 2006
610.73'076—dc22

2005011214

I dedicate this book —

To my husband, Tom —

You are a course in Enthusiasm 101, exactly what I needed in easing the stressful confluence of roles as a parent, as a family member, and as the author/editor of the latest seven nursing books. Your ability to search the day for what is beautiful, marvel at ordinary "stuff," and embrace all with kindness, patience, and harmony was my beacon.

Your "broad shoulders" and "strong back" qualities have sustained as well as inspired me to feel the joy of achievement.

The wonder and wisdom of you, your gentle yet strong, caring ways are boundless.

You are a gift, a *makana*, in the Hawaiian sense.

To our daughter, Elana —

You have a remarkable, beautiful ability to put yourself in the mind, heart, and soul of another. Your compassion has taken me on my own journey of greater understanding, and the celebration of sharing motherhood has brought a healing touch to my life.

I am so proud of your and Dan's loving ways in raising Kaya. I am equally proud and excited to see your creative arts team projects be so rewarding. Your enthusiasm and talents glow!

To Dan —

You are our son-in-law who has become deeply respected and appreciated not only for your incredible ability to meet the challenge of making our joint electronic projects a success but also for reaching out, offering me a "compass" with a balanced perspective, and fostering good humor with your quick insightful wit.

To Kaya, our first grandchild —

May your happy spirit, your love of books, music, and dance, your amazing language and cognitive development continue to delight us all.

Being with you two days a week during your first two years has brought us the joys of participating in your growth and development.

A wish for your future — may your boundless curiosity and joyfulness touch the lives of those around you so that you continue to make a difference.

To our son, Kalen —

As you move on, may your adventure take you on your own journey of great joy in achieving new milestones—both professionally and personally (as you celebrate your first anniversary with Lara).

I look back with love and appreciation for the years of your devotion to us as our family member as well as for your many significant contributions (marketing, sales, management, and electronics) to making Review for Nurses what it is today.

To my mother, Sonia Lambert —

Your ninety-second birthday year was a gift for us all as we celebrated four generations of being together. *L'chaim!*

To Bonnie Bergstrom — my friend, our very own special editor who understands what I'm trying to say and says it better! And who can even read my writing!

Contact with you is always a gift. This is our seventh book together! And it would not have become a reality without you—once again!

There is no one quite like you when it comes to giving "your all," your devotion to excellence, your editing expertise, your sense of balance, and your kindness and patience with us all.

You built and sustained a "road map" for all of us authors to help us navigate through the complexities of this book—from conception to delivery, from infancy to coming-of-age, from coping with changes (and delays!), to your determination to resolve some of our manuscript preparation problems (both acute and chronic).

The outcome—this book—is a grateful tribute to you, to be used by those who are entering, returning to, or staying in the nursing profession.

—Sally Lambert Lagerquist

To my husband Mike, my best friend and humorist, who kept me from taking myself too seriously. Thank you for turning off my laptop when I was too tired or stressed to do it myself. I am blessed by God with your endless love and devotion. Thanks for sticking with me through "the dark years." Thank you for pretending to be enthralled by my fascinating nursing stories. To my daughter, Rachel, who gives me joy. I am so proud of the woman and future nurse you are becoming. To my son, Justin, I hope you find your path in life; you have so much potential!

To my parents, John and La Verne Mahony, who expected the best in me and knew I had the talent and ability to achieve my goals.

To my big brother, John, for the life lessons including selling me "H_2O" from the tap, and my brother Brian, who has been making God and all of heaven laugh for the last 10 years.

I am forever indebted to my mentors, Dr. Mollyn Bohnen and Dr. Louise Timmer. Thank you for your wisdom and encouragement. I can only hope to fill your huge shoes.

To my nursing students, whose enthusiasm and joy in learning inspire me. Each time I see the excitement of a nursing student participating in a birth for the first time, I recognize myself and remember why I became a perinatal nurse. I have never grown tired of my choice to be a nurse. Be proud of being a nurse, and never forget "where you came from" when you have the responsibility of mentoring the next generation of nurses.

Lastly, I thank the Lord every day for His marvelous grace abundantly poured upon me.

—Jan McMillin

The need for nurses has never been greater than it is now. It has been said that we face a public health crisis when there is a shortage of qualified professional nurses. This book is dedicated to the future of professional nursing — those of you who have chosen nursing and who are preparing for the licensure examination. May this book assist you in preparing for the exam that will enable you to offer a lifetime of professional service to others and in return receive personal rewards unmatched by many career choices.

My husband Dean, our daughters Tina and Kelly, their husbands Bob and Ben, my mother Patty, and my most precious grandsons Stirling and Sage will have better lives because of the contributions you will make to the health of your communities, and potentially to their personal health. Thank you for caring — thank you for choosing nursing!

—Robyn M. Nelson

This book is gratefully dedicated:

To Terry Oleson, PhD. Thank you for your endless patience and guidance in helping me find the answers to my life's questions.

To my nursing instructors, religious and secular, who taught me that I wanted to be a pediatric nurse and had the "right stuff" with which to do it.

To my pediatric patients and their families who taught me how to be a pediatric nurse.

To my pediatric nursing students who taught me how to teach pediatric nursing.

To my friends and colleagues in the pediatric community who, with their combined experience and wisdom, gave me insight into the writing of pediatric content and taught me that there is always a "light at the end of the tunnel" and that this book was not an everlasting project.

And, finally, to Steevio Bardakjian, my resident computer genius and guru who taught me the mysteries of the computer world.

Thank You!

—Kathy Snider

Sally Lambert Lagerquist, RN, MS, is the author and editor of four editions of *Practice Questions and Answers for NCLEX-RN*, published by Review for Nurses Tapes Co.; *How to Pass Nursing Exams,* published by Review Press; four editions of Addison Wesley's *Nursing Examination Reviews* (1977–1991); four books for NURSENOTES series: *Psychiatric-Mental Health, Maternal-Newborn, Pediatrics, Medical-Surgical,* published by Lippincott; Little, Brown's *NCLEX-RN Examination Review,* and Little, Brown's *Nursing Q&A: Critical-Thinking Exercises,* published by Little, Brown and Company. She is president and course coordinator of Review for Nurses, Inc. She has coordinated RN licensure exam review courses on campuses nationwide since 1976. She is presently a lecturer on test-taking techniques at workshops held for graduating senior nursing students. She has produced and developed the **NCLEX-RN Board Game** and audio tapes, CD-ROMs, DVDs, and video tapes on Nursing Review and Successful Test-Taking Techniques for Nurses. She originated, developed, and has presented national **satellite telecourses** for NCLEX-RN review since June 1989. She has developed an **online** NCLEX-RN® review course and an online **Pre-NCLEX-RN®** Assessment Series for Success (PASS™) to help candidates assess and fill in gaps in knowledge as well as increase their test-taking skills. She has been a marriage, family, and child counselor and is a member of Sigma Theta Tau. She has been a faculty member at the University of California at San Francisco School of Nursing for over 10 years, where she also received her BS and MS degrees.

Janice Lloyd McMillin, RN, MSN, EdD, is a lecturer in perinatal nursing in the Division of Nursing at California State University, Sacramento. In addition, she currently works in Labor and Delivery at Methodist hospital in Sacramento. She has been a lecturer for several years for Review for Nurses, Inc. She received her BA in Biology, BS in Nursing, and MS in Nursing from CSU, Sacramento. She completed her doctorate at the University of San Francisco. Her dissertation study examines the transition experiences of first-year labor and delivery nurses. She has been a perinatal nurse for over 20 years.

Robyn M. Nelson, DNSc, RN, is chairperson and professor in the Division of Nursing at California State University, Sacramento. Additionally, she currently teaches research and issues and ethics at the graduate level over distance education and the Web. She received her BS in Nursing from Loma Linda University, her MS from Boston University, and a Doctor of Nursing Science degree from the University of California, San Francisco. In addition to *Davis's NCLEX-RN® Success,* she was coauthor of NURSENOTES: *Medical-Surgical Nursing* (Lippincott) and a contributor to *Nursing Q and A* (Lippincott) and has developed a number of audio and visual aids for students preparing for the licensure examination. Dr. Nelson has been a lecturer for Review for Nurses, Inc., for 20 years, both at on-site national review courses and as one of the faculty for the "first ever" nationally televised satellite review course that was offered for 7 years. She holds memberships in Sigma Theta Tau International, ANA, ANA/California, and Phi Kappa Phi. Dr. Nelson is a member of the Bioethics Committee of Sutter Community Medical Center and on the boards of the Association of California Nurse Leaders (ACNL); Blood Source, Northern California's leader in blood banking; and *Nurse Week* (California). In January 2006, Dr. Nelson will assume the position of Dean, College of Health and Human Services for Touro University–Nevada in Las Vegas.

Kathy Snider, RN, MSN, CNS, has been a pediatric nurse for over 35 years and has a broad range of clinical and educational experience. She received her diploma in nursing from Saint Vincent's College of Nursing, Los Angeles; her baccalaureate in nursing from Mount Saint Mary's College, Los Angeles; and her master's degree in nursing from California State University, Los Angeles. She has been teaching pediatric nursing since 1976 in diploma, associate of arts, and baccalaureate nursing programs. She began teaching national licensure examination reviews in the mid-1980s and has remained active in that area ever since. She is a contributing author to two editions of *Davis's NCLEX-RN® Success* book and to Lippincott's NURSENOTES: *Pediatrics, Core Content At-A-Glance.* She also served as a reviewer for the 1996 Little, Brown's *Nursing Q & A Critical-Thinking Exercises* book. Kathy is currently a professor of nursing at Los Angeles Valley College, Valley Glen, California, and teaches pediatric nursing, theory, and clinical to associate of arts nursing students. She is an active member in the American and California Nurses Associations, in national and local chapters of the Association of Pediatric Nurse Practitioners, and in the Los Angeles County School Nurses Association. She has served as a District Academic Senator for the Los Angeles Community College District and is currently serving as an Academic Senator at Los Angeles Valley College. In 1999 she received the "One of Our Own" award from the National Association of Pediatric Nurse Associates and Practitioners, Los Angeles Chapter, for service and excellence in pediatric nursing.

Contributing Authors to This Edition

Debra Brady, RN, MS
(Special reviewer, contributing author to Unit 7)
Assistant Professor, Division of Nursing,
California State University, Sacramento

Mary St. Jonn Seed, RN, PhD
(Contributor of selected sections)
Associate Professor, School of Nursing, Department of
Community Mental Health, University of San Francisco
San Francisco, California

NEW TEST ITEM WRITERS FOR THIS EDITION

Debra Brady, RN, MS
Assistant Professor, Division of Nursing, California State
University, Sacramento

Christine Hooper, RN, EdD
Associate Professor, San Jose State University School of
Nursing,
San Jose, California

Cheryl Osborne, RN, EdD
Professor, Division of Nursing, Director of Gerontology
Program,
California State University, Sacramento

Carolyn Van Couwenberghe, RN, PhD
Professor, Division of Nursing,
California State University, Sacramento

Contributing Authors and Test Item Writers for the Disk in Previous Editions

Irene M. Bobak, RN, PhD, FAAN
Professor Emerita, Women's Health and Maternity Nursing, San Francisco State University, San Francisco

Geraldine C. Colombraro, RN, MA, PhD
Assistant Dean for Administration
Lienhard School of Nursing, Pace University, Pleasantville, New York

Eileen Hackett, RN, MA
Professor of Nursing and Assistant Director of Nursing, College of the Desert, Palm Desert, California

Rosemary J. Mann, RN, JD, PhD
Assistant Professor, San Jose State University School of Nursing, San Jose, California

Bobbi Morrison, ARNP, MN, PhD
Women's Health Nurse Practitioner; Instructor, Intercollegiate Center for Nursing Education, Washington State University College of Nursing, Spokane, Washington

Lynda Schweid, MS, RN
Assistant Dean, Health Sciences, Contra Costa College, San Pablo, California

Janice Horman Stecchi, RN, EdD
Dean Emerita, College of Health Professions, University of Massachusetts, Lowell, Massachusetts

Acknowledgments

A special note of appreciation to Carina Mifuel, who single-handedly and skillfully filled the many roles needed to keep Review for Nurses, Inc. (our nursing seminar company) going at full speed while I worked on this book for over a year! You were our Registrar, Conference Coordinator, Special Projects Director, and Product and Office Manager while at the same time doing marketing and on-going projects for our Web site. I deeply appreciate your energy, caring, and willingness to see a need and fill it. Your unique contribution was your upbeat spirit and *always* being available to us. You had the gift of making me feel valued and that this book was important to you also.

Thank you also to Alan Sorkowitz, Bob Butler, and the editorial and production people of F.A.Davis for their help in shepherding this book through its labor-intensive phases of manuscript preparation, copy-editing, proofing, and backtracking a number of times with changes as we needed to make this second edition the best possible and unique resource for nurses preparing to take and pass the NCLEX-RN® licensure exam.

What's New and Different

- New! This book and its accompanying disk both have questions in ALTERNATE ITEM FORMAT.
- Totally **new Pre Test** with 500 questions, each with rationale and unique test-taking tips.
- Newly expanded and reorganized **management of care** section including: *delegation*, establishing *priorities*, *HIPAA* rules, *emergency response plan* (fire safety and preparedness).
- **Infection control:** animal-borne diseases (SARS, West Nile virus, mad cow, monkeypox, Lyme, rabies, salmonella).
- **Bioterrorism agents and associated syndromes** (anthrax, botulism, plague, smallpox, tularemia, Ebola, Lassa, hantavirus).
- **Herbal medicines:** dietary supplements and herbal products used for psychiatric conditions; herbs and potential dangers.
- Complementary and alternative therapies.
- Pediatric safety and injury prevention chart.
- Updated CPR.
- **Calculations and conversions** in medication administration.
- An index to help you find questions coded for *cognitive level* of difficulty and the four client needs and six client subneeds categories based on NCLEX-RN® official Test Plan.
- New conditions covered: pheochromocytoma, Guillain-Barré, Raynaud's, obesity.
- All new questions in *The Older Adult* unit.
- New *Clinical Pathway in Pediatrics* (emergency appendectomy).

We are very pleased that you have selected our book to help you on your path to success on NCLEX-RN®.

Our aim is to lead you all the way, to have PASSING NCLEX-RN® MADE EASY for you—the *first-time test-taker*, the *international* nurse, and the *repeat test-taker.*

With a conceptual framework based on the components of the current NCLEX-RN® Test Plan (four client needs and their six subcategories), this book differs significantly from other nursing review books. **It is the only nursing review book that thoroughly covers the content in the current NCLEX-RN® Test Plan and has a test tip for each of the more than 2500 questions!**

Each unit incorporates all the components of the most current test plan. In addition, **Unit 3** specifically includes content that focuses on **Safe, Effective Care Environment** (with **Management of Care**). **Units 4** and **5** emphasize **Health Promotion and Maintenance** (*growth and development, prevention and early detection of disease,* and **Safety and Infection Control**). **Unit 6** focuses specifically on **Psychosocial Integrity** (*coping and adaptation*). **Units 7, 8, 9,** and **10** emphasize **Physiological Integrity** (with **Unit 7** specifically addressing **Basic Care and Comfort** and **Physiological Adaptation**) and cover additional aspects of

Infection Control and prevention and early detection of disease. **Unit 9** is on *Nutrition and Diet Therapy;* **Unit 10** is devoted to **Pharmacological and Parenteral Therapies;** and **Unit 11** specifically emphasizes **Reduction of Risk Potential.**

In addition, **Unit 2** is a unique unit that addresses the needs of **international nurses** and **repeat test-takers;** and **Unit 8** addresses the special *needs of the Older Adult.*

To locate where in the book you will find the *theory* and *practice questions* for each of the above-named subcategories of client needs that are tested on the exam, see **Appendixes C, D,** and **E.**

Proven Results

This is the only review book for NCLEX-RN® that has evolved from and been tested with over 300,000 NCLEX-RN® candidates who have taken our national nursing exam review courses over the last **35 years and passed!** These courses emphasize a comprehensive review of *commonalities* in client care throughout the life span and in a variety of clinical settings. The content, the framework, the sequence of topics, the test-taking guidelines, and the practice exam questions and answers in this book have been tested during the last 35 years with *examination candidates* who have passed the RN licensure exam with highly successful results. **This gives the material an authenticity and relevance that is difficult to attain any other way.**

Conceptual Framework

The conceptual framework of this book concentrates on nursing concerns for *client needs* and the essential requirements for safe, effective, competent nursing care. The text emphasizes *practical application* of clinically relevant data. Each unit is organized in terms of the eight areas of human functions (which are subtopics of the client needs): (1) Protective; (2) Sensory-Perceptual; (3) Comfort, Rest, Activity, and Mobility; (4) Nutrition; (5) Growth and Development; (6) Fluid-Gas Transport; (7) Psychosocial-Cultural; and (8) Elimination functions. (See **Appendix H** for definitions of these key terms and **Appendixes I** and **J** for an index to content [theory] in these key categories in the **text** and **test questions.**) Separate units emphasize the content areas of **nutrition; pharmacology; common diagnostic procedures, treatments, and nursing care;** and **management of care,** including **ethical and legal aspects in nursing.** A separate unit features the *older adult.*

Special Features

There are many special features in this *abundantly illustrated* book (over 190 charts, tables, and illustrations) that make it **stand out from all other nursing review books.** The unique features that help you prepare for exams are: **test-taking tips** for **each of the questions,** an *expanded* section on **memory aids** (**Appendix N**), lists of **common abbreviations and clinical signs** (**Appendixes L** and **M**), and a **one-of-a-kind** index to guide you to where in the book you will find the theory (topics) and practice questions that specifically relate to the official NCLEX-RN® Test Plan (**Appendixes C, E,** and **K**). These features provide quick, easy, and interesting ways to review. **This is the only NCLEX-RN® review book that has** 14 detailed examples of *Clinical Pathways* (also known as *Critical Pathways* or *Patient Care Management Plans*). In the **Orientation** section of **Unit 1,** you'll also find **study tips and relaxation exercises,** along with memorizing ideas.

Other Features

- A practice **computer test** (CD-ROM) for self-assessment and familiarization with the NCLEX-RN® computer testing format now includes **test-taking tips with each answer.**
- Many **easy-to-find and easy-to-use tables** summarize information for *quick* review and emphasize nursing responsibilities in *a visual way.*
- **Boxed lab data, diagnostic tests** indicated by a ✎, **drug information** indicated by a ⬤, **diets** indicated by a 🍴, **position** indicated by a ◥, **standard precautions** indicated by a ✚, **mnemonic memory aids** indicated by a 💡, **nursing process** indicated by a ◆, and hands-on nursing care indicated by a ▶, in the margin for quick reference. Also, **nursing diagnoses, positions, diets,** and **nursing procedures** are *italicized* for visual reinforcement.
- Easy-to-find **content divisions** are marked with black page tabs at the outer margin of each page.
- Unique **indexes to content and test questions** related to **six specific subcategories** of **client needs** (**Appendixes C** and **E**) and **four general (broad) client needs** (**Appendix D**) as well as an index to **test questions** found at the end of each unit that cover specific steps of the **nursing process** (**Appendix G**). These indexes are based on the official NCLEX-RN® Test Plan and are especially useful in facilitating review for **repeat exam-takers.**
- Emphasis is given to all **five steps of the nursing process,** especially *health teaching* and specific *outcome criteria for evaluation* of the effectiveness of nursing care.
- Current NANDA-approved *nursing diagnoses* are provided as a structure for presenting nursing interventions.
- A thorough **question-and-answer review** at the end of *each unit,* in a nursing process format, reflects **diverse cultural influences.**

This review book has been updated and revised to incorporate the latest knowledge and current trends in nursing practice and to parallel the **latest NCLEX-RN® Test Plan.** All content has been submitted to outstanding educators and nursing practitioners for their review and critique. We would like to express our appreciation to this editorial review panel for their contributions, which make this book the best to use for complete nursing review.

In **Unit 1, Orientation and Pre Test,** you will find suggestions on how to use this book and how to plan your study,

information about the NCLEX-RN®, *study tips and strategies,* help with memorization, and relaxation exercises. At the end of this unit is a **new 500-question Pre Test** to use as self-assessment before reading the nursing content units that follow. This special assessment section is completely new and visually different:

- We wanted to give candidates a 500-item **Pre Test** that comprehensively covers and is *directly based* on (and coded for) all *content* areas under the four general client needs and six subcategories in the latest official NCLEX-RN® Test Plan.
- The rationale for each option is by chronological order, with the entire rationale for the correct answer in **bold-face,** for emphasis as well as to help make the best answer easy to find and make it easier to focus on the most relevant information.

Unit 2, Guidelines and Tips for International Nurses and Repeat Test-takers, is unique. *No other book* addresses the special concerns of candidates who have taken the test more than once or who are graduates of nursing programs outside the United States. **Unit 2** covers:

- **Risk factors** for not passing the first time
- Five steps on **what to do to pass next time**
- **How to know if you are prepared** to take the exam again
- **Sixty test-taking tips and guidelines** to use in answering questions

Unit 3 has been reorganized, with special focus on **Management of Care, Cultural Diversity, Ethical and Legal Aspects,** and **Nursing Trends. New** content includes: safe use of equipment, *delegation,* establishing *priorities,* emergency response plan, and new **HIPAA** law. Expanded content has been added: *cultural diversity* relevant to nursing practice as well as *religious* and *spiritual* influences on health. Also included are: advance directives, advocacy, organ donation; bioethics and client rights; and concepts of *management:* case management, quality assurance, variance reports, resource management, supervision, disaster planning. A review of client restraints and nursing responsibilities is also included.

All questions and answers have *test-taking tips* in addition to a complete rationale.

Unit 4, Nursing Care of the Childbearing Family, is streamlined, visually enhanced, and up-to-date; it contains the most exam-relevant content for both pregnancy and care of the neonate. This is the only nursing review book that features **clinical pathways** (intrapartum, postpartum, newborn). This unit includes *detailed* information regarding many important *diagnostic tests,* such as chorionic villi sampling and biophysical profile testing, to identify the woman and fetus at risk. *Numerous illustrations* are included (e.g., amniocentesis, fetal circulation, and ectopic pregnancy). We include the latest information on *emergency care* in labor and birth, perinatal acquired immune deficiency syndrome, sexually transmitted diseases, and *preterm labor.* We have *updated* pharmacological information regarding new drug therapies during the perinatal period recommended for the at-risk infant, as well as **new** trends and new modes for *contraception* delivery. Updated information is included on intrapartum *complications* and *risk factors*. **New** content has been added on *hepatitis* and *TB* in *pregnancy*. *Client teaching* and *nursing interventions* are delineated for each of these areas of practice. The question and answer sections also address these advances in technology and care.

Unit 5, Nursing Care of Children and Families, has **new** content on the role of the pediatric nurse in *management of care* of infants, children, and adolescents; in *safety and infection control* (a **new table** plus updated immunization information); in *prevention and early detection of disease* (an expanded table: *Preventive Care Timeline*); pediatric *emergencies* (revised airway, CPR, and Heimlich maneuver tables); and updated information (nursing care, medications, tests, etc.) concerning all major physical systems of the body. Much of this information has been synthesized into table format for *easier reading, recall,* and *application* to client care. **Diagrams** show genetic transmission of sickle cell anemia and hemophilia. **Illustrations** depict five cardiac defects, airway, CPR and Heimlich maneuver, TEF and esophageal atresia, developmental hip dysplasia, and scoliosis. Coverage is provided for Reye syndrome, Kawasaki disease, and salicylate, Tylenol, and lead poisoning. Content includes greatly expanded coverage in all areas of physical growth and assessment, normal development concerns, and parental counseling as well as appreciation of **cultural diversity** in assessment and nursing interventions. Additional **new** content includes *spiritual* development in children in **new table format;** a pediatric-focused **clinical pathway;** and advantages and disadvantages of various oxygen-delivery systems. *Updated tables* include: one- and two-rescuer CPR for children, acute post-streptococcal glomerulonephritis (APSGN), pediatric respiratory infections, and juvenile rheumatoid arthritis.

Unit 6, Nursing Care of Behavioral and Emotional Problems Throughout the Life Span (Client Need: *Psychosocial Integrity),* presents psychiatric disorders that have been organized under DSM-IV-TR guidelines. We have included *thorough* coverage of suicide precautions, *midlife* crises, mental health of the *elderly,* substance abuse, panic disorders, post-traumatic disorder, amnestic disorders, personality disorders, sleep and eating disturbances, and affective disorders. Content includes a detailed section on psychiatric *emergencies* and therapeutic communication techniques. The theoretical model section has been greatly expanded to include Piaget's age-specific developmental levels, Duvall's Family Development, and Kaplan's mental health model.

Also, three developmental sections have been included: a table on development of *body image* (includes disturbances and four phases of crises), *human sexuality* throughout the life cycle (with causes of dysfunction, sexual health counseling, and sexual assessment interview format), and a *table on emotional disturbances in children,* with updated sections on autistic spectrum disorder, attention deficit hyperactivity disorder, and child abuse.

A *unique* feature is the inclusion of **six clinical pathways** (on eating disorders, alcohol withdrawal, post-trauma, depression, manic behavior, and schizophrenic psychoses).

Nine important sections are: *domestic violence* (abused woman and child; elder abuse/neglect), *diagnostic tests* (for dementia/cognitive disorders and alcohol abuse); mental

status assessment (individual, cultural); interviewing, general principles of health teaching; self-concept; coping mechanisms; treatment modes with a **new** section on **complementary and alternative methods.** There is also an extensive glossary.

Unit 7, Nursing Care of the Acutely Ill and the Chronically Ill Adult, presents content under appropriate categories of human functions. *Risk factors* have been identified for all conditions, *goals of nursing* are clearly stated, five sample **clinical pathways** are included (MI, CHF, stroke, spinal fusion, and hip arthroplasty), and a brief description of *pathophysiology* is incorporated with each condition.

New tables have been added: Factors Affecting Vital Signs, SIADH Versus Diabetes Insipidus, Bioterrorism, and Infectious Diseases (including animal-borne). Other *tables* on fluid and electrolyte imbalances, acid-base disorders, assessment differences with valvular defects, hazards of immobility, complications of diabetes, and malignant disorders supplement the *condensed* and *consolidated* content.

New content includes: management of PICC lines, use of metered-dose inhalers, pneumonia severity, pheochromocytoma, Raynaud's disease, SARS, and Guillain-Barré syndrome. The up-to-date content also includes acquired immune deficiency syndrome, GERD, latex allergies, JCAHO Requirements for Pain Assessment, Lyme disease, compartment syndrome, Crohn's disease, ulcers, external fixation devices for fractures, and lithotripsy. **Illustrations** include: 12 types of fractures, 8 skin and skeletal tractions, and breast and testicular self-exam. The *many other tables, charts,* and *diagrams* include cardiac dysrhythmias (**new** content on atrial flutter), comparison of causes of chest pain, burn care, the Glasgow Coma scale, chest drainage, comparison of hepatitis types, postoperative complications, enteric and standard precautions, respiratory isolation, care of the adult client with medical and surgical emergencies, preventing TPN complications, and TPN dressing changes. *Nursing interventions* are grouped according to the goal of care and identify appropriate treatments and drug therapies. More detailed discussions follow in two special units on *pharmacology* (**Unit 10**) and *diagnostic procedures* and *treatments* (**Unit 11**).

Unit 8, The Older Adult, has all **new questions** at the end. This concise and highly readable unit synthesizes 12 key problems associated with care of the older adult. There is an expanded section on *assessment of the older adult* that includes material on normal changes of aging, including a **new table** summarizing common concerns in the older adult. *Five functional rating scales* and *a functional screening* exam are included to make management of care easier:

- Social resources rating scale
- Economic resources rating scale
- Mental health rating scale
- Physical health rating scale
- Performance rating scale for activities of daily living

Unit 9, Review of Nutrition, contains unique information regarding *ethnic* food patterns, eating problems, nutritional needs of the *elderly, religious* and *ethnic* food preferences, and *cultural* disease treatments involving food. *Special* and *therapeutic diets* are featured. **New content** has been added on medical conditions with dietary management; Dietary Reference Intakes; high *phosphorus* and *lactose-free* diets; and *anticancer nutrients*.

Unit 10, Review of Pharmacology, contains drug classifications and drug treatments with emphasis on **nursing implications. New content** has been added on drug conversions and calculations. Pediatric medication administration, obstetric analgesia, and psychotropic and mind-altering substances are included; and 18 **new drugs** have been added, as well as **new tables** on herbal therapies (with potential dangers).

Unit 11, Common Diagnostic Procedures, Intravenous and Oxygen Therapy, Infection Control/Isolation Precautions, and Hands-on Nursing Care, includes content on commonly used *tubes, fluid and electrolyte therapy*, **new content** on oxygen delivery equipment, and colostomy care as well as many diagnostic procedures commonly tested on NCLEX-RN®. **New tables** include *Types of Precautions* and *Illnesses Requiring the Precautions*, and *Infection Control Conditions that Need Additional Precautions*. Also included are diagnostic tests to evaluate *fetal well-being, newborn screening* procedures (**new** content on Tay-Sachs screening), *bladder* and *bowel* training, guidelines for *isolation* precautions, and commonly used *IV fluids*. Common client *positions* and *intubation* and *ventilation* are illustrated.

Appendixes in this book include indexes to content and test questions related to **four general client needs** (**Appendixes C** and **D**) and their **six subcategories** (**Appendix E**). These indexes, **which are not found in any other book,** provide immediate, easy reference to topics from the NCLEX-RN Test Plan that are covered in this book. Other appendixes cover: complementary and alternative therapies (**new**), *lab values,* common abbreviations and clinical signs, and fun-to-use **memory aids.**

Four Unique Self-Evaluation Tools—Over 2500 Test Questions and Test-Taking Tips

This book contains four special, *integrated* tests to help you assess your knowledge before taking the NCLEX-RN®. The special **new** 500-item integrated **Pre Test** at the end of **Unit 1** is intended for students to take *after* reading the **Orientation** section but *before* reading the rest of this book. It is a preassessment tool to let you find your areas of strength and weakness based on the 10 client needs/subneeds of the NCLEX-RN® Test Plan before beginning focused study. The integrated **Practice Test** is intended to be taken *after* reviewing the material in this book to evaluate your progress. The **Final Test,** the third integrated exam tool, will assess your readiness to take NCLEX-RN® and identify any last-minute knowledge gaps.

Use the practice **Computer Test** on the CD-ROM anytime in your preparation when you need extra practice or when you want to become familiar with the NCLEX-RN® testing format.

In addition to these four tests, there are different review **questions and answers following each unit.** Their purpose is to help students *review each content area separately* before taking the integrated tests. All questions at the *end of units* and in the integrated tests have been field-tested for several years with students—a diverse group of candidates who have successfully passed the exam—from all over the United States. These questions have also been reviewed by an editorial panel for appropriateness. The Answers/ Rationales/Tips sections in each unit contain detailed explanations about why a particular answer is *best* and *why the other* options are incorrect, with a **test-taking tip for each question.** We expect that these special integrated tests, end-of-unit review questions, and corresponding answer sections will prove to be invaluable review tools for each and every student.

In the answers for each of the end-of-unit review question sections, as well as for the **Pre Test, Practice Test, Final Test,** and **Computer Test,** you will find a six-part code to help you understand exactly what is being tested by each question. The code refers to the step of the *nursing process,* the *cognitive level* (level of difficulty of the item), the *category of human function,* the *clinical/subject area,* the *client need,* and the *subcategory of client need* that applies to that question. See the code legend on the first page of each Answers/Rationale/Tips section. The **Computer Test** will track these codes for you to identify your problem areas. Use these codes as a guide for review when you find you did not select the best answer. The **test-taking tips** and **codes are unique to this book;** they are an added study tool to help you assess your strengths and pinpoint problem areas as you prepare for the NCLEX-RN®.

SLL
JLM
RMN
KS

Money Back Guarantee

If you are a graduate of a nursing program accredited in the United States, are taking the NCLEX-RN® for the first time, and do not pass after using *Davis's NCLEX-RN Success,* return the book to F.A. Davis Company, Customer Service, 404-420 N. 2nd Street, Philadelphia, PA 19123. Enclose your original receipt for purchase of the book, a copy of your official test results notification, and a copy of your certification of graduation. We will refund the price you paid for the book. If you have any questions, please call 800-323-3555.

List of Tables

List of Figures

Contents

Unit 1

Orientation and Pre Test

Sally L. Lagerquist • Debra Brady • Christine Hooper • Janice McMillin
• Robyn Nelson • Cheryl Osborne • Mary St. Jonn Seed
• Kathleen Snider • Carolyn VanCouwenberghe

ORIENTATION

How to Use This Review Book as a Study Guide

Although nursing students may know that they are academically prepared to take the computer adaptive National Council Licensure Examination (NCLEX-RN)®, many find that reviewing nursing content for the licensure examination itself presents special concerns about *what* and *how* to study.

Some typical concerns about **what to study** are reflected in the following questions:

- Considering that there will be up to 265 questions on the exam, and every candidate gets a different exam, how does one select what is the most important content for review? How does one narrow the focus of study and distinguish the relevant from the irrelevant material?
- What areas should be emphasized?
- How detailed should the review be?
- How does one know what areas to review first?
- Should basic sciences, such as anatomy, physiology, microbiology, and nutrition, be included in the study?

Concerns relating to **how to study** include:

- How does one make the best of limited review time to go over content that may be in lecture and clinical notes compiled during 2–4 years of schooling?
- Is it best to review from all the major textbooks used in nursing school?
- Should material be memorized, or should one study from broad principles and concepts?

We have written this nursing review book with the *general* intent of assisting nurses in identifying what they need to study in a format designed to use their study time effectively, productively, and efficiently while preparing for the examination.

The contributing authors have selected content and developed a style of presentation that has been tested by thousands of nursing students attending review courses coordinated by the editor in various cities throughout the United States. This book is the result of this study.

This review book can be used in a variety of ways: (a) as a *starting point* for review of essential content specifically aimed at NCLEX® or Canadian exam preparation, (b) as an *end point* of studying for the examinations, (c) as an *anxiety-reduction tool,* (d) as a general guide and *refresher* for nurses not presently in practice, and (e) as a guide for graduates of nursing schools *outside of the United States,* as well as *repeat test-takers* (see **Unit 2**).

As a Starting Point

This text can be used in early review when a longer study period is needed to *fill in gaps* of knowledge. One cannot remember something if one does not know or understand it. A lengthy review before the exam allows students time to rework and organize notes accumulated during 2–4 years of basic nursing education. In addition, an early review allows time for *self-evaluation*. We have provided questions and answers to help students identify areas requiring further study and to help them *integrate* unfamiliar material with what they already know.

As an End Point

This text can also be used for a *quick review* (a) to *promote retention and recall* and (b) to aid in determining *nursing actions* appropriate to specific health situations. During the time immediately preceding the examination, the main objective might be to *strengthen previous learning* by refreshing the memory. Or a brief overview may serve to *draw together* the isolated points under key concepts and principles in a way that shows their relationships and relative importance.

As an Anxiety-Reduction Tool

In some students, anxiety related to taking examinations in general may reach such levels that it causes students to be unproductive in study and to function at a lower level during the actual examination. Sections of this unit are directed toward this problem and provide simple, *practical approaches to the reduction of general anxiety.* For anxiety specifically related to unknown aspects of the licensure examination itself, the section on the *structure, format, and mechanics of the RN examination* might bring relief through its focus on basic examination information (see **pp. 3–7**).

For anxiety related to lack of confidence or skill in test-taking "know-how," the special section on *test-taking techniques* may be helpful (see **Unit 2**).

As a General Study Guide and as a Refresher for Nurses Not Presently in Practice

Many nursing students will find this review book useful throughout their education as a general study guide as they prepare client care plans and study for midterm and final exams. It will help them put information into perspective as they learn it. And nurses who have not been in practice for several years will find it a useful reference tool and review device.

Where to Begin

In using this review book to prepare for the licensure examination, the nurse must:

1. Be prepared mentally.
   a. Know the purpose of the examination.
   b. Know the purpose of reviewing.
   c. Anticipate what is to come.
   d. Decide on a good study method—set a study goal before beginning a particular subject area (number of pages, for example); plan the length of the review period by the amount of material to be covered, not by the clock.
2. Plan the work to be done.
   a. Select one subject at a time for review, and establish and follow a sequence for review of each subject.
      (1) Answer the practice questions following the outline of the selected subject area. (Set a time limit, because pacing is important.)
      (2) Compare your answers with those provided following the questions as a means of evaluating areas of competence.
   b. Identify those subjects that will require additional concentrated study in this review book as well as in basic textbooks.
   c. Study the review text outlines, noting headings, subheadings, and *italics* and **boldface** type for emphasis of relative importance.
   d. Study the content presented in the shaded boxes and chart format to facilitate memorization, understanding, and application.
   e. Repeat the self-evaluation process by taking the test again.
   f. Look up the answers for the correct response to the multiple choice questions. Do not memorize the answers. Read the rationale explaining *why* it was the correct response. (These explanations serve to correct as well as reinforce. Understanding the underlying principles also serves as an aid in applying the same

principles to questions that may be based on similar rationale, but phrased differently on the actual examination.)
   g. If necessary, refer to basic textbooks to relearn any unclear aspects of anatomy, physiology, nutrition, or basic nursing procedures. Look up unfamiliar terminology in a medical dictionary.

While Reviewing

1. Scan the outline for main ideas and topics.
   a. Do not try to remember verbatim what is on each page.
   b. Paraphrase or explain this material to another person.
2. Refer to basic textbooks for details and illustrations as necessary to recall specific information related to basic sciences.
3. Integrate reading with experience.
   a. Think of examples that illustrate the key concepts and principles.
   b. Make meaningful associations.
   c. Look for implications for nursing actions as concepts are reviewed.
4. Take notes on the review outline—use stars and arrows, underscore, highlight with highlighter pens, and write comments in margins, such as "most important" and "memorize," to reinforce the relative importance of points of information.

After Reviewing

1. Repeat the self-evaluation process as often as necessary to gain mastery of content essential to safe nursing practice.
2. Continue to refer to major textbooks to fill in gaps where greater detail or in-depth comprehension is required.
3. Look for patterns in your selection of responses to the multiple choice practice questions—identify sources of difficulty in choosing the most appropriate answers.
4. Review test-taking strategies (see **Unit 2, pp. 113–117**).

Key Points to Recall for Better Study

1. *Schedule*—study time should be scheduled so that review begins close to the time at which it will be used. Retention is much better following a well-spaced review. It may be helpful to group material into small learning segments. Study goals should be set before beginning each period of study (number of pages, for example).
2. *Organize*—many students have better retention of material after they have reorganized and relearned it.
3. *Rephrase and explain*—try to rephrase material in your own words or explain it to another person. Reinforce learning through repetition and usage.
4. *Decide on order of importance*—organize study time in terms of importance and familiarity.
5. *Use mechanical memory aids*—mnemonic (memory) devices simplify recall. For example, in "On Old Olympus's Towering Top a Finn and German Viewed Some Hops," the first letter of each word identifies the first letter of a cranial nerve (see **Appendix N**).

6. *Association*—associate new material with related concepts and principles from past experience.
7. *Original learning*—if an unfamiliar topic is presented, do more than review. Seek out sources of additional information.
8. *Make notes*—look for key words, phrases, and sentences in the outlined review material, and mark them for later reference.
9. *Definitions*—look up unfamiliar terms in a dictionary or the glossary of a basic text, or in **Appendix L.**
10. *Additional study*—refer to other textbook references for more detailed information.
11. *Distractors*—keep a pad of paper on hand to jot down extraneous thoughts; get them out of the mind and onto the paper.

Memorization: Purpose and Strategies

You'll need to memorize some items before you can rapidly assess or apply that knowledge to a particular situation; for example, you need to be able to recall the standard and lethal doses of a drug before deciding to administer it. Items you should memorize include, but are not limited to:

1. Names of common drugs.
2. Lethal and therapeutic doses.
3. Lab norms and values.
4. Growth and development norms.
5. Foods high or low in iron, protein, sodium, potassium, or carbohydrates.
6. Conversion formulas.
7. Anatomical names.
8. List of cranial nerves and their innervations.
9. Definitions of defense mechanisms.

To facilitate memorizing these and other essentials, here are some strategies.

1. Before you work on training your mind to remember, you must *want* to remember the material.
2. You cannot memorize something that you do not understand; therefore, *know* your material.
3. Visualize what you want to memorize; picture it; draw a picture.
4. Use the familiar to provide vivid mental pictures, to peg the unfamiliar.
   a. When needing to remember a *sequence,* use your body to turn material into a picture. Draw a person, then list the first item to be memorized on top of the head, the next item on the forehead, and so on for nose, mouth, neck, chest, abdomen, thighs, knees, and feet.
   b. Use what you already know to tie in with what you want to remember; make it memorable.
   c. Use as pegs the unexpected, the exaggerated. Weird imagery is easiest to recall.
5. Use the blank-paper technique:
   a. Place a large blank sheet on the wall.
   b. After you have studied, draw on the blank paper what you remember.
   c. When you have drawn all that you can recall, check

with the book and study what you did correctly and incorrectly.
   d. Take another sheet and do it again. Purpose: to reinforce what you already know and work with what you want to remember.
6. Make up and use mnemonic devices to help you remember the important elements (see **Appendix N**).
7. Repetitively explain to another person the material you want to memorize.
8. Saturate your environment with the material you want to memorize.
   a. Purpose: to overcome the mind's tendency to ignore.
   b. Tape facts, formulas, concepts on walls.
9. Above all, feel confident in your ability to memorize!

The Mechanics of the National Council Licensure Examination for Registered Nurses–Computer Adaptive Test (NCLEX-RN®)

Since 1994, the licensure examination for registered nurses has been administered year-round by computer, in an adaptive format: NCLEX-RN®. Frequently, candidates for the exam have many questions about the structure and format of the test itself and the rules and regulations concerning the examination procedure.

As an aid to reducing apprehension and time spent on speculation, this section is intended to provide information that candidates need, in outline form; the last segment offers a "question-and-answer" format for specific questions frequently asked by nursing students.

This information was verified as correct at the time that it was compiled from information provided by the National Council of State Boards of Nursing, Inc., and other parties involved in the testing. If you have further questions, contact the board of nursing in your state (see **Appendix O**).

I. **What NCLEX® is**
    A. National Council Licensure Examination, developed and administered by the National Council of State Boards of Nursing, Inc., with services provided by VUE (Virtual University Enterprises), an NCS (National Computer Systems) Pearson Company.
    B. Tests for minimum nursing competence according to a national standard.
    C. Pass/fail result; must pass to be issued license from state board of registered nursing.
    D. National exam. Application procedure and licensing requirements are determined by each state board and may differ from state to state.

II. **CAT: How it works**
    A. Stands for "computer adaptive testing."
    B. "Adaptive" because the computer estimates the candidate's ability after each question; the next question is chosen based on the candidate's estimated ability so far. The test is therefore "adapted" to each candidate; everyone takes a different, "customized" test.

C. Estimated ability is recalculated after each question until it is precise enough to determine whether the candidate is above or below minimum competence level, in all areas of the test plan. The test will stop as soon as this is determined.

D. Example: The first question is at a fairly easy level. The candidate answers correctly, so the computer estimates that the candidate's ability level is above the level of this question and selects a harder question; or if the candidate answers incorrectly, it selects an easier question, to pinpoint where the candidate's ability level lies, in each area of the test plan.

III. **Some specifics**

A. Format

1. Most questions will be multiple choice, each with four options from which you choose only one option. Some "alternate items" may direct you to "select all that apply," fill in the blank, or point and click (also known as "hot spot" items); others may have diagrams or charts, or require numerical entry or ordered response.

2. One question at a time appears on screen (**Figure 1.1**).

3. Each question stands alone (no "scenarios" with several spin-off questions); no question will relate to information given in *previous* questions.

B. Answering

1. As candidate chooses the answer to each question, he or she will be asked to confirm that answer by pressing the <NEXT> button, *or* can change that answer before confirming.

2. Must answer every question (no penalty for guessing; will simply count as a correct or incorrect answer and adjust difficulty of next question accordingly).

3. Cannot go back to previous questions either to review or change answers (because the level of *subsequent* questions administered is based on *previous* answers).

C. Number of questions

1. 75–265, including about 15 "tryout" questions that are not scored (these are questions being field tested for use on future exams).

2. Depends on number needed to determine whether candidate is definitely above or definitely below minimum competence level.

3. Taking only the minimum can mean **either pass or fail;** it indicates that it took fewer questions to determine whether this candidate is above or below minimum competence, but does not indicate which!

D. Timing

1. No time limit for each question.

2. Maximum time for test is 6 hours.

3. A preprogrammed optional break is given after 2 hours; a second preprogrammed optional break may be taken after another $1\frac{1}{2}$ hours.

E. The test will stop when any *one* of the following occurs:

1. A "pass" or "fail" determination can be made.

2. The maximum number of questions has been taken (265).

3. The test has lasted for 6 hours, including exam instructions, sample items, and all rest breaks).

F. The computer

1. Computer experience will not be necessary.

2. A mouse is used to move down the list of options and select and confirm answer choice by pressing the <NEXT> button; all keys will be "turned off."

3. An on-screen calculator will be available.

4. Candidate receives a brief orientation in the use of the mouse and on-screen calculator with sample questions before beginning the exam.

IV. **Administration**

A. Application and scheduling

1. Involves three parties: the state board of nursing, VUE, and Pearson Professional Center.

2. Candidate applies to the board of nursing in the state in which licensing is desired; must meet requirements of that state board. (There is a test fee and some state boards may also require an administrative fee.)

3. After state board determines eligibility and fees are received, candidate will be mailed an *Authorization to Test (ATT)* and information on available Pearson Professional Test Centers, which serve as testing sites (at least one per state; some states have many more).

4. Candidate must schedule an appointment to take the exam by calling NCLEX® Candidate Services or going to the NCLEX® Candidate Website. (*Note*: These procedures differ in some states, such as Massachusetts. Candidates should follow instructions from state board.)

5. Candidate contacts Pearson Professional Test Center (or other designated test site) to set up testing appointment (5 days/wk, 15 hr/day, in 6-hour time slots). Candidates may test at any test center in any state (they do not have to take the test in the same state to which they have applied for licensure).

6. After testing, results are communicated to state board to which the candidate applied, which

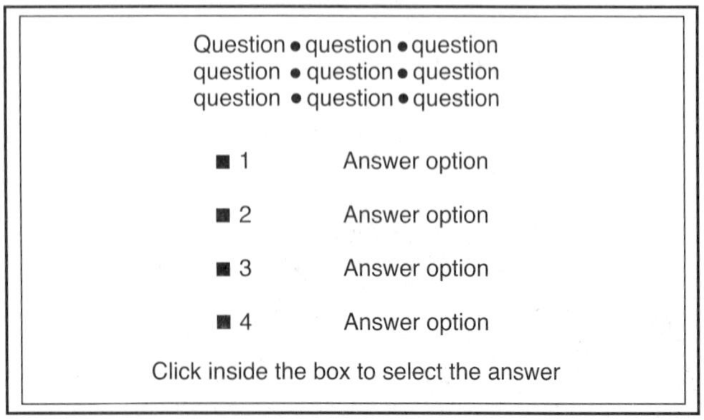

```
        Question • question • question
        question • question • question
        question • question • question

          ■ 1        Answer option

          ■ 2        Answer option

          ■ 3        Answer option

          ■ 4        Answer option

      Click inside the box to select the answer
```

FIGURE 1.1   Computer screen.

mails results to candidate (time frame will differ by state). Candidates who do not pass will receive a Candidate Performance Report, indicating performance in each area of the test plan relative to the passing standard, and information about retesting.

B. Test environment: Pearson Professional Test Center test sites
   1. Up to 30 workstations, each with computer terminal, desk lamp, work surface, and scratch paper.
   2. Designed for security, monitored by a proctor and by videotape.
   3. Candidate must present *Authorization to Test* and two signed pieces of identification, one with picture; candidate must sign in and be fingerprinted and photographed.
   4. Lockers or other secured storage provided; personal items restricted in testing room.

V. **Test plan, development**
   A. Test plan*
      1. *Client needs* are the bases, or "dimensions," for the test plan (**Table 1.1**).
      2. Health needs of clients: The test plan primarily emphasizes meeting the clients' physical needs in actual or potentially life-threatening, chronic, or recurring *physiological* conditions and the needs of clients who are at risk for complications or untoward effects of treatment. Subneeds include (1) basic care and comfort (6%–12%), (2) pharmacological and parenteral therapies (13%–19%), (3) reduction of risk potential (13%–19%), and (4) physiological adaptation (11%–17%).

         The second highest category of emphasis is *safe, effective care environment,* which focuses on (1) management of care (13%–19%) and (2) safety and infection control (8%–14%). *Health promotion and maintenance* (6%–12%) covers growth and development throughout the life span and prevention and early detection of disease. *Psychosocial integrity* (6%–12%) concerns coping and adaptation in stress- and crisis-related situations throughout the life cycle.

   3. *Nursing process* (nursing behaviors): The exam integrates steps of the nursing process, as applied to client situations from all stages in the life cycle and to common health problems in all the major health areas and based on current morbidity studies. It is a problem-solving approach to client care that includes data collection (assessment, analysis), planning, implementation, and evaluation.
   4. Levels of *cognitive ability*: Most items are at the levels of *application* (application of rules, procedures, principles, ideas, and theories, and using a concept in a new situation) and *analysis* (analysis of data to set priorities and see relationships). Some items include knowledge and comprehension (simple recognition or recall of material; restating or reorganizing material to show understanding).
   5. Categories of nursing knowledge and other concepts that are commonly tested:
      a. **Caring** ways by which nursing can assist individuals to maintain health and cope with health problems. It involves interaction between nurse and client in a collaborative environment, with mutual respect and trust. The nurse provides hope, support, and compassion to achieve desired outcomes. (See *nursing care plan/implementation* sections in *each* unit.)
      b. **Communication** (see **Unit 6**).
      c. Effect of age, sex, culture, ethnicity, and religion on health needs (sociocultural components) are integrated into all units; for special emphasis see **Units 3 and 9** (dietary implications).
      d. **Documentation;** legal and ethical aspects of nursing, accountability (see **Unit 3**).
      e. Self-care.
      f. **Teaching-learning;** helping client and significant others to acquire knowledge, skills, and attitudes that facilitate changes in behavior. (See *health teaching* sections [after the conditions] that are part of **Nursing care plan/implementation.**)
      g. Nursing fundamentals (see **Unit 11**).
      h. Nutrition and diet therapy (see **Unit 9**).
      i. Pharmacology (see **Unit 10**).
      j. Communicable diseases (see **Units 5 and 7**).
      k. Natural and behavioral sciences (integrated into all units).
      l. Normal growth and development (see **Units 4, 5, and 6**).
      m. Basic human needs (see **Unit 6**).
      n. Individual coping mechanisms (see **Unit 6**).
      o. Actual or potential health problems (see **Units 4, 5, 7, and 8**).
      p. Life cycle (consult the **Table of Contents** to

TABLE 1.1	Exam Weight Given to Each Category of Health Needs of Clients Based on Current Practice Analysis Study
Client Health Needs Tested (subneeds)	**Total Percentage of Test**
Safe, effective care environment (Management of Care, Safety and Infection Control)	21–33
Health promotion and maintenance	6–12
Psychosocial integrity	6–12
Physiological integrity (Basic Care and Comfort, Pharmacological Parenteral Therapies, Reduction of Risk Potential, Physiological Adaptation)	43–67

*Source: National Council of State Boards of Nursing.

see how the conceptual framework for this book is organized by life cycle).

    q. Client environment (there is continual reference throughout this book related to protection from harm against airborne irritants, cold, and heat; identification of environmental discomforts such as noise, odors, dust, and poor ventilation; elimination of potential *safety hazards;* maintenance of environmental order; and *cleanliness*).

B. Development

1. The Examination Committee of the National Council prepares the test plan, which is approved by the delegates representing the state boards of nursing. It is designed to reflect the knowledge and skills needed for *minimum competence by a newly licensed nurse to be a safe and effective practitioner in entry-level nursing,* as determined by studies of nursing practice (performed every 3 years to reflect current nursing practice).

2. State boards take turns nominating item writers (faculty, clinical nurse specialists, or beginning practitioners); the Board of Directors of the National Council then selects from this group those who meet the criteria for item writing based on expertise in a particular area of nursing, type of nursing program, credentials, regional balance, etc. The item writers write questions based on common clinical situations and according to the test plan. Then the questions are researched and reviewed by a panel of experts (nominated by the state boards), by those state boards that choose to review, and by the National Council's Examination Committee.

3. Finally, the questions are field tested to eliminate questions that may be ambiguous, irrelevant, or not equally applicable to all regions of the United States. (Each candidate taking NCLEX® will take 15 of these "tryout" questions, mixed in with the regular questions; they will *not* count toward that candidate's performance.) The data gained through field testing are also used to analyze and determine the difficulty level of a question.

C. Passing standard: The passing standard is *criterion referenced;* this means that there is no fixed percentage of candidates that pass or fail. Passing depends solely on performance in relation to the level of minimum competence. The passing standard is reviewed every 3 years.

VI. Frequently asked questions and answers about NCLEX-RN®

A. Test questions, test plan

1. *How many questions will there be?* You will take anywhere from 75 to 265 questions (see **III. Some specifics, p. 4**).

2. *Where do the questions come from?* The state boards of nursing nominate item writers, who must meet various criteria (see **V. B. Development,** above).

3. *Will there be questions involving conditions with*

which I may not have had experience in my nursing program? Most of the questions are about clients with conditions familiar to you and are representative of common health problems on a national basis. Some questions may relate to nursing problems with which you may not have had prior experience; their purpose is to test your ability to *apply* knowledge of specific principles from the physical, biological, and social sciences to *new* situations.

4. *Can some questions have more than one answer?* Yes. In some questions, only *one* of the four options is the *best* answer. In alternate items, you may be asked to choose more than one option as your answer.

5. *Will I get partial credit for selecting the next-to-the-best answer?* No. Your answer will be treated only as correct or incorrect.

6. *If everyone takes a different test, how can it be fair?* Each candidate is tested according to the *same test plan,* and the *same passing standard.* It may simply require more items to reach a stable pass/fail determination for one candidate, while another may require fewer questions to demonstrate competence level.

7. *Do diploma, associate, and baccalaureate graduates all take the same test? What about graduates from schools outside the United States?* All candidates are held to the *same test plan and passing standard,* and take the "same test." (Of course, due to the nature of CAT, each will receive an "individualized" test, without regard to degree, or to state or country of education.)

8. *Does the exam differ by state?* The exam is a national exam; all candidates are held to the *same test plan and passing standard,* and take questions from the same pool. (Again, through CAT, each candidate receives an "individualized" test, but without regard to state.)

B. Taking the test/after the test

1. *Can I skip questions?* No. You must answer each question in order to move on to the next. You also will not be able to return to previous questions to try them again or change the answer (because the level of *subsequent* questions administered is based on *previous* answers).

2. *What if I just don't know the answer?* Use the tips in **Sixty Strategies to Use in Answering Questions, Unit 2, pp. 113–117,** to make your best guess. You will need to answer the question in order to move on to the next question.

3. *When will I know my results? Will the computer tell me?* You will not learn your pass/fail status at the testing center; the results will be communicated directly to your state board of nursing, who will mail the results to you. The time frame may differ from state to state, but most candidates should receive their results within 2–4 weeks after taking the exam. Some states provide a Results-by-Phone Service, where unofficial

results are available 3 business days after taking the exam. There is a flat fee for this service. **Note:** Taking only the minimum number of questions, or taking the maximum, is not an indication of whether you have passed or failed. It merely indicates that a lesser, or greater, number of items was required to reach a determination.

4. *What percentage must I answer correctly to pass?* Because of the nature of CAT, a percentage rate is *not* used to determine passing or failure. The test determines whether you are above or below standard competence by determining not the *number* of questions you answer correctly, but rather the *difficulty level* you can *consistently* answer correctly. The process of administering harder or easier questions, as described in **II. CAT: How it works, pp. 3–4,** continues until you reach the level where you answer approximately 50% of the complex questions correctly. **NOTE:** When practicing with questions of mixed difficulty, such as those in this book, you may wish to use 80% correct as a "benchmark" goal for yourself.

5. *If I do not pass, can I retest only those areas of the test plan in which I tested poorly?* No. The whole exam is on a pass/fail basis.

6. *Can I repeat the exam before I get my results?* No.

7. *How many times can the exam be repeated, and when?* The National Council allows you to repeat the exam not more than once in any 45-day period; however, each state board may set its own, more restrictive time limits and retake requirements. At present, most states allow the exam to be repeated after 45 days; other states still require a 91-day waiting period before repeating the exam.

8. *Who grants the nursing license?* The license is granted by the state board of nursing to which you applied and for which you took the exam.

C. Testing facilities

1. *Can I bring any materials into the examination room?* There are severe restrictions on personal items allowed in the examination room; you will be provided with a locker or other secure place for your belongings. Do *not* take any study materials (books, notes, calculators, etc.), pens, pencils, candy, chewing gum, drinks, food, watches, pagers, cell phones, note pads or Post-it notes, purses, wallets, or cameras into the examination building.

2. *How many people will take the test at the same time?* Up to 30 people may be at computer workstations in your testing room; however, they may not all be taking the NCLEX®, because Pearson Professional Test Centers also offer other services.

3. *When and where will I take the test?* As soon as you receive your authorization (ATT), you must contact a Pearson Professional Center facility to set up your own testing appointment (5 days/wk, 15 hr/day, in 6-hr time slots). There is at least one facility per state, although most states have many

more. A candidate must test within the validity dates of the ATT. These dates cannot be extended. If the ATT expires, you may be required to re-register and repay to test.

4. *What accommodations are available for candidates with disabilities?* All test centers are accessible to candidates with disabilities. Other accommodations will be made only with the prior authorization of the board of nursing; contact your state board *before* submitting your application.

How to Prepare for and Score Higher on Exams

The Psychology of Test Taking

Many nursing students know the nursing material on which they are being tested, and can demonstrate their nursing skills in practice, but do not know how to prepare themselves for taking and passing examinations.

It is not just a matter of taking exams but of *knowing how* to take them, taking steps to ensure you can function at full capacity, and using the allotted time in the most productive way. You must learn to use strategy and judgment in answering questions, and to make educated guesses when you are not sure of the right answer.

This section offers practical suggestions to help ensure that you are "at your best" on exam day, and discusses practical strategies for eliminating wrong answers and for increasing your chances of selecting the best ones.

Prepare Physically and Mentally

1. *On the morning of an exam, avoid excessive oral intake of products that act as diuretics for you.* If you know that coffee or cigarettes, for example, increase urgency and frequency, it is best to limit their intake. Undue physiological discomforts can distract your focus from the exam at hand.

2. *Increase your oral intake of foods high in glucose and protein.* These foods reportedly have been helpful to some examinees for keeping up their blood-sugar level. This may enhance your concentration and problem-solving ability at the times when you most need to function at a high level. On the other hand, avoid carbohydrates such as doughnuts, which slow down thinking.

3. *Before examination days, avoid eating exotic or highly seasoned foods to which your system may not be accustomed.* Avoid possible gastrointestinal distress when you least need it!

4. *Use hard candy or something similar* prior to entering the exam room, to help relieve the discomfort of a dry mouth related to a state of anxiety.

5. *Wear comfortable clothes that you have worn before.* The day of an exam is not a good time to wear new clothes or footwear that may prove to be constricting, binding, or uncomfortable, especially at the waistline and shoulder seams.

6. Anxiety states can bring about rapid increases and decreases in body temperature. *Wear clothing that can be*

shed or added on. For example, you might bring a sweater that can be put on when you feel chilled or removed when your body temperature fluctuates again.

7. *Women need to be prepared for late, irregular, or unanticipated early onset of menses* on exam day, a time of stress.

8. Exam jitters can elicit anxiety-like reactions, both physiological and emotional. Because anxiety tends to be contagious, *try to limit your contacts with those who are also experiencing exam-related anxiety or who elicit those feelings in you.*

9. *The night before an exam is a good time to engage in a pleasurable activity* as a means of anxiety reduction. You need stamina and endurance for sitting, thinking, and reacting. Give yourself a chance for restful, not energy- or emotion-draining, activities in the days before an exam.

10. *Try a relaxation process* if anxiety reaches an uncomfortable level that cannot be channeled into the service of learning (see **How To Reduce Anxiety** below).

11. When you arrive home after an exam, *jot down content areas that were unfamiliar to you.* This may serve as a key focus for review.

Tips for NCLEX-RN®

1. Get an early start on the day you take the examination, to avoid raising your anxiety level before the actual exam starts. Allow yourself time for delays in traffic and in public transportation or for finding a parking place. Even allow for a dead battery, flooded engine, flat tire, or bus breakdown. If you are unfamiliar with the area in which the test center is located, find it the day before.

2. Remember that *you do not need to get all the answers right to pass.* The exam is designed to test for *minimum* competence; demonstrating a higher level will not earn a special designation on your license, or any other bonus. Moreover, due to the adaptive nature of the test, you will probably reach a level where you are answering only 50% of the questions correctly; this is *normal* for this test and *should not* in itself be taken as an indication of poor performance (you may be answering 50% of the *very difficult* questions correctly)!

3. Because you cannot skip questions and go back to them, or go back to change answers, it is important that you simply *do the best you can* on a particular question, using the **Sixty Strategies to Use in Answering Questions, Unit 2, pp. 113–117,** and *move on.* The adaptive test will give you another chance to show your competence, should you get that question wrong.

4. Remember that although you cannot change answers you have already "confirmed," you *may change your answer during the selection process.* As you make your answer selection, you will *choose* an answer (by pressing the enter key once) and then *confirm* it (by pressing the <NEXT> key); you will be able to change your mind *before confirming* your answer choice.

5. Although the exam uses different levels of difficulty to estimate your competence level, *do not try to figure out the difficulty level* of each question; likewise, do not try to keep track of the number of questions you are answering.

You will only distract yourself and raise your anxiety. Again, simply answer each question to the best of your ability and move on.

6. When taking practice questions, it is a good idea to *aim for an average of 1 minute per question,* so that you will be at a speed to finish the exam even if you *do* need to take the maximum number of questions. For the actual exam, however, the 6-hour time limit is not a problem for most candidates, so go ahead and *take the time to work through a difficult problem,* and make use of the scratch paper provided (but *don't* dwell on a question you "just can't get!").

Tips for Other (Pencil-and-Paper) Tests and Exams

1. *Answer the easy questions first.* Too often students focus on 1 question for 10 minutes; for example, instead of going on to answer 20 additional questions during this time. The main goal in this type of exam is to answer correctly as many questions as possible.

2. *Your first hunch is usually a good one.* Pay attention to your intuition, which may indicate which answer "feels" best.

3. *Be wise about the timing.* Divide your time. For example, if you have 90 questions and $1\frac{1}{2}$ hours for the test, aim for an average of 1 question per minute. Keep working! Do not lose time looking back at your answers.

4. *If you cannot decide between two multiple-choice answers, make a note of the numbers of the two choices.* This will narrow down your focus when you come back to this question. Leave the question; do not spend much time on those in doubt. When you have completed the test, go back and spend more time on those with which you had trouble.

5. *Exercise care and caution when using electronically scored answer sheets or booklets.* It is essential that you use only the type of pencil or ink specified in the instructions. If erasing is possible, be sure to erase completely; a mere trace might throw out the answer.

6. When using a separate answer sheet or booklet, be especially careful to *mark your answer in the space for the correct question number.* It might be helpful to say to yourself as you answer each question, "Choice No. 4 to question No. 3," to make sure that the right answer goes with each question number.

7. *Stay the entire time allotted.* If you complete the test early, check your answers. On a second look, after you have completed the test, you may find something that you are *now sure* you marked in error the first time. If you were undecided between two possible answers on any questions, use leftover time to reconsider those answers. (Also, look for and erase stray marks, if using electronically scored answer sheets.)

How to Reduce Anxiety

Most people have untapped inner resources for achieving relaxation and tension-release in stressful situations (such as during an examination) when they need to function at their highest potential. The goal of this discussion is to help you experience a self-guided approach to reducing your anxiety level to one that is compatible with learning and high performance.

In anxiety-producing settings whenever you feel overwhelmed or blocked, a fantasy experience can be of help in mastering the rising anxiety by promoting a feeling of calm, detached awareness, and a sense of deeper personal coping resources. Through the fantasy you can gain access to a zone of *tranquility* in the center of your being. Guided imagery often carries with it feelings of serenity, warmth, and comfort.

Fantasy experiences are, of course, highly individual. Techniques that help one person experience serenity may frustrate another. Try out the self-guided experiences suggested here, make up your own, and select ones that are best for you. There are endless possibilities for fantasy journeys. The best approach is to work with whatever fantasy occurs to you at the moment. The ideas for a journey presented here are meant to be a springboard for variations of your own.

A fantasy will be more effective if you take as comfortable a physical position as possible, with eyes closed and attention focused on the inner experience. Get in touch with physical sensations, your pattern and rate of breathing, your heartbeat, and pressure points of your body as it comes in contact with the chair and floor.

When you take a fantasy journey by yourself, it is important for you to read over the instructions several times so that you will be able to recall the overall structure of the fantasy. *Then,* close your eyes and take your trip without concern for following the instructions in detail.

Progressive Relaxation

Relaxation approaches are used in a variety of anxiety states whenever stress interferes with the ability to function.

Progressive relaxation training was originated in 1929 by Dr. Edmund Jacobson. It is a technique for attaining self-control over skeletal muscles in order to induce low-level tonus in the major muscle groups. The approach involves learning systematically and sequentially to tense and relax various muscle groups throughout the body.

The *objectives* of this approach are to soothe nerves, combat hypertonus in muscles, and substitute relaxing activities for stressful ones in order to feel comfortable in and more alert to the internal and external environments.

The *theory* behind this method takes as its basis the idea that muscular relaxation and anxiety states produce directly opposite physiological effects and thus cannot coexist. In other words, it is not possible to be tense in any body part that is completely relaxed.

The *physiological changes* during relaxation include decreased oxygen consumption, decreased carbon dioxide elimination, and decreased respiratory rate.

The basic factors vital to eliciting a relaxation response include the following:

1. *Quiet setting*—eliminate unnecessary internal and external stimuli.

2. *Passive, "let-it-happen" attitude*—empty your mind of thoughts and distractions.
3. *Comfortable position*—sit or recline in one position for 20 minutes or so.
4. *Constant stimulus on which to focus*—a repetitive sound, constant gaze on an object or image, or attention to one's own breathing pattern.

Relaxation training is a procedure that can be defined, specified, and memorized until you can go through the exercises mechanically. If you regularly practice relaxation, you will be able to cope more effectively with difficult situations by reaping the physiological and psychological benefits of a balanced and relaxed state.

Instructions

- Sit comfortably in a chair. Shut your eyes and chase your thoughts for a minute; go where your thoughts go.
- Then, let the words go. Become aware of how you *feel,* here and now, not how you would like to feel.
- Shift your awareness to your feet. Do not move them. Become aware of what they are doing.
- Spend 20 to 30 seconds focusing progressively on different parts of your body. Relax each part in turn:

Relax each of your toes; the tops of your feet; the arch of each foot; the insteps, balls, and heels; and your ankles, calves, knees, thighs, and buttocks. Become aware of how your body is contacting the chair in which you are sitting. Let go of your abdominal and chest muscles; relax your back. Release the tension in your shoulders, arms, elbows, forearms, wrists, hands, and each finger in turn; relax the muscles in your throat, lips, and cheeks. Wrinkle your nose; relax your eyelids and eyebrows (first one and then the other); relax the muscles in your forehead and top and back of your head. Relax your whole body.

Concentrate on your breathing; become aware of how you breathe. Allow yourself to inhale and exhale in your usual way. Become aware of the depth of your breathing. Are you expanding the lungs all the way? Or is your breathing shallow? Increase your depth of breathing. Now focus on the rate at which you are breathing. See if you can slow the rate down. When you breathe in, can you feel an inflow of energy that fills your entire body?

- Now concentrate on the sounds in the room.
- Focus on how you feel right now.
- Slowly open your eyes.

Suggestions for Additional Experiential Vignettes

- Imagine yourself leaving the room. In your mind's eye go through the city and over the fields. Come to a meadow covered with fresh, new grass and flowers. Look out on the meadow and focus on what you see, hear, smell, and feel. Walk through the meadow. See the length and greenness of the grass; see the brilliance and feel the warmth of the sunlight.
- For a more expansive feeling, visualize a mountain in the distance. Fantasize going to the country and slowly ascending a mountain. Walk through a forest. Climb to the

top until at last you reach a height where you can see forever. Experience your awareness.

- Focus on a memory of a beautiful place you have been to, enjoyed, and would like to enjoy again. Be there; experience it.
- Imagine that you are floating on your back down a river. It may help at first to breathe deeply and feel yourself sinking. Visualize that you are coming out on a gentle river that is slowly winding its way through a beautiful forest. The sun is out and the rays feel warm on your skin. You pass trees and meadows of beautiful flowers. Smell the grass and flowers. Hear the birds. Look up in the blue sky; see the lazy tufts of clouds floating by. Leave the river and walk across the meadow. Enjoy the grass around your ankles. Come to a large tree...

Fill in the rest of the trip—what do you see now? Where do you want to go from here?

Sally L. Lagerquist

PRE TEST

Introduction

This **Pre Test** is unique—it provides you with a special roadmap to your exam success with 500 challenging assessment questions (50 are in alternate item format).

The **Pre Test** is an *initial assessment* tool intended to help you to assess your strengths and weaknesses in your ability to apply the material you have learned in specific clinical areas to any nursing situation. By taking the **Pre Test,** you can focus your subsequent review of content, based on your own analysis of your results.

We suggest that you take the **Pre Test** before you read any of the content units in this book. After taking the **Pre Test,** you should:

1. Score your answers.
2. Take another look at the questions where your answer was wrong.
3. Identify the **clinical** areas where you need further review (e.g., Childhood and Adolescence, Behavioral and Emotional, Med-Surg, Maternity/Newborn).
4. Read those specific *content* units in detail (Units 4–8).
5. Then test yourself again on the **Pre Test.**

This time, take all the questions by one **clinical** area at a time (starting with the one you missed the most).

If you are repeating the NCLEX-RN®, also use the **Pre Test** a second time but take questions by client needs/ subneeds where you scored **below the passing standard** and/or **near the passing standard**.

Questions

Select the one answer that is best for each question, unless otherwise directed.

1. A client has just returned from surgery. Twenty minutes later the client is observed trying to get out of bed, trailing the intravenous line and the wound drain. The nurse's best action would be to:
   1. Put a jacket restraint on the client and leave a note in the client's chart for the physician.
   2. Call the nursing supervisor to have a sitter assigned to this client immediately.
   3. Reorient the client, make sure the call light is within reach, and move the client to a room closer to the nurse's station if possible.
   4. Put a jacket restraint on the client and place client in a wheelchair next to the nurse's station.

2. Which client has special risk factors that warrant testing for tuberculosis?
   1. 45-year-old Caucasian man who has been homeless for 2 years.
   2. 15-year-old Caucasian woman with asthma.
   3. 72-year-old woman who is a recent immigrant from Russia.
   4. 50-year-old Iowa farmer.

3. A 10-year-old child has juvenile rheumatoid arthritis. Which action taken by the child best indicates to the nurse that the child has understood the nurse's teaching regarding measures that would reduce the risk for activity intolerance?
   1. Delaying eating breakfast until after morning medications are taken.
   2. Increasing fluid intake.
   3. Taking a warm bath prior to going to school.
   4. Continuing to participate in activities of daily living (ADLs) despite fatigue and persistent pain.

4. When auscultating heart sounds, the nurse knows that the first heart sound (S_1) is best heard:
   1. Using the bell of the stethoscope
   2. With the client lying on the right side
   3. At the second intercostal space, right sternal border
   4. At the fifth intercostal space, left sternal border.

5. A client, 25 weeks pregnant, complains of frequent urination, lower abdominal cramping, backache and dysuria. The most likely reason is:
   1. Kidney stones.
   2. Urinary tract infection.
   3. Preterm labor.
   4. Cervical incompetence.

6. When auscultating heart sounds, the nurse detects an irregular rhythm. The nurse should *first*:
   1. Call for a STAT ECG.
   2. Reposition the client to a left side-lying position, and auscultate further.
   3. Compare the apical pulse to the radial pulse.
   4. Prepare to administer Lidocaine intravenously.

7. A 24-month-old child is diagnosed with intussusception and scheduled for a barium enema. Which nursing action would best demonstrate the procedure to the child?
   1. Blow air through a straw, and then encourage the child to perform the action.
   2. Show the child a picture of the barium enema equipment.
   3. Explain the procedure to the child using short, simple sentences.
   4. Instruct the child to mentally picture a garden hose watering the lawn.

8. An 80-year-old client has returned to the room after surgery with general anesthesia. The nurse needs to:
   1. Put the bed into slight Trendelenburg to counteract potential hypotension.
   2. Infrequently reposition the client to allow for rest.
   3. Maintain IV therapy and accurate I&O to ensure adequate renal perfusion.
   4. Loosely apply soft wrist restraints in case of postoperative confusion.

9. A newborn infant, 37 weeks gestation, displays tremors, lethargy and a high-pitched shrill cry. What action should the nurse take *first*?
   1. Pick up the infant to provide comfort.
   2. Stimulate the infant by rubbing the back and soles of the feet.
   3. Perform a heelstick to check the blood glucose level.
   4. Collect cord blood specimen to check for chromosomal abnormalities.

10. Which health-care provider should the nurse assign to assess a client with major depression who is to be discharged from the hospital that day?
    1. Physician.
    2. Licensed vocational nurse/licensed practical nurse (LVN/LPN).
    3. Certified nursing assistant (CNA).
    4. Registered nurse (RN).

11. A child with juvenile rheumatoid arthritis must take long-term steroids. Through health teaching on the nurse's part, which adverse effect of the medication can be prevented?
    1. Hyperglycemia.
    2. Hirsutism.
    3. Infection.
    4. Delayed growth.

12. The best place to assess for dehydration by checking skin turgor in older adults is on the:
    1. Dorsal aspect of the forearm
    2. Anterior chest, below the clavicle
    3. Back of the hand
    4. Abdomen

13. The nurse is conducting a physical assessment on a 76-year-old woman. The nurse should:
    1. Dim the lights in the room.
    2. Conduct the exam quickly.
    3. Raise her voice to say "good morning."
    4. Increase the temperature in the exam room slightly and provide a blanket.

14. A client is admitted to the hospital with a diagnosis of severe PIH. Her treatment would include:
    1. Complete bedrest, limited oral intake, and magnesium sulfate.
    2. Modified bedrest, limited salt diet, and magnesium sulfate.
    3. Limited stimulation, increased protein diet, and Valium.
    4. Modified bedrest, strict intake and output, and magnesium sulfate.

15. When assessing a client, the nurse notes retinal hemorrhages. The nurse should further assess for:
    1. Glaucoma
    2. Impairment of cranial nerve III, the oculomotor nerve.
    3. Hypertension.
    4. The client's need for corrective lenses.

16. What would the nurse in a newborn nursery be sure to provide for an infant of a mother who is drug-addicted?
    1. Tight blanket wrap
    2. Stimulation to enhance development
    3. Loose blanket wrap
    4. Frequent feedings

17. The nurse counsels an 11-year-old child with asthma and the family that the most therapeutic exercise for this child is:
    1. Lawn croquet.
    2. Ping-pong.
    3. Bowling.
    4. Checkers.

18. A client with acute pulmonary edema secondary to congestive heart failure has continuous monitoring of central venous pressure. Which statement about central venous pressure indicates that the client's treatment regimen is effective?
    1. Central venous pressure increases.
    2. Central venous pressure decreases.

3. There is no change in the central venous pressure.
   4. Central venous pressure is not a useful measure for this client.

19. Thirty minutes after left-heart catheterization the client's blood pressure begins to drop. Which potential complication explains this?
    1. Absent distal pulses.
    2. Increased pain at puncture site.
    3. Nausea.
    4. Bleeding or hematoma at the puncture site.

20. How often should a nurse remove restraints that have been applied to a client who is combative?
    Fill in the blank.
    At least every _____ hour(s)

21. A school-age child with asthma inhales a steroid via a metered dose inhaler (MDI) 3 times a day. The nurse's *priority* health teaching regarding the use of the steroid is:
    1. Handwashing before and after taking the medication.
    2. "Swish and spit" with water after taking the medication.
    3. Gargle with mouthwash after taking the medication.
    4. Suck on a piece of hard candy to alleviate the dry mouth that accompanies the use of this medication.

22. An appropriate nursing diagnosis for a client undergoing a cardiac catheterization is:
    1. *Risk for altered tissue perfusion* related to bleeding or thrombosis.
    2. *Risk for altered fluid balance* related to diuretic action of dye used during the procedure.
    3. *Risk for altered acid/base balance* related to vomiting post-procedure.
    4. *Body image disturbance* related to puncture site and post-procedure limitations.

23. A client receiving magnesium sulfate states to the nurse that she "feels like an elephant is sitting on my chest." The nurse knows that this is most likely caused by:
    1. A pulmonary embolism.
    2. A myocardial infarction.
    3. Asthma.
    4. Increased blood serum level of magnesium.

24. The client returned from thoracic surgery 3 hours ago with two chest tubes placed at 20 cm suction. Which finding would be considered abnormal?
    1. Bubbling in the suction control chamber.
    2. 350 cc of sanguineous drainage in the drainage chamber over the last 3 hours.
    3. No fluctuation in the water seal chamber.
    4. Small amount of sanguineous drainage on the chest tube dressing.

25. The client with a new ileostomy has received discharge teaching. Which dinner menu selected by the client indicates understanding of an appropriate diet for a new ileostomy?
    1. Baked chicken, whole grain biscuit, corn on the cob, canned peaches.
    2. Baked chicken, mashed potato, cooked carrots, angel food cake.
    3. Ham, mashed potato, salad with raw carrots, canned peaches.
    4. Roast beef, pasta with butter and garlic, split pea soup, 2 chocolate chip cookies with walnuts.

26. What important observation would the nurse look for in a newborn 24–48 hours after birth?
    1. Decrease in size of caput succedaneum.
    2. Passage of meconium stool.
    3. Presence of milia.
    4. Decrease in vernix.

27. A client with mitral stenosis has a murmur. The nurse may also find:
    1. Dyspnea on exertion.
    2. Jugular vein distention.

3. Syncope on exertion.

4. Angina

28. The nurse knows that the client understands how to live with his new implanted pacemaker when he says:
   1. "I should wear a Medic Alert bracelet and carry an identification card."
   2. "I guess this means I have to get rid of my microwave oven."
   3. "I can't travel by airplane anymore because I will set off the metal detectors."
   4. "The only time I need to call the doctor is if my pulse is too fast or too slow."

29. The parents of an adolescent with hemophilia seek counseling from the nurse. The mother states, "We just can't put up with any more of his risk-taking behaviors. We don't know what to do with him!" After the nurse discusses options with the parents, which statement indicates continued coping difficulties on the parent's part?
   1. "We will rejoin the hemophilia support group."
   2. "We will ask our in-laws to supervise him 1 night a week so that we can go out for dinner together."
   3. "We will talk to his favorite teacher at school and ask her to talk to him about his behaviors."
   4. "We will back off and make him be more responsible for his own care."

30. The nurse working on a psychiatric unit recognizes the need for further teaching when a staff person is overheard saying on the telephone:
   1. "I cannot acknowledge that the client has been admitted to the hospital."
   2. "Yes, Mr. Smith was admitted to the hospital today."
   3. "Clients admitted to this unit have a right to privacy."
   4. "I can take your name and number and give it to the client, if the client is here."

31. Which woman would be most at risk for cervical cancer?
   1. A 40-year-old who has never had any children.
   2. A 27-year-old woman who is sexually active with multiple partners.
   3. A 56-year-old woman who is postmenopausal and who started menstruation at age 10.
   4. A woman who had a child at age 20 and breast-fed for 2 years.

32. The nurse notes that the client's ECG has a rate of 78 bpm, normal P waves that precede each QRS complex, PR intervals of 0.16 seconds, and a regular pattern of shortening and lengthening of P-P and R-R intervals. The nurse should:
   1. Notify the physician STAT.
   2. Call for a STAT 12-lead ECG.
   3. Prepare the client for a cardiac catheterization.
   4. Document the client as having sinus arrhythmia.

33. When entering the client's room, the nurse notices a flat line on the client's ECG monitor and the ECG alarm is sounding. What should the nurse do *first*?
   1. Call a code.
   2. Assess the client for responsiveness.
   3. Notify the physician STAT.
   4. Begin CPR.

34. A client has been in a motor vehicle accident and is transported to the emergency department. The nurse must complete a primary survey. What does the nurse do *first*?
   1. Check the carotid pulse.
   2. Auscultate the lungs.
   3. Determine the need for an oral airway.
   4. Assess level of consciousness.

35. Which nursing action would be most effective in teaching a 6-year-old child with asthma how to identify asthma triggers?
   1. Have the child watch a video dealing with asthma triggers.
   2. Read a pamphlet dealing with asthma triggers to the child.

3. Have the child participate in an activity such as a nature walk to learn about asthma triggers.

4. Provide the child with crayons and a coloring book that deals with with asthma triggers.

36. The nurse is teaching a new mother how to breastfeed her child. The nurse knows that the newborn is feeding well when:
   1. The newborn makes a smacking sound.
   2. The mother has to pull the newborn off the nipple
   3. The breast completely covers the newborn's face
   4. The newborn makes a soft puffing sound.

37. A client arrives at the emergency department via ambulance. Assessment of the client reveals flushed, dry skin; rapid, labored respirations; breath odor of acetone; confusion; and a fingerstick blood glucose of 360. The nurse should *immediately* expect to:
   1. Auscultate the client's lungs for fluid overload.
   2. Call for a STAT 12-lead ECG.
   3. Administer sodium bicarbonate.
   4. Begin an IV infusion of normal saline.

38. A camp nurse prepares to orient a group of school-age children with sickle cell anemia to their first summer camping experience. The *priority* information that the nurse will emphasize to the children is to:
   1. Avoid other campers who may be ill.
   2. Turn in their immunization records as soon as possible.
   3. Adhere to their medication schedules.
   4. Consume extra fluids.

39. A client has had a cuffed endotracheal tube for 3 days. When the nurse goes to the bedside, the nurse hears the client say "good morning." This indicates:
   1. The client is feeling better, is more alert, and is appropriately responsive.
   2. The cuff on the endotracheal tube is deflated, or the tube is misplaced and the nurse should act immediately.
   3. The endotracheal tube needs to be replaced immediately.
   4. The endotracheal tube has migrated to the right mainstem bronchus and the nurse should obtain a STAT chest x-ray.

40. The staff nurse notes a new order for fluoxetine (Prozac) 20 mg/q A. M. in the client's chart. The medication is included in the client's morning medications. After administrating the medication, the nurse sees that the client has not given consent to take the medication. The nurse immediately notifies the physician that the client was given Prozac that morning. What should be the next step taken by the nurse?
   1. Report the incident to the supervisor.
   2. Fill out an incident report.
   3. Bring the issue to the next staff meeting to prevent reoccurrences.
   4. Tell the client to question medications that are new.

41. A 2-year-old child is brought into the emergency department in a postictal state. This was the child's first seizure which was tonic-clonic in nature. As soon as it is safe to do so, which *priority* action will the nurse take during the initial assessment and stabilization of the child?
   1. Take the child's blood pressure.
   2. Take the child's respirations.
   3. Take the child's temperature.
   4. Take the child's heart rate.

42. To maintain correct placement of an endotracheal tube, the nurse should:
   1. Check cuff pressure periodically.
   2. Suction the client prn.
   3. X-ray the tube every day.
   4. Mark the tube at its insertion point into the client's mouth or nose.

43. A client with a cuffed endotracheal tube is on mechanical ventilation at a rate of 16 breaths per minute, a tidal volume of 900 mL, and an FiO_2 of 0.6. The client's blood gases are as follows: pH 7.48; PaO_2 100; $PaCO_2$ 30; SaO_2 98%. Which change in ventilator settings would be appropriate?
   1. Increase the FiO_2.
   2. Increase the rate of ventilations.
   3. Decrease the rate of ventilations.
   4. Decrease the tidal volume.

44. A client is on a mechanical ventilator with a cuffed endotracheal tube. One of the alarms on the ventilator sounds. The nurse should *immediately*:
   1. Auscultate lung sounds.
   2. Obtain STAT arterial blood gases.
   3. Check the tubing for accidental disconnection.
   4. Check the client for respiratory distress.

45. A woman comes to the clinic for a prenatal visit but she does not want to be tested for gonorrhea. The nurse advises her that the purpose of the test is to:
   1. Prevent neonatal ophthalmic infections from passage through the birth canal.
   2. Decrease incidence of preterm labor, premature rupture of membranes (PROM), and preterm delivery.
   3. Prevent reinfection of sexual partners exposed to sexually transmitted diseases.
   4. Avoid congenital heart defects associated with congenital gonorrhea.

46. A woman who delivered 2 days ago is preparing for discharge from the hospital. The woman's prenatal history shows she is not immune to rubella. The nurse instructs the woman that the purpose of the vaccination is:
   1. To prevent fetal heart defects and hearing loss during her next pregnancy.
   2. To prevent contracting rubella infection while breastfeeding.
   3. To avoid transmitting rubella to the newborn infant.
   4. To prevent fetal hydrops in her next pregnancy.

47. A client had a cuffed tracheostomy tube placed 4 weeks ago. The client is going to begin eating by mouth, with the tracheostomy tube in place. To prevent aspiration, the nurse will:
   Select all that apply.
   1. Raise the head of the bed to high Fowler's.
   2. Increase the client's FiO_2.
   3. Deflate the cuff on the tracheostomy tube.
   4. Suction the client before eating.
   5. Assess gag and swallow ability.
   6. Replace the tracheostomy ties.

48. A preschooler ingested a toxic dose of acetaminophen/Tylenol and was admitted to the pediatric unit for acetylcysteine/Mucomyst therapy via nasogastric tube. The preschooler receives 5 doses of the medication and pulls the nasogastric out. The decision is made by the pediatrician to give the remaining doses of the medication by mouth. To achieve this goal, the nurse would gather the following item(s):
   Select all that apply.
   1. Water or milk.
   2. A sweet beverage such as Coca-Cola.
   3. A covered cup.
   4. A drinking straw.

49. The client is scheduled for a percutaneous renal biopsy to diagnose the presence of a benign or malignant mass. Which actions should the nurse implement following the procedure?
   Select all that apply.
   1. Check urine for presence of hematuria.
   2. Restrict fluids for 24 hours.
   3. Maintain bedrest for at least 4 hours.
   4. Maintain pressure over the puncture site.

5. Perform passive range of motion to extremities.
6. Keep head of bed elevated greater than 45 degrees.

50. It is most important for the nurse to ensure that a client with schizophrenia-paranoid type disorder has a room that is:
   1. Quiet and away from conversation.
   2. Close to the nurse's station.
   3. Near the community room.
   4. With another client who is paranoid.

51. A clinic nurse reviews information regarding the at-home administration of antihemophilic factor with a school-age child with hemophilia and the parents. The nurse's *priority* assessment of their knowledge base would focus on:
   1. Their understanding of the signs and symptoms of transfusion-like reactions.
   2. Their understanding of the signs and symptoms of fluid overload.
   3. Their understanding of the signs and symptoms of infiltration at the IV insertion site.
   4. Their understanding of the signs and symptoms of hepatitis and HIV.

52. The client has bloody urine and comes to the clinic for a cystoscopy without cystography. The appropriate nursing action prior to the procedure is to:
   1. Check the client history for allergy to seafood or shellfish.
   2. Drape the client's groin area with a lead apron.
   3. Instruct the client on what to expect during the procedure.
   4. Remove loose metal objects and jewelry.

53. A woman is in active labor. In checking the fetal heart rate (FHR), what would alert the nurse that something is wrong?
   1. Persistent fetal heart rate of 120 bpm.
   2. Increase in baseline fetal heart rate from 140 bpm to 180 bpm.
   3. An abrupt decrease of 20 bpm below baseline 2 times in the last 30 minutes.
   4. An increase of 20 bpm over the baseline 3 times in the past 30 minutes.

54. The client is scheduled for an intravenous pyelogram (IVP) to evaluate possible obstruction in the urinary tract. To prepare the client, the nurse will:
   Select all that apply.
   1. Give a laxative and/or enemas starting the night before the procedure.
   2. Force fluids orally or by IV at least 4 hours before the test.
   3. Verify that an informed consent has been signed.
   4. Explain that there might be a salty taste in the mouth from the dye.
   5. Drape a lead apron over the pelvic area for radiation protection.
   6. Instruct the client to drink plenty of fluids after the procedure.

55. IV orders for a 78-year-old client include D5 $^1/_2$ NS with 20 mEq KCl at 75 cc/hr. At 6:00 A.M. a new bag of 1000 mL was hung. At 8:00 A.M. the nurse sees that only 200 mL remains. The *first* action by the nurse would be to:
   1. Check the site for infiltration and elevate the extremity if needed.
   2. Order an infusion pump to provide better control of the rate.
   3. Slow the IV to "keep open" and check the client for lung crackles.
   4. Assist the client to the bathroom to void.

56. A woman with gestational diabetes tells the nurse, "Sometimes I forget to take my insulin." The nurse knows that the client and her fetus are at risk for which complications?
   Select all that apply.
   1. Oligohydramnios.
   2. Macrosomia.
   3. Pregnancy-induced hypertension (PIH).

4. Polyhydramnios.
5. Hypoglycemia.
6. Microcephaly.

57. Discharge teaching for a client who had a thyroidectomy would include:
    1. Calling health-care provider if lethargy, headache, or weak muscles occur.
    2. Calling health-care provider if experiencing numbness or tingling around mouth.
    3. Maintaining a high potassium diet including bananas, broccoli, and tomatoes.
    4. Avoiding high calcium foods such as tofu, milk, kale, and collard greens.

58. Which information should the nurse give a client with diabetes to prevent a foot infection?
    1. Trim the toenails if soft and thin.
    2. Soak feet in warm water as needed.
    3. Apply moisturizing lotion on soles and between toes.
    4. Remove calluses with a safety razor.

59. A school-aged child with hemophilia is thrown from his bicycle and is seriously injured. He is admitted to the emergency department. To expedite the management of his care, the nurse manager of the emergency department would assign a nurse to this child who can:
    Select all that apply.
    1. Interact effectively with a child who is acutely ill.
    2. Interact effectively with a child who is chronically ill.
    3. Interact effectively with family who are anxious.
    4. Interact effectively with personnel in the blood bank of the hospital.

60. A nurse receives a referral to make a home visit to a client who has schizophrenia and complains of hearing voices. The mother lives alone with an 8-month-old infant in subsidized housing, and does not have any baby furniture in the apartment. Which nursing observation will have the greatest priority in planning the care for this mother and infant?
    1. The electrical outlets which do not have protected sockets.
    2. The mother lacks knowledge about the infant's cognitive development.
    3. There are many small items of trash and garbage on the floor.
    4. The mother's medications will run out in 2 days.

61. The newborn infant's heart rate is 90, with irregular gasping respirations, central cyanosis, limp muscle tone, and a grimace with stimulation. The APGAR score is:
    Fill in the blank.

    _____

62. A client with diabetes complains of feeing full and nauseated after meals. The appropriate nursing action to manage this problem is to :
    1. Place the head of the bed flat for 30 minutes after meals.
    2. Give metoclopramide (Reglan) as ordered before meals.
    3. Change from oral to parenteral nutrition.
    4. Check to see if client is swallowing air while eating.

63. A person who has diabetes and is insulin-dependent is vomiting frequently. Which physician order(s) would the nurse question?
    Select all that apply.
    1. Give insulin and monitor blood glucose levels every 1–2 hours.
    2. Hold next scheduled dose of insulin and check blood glucose in 6 hours.
    3. Give acarbose (Precose) as ordered, and check urine sugar and acetone.
    4. Hold scheduled dose of acarbose (Precose) and give sublingual sugar.
    5. Give Compazine by mouth between episodes of vomiting.

64. An adolescent with hemophilia is being discharged from the pediatric unit following a bleeding episode into a joint

(hemarthrosis). Which discharge instruction, written by the pediatrician, should the charge nurse question?
1. "No aspirin or aspirin-related products."
2. "Tylenol 480 mg po q4–6h prn for pain."
3. "May resume adaptive physical education class upon return to school."
4. "May resume taking prophylactic antihemophilic factor at home and at H.S."

65. The nurse tells the client that the potential risk of blindness is minimized by:
    1. Keeping the corneas moist with artificial tears.
    2. Keeping the blood sugar below 120 mg/dL.
    3. Increasing the intake of foods rich in beta carotene.
    4. Planning early surgical removal of developing cataracts.

66. Which statement made by an 11-year-old child with mild hemophilia would validate the effectiveness of the nurse's teaching?
    1. "I will take extra factor when I know that I'm going to increase my activity level."
    2. "I will take extra factor after strenuous exercise."
    3. "I will apply warm compresses to ease my pain following a joint injury."
    4. "I will wear my splints all the time."

67. A 50-year-old man who is diabetic admits to difficulty obtaining and maintaining penile erection. The nurse would instruct the client to:
    1. Maintain blood sugar levels in the 150–250 mg/dL range.
    2. Drink 2–3 glasses of red wine before sexual intercourse.
    3. Perform 50–100 sets of pelvic floor contractions twice a day.
    4. Avoid smoking particularly before sexual intercourse.

68. A client who is 8 weeks pregnant, comes to the clinic with severe lower abdominal pain, feels faint, has shoulder pain, is afebrile, and has no vaginal bleeding. The most likely reason for her current condition is:
    1. Pelvic inflammatory disease.
    2. Ruptured tubal pregnancy.
    3. Urinary tract infection.
    4. Imminent spontaneous abortion.

69. The nurse receives notification from the laboratory that the client, who is diabetic, has an $HgbA_{1c}$ of 6%. The best action by the nurse would be to:
    1. Counsel the client on the need for better glycemic control.
    2. Document the results in the client record.
    3. Encourage a diet with more red meat and green leafy vegetables.
    4. Acknowledge the client's successful glycemic control.

70. A client comes to the clinic and reports, "hearing voices inside my head." To determine the next nursing action, which question should the nurse ask *first*?
    1. "What do the voices say to you?"
    2. "Do you hear the voices often?"
    3. "At what time of the day are the voices worse?"
    4. "Have you recently experienced a change in your life?"

71. A client delivered a 38-week-gestation infant. The most critical physiological change in the infant is:
    1. Immune system defense at birth.
    2. Temperature maintenance.
    3. Respirations initiated and maintained.
    4. Closure of the fetal circulatory bypasses.

72. A client is admitted with a blood glucose of 140 mg/dL, total carbon dioxide (bicarbonate) is 28 mEq/L, blood pressure is 148/94, and pulse is 88. The *first* nursing priority would be to:
    1. Give 40 units of regular insulin.
    2. Check urine for sugar and acetone.
    3. Encourage deep, slow breaths.
    4. Record the admitting baseline data.

73. A client with diabetes complains of bilateral foot and lower leg pain. The best action by the nurse would be to:

1. Apply continuous heat to the extremities.
2. Perform range of motion with the feet dependent to knees.
3. Give Neurontin around the clock.
4. Give morphine as needed for the pain.

74. The best nursing actions for a client with acute pancreatitis would be:
    1. NPO, bedrest, side-lying with knees flexed, and pain medication as ordered.
    2. Low protein diet, Metamucil mixed with minimal water, and ambulation prn.
    3. Prednisone and sulfasalazine as ordered, and ambulation tid.
    4. Dressing change bid, pancreatic enzyme, and pain medication as ordered.

75. The parents of a newborn infant do not want antibiotic ointment placed in the infant's eyes after birth. The nurse advises the parents that the ointment is used to:
    1. Treat any swelling of the infant's eyelids and facilitate vision.
    2. Facilitate formation of tears and provide lubrication for the eyes.
    3. Destroy infectious organisms transmitted during passage through the birth canal.
    4. Treat newborn for infectious organisms present in the hospital during the birth.

76. Which nursing action would be most effective when dealing with a preschooler with Kawasaki disease who is irritable?
    1. Sedate the preschooler until the irritability subsides.
    2. Set limits regarding acceptable behavior.
    3. Provide age-appropriate diversional activities.
    4. Reason with the child regarding the need for cooperation.

77. A client had a positive fecal occult blood test during a health screening. The nursing assessment would include:
    Select all that apply.
    1. Orthostatic (postural) blood pressure and pulse.
    2. STAT request for hemoglobin and hematocrit.
    3. Description of stool volume, color, and consistency.
    4. Diet history of raw meat consumption.
    5. Regular use of aspirin or NSAIDs.
    6. Vitamin C, 250 mg tablets, before the test.

78. In the recovery room, the nurse is unable to detect any bowel sounds in the abdomen of a client following a gastrojejunostomy (Billroth II). Which action would the nurse take *first*?
    1. Notify the surgeon ASAP because the anastomosis may be leaking.
    2. Check VS and urine output; client may be bleeding internally.
    3. Gently massage the abdomen, and recheck bowel sounds.
    4. Continue to monitor recovery, and position for comfort.

79. A preschooler hospitalized with Kawasaki disease tearfully tells the nurse that there are "bees in my ears." The nurse would correctly interpret this statement as being:
    1. A statement that must be reported to the child's pediatrician.
    2. A way of getting attention by the child.
    3. An example of an overactive imagination.
    4. A normal preschool fear.

80. A nurse is visiting a client with chronic schizophrenia in a group home. The client is actively hallucinating, unable to follow directions, and is agitated by voices. The client is not taking antipsychotic medications. The nurse calls the client's physician to report the findings, and an order for chlorpromazine HCl (Thorazine) is given. The nurse would question the order if the client had a history of:
    1. Extrapyramidal symptoms (EPS).
    2. Neuroleptic malignant syndrome (NMS).
    3. Substance abuse.
    4. Dystonia and akathisia.

81. A client wished to breastfeed immediately after birth. She notices that her milk is yellowish in color. She states to the nurse that the milk does not look good enough to feed to the baby. What would be the best explanation by the nurse?
    1. Poor nutrition during pregnancy produced this milk deficiency.
    2. The yellow color indicates a possible infection and should not be fed to the infant.
    3. The first milk is usually bluish, and the yellow color indicates a lack of nutrients.
    4. The first milk is normally yellowish and contains antibodies for the infant.

82. The best nursing action for a client diagnosed with chronic fatigue syndrome is to:
    1. Eliminate protein and fat-soluble vitamins (A, D, E, and K) from the diet.
    2. Give low doses of systemic glucocorticoids as ordered daily.
    3. Teach visualization to overcome psychosomatic symptoms.
    4. Plan regular periods of daily exercise and rest.

83. The appropriate nursing action when inserting a nasoduodenal (e.g., Dobhoff) tube would be to:
    1. Have client take a deep breath as the tube is advanced past the oral pharynx.
    2. Tip the client's head back as the tube is advanced into the esophagus.
    3. Measure from xyphoid to ear to nose to determine correct insertion point.
    4. Have the client swallow as the tube is advanced through the esophagus.

84. When palpating a woman's fundus on the second postpartum day, the nurse observes that the fundus is above the umbilicus and displaced to the right. The nurse evaluates that she probably has:
    1. Retained placental fragments.
    2. Overstretched uterine ligaments.
    3. A slow rate of involution.
    4. A full, overdistended bladder.

85. The nurse reviews the chart of a client following cardiac catheterization and notes the ejection fraction is 0.3 or 30% of normal. The nurse would expect the plan of care to focus on:
    1. Management of pain from anginal episodes.
    2. Inability to perform self-care caused by fatigue.
    3. Impaired motor and sensory function in extremities.
    4. Reducing risk of stroke (brain attack) from hypertension.

86. A nurse from the float pool is assigned to care for a child with Kawasaki disease. The *priority* action for the nurse to take before initiating care is to:
    1. Check that protamine sulfate is in the child's medication cassette.
    2. Check that phytonadione is in the child's medication cassette.
    3. Check that deferoxamine mesylate is in the child's medication cassette.
    4. Check the child's menu to make sure that food sources rich in vitamin K have been ordered by the parents.

87. During report from the night shift, the day nurse receives information on four clients. Which client should the nurse assess *first*?
    1. 78-year-old client 3 days after knee surgery whose pain level at 6:00 A.M. was 3 out of 10.
    2. 45-year-old client with diverticulosis who is scheduled for bowel surgery at 8:00 A.M.
    3. 18-year-old client with multiple fractures whose Hct is 32, which is down from 32.5 of the previous day.
    4. 62-year-old client 2 days following bladder surgery whose WBC is 11,000.

88. The best indication that a client has recovered fully from general anesthesia is:
    1. The blood oxygen level is normal.
    2. The client is able to lift legs off the bed.
    3. The client is awake and oriented.
    4. The blood pressure and pulse are normal.

89. A school-age child with sickle cell anemia develops osteomyelitis and is admitted to the pediatric unit for long-term IV antibiotics. The mother of the child comes out to the nurse's station and informs the charge nurse that the child's IV is leaking. The charge nurse's *first* action is to:
    1. Go directly to the child's room and assess the IV.
    2. Notify the nurse who is caring for the child that the IV is leaking.
    3. Instruct the mother to return to the child's room and turn on the call light.
    4. Ask the nursing student who is caring for the child to assess the IV.

90. Because an 80-year-old client with dementia has a history of falls, which nursing measure will be essential to the plan of care?
    1. Use soft restraints when the client is sitting in a chair.
    2. Allow the client freedom to roam anywhere on the unit.
    3. Have the client sit in the dayroom with other clients for observation.
    4. Provide the client with a recliner or a deep seated chair in front of the nurse's station.

91. While making a home visit, the client tells the nurse that the cefuroxime has been taken daily the first 3 days, twice a day for 3 days, and now 3 times a day. The best response by the nurse would be:
    1. "Were you able to tolerate the side effects as the dose was increased?"
    2. "May I see the directions on the bottle? That's an unusual schedule."
    3. "Have you had any rashes or difficulty breathing with the drug?"
    4. "Will you increase the dose again or stay at 3 tablets each day?"

92. A client who is pregnant has class III cardiac disease. Nursing care for her in labor would include:
    1. Preparing her for a cesarean section to avoid stress during labor.
    2. Preparing her for an epidural anesthetic to avoid pain during labor.
    3. Helping her during labor, without an epidural, to increase sensation during pushing.
    4. Encouraging Valsalva pushing to decrease the length of the second stage of labor.

93. The client's chart indicates an allergy to penicillin. Which drug would be inappropriate for the client to have?
    1. Acetaminophen.
    2. Diphenhydramine.
    3. Vitamin C.
    4. Ceftriaxone.

94. A school-age child with Legg-Calvé-Perthes disease is placed on prolonged bedrest. Which potential outcome of this therapy would be most detrimental to the child?
    1. Obesity.
    2. Constipation.
    3. Social isolation.
    4. Pressure ulcers.

95. It is very important to anticipate drug interactions. Which medication order(s) would the nurse question?
    Select all that apply.
    1. Atenolol 50 mg PO daily for a client with a pulse of 50 bpm.
    2. Furosemide 20 mg for a client with high serum potassium.
    3. Birth control pills for a 40-year-old client who smokes.
    4. Albuterol for a client with asthma.
    5. Insulin IV for a client with elevated serum potassium.
    6. Aspirin 81 mg daily for a client at risk for brain attacks (strokes).
    7. Levothyroxine 150 µg for a client with a recent MI.
    8. Docusate sodium bid for a client taking morphine for pain.

96. One day after knee surgery the client is started on both heparin and warfarin. The nurse tells the client both are needed because:
    1. Heparin works rapidly to provide anticoagulation until the warfarin takes effect in several days.
    2. Warfarin works rapidly to provide anticoagulation until the heparin takes effect in several days.
    3. Warfarin will reduce the risk of bleeding from the heparin.
    4. Heparin will reduce the risk of bleeding from the warfarin.

97. The charge nurse is observing a new graduate on the pediatric unit. Which behavior on the part of the new graduate would warrant remedial instruction by the charge nurse?
    1. The new graduate uses latex gloves while implementing enteric precautions when caring for an infant with acute gastroenteritis.
    2. The new graduate uses latex gloves while changing a diaper on an infant with a suspected urinary tract infection.
    3. The new graduate uses latex gloves while drawing a blood specimen from an infant with a myelomeningocele.
    4. The new nurse graduate uses latex gloves while using an oral bulb to suction a child with bronchiolitis.

98. A client with gestational diabetes asks about her insulin dose. The nurse knows the client understands her teaching when she states:
    1. "I know I will need to take more insulin during the later part of my pregnancy."
    2. "The insulin dosage should decrease each week after the first trimester."
    3. "The insulin dosage will increase after I deliver the baby."
    4. "The insulin dosage should be about the same throughout my pregnancy."

99. Which assessment is of primary importance when caring for a client with Guillain-Barré syndrome?
    1. Pain.
    2. Corneal reflex.
    3. Rate, depth, and quality of respirations.
    4. Arterial blood gases.

100. After using alternative interventions, the nurse determines that a client who is agitated requires the application of restraints. Which direction by a staff nurse to an LVN/LPN applying the restraints indicates the need for further teaching?
    1. "Secure the restraints to the bedrails for easy removal."
    2. "Place padding around the restraints to protect the skin."
    3. "Use knots with hitches for easy removal."
    4. "Secure restraints to parts of the bed that move with the client."

101. A school nurse returns from lunch and finds four children waiting to be seen in the school health office. Which child could the school nurse safely assign to the school health office aide?
    1. A child with hemophilia who has a reddened elbow.
    2. A child complaining of a persistent cough who had a tonsillectomy 5 days ago.
    3. A child with asthma who is wheezing.
    4. A child with scoliosis who is complaining of itching under the Boston brace.

102. A client with a complete spinal cord injury at the C5 level is complaining of a headache. The nurse should:

1. Give the client 650 mg of acetaminophen.
2. Catheterize the client's bladder.
3. Call the physician STAT.
4. Immediately assess the client's blood pressure.

103. Discharge teaching for the client with a total hip replacement should include:
   1. Use of a raised toilet seat.
   2. Daily monitoring of coagulation status if the client will be self-administering enoxaparin at home.
   3. A gentle program of jogging to strengthen the quadriceps muscles.
   4. Active range of motion exercises that include 90° flexion at the hip.

104. A UAP reports to the registered nurse caring for a 5-year-old child who had a tonsillectomy 6 hours ago that the child is repeatedly blowing his nose. The *first* action on the part of the registered nurse is to:
   1. Reassure the UAP that this is a normal behavior and to be expected.
   2. Instruct the UAP to ask the child not to blow his nose.
   3. Call the pediatrician and report the behavior.
   4. Inform the UAP that the registered nurse will talk to the child as soon as possible.

105. A client comes to labor and delivery at 28 weeks gestation with severe abdominal pain, vaginal bleeding, sweating, and tachycardia. What should the nurse do *first*?
   1. Place the client on a fetal monitor to check fetal heart tones.
   2. Perform a vaginal exam to determine dilation of the cervix.
   3. Start an IV to administer tocolytics.
   4. Call the physician to obtain orders for pain medication.

106. While assessing an 82-year-old client in cardiac rehabilitation, the nurse can expect to find:
   1. A resting respiratory rate of 8–10 breaths per minute.
   2. A maximum exercise heart rate of 120 bpm.
   3. A blood pressure of 110/60.
   4. Increased vital capacity and chest excursion.

107. The nurse determines that a 78-year-old client is experiencing the occasional forgetfulness that normally occurs as people age when the client:
   1. Does not know the day or month.
   2. Forgets people who are important, such as children and siblings.
   3. Needs to use a pill box marked with the days of the week.
   4. Repeats the same question only a few minutes later.

108. A client is admitted with a diagnosis of HELLP syndrome. The nurse explains to the client that magnesium sulfate is administered to:
   1. Decrease risk for developing seizures.
   2. Prevent neonatal respiratory distress.
   3. Decrease blood pressure.
   4. Improve perfusion to the liver and uterus.

109. A registered nurse returns to the pediatric unit from dinner break and receives the following report from the LVN/LPN. Which child should the registered nurse attend to *first*?
   1. A child with epiglottitis and a tracheostomy with a neck dressing that is wet and soiled.
   2. A child with acute glomerulonephritis whose urine is bloody.
   3. A child with sickle cell anemia whose PCA (patient-controlled analgesia) medication cassette is empty.
   4. A child with pyloric stenosis who has vomited.

110. A client with a 9-month-old infant comes to the clinic for the first time and asks the nurse why the infant is not afraid of strangers. Which response by the nurse would be most appropriate at this time?
   1. Reassure the client that many infants do not experience stranger anxiety.

2. Refer the client to developmental education that includes parenting strategies.
3. Assess the infant's and mother's attachment behaviors.
4. Show concern and reassure the parent that there is no need to worry.

111. The nurse is caring for an 80-year-old Filipino client who was admitted to the hospital yesterday with cellulitis of the left foot. The nurse knows it is important to:
   1. Create a calm, restful environment by discouraging visitors in the room.
   2. Encourage the client to speak English to facilitate communication.
   3. Discourage consumption of ethnic foods because they are often high in fat, sodium, or sugar.
   4. Allow the client to keep rosary beads and crucifix next to the bed.

112. The nurse is teaching a 78-year-old client how to give himself enoxaparin shots at home after he is discharged from the hospital following a total knee replacement. The nurse knows that the client's discharge teaching will be most successful if the nurse:
   1. Explains that the shots are a necessary part of the client's recovery and it is essential for him to learn to give them.
   2. Schedules a short teaching session because clients who are elderly have a shorter attention span.
   3. Invites the client's wife and three daughters to attend the teaching session.
   4. Keeps instructions simple and repeats them often.

113. A school bus is involved in a traffic accident at 7:30 A.M. en route to delivering a group of children with "special needs" to school. A pediatric emergency team is dispatched to the scene of the accident. The registered nurse will give greatest *priority* to:
   1. The child with epilepsy who is complaining of a headache.
   2. The child with diabetes mellitus who is complaining of feeling scared and shaky.
   3. The child with rheumatoid arthritis who is complaining of feeling stiff and sore.
   4. The child with scoliosis who is wearing a Milwaukee brace and complaining of shoulder level pain.

114. A cesarean section is always performed when the client has current:
   1. Pelvic inflammatory disease
   2. Outbreak of herpes on her genitalia.
   3. Outbreak of herpes on her upper lip.
   4. Group B beta streptococcal infection.

115. A nurse is reading the results of a TB skin test on a 72-year-old client who has never had a TB skin test. There is no induration around the injection site. The nurse should document the test as negative and:
   1. State that the client does not have TB.
   2. Have the client repeat the skin test in 2 weeks.
   3. Schedule the client for a follow-up chest x-ray.
   4. Start the client on prophylactic TB medications because the client is in a high-risk group.

116. An 85-year-old client who is Chinese is admitted to the hospital for treatment of acute congestive heart failure. The family states that they practice traditional Chinese medicine, and had difficulty getting the client to come to the emergency department. When planning care, the nurse needs to:
   1. Obtain a list of the herbal medicines the client takes, so that drug interactions can be prevented.
   2. Consider that treatment for this client is likely to be unsuccessful because the client does not believe in Western medicine.
   3. Allow the client to continue taking herbal remedies because they are safe.
   4. Position the client in Fowler's to maintain the flow of *qi*.

117. A 45-year-old client is admitted for an emergency appendectomy. The client has a current history of alcoholism. The nurse will:
    1. Administer pain medications sparingly to avoid interaction with any alcohol in the client's system.
    2. Put the client in jacket and wrist restraints immediately after surgery to prevent injury to self or others due to delirium tremens.
    3. Turn the lights on and close the client's door.
    4. Admit the client to an alcohol recovery program.

118. Chorioamnionitis is suspected in a client who is 38 weeks pregnant. *Select all the symptoms she will likely exhibit:*
    1. Tachypnea.
    2. Fetal heart rate bradycardia.
    3. Uterine contractions.
    4. Hyperglycemia.
    5. Tachycardia.

119. The hospital's disaster system alert is activated. The charge nurse on the pediatric unit prepares the pediatric nursing staff to evacuate. Prior to evacuating the pediatric unit, the charge nurse will want to obtain additional support personnel to assist in transporting/caring for:
    1. A child with an oxygen saturation of 88%.
    2. A child with a nasogastric tube connected to intermittent decompression.
    3. A child with a continuous nasogastric feeding.
    4. A child with a PCA (patient-controlled analgesia).

120. The nurse is conducting a parenting class for a group of parents with toddlers (1–3 yrs). What guidance would be most important for the nurse to offer?
    1. Children at this age may not be able to tolerate long periods of separation.
    2. Need to set limits with negative reinforcement when the child throws temper tantrums.
    3. Learning when and how to say "no" is an important part of the toddler's communication.
    4. Offering opportunities to play with other toddlers without supervision.

121. A 57-year-old client is admitted to the hospital with shortness of breath, hemoptysis, and weight loss. The family actively encourages the client to comply with tests and treatments. The client does not want aggressive treatment if the diagnosis is lung cancer. The nurse should:
    1. Tell the client that it is too soon to make any decisions; the diagnosis isn't even known yet.
    2. Support the family in encouraging the client to comply with tests and treatment.
    3. Suggest to the physician that the client be made a "no code."
    4. Make sure that the client has an advance directive in the chart.

122. A hospitalized 4-year-old calls out repeatedly for the mother who is unable to visit her child until after work. The nurse's best response would be:
    1. "Stop crying and I'll take you to the playroom."
    2. "Mommy will come back later."
    3. "Mommy will come back after dinner."
    4. "Mommy is at work right now."

123. The nurse asks the licensed practical/vocational nurse (LPN/LVN) to check the vital signs and puncture site on a client who returned 1 hour ago from a cardiac catheterization. Who is accountable for this task?
    1. The nurse.
    2. The practical/vocational nurse.
    3. The physician.
    4. The hospital.

124. A 52-year-old client with a 6-year history of diabetes mellitus, type 2, is being seen for a routine checkup. A blood test reveals an HgbA$_{1c}$ of 8%. It is important for the nurse to *first:*
    1. Assess what the client already knows.
    2. Increase the daily dose of antihyperglycemic medication.
    3. Enroll the client in classes on managing diabetes.
    4. Inform the client that diabetes is being poorly controlled, which will lead to complications.

125. Cocaine use is suspected in a client who is 34 weeks gestation. For what complications is the fetus at high risk?
    1. Late decelerations.
    2. Polyhydramnios.
    3. Macrosomia.
    4. Hyperbilirubinemia.

126. The client, a high school teacher, has been admitted for a modified radical mastectomy to be performed on the following day. This is the client's first hospitalization. The nurse attempts to teach the client how to use an incentive spirometer, but the client waves the nurse away and does not want to learn that now. Which factor most likely led to this unsuccessful teaching session?
    1. The client's intelligence and educational level.
    2. The client's occupation as a high school teacher.
    3. The client's perception of the need to learn to use an incentive spirometer.
    4. The fact that the client lives at home with a husband and three children.

127. A middle-school teacher questions the school nurse about why the girls in her class are more developed than the boys. The nurse's best response would be:
    1. "This is normal. Girls begin puberty before boys and as a result are taller, heavier, and more developed than the boys."
    2. "This is abnormal. Boys begin puberty before girls and as a result should be taller, heavier, and more developed than the girls. I will pay a visit to your classroom and assess your students."
    3. "I will consult with the school physician about your observations and get back to you."
    4. "What is the ethnic mix in your classroom?"

128. The nurse is caring for a client in the intensive care unit who is terminally ill and comatose. The client's family, who are Chinese, wants to give the client herbal medicines via the nasogastric tube. The nurse is unsure if this would be ethically correct. To resolve this ethical dilemma, the nurse should:
    1. Give the herbs because the client is terminally ill and comatose.
    2. Refuse to give the herbs because the herbs may interact with the client's other medications and cause harm.
    3. Collect more information to determine the medically and ethically correct thing to do.
    4. Confer with other staff members about the situation.

129. A woman is complaining of sore nipples while breastfeeding. The nurse instructs her to:
    1. Wait to latch the infant until the infant is really hungry.
    2. Put warm compresses on the breasts and express the breastmilk.
    3. Put ice packs on the breasts and do not stimulate them.
    4. When latching, be sure the infant has a large amount of the areola in the mouth.

130. Which finding in an 82-year-old client would the nurse consider a normal characteristic?
    1. Not being able to tell the nurse everything that was eaten that morning for breakfast.
    2. Changing the exercise from bicycling to walking 3 times per week.
    3. Reducing contact with friends.
    4. Ignoring signs of aging.

131. The nurse realizes that the wrong medication was given to a client. The nurse immediately informs the nursing supervi-

sor and begins the hospital's protocol regarding medication errors. The nurse is demonstrating:
1. Competence.
2. Professionalism.
3. Reliability.
4. Accountability.

132. When faced with an ethical dilemma in the care of a client, what should guide the nurse's actions?
1. Strong religious beliefs.
2. Respect for client autonomy.
3. Thorough understanding of the law.
4. The physician's orders.

133. A client who recently had a positive pregnancy test states she has a history of frequent urinary tract infections. When planning teaching interventions, the nurse understands the client is at high risk for developing:
1. Chorioamnionitis
2. Pelvic inflammatory disease
3. Preterm labor
4. Kidney stones

134. A client who is confused and agitated is refusing to take PO medications. The nurse can:
1. Inform the physician.
2. Explain to the client the benefits of taking the medications and the consequences of not taking them.
3. Withhold the medications, document them as not given, and try to give them later when the client is calmer.
4. Ask several other nurses to help restrain the client while the nurse puts the pills in the client's mouth.

135. The mother of a 4-year-old child is worried because her child is a finicky eater who wants her to buy the junk food advertised in commercials on television. The mother expresses her concerns to the nurse about her child's lack of a balanced diet. The nurse's *priority* action would be to:
1. Provide the mother with literature regarding a preschooler's nutritional needs.
2. Review the basic food groups with the mother.
3. Suggest to the mother that she allow the child to self-select food.
4. Assess the child's daily eating pattern.

136. In which situation does the nurse need to fill out a quality assurance or unusual occurrence report?
1. While ambulating in the hall with the nursing assistant, the client gets dizzy and has to sit down.
2. The client gets up to go to the bathroom and slips and falls.
3. The client's skin becomes red and itchy where the IV was taped.
4. The client eats a cheeseburger and French fries brought in by the family.

137. A nurse is assigning clients on the postpartum unit. Which client should not be assigned to the LVN/LPN?
1. A client with a cesarean section, wound infection, and on IV antibiotics.
2. A client with a vacuum-assisted vaginal delivery and a third-degree laceration.
3. A client with pregnancy-induced hypertension and on magnesium sulfate.
4. A client with hyperemesis of pregnancy and on IV hydration.

138. For what reason would the nurse make out an unusual occurrence report?
1. To determine how client-care problems can be prevented in the future.
2. To protect the hospital in case of a lawsuit.
3. To evaluate the nurse's performance.
4. To provide documentation of the nurse's negligence.

139. The clinic nurse is beginning to administer the DDST (Denver Developmental Screening Test) to a small child when the mother says, "Can you tell me again what this DDST is?" The nurse's best response would be:
1. "It is an excellent way to see if a child's development is normal."
2. "It is a test given to measure a child's development."
3. "It tells us what a child can do at a particular age."
4. "It is a simple intelligence test for young children."

140. A couple comes to the mental health clinic, stating they are "afraid of how things will be now that the children are out of the house." Which response by the nurse indicates an understanding of the normal changes that occur in midlife?
1. "I don't blame you for being afraid; many people feel the same way."
2. "Try not to worry; you will adjust in time."
3. "You will begin to experience many losses as life goes on."
4. "Usually husbands and wives tend to become closer after the children leave."

141. A woman who is primigravida and 29 weeks pregnant is 3 centimeters dilated. She is having back pain and whitish, creamy vaginal discharge. The most likely treatment for her is:
1. Strict bedrest, tocolytics, and IV hydration.
2. Strict bedrest, oral hydration, and tocolytics.
3. IV hydration, bedrest, and tocolytics.
4. IV hydration, cervical cerclage, and bedrest.

142. On her first visit to the prenatal clinic, a woman states she has been pregnant 5 times, 1 delivery at 27 weeks gestation , 1 elective abortion at 6 weeks gestation, and 2 spontaneous abortions at 8 and 12 weeks gestation. The correct designation for her obstetrical history would be:
1. G5 P1 T0 AB3
2. G6 P3 T0 AB1
3. G5 P0 T1 AB3
4. G6 P1 T0 AB3

143. The nurse is developing a discharge plan for a client with a new ileostomy. The client is 32 years old, mentally competent, lives with her husband of 3 years, and works outside her home. Which nursing diagnoses are important to include in the discharge plan?
Select all that apply.
1. *Risk for fluid volume deficit.*
2. *Risk for fluid volume excess.*
3. *Risk for constipation.*
4. *Risk for impaired skin integrity.*
5. *Altered nutrition: more than body requirements.*
6. *Altered sexuality patterns.*

144. Which situations violate the client's rights?
Select all that apply.
1. While charting the client's 9:00 A.M. medications, the nurse briefly leaves the computer screen to speak to a visitor. The computer screen shows a list of the client's medications.
2. The client refuses surgery for colon cancer, despite being informed of the need, benefits, and risks of the surgery.
3. When asked about allergies, the client does not inform the health-care team about allergy to penicillin, and suffers a severe reaction when the drug is administered.
4. The physician is standing outside the client's room and asks the nurse at the nurse's station what the client's latest hemoglobin and hematocrit are. From the nurse's station, the nurse tells the physician what the lab values are.
5. Three nursing students discuss their assigned clients over lunch in the cafeteria.
6. The client has five visitors in the room. The nurse asks them to leave.

145. The client has a severe systemic infection. The physician has ordered gentamicin to be given intravenously every 8 hours. The recommended dose of gentamicin is 3–5 mg/kg/d. If the client weighs 165 lb, what is the correct range for a single dose of gentamicin?
Fill in the blank.
_____ mg q8h

146. The mother of a preschool-age child is concerned because her child has recently had trouble going to sleep at night. The child says, "a mean dog comes into my room and tries to bite me." The family does not have a pet dog. When counseling the mother, the nurse's *first* action would be to:
1. Suggest that the child be seen by a psychiatrist for evaluation.
2. Suggest that the child stop watching television prior to bedtime.
3. Suggest that the child be given a night light for the bedroom.
4. Suggest that the child be enrolled in a pet therapy program.

147. A school-age child sustains multiple fractures in an accident and is hospitalized for prolonged traction. The most effective nursing intervention to assist the child in maintaining a sense of control while hospitalized is to:
1. Have friends and classmates visit.
2. Have the child life specialist visit the child on a daily basis.
3. Allow the child to make as many choices as possible.
4. Allow the child to freely pick and choose what to do or not do.

148. The client is in the intensive care unit after coronary artery bypass surgery. One of the many post-op orders reads: "give potassium 2 mEq IV for each 0.1 mEq serum K+ less than 5.5." The nurse has on hand a solution of potassium that contains 2 mEq in each milliliter. If the client's potassium level is 3.2 mEq/L, how many milliliters of potassium will the nurse give?
Fill in the blank.
_____ mL

149. The nurse is counseling a client with chronic renal failure on hemodialysis. The client demonstrates understanding of an appropriate diet when choosing which food items for lunch:
Select all that apply.
1. 2 boneless, skinless chicken breasts.
2. 8 ounces of tomato juice.
3. 4 ounces of milk.
4. Lettuce and cucumber.
5. 2 tablespoons of mayonnaise.
6. 2 slices of bread.

150. In assessing a client, which behavior would indicate that the client is experiencing normal changes associated with adolescence?
1. Behavior is moody, unpredictable, and inconsistent.
2. Worries about accomplishing tasks.
3. Develops a strong relationship with one parent.
4. Cries frequently for unknown reasons.

151. Client education should include strategies to manage which long-term side effect from narcotic use?
1. Confusion.
2. Low blood pressure.
3. Constipation.
4. Respiratory depression.

152. A woman who is pregnant is given health teaching during her prenatal visit. When will the nurse instruct the client to seek medical immediate attention?
Select all that apply.
1. When she has swelling of the face, feet, and hands.
2. When uterine contractions occur during position changes.
3. When there is decreased vaginal discharge.
4. When she has a headache that is unrelieved by acetaminophen.
5. When there is increased fetal movement.

153. The best technique for preventing foot drop in a client who is immobilized following a brain attack (stroke) is:
1. Applying dorsiflexion boots or high top shoes.
2. Using a linen cradle to hold the sheets off the feet.
3. Turning side to back to side every 2 hours.
4. Placing a pillow under the lower leg to raise heels.

154. A client during postpartum has a temperature of 101°F, foul-smelling lochia, a tender uterus on palpation, and tachycardia. The client is at high risk for:
1. Urinary tract infection
2. Endometriosis
3. Bacterial vaginosis
4. Endometritis

155. Following a cleft-palate repair, a toddler is refusing to drink despite being offered a variety of fluids by the nurse. When the nurse weighs the toddler, no weight loss is noted. The nurse's best action is to:
1. Notify the pediatrician.
2. Wait until the toddler's mother comes to visit and enlist her assistance.
3. Document the toddler's I&O.
4. Ask the child life specialist to make a game out of drinking.

156. Which nursing action would be inappropriate for a client with heart failure?
1. Placing the client in modified-Trendelenburg to minimize ankle edema while sleeping.
2. Teaching about adequate nutritional intake within dietary limitations.
3. Teaching about the signs and symptoms to report to physician.
4. Providing opportunity to discuss concerns about the diagnosis.

157. The client is admitted with symptoms of peptic ulcer disease and a hematocrit (Hct) of 23%. The nurse knows that the lab value indicates:
1. Hemoconcentration has resulted to compensate for blood loss.
2. A normal level, and there is no active bleeding currently.
3. A slight drop, and the test should be repeated in 8 hours.
4. A very low level; vital signs should be checked immediately.

158. Following a laparoscopic cholecystectomy, the nurse tells the client that it is important to remain flat to prevent:
1. Pneumonia, from pressure on the diaphragm and shallow breathing.
2. Shoulder pain, from the carbon dioxide pressing on the diaphragm.
3. A headache following spinal anesthesia.
4. Blockage of the bile drainage from the T tube in the common bile duct.

159. The nurse prepares to remove a nasogastric tube from a 3-year-old child who had abdominal surgery for intussusception. The child begins to cry and says, "You're taking my insides out!" The nurse's initial response to the child should be to:
1. Ask the child to assist with the removal of the nasogastric tube.
2. Stop and reassure the child.
3. Ask the mother to assist with the removal of the nasogastric tube.
4. Notify the pediatrician and request an order for sedation.

160. A client who is 6 weeks pregnant asks the nurse if schizophrenia can be prevented. Which statement by the nurse is the most accurate?

1. "Schizophrenia is a genetic brain disease with neuro-chemical imbalances of serotonin, and a study by Smith has proven it cannot be prevented."
2. "Try not to worry. The chances of your baby having schizophrenia are low; in fact it is just one percent."
3. "Why do you want to know? I haven't been asked a question like that before."
4. "Research indicates that preventing the flu during pregnancy may prevent schizophrenia in the baby."

161. In the first trimester of pregnancy a physician orders a Pap smear. The client asks the nurse the reason for this test. The nurse responds that the test is to:
    1. Determine the presence of chlamydia that can affect the fetal growth and development.
    2. Detect the presence of fetal proteins which may indicate a neural tube defect.
    3. Check for abnormal cervical cells that may be precursors to cervical cancer.
    4. Obtain fetal cells to test for chromosomal abnormalities.

162. Following an MI, the client has begun a gradual exercise program. The nurse tells the client not to expect:
    1. Improved stamina and strength.
    2. A lowering of the high density lipid levels.
    3. Increased peripheral vascular blood flow.
    4. Decreased physical and psychological stress.

163. Which nursing action will be most effective in treating peptic ulcer disease?
    1. Giving alternating doses of magnesium and aluminum antacids every 2–4 hours.
    2. Giving antibiotics and HCl secretion inhibitors daily as ordered for one week.
    3. Obtaining information on enrollment in a stress management class.
    4. Explaining procedure for insertion of Minnesota or Blakemore tube with traction.

164. A client with a fourth degree episiotomy is receiving discharge teaching from the nurse. The nurse gives the client instructions to:
    1. Decrease the roughage in the diet for 2–3 weeks.
    2. Use hot packs to assist in healing.
    3. Use ice packs to decrease soreness.
    4. Take stool softeners and increase fluid intake to avoid constipation.

165. A client who is obese has begun a diet that includes protein, fats, and no carbohydrates. The best response by the nurse to this client would be:
    1. "If it works I'll recommend it to other clients."
    2. "Sufficient fluids will be needed to prevent acidosis."
    3. "Any plan you think might work will be supported."
    4. "Another client lost 90 pounds on the same diet."

166. Upon admission to the emergency department, racemic epinephrine was administered to a 2-year-old child with laryngotracheobronchitis. The child is to be admitted to the pediatric unit but there will be a wait of several hours because of lack of available pediatric beds. While waiting, the emergency department nurse who is caring for the child will focus on:
    1. Encouraging the child to take oral fluids.
    2. Administering oxygen as ordered to the child.
    3. Assessing the child's respiratory status and stability.
    4. Measuring the child's oxygen saturation level.

167. The client has begun a low carbohydrate diet for weight loss. Which group of foods would the nurse recommend for the diet?
    1. Ham, butter, cheese, and lettuce.
    2. Bread, pasta, corn, and milk.
    3. Oatmeal, split pea soup, and canned pears.
    4. Fruitcake, applesauce, and lima beans.

168. An infant is returned to the pediatric unit after a pyloromyotomy for the correction of pyloric stenosis. Which postoperative order would the nurse immediately question?
    1. "Begin incremental glucose water feedings when fully awake."
    2. "Notify pediatrician when bowel sounds return for feeding instructions."
    3. "Routine vital signs."
    4. "Strict I&O."

169. The client is complaining of a sudden steady epigastric pain. This pain description would be most consistent with a history of:
    1. Cholelithiasis.
    2. Endometriosis.
    3. Irritable bowel syndrome.
    4. Crohn's disease.

170. In assessing a client, which prodromal symptoms would indicate that the client is beginning to show signs of a psychotic break?
    Select all that apply.
    1. Withdrawing from friends.
    2. Magical thinking.
    3. Hallucinations.
    4. Delusions.
    5. Sensing the presence of a force.
    6. Grades dropping in school.

171. What is a correct statement made by a nursing student in a clinical conference about gonorrhea and pregnancy?
    1. Most clients who are pregnant know they have gonorrhea because they have profound symptoms of burning and vaginal itching.
    2. Gonorrhea can be passed from mother to infant during birth, infecting the infant's genital tract.
    3. It is difficult to treat gonorrhea in clients who are pregnant because the antibiotics cause fetal malformations.
    4. Prophylactic antibiotic eye ointment is administered at birth to prevent the eye damage caused by undiagnosed gonorrhea.

172. The nurse explains to the client that following a laparoscopic cholecystectomy there will be:
    1. A drainage tube inserted for 48 hours in case there are stones in the bile duct.
    2. A stoma will be created to drain the bile into a bag until the swelling resolves.
    3. Several small incisions on the abdomen each about $1/2$ inch in length.
    4. An upper midline incision in order to explore the common bile duct.

173. The client is scheduled for an abdominal CT scan with contrast agent. The nurse explains that the procedure requires:
    1. Lidocaine spray to the throat to reduce the gag reflex during tube insertion.
    2. A low fat diet for 48 hours before the test to enhance visualization.
    3. No history of allergic reactions to seafood and iodine.
    4. A lead apron over the abdomen before entry into the scanner.

174. A client with a possible diagnosis of colon cancer is scheduled for a barium enema. Client teaching will include:
    1. Cleansing the intestines before the test.
    2. Drinking the barium solution 24 hours before the test.
    3. Drinking the barium solution in radiology just before the test.
    4. Eating a high protein meal 2 hours before the test.

175. Hirschsprung's disease is suspected in a newborn. When admitting the newborn to the pediatric unit, the, nurse's most important assessment will be the newborn's:

1. Weight.
2. Hydration status.
3. Abdominal circumference.
4. Laboratory value.

176. A client has recently been diagnosed with breast cancer. The nurse knows most women with breast cancer have:
    1. Blood relatives with breast cancer.
    2. Not breastfed any children.
    3. No identified risk factors for breast cancer.
    4. Not routinely performed breast self-examination.

177. While working in an AIDS clinic, the nurse discards a used syringe in the sharps container which is overfilled, and she is stuck with a needle already in the box. What would be the recommended management of this exposure?
    1. A single dose each of ddI (didanosine) and d4T (stavudine) within 2 hours of exposure.
    2. A single dose of ZDV (zidovudine) within 2 hours of exposure.
    3. Take zidovudine and 3TC (lamivudine) for 4 weeks after exposure.
    4. No treatment is required now, but a test for HIV should be done in 6 months.

178. A client with hypothyroidism is admitted to the emergency department with T-33.4°C; P-72; BP-110/58; and R-16. The *first* action by the nurse would be to:
    1. Start 2 large-bore intravenous access lines.
    2. Give levothyroxine per order.
    3. Draw blood to test the T3 and T4 levels.
    4. Cover with warm blankets.

179. An 11-month-old infant with hydrocephalus is admitted to the pediatric unit for revision of a malfunctioning ventriculoperitoneal shunt. On physical assessment, the nurse would expect to find:
    1. An increasing head circumference.
    2. An increasing abdominal circumference.
    3. Difficulty in sucking and feeding.
    4. Hyperactivity.

180. Which statement by a 14-year-old girl indicates that the client is at a high risk for developing an eating disorder?
    1. "I hate my body and spend hours each day in front of the mirror trying to look like the models in magazines."
    2. "My body is starting to attract attention from boys at school and many other girls are jealous."
    3. "I notice that other girls at school are thinner with more curves in their body. It makes me nervous."
    4. "My body is strange. Many of my girlfriends are changing too. It's kind of scary."

181. A client is to receive radioactive iodine therapy. What should the nurse teach the client before therapy begins?
    1. Children and women who are pregnant should not visit during therapy.
    2. Do not take acetaminophen until normal liver function is determined.
    3. Flush the toilet twice after urinating and wash hands carefully.
    4. Avoid tight clothing over the area being radiated and keep skin moist.

182. A doctor has ordered a contraction stress test (CST) for a client who is 41 weeks pregnant. The nurse knows that the fetal has adequate oxygenation when the CST test results are:
    1. Negative, nonreactive CST
    2. Positive, reactive CST.
    3. Positive, nonreactive CST.
    4. Negative, reactive CST

183. The nurse is evaluating a fetal monitor strip. Which pattern requires *immediate* nursing intervention?
    1. Early decelerations with increased baseline variability.
    2. Variable decelerations with average baseline variability.
    3. Variable decelerations with increased baseline variability.
    4. Late decelerations with decreased baseline variability.

184. The client has only one intravenous access line and several drugs are ordered. Which drug should be given *first*?
    1. Morphine 2 mg prn.
    2. Vancomycin 1 g q12h.
    3. Phenytoin 100 mg q8h.
    4. Metronidazole 500 mg q6h.

185. An 84-year-old woman with a history of urinary methicillin-resistant staphylococcal aureus (MRSA) infection is to be admitted for dehydration. Which client is the most appropriate roommate?
    1. A 34-year-old woman with HIV infection.
    2. A 68-year-old woman 10 days post chemotherapy.
    3. A 68-year-old woman with community-acquired pneumonia.
    4. A 76-year-old-woman postoperative with a tracheostomy.

186. The nurse observes a nursing student caring for an infant with hydrocephalus and a newly revised ventriculoperitoneal shunt. Which action on the part of the nursing student requires *immediate* intervention by the nurse?
    1. The nursing student places the infant on the nonoperative side.
    2. The nursing student maintains the infant flat in bed for the first 24 postoperative hours.
    3. The nursing student places the infant in a slightly head-down position.
    4. The nursing student gradually increases the angle of the head of the bed with each postoperative day.

187. Which nursing action promotes a client's first line of defense against infection?
    1. Turn the client who is immobilized every 2 hours so the skin does not break down.
    2. Collect an immunization history on the client.
    3. Apply heat immediately after an injury.
    4. Desensitize the client by providing small doses of allergen.

188. A school-age child is admitted to the emergency department with suspected appendicitis. Which statement made by the child should the nurse *immediately* report to the child's pediatrician?
    1. "My right side really hurts!"
    2. "My right side isn't hurting me anymore!"
    3. "I'm so thirsty. Can I have a drink of water?"
    4. "I'm so hot. Can you take the blanket off me?"

189. A client has had the spleen removed after a traumatic abdominal injury. The nurse instructs the client that it will be most important to avoid:
    1. Carcinogens such as smoking.
    2. Animal dander causing allergies.
    3. Cuts leading to bloodstream infections.
    4. Irritants causing dermatitis.

190. Which measure, if used by the nurse, would be most effective in preventing the development of depression in clients who are adolescents?
    1. Advocating for a teen-led suicide crisis phone line at the local high school.
    2. Developing a music workshop for 10-year-old boys who are not interested in sports.
    3. Educating parents of adolescent children how to recognize the signs of depression.
    4. Informing high school staff of a new adolescent depression screening tool available online.

191. The nurse would determine that amoxicillin was having the desired effect if the:
    1. Client's temperature is below 37.5°C.
    2. Drug blood levels are within normal limits.
    3. Client denies itching.
    4. The full course of antibiotic was completed.

192. What is the most important nursing action for a client with a neutrophil count of 500/mm³?
    1. Place client with a roommate who is infection-free.
    2. Have the client wear a mask when out of the room.
    3. Order a diet high in fresh fruits and vegetables.
    4. Use hypoallergenic sheets on the bed.

193. The parents of a toddler with cerebral palsy seek information from the nurse regarding feeding techniques. The toddler has a history of aspiration when feeding. The nurse's best response would be:
    Select all that apply.
    1. Feed the toddler in an upright position while stabilizing the jaw.
    2. Feed the toddler slowly.
    3. Feed the toddler using specialized utensils.
    4. Feed the toddler through a gastrostomy tube.

194. A preschool-age child with nephrotic syndrome is admitted to the pediatric unit. The charge nurse would be correct in assigning the child to a room with:
    1. A preschool-age child waiting for a hypospadias repair.
    2. A preschool-age child with pneumonia.
    3. A preschool-age child with tonsillitis.
    4. No other child.

195. The client complains that every time she sneezes or coughs she urinates a small amount. Which action will be best in helping the client manage this problem?
    1. Doing pelvic muscle exercises twice a day for 3–4 months.
    2. Obtaining a prescription for tolterodine or oxybutynin.
    3. Application of an external urethral barrier with adhesive.
    4. Avoiding strenuous physical activity.

196. A client, gravida 2, para 1, has come to the prenatal clinic for her first prenatal visit. Review of her records reveals she is O negative and the father of the infant is B positive. The client states her first child is AB+ and she was given RhoGAM. The client asks if she will need to receive RhoGAM this pregnancy. The nurse correctly states:
    1. "You do not need to get RhoGAM this pregnancy because you had a shot last pregnancy, which protected this baby."
    2. "You will need to get a RhoGAM injection after delivery if the baby is Rh-negative, to protect the next pregnancy."
    3. "You will need to receive an injection of RhoGAM during the third trimester of pregnancy to protect the next pregnancy."
    4. "You will need to get a RhoGAM injection after delivery if the baby is Rh-positive, to protect the next pregnancy."

197. A 52-year-old woman has been experiencing sudden urges to urinate accompanied by incontinence. What is the best action to manage this problem?
    1. Insert an indwelling bladder catheter.
    2. Perform an in-and-out catheterization every 6 hours.
    3. Void every 2 hours for 1 week and then increase the interval.
    4. Restrict overall daily fluid intake to no more than 1.5 liters.

198. The nurse finds the client's IV bag empty at change of shift. The RN on the previous shift reported that a new 1000-mL bag would be hung. The client is in no apparent distress. What is the *first* priority?
    1. Maintain patency of the IV site with a new bag of solution.
    2. Check the IV record to see if a new bag was charted.
    3. Assess heart and lungs for signs of fluid overload.
    4. Complete an incident report and notify physician of error.

199. A client is admitted with a diagnosis of severe pregnancy-induced hypertension (PIH). Which assessment findings indicate severe pregnancy-induced hypertension?

    1. A weight gain of 3 pounds per week during the previous 2 weeks.
    2. Severe pedal and facial edema, BP 170/98, 4+ protein on urine dipstick.
    3. Constant headache with visual changes, BP 140/100, trace proteinuria.
    4. Urine dipstick with 2+ protein, BP 100/64, slight pedal edema.

200. A woman brings her 86-year-old mother with Alzheimer's to the mental health clinic for a routine examination. She says to the nurse during the assessment interview, "At times I get so frustrated and I feel like hitting her when she doesn't cooperate." Which response by the nurse would be the most appropriate at this time?
    1. "If you hit your mother, I will have to report it to adult protective services."
    2. "It must be frustrating to not have her cooperation. She will get better."
    3. "Tell me what is going on for you when you have these feelings."
    4. "Hitting her would be the wrong thing to do. I am glad you resist the impulse."

201. An infant with acute gastroenteritis is admitted to the pediatric unit. The infant is in stable condition. The parents question the nurse about why their baby is being disturbed while napping and during the night to take vital signs every 2 hours. The nurse's best response would be:
    1. "Because your baby is so stable, I'll ask the pediatrician to change the orders so that your baby can get more rest."
    2. "It is policy on the pediatric unit to take vital signs every 2 hours."
    3. "Please discuss this with your pediatrician. I have to do what has been ordered for your baby."
    4. "A baby's status can change rapidly. We need to continue to monitor your baby frequently in order to detect any changes."

202. If a client who is pregnant develops HELLP syndrome, the laboratory tests should demonstrate:
    1. Increased HgB, increased platelets, decreased liver enzymes.
    2. Hemolysis of RBCs, elevated liver enzymes, and decreased platelet count.
    3. Hemoconcentration, decreased platelet count, and elevated liver enzymes.
    4. Hemolysis of RBCs, decreased liver enzymes, and decreased platelet count.

203. The nurse is demonstrating the use of surgical asepsis when:
    1. Wearing clean gloves to change linen.
    2. Cleaning the client's skin with povidone/iodine and alcohol before inserting an intravenous catheter.
    3. Putting on a HEPA mask when entering the room of a client with tuberculosis.
    4. Placing a used syringe in a sharps container.

204. The nurse uses sterile technique to change a soiled dressing on a surgical wound. Which element of the chain of infection is broken?
    1. Transmission.
    2. Infectious agent.
    3. Host.
    4. Reservoir.

205. A client who is primigravida is diagnosed with severe pregnancy-induced hypertension at 32 weeks gestation. The client asks the nurse if there is a cure for pregnancy-induced hypertension. The nurse replies that the only cure is:
    1. Magnesium sulfate.
    2. Aldomet.
    3. Delivery of the fetus.
    4. A high protein, low sodium diet and diuretics.

206. Which nursing action is intended to prevent a nosocomial infection?
    1. Wearing a mask when changing the dressing on the client's central line.
    2. Rinsing the suction catheter with normal saline after suctioning the client's tracheostomy tube.
    3. Wearing clean gloves to remove the lunch tray of a client with hepatitis A.
    4. Wearing clean gloves to empty a wound drain.

207. Which characteristic of aging puts the client at increased risk for infection?
    1. Increased production of saliva.
    2. Increased cough effort.
    3. Increased cell-mediated immunity.
    4. Thinning of the skin.

208. A school-age child with leukemia has a central line in place for the administration of chemotherapy. The nurse observes that the intravenous site is reddened and the child states, "It hurts!" The nurse's *first* action is to:
    1. Begin the chemotherapy infusion and see if signs of infiltration develop at the site.
    2. Flush the line with heparin followed by normal saline.
    3. Withhold administering any IV fluids and notify the pediatrician.
    4. Remove the central line dressing and observe the insertion site for signs of infection.

209. Which client is at greatest risk for infection?
    1. 18-year-old client with a surgical repair of a torn knee ligament.
    2. 45-year-old client with an uncomplicated appendectomy.
    3. 52-year-old client with diabetes.
    4. 67-year-old client with a broken hip.

210. A client who was diagnosed with Alzheimer's disease 5 years ago has recently moved in with her 40-year-old daughter, the daughter's husband, and their 16-year-old son. Which statement by the daughter indicates that the family is adjusting to the new living arrangements?
    1. "My husband and I are afraid to leave my son home alone with my mother."
    2. "I will no longer be able to work outside the home, and my husband is worried."
    3. "We have arranged for our son to have a private place in the house to see his friends."
    4. "My son has become very silent; he doesn't want to bother my mother."

211. Which client should be in a private room with negative airflow?
    1. 53-year-old client with MRSA in his wound.
    2. 23-year-old client who is neutropenic.
    3. 36-year-old client with chickenpox.
    4. 64-year-old client with an infected, draining wound.

212. What are the primary causes of antepartum third trimester bleeding?
    1. Spontaneous abortion, molar pregnancy.
    2. Retained placenta, placenta previa.
    3. Placenta previa, abruptio placenta.
    4. Abruptio placenta, ectopic pregnancy.

213. Following a course of chemotherapy, a school-age child has experienced hair loss. The child tells the nurse, "I don't want to be bald like my grandpa! I want my hair back!" The nurse's best response is:
    1. "We can cover up your head with a baseball cap and no one will know that you have lost your hair."
    2. "Would you like to get a wig to wear to school?"
    3. "You lost your hair for a different reason than your grandpa's. Your hair will come back, but it might be a different color."
    4. "I know that this is hard for you but you are getting better every day. Remember when you were so sick from the chemotherapy?"

214. The charge nurse prepares discharge instructions for a preschool-age child with leukemia. The charge nurse will want to emphasize that:
    1. The parents should notify the pediatrician immediately if the child is fussy or irritable.
    2. The parents should notify the pediatrician immediately if the child has difficulty getting to sleep at nighttime.
    3. The parents should notify the pediatrician immediately if the child has persistent vomiting and diarrhea.
    4. The parents should notify the pediatrician immediately if the child is not eating well.

215. A 16-year-old client is unconscious in intensive care after sustaining a head injury in a river-rafting accident. The best assessment tool to evaluate the neurological status of this client is the:
    1. Mini Mental State Exam.
    2. 4 Unrelated Words test.
    3. Glasgow Coma Scale.
    4. PERRLA test.

216. The nurse is assessing the mental status of a 15-year-old client. The client is wearing a full-length leather coat on a hot summer day, black lace underwear over her clothes, and has multiple body piercings. The nurse:
    1. Determines that the client has impaired self-concept.
    2. Knows that more data must be collected before mental status can be accurately determined.
    3. Concludes that the client suffers from bipolar disorder.
    4. Should develop a care plan that includes teaching about personal hygiene and the risks of body piercing.

217. When the nurse assesses the client's capacity for abstract thinking, the nurse asks the client to:
    1. Interpret the phrase "Losers weepers, finders keepers."
    2. Describe what the client would do if the client found an addressed, stamped envelope lying in the street.
    3. Repeat 4 unrelated words that the nurse verbalized 5 minutes ago.
    4. Name 3 objects in the room to which the nurse points.

218. An 82-year-old man with Alzheimer's lives with his daughter and her family. The client has become progressively debilitated, needing constant supervision. After wandering out of the house at night several times, the family is reluctantly considering placing the client in a residential care center. An appropriate nursing diagnosis would be:
    1. *Neglect.*
    2. *Hopelessness.*
    3. *Caregiver role strain.*
    4. *Ineffective family coping.*

219. A client with insulin-dependent gestational diabetes presents to labor and delivery at 29 weeks gestation with nausea, vomiting, polyuria, and uterine cramping. She is disoriented and does not remember her insulin dosage. The nurse assesses that her skin is warm and dry, with poor turgor. The client's vital signs are: T 100.1°F; P 102; R 24; BP 96/58; her fingerstick blood sugar results were 350. Her current condition is likely a result of:
    1. An overdose of insulin.
    2. Illicit use of heroin.
    3. Pregnancy-induced hypertension.
    4. Dehydration caused by nausea and vomiting.

220. Which ego defense mechanisms are normal psychological reactions when a client has a need to soothe emotional conflict or reduce extreme anxiety?
    Select all that apply.
    1. Displacement.
    2. Denial.
    3. Projection.
    4. Suicide.
    5. Identification.
    6. Rationalization.

221. A 37-year-old man with ulcerative colitis has a new ileostomy. To promote a positive self-image for the client, the nurse will:
1. Teach the client to inspect the stoma daily.
2. Invite the client's wife and two sons to observe while the client changes the ostomy appliance.
3. Support the client in changing the ostomy appliance, but realize he may not like it.
4. Acknowledge the presence of odor during ostomy appliance changes by holding her breath.

222. During labor, a client, with spontaneous rupture of membranes, has frequent vaginal exams to determine progression of labor. Frequent vaginal exams place the client at high risk for development of:
1. Pelvic inflammatory disease.
2. Endometriosis.
3. Chorioamnionitis.
4. Premature rupture of membranes.

223. The parents of a child with myelomeningocele inform the nurse that their child has developed an allergy to latex products. The emphasis of the nurse's teaching regarding the latex allergy will be on the need to:
1. Obtain a kit containing premeasured adrenalin for emergency treatment of anaphylaxis.
2. Obtain the Spina Bifida Association's list of products containing latex and potential substitutes.
3. Read all labels carefully before purchasing and/or using the product.
4. Purchase a Medic-Alert bracelet for the child.

224. The client had surgery on the back 8 months ago and continues to use narcotic analgesics for pain. Which statement by the client suggests drug dependency?
1. The client was arrested twice in the last 6 months for driving under the influence of narcotics.
2. The client is taking larger and larger doses to obtain relief from pain.
3. The client is on probation at work because of excessive absences.
4. The client became intoxicated at a family gathering 4 months ago and had an argument with the family about this.

225. Which statement is true about the elderly population and drug abuse?
1. Use of illegal drugs is higher in the elderly population than in younger populations.
2. The elderly client who has been drinking for many years will experience fewer drug-alcohol interactions than the elderly client who has recently begun drinking.
3. The effects of drug abuse in the elderly population are the same as those in younger populations.
4. The elderly population has a higher use of over-the-counter drugs simultaneously with prescription drugs.

226. The client is admitted to the hospital for incision and drainage of an abscess. The client has a current history of addiction to narcotics. Which symptom of withdrawal can the nurse expect?
1. Flu-like symptoms.
2. Delirium.
3. Seizures.
4. Depression.

227. Which statement made by the mother of a 2-month-old infant with hip dysplasia being treated with a Pavlik harness warrants further evaluation and possible teaching on the part of the nurse?
1. "I'll put a shirt and socks on my baby under the harness."
2. "I'll remove the harness just for diaper changes."
3. "I'll change my baby's position frequently."
4. "I'll keep my baby's hips abducted when I take the harness off."

228. A definitive diagnosis of gestational diabetes is based upon:
1. An abnormal 1-hour glucola test in the first trimester of pregnancy.
2. An abnormal 3-hour glucola test in the third trimester of pregnancy.
3. An abnormal 1-hour glucola test in the third trimester of pregnancy.
4. Family history of gestational diabetes.

229. A client who is elderly is brought to the emergency department by the daughter. The client's left wrist is swollen, bruised, painful, and restricted in motion. The injury to the client's wrist occurred 3 days ago. It is most important that the nurse observe the client's:
1. Grooming.
2. Relationship and interaction with the daughter.
3. Mood and affect.
4. Nutritional status.

230. The nurse enters the room of a 35-year-old man who was admitted with a diagnosis of bipolar disorder–manic phase and finds the client having sexual intercourse with a woman visitor. Which response by the nurse would be most appropriate?
1. Wait outside the room and talk to the client and visitor after the incident to explain the agency's rules about sexual behavior.
2. Talk to the visitor as she leaves the unit and explain to her that the client's illness prevents him from using sound judgment.
3. Stop the sexual activity and set limits on the behavior by telling the couple that the behavior is inappropriate in the hospital.
4. After the incident, encourage the client to express any anger that he may be acting out by breaking the hospital rules.

231. The client is experiencing a crisis. The nurse should *first*:
1. Formulate a nursing care plan with long-term goals for stress reduction.
2. Thoroughly evaluate the stressors in the client's life and the client's responses.
3. Focus on immediate stress reduction techniques.
4. Allow the client to independently work through the crisis.

232. The client has terminal cancer and has a feeding tube. The client and family have talked about removing the feeding tube. The nurse who cares for the client and family needs to know that a key difference between active and passive euthanasia is that:
1. Passive euthanasia is illegal in all 50 states.
2. Active euthanasia is a client right guaranteed by the U.S. constitution.
3. Passive euthanasia is governed by the principles of informed consent and the client's right to refuse treatment.
4. Active euthanasia involves a lack of action that results in the death of the client.

233. The client has an arteriovenous fistula (AV fistula) for hemodialysis. Care of this hemodialysis access includes:
1. Appling a pressure dressing after every blood draw from the AV fistula.
2. Flushing the AV fistula with heparin solution every shift to maintain patency.
3. Irrigating the tubing every 4 hours with normal saline.
4. Assessing the AV fistula for thrill and bruit every shift.

234. Infants of mothers with gestational diabetes, who delivered at full-term gestation, are at a higher risk of developing:
1. Hypothermia.
2. Hypotension.
3. Hyperglycemia.
4. Hypoglycemia.

235. The nurse is using palpation to assess the uterine contraction pattern of a client in labor. How would the nurse appropriately use palpation to assess contractions?

1. Place fingertips below the umbilicus and palpate the contraction frequency with the fingertips.
2. Assess the duration of a contraction by timing the beginning of one contraction to the beginning of the next contraction.
3. Assess the frequency of the contractions by timing from the end of one contraction until the start of the next contraction.
4. Determine contraction duration by pressing fingertips over the fundus of the uterus.

236. A teaching plan for a client with cholelithiasis should include:
    1. Low fat diet.
    2. Morphine for severe pain associated with attacks.
    3. Preparation for cholecystectomy, which is inevitable.
    4. A diet high in dairy products to provide protein and calcium.

237. Nutritional counseling for a client with Ménière's disease should include recommendations for:
    1. Low fat diet.
    2. Megavitamin therapy.
    3. Low sodium diet.
    4. A glass of wine with dinner every day.

238. A child with attention deficit-hyperactivity disorder is experiencing the side effects of decreased appetite and weight loss from the psychostimulants prescribed by the pediatrician. The nurse should counsel the parents to provide additional calories in the form of nutritious snacks to be eaten in the:
    1. Morning.
    2. Mid-morning.
    3. Mid-afternoon.
    4. Evening.

239. A widowed grandmother is raising her grandson who has attention deficit-hyperactivity disorder. In planning care for this family, the nurse would be most concerned about which nursing diagnosis?
    1. *Risk for injury.*
    2. *Risk for impaired social interaction.*
    3. *Risk for noncompliance.*
    4. *Risk for caregiver role strain.*

240. While on a home visit, which action from an adult child of a client in the middle phase of Alzheimer's is a *priority* concern for the nurse?
    1. Locks are placed on the top of all outside doors.
    2. The adult child cries when the parent doesn't recognize him.
    3. The car has been taken away from the client without permission.
    4. The adult child asks for help on how to prevent the client from undressing in public.

241. The nurse palpates a newborn infant's head and feels a soft lump over the occiput extending across the sagittal suture line. The nurse correctly identifies this finding as:
    1. Cephalosuccadeum
    2. Hemangioma
    3. Caput succedaneum.
    4. Cephalohematoma.

242. The nurse is providing nutrition information to the wife of a 67-year-old man with Parkinson's disease. What should the nurse include?
    1. Restrict fluid to reduce the risk of aspiration.
    2. Provide 5 or 6 small meals per day, which includes foods the client likes, and cut food into small pieces.
    3. Include red meat and chicken for extra protein calories, and raw vegetable for roughage.
    4. Weigh the client daily to monitor nutritional status.

243. What would the nurse include in teaching the client about taking valproic acid (Depakene)?

1. The client may continue a regimen of 1 aspirin a day to prevent heart attack and stroke.
2. Driving and operating heavy machinery is acceptable while taking valproic acid.
3. Valproic acid may be taken prn, and discontinued when symptoms subside.
4. Physical dependence may occur with long-term use of valproic acid.

244. A 42-year-old mother of three has just been diagnosed with ovarian cancer. Which actions are appropriate for the nurse to recommend to help the client deal with the stress of this diagnosis?
    Select all that apply.
    1. Prioritizing the client's treatment options.
    2. Using sedatives such as diazepam.
    3. Reading a funny book, or see a funny movie.
    4. Engaging in meditation or prayer.
    5. Canceling her social engagements to preserve energy.
    6. Canceling her Tai Chi class to preserve energy.

245. The mother of a school-age child who was just diagnosed with attention deficit-hyperactivity disorder is concerned that the prescribed medication regime ultimately will cause the child to become a "drug abuser." The nurse can correctly counsel the mother that:
    1. This is a high risk potential outcome of the medication regime.
    2. This is an unlikely outcome of the medication regime.
    3. Taking "drug holidays" on weekends and school vacations will prevent this from happening.
    4. This can be prevented if the mother administers the medication to the child.

246. The nurse is aware that many myths exist regarding pain. Which statements are true?
    Select all that apply.
    1. The intensity of pain experienced by a client directly indicates the degree of tissue injury.
    2. Consistently administering analgesics to the client at regular intervals can lead to drug addiction.
    3. Pain is whatever the client describes it as, and whenever the client says it occurs.
    4. Psychogenic pain, such as the phantom pain experienced after an amputation, is not real.
    5. If the client is able to sleep, then the client is not really in pain.
    6. Pain is a protective mechanism.

247. A 1-year-old infant comes into the pediatrician's office for a well-child checkup. The infant's birth weight was 3400 g. The office nurse realizes that the infant should now weigh approximately how many pounds?
    Fill in the blank.

    _____ lbs

248. The client is admitted to the hospital with an acute episode of asthma. One of the physician's orders reads: "Aminophylline drip, 30 mg/hr, IV for 12 hours." The pharmacy sends an IV bottle with 1 gram of aminophylline in 500 mL of D_5W. At how many mL/hr will the nurse program the IV pump to run?
    Fill in the blank.

    _____ mL/hr

249. The nurse performs a physical assessment on a newborn infant. Which finding requires that the pediatrician be notified?
    1. Small, peach-colored crystals in the diaper.
    2. Mongolian spots across the buttocks.
    3. Firm skull with overlapping sutures.
    4. Unequal leg creases.

250. Which statement indicates to the nurse that a client who is dying is coping with the end-of-life process?

1. "I am going to stay positive and look to the future."
2. "I do not want to talk about my death with my family."
3. "I am going to fight until the doctors find a cure."
4. "I let myself cry often. When will this change?"

251. A client with a spinal cord injury has a post-void residual of 250 mL. The best response by the nurse would be to:
    1. Restrict fluids.
    2. Apply bladder pressure.
    3. Catheterize intermittently.
    4. Give tolterodine or oxybutynin.

252. A 12-year-old girl comes into the pediatrician's office for a back-to-school checkup. The office nurse's *priority* assessment would be:
    1. Development of 32 teeth.
    2. Development of adult-like vital signs.
    3. Onset of menstruation.
    4. Changes in nipples and areola.

253. A nurse on the postpartum unit is working with an LVN/LPN. Which client should be seen *first* by the RN?
    1. A client who delivered 4 hours ago, with a history of thrombophlebitis, and is being treated with heparin.
    2. A client who delivered vaginally 24 hours ago, and is experiencing difficulty having the newborn latch on.
    3. A client who is 27 weeks pregnant, with pyelonephritis and is being treated with IV antibiotics.
    4. A client who delivered 2 hours ago and is unable to void after delivery.

254. An 82-year-old woman with a fractured hip is scheduled for surgery. Preoperative lab values include: WBC 10,000; Hct 37; INR 3; Na$^+$ 134; K$^+$ 4.2. The nurse's response to these labs is that:
    1. These values are essentially normal for preoperative status.
    2. Oxygenation may be impaired and a transfusion required.
    3. There is a high risk for clotting disorders during and following surgery.
    4. Sodium level is low, but with K$^+$ replacement the level will improve.

255. The client returns to the PACU following GI surgery. Postoperative lab values include: O$_2$ saturation 99%; WBC 11,500; Hct 35; Na$^+$ 139; K$^+$ 3.9; glucose 51. The *first* priority of the nurse would be to:
    1. Assess the postoperative wound for infection.
    2. Obtain an order for dextrose solution IV.
    3. Increase nasal O$_2$ to improve oxygen delivery.
    4. Decrease amount of K$^+$ in IV to avoid arrhythmias.

256. A client who was previously healthy was involved in a motor vehicle accident. Lab values 4 days after surgery are: O$_2$ saturation 99%; WBC 19,000; Hct 19; Hgb 6; PTT 30 sec. The nurse will expect to:
    1. Give vitamin K to correct a clotting problem.
    2. Start a unit of blood which has been filtered to remove the WBC.
    3. Assess for a worsening of the condition.
    4. Start IV antibiotics and a unit of packed red blood cells.

257. Discharge teaching for a client recently hospitalized with pneumonia who has a complement deficiency should include:
    1. "Take the full course of the prescribed diphenhydramine (Benadryl)."
    2. "Report early any signs of infection to the health-care provider."
    3. "Eat a diet high in protein to improve resistance."
    4. "Avoid meningococcal, pneumococcal, and influenza vaccinations."

258. A client who is 3 days postpartum asks her nurse why she is voiding so frequently. The nurse bases her response on the knowledge that the frequent voiding is a result of:
    1. A urinary tract infection.
    2. Drinking an increased amount of fluids after delivery.
    3. Normal diuresis after delivery.
    4. Increased tone of the bladder and ureters after delivery.

259. While conducting a Denver Developmental Screening Test (DDST), the nurse would anticipate that a 1-year-old infant could be expected to:
    1. Jabber.
    2. Say "da da" and "ma ma."
    3. Point to at least one named body part.
    4. Combine 2 or 3 words.

260. The nurse knows that the average duration of Alzheimer's disease from onset of symptoms to death is:
    Fill in the blank.

    _____ years

261. A client with a diagnosis of neutropenia has been admitted from the emergency department. What is the *most important* nursing action when admitting the client to the unit?
    1. Thorough hand-washing before any client contact.
    2. Start 2 or more large bores for rapid infusions.
    3. Give pain medication as ordered.
    4. Request hypoallergenic sheets from the laundry.

262. A woman delivered a 9 pound-3 ounce infant vaginally 6 hours ago. The nurse checks her vaginal bleeding and finds that the client soaked through two pads in the past hour. What is the *first* action the nurse should take?
    1. Call the doctor for an order of Pitocin.
    2. Get the client up to go to the bathroom to void.
    3. Change her pads, as this is a normal amount of bleeding.
    4. Massage her uterus to expel any clots.

263. A client with cancer is immunosuppressed and malnourished due to decreased intake because of nausea, anorexia, and a feeling of fullness. A Salem sump tube had been draining the stomach and has been discontinued. The *initial* nursing action to manage malnutrition would be:
    1. Teach the client about total parenteral nutrition (TPN).
    2. Assist with insertion of a PEG tube.
    3. Give an antiemetic before serving small, frequent meals.
    4. Give an aluminum hydroxide antacid with meals.

264. The nurse in a well-child clinic is assessing the coping abilities of a mother of a two-year-old toddler. Which statement indicates coping difficulties on the mother's part?
    1. "I put a plastic sheet on the floor under the high chair during mealtimes."
    2. "I only offer choices that are already acceptable to me."
    3. "I'm frustrated with fighting over toys between my toddler and my preschooler."
    4. "I expect sharing of snacks between my toddler and my preschooler."

265. Which nursing action would best assist a client with rheumatoid arthritis to maintain independence with activities of daily living?
    1. Bathe and dress the client to conserve strength.
    2. Offer assistive devices such as utensils with large handles.
    3. Apply ice packs continuously at night to lessen pain.
    4. Wrap hands in a flexed position for 30 minutes bid to improve function.

266. A client comes to labor and delivery at 39 weeks gestation with a severe headache for the past 2 days, nausea, right upper quadrant pain, and visual changes including flashes of light. What should the nurse do *first*?
    1. Check client's vital signs and reflexes.
    2. Perform a vaginal exam for cervical dilation.
    3. Administer acetaminophen for the headache pain.
    4. Ask if the client has uterine contractions.

267. The nurse tells the client with discoid lupus erythematosus that the most effective treatment for the skin rash is:
    1. Application of warm moist compresses.
    2. Glucocorticoid cream and sunscreen before sun exposure.

3. Application of hypoallergenic cosmetics after using a moisturizer
4. Vitamin D, rubbing alcohol, and 15 minutes of a light treatment.

268. A staff nurse informs the charge nurse that she has a child who is sick at home with the chickenpox. Which clients must the charge nurse assign to the staff nurse?
   1. None, because the staff nurse must be sent home.
   2. Any client on the floor as long as the staff nurse wears a face mask while giving nursing care.
   3. Clients who are not immunocompromised.
   4. Clients who have previously had the chickenpox.

269. The client is scheduled for a carotid endarterectomy. The preoperative aPTT is 120. The best interpretation by the nurse would be that:
   1. It is necessary to repeat the test and notify the surgeon.
   2. Clotting after surgery will be normal.
   3. The therapeutic level of heparin has been achieved.
   4. The therapeutic level of warfarin has been achieved.

270. Which nursing diagnosis has the *highest priority* for a client with bipolar disorder-manic phase?
   1. *Impaired social interaction.*
   2. *Self-care deficit.*
   3. *Sexual dysfunction.*
   4. *Sleep pattern disturbance.*

271. A client comes to labor and delivery at 34 weeks gestation with a moderate amount of painless vaginal bleeding. Which question should the nurse ask the client *first*?
   1. "Have you had intercourse in the past 24 hours?"
   2. "Do you have any uterine contractions?"
   3. "Have you had an ultrasound exam?"
   4. "Has your doctor checked your cervix?"

272. The nurse is concerned that a client is a victim of elder abuse. When talking with the client, the nurse asks questions to gain information about who may be the source of the abuse. The nurse knows the most likely abuser of an elder is a:
   1. Friend.
   2. Stranger.
   3. Family member.
   4. Health-care professional.

273. The charge nurse in the emergency department observes a new graduate attempting to care for a child with acute epiglottitis. Which potential action taken by the new graduate would indicate to the charge nurse that immediate intervention is needed?
   1. Placing the child NPO.
   2. Maintaining a patent IV line.
   3. Removing the tongue blade from the examination tray.
   4. Notifying radiology that the new graduate will transport the child for a lateral neck x-ray within the next 10 minutes.

274. The nurse is discussing with the mother ways of preventing bacterial meningitis in an infant. Which statement(s) made by the mother indicate that the nurse's teaching has been effective?
   Select all that apply.
   1. "I will make sure that my baby gets all of the HIB immunizations."
   2. "If my baby starts tugging at an ear, I'll get an appointment with the pediatrician right away."
   3. "I won't prop the bottle in the crib with the baby anymore."
   4. "I'll hold the baby lying down in my arms when feeding so that choking won't happen."

275. Three days following surgery for bilateral fractured tibias, the client is scheduled for discharge. The client seems quite anxious and complains of chest pain. Vital signs are: BP 134/78; T 37.8° C; P 112; R 28; O₂ Sat. 84% on room air. The nurse would *first*:

1. Give pain medication, document the EKG pattern and call the physician.
2. Call the discharge planner to reevaluate sending the client home.
3. Give O₂ by mask and call the physician.
4. Call the physician to get a STAT ultrasound of the legs.

276. On the morning of surgery for a hernia repair, the client's vital signs are: T 37.3° C; P 98; R 22; BP 112/76; O₂ Sat. 97% on room air. The client reports pain is 2 on a scale of 10. The nurse would interpret these vital signs as:
   1. Signs that some degree of anxiety is present, although not a concern for increased surgical risk.
   2. An indication that an infection exists that could postpone surgery; notify the surgeon.
   3. An increased risk for fluid volume deficit may exist post-operatively.
   4. Oxygen will be needed as well as analgesia to eliminate pain.

277. A client has just returned to the PACU following an open reduction of a left leg fracture and general anesthesia. The nurse's *priority* assessment would be to:
   1. Auscultate for return of bowel sounds.
   2. Determine level of consciousness and wakefulness.
   3. Check the circulation, sensation and movement of feet.
   4. Palpate bladder for distention and inability to void spontaneously.

278. A 3-day-old infant has been exclusively breastfed since birth. The infant now has developed lethargy and appears icteric. What is the probable cause of the infant's current condition?
   1. Physiological jaundice
   2. Liver failure
   3. Neonatal sepsis
   4. Blood incompatibility

279. A client with sinusitis is going home with an antibiotic prescription. Discharge teaching should include:
   1. "Go to the emergency department immediately if any headaches occur."
   2. "Breathe in cool air via humidifier every 2 hours."
   3. "Use decongestants and antihistamines conservatively."
   4. "Follow fluid restriction guidelines."

280. Which assessment question would indicate that the nurse understands the major symptoms associated with mania?
   1. "Do you have feelings of hopelessness or doom?"
   2. "Are you hearing voices inside your head?"
   3. "What does your family think about your spending habits?"
   4. "Have you been isolating yourself from your friends?"

281. A client came to the clinic with epistaxis, nasal packing was done, and the client was later transferred to the hospital for observation. What teaching should be done?
   1. "Remove packing and exhale rapidly through the nose to clear clots 4 times a day."
   2. "Keep head of bed elevated (high Fowler's) to avoid aspiration of blood."
   3. "Avoid solid food because it is poorly tolerated due to blood in the stomach."
   4. "Keep the head straight, not turned, to avoid plugging eustachian tubes."

282. The nurse in charge of a daycare center is assessing the children. Which infant/child is at high risk for developing meningitis?
   1. A 3-month-old infant who is bottlefed.
   2. A 5-month-old infant who is breastfed.
   3. A 2-year-old child with quadriplegia due to cerebral palsy.
   4. A 3-year-old child who lives with parents who smoke cigarettes.

283. The charge nurse on the pediatric unit observes a new graduate preparing to enter the room of a child with chickenpox who is in isolation. Which action taken by the new graduate

would indicate to the charge nurse that additional teaching is needed?

1. Removes silverware from meal tray and substitutes plastic eating utensils.
2. Obtains a disposable stethoscope.
3. Puts on gown and gloves prior to entering the room.
4. Places a covered waste container directly outside of the room.

284. Upon assessment, the nurse finds the client, who is 3 days postpartum, crying that her breasts hurt, and her infant won't eat. The nurse's best response is:

1. "Put ice packs on your breasts, and give the baby some formula."
2. "Express some milk, put warm packs on your breasts, and feed the baby frequently."
3. "Put ice packs on your breasts for 10 minutes, and try feeding the baby again."
4. "Take some acetaminophen, put warm compresses on your breasts, and give the baby formula."

285. A 38-year-old client had a cesarean section yesterday. She is 5′3″ and weighs 235 pounds. Which is the most important nursing action for this client?

1. Early ambulation
2. Incentive spirometer
3. Pain control
4. Intake and output measurements

286. The *most important* information to include when teaching a client who recently began antituberculin drugs for a TB skin test conversion is:

1. Effect of prednisone on urine color.
2. Use of the incentive spirometer tid for congestion.
3. Importance of taking anti-TB drugs for several months.
4. Repeating skin test 30 days after the start of therapy.

287. A client had required 100 mg of IV morphine for baseline pain control over the last 24 hours. The physician has ordered a fentanyl patch. According to the equianalgesic table, the appropriate hourly fentanyl dose for this client would be:
Fill in the blank.

_____ μg/hr

EQUIANALGESIC TABLE

Analgesic	Parenteral (mg)	PO (mg)
Morphine (MS)	10	30
Codeine	130	200 (not recommended)
Fentanyl	100 μg/hr— 4 mg/h MS IV	
Hydromorphone	2	7
Methadone	10	20
Oxycodone	NA	20

288. Pain is commonly managed with Vicodin (hydrocodone 5 mg and acetaminophen 500 mg). Sometimes clients on Vicodin also want to take additional Tylenol (acetaminophen). Toxicity can occur if the dose of acetaminophen exceeds 4 g/day. If a client is taking 2 Vicodin every 6 hours, how many additional 500 mg Tylenol tablets can the client safely take?
Fill in the blank.

_____ tablets

289. The client is receiving hydromorphone by patient-controlled analgesia (PCA) pump. The syringe has 0.2 mg/mL. Each time the client receives a dose, 1 mL is given. If the client can receive a dose every 6 minutes, what is the maximum dose (in mg) of drug the client can receive in 1 hour?
Fill in the blank.

_____mg

290. A client is seen at the mental health clinic with a nursing diagnosis of *altered thought process*. When taking the history, the nurse would expect the client to express:

1. Auditory hallucinations.
2. Delusions.
3. Anxiety.
4. Depression.

291. When reconstituting azithromycin oral suspension, the directions instruct the nurse to add 12 mL of water to 900 mg of medication for a total volume of 22.5 mL.
Fill in the blank.
To give 200 mg, the nurse would draw up _____ mL.

292. A client with myasthenia gravis is admitted with severe muscular weakness and a diagnosis of myasthenic versus cholinergic crisis. The family asks the nurse to explain how the cause of the weakness will be determined. The correct explanation would be:

1. A CT scan will be done to differentiate between the two diagnoses.
2. A V/Q scan will be done to confirm the cause of the weakness.
3. Edrophonium (Tensilon) is usually given to make the determination.
4. A 24-hour urine catecholamines will be collected to determine the cause.

293. The staff nurse is caring for a 6-year-old child with glomerulonephritis. Which statement indicates to the nurse that the child understands why he is sick?

1. "I was bad and I got sick."
2. "I got a germ in my throat and it made me sick."
3. "I got a germ in my pee-pee and it made me sick."
4. "I played with a sick friend after school and then I got sick."

294. Nurses must know about elder abuse prevalence in order to correctly address client needs. The nurse knows elder abuse is:

1. Most common in non-white cultures.
2. Present in all cultures and sub groups.
3. Most common in white cultures.
4. Almost never seen in people of color.

295. The client in receiving heparin IV at 1000 units/hr. In the morning aPTT was 24 sec. There is a new order to give a 2000 unit bolus of heparin and increase the IV rate to 1200 units/hr. The IV bag has 100 units heparin per mL. The bolus solution has 10,000 units of heparin per mL. The nurse would:

1. Give 0.2 mL of the bolus solution. Increase rate of IV from 10 to 12 mL/hr.
2. Increase the rate of the drip to 20 mL/hr for one hour; then reduce to 10 mL/hr.
3. Increase the rate of the drip to 20 mL/hr for one hour; then reduce to 12 mL/hr.
4. Know the desired goal for the aPTT; request a repeat test before any change.

296. A nurse working on the maternal-infant unit is responsible for the following clients. Which client is identified by the nurse to be the most at-risk for a postpartum hemorrhage?

1. G5, P2, who delivered a 7-lb infant after 6 hours in active labor.
2. G2, P1, who delivered a 7-lb infant by a repeat cesarean section.
3. G8, P6, who delivered a 9-lb infant over an intact perineum.
4. G4, P3, who delivered an 8-lb infant using a vacuum-assisted delivery.

297. A 9-year-old child is hospitalized with a pain episode secondary to sickle cell anemia. The pediatrician has ordered warm compresses to the affected areas and pain medication every 4 hours. As the nurse assesses the child in the morning after admission to the hospital, the child states: "I don't hurt any more, and I don't want any more pain medication." The nurse's best response to this would be:

1. "I won't give you any more warm compresses."
2. "I won't give you any more pain medication."
3. "You have to continue with the pain medication because the pediatrician ordered it."
4. "Let's talk to your pediatrician about another way to take care of your pain."

298. The client with multiple sclerosis is complaining of diplopia. The nurse suggests:
   1. Visually scanning the room before moving through the room, to reduce the risk of falls.
   2. Pureed foods to increase the ease of swallowing.
   3. Putting an eye patch on one eye to control the problem.
   4. Applying topical steroid eye drops as prescribed to improve vision.

299. A home health nurse is planning her schedule for visiting clients. Which client should the home health nurse visit *first*?
   1. An infant who is 4 days old, with a total bilirubin level of 20.2, with orders to begin phototherapy
   2. An infant who is premature at risk for contracting a respiratory infection who needs an antiviral injection.
   3. A client who is 5 days postpartum, who was delivered by cesarean section and who has a wound infection.
   4. A client who is 10 weeks pregnant with a diagnosis of hyperemesis who needs IV hydration.

300. The nurse explains to a client in the detoxification phase of treatment for alcohol dependency that the purpose of administering benzodiazepines is to control:
   Select all that apply.
   1. Insomnia.
   2. Relapse.
   3. Agitation.
   4. Weight loss.
   5. Seizures.
   6. Suicide.

301. A client in the hospital has just started receiving total parenteral nutrition (TPN) via a central venous catheter. Which action is best to prevent hyper- or hypoglycemia?
   1. Add 1000 units of NPH insulin to the first container only of TPN solution.
   2. Check the client's fingerstick blood glucose once a day.
   3. Teach the client to monitor and adjust the TPN flow rate as needed.
   4. Maintain the TPN at the ordered rate; neither slow it down, nor speed it up.

302. The nurse would expect a client using albuterol for bronchial asthma to be cautious about also taking:
   1. Fluoxetine.
   2. Beta-adrenergic blockers.
   3. Ranitidine.
   4. Ipratropium.

303. A client is receiving discharge instructions concerning infant care. Which statement by the nurse is accurate when teaching about umbilical cord care?
   1. Separation of the umbilical cord usually happens during the first 2 weeks of life.
   2. A sterile dressing is recommended for the umbilical stump.
   3. Applying antibiotic ointment several times a day will help the umbilical cord to separate.
   4. It is necessary to apply a Betadine solution to the umbilical stump after each diaper change.

304. What is an appropriate nursing intervention for a newborn infant immediately after birth?
   Select all that apply.
   1. The infant should be dried promptly to decrease heat loss.
   2. The infant should be given vitamin K and eye prophylaxis within 10 minutes after birth.
   3. The vernix should be removed to prevent infection.
   4. The newborn should be handled as much as possible to enhance bonding.
   5. The newborn should be bathed after the temperature has stabilized.

305. The charge nurse on the pediatric unit observes an LVN/LPN caring for an infant with severe pruritus secondary to eczema. Which action on the part of the LVN/LPN calls for *immediate* intervention by the charge nurse?
   1. The LVN/LPN prepares a tepid bath for the infant.
   2. The LVN/LPN applies an over-the-counter lotion to the infant's skin.
   3. The LVN/LPN wears gloves when caring for the infant.
   4. The LVN/LPN places cotton socks over the infant's hands.

306. The nurse knows that the best way to prevent a transfusion reaction when administering packed red blood cells to a client is to:
   1. Verify the client, unit and donor numbers, type of blood product, and expiration date with another RN before hanging the blood.
   2. Run the blood slowly for the first 15 minutes.
   3. Use y-type tubing to administer the blood.
   4. Monitor vital signs frequently while the blood is infusing.

307. The charge nurse on the pediatric unit receives a fax from the pediatrician's office regarding a child who is to be admitted to the hospital for hydration secondary to the measles. In reviewing the pediatrician's history and physical on the child, the nurse would specifically look for:
   1. Fever and general malaise.
   2. Rash on face, trunk, and limbs.
   3. Red spots with a white center on the buccal mucosa.
   4. Dry cough.

308. Nursing care for the client who is acutely ill with Cushing's syndrome includes:
   1. Consistent administration of corticosteroids.
   2. Daily blood glucose monitoring.
   3. Reverse isolation to protect against infection.
   4. Encouraging good grooming to improve self-image.

309. Long-term management of a client with Addison's disease includes:
   1. Diligently maintaining consistent doses of corticosteroids.
   2. Decreasing the dose of corticosteroids during times of stress.
   3. Increasing the dose of corticosteroids during times of stress.
   4. Gradually weaning the dose of corticosteroids until the client is no longer taking any.

310. In looking at the client's chart with a diagnosis of schizophrenia, the nurse would expect to note that the onset of symptoms for this disorder would occur between what ages?
   Fill in the blank.
   _____ years of age

311. The nurse knows that syndrome of inappropriate antidiuretic hormone (SIADH) is characterized by:
   1. Increased cellular resistance to insulin.
   2. Fluid retention and decreased serum osmolality.
   3. Decreased body weight and fluid volume deficit.
   4. Increased urinary output and hypernatremia.

312. A child is admitted to the pediatric unit with scarlet fever. After completing the initial admission assessment, the nurse's charting should include:
   Select all that apply.
   1. Strawberry-like tongue.
   2. Sore throat.
   3. Circumoral pallor.
   4. Crusted lesions.

313. A staff nurse reports for duty on the infectious disease section of the pediatric unit. After hearing the report, which child would the nurse assess *first*?

1. A child with fifth disease.
2. A child with diphtheria.
3. A child with pertussis.
4. A child with measles.

314. A 47-year-old with chest trauma secondary to a motor vehicle accident is in the intensive care unit after surgery. The client is receiving mechanical ventilation with an FiO_2 of 40%. Which findings of a respiratory assessment are consistent with acute respiratory distress syndrome (ARDS)?
    1. Po_2 40 mm Hg; normal pulmonary artery wedge pressure; O_2 saturation 85%; diffuse crackles.
    2. Po_2 40 mm Hg; increased pulmonary artery wedge pressure; O_2 saturation 90%; diffuse crackles.
    3. Po_2 90 mm Hg; increased pulmonary artery wedge pressure; O_2 saturation 92%; scattered wheezes.
    4. Po_2 96 mm Hg; increased pulmonary artery wedge pressure; O_2 saturation 95%; scattered wheezes.

315. A newborn infant has poor respiratory effort at birth. Which action should the nurse take to stimulate the infant to breathe?
    1. Vigorous suctioning of the mouth and nose.
    2. Rubbing the infant's back.
    3. Shaking the infant.
    4. Dilating the anal sphincter with a thermometer.

316. When performing a cardioversion on a client who is unconscious and in ventricular tachycardia, it is most important to:
    1. Place alcohol pads on the client's chest to improve electrical conduction.
    2. Premedicate the client with diazepam so the cardioversion is less uncomfortable.
    3. Administer a bolus of lidocaine intravenously.
    4. Make sure all personnel, including the person doing the cardioversion, stand away from the client's bed to avoid electric shock.

317. Preoperative care for the client undergoing transurethral resection of the prostate (TURP) includes:
    1. Fluid restriction.
    2. Counseling regarding the complete loss of sexual function that will occur as a result of the surgery.
    3. Administering IV fluids and antibiotics as ordered.
    4. Catheterizing the client with a 16 Fr, or larger, urinary catheter to empty the bladder and relieve the discomfort of urinary retention.

318. An Apgar score of 6 is assigned to a newborn infant at 1 minute of age. This Apgar score indicates the infant:
    1. Needs immediate resuscitation.
    2. Needs additional observation during transition to extrauterine life.
    3. Will likely develop cerebral palsy.
    4. Has a low Apgar due to asphyxia and will likely suffer long-term neurological damage.

319. The nurse caring for the client who has just undergone a left pneumonectomy knows that the client should be positioned on:
    1. The back with the head of the bed flat.
    2. The left side with the head of the bed flat.
    3. The left side with the head of the bed elevated.
    4. The right side with the head of the bed elevated.

320. Which nonpharmacological intervention would be most effective in helping a client with a nursing diagnosis of *sleep pattern disturbance*?
    1. Administering hypnotic medication with the routine h.s. medication.
    2. Encouraging exercise during the day and discouraging afternoon naps.
    3. Having the client lie down in bed 30 minutes prior to taking hypnotic medication.
    4. Suggesting that the client drink 2–3 glasses of wine before bedtime to relax.

321. The mother of a toddler who is newly diagnosed with sickle cell anemia asks the nurse for suggestions for the best way to care for the toddler. The nurse's most important response would be:
    1. Encourage the toddler to eat a balanced diet.
    2. Encourage the toddler to engage in nonstrenuous play activities.
    3. Protect the toddler from excessive exposure to the sun.
    4. Protect the toddler by keeping all immunizations up to date.

322. A new client comes to the prenatal clinic asking questions about common pregnancy symptoms. The nurse's teaching plan is based on the knowledge that:
    Select all that apply.
    1. Morning sickness usually subsides after 12 to 16 weeks of pregnancy.
    2. Sensations of fetal movement are usually felt by 18 weeks gestation.
    3. Urinary frequency is a result of increased susceptibility to urinary tract infections.
    4. Easy fatigability is characteristic of third trimester pregnancy.
    5. Moderate bleeding is common in the first trimester of pregnancy.

323. Which findings are consistent with Raynaud's phenomenon?
    1. Absent radial and ulnar pulses.
    2. Mild pain with no numbness or tingling.
    3. Hyperemia of affected areas.
    4. Underlying collagen disease.

324. The nurse recognizes that the client needs more teaching about hypertension when the client says:
    1. "I will walk at least 1 mile a day."
    2. "I will not add salt to my food."
    3. "I must take my medications regularly because that is the only way I can lower my blood pressure."
    4. "I will learn yoga to decrease stress."

325. Which risk factors are major, modifiable risk factors for coronary artery disease?
    1. Elevated serum lipids, hypertension, smoking.
    2. Elevated serum lipids, gender, diabetes mellitus.
    3. Hypertension, family history, obesity.
    4. Obesity, diabetes mellitus, age.

326. After spilling 20 cc of a chemotherapeutic agent on the floor in the client's room, the nurse should:
    1. Call housekeeping.
    2. Immediately exit the room.
    3. Use the "spill kit" to contain the medication.
    4. Notify the fire department.

327. A woman in active labor asks the nurse, "Is my baby getting enough oxygen?" The explanation is based on the knowledge that:
    1. The oxygen saturation of maternal blood in the intervillous space is greater than the maternal arterial blood.
    2. The oxygen saturation of maternal blood in the intervillous spaces is about the same as maternal capillary blood.
    3. The average oxygen saturation in the intervillous space is about 96%.
    4. The oxygen saturation in the intervillous space is greater than maternal capillary blood.

328. A 6-year-old child is being evaluated for attention deficit-hyperactivity disorder. The child lives in a house built in the 1920s which is being remodeled. The nurse's *priority* assessment is:
    1. The type of paint originally used in the house.
    2. The types of foods and fluids served to the child on a daily basis.
    3. The type of discipline used by the parents.
    4. The type of personal and social problems the child is experiencing at school.

329. The nurse is counseling a 67-year-old woman with a family history of bladder cancer about risk factors for bladder cancer. The nurse knows that risk factors for this client include:
    1. Low fiber diet.
    2. Smoking cigarettes.
    3. Hysterectomy at age 42.
    4. History of occasional urinary tract infections.

330. Which measure, if used by the nurse, would be most effective in preventing childhood obesity?
    1. Alleviating the guilt associated with being obese.
    2. Promoting awareness of stressful events.
    3. Helping mothers not to overfeed their infants with formula.
    4. Encouraging diets low in carbohydrates.

331. When assessing the client for pain, the nurse knows that the most accurate indicator of pain is the:
    1. Client's vital signs.
    2. Client's diagnosis or type of surgery.
    3. Nurse's observation of the client's body language.
    4. Client's own report of pain.

332. According to the World Health Organization (WHO), which category of drugs is considered adjuvant analgesics?
    1. Tricyclic antidepressants.
    2. Nonsteroidal antiinflammatory drugs.
    3. Nonopioid analgesics.
    4. Narcotic agonist analgesics.

333. A client, 36 weeks pregnant, states that her 2-year-old ran into her abdomen with both hands. She wants to know if the baby will be harmed from the impact. The nurse's response is based on the understanding that:
    Select all that apply.
    1. The amniotic fluid prevents bacterial infections from affecting the fetus
    2. The amniotic fluid helps protect the fetus from harm by trauma.
    3. The purpose of the amniotic fluid is to provide oxygen to the fetus.
    4. The amniotic fluid causes dilation of the cervical canal during labor.
    5. The amniotic fluid provides cushioning to the fetus against injury

334. The staff nurse on the pediatric unit has just finished listening to the end-of-shift report. Which client should the staff nurse assess *first*?
    1. A child with sickle cell anemia who is complaining of chest pain.
    2. A toddler who had surgery for phimosis and is incontinent.
    3. An infant with acute gastroenteritis who has green, liquid stools.
    4. A child with asthma who has retractions.

335. An important measure for a client on a cooling blanket to reduce fever is to:
    1. Sponge the client with tepid water and alcohol to augment the effect of the cooling blanket.
    2. Leave the cooling blanket on until the client exhibits mild shivering.
    3. Wrap the client's fingers and toes to prevent "freeze burn."
    4. Turn a fan on the client to enhance the effect of the cooling blanket.

336. A client, gravida 1, para 0, is in labor and delivery with irregular contractions at 39 weeks gestation. Her cervical exam reveals that the cervix is dilated 1 cm and she is 50% effaced. After two hours of observation, her contractions remain irregular and her cervix has not changed. The best explanation of her current condition is:
    1. The client has failure-to-progress and needs a cesarean section.
    2. The client is experiencing prolonged latent phase of labor.
    3. The client has an arrest of second stage of labor.
    4. The client is experiencing a protracted active phase of labor.

337. The nurse triages clients in the emergency department. Which client should the nurse treat *first*?
    1. A 27-year-old man with right-side chest pain, shortness of breath, and unequal chest excursion who was in a motor vehicle accident.
    2. A 7-year-old child who sustained a scalp laceration in a soccer game. The child is awake and crying.
    3. An 82-year-old man with chest pain who is pale and diaphoretic.
    4. A 35-year-old woman with a compound tibial fracture.

338. The pediatric unit conducts a mock disaster drill. The nurse in charge of the disaster team must decide which client can be safely discharged home in order to make room for a client being admitted from the scene of the disaster. The client who could be safely discharged is:
    1. A child with glomerulonephritis who has an elevated albumin level.
    2. A child with fifth disease who is not immunosuppressed.
    3. A child with osteomyelitis who is on long-term IV antibiotic therapy.
    4. A child with asthma who has retractions.

339. In general, a client with a fracture should be positioned:
    1. With the fracture below the level of the heart to promote arterial circulation.
    2. With 10, or more, pounds of traction weight.
    3. Above the level of the heart to promote venous return.
    4. At heart level to prevent compartment syndrome.

340. Which short-term outcome would the nurse consider most important for a client with bulimia?
    1. Absence of signs and symptoms of dehydration.
    2. A gain of 3 pounds per week as indicated.
    3. Demonstration of insight into binging and purging.
    4. Expression of genuine feelings in group therapy.

341. A client is given a prescription for iron supplements during her pregnancy. When providing teaching about her medications, the nurse bases her explanation to the client on the knowledge that:
    1. Exogenous supplements are usually not required in pregnancy.
    2. Absorption of iron from the intestine is increased in pregnancy.
    3. The hemoglobin production of the fetus will be blocked if the client is iron-deficient.
    4. The maternal hemoglobin rises during the second half of pregnancy without iron supplementation.

342. The client is receiving lactulose by mouth. The nurse knows the medication is effective when the client:
    1. Becomes constipated.
    2. Has diarrhea.
    3. Has a decrease in potassium level.
    4. States pain is diminished or relieved.

343. A client with COPD undergoes surgical repair of an inguinal hernia. Preoperative arterial blood gases were: pH 7.36; Pco_2 54; and Po_2 70 on room air. After surgery arterial blood gases were: pH 7.35; Pco_2 60; and Po_2 65 on oxygen at 2 L/min via nasal cannula. What is the nurse's best action?
    1. Increase the client's oxygen to 4 L/min.
    2. Suction the client.
    3. Order a nebulizer treatment.
    4. Have the client cough and deep breathe.

344. A toddler is to have a cardiac catheterization. The most appropriate preparatory nursing intervention would be to:
    1. Explain the procedure to the toddler in simple sentences just before giving the preoperative sedation.
    2. Bring a puppet in the evening before the procedure and show the toddler where the catheter will be inserted.

3. Read a story to the toddler about a child who has a cardiac catheterization.

4. Show the toddler a model of the heart.

345. Which client is at greatest risk for developing hypertension?

1. A 52-year-old Caucasian man with a family history of hypertension and heart disease.

2. A 40-year-old African-American woman who is 24 pounds overweight.

3. A 52-year-old African-American man who smokes cigarettes.

4. A 67-year-old Caucasian man with diabetes.

346. When assisting with a cardioversion, which item should the nurse ensure is available?

1. Back board for chest compressions.

2. EKG monitor.

3. Alcohol pads.

4. Sodium bicarbonate

347. Immediately after delivery, a client is concerned about the oblong, lumpy shape of her newborn baby's head. The nurse's teaching would include:

1. Reassurance that the infant's head will return to a normal, round shape within a couple of days.

2. Assurance that the infant will be examined by the physician to determine the extent of trauma.

3. Information that the infant will have brain damage due to intracranial pressure.

4. Referral to a support group for mothers with children who are hydrocephalic.

348. The physician has ordered the client to be transfused with 2 units of packed red blood cells over 4 hours. Each unit contains 350 cc. If the drop factor of the blood tubing is 10 gtt/mL, the nurse should set the blood transfusion drip rate at:

Fill in the blank.

_____ gtt/min

349. The nurse is discussing toddler growth and development with the parent. Which suggestion by the nurse to the parent would foster development of autonomy?

1. Assist the toddler to learn the difference between right and wrong.

2. Provide the toddler with opportunities to play with other children.

3. Encourage the toddler to take appropriate actions independently.

4. Help the toddler to complete tasks.

350. Before planning a high protein diet for a client who has just been admitted for alcohol withdrawal, which lab value should the nurse check?

1. CBC.

2. Liver function tests.

3. Hemoglobin.

4. Urinalysis.

351. The client with myasthenia gravis is experiencing dysphagia related to muscle weakness. The most appropriate nursing action would include:

1. Minimizing distraction during mealtime so client can focus on swallowing.

2. Using a voice amplifier so client can be heard without straining the voice.

3. Offering nutritious thin liquids to prevent aspiration and malnourishment.

4. Turning the plate around halfway during the meal so all food can be seen.

352. The employee health nurse decides to survey staff to screen for cardiovascular risks that can be modified with teaching. Which question would most likely identify an "at risk" population that can be helped?

1. "Do you take medicine for high blood pressure?"

2. "Have you ever been told your cholesterol is under 240 mg/dL?"

3. "Do you smoke or do you live with people who smoke?"

4. "What is your age?"

353. When conducting a Denver Developmental Screening Test (DDST), the nurse would anticipate that a 4-month-old infant could be expected to:

1. Reach for objects.

2. Demonstrate a pincer grasp.

3. Lift head 45–90 degrees while on stomach.

4. Pull self up into sitting position.

354. A client who is 12 weeks pregnant has a history of class II heart disease. In planning her care, which statement about class II heart disease and pregnancy are correct?

Select all that apply.

1. The woman should be counseled to have an abortion to reduce the risk of maternal death during labor.

2. The woman should perform daily fetal kick counts to monitor fetal well-being.

3. The woman should be hospitalized throughout her pregnancy to monitor her and her fetus.

4. The woman should plan for maximum rest and minimum work throughout her pregnancy.

5. The woman should be delivered by cesarean section to decrease the stress of labor.

355. A client recently diagnosed with gestational diabetes is at 32 weeks' gestation. Her physician has ordered her to begin insulin injections. What instructions will the nurse include in teaching the client?

1. Directions to administer the insulin injections in her abdomen.

2. The importance of administering her insulin injections as soon as she had finished her breakfast.

3. The importance of starting an exercise program to help utilize the insulin she is injecting.

4. If the client follows her diet carefully, the insulin will be discontinued in a couple of weeks.

356. The nurse in a well baby clinic is preparing to immunize a 4-month-old infant. Which of the pediatrician's standing orders should the nurse question?

1. "Administer hepatitis B vaccine (HEP B) at 4-month-old visit."

2. "Administer inactivated polio vaccine (IPV) at 4-month-old visit."

3. "Administer pneumococcal vaccine (PCV) at 4-month-old visit."

4. "Administer measles, mumps, and rubella vaccine (MMR) at 4-month-old visit."

357. When caring for clients who are elderly in a skilled nursing facility, the nurse should assess for documentation of which routine vaccinations?

Select all that apply.

1. Pneumococcal, one dose after age 65.

2. Meningococcal, every 5 years.

3. Influenza, once each fall.

4. Tetanus, every 10 years.

5. Varicella, two doses.

6. Hepatitis B, series of 3.

358. A client is placed in a hard neck brace to immobilize the spine following trauma to the neck. X-rays are inconclusive because of swelling. To assess and care for the skin under the collar, the nurse should:

1. Place the client flat and supine, remove the anterior section of the collar, turning the head to the right or left to remove the back section.

2. Have the client sit up in a chair to remove the front and back sections without turning the head from side to side.

3. Have at least one nurse stabilize the head in line with the torso, while the other nurse removes the collar sections.

4. Wait until the x-rays are conclusive for any trauma before assessing the skin, or providing skin care under the collar.

359. A client was placed on spinal precautions. The *first* priority in caring for this client is:
1. Having other nurses assist with logrolling the client.
2. Giving corticosteroids for the first 48 hours.
3. Keeping the head of the bed elevated 30–60 degrees.
4. Assessing the extremities for numbness or weaknesses q4h.

360. A community health nurse visits a client with obsessive-compulsive disorder who has recently been started on lorazepam (Ativan) prn. for severe anxiety. It would be most important for the nurse to explain that the medication:
1. Can result in drowsiness and motor coordination.
2. Is habit forming and is to be used only as needed.
3. Always controls anxiety for up to 4 hours.
4. May need to be abruptly discontinued.

361. The indwelling Foley catheter was removed following an episode of prostatitis, but the client did not void for the next 8 hours, even when allowed to stand. The best action for the nurse to take is to:
1. Ask the physician for a prostate evaluation.
2. Wait another 8 hours and encourage frequent attempts.
3. Ask the physician for orders to catheterize the bladder.
4. Encourage oral fluids and hot baths to relax the sphincter.

362. A client with terminal cancer has been receiving fentanyl by a transdermal patch at 50 μ/hr. Each 3600 μ patch lasts for 3 days. Exactly 48 hours after applying the patch the client died. The nurse should:
1. Document the transfer of a 50 μ/hr fentanyl patch to the morgue.
2. Have another nurse witness disposal of 1200 μ of fentanyl.
3. Remove the patch and place it with the client's belongings.
4. Remove the patch, return to the pharmacy, and chart 2400 μ given.

363. A client is concerned about the possible side effects of an intrauterine device (IUD). When explaining the possible complications, the nurse knows which of the following is associated with the use of an IUD?
Select all that apply.
1. There is an increased incidence of pelvic inflammatory disease (PID) with the use of an IUD.
2. It is common to have a longer menstrual period, with more cramping, with an IUD in place.
3. Women who have an IUD in place have a higher risk of mortality than those using oral contraceptives.
4. Uterine perforation is common with the use of an IUD.
5. Women who smoke are discouraged from using an IUD.

364. A client is planning to breastfeed and is asking the nurse about contraception. What will be a correct statement about breastfeeding and contraception that the nurse will make?
1. Breastfeeding has been shown to be an effective method of contraception until the first menstrual period after delivery.
2. An IUD should not be used by a woman who is breastfeeding.
3. A woman who is breastfeeding will not ovulate until her infant is weaned.
4. It is important for the woman to be refitted for a diaphragm after delivery of an infant.

365. The client comes to the emergency department with complaints of frequent nosebleeds, headaches in the morning, fatigue, shortness of breath on exertion, and blurred vision. Which action should the nurse take *first*?
1. Check the client's O₂ saturation.
2. Collect a urine specimen for ketone dumping.
3. Check the client's blood pressure.
4. Assess for neurological impairment.

366. Prior to the use of a newly placed peripherally inserted central catheter (PICC), which action should the nurse take to verify placement?
1. Flush catheter with a 50 mL of normal saline.
2. Call for x-ray to confirm placement in superior vena cava (SVC).
3. Order an ultrasound to confirm right ventricle placement.
4. Aspirate 10 mL of blood from catheter.

367. The grandparents of a toddler with meningitis ask the nurse what type of toy they should purchase for the toddler to play with while hospitalized. The nurse's best response would be:
1. A wagon.
2. Blocks in multiple shapes, sizes, and colors.
3. Crayons and finger paints.
4. A storybook.

368. A 15-year-old adolescent was diagnosed with diabetes mellitus at 7 years of age. The adolescent now has the opportunity to travel to Washington, DC, on an honor's history class field trip. The parents will not be accompanying the adolescent on the trip. Which test would best assess that diabetes mellitus is under control in order to allow the adolescent to participate in this activity?
1. Self-monitoring of blood glucose on a scheduled basis.
2. Urine testing for glucose.
3. Fasting glucose level.
4. Glycosylated hemoglobin.

369. The physician has ordered a STAT chemistry panel followed by placement of a peripherally inserted central catheter (PICC) and TPN IV infusion. Which site for PICC placement would the nurse plan to reserve?
1. Left hand.
2. Left lower forearm.
3. Right antecubital.
4. Right hand.

370. Which goal has the *highest* priority for a client who is receiving paroxetine (Paxil)?
1. Client will not hurt self.
2. Improvement in mood.
3. Reduction in insomnia.
4. Increase in the client's appetite.

371. In calculating the gestational age of a fetus, the nurse would start from:
1. The first day of the last menstrual period.
2. The day of conception.
3. The last day of the last menstrual period.
4. The day of ovulation.

372. The client admitted with an acute myocardial infarction (MI) has been placed on a beta-blocker medication. The first dose of the beta-blocker is to be given STAT. The nurse knows that the beta-blocker on the list of medications ordered is:
1. Famotidine 20 mg PO bid.
2. Metoprolol 50 mg PO bid.
3. Diazepam 2 mg PO q6h.
4. Furosemide (Lasix) 40 mg IV qd.

373. The charge nurse in a well-baby clinic questions a new graduate preparing to assess a 10-month-old infant as to what physical findings the new graduate will look for in the assessment. Which response made by the new graduate would indicate to the charge nurse that additional teaching is needed?
Select all that apply.
1. The presence of Ortolani's click.
2. The presence of 4 teeth.
3. The presence of an open anterior fontanel.
4. The presence of Babinski's sign.

374. The client with newly diagnosed hypertension has been placed on a beta-blocker. The nurse knows that discharge medication instructions for beta-blockers should include:

1. Taking the pulse daily and knowing the symptoms of hypotension.
2. Avoiding eating dark leafy green vegetables.
3. Potential for potassium depletion with increased urine output.
4. Taking the medication with food only.

375. The client is admitted for acute respiratory distress. A B-type natriuretic peptide (BNP) is included in the laboratory orders. In providing education to the client about the purpose of the lab test, the nurse tells the client that the test helps evaluate:
1. Pancreatic function.
2. Pleural effusion.
3. Kidney function.
4. Heart failure.

376. The nurse is performing a vaginal exam on a woman in the active phase of labor. Which landmarks would the nurse use to determine the position of the fetal head?
1. The sagittal suture and fontanels of the fetal head.
2. The pelvic inlet of the mother.
3. The ischial spines of the mother's pelvis.
4. The temporal suture and fontanels of the fetal head.

377. The client is admitted for a recent onset (less then 2 hours) of left hemiparesis, facial droop, field cut, and an imaging report indicating a positive computed tomography (CT) scan of the head. The RN knows that this indicates:
1. A hemorrhagic brain attack and should receive a thrombolytic agent.
2. An ischemic brain attack and should have a thrombolytic agent.
3. A hemorrhagic brain attack and should not receive a thrombolytic agent.
4. An ischemic brain attack and should not receive a thrombolytic agent.

378. The mother of a 3-week-old infant comes to the emergency department after being seen earlier that day in a well-baby clinic. The mother was instructed by the staff in the well baby clinic to seek immediate acute care for the infant. The mother informs the nurse that the infant began vomiting after every meal about 1 week after being discharged from the hospital as a newborn. The nurse's *first* action is to obtain the infant's weight to determine the state of dehydration. *Fill in the blank.*
Severe dehydration would be a weight *loss of* _____ *percent.*

379. The client is in the hospital for syncope related to atrial arrhythmias. Prior to the administration of oral diltiazem (Cardizem), it is most important for the nurse to assess:
1. Blood pressure.
2. Heart rate.
3. Peripheral pulses.
4. Urine output.

380. A community health nurse is planning to visit 4 clients who live 5 miles from each other. Who should the nurse plan to visit *first*?
1. A client who is manic and has been taking lithium carbonate (Eskalith) and valproic acid (Depakote) for 3 weeks.
2. A client who is psychotic and was started on haloperidol (Haldol) and trihexyphenidyl (Artane) yesterday.
3. A client discharged from a psychiatric unit yesterday with major depression who was started on imipramine (Tofranil) 2 weeks ago.
4. A client who is an alcoholic, in the first month of recovery, taking disulfiram (Antabuse) and who is refusing to attend Alcoholics Anonymous (AA) meetings.

381. A client is 37 weeks pregnant with a fundal height of 32 cm. The nurse knows the most likely explanation for this assessment is:

1. The client has a fetus with macrosomia.
2. The client has polyhydramnios.
3. The client has maternal diabetes.
4. The client has severe pregnancy-induced hypertension.

382. Two hours ago the client had a left thoracotomy with a lobe resection. The sanguinous drainage in the chest tube collection chamber is 325 mL. The nurse recognizes that this is:
1. Normal chest tube drainage.
2. Indicative of a pneumothorax.
3. Chyle drainage.
4. A sign of hemorrhage.

383. A nursing student who is preparing for a clinical conference on fetal development needs to know that fetal circulation is characterized by:
1. High pulmonary vascular resistance.
2. High pulmonary blood flow.
3. High resistance of the ductus arteriosis.
4. High umbilicoplacental resistance.

384. A client admitted for decreased level of consciousness and dehydration is receiving an IV of $D_5 \frac{1}{2}$ NS with 40 mEq KCl/L infusing at 100 cc/hr. The client's potassium level is 5.9. The nurse knows to:
1. Recheck the potassium level 6 hours after the blood is drawn in the morning.
2. Stop the IV, maintain the site, notify the physician about the lab level.
3. Decrease the IV rate to 50 cc/hr and notify the physician when the physician is on rounds.
4. Assess the IV site and continue with the current order.

385. A client is admitted for closed head injury following a motor vehicle accident (MVA). Which intervention should the nurse plan that would minimize increased intracranial pressure?
1. Maintain the head of the bed (HOB) at less than 10 degrees.
2. Group all nursing activities and leave the client undisturbed for 2 hours.
3. Maintain alignment of the head and neck.
4. Elevate the client's legs.

386. The client has just undergone gastric resection and is being transferred to the postanesthesia recovery room. The *first* assessment priority in caring for this client is:
1. Blood pressure and heart rate.
2. Temperature.
3. Respiratory rate and oxygen saturation.
4. Pain.

387. The nurse in a well-child clinic observes the mother of a 4-year-old child slap the child in the face. The 4-year-old child has been teasing a 2-year-old sibling while waiting to see the pediatrician. The mother had repeatedly warned the 4-year-old child to "stop doing that." The nurse should:
Select all that apply.
1. Review the 4-year-old child's chart for signs and symptoms of previous abuse.
2. Notify the nursing supervisor of the mother's action.
3. Take the mother aside privately and offer to watch the 4-year-old child for a few minutes.
4. Discuss alternate discipline strategies with the mother.

388. The mother of a 9-month-old infant receives an updated food list from the nurse during a well-child checkup. The mother questions the nurse as to why the infant may now start eating egg yolk but not egg white. The nurse's best reply would be:
1. "Babies like the taste of egg yolk better than egg white."
2. "Babies like visually stimulating food, such as an egg yolk, better than visually bland food, such as egg white."

3. "The slippery texture of egg white could lead to the baby's choking or aspiration; the semi-solid texture of egg yolk is safer."
4. "Egg white is a potential cause of allergy development in a baby."

389. While assessing the client who has just had a chest tube placed, the nurse notes fluctuations (tidaling) in the water-seal chamber. The nurse knows that this indicates:
1. Expected fluid movement with respiration.
2. An air leak.
3. Presence of subcutaneous emphysema.
4. Appropriate suction level.

390. In caring for a client who is psychotic and who recently started taking haloperidol (Haldol) 10 mg bid, for which side effects should the nurse look?
Select all that apply.
1. Motor restlessness.
2. Limb and neck spasms.
3. Cogwheeling rigidity.
4. Tardive dyskinesia.
5. Shuffling gait.
6. ECG changes.

391. A client with a spontaneous pneumothorax has had a chest tube for 3 days. On morning rounds, the physician clamped the chest tube to determine the client's readiness to have the chest tube discontinued. Two hours after having the chest tube clamped, the client began to have difficulty breathing. What action should the nurse take *first*?
1. Notify the physician.
2. Unclamp the chest tube.
3. Assess the client for subcutaneous emphysema.
4. Place the client on 2 L nasal cannula oxygen.

392. While assessing the client who has a chest tube, the nurse notes that the tubing is kinked between the bedrails. The nurse knows that this places the client at increased risk for:
1. Tension pneumothorax.
2. Air leak.
3. Hemorrhage.
4. Cardiac tamponade.

393. A client is admitted for acute myocardial infarction (MI) and has undergone heart catheterization, angiography, and coronary angioplasty with stents. The client is receiving antiplatelet agents (aspirin and Plavix), a proton pump inhibitor (Prevacid), potassium supplement (K-Dur), and a stool softener (Colace). Prior to the administration of these medications, it is *most important* for the nurse to assess:
1. Blood pressure.
2. Serum troponin level.
3. Serum potassium level.
4. Peripheral pulses.

394. A client with chronic renal insufficiency has been admitted for acute myocardial infarction (MI) and has had a coronary angiography. The angiography results indicated that the client requires coronary artery bypass surgery. After heart catheterization was done, the nurse reviews the laboratory values. Which change would be of greatest concern before surgery?
1. Serum troponin from 0.7 ng/mL to 0.85 ng/mL.
2. Serum WBC from 6000/mm³ to 11,000/mm³.
3. Serum CPK-MB from 5.5 ng/mL to 6.7 ng/mL.
4. Serum creatinine from 1.8 mg/dL to 2.8 mg/dL.

395. The client's arterial blood gases on room air are: pH 7.33; P_{O_2} 77; P_{CO_2} 50; H_{CO_3} 23. The nurse would instruct the client to:
1. Try to breathe more slowly.
2. Use the bedside inspirometer hourly when awake.
3. Wear nasal cannula oxygen at 6 L/min.
4. Increase fluid intake to flush the kidneys.

396. The school nurse plans to present a sex education program to a group of 11 year old boys. The program will be conducted during the school semester at regularly scheduled intervals. The school nurse would best demonstrate knowledge of the learning needs of late school-age children by scheduling which topic *first*?
1. How the penis becomes erect.
2. How diseases are sexually transmitted.
3. How to be sexually responsible.
4. How AIDS is acquired.

397. A nursing student is enrolled in the pediatric rotation of the nursing program. The nursing student is to attend a one-day experience in a child development center. The nursing student is assigned to devise an activity plan for a group of 5-year-old children which will promote gross motor development as well as social skills. The nursing student should select:
1. Finger painting.
2. Playing house.
3. Walking along a nature trail.
4. Playing soccer.

398. What is an accurate statement about the fetus of a mother who is diabetic?
1. The insulin produced by the fetus helps to meet the insulin requirements of a mother who is diabetic.
2. At birth, the blood insulin levels are low in infants of a mother who is diabetic.
3. The fetus produces additional insulin in response to maternal hyperglycemia.
4. The insulin needed by the fetus is produced by the mother's pancreas and transported to the fetus.

399. What is accurate information about fetal respirations in utero?
1. A healthy fetus makes no respiratory movements before birth.
2. Fetal crying in utero is a common occurrence.
3. A normal fetus demonstrates irregular respiratory motions in utero.
4. Asphyxia in utero results in decreased respiratory effort.

400. A nurse is making a home visit to a 10-year-old child who is taking desipramine HCl (Norpramin) 50 mg bid for depression. The child has been vomiting and has a temperature of 101°F. An older child in the family just recovered from a stomach flu that lasted 3 days. Which response from the nurse would be most appropriate regarding the prescribed medication?
1. Have the parent hold the medication until the vomiting subsides.
2. Ask the parent to hold the medication for 24 hours and call the doctor.
3. Instruct the parent to continue giving the medication with food.
4. Instruct the parent to give 1 tbs clear liquids q 15 min and continue the medication.

401. Which doctor's order should the nurse question?
1. Amitriptyline is prescribed for a client who has chronic back pain.
2. Enoxaparin is prescribed for a client who has had a total hip replacement.
3. Propranolol is prescribed for a client with COPD.
4. Lovastatin is prescribed for a client with hypercholesterolemia.

402. A client with chronic sinusitis has had pneumonia 3 times in the last year. The nurse should suggest:
1. Salt water gargle.
2. Cool humidifier.
3. Classic antihistamines such as diphenhydramine.
4. Oral corticosteroids.

403. A teen client is concerned about developing stretch marks during her pregnancy. The nurse develops her teaching plan for this client based on the knowledge that:
    1. Stretch marks occur in all pregnancies. They are indicators of good fetal growth.
    2. Stretch marks are uncommon in nulliparous women.
    3. Stretch marks will completely disappear after delivery.
    4. Stretch marks may occur and will change to silvery streaks after delivery.

404. The client has a nasogastric tube connected to low continuous suction for abdominal decompression. The nurse notes that gastric fluid in the suction tubing is not moving and the client's abdomen is becoming distended. The nurse's best action is to:
    1. Pull out the NG tube and insert a new one.
    2. Irrigate the tube with 30 cc of water.
    3. Tell the client to take a few deep breaths.
    4. Turn the suction higher.

405. What assessment finding would alert the nurse that the client has a bowel obstruction?
    1. High-pitched bowel sounds above the site of the obstruction.
    2. High-pitched bowel sounds below the site of the obstruction.
    3. Absence of bowel sounds.
    4. Fever of 101°F or greater.

406. The nurse prepares to assess a healthy, 2-week-old infant. Which physical finding would the nurse consider to be normal?
    1. When suspended in a horizontal prone position and suddenly thrust downward, hands and fingers extend forward.
    2. When suspended in a horizontal prone position, the head is raised and legs and spine are extended.
    3. When stroking the back alongside spine, hips move toward stimulated side.
    4. When supine, head is turned to one side and shoulder, trunk and pelvis will turn toward that side.

407. The client is undergoing treatment for pheochromocytoma. What is most important for the nurse to carefully monitor?
    1. Pulse rate.
    2. Blood sugar.
    3. Blood pressure.
    4. Urine output.

408. The charge nurse on a pediatric unit is teaching a class on general safety to a group of new UAPs (unlicensed assistive personnel). The charge nurse should stress:
    Select all that apply.
    1. "Baby walkers" may not be brought in from home by the parent.
    2. Unoccupied cribs must have the crib rails in the up position at all times.
    3. Latex balloons are not permitted on the pediatric unit.
    4. Infants may be transported to other areas in the hospital in bassinets or cribs.

409. What is an accurate statement about the relationship between pregnancy and maternal blood volume?
    1. The maternal blood volume increases steadily throughout the pregnancy.
    2. The maternal blood volume increase results from an increase in both plasma and erythrocytes.
    3. The maternal blood volume increases by an average of 75% over prepregnancy values.
    4. The maternal blood volume increases are caused by a doubling of plasma volume.

410. The physician prescribes lithium carbonate (Lithobid). Before initiating the prescription, it is most important for the nurse to check:
    1. Renal function tests.
    2. History of alcohol use.
    3. Liver function tests.
    4. The client's diet.

411. A client with myasthenia gravis is given a Tensilon test. Forty minutes after the test, the client develops severe weakness and ptosis. The nurse should be prepared to:
    1. Administer atropine.
    2. Administer pyridostigmine.
    3. Check for constricted pupils.
    4. Intubate the client.

412. The nurse knows that the S_1 heart sound is best heard at the:
    1. Second intercostal space, right sternal border.
    2. Second intercostal space, left sternal border.
    3. Third intercostal space, left sternal border.
    4. Fifth intercostal space, left midclavicular line

413. A client, 6 weeks pregnant with a history of class I heart disease, denies any other medical problems. In planning her care, the nurse knows that the client's cardiac output during pregnancy:
    1. Increases during the first trimester and decreases during the second and third trimester.
    2. Is greater in the supine position than in a lateral position in late pregnancy.
    3. Is increased during the first stage of labor and decreased during the second stage of labor.
    4. Steadily increases during the first trimester and remains elevated throughout pregnancy.

414. A client with mild hypertension, and no additional risk factors, runs several times a week for exercise. What would the nurse advise this client?
    1. Increase running to 5 miles, 6 times per week.
    2. Enroll in stress reduction or biofeedback courses.
    3. Eliminate caffeine from the diet.
    4. Maintain dietary intake of potassium and calcium.

415. What is the correct nursing procedure for tracheal suctioning?
    1. Place 10 cc sterile saline down the trachea before suctioning.
    2. Set wall suction at 120 mm Hg
    3. Suction for 20–30 seconds to get all secretions.
    4. Deflate the cuff on the airway just before suctioning.

416. A client in active labor is lying in a supine position. The nurse knows that by encouraging this position in labor, it may lead to:
    1. Increased venous return.
    2. Increased cardiac output.
    3. Increased blood flow to the lower extremities.
    4. Arterial hypotension.

417. The client is having a central line inserted into the right subclavian vein. Which assessment should be reported to the physician during the procedure?
    1. Dark red blood flowing briskly from the catheter hub just prior to attaching the IV tubing.
    2. Coughing.
    3. Mild pain at the insertion site.
    4. Sinus rhythm.

418. A home health nurse is assessing potential health hazards in homes with "at-home-care" infants and children. Which situation requires the nurse's intervention?
    1. An 8-month-old infant is removed from the apnea monitor during feedings.
    2. A 5-year-old child with a neurogenic bladder is on clean intermittent catheterization (CIC) guidelines.
    3. A newborn with developmental hip dysplasia is wearing a Pavlik harness 23 hours a day.
    4. A 12-year-old child with hemophilia is self-administering the IV clotting factor.

419. The staff nurse on a pediatric unit is preparing to discharge a mother with a 5-day-old infant who was hospitalized with

physiological jaundice. What critical information must the mother understand prior to going home?
1. The need to purchase a musical mobile and keep it suspended above the newborn's crib to provide auditory stimulation.
2. The need to assess the fit of the crib mattress to the crib frame and allow a maximum of two adult fingerbreadths between the crib mattress and the crib frame.
3. The need to place the newborn's car seat in the backseat of the car and facing the rear of the car.
4. The need to purchase a sturdy, one-piece pacifier to provide oral stimulation.

420. In assessing a client with bipolar disorder-manic taking lithium carbonate (Lithobid), what lithium blood level in mEq/L would indicate that the client is at high risk for lithium toxicity?
Fill in the blank.
_____ mEq/L

421. What is the nurse's *primary* concern when initially caring for a client with second- and third-degree burns on both arms?
1. Administering parenteral antibiotics.
2. Starting range-of-motion exercises.
3. Maintaining a patent IV.
4. Pain management.

422. What lab value should the nurse be most concerned about?
1. Na$^+$ 120.
2. Hct 31%.
3. Platelets of 100,000.
4. K$^+$ 4.7.

423. A client in active labor is having contractions every 3–4 minutes, lasting 60–90 seconds. The contractions are palpated as being moderate in strength. The client is complaining of lower back pain during contractions. The best position for this client during labor is:
1. Semi-Fowler's.
2. Left lateral.
3. Knee-chest.
4. Trendelenburg.

424. The client understands postileostomy care when the client states:
1. "I empty my bag when it gets too heavy."
2. "I empty my bag before it is half full."
3. "I empty my bag before it is one-third full."
4. "I don't need to wear a bag all the time."

425. The nurse is assessing the function of the third cranial nerve. This assessment would be performed by:
1. Touching the client's cheeks with a piece of cotton.
2. Moving a pen light from the side, toward the client's pupils.
3. Asking the client to stick out the tongue.
4. Asking the client to identify the odor of peppermint, with eyes closed.

426. The nurse assigned to a day-care center is discussing toddler car safety with a group of mothers. The nurse would correctly inform the mothers to place the toddler's car seat:
1. In the rear-facing position in the middle of the back seat of the car.
2. In the front-facing position in the middle of the back seat of the car.
3. As close to the car's air bags as possible.
4. In the front-facing position in the front of the car with the passenger-side air bag switched to the off position.

427. A school nurse assigned to multiple schools notices skin lesions on some of the students. Which skin lesions require *immediate* notification to the school pediatrician by the school nurse?

1. Slightly elevated, crusted lesions on the pinna of the ear of a 2-year-old toddler in a developmental center.
2. Superficial but elevated pustules on the cheeks of a 16-year-old adolescent in high school.
3. Elevated vesicles on the palms of the hands of a 7-year-old child in elementary school.
4. Flat, pinkish-red macules on the face, neck and trunk of a 5-year-old child in kindergarten.

428. A case management nurse in an acute care facility has been assigned four clients. Which client will require the most complex case management?
1. A client who is 25 years old with testicular cancer and a recent orchiectomy.
2. A client who is 63 years old who had a recent brain attack.
3. A client who is 18 years old who had a ruptured appendix.
4. A client who is 37 years old with diabetes and a below-the-knee amputation.

429. A client is in the fourth stage of labor. What assessment would the nurse make?
1. Fetal heart rate, fetal position and, station.
2. Dilation, effacement, and station.
3. Fundal location, lochia, and perineum.
4. Placental separation, fundal location, and uterine tone.

430. The nurse would be correct in telling a 16-year-old adolescent that intoxication occurs when a blood-alcohol level is at or above what percent?
Fill in the blank.
_____ percent

431. The client has a complete loss of vision. What should the nurse do to establish effective communication with this client?
1. Speak loudly, directly into the client's ear.
2. Speak very softly.
3. Speak directly in front of the client.
4. Speak with a smile.

432. Four weeks ago, while on a family camping trip to the northeastern United States, a child sustained several tick bites and now has a large circumferential ring with a raised, edematous doughnut-like border in the groin area. The child is "tired all of the time" and describes the lesion as "burning." The infectious disease nurse would correctly identify the child as being in what stage of Lyme disease?
1. Stage 1.
2. Stage 2.
3. Stage 3.
4. Stage 4.

433. What breathing technique would be helpful to teach a client with chronic obstructive pulmonary disease (COPD)?
1. Inhale deeply through the mouth.
2. Exhale through pursed lips.
3. Exhale approximately one third as long as inhaling.
4. Use the neck and upper chest muscles to improve chest wall expansion.

434. A client who is postpartum asks the nurse, "When will my body be back in shape?" The best response by the nurse is:
1. "Nothing is ever the same after you have a baby. Your new image is a mother."
2. "Your uterus will be back to its prepregnancy size by about 1 to 2 weeks postpartum."
3. "Exercise is the only way you can regain your shape. You can start vigorous exercise as soon as you like."
4. "Your body has been through many changes. It takes time for your body to regain its shape."

435. The client has begun breastfeeding for the first time after delivery of her infant. Her breasts are leaking colostrum. The nurse informs the client that her colostrum:

1. Will be secreted during the first week postpartum.
2. Contains a large amount of fat, but no vitamins.
3. Contains immunoglobulins that protect the infant against infection.
4. Contains minerals and antigens that protect the infant against infection.

436. The nurse needs to take a client with active respiratory TB to radiology for a chest x-ray. Before leaving the client's room, the nurse should:
    1. Put on a HEPA mask.
    2. Put a HEPA mask on the client.
    3. Put a gown and gloves on the client.
    4. Call ahead to radiology to let them know the nurse is coming with the client.

437. A family with school-age children is planning to take a 10-day camping trip in the northeastern United States. Prior to their departure, the parents contact the nurse in the pediatrician's office about ways to prevent Lyme disease while camping. The nurse should emphasize:
    1. Walking in the center of hiking trails.
    2. Wearing dark-colored clothing.
    3. Manually removing any observed ticks.
    4. Spraying the children with an insect repellent containing DEET or permethrin.

438. A charge nurse on a medical/surgical floor observes a nurse's aide taking care of a client with chronic arterial occlusive disease in the lower extremities. Which behavior requires intervention by the charge nurse?
    1. The aide soaks the client's feet in warm water.
    2. The aide places the client's bed in reverse Trendelenburg at 10 degrees.
    3. The aide places sheepskin between overlapped toes.
    4. The aide walks with the client just until the client complains of pain in the lower extremities.

439. The nurse caring for a client who was admitted 36 hours ago with a myocardial infarction (MI) hears a new murmur not previously noted. What should the nurse ask this client?
    1. "Has anyone in your family ever had a heart murmur?"
    2. "Are you having chest pain?"
    3. "Did you just walk to the restroom?"
    4. "How long ago did you take your Inderal?"

440. A client is to receive the first electroconvulsive therapy treatment. The nurse would be correct in explaining to the family that they should:
    1. Expect to see confusion initially after the treatment.
    2. Not tell the client the number of treatments needed.
    3. Wait until the client is in contact with reality before having a conversation.
    4. See the client's mood improve after 6 treatments.

441. A client is in the emergency department with a pneumothorax secondary to a gunshot wound. The client complains of shortness of breath and exhibits tracheal and mediastinal shifts to the left. For what procedure should the nurse prepare?
    1. Intubation with an endotracheal tube.
    2. Insertion of a closed chest drainage tube.
    3. Paracentesis.
    4. MRI of the chest.

442. A client delivered a 9 lb 5 oz infant with the use of outlet forceps 8 hours ago. The client had an epidural for pain control in labor and has been unable to void spontaneously. The most likely reason for the client's condition is:
    1. Delivery has resulted in an edematous bladder with an increased capacity.
    2. She has damage to the nerves caused by the epidural analgesia.

3. She has urinary tract damage caused by the forceps delivery.
4. The client is dehydrated after delivery and needs additional oral fluid intake.

443. A school-age child with celiac disease tells the nurse in the pediatrician's office, "I want to have a birthday cake like all of the other kids in my class." The nurse's best response would be:
    1. "Let's ask doctor if you can get off your diet just this once. After all, it is your birthday."
    2. "I know that you are disappointed but the diet is for your own good."
    3. "Have your ever had an ice cream cake? You could have that for your birthday!"
    4. "Let's build a special cake out of popcorn balls. All of the kids at your birthday party can help make it!"

444. The nurse knows the client understands treatment with the drug Isordil when the client says:
    1. "I can take a lower dose of this drug if the headaches get too bad."
    2. "I should take this drug only when I have chest pain."
    3. "I should let someone else drive for a while."
    4. "It's OK to have a couple of cocktails in the evening."

445. A client needs to be admitted to a nursing unit after having an appendectomy. Which client can be discharged in order to make room for this client?
    1. A client who is 18 years old, admitted one day ago with a diagnosis of diabetes, type 2, and who lives in a college dorm.
    2. A client who is 40 hours post-myocardial infarction (MI) with CK-MB of 8.2 ng/mL.
    3. A client with chronic asthma who has acute bronchitis with an oxygen saturation of 90% on 3 liters/minute via nasal cannula.
    4. A 61-year-old client with osteoarthritis who lives in a nursing home, is scheduled for a total hip replacement.

446. A hospital is preparing for emergency admission of clients who were in a bus accident. Which client can be discharged to make room for the new admissions?
    1. A client with a fractured femur and suspected fat embolus.
    2. A client with bronchial asthma with 95% oxygen saturation on room air.
    3. An elderly client with dementia who was admitted the day before with congestive heart failure.
    4. A client admitted 3 days ago with small bowel obstruction who has a nasogastric tube in place.

447. The community health nurse must report to the public health department a client who is diagnosed with:
    1. Acid fast bacilli.
    2. Scabies.
    3. Rubella.
    4. Strep throat.

448. When counseling a school-age child with celiac disease, the nurse would anticipate the difficulty that compliance with prescribed food restrictions at meals and snacks presents. Which meal or snack time would present the most difficulty with compliance for the school-age child?
    1. Breakfast.
    2. Lunch.
    3. Dinner.
    4. Bedtime snack.

449. A client delivered a normal full-term infant vaginally, with a medial episiotomy 4 hours ago. She has been medicated one hour ago with codeine for episiotomy pain rated at that time by the client to be 8/10 on the pain scale. Upon assessment, after medication was given, the nurse asked the client to rate her pain on a scale of 1 to 10. The client stated that her pain

was unrelieved by the codeine and is currently a 10/10 on the pain scale. The client is visibly uncomfortable and unable to sit in a chair. What is the *first* action the nurse should take?
1. Call the physician to obtain additional orders for pain medication.
2. Assess the client's episiotomy to see if the client has an infection.
3. Assess her fundus to ensure that she doesn't have excessive bleeding.
4. Check the client's perineum for hematoma formation.

450. A 30-year-old client is admitted to a psychiatric unit for severe depression. The client is started on antidepressant medication. Which information should the evening charge nurse communicate *immediately* to the physician?
1. Urine drug screen positive for benzodiazepines.
2. History of sexual abuse.
3. Elevated thyroid-stimulating hormone (TSH).
4. A family member visits while intoxicated.

451. The 30-year-old client with asthma is brought into the emergency department by a friend because of difficulty breathing throughout the day and is now confused. The client's arterial blood gases (ABGs) are: pH 7.19; PaO_2 46; PCO_2 88; HCO_3 25. The nurse would anticipate that the client's *immediate* treatment will be directed at:
1. Increasing O_2 via nasal cannula to maintain pulse oximetry saturation greater than 94%.
2. Starting IV with Solu-Medrol.
3. Intubation and mechanical ventilation.
4. Administration of STAT bronchodilator via hand-held nebulizer.

452. The client comes to the emergency department with complaints of cough and difficulty breathing. The nurse assesses the client and notes decreased breath sounds in the right lower lobe, crackles in the right middle lobe, and exaggerated breath sounds on the left side. The client is most likely exhibiting symptoms of:
1. Pneumonia.
2. Cardiac tamponade.
3. Pulmonary edema.
4. Pleural friction rub.

453. The client who is 6 weeks pregnant comes to the clinic for her first prenatal visit. In doing health teaching, the nurse tells the client that each prenatal visit will include:
1. Cervical dilation, weight gain, and fundal height.
2. Blood pressure, weight gain, and fundal height.
3. Blood pressure, fundal height, and cervical dilation.
4. Blood pressure, weight gain, and measurement of the pelvic diameter.

454. The heart rate alarm for the client admitted for acute myocardial infarction (MI) rings suddenly at the nurses' station. The heart rate is 168 according to the monitor. What action should the nurse take *first*?
1. Monitor the EKG to determine if the rhythm is atrial fibrillation.
2. Assess the client's blood pressure and level of consciousness.
3. Notify the physician STAT of the rapid heart rate and obtain an order for a 12-lead EKG.
4. Check the client's recent potassium and magnesium levels.

455. The staff nurse on a pediatric unit prepares to admit a 2-year-old toddler for chelation therapy to treat long-term lead ingestion. The most necessary piece of equipment or article that the staff nurse will place at the bedside of the toddler is:
1. An IV pole.
2. An intake and output (I&O) form.

3. An oral airway.
4. An age-appropriate pain assessment scale.

456. A client with sepsis is to receive an aminoglycoside antibiotic (Vancomycin) 1 g IV every 24 hours. Which lab value is most important for the nurse to monitor for adverse/toxic effect of this drug?
1. Serum creatinine.
2. Serum amylase.
3. Serum troponin.
4. Serum white blood cell (WBC) count.

457. A 4-year-old child is hospitalized on the pediatric unit with nephrotic syndrome. Which food item ordered for the child by the child's mother indicates the need for further dietary teaching on the staff nurse's part?
1. A scrambled egg.
2. A glass of milk.
3. A peanut butter and jelly sandwich.
4. A slice of melon.

458. A client is 6 weeks pregnant. During her first prenatal visit, she tells the nurse she was on vacation when she got pregnant, and she consumed 4 alcohol drinks per day for a 1-week period. The teaching plan for the client is influenced by the knowledge that excessive alcohol consumption during pregnancy can lead to:
1. Anomalies in the fetus including craniofacial and limb defects.
2. Macrosomia and polyhydramnios.
3. Hydrops and fetal erythrocyte destruction.
4. Hydrocephalus and spina bifida.

459. A 70-year-old client with a history of smoking for 40 years is intubated and on a mechanical ventilator following an extensive bowel resection for a perforated bowel. Blood cultures indicate gram negative sepsis. For 3 hours after surgery there have been increased crackles in both lungs, FiO_2 has been increased from 50% to 80% to keep the PaO_2 at 70%. The recent chest x-ray shows bilateral patchy infiltrates throughout both lung fields. These changes are most consistent with the development of:
1. Pulmonary embolism.
2. Chronic obstructive pulmonary disease (COPD).
3. Acute respiratory distress syndrome (ARDS).
4. Pneumothorax.

460. In caring for a client with anorexia nervosa, for which electrolyte imbalances should the nurse be alert?
1. Hyperkalemia, hypermagnesium, hypernatremia.
2. Hyperkalemia, hyponatremia, increased magnesium.
3. Hypokalemia, hyponatremia, hypermagnesium.
4. Hypokalemia, hyponatremia, decreased magnesium.

461. A client at 37 weeks' gestation is admitted to the labor and delivery unit with uterine contractions. On admission, the client states she has had a previous cesarean section for breech position. Which assessment should the nurse do *first*?
1. Measure fundal height and cervical dilation.
2. Review history for type of previous cesarean section.
3. Obtain urine specimen and check cervical dilation.
4. Perform Leopold's maneuvers and obtain vital signs.

462. A 5-year-old child who was hospitalized for recurrence of nephrotic syndrome is being discharged on steroids from the pediatric unit. The nurse's *priority* for at-home-care teaching is:
1. Compliance with a low sodium diet.
2. The appetite stimulant effects of the steroids.
3. Monitoring the weight on a weekly basis.
4. Updating immunizations.

463. The client who was admitted for multiple fractures of the right femur and right arm following a mountain climbing accident suddenly becomes very anxious and complains of difficulty breathing and sharp chest pain on inspiration.

Assessment findings include: rapid and shallow respirations, tachycardia and crackles with a pleural rub in the left lung, and a drop in blood pressure to 90/45. The nurse knows that these subjective and objective assessment data are most consistent with:
1. Cardiac tamponade.
2. Pulmonary emboli.
3. Pneumothorax.
4. Pulmonary edema.

464. The client is admitted for heart failure. The nurse gives furosemide (Lasix) 40 mg via IV push. Two hours later the nurse notes frequent preventricular complexes (PVCs) on the monitor. The most appropriate lab test to determine the cause would be:
1. Serum potassium.
2. Serum creatinine.
3. Troponin.
4. WBC.

465. Polypharmacy and inappropriate dosing are major issues for elders. The four clients in room 333 talk about taking medications at home. About which client would the nurse be least concerned?
1. "I get all my medications at Joe's Pharmacy."
2. "My friend is *so* thoughtful; she gave me some of her 'water pills' when I ran out and couldn't get to the store."
3. "I sometimes forget which medication was ordered to be taken at which time."
4. "My sight is getting worse so it's hard to read what the bottles say."

466. A 16-year-old adolescent boy was diagnosed with cystic fibrosis 14 years ago but has managed the disease well. The nurse prepares to update the adolescent's understanding of the disease. What new information based on the adolescent's developmental milestone should the nurse place greatest emphasis?
1. The probable onset of diabetes mellitus.
2. Quality of life and end-of-life issues.
3. Lung transplantation.
4. Sexuality.

467. Which client is most at risk for a puerperal infection?
1. The client who had ruptured membranes for more than 24 hours prior to delivery.
2. The client who had a prolonged latent phase of labor.
3. The client who had two vaginal exams before delivery.
4. The client who had a first degree perineal laceration.

468. When giving medications to older adults the nurse knows that medication dosages should generally be:
1. One-half to two-thirds of the dose used for younger people.
2. The same as used for younger people.
3. One-third to one-half of the dose used for younger people.
4. Three-fourths of the dose used for younger people.

469. When giving medications to older adults, which response should the nurse anticipate?
1. Self-maintenance problems may result.
2. Side effects are similar to those seen in younger clients.
3. Mental changes are unlikely to occur.
4. Therapeutic effects are predictable.

470. A client who is psychotic has just seriously cut his throat with a plastic knife after hearing voices telling him to kill himself in this fashion. Which short-term goal would the nurse consider the *priority* at this time?
1. The client will not harm self.
2. The client will be free of auditory hallucinations.
3. The physical condition will stabilize.
4. The client will identify new coping strategies.

471. The nurse knows that the greatest risk for falls in the client who is elderly will be associated with a client who:
1. Has frequent drop attacks.
2. Takes medications to control postural HTN.
3. Has mild cognitive impairment.
4. Continues to drink one glass of wine per day.

472. When teaching older adult clients about falls, which recommendation demonstrates the nurse's understanding about the greatest risk?
1. "Be sure to pay close attention when you are walking on uneven pavement."
2. "You are most likely to fall while taking a shower."
3. "You are most likely to fall when you are getting up or down from the toilet or bed."
4. "You are most likely to fall because of your throw rugs."

473. A client is a gravida 1 para 0 at 42 weeks' gestation. The nurse knows that the client and her fetus are most at risk for:
1. Oligohydramnios, meconium aspiration, and macrosomia.
2. Polyhydramnios, meconium aspiration, and fetal demise.
3. Umbilical cord compression, precipitous delivery, and meconium aspiration.
4. Placenta previa, oligohydramnios, and meconium aspiration.

474. In the first 4–6 hours after delivery of an infant, the most important nursing intervention for the new mother is:
1. Assisting the woman to begin breastfeeding, to help uterine involution.
2. Encourage parental involvement in the care of the infant, to enhance bonding.
3. Frequent assessment of the fundus, to avoid uterine atony.
4. Careful perineal care, to avoid puerperal infection.

475. A school nurse pays special attention to several students in the elementary school who have cystic fibrosis. One of the school nurse's concerns for these students is proper physical growth and development. The school nurse could best assess this by:
1. Weighing each student at the beginning and end of each semester.
2. Asking the parents to submit a weekly food intake diary.
3. Plotting each student's height and weight on a growth curve form.
4. Arranging for a dietitian to evaluate each student.

476. The mother of a 2-year-old toddler informs the nurse in the pediatrician's office that the toddler doesn't eat all of the food that the mother prepares. In order to determine the most likely cause for the toddler's behavior, which question should the nurse ask the mother?
1. "Does your toddler eat a variety of foods?"
2. "What is your toddler's usual eating pattern?"
3. "Is your toddler eating meals with the rest of the family?"
4. "What serving size do you give to your toddler?"

477. Which assessment finding would the nurse expect in an 85-year-old with pneumonia?
1. A temperature of 102°F.
2. An oral temperature of 98°–99°F.
3. Excessive sweating.
4. Increased thirst.

478. Which intervention should the nurse suggest to caregivers to help them decrease and manage caregiver burden?
1. Encourage sameness in daily routines.
2. Focus on the past.
3. Retell why they chose to become caregivers.
4. Ask for respite care when life gets hard.

479. A caregiver asks, "What can I do? I'm having difficulty caring for my husband who has Parkinson's disease." What nursing action would best support the caregiver during this final stage in caregiving?

1. Encourage attendance at a support group, and write thoughts, and feelings in a journal.
2. Provide resources to assist the caregiver to find respite care.
3. Encourage the caregiver to let her husband make the decisions regarding care.
4. Provide resources to assist the caregiver to learn more about Parkinson's.

480. Which psychiatric condition would most likely have a *priority* nursing diagnosis of *fluid volume deficit*?
Select all that apply.
1. Depression.
2. Anorexia nervosa.
3. Bulimia.
4. Schizophrenia-catatonia.
5. Dementia.
6. Borderline personality disorder.

481. What is the most important nursing action when initially planning care for an elderly client with increasing symptoms of hearing loss?
1. Ask people to speak louder when near the client.
2. Check the amount of cerumen in the client's ears.
3. Ask people to speak slower and in a lower tone when near the client.
4. Get enough light on the speaker's face.

482. The pediatrician informs the mother of a child with cerebral palsy that the child is a candidate for botulinum toxin type A (Botox) therapy. The mother agrees to think it over. Later that day the mother asks the nurse, "Botox is that stuff they use to get rid of wrinkles, isn't it? What good will it do for my child who has cerebral palsy?" The nurse's best response would be to:
1. Explain that the medication does have a role in the treatment of cerebral palsy.
2. Reassure the mother that a miscommunication has occurred between the mother and the pediatrician.
3. Instruct the mother to ask the pediatrician for additional information.
4. Inform the mother that other oral muscle relaxants are also available.

483. The nurse explains to a client that presbycusis is a common reason that older persons have difficulty hearing. Hearing is made difficult because of:
1. A decreased ability to hear high-pitched sounds and sibilant consonants.
2. A decreased ability to hear low-pitched sounds and consonants.
3. An elder's disinterest in the conversation.
4. A decreased ability to discriminate words.

484. A client delivered a full-term infant yesterday. Upon assessment, the nurse notes small, reddish blisters on the client's breasts. Which nursing intervention would be the most supportive for this client?
1. Ask the mother how long she is nursing on each side. The blisters may be a result of nursing for too long.
2. Check the infant's mouth for presence of white patches of thrush causing the nipple blisters.
3. Take the mother's temperature to determine if she is developing mastitis.
4. Observe the client breastfeeding to assess the latch and position since these are common causes of blisters.

485. When deciding to institutionalize an individual, one of the primary deciding factors is the individual's ability to remain continent. Which is the least likely reason older adults are at higher risk for incontinence?
1. Tissue changes, environmental factors, and medications.
2. Decreased muscle tone, acute infections, and decreased independence.
3. Estrogen deficiency, 400-mL bladder capacity, and increased muscle tone.

4. Prostatic enlargement, decreased bladder capacity, and limited mobility

486. A client is 4 months pregnant. She has been using marijuana daily for the past 2 years. In discussing the client's drug use and fetal development, the nurse's teaching would be influenced by the knowledge that:
1. The first trimester is the most important for teratological damage to the fetus.
2. The second trimester is the most important for preventing congenital malformations.
3. After the first trimester, the placental acts as a barrier for all substances harmful to the developing fetus.
4. The second trimester is the most important for avoiding damage to the fetus caused by drug use.

487. When teaching about managing incontinence in the elderly, what should be included as the two most common reasons?
1. Age and family history.
2. Impaired thinking and immobility.
3. Family history and medications.
4. Medications and disease.

488. The client who is most likely to have improved continence with bladder training is one who:
1. Moves slowly and uses a walker.
2. Has fewer than 6 incontinence episodes in 24 hours.
3. Has a history of urge incontinence.
4. Recently had surgery to tighten the bladder.

489. A child with spastic cerebral palsy is implanted with the Baclofen pump. When educating the family about the pump, the nurse would emphasize:
1. The need to keep regularly scheduled appointments to add additional medication to the pump.
2. The need for the parents to learn to regulate the dosage of the medication delivered by the pump.
3. The child's ability to participate in age-appropriate physical activities after the implantation of the pump.
4. The signs and symptoms of pump rejection.

490. A client who is alcoholic and on day 2 of detoxification, complains of seeing bugs crawling on the bed. Which action should the nurse take *first*?
1. Place the client on seizure precautions.
2. Administer prn chlordiazepoxide (Librium) as ordered.
3. Check the client's blood pressure.
4. Initiate intravenous fluids.

491. The best ongoing nursing intervention for dealing with night incontinence in an older adult who is frail is to:
1. Limit fluid intake throughout the day.
2. Encourage client to wear paper protectors at night.
3. Limit fluids after dinner.
4. Refer client to NP/MD.

492. When teaching elder clients about improving their reading ability, the nurse needs to include suggestions for:
1. Using sunglasses that have blue or gray lenses when reading outside.
2. Buying light bulbs with three times more intensity than what was used before.
3. Using bright lighting when reading inside.
4. Buying light bulbs four times more the intensity than before.

493. Which concept guides the nurse's interventions for nighttime sleep when planning activities for the elder client with moderate cognitive impairment?
1. It is best for the client to take multiple daytime naps.
2. The nighttime sleep of elders who are cognitively impaired is commonly heavy and efficient.
3. Nurses should encourage the client to be more active before and after peak nap times.
4. It is best to plan activities to occur during the client's peak daytime nap.

494. Five weeks after her husband's sudden death, the client says she is sometimes still very tearful and sometimes just sits and stares out the window. The nurse knows that this is:
1. Unhealthy.
2. Common in the grieving process.
3. Suggestive of need for psychiatric intervention.
4. Unusual, considering that it's been quite a while since the husband's death.

495. The physician orders a bolus of magnesium sulfate for a client with a diagnosis of pregnancy-induced hypertension. The written order: "Give a 6-gram loading dose over a 30-minute period using an IV infusion pump." There are 40 g in 1000 mL of lactated Ringer's solution.
Fill in the blanks.
The nurse should administer _____mL of magnesium sulfate solution at a rate of _____ mL/hr via IV pump.

496. The client has been restrained per order to ensure that the IV and NG tubes do not get pulled out. The nurse's greatest concern with the older adult who is restrained is
1. Increased agitation.
2. Bone loss.
3. Physical injury.
4. Risk for falls.

497. A nurse must report neglect and abuse when:
1. A high index of suspicion of abuse exists.
2. Abuse is described by a client.
3. Signs of abuse are observed.
4. Physical symptoms are seen.

498. An 11-year-old child with long-term diabetes mellitus (type 1) receives an insulin pump. The child tells the nurse, "I'm so mad!! I love the pump. Why didn't I get one a long time ago?" The nurse's best response would be:
1. "You weren't on the type of insulin that the pump is able to deliver."
2. "You were well maintained on oral hypoglycemic agents and the pump wasn't necessary."
3. "You weren't able to do the necessary math that having the pump requires."
4. "You were too young to know what to do when the pump's alarm system would have activated."

499. A client with acute heart failure is receiving digoxin and furosemide. What is the *best* indicator that this regimen is effective in removing excess fluid?
1. Decreased weight
2. Therapeutic digoxin level.
3. Decreased swelling of the ankles.
4. Pulse rate decreases to 84.

500. A client with anorexia nervosa is admitted with a nursing diagnosis of *altered nutrition, less than body requirements.* For which physiological symptom(s) should the nurse be alert?
1. T-wave inversion reading on the electrocardiogram (EKG).
2. Hyperglycemia and anemia
3. Feelings of dread regarding weight gain.
4. Metabolic acidosis.

Answers/Rationales/Tips

1. **(3) It is appropriate to use conservative measures first, such as frequent checks and reorientation, moving the client closer to the nurse's station, or bed alarms before resorting to restraints. Answer 1** is incorrect because the nurse should apply a restraint only as a last resort, to keep the client from injuring himself, and should notify the physician immediately if restraints are applied. **Answer 2** is incorrect because more conservative measures such as placing the call light within easy reach, frequently reorienting the client, and placing the client

near the nurse's station are appropriate, unless it is determined through assessment that conservative measures are inadequate. **Answer 4** is incorrect because the nurse should apply a restraint only as a last resort, to keep the client from injuring himself. In addition, it is probably safe to assume that a client who is newly postoperative is not ready yet to sit up in a wheelchair for an indeterminate length of time.

TEST-TAKING TIP—Notice that the question asks for the nurse's *best* action. Eliminate **Answers 1** and **4** because they involve the immediate use of restraints, rather than assessment and conservative measures. **Answers 2** and **3** are both potentially correct; however, **Answer 2** involves significantly increased costs and is not warranted in this situation.
IMP, APP, 1, M/S: Postop, SECE, Safety and Infection Control

2. **(1) People who are homeless are at high risk for TB due to their lack of access to the health-care system and the difficulty health-care providers have in monitoring treatment. In addition, foreign-born individuals particularly from Southeast Asia and Haiti, older adults, all socioeconomically disadvantaged and medically underserved populations, and individuals in prisons and nursing homes are at risk.** **Answer 2** is incorrect because young people with asthma are not necessarily at high risk for TB. **Answer 3** is incorrect because people immigrating from Russia and Europe are not necessarily at high risk for TB. **Answer 4** is incorrect because this person does not fit into a high-risk group.

TEST-TAKING TIP—To answer this question, it is helpful to evaluate each individual's risk for TB according to the known high-risk categories. In this case, it is *not* gender, race, or occupation.
AN, ANL, 1, M/S: CD, HPM, Health Promotion and Maintenance

3. **(3) The warmth of the water will reduce the morning stiffness of the joints and thus increase mobility. Answer 1** is incorrect because this action could contribute to the child being at *risk for injury* due to the irritating nature on the gastrointestinal tract by the medications taken to treat juvenile rheumatoid arthritis. **Answer 2** is incorrect because this action, while correct in itself, correlates with reducing the *risk for injury* rather than *activity intolerance.* Increasing fluid will decrease the risk for the formation of renal calculi brought about by immobility. **Answer 4** is incorrect because this action would contribute to the child being at *risk for injury.* Activities of daily living (ADLs) should be temporarily discontinued in the presence of fatigue and persistent pain.

TEST-TAKING TIP—Look for similarities in responses. Three of the four responses dealt with preventing *injury.*
EV, ANL, 3, PEDS, PhI, Basic Care and Comfort

4. **(4) The closing of the mitral and tricuspid valves, which constitute the S_1 sound, is best heard at the fifth intercostal space, left sternal border. Answer 1** is incorrect because

KEY TO CODES FOLLOWING RATIONALES:

Nursing process: **AS,** assessment; **AN,** analysis; **PL,** plan; **IMP,** implementation; **EV,** evaluation. *Cognitive level:* **KNOW,** knowledge; **COM,** comprehension; **APP,** application; **ANL,** analysis. *Category of human function:* **1,** protective; **2,** sensory-perceptual; **3,** comfort, rest, activity, and mobility; **4,** nutrition; **5,** growth and development; **6,** fluid-gas transport; **7,** psychosocial-cultural; **8,** elimination. *Client need:* **SECE,** safe, effective care environment; **HPM,** health promotion/maintenance; **PsI,** psychosocial integrity; **PhI,** physiological integrity. (Client subneed appears after Client need code.) See appendices for full explanation.

normal heart sounds, S_1 and S_2, are best heard using the *diaphragm* of the stethoscope. The bell is used when auscultating for extra heart sounds and murmurs. **Answer 2** is incorrect because right side-lying is not an appropriate position for auscultating heart sounds. **Answer 3** is incorrect because the *second* heart sound, S_2, is best heard at the second intercostal space, right sternal border.

TEST-TAKING TIP—To answer this question, it is helpful to visualize chest anatomy and the landmarks for listening at the aortic, pulmonic, mitral, and tricuspid areas.
IMP, APP, 6, M/S: Cardiac, HPM, Health Promotion and Maintenance

5. **(2) Urinary tract infections cause *all* of the symptoms listed.** **Answer 1** is incorrect because kidney stones cause severe back pain, but do *not* cause uterine cramping or dysuria. **Answer 3** is incorrect because pre-term labor is characterized by uterine contractions and backache, but *not* dysuria. **Answer 4** is incorrect because cervical incompetence does *not* have any of the symptoms listed. It is characterized by *painless* cervical dilation.

TEST-TAKING TIP—Turn each symptom into true-false alternatives; first, think of each condition. Does each individual symptom fit the condition? If a symptom is not part of that condition, eliminate the answer.
AN, ANL, 8, Maternity, PhI, Reduction of Risk Potential

6. **(3) It is appropriate to compare apical and radial pulses when an irregular rhythm is detected to determine if there is a pulse deficit.** **Answer 1** is incorrect because there is *no apparent emergency* in this situation. The nurse should continue with the assessment. **Answer 2** is incorrect at this time. Auscultating heart sounds while the client is lying on the left side often provides useful information about *extra* heart sounds, but will not provide useful information about the *irregularity*. **Answer 4** is incorrect because the type of irregularity is unknown and it would be premature to treat until more data are gathered.

TEST-TAKING TIP—There is nothing in the scenario to indicate an emergency; many heart rhythm irregularities are non-life threatening. Therefore, **Answers 1** and **4** can be eliminated. **Answers 2** and **3** are both potentially correct; however, only **Answer 3** will provide information specifically about the irregularity.
IMP, APP, 6, M/S: Cardiac, PhI, Reduction of Risk Potential

7. **(1) A 24-month-old child is in the developmental stage of autonomy and needs to "taste, hold and feel" in order to comprehend. Also, the barium enema will involve "air being blown through a tube" and will realistically prepare the child for the procedure.** **Answer 2** is incorrect because a 24-month-old child could not comprehend and then correlate the picture with the procedure. **Answer 3** is incorrect because a 24-month-old child lacks the attention span to listen to and then comprehend this type of information. **Answer 4** is incorrect because a 24-month-old child lacks the abstract reasoning ability to mentally picture objects.

TEST-TAKING TIP—Knowing the developmental milestone of autonomy for a 24-month-old child is the key to answering this question correctly.
IMP, APP, 5, PEDS, HPM , Health Promotion and Maintenance

8. **(3) Decreased glomerular filtration is a consequence of aging; therefore, anesthetic and postoperative medications will take longer to clear.** **Answer 1** is incorrect because arterial elasticity decreases with age, predisposing the client to *hyper*tension, rather than hypotension. **Answer 2** is incorrect because aging

skin has less subcutaneous tissue and is more fragile, which puts the client at risk for skin tears and pressure ulcers. Frequent repositioning is important. **Answer 4** is incorrect because it is inappropriate to apply restraints before the client's behavior warrants it.

TEST-TAKING TIP—Eliminate **Answers 1, 2,** and **4** because they are *theoretically* wrong. **Answer 3** represents a correct nursing intervention.
PL, APP, 1, M/S: Postop, PhI, Reduction of Risk Potential

9. **(3) The infant is displaying symptoms of hypoglycemia. A heel stick glucose level will confirm that the symptoms are caused by low blood sugar.** **Answer 1** is incorrect because the symptoms are *not* primarily caused by discomfort. The symptoms are most consistent with hypoglycemia. Lethargy and tremors are not indicative of infant discomfort. **Answer 2** is incorrect because tactile stimulation will cause the infant *additional* stress, utilizing more glucose reserves. **Answer 4** is incorrect because this action would *not be the first* action taken by the nurse. The question asks about prioritizing nursing actions.

TEST-TAKING TIP—The key to this question is to select the option the nurse would do first.
IMP, ANL, 4, Newborn, PhI, Physiological Adaptation

10. **(4) The registered nurse needs to fully assess and document the client's mental status and the health teaching that was performed at the time of discharge.** **Answer 1** is incorrect because the nurse does not make assignments to the physician. **Answer 2** is incorrect because a Licensed Vocational/Practical Nurse (LVN/LPN) cannot do assessments or discharge planning. **Answer 3** is incorrect because a certified nursing assistant cannot do assessments or discharge planning.

TEST-TAKING TIP—Do not delegate functions of *assessment* to an LVN or CNA. Do not "pass the buck" to the physician.
AS, APP, 7, Psych, SECE, Management of Care

11. **(3) Although immunosuppression is an adverse effect of long-term steroid usage, measures such as handwashing and staying away from others who are ill, can prevent infection from occurring.** **Answer 1** is incorrect because hyperglycemia is an unpreventable adverse effect of long-term steroid usage. For this reason, insulin therapy is often initiated with high dose, long-term steroid usage. **Answer 2** is incorrect because hirsutism (excessive hair growth) is an unpreventable adverse effect of long-term steroid usage. Usually, upon discontinuance of the steroid, this problem resolves independently. **Answer 4** is incorrect because delay in linear growth is an unpreventable adverse effect of long-term steroid usage. Usually, upon discontinuance of the steroid, this problem will resolve, although sometimes the child does not achieve full growth potential following discontinuance of the steroid.

TEST-TAKING TIP—Only one of the responses can be resolved by an independent nursing intervention. Select that response.
IMP, ANL, 1, PEDS, PhI, Pharmacological and Parenteral Therapies

12. **(2) The anterior chest, below the clavicle, is the preferred site for checking skin turgor in adults because it is less subject to deterioration of connective tissue.** **Answer 1** is incorrect because the dorsal aspect of the forearm may show signs of skin tenting simply as a result of *aging*. **Answer 3** is incorrect because the back of the hand may show signs of skin tenting simply as a result of *aging*. **Answer 4** is incorrect because the abdomen is an appropriate place to check skin turgor in *babies*, not adults.

TEST-TAKING TIP—Notice that the question asks about the *best* place to assess for dehydration in *older* adults. The dorsal surfaces of the hand and forearm can often be used to check skin turgor in adults; however older adults often exhibit skin tenting on these sites because of the loss of elasticity that occurs with *aging* and *not* from dehydration; therefore, **Answer 2** is the *best* choice.
AS, APP, 5, M/S: GI, HPM, Health Promotion and Maintenance

13. **(4) Diminished peripheral vascularity in the aging client often results in chilling easily and calls for providing warmth. Answer 1** is incorrect because aging results in decreased capacity to adapt to darkness; the aging adult needs *more light*, not less. **Answer 2** is incorrect because the exam should be paced to accommodate the possible *slowed* pace of the aging client. **Answer 3** is incorrect because the aging client *may not* be hard of hearing, although loss of hearing is common. It is more appropriate to speak clearly and directly to clients to determine if they are hard of hearing, rather than assuming they are hard of hearing.

TEST-TAKING TIP—Answering this question requires knowledge of the common consequences of aging that affect vision, cognitive abilities, hearing, and the peripheral vascular system. Focus on the 2 choices that relate to the physical environment (**Answers 1** and **4**) and select the answer that prevents a problem (chilling).
PL, APP, 5, M/S: Geriatrics, HPM, Health Promotion and Maintenance

14. **(4) All these treatments are important in managing clients with PIH. Modified bedrest increases the perfusion to the placenta and decreases some of the edema. Strict intake and output is important because decreasing output is indicative of worsening PIH; and magnesium sulfate is used to prevent the complication of seizures in clients with PIH. Answer 1** is incorrect because complete bedrest can lead to life-threatening thrombophlebitis. **Answer 2** is incorrect because a limited salt diet has not been shown to decrease the severity of PIH and the associated edema. **Answer 3** is incorrect because increased protein in the diet has not been shown to be an effective treatment in clients with PIH.

TEST-TAKING TIP—Bedrest is indicated in clients with PIH, but *complete* bedrest can lead to complications; therefore eliminate **Answer 1**. Eliminate **Answer 3** because magnesium sulfate is used, *not* Valium. **Select Answer 4** because of *strict* I&O.
PL, APP, 1, Maternity, PhI, Reduction of Risk Potential

15. **(3) Retinal hemorrhage is often associated with hypertension, and alerts the health-care provider to assess the client further. Answer 1** is incorrect because retinal hemorrhage is not associated with glaucoma. **Answer 2** is incorrect because retinal hemorrhage is not associated with impairment of cranial nerve III. **Answer 4** is incorrect because corrective lenses would not correct a problem of retinal hemorrhage.

TEST-TAKING TIP—Consider the nature of hypertension: it is a disease affecting arteries, including retinal arteries. Choose the answer that is different than the others: 3 answers (**Answers 1, 2,** and **4**) focus specifically on the eyes, whereas **Answer 3** focuses on a broader, systemic cause.
AN, ANL, 6, M/S: Eye, HPM, Health Promotion and Maintenance

16. **(1) Drug-exposed infants need the security of being tightly wrapped. Infants experiencing drug withdrawal are very irritable, hard to comfort, and hypersensitive to lights, sounds** and tactile sensations like air, water or cloth on their skin. For infants who may be opiate-addicted, tight swaddling keeps them from shaking. **Answer 2** is incorrect because overstimulation can lead to complications, such as apnea and oxygen desaturation; it does *not* enhance development. **Answer 3** is incorrect because the drug-exposed infant needs to be secure, and loose wrap will not be effective for the infant's needs. **Answer 4** is incorrect because frequent feeding require additional handling of the infant, causing *overstimulation.*

TEST-TAKING TIP—Look at the wording of the question. Does stimulation enhance development? Eliminate that answer and concentrate on the other options. When there are two contradictory options, focus on those: tight swaddling or loose wrapping?
PL, APP, 5, Newborn, HPM, Health Promotion and Maintenance

17. **(3) Bowling does generate enough activity to stimulate the desired lung expansion in a child with asthma. Bowling alleys are now smoke-free areas and thus safe for the child with asthma. Answer 1** is incorrect because lawn croquet is played outdoors on the grass. Triggers in the air and from the grass could initiate an asthmatic episode. **Answer 2** is incorrect because playing ping-pong does not generate enough activity to stimulate the desired lung expansion in a child with asthma. **Answer 4** is incorrect because checkers is a quiet, sedentary activity and does not generate enough activity to stimulate the desired lung expansion in a child with asthma.

TEST-TAKING TIP—When all of the answers are developmentally appropriate for the age of the child, look for the one answer that is specific to some aspect of the disease. In this case, it is "therapeutic" activity in relation to asthma.
IMP, APP, 3, PEDS, HPM, Health Promotion and Maintenance

18. **(2) Decreased central venous pressure indicates *decreased* fluid in the vascular space, one of the goals of treatment for this client. Answer 1** is incorrect because increased central venous pressure indicates increased fluid in the vascular space, which is *not* the desired goal. **Answer 3** is incorrect because no change in central venous pressure indicates *no change* in vascular fluid volume. **Answer 4** is incorrect because, along with other measures, central venous pressure is an accepted indicator of vascular fluid status.

TEST-TAKING TIP—Answering this question correctly requires knowledge of fluid dynamics. Focus on 2 options that are opposites: "increases" (**Answer 1**), and "decreases" (**Answer 2**). Pulmonary edema and congestive heart failure are generally accompanied by increased pressure in the right side of the heart. If one of the goals of treatment is to *reduce* this pressure, then the only acceptable answer is the one that indicates a *decreased* central venous pressure.
EV, ANL, 6, M/S: Cardiopulmonary, PhI, Physiological Adaptation

19. **(4) Loss of circulating volume from the puncture site or into tissues surrounding the site can result in decreased blood pressure. Answer 1** is incorrect because absent distal pulses indicate a blockage in the artery, but will not necessarily be accompanied by decreased blood pressure. **Answer 2** is incorrect because increased pain is more likely to result in *increased* blood pressure. **Answer 3** is incorrect because nausea is more likely to result in *increased* blood pressure.

TEST-TAKING TIP—All of the answers are potential complications, but **Answer 4** is the only one associated with decreased blood pressure.
AN, ANL, 7, M/S: Cardiac, PhI, Reduction of Risk Potential

20. **(2) At least every 2 hours, to allow for activites of daily living for a client who may cause harm to self or others (or in a psychiatric emergency).**

> **TEST-TAKING TIP**—It is important to use restraints only in an emergency for a limited time (not longer than 24 hours) for the limited purpose of protecting the client from injury. Check frequently to ensure that there is no circulatory impairment. Remove restraints at the first opportunity.
> **IMP, COM, 7, Psych, SECE, Management of Care**

21. **(2) A side effect of steroids is to reduce normal flora which predisposes the child to opportunistic infections. This is true no matter what route the steroid is administered by. A quick "swish and spit" (AKA "S&S") after each inhalation will reduce the chance of this happening by removing the steroid residual from the mouth.** Answer 1 is incorrect because, while teaching handwashing is always an appropriate intervention, it is *not* the priority intervention. **Answer 3** is incorrect because it is unlikely that the child would have access to mouthwash after each inhalation nor is the child likely to comply. School-age children want to be "just like" their peers and this activity would make them "different." A quick gargle with water is less likely to set them apart from their peers. Mouthwash is also an unnecessary expense when water is just as effective. **Answer 4** is incorrect because sucking on hard candy will promote the formation of dental caries.

> **TEST-TAKING TIP**—Know the side effects of the medication and correlate them with the desired outcome of the nurse's teaching.
> **IMP, ANL, 1, PEDS, PhI, Pharmacological and Parenteral Therapies**

22. **(1) A major artery, usually the femoral artery, is punctured to perform this procedure; bleeding and thrombosis are 2 of the major risk factors for cardiac catheterization.** Answer 2 is incorrect because *IV fluid* is administered to the client during the procedure, the client is generally allowed *to eat* after the procedure, and *PO fluids are encouraged* to flush the dye out of the client's system. **Answer 3** is incorrect because vomiting is *not* a common reaction to cardiac catheterization; and, if it occurs, can be relieved with adequate fluid and antiemetics. **Answer 4** is incorrect because body image disturbance is *not* generally associated with cardiac catheterization.

> **TEST-TAKING TIP**—Focus on the option that is most critical, or potentially life-threatening: bleeding and thrombosis (**Answer 1**). Although fluid imbalance due to the diuretic action of the dye that is used during the procedure (**Answer 2**), and nausea and vomiting occasionally occur (**Answer 3**), neither of these conditions is immediately life-threatening.
> **AN, ANL, 6, M/S: Cardiac, PhI, Reduction of Risk Potential**

23. **(4) Chest heaviness is common when the magnesium level becomes higher than a therapeutic level.** Answer 1 is incorrect because a client with a pulmonary embolism will *also* likely experience shortness of breath and severe "stabbing-like" pain *rather than* heaviness in the chest. **Answer 2** is incorrect because a woman who is young and healthy is at lower risk for a myocardial infarction. If it was a myocardial infarction, her symptoms might *also include* diaphoresis and chest pain, *rather than* overall chest pressure. **Answer 3** is incorrect because asthma *also* results in shortness of breath and wheezing.

> **TEST-TAKING TIP**—Think about the risk factors in the client. Specifically, this is a woman who is young, pregnant, and on magnesium sulfate, without any history of previous respiratory or cardiovascular diseases. The question is looking for the side effects of too much magnesium sulfate.
> **EV, ANL, 1, Maternity, PhI, Pharmacological and Parenteral Therapies**

24. **(3) Some fluctuation in the water seal is expected after thoracic surgery. Absence of fluctuation indicates a problem.** Answer 1 is incorrect because bubbling in the suction control chamber indicates that suction is present to remove air and fluid from the chest and *is expected* after thoracic surgery. **Answer 2** is incorrect because sanguineous drainage from the chest tubes *is expected* after thoracic surgery, as long as it does not exceed 200 cc/hr. **Answer 4** is incorrect because a small amount of drainage on the dressing immediately after surgery is *not unusual*.

> **TEST-TAKING TIP**—Choose the answer that is different than the others: 3 options include bubbling or drainage: one option has neither.
> **AN, ANL, 1, M/S: Thoracic, PhI, Physiological Adaptation**

25. **(2) The menu contains no food items that are initially contraindicated for a client with an ileostomy.** Answer 1 is incorrect because whole grains and corn are considered high-fiber and may cause blockages in the client with an ileostomy. **Answer 3** is incorrect because raw vegetables are considered high-fiber and may cause blockages in the client with an ileostomy. **Answer 4** is incorrect because peas and nuts are considered high-fiber and may cause blockages in the client with an ileostomy. In addition, the garlic may produce odor that is unpleasant to the client.

> **TEST-TAKING TIP**– Notice that the question specified a client with a *new* ileostomy. Remember that the recommended diet for a client with a *new* ileostomy is low fiber; therefore nuts, whole grains, raw vegetables, peas, and corn are *initially discouraged*. The client may add these items to the diet gradually, one at a time, to determine if they are problematic.
> **EV, ANL, 4, M/S: GI, PhI, Basic Care and Comfort**

26. **(2) Passage of meconium stool reassures the nurse that the anus is patent and the GI tract is functional. This is the most important observation among the choices for this question.** Answer 1 is incorrect because a reduction in the edema of the scalp *is an expected* occurrence; while important, it is *not* the most important observation during this time period. **Answer 3** is incorrect because milia are a *normal* finding and require no intervention. **Answer 4** is incorrect because the absorption of vernix is a *normal* finding and requires no additional intervention.

> **TEST-TAKING TIP**—Think about the normal newborn assessment. Three of the options are normal findings, and do not lead to additional problems. Blockage of the intestinal tract *is* a possibility if there is no passage of meconium.
> **AS, APP, 5, Newborn, HPM, Health Promotion and Maintenance**

27. **(2) Mitral stenosis results in enlargement of the left atrium, which over time, results in increased pulmonary pressure and jugular venous distention.** Answer 1 is incorrect because dyspnea on exertion is associated with *aortic* valve abnormalities. **Answer 3** is incorrect because syncope is associated with *aortic* valve abnormalities. **Answer 4** is incorrect because angina is associated with *aortic* stenosis.

> **TEST-TAKING TIP**—It is helpful to consider the flow of blood through the heart; specifically forward flow and backward flow. The *aortic* valve is associated with abnormalities of *forward* flow: angina, syncope, and dyspnea on exertion.

On the other hand, *mitral* valve abnormalities are associated with problems of *backward* flow: orthopnea, paroxysmal nocturnal dyspnea, pulmonary edema, and jugular vein distention.
AS, APP, 6, M/S: Cardiac, PhI, Physiological Adaptation

28. **(1) The client with a pacemaker should carry an information card at all times that provides information about the type of pacemaker as well as the settings. Answer 2** is incorrect because microwave ovens are safe to use and do not present a hazard to clients with pacemakers. **Answer 3** is incorrect because the client with a pacemaker *can travel* by airplane, but should carry an identification card to document presence of the pacemaker; implanted pacemakers can set off metal detectors, although this is rare. **Answer 4** is incorrect because insertion of a permanent pacemaker is a surgical procedure, and the client *should* receive pertinent information, such as calling the physician if a fever develops or if the incision starts to drain.

TEST-TAKING TIP—**Answer 1** is the only theoretically correct answer. **Answers 2** and **3** represent common misconceptions about implanted pacemakers, and **Answer 4** indicates that the client received incomplete discharge teaching; the client should also notify the physician about drainage or bleeding from the insertion site, or presence of a fever.
EV, ANL, 1, M/S: Cardiac, HPM, Health Promotion and Maintenance

29. **(4) The adolescent is unlikely to become more compliant with his medical regime with less supervision and structure. The parents must remain vigilant and in control until the adolescent demonstrates positive behaviors regarding the management of his hemophilia. In matters of health and safety, the parents must always have the final "say" regardless of the child's/adolescent's age. Answer 1** is incorrect because rejoining the hemophilia support group is a positive coping strategy on the parents' part. **Answer 2** is incorrect because enlisting the assistance and support of family members is a positive coping strategy on the parents' part. **Answer 3** is incorrect because requesting assistance from another adult, whom the adolescent likes and might listen to, is a positive coping strategy on the parents' part.

TEST-TAKING TIP—Key words in the stem: "continued coping difficulties."
EV, ANL, 7, PEDS, PsI, Psychosocial Integrity

30. **(2) The staff person on a psychiatric unit needs to maintain confidentiality of the client's admission. Answer 1** is incorrect because the staff person *should not* identify that a client has been admitted to a psychiatric unit. **Answer 3** is incorrect because this statement by a staff person *is* correct. **Answer 4** is incorrect because this *is* an appropriate alternative to helping the caller make contact with the client while maintaining the client's confidentiality. The client has the right to notify others of admission to the hospital, and the caller may be an important support person for the client.

TEST-TAKING TIP—Look for the answer that is different from the others. Read the question carefully or reword the stem; this question asks for the *wrong* response from the staff person.
AS, ANL, 1, Psych, SECE, Management of Care

31. **(2) Exposure to multiple sexual partners increases the chance of contracting genital warts, which is a high-risk factor for the development of cervical cancer. Answer 1** is incorrect because her risk for cervical cancer is no greater than average. She is at slightly higher risk for *breast* cancer,

having never had any children. **Answer 3** is incorrect because she is also an average risk for cervical cancer. None of her stated risk factors increases the chance of cervical cancer. Early onset of menarche has been associated with a higher risk of *breast* cancer. **Answer 4** is incorrect because this client has *no* risk factors that are associated with an increased risk of cervical cancer.

TEST-TAKING TIP—Review risk factors for development of cancer. Think which factors are associated with increased risk of cervical cancer. Read carefully and don't be distracted by **Answers 1** and **3**, where the client has risk factors for *breast* cancer.
AN, APP, 5, Women's Health, HPM, Health Promotion and Maintenance

32. **(4) The characteristics described are consistent with sinus arrhythmia, a common and non-life-threatening arrhythmia. Answer 1** is incorrect because there is *no emergency* in this situation. The characteristics described are consistent with a sinus arrhythmia. **Answer 2** is incorrect because there is *no emergency* in this situation. The characteristics described are consistent with sinus arrhythmia. **Answer 3** is incorrect because the characteristics described do not warrant cardiac catheterization.

TEST-TAKING TIP—Notice that there is a pattern of responses to this question and focus on the option that does not fit the pattern. Three of the options (**Answers 1, 2,** and **3**), call for urgent action while **Answer 4** does not.
AN, ANL, 6, M/S: Cardiac, HPM, Health Promotion and Maintenance

33. **(2) The nurse should *first assess* the client to determine if an emergency actually exists, or if one of the EKG leads has simply fallen off. Answer 1** is incorrect because the nurse should *first assess* the client before instituting emergency procedures. **Answer 3** is incorrect because the nurse has no pertinent data regarding the client's actual condition at this time. **Answer 4** is incorrect because *checking for responsiveness* is always the first step in CPR.

TEST-TAKING TIP—Notice that the question asks what the nurse should do *first*. Recall that *assessment* is the first step of the nursing process.
IMP, APP, 6, M/S: Cardiac, PhI, Reduction of Risk Potential

34. **(3) It addresses the client's airway, which is always the first step in a primary survey. Answer 1** is incorrect as a first action, although it is a necessary part of the client assessment. **Answer 2** is incorrect as a first action, although it will be necessary *later* in the client assessment. **Answer 4** is incorrect as a first action, although it is a necessary part of the client assessment.

TEST-TAKING TIP—When performing a primary survey of almost any client, the first priority is airway, then breathing, then circulation (just as is taught in basic cardiopulmonary resuscitation). While all of the answers are important to assess, **Answer 3** is the only one that addresses airway.
IMP, APP, 1, M/S: Trauma, PhI, Reduction of Risk Potential

35. **(4) This child is in the stage of industry and would be eager to learn by doing. An activity book that contains pictures of asthma triggers for the child to color would be both accepted by the child as well as developmentally appropriate. Answer 1** is incorrect because a 6-year-old child would not have the attention span necessary to watch and comprehend such technical information. **Answer 2** is incorrect

because a 6-year-old child would not have the attention span necessary to listen to and comprehend such technical information. **Answer 3** is incorrect because this type of activity might unnecessarily expose the child to asthma triggers.

TEST-TAKING TIP—Knowing the developmental milestone of industry for a 6-year-old child is the key to answering this question correctly.
IMP, APP, 5, PEDS, HPM, Health Promotion and Maintenance

36. **(4) A soft, puffing sound indicates swallowing, a sign of good breastfeeding. Answer 1** is incorrect because it indicates a poor latch; a newborn should *not* make any smacking or sucking noises while breastfeeding. **Answer 2** is incorrect because the mother should *not* pull the infant off the nipple. She should first break the suction, then remove the nipple; it is not an indicator of the quality of the newborn feeding. **Answer 3** is incorrect because the newborn's nose and chin should *touch* the mother's breast, but n*ot* completely cover the face, which may interfere with the respirations of the newborn.

TEST-TAKING TIP—Look at the words "completely covers" in **Answer 3**, and think about proper positioning and latching for breastfeeding. Visualize what the infant looks like while properly positioned and latched on to the breast.
EV, APP, 4, Newborn, HPM, Health Promotion and Maintenance

37. **(4) An IV of normal saline is priority treatment for a client in diabetic ketoacidosis. Answer 1** is incorrect because lung sounds are *not* an immediate need, although they will be important later in the client's treatment. **Answer 2** is incorrect because, while monitoring the client's heart rhythm is important, a 12-lead ECG is *not* a first priority; managing the ketoacidosis is. **Answer 3** is incorrect because sodium bicarbonate would *not* be administered until the client's actual blood pH was determined.

TEST-TAKING TIP—Although medical diagnosis is not part of the nurse's scope of practice, a client in diabetic ketoacidosis should be obvious. Notice that the question asks what the nurse should do *immediately*. While all of the options involve potential nursing actions for this client, **Answer 4** addresses an *immediate* action.
IMP, ANL, 6, M/S: Endocrine, PhI, Pharmacological and Parenteral Therapies

38. **(4) A child with sickle cell anemia needs to consume additional fluids on a regular basis to prevent sickling episodes. This would be even more important than usual when the child is at summer camp and temperatures are usually higher in the summer, thus increasing the need for additional fluids. Answer 1** is incorrect because a child who is ill would not be allowed to participate in a camping experience. A child who has become ill while at camp would be separated from the general population of campers and sent home. **Answer 2** is incorrect because the immunization records would have been supplied to the camp nurse by the parents when applying for the child to attend camp. Delinquent immunizations would have been updated prior to accepting the child for the camping experience. **Answer 3** is incorrect because, in the interest of safety, all medications would have been turned into the camp nurse by the parents when the child was brought to camp. In a camping situation, the camp nurse would administer all medications to the child, even if the child self-medicates at home.

TEST-TAKING TIP—The key word in this question is "summer." Think "hot weather" and correlate it with fluid requirements in a child with sickle cell anemia.
IMP, ANL, 6, PEDS, PhI, Basic Care and Comfort

39. **(2) Being able to hear the client's voice indicates that the cuff on the tube is deflated, or the tube is misplaced. Answer 1** is incorrect because the client should not be able to audibly speak if the cuff on the endotracheal tube has adequately sealed the trachea, and if the tube is correctly placed just above the carina. **Answer 3** is incorrect because, in this case, the cuff *pressure* should be checked *first*, and position of the tube evaluated to determine the need for a new tube. **Answer 4** is incorrect because the client would more likely not exhibit, or have greatly diminished breath sounds on the left, if the tube had migrated to the right side of the lung.

TEST-TAKING TIP—Recalling upper respiratory anatomy is helpful to answer this question. The purpose of a cuff on a tracheal tube is to seal the trachea, so that air flows only through the tube. Therefore, no air flows past the vocal cords and the client cannot speak. Part of the nurse's responsibility for caring for a client with a tracheal airway is to monitor placement of the tube and cuff pressure.
AN, ANL, 6, M/S: Resp., PhI, Physiological Adaptation

40. **(2) It is the nurse's responsibility to complete an incident report when a medication error is made after the physician and client are notified. Answer 1** is incorrect because the client is *not* in immediate danger, and the incident report will be read by the *nurse manager* of the unit. **Answer 3** is incorrect because it is *not the next step* taken by the staff nurse and it is *not* the staff nurse's responsibility to determine if other staff are making the same medication error. If the *nurse manager* determines that it is a staff issue, then it can be discussed at the staff meeting by the manager. **Answer 4** is incorrect because it is *not appropriate* for the nurse to imply that the client had responsibility for the medication error by telling the client to be more careful. Encouraging the client to *be aware* of their medications is an important part of medication teaching, but can be done *after* the incident report is complete.

TEST-TAKING TIP—Choose the answer that is a legal priority. Avoid answers that talk down or "tell" the client.
IMP, APP, 7, Psych, SECE, Management of Care

41. **(3) Children in this age group often experience a first seizure in the presence of a high fever. Obtaining the child's temperature will provide an immediate clue as to the cause of the seizure. Answer 1** is incorrect because, while this is useful information and an important aspect of basic assessment, it will not provide a clue as to the nature of the seizure. **Answer 2** is incorrect because, while this is useful information and an important aspect of basic assessment, it will not provide a clue as to the nature of the seizure. **Answer 4** is incorrect because while, this is useful information and an important aspect of basic assessment, it will not provide a clue as to the nature of the seizure.

TEST-TAKING TIP—First onset seizures in children between 6 months and 3 years of age are usually febrile in nature.
IMP, ANL, 2, PEDS, PhI, Physiological Adaptation

42. **(4) Marking the insertion point of the tube provides a reference point for determining if the tube has moved in or out. Answer 1** is incorrect because measuring cuff pressure verifies that the cuff is inflated to the correct pressure; it gives

no information about placement of the tube. **Answer 2** is incorrect because suctioning the client does not help maintain placement of the tube. **Answer 3** is incorrect because x-raying the tube is done after initial placement of the tube, or if there is reason to suspect that the tube is misplaced.

> **TEST-TAKING TIP**—Focus on the two options that specifically address placement of the tube; **Answers 3** and **4**. Of these 2 options, **Answer 4** offers a method of checking tube placement that is simple and reliable, while **Answer 3** involves a method that is costly, impractical, and subjects the client to needless risk.
> **IMP, APP, 6, M/S: Resp., PhI, Reduction of Risk Potential**

43. **(3)** The blood gases indicate *respiratory alkalosis*, which is caused by *hyperventilation*. **Answer 1** is incorrect because the client appears to be *well oxygenated* with a Pao$_2$ of 100 and SaO$_2$ of 98%. **Answer 2** is incorrect because this would *increase* the client's *hyperventilation*. **Answer 4** is incorrect because there are *no data* to suggest that decreasing tidal volume would be a desirable action.

> **TEST-TAKING TIP**—Note: *Increase rate* (**Answer 2**) vs. *decrease rate* (**Answer 3**). Choose **Answer 3** because the client's blood gases indicate respiratory alkalosis, which is generally caused by hyperventilation. It makes sense, therefore, to reduce the client's rate of ventilations.
> **EV, ANL, 6, M/S: Resp., PhI, Physiological Adaptation**

44. **(4)** The client's status determines the nurse's next course of action: if the client is in respiratory distress, it is acceptable to provide an alternate source of oxygen, such as an Ambu-bag, until the source of the alarm is discovered and corrected. If the client is not in respiratory distress, the nurse has more time to investigate other possibilities, such as accidental tube disconnection. **Answer 1** is incorrect because lung sounds are not an immediate concern; other assessments need to be made first. **Answer 2** is incorrect because arterial blood gases would not provide information about the cause of the ventilator alarm. **Answer 3** is incorrect because, even though this may be the cause of the alarm, the client's status is most important.

> **TEST-TAKING TIP**—Focus on the option that addresses the client's immediate status (**Answer 4**). While disconnection of the tubing is a likely cause of the ventilator alarm, the nurse must act quickly if the client is in respiratory distress.
> **IMP, ANL, 6, M/S: Resp., PhI, Reduction of Risk Potential**

45. **(2)** A pregnant woman with a gonorrhea infection is at a higher risk for premature rupture of membranes, preterm labor and delivery. **Answer 1** is incorrect because all newborns are routinely given a prophylactic dose of antibiotic ointment at birth to prevent eye infections transmitted at birth. **Answer 3** is incorrect because the purpose of the test is *not to treat sexual partners*; the individuals exposed must also be tested for the presence of gonorrhea. **Answer 4** is incorrect because congenital heart defects are associated with *rubella* infection, *not* gonorrhea infection.

> **TEST-TAKING TIP**—Focus on the *woman*, not the neonate (**Answers 1** and **4**), nor partners (**Answer 3**). Think about what the question is asking. What is the purpose of having the client who is *pregnant* tested for gonorrhea? It is to prevent problems with the *pregnancy* when a *client* has an undiagnosed gonorrhea infection, including preterm labor and delivery.
> **PL, APP, 1, Maternity, HPM, Health Promotion and Maintenance**

46. **(1)** Infection with rubella during pregnancy can lead to fetal congenital anomalies, including heart defects and hearing loss. **Answer 2** is incorrect because rubella virus does *not pass* in the breastmilk. **Answer 3** is incorrect because the purpose of the vaccine is to prevent congenital *malformations*, *not* prevent *transmission* to the *newborn*. **Answer 4** is incorrect because hydrops is a result of fetal erythrocyte breakdown and anemia caused by *Rh sensitization* in utero.

> **TEST-TAKING TIP**— What is the purpose of the vaccine *after* delivery of an infant? Therefore, eliminate **Answers 2 and 3**. The purpose is prevention of the possible congenital malformations in the fetus in the *next* pregnancy. The mother also needs to be instructed to avoid pregnancy for at least 3 months after receiving the vaccine to avoid exposure of the fetus to the virus present in the vaccination.
> **PL, COM, 1, Maternity, HPM, Health Promotion and Maintenance**

47. **(1, 3, 4, 5)** **Answer 1** is correct because by raising the head of the bed, gravity helps the client swallow and helps prevent aspiration. **Answer 3** is correct because the cuff should initially be deflated to assess gag and swallowing ability. In addition, some clients find it *more difficult* to swallow with the *cuff inflated*. **Answer 4** is correct because the client's airway should be patent, and secretions removed before deflating the cuff. **Answer 5** is correct because assessing the client's gag and swallowing ability is crucial before starting the client on PO food and fluids. **Answer 2** is incorrect because there is no reason to increase the FiO$_2$. **Answer 6** is incorrect because it is not necessary to replace the tracheostomy ties before the client eats, unless they are noted to be soiled or loose.

> **TEST-TAKING TIP**—Aspiration is a major concern when a client with a tracheostomy begins to learn to take food and fluids by mouth. Nursing actions center around preventing aspiration.
> **IMP, APP, 4, M/S: Resp., PhI, Basic Care and Comfort**

48. **(2, 3, 4)** **Answer 2** is correct because a sweet, flavored beverage such as Coca Cola would camouflage the taste and odor of the medication. **Answer 3** is correct because a covered cup would camouflage the odor of the medication. **Answer 4** is correct because a drinking straw would camouflage the taste of the medication. **Answer 1** is incorrect because acetylcystein/Mucomyst has an offensive taste and odor (i.e., rotten eggs). In order to convince the preschooler to drink the medication, it would be necessary to camouflage these characteristics. Diluting the medication with water or milk would not accomplish this goal.

> **TEST-TAKING TIP**—Preschoolers are notoriously picky eaters. Eliminate **Answer 1** because it is the only option that would not cover up the taste and smell of the drug.
> **IMP, ANL, 5, PEDS, PhI, Pharmacological and Parenteral Therapies**

49. **(1, 3, 4)** **Answer 1** is correct because the kidney has been punctured with a biopsy trocar. Although some type of guided imaging is used to avoid large blood vessels, hemorrhage is a possible complication. The hematocrit is also usually monitored following a biopsy. **Answer 3** is correct because the puncture site must be observed for bleeding and the vital signs assessed. The time for bedrest may range from 4–24 hours depending on the physician. Activity should be limited for at least 24 hours after the procedure. **Answer 4** is correct because pressure must be applied to the puncture site for 20 minutes to prevent bleeding. The client may lie on a sandbag positioned against the puncture site.

Answer 2 is incorrect because fluids are *forced* to promote urination and prevent clot formation which could obstruct urination. **Answer 5** is incorrect because activity should be limited for the first 24 hours to prevent bleeding. ROM would *not* be indicated if on bedrest. **Answer 6** is incorrect because head elevation will likely make it more difficult to apply the needed pressure to the puncture site. Flat or with a pillow would be more appropriate.

> **TEST-TAKING TIP**—Think about the location and what was done—puncture → bleeding.
> **IMP, APP, 8, M/S: Renal, PhI, Reduction of Risk Potential**

50. **(1) A client who is paranoid can easily misinterpret other conversation.** **Answer 2** is incorrect because nursing stations can be loud with conversation between nurses and between nurses and other clients. **Answer 3** is incorrect because the community room is a place for conversation between and with clients and there is noise from the television which may be misinterpreted by the client. **Answer 4** is incorrect because placing two clients who are paranoid in the same room would not be therapeutic because fear is contagious.

> **TEST-TAKING TIP**—Eliminate the answers that involve other people (**Answers 2, 3,** and **4**). Choose the answer that is different from the others: "quiet" is the opposite of "noise" (**Answers 2, 3, 4**).
> **PL, APP, 7, Psych, SECE, Management of Care**

51. **(1) Antihemophilic factor is prepared from the plasma of multiple donors, and a transfusion-like reaction is always a possibility, especially with repeated administration of the medication. It is also the most immediately life-threatening of the responses and therefore the focus of the nurse's greatest concern.** **Answer 2** is incorrect because, while the factor is administered via the IV route, it is a powder in a single dose vial that is diluted with small amounts of (usually 10–30 mL) of IV fluid. Thus fluid overload is *not* a priority concern. **Answer 3** is incorrect because, while IV infiltration is always a concern, it is *not* a life-threatening event in itself. **Answer 4** is incorrect because, while contracting hepatitis and HIV from blood by-products is always a concern, it is a long-term concern related to multiple administrations of the medication. For this reason, children with hemophilia are immunized against Hepatitis B prior to starting this medication, and screened for HIV on a regular basis.

> **TEST-TAKING TIP**—A response involving an immediate life-threatening event would always take priority over other responses, which while serious in themselves, would not be immediately life-threatening.
> **AS, ANL, 1, PEDS, SECE, Safety and Infection Control**

52. **(3) The nurse should confirm that the client understands the positioning, method for sedation, and if there will a need for analgesia during the procedure.** **Answer 1** is incorrect because the procedure does not involve any dye or contrast medium that might result in an allergic reaction to iodine. A cystoscopy is a diagnostic visualization of the urinary tract. **Answer 2** is incorrect because the procedure does not involve any radiation; consequently, protection of the pelvis or groin is not needed. **Answer 4** is incorrect because the procedure does not involve any magnetic imaging where loose metal objects could cause injury if pulled into the machine.

> **TEST-TAKING TIP**—Look for patterns—choose an option that is directed at the client.
> **IMP, APP, 8, M/S: Renal, PhI, Reduction of Risk Potential**

53. **(2) A normal baseline for fetal heart rate is 120–160 bpm. A baseline of 180 is tachycardia, an indicator of possible fetal**

distress or a maternal fever. It is never a normal part of active labor to have a baseline fetal heart rate of 180 bpm. **Answer 1** is incorrect because a fetal heart rate baseline of 120 bpm is within the *normal* 120–160 bpm range. **Answer 3** is incorrect because in active labor, abrupt decreases in heart rate can be part of a *normal* heart rate pattern. **Answer 4** is incorrect because increases in the fetal heart rate are accelerations, a part of a *normal* fetal rate pattern in a fetus who is healthy.

> **TEST-TAKING TIP**— "Baseline" is the key word in the correct option. Ask "what is the normal fetal heart rate baseline?" Picture what the patterns of variable, early and late decelerations look like. Accelerations are normal and abrupt variable decelerations can be a normal part of a healthy fetal heart rate in active labor.
> **EV, APP, 6, Maternity, PhI, Reduction of Risk Potential**

54. **(1, 3, 4, 6)** **Answer 1** is correct because the bowel must be cleansed because stool could obscure the movement of the dye through the kidneys and bladder. **Answer 3** is correct because there are risks associated with the procedure, and the nurse should always verify that the physician informed the client about the procedure. **Answer 4** is correct because a metallic taste, as well as flushing and burning, can occur when the dye is injected. **Answer 6** is correct because hydration is important if the kidney is going to be able to excrete the dye. Poor renal function is a contraindication for use of the dye. **Answer 2** is incorrect because the client is NPO for several hours before the test. If mildly dehydrated, the dye will be more concentrated during the test and there will be better visualization of the kidneys and bladder. **Answer 5** is incorrect because a lead apron would prevent visualization of the area of interest.

> **TEST-TAKING TIP**—Know common diagnostic tests. Think about the desired outcome after the test.
> **IMP, APP, 8, M/S: GU, PhI, Reduction of Risk Potential**

55. **(3) The first priority is to assess the effect on an elderly client from the rapid infusion of 800 mL of fluid. The older adult is at greater risk for signs and symptoms of volume overload (shortness of breath, crackles, decreased oxygen saturation) particularly with a history of heart failure.** **Answer 1** is incorrect because the first priority is to assess the effect on an elderly client from the rapid infusion of 800 mL of fluid. The volume infused would not have been as great if the IV had infiltrated. **Answer 2** is incorrect because the first priority is to assess the effect on an elderly client from the rapid infusion of 800 mL of fluid. Using an infusion pump would have likely *prevented* this problem and should be a consideration in clients at risk for complications from sudden changes in fluid volume. **Answer 4** is incorrect because the *first priority* is to assess the *effect* on an elderly client from the rapid infusion of 800 mL of fluid. If the client does not have a history of heart failure or compromised renal function, the client will need to void.

> **TEST-TAKING TIP**—A priority question—IV access is important in the event medication would be needed to reverse the effects of rapid infusion of fluids.
> **IMP, ANL, 6, M/S: Geriatrics, PhI, Physiological Adaptation**

56. **(2, 3, 4)** **Answer 2** is correct because infants of mothers who are diabetic have a higher circulating blood glucose, which is stored as fat, causing macrosomia, increased weight at birth. **Answer 3** is correct because diabetes is a vascular disease affecting all maternal organ systems, and predisposes a client with diabetes to develop pregnancy-induced

hypertension. **Answer 4 is correct because an infant of a mother with high blood glucose due to uncontrolled diabetes voids more frequently, resulting in polyhydramnios. Answer 1** is incorrect because oligohydramnios is not associated with uncontrolled diabetes. It is associated with *maternal dehydration* and *fetal renal agenesis.* **Answer 5** is incorrect because the question asks about the *client, not the* infant. The client would have hyperglycemia, the *infant* would have hypoglycemia *after delivery.* **Answer 6** is incorrect because microcephaly is *not* a result of maternal diabetes. It is a result of *fetal alcohol syndrome.*

> **TEST-TAKING TIP**—When answering a "multiple-multiple choice" type of question, ask a separate true-false question of each possible answer. If it is true, choose the answer; if it is false, eliminate the answer.
> **AS, ANL, 1, Maternity, PhI, Physiological Adaptation**

57. **(2) The client is at risk to develop hypocalcium from accidental removal or injury to the parathyroid gland. The parathyroid hormone increases calcium absorption, leading to numbness and tingling around the mouth, as well as in toes and fingers. Answer 1** is incorrect because the client is at risk to develop *hypocalcium* from accidental removal or injury to the parathyroid gland. These signs and symptoms would be characteristic of a *sodium or potassium imbalance.* **Answer 3** is incorrect because any special diet would be to treat hypoparathyroidism and the foods would be high in *calcium* (e.g., tofu, milk, kale, and collard greens). **Answer 4** is incorrect because if the client experienced symptoms of hypoparathyroidism, the diet *would be* high in calcium-rich foods such as tofu, milk, kale, and collard greens.

> **TEST-TAKING TIP**—Think long-term complication—accidental removal of the parathyroid gland.
> **IMP, APP, 3, M/S: Endocrine, PhI, Reduction of Risk Potential**

58. **(1) Toenails may be trimmed by the client or family if the nails are soft and thin. Corners and rough edges should be gently filed. The risk of a foot infection is great in a person with diabetes and may result in an amputation. If the toenails are thick or brittle, they should be trimmed by a podiatrist. Answer 2** is incorrect because soaking the feet promotes a moist environment between the toes, which is more conducive to infection. **Answer 3** is incorrect because applying lotion between the toes promotes a moist environment between the toes, which is more conducive to infection. **Answer 4** is incorrect because calluses should be removed only by an expert in foot care. Using a razor blade will increase the risk of a cut. Healing is poor in a person with diabetes, and the cut may become infected.

> **TEST-TAKING TIP**—Look for patterns. Only one choice does not affect the skin—the first line of defense for infection.
> **IMP, COM, 1, M/S: Endocrine, HPM, Health Promotion and Maintenance**

59. **(1, 2, 3, 4)** Answer 1 is correct because, although hemophilia is a chronic condition, the child is now acutely ill due to his injuries. A child with well-managed hemophilia may have had little or no experience with trauma and emergency departments, and, thus, may need the same type and amount of reassurance that a child with a first time admission to the emergency department would warrant. Answer 2 is correct because hemophilia is a chronic condition. Children with chronic conditions tend to become "disease-wise" and are often used to being highly involved in their care. Attention must be paid to the child's feelings about being in a depend-

ent role while acutely ill and in the emergency department. Answer 3 is correct because, while the family of a child with hemophilia would undoubtedly be highly knowledgeable regarding their child's at-home medical needs, they might lack knowledge in an acute care situation and thus be anxious in this new experience. Answer 4 is correct because it is reasonable to anticipate that this child will have lost blood due to his injuries and be in need of blood replacement. The nurse assigned to care for this child would need to be able to effectively communicate to the blood bank that this child should be evaluated as a "high priority" client.

> **TEST-TAKING TIP**—It is important to remember that a child who is chronically ill can become acutely ill and vice-versa. The nurse assigned to such a child must be skilled in both areas.
> **AS, ANL, 7, PEDS, SECE, Management of Care**

60. **(3) Infants who are crawling can and will put items into their mouth, which could lead to choking or poisoning. It is the priority plan of care. Answer 1** is incorrect because 8-month-old infants are beginning to crawl and do not have the fine motor coordination to stick items into electrical sockets. It is important health teaching for the mother but is *not the priority plan* of care. **Answer 2** is incorrect because it is *not the priority* intervention for the mother and infant at this time. Providing cognitive stimuli to the infant, such as by reading frequently to the infant, is health teaching that can come *later* in the therapeutic relationship. **Answer 4** is incorrect because it is not a priority. The mother's medications can be refilled over the next few days. Assessing compliance with medication is an important intervention, but is *not* a safety priority.

> **TEST-TAKING TIP**—Think safety when the question calls for a priority or immediate response; safety first. Focus on the age-appropriate answer.
> **PL, ANL, 1, Psych, SECE, Safety**

61. **3.** This infant has an Apgar of 3. Give 1 point for heart rate, 1 point for gasping respirations, 0 points for central cyanosis, 0 points for limp muscle tone, and 1 point for a grimace with stimulation. Total score is 3 points out of a possible 10 points.

> **TEST-TAKING TIP**—*Visualize* what the described infant looks like: cyanotic, floppy, poor tone, respiratory effort, and a heart rate less than 100. This infant is depressed at birth; therefore, the Apgar score must be low. Each of the five descriptions given was a scoring parameter for the total APGAR score.
> **AN, APP, 5, Newborn, PhI, Physiological Adaptation**

62. **(2) Metoclopramide given before meals will stimulate peristalsis and reduce nausea. Answer 1** is incorrect because gastroparesis resulting in gastric emptying exists. A flat position increases the risk of aspiration when the stomach is full. **Answer 3** is incorrect because parenteral nutrition adds potential complications, and would limit the client's ability to resume as normal a life as possible. Drug therapy is a more appropriate choice. **Answer 4** is incorrect because the fullness is not related to swallowing air, but is due to delayed gastric emptying.

> **TEST-TAKING TIP**—The goal—continue oral intake and facilitate motility.
> **IMP, APP, 4, M/S: Endocrine, PhI, Basic Care and Comfort**

63. **(2, 3, 4, 5)** Answer 2 should be questioned because insulin is needed to prevent metabolism of fat and acidosis. Blood glucose must be monitored *more often.* Answer 3 should be questioned because acarbose is normally taken with food to slow absorption of glucose from the intestine. The client is

unable to retain any oral food. Urine sugar and acetone are indirect measures of blood glucose and not as accurate as a measurement of the blood glucose level. **Answer 4** should be questioned because sublingual sugar is not indicated at this point, although holding the acarbose is appropriate. **Answer 5** should be questioned because an oral antiemetic may stimulate vomiting. A suppository will likely be ordered. **Answer 1** is incorrect because the nurse *would* expect a client who has diabetes, type 1, to need some insulin even if not eating, or the body will metabolize fats and become acidotic. The dose will most likely be reduced.

> **TEST-TAKING TIP**—Anything oral would be questioned. Delaying assessment puts client at risk.
> **AN, ANL, 4, M/S: Endocrine, PhI, Reduction of Risk Potential**

64. **(4) Although many children with hemophilia do take anti-hemophilic factor on a regular basis to prevent bleeding episodes, the factor (which has a short half-life) should be taken in the *morning* so that factor levels can be highest when the child is most active and prone to injury. Answer 1** is incorrect because children with hemophilia *are* taught to avoid taking aspirin or aspirin-related/containing products due to the natural anticoagulation properties of this medication. **Answer 2** is incorrect because children with hemophilia *are* taught to take acetaminophen/Tylenol for mild to moderate pain. This medication does not interfere with coagulation. Children over 12 years of age may take up to 480 mg/dose or 4 g/24 hr so the ordered dose is safe and does not need to be questioned. **Answer 3** is incorrect because children with hemophilia *are* restricted from regular physical education classes which may involve contact sports that could cause injury and precipitate a bleeding episode. Adaptive physical education classes feature non-contact sports such as swimming and golf.

> **TEST-TAKING TIP**—The key words here are "should … question," meaning the order is not right. Also, the half-life of a medication provides a guide to the timing of the administration and number of doses of a medication.
> **EV, APP, 1, PEDS, SECE, Management of Care**

65. **(2) Diabetic retinopathy is associated with the lack of glycemic control and the development of microvascular changes. Keeping blood glucose in the normal range ($<$120 mg/dL) is important in preventing blindness. Answer 1** is incorrect because the cause of blindness is not corneal dryness, but is the result of microangiopathy and retinopathy. **Answer 3** is incorrect because no amount of beta carotene will prevent retinopathy. Only glycemic control can prevent blindness. **Answer 4** is incorrect because the blindness is related to retinal changes, not corneal opacity with cataracts. Cataracts impair vision but vision is improved with cataract removal. Blindness from diabetic retinopathy is not reversible.

> **TEST-TAKING TIP**—Think prevention, not treatment.
> **PL, APP, 2, M/S: Eye, PhI, Reduction of Risk Potential**

66. **(1) The antihemophilic factor is a prophylactic medication in mild cases of hemophilia. It can be taken at regularly scheduled intervals throughout the week, or before an anticipated increase in activity level to prevent bleeding episodes. Answer 2** is incorrect because the antihemophilic factor should be taken prophylactically or *before* the possibility that increased or strenuous exercise could lead to injury and subsequent bleeding episodes. **Answer 3** is incorrect because ice (*cold* = vasoconstriction) should immediately be applied to the joint following injury to assist in controlling the bleeding. Warmth/ heat = vasodilatation, which can prolong bleeding episodes. **Answer 4** is incorrect because *prolonged*

immobility from braces and splints can lead to permanent deformities and loss of mobility. Such devices should be worn as recommended by the pediatrician and/or physical therapist.

> **TEST-TAKING TIP**—The primary focus in caring for a child with hemophilia is to *prevent* and/or control bleeding. Select the answer that would best accomplish this goal.
> **EV, ANL, 3, PEDS, PhI, Reduction of Risk Potential**

67. **(4) Cigarette smoking causes vasoconstriction and affects an erection, which needs vasodilation for penile engorgement. Impotence occurs in 50% of men with diabetes by the age of 50. Answer 1** is incorrect because impotence in the person with diabetes can be managed with strict control of the blood sugar, maintaining the level between 90–120 mg/dL. **Answer 2** is incorrect because alcohol intake will *worsen* impotence. **Answer 3** is incorrect because pelvic floor exercises will manage incontinence, *not* impotence.

> **TEST-TAKING TIP**—Know the modifiable lifestyle choices ("avoid…") with an immediate effect.
> **IMP, APP, 5, M/S: GU, PhI, Physiological Adaptation**

68. **(2) The blood loss caused by a ruptured tubal pregnancy would cause shoulder pain, which is referred pain from the abdominal blood, as well as symptoms associated with shock, such as feeling faint. The blood would *not* be seen *vaginally*, since the site of bleeding is the fallopian tube. Answer 1** is incorrect because a client with pelvic inflammatory disease would have a abdominal pain and *fever*. She would *not* have shoulder pain or a feeling of faintness. **Answer 3** is incorrect because the client would have symptoms of *dysuria*, uterine cramping, and possible fever. Symptoms of shock would not be consistent with a urinary tract infection. **Answer 4** is incorrect because an imminent spontaneous abortion *would have* vaginal bleeding.

> **TEST-TAKING TIP**—Think about each of the symptoms and use the true-false alternative. For example, if the client has a urinary tract infection, would she have abdominal pain (maybe) and shoulder pain (probably no); if no, eliminate that alternative.
> **AN, ANL, 1, Maternity, HPM, Health Promotion and Maintenance**

69. **(4) The client needs reinforcement and positive feedback that the current diabetic management is achieving the desired goal of HgbA$_{1c}$ below 7%. Answer 1** is incorrect because the HgbA$_{1c}$ result is below 7%, which indicates glycemic control. HgbA$_{1c}$ indicates the average daily blood sugar level by showing how much sugar is attached to the hemoglobin. **Answer 2** is incorrect because the best response would be to offer positive feedback to the client. The report will eventually be placed in the client record. **Answer 3** is incorrect because meat and leafy green vegetables are high in iron; the laboratory value is not measuring hemoglobin, but rather the average daily blood sugar level.

> **TEST-TAKING TIP**—The question asks for the best action—know the desired outcome.
> **IMP, ANL, 4, M/S: Endocrine, PhI, Physiological Adaptation**

70. **(1) It is important to assess the content of the voices in order to determine if the voices are telling the client to hurt himself or another person. The question is open-ended and encourages self expression. Answer 2** is incorrect because frequency is not the priority question that needs to be asked first, and it requires a "yes/no" response. **Answer 3** is incorrect because time frame is *not* the priority question, but it is a question that can be asked *later* in the assessment. **Answer 4**

is incorrect because it is *not* a priority, and can be asked *later* in the assessment.

> **TEST-TAKING TIP**—Think safety when the question calls for a priority or immediate response, Safety first. Choose open-ended questions that encourage elaboration and expression of feelings.
> **AS, APP, 2, Psych, SECE, Safety**

71. **(3) Respirations are the most critical physiological change. Without respirations, oxygen is not transported to the brain tissues and damage can occur. Answer 1** is incorrect because immunity is *not the most critical* physiological change at birth. **Answer 2** is incorrect because temperature regulation is important to decrease stress in the newborn, but it is *not the most critical* physiological change at birth. **Answer 4** is incorrect because closure of the circulatory bypasses is an important part of the newborn transition, but the first breath of air starts all the changes at birth.

> **TEST-TAKING TIP**—think about the ABCs. Airway and initiating respirations is the most critical component for a newborn to transition to extrauterine life.
> **AN, APP, 5, Newborn, HPM, Health Promotion and Maintenance**

72. **(4) There are no indications of an urgent need for treatment. The data should be recorded and the client observed for changes. Answer 1** is incorrect because the blood glucose level is *not high enough* to be the priority response. The elevated blood sugar may be a response to illness and the stress of hospitalization. **Answer 2** is incorrect because the urine is generally negative until the blood sugar is over 250 mg/dL. This data would not be useful and not a priority. **Answer 3** is incorrect because the bicarbonate level, which evaluates for metabolic acidosis, is within the *normal* range. No immediate treatment is required.

> **TEST-TAKING TIP**—Don't jump to conclusions that something must be done urgently.
> **IMP, ANL, 4, M/S: Endocrine, PhI, Physiological Adaptation**

73. **(3) An antiseizure drug, such as Neurontin, acts directly on the nerves to minimize the pain from peripheral neuropathy. Answer 1** is incorrect because heat is effective with inflammation; the pathology producing the pain is peripheral neuropathy. Heat is also potentially dangerous for a person who is diabetic with peripheral neuropathy, since sensation is reduced and burns can result. **Answer 2** is incorrect because range of motion is not effective in reducing neuropathic pain. ROM would promote arterial circulation, and lessen the pain from intermittent claudication. **Answer 4** is incorrect because peripheral neuropathy is typically unresponsive to narcotics.

> **TEST-TAKING TIP**—Look for a choice that includes "neuro" in the option.
> **IMP, APP, 3, M/S: Pain, PhI, Basic Care and Comfort**

74. **(1) The priority is rest—for both the client and the inflamed organ. Nothing by mouth rests the gastrointestinal tract, reduces pancreatic stimulation, and decreases the pain. Side-lying with knees flexed and a pillow against the abdomen or sitting with the trunk flexed are positions of comfort. Timely administration of pain medication, meperidine (Demerol) as the drug of choice, is a priority. Answer 2** is incorrect because the priority is rest for the GI tract and the client. *Nothing by mouth* and bedrest are indicated for acute pancreatitis. **Answer 3** is incorrect because the drugs of choice are non-opiate analgesics (particularly Demerol), and possibly anticholinergics or histamine-receptor antagonists to quiet the pancreas and decrease enzyme

secretion. **Answer 4** is incorrect because surgical management would only be indicated if the client did not respond to the pharmacological and non-pharmacological treatments. The option is *partially* correct: pain management *is* a priority. Supplemental pancreatic enzymes would *not* be appropriate during acute pancreatitis.

> **TEST-TAKING TIP**—Look for an action that rests an "itis."
> **IMP, APP, 3, M/S: GI, PhI, Basic Care and Comfort**

75. **(3) The purpose of the eye prophylaxis is to destroy organisms that can be transmitted from the mother to the infant's eyes during the birth process. Answer 1** is incorrect because the swelling of the eyelids is a normal result of the birth process. Antibiotic ointment does *nothing* to decrease this swelling or facilitate vision. **Answer 2** is incorrect because antibiotic ointment does *not* aid in the formation of tears. The ointment acts as a lubricant, but newborns do not require lubrication. **Answer 4** is incorrect because antibiotic eye ointment is *not* effective against nosocomial infections that may be transmitted to the infant in the hospital environment.

> **TEST-TAKING TIP**—The purpose of antibiotics is to *destroy* microorganisms. Eliminate **Answers 1** and **2** that do not include this purpose.
> **PL, APP, 1, Newborn, SECE, Safety and Infection Control**

76. **(3) Diversional activities, such as playing with puppets or dolls, coloring with crayons, doing arts and crafts projects, would help the child focus on pleasant, enjoyable tasks, and draw attention away from discomfort and the stress of being hospitalized. Answer 1** is incorrect because the irritability accompanying Kawasaki disease persists through the acute and subacute phases of the disease, and begins to subside in the convalescent phase of the disease. These phases can collectively last up to 6–8 weeks from the onset of the disease. This makes sedating the child, for this extended period of time, unrealistic. It is not a generally accepted policy in pediatrics to sedate children in order to elicit desirable behavior. **Answer 2** is incorrect because the irritability accompanying Kawasaki disease causes the child to be nearly inconsolable. Setting limits is always a good idea with any child, hospitalized or nonhospitalized; but, in this case, it is unlikely to elicit desirable behavior. **Answer 4** is incorrect because a preschooler does not have the fully developed use of reason and logic and is, therefore, unlikely to cooperate with the desired plan of care and demonstrate desirable behavior.

> **TEST-TAKING TIP**—Three of these answers involve the nurse doing something to the child to bring about desired behavior. The remaining answer allows the child to self-modify behavior.
> **IMP, APP, 5, PEDS, PsI, Psychosocial Integrity**

77. **(1, 3, 4, 5, 6) Answer 1 is correct because inadequate volume from a significant blood loss will result in a drop of the systolic blood pressure >25 mm Hg, the diastolic value >20 mm Hg, and an increase in the pulse rate of 30 bpm when the client goes from flat to sitting/standing. Answer 3 is correct because the nursing assessment would include a description of the characteristics of the stool as a basis for a nursing diagnosis. Answer 4 is correct because eating red meat prior to the test may result in a false positive finding. Answer 5 is correct because it should be known if the client has a history of frequent and high doses of drugs known to cause GI irritation and bleeding. Answer 6 is correct because taking vitamin C within 48 hours and just before a fecal occult blood test will cause a false positive reading. Answer 2** is incorrect because ordering laboratory tests is not part of the nursing assessment.

TEST-TAKING TIP—Think cause and effect.
AS, COM, 3, M/S:GI, PhI, Reduction of Risk Potential

78. **(4) Absent bowel sounds are normal. A side effect of general anesthesia is decreased motility (the absence of peristalsis). The nurse should monitor for signs of hemorrhage and manage the client's pain. Answer 1** is incorrect because bowel sounds *will be absent* after gastric surgery. A nasogastric tube will be present to prevent distention. **Answer 2** is incorrect because absence of bowel sounds is *normal* postoperatively and does not indicate bleeding. Bright red NG drainage is *normal* immediately following surgery. **Answer 3** is incorrect because massaging the abdomen *could cause* bleeding from the suture line of the anastomosis and also move the placement of the NG tube, which is over the suture line to prevent pressure at that site.

TEST-TAKING TIP—A priority question based on knowledge of the effects of general anesthesia.
PL, ANL, 8, M/S: GI, PhI, Reduction of Risk Potential

79. **(1) High-dose aspirin therapy is administered to control the fever and inflammation accompanying Kawasaki disease. A potential side effect of this therapy is tinnitus or a ringing/buzzing in the ears. It would be reasonable that a preschooler would describe the sensation in this manner. This finding should be reported to the child's pediatrician immediately because dosage readjustment may be necessary. Answer 2** is incorrect because, although a preschooler is highly creative child, it is unlikely that this statement would be used as a way of getting attention. **Answer 3** is incorrect because, although a preschooler does have an active imagination, it is unlikely that this statement would be made unless the preschooler is actually experiencing the sensation. **Answer 4** is incorrect because, although a preschooler does have many normal fears, they are usually about monsters, the dark, and being hurt, rather than "bees in my ears."

TEST-TAKING TIP—Three of these responses involve *normal* aspects of preschool growth and development, but are *not* relevant for the condition and possible side effect. Think like a preschooler and recognize that "bees in my ears" is a reasonable way to express the sensation of *tinnitus* which must be reported to the child's pediatrician.
AN, ANL, 2, PEDS, HPM, Health Promotion and Maintenance

80. **(2) NMS is a serious adverse reaction to antipsychotic medications that have high mortality rates. Clients with a history of NMS can no longer take antipsychotic medications. Answer 1** is incorrect because EPS *can* be treated with an antiparkinsonian agent. If the physician does not order an antiparkinsonian agent, the nurse can remind the doctor of the client's history of EPS. **Answer 3** is incorrect because a history of substance abuse would *not* affect drug treatment with antipsychotic medications. **Answer 4** is incorrect because dystonia and akathisia are extrapyramidal symptoms that can be treated with an antiparkinsonian agent.

TEST-TAKING TIP—Note the word "malignant" in **Answer 2** and think "serious" problem. If two answers cover the same points (**Answers 1 and 4**), eliminate both of the answers.
AN, ANL, 1, Psych, SECE, Safety

81. **(4) The first milk is called colostrum and is yellowish in color and has antibodies from the mother. Answer 1** is incorrect because poor nutrition does *not* affect the quality and color of the milk. **Answer 2** is incorrect because a breast infection does not result in yellowish milk. The

symptoms are a red, hard spot on the breast and a fever. The milk does *not* look infected. **Answer 3** is incorrect because the *first milk is a yellowish color, more mature milk is the bluish* color. The yellow color is *not* a result of lack of nutrients.

TEST-TAKING TIP—**Answers 1 and 3** state similar information about the milk lacking in nutrients; when the same information is stated in different ways, both can not be correct; therefore, eliminate them. Choose the 1 option that is different from the others: 3 answers focus on a *problem*, 1 option states it is *normal*.
IMP, APP, 4, Maternity, HPM, Health Promotion and Maintenance

82. **(4) Exercise is important or the client will become even weaker. The syndrome often follows periods of infection or stress and is associated with fibromyalgia. The plan of care should include a balance of exercise and rest. Answer 1** is incorrect because chronic fatigue has no known cause. Diet modifications would not be a specific treatment and there are *no known* restrictions. A balanced diet is important to maintain energy. **Answer 2** is incorrect because chronic fatigue has no specific causation. While generalized aching is present, treatment with steroids would *not* be standard. **Answer 3** is incorrect because the syndrome is a *real* physical disability—not an emotional response to stress.

TEST-TAKING TIP—The priority should be something the nurse does directly with/for the client.
IMP, APP, 3, M/S: NM, PhI, Basic Care and Comfort

83. **(4) Swallowing helps to carry the tube down into the stomach. There needs to be slack in the tube if the tip is going to be carried postpyloric. Answer 1** is incorrect because deep breathing increases the likelihood of inserting the tube into the *lung*. **Answer 2** is incorrect because tipping the head back increase the likelihood of inserting the tube into the *lung*. **Answer 3** is incorrect because the measurements would result in a *gastric* placement of the tube. There needs to be more length for the tube to be placed post-pyloric.

TEST-TAKING TIP—Think client safety—what will ensure accurate tube placement?
IMP, APP, 4, M/S:GI, PhI, Reduction of Risk Potential

84. **(4) The bladder competes for space with the uterus, and a full bladder will push the fundus to the right. Answer 1** is incorrect because retained placental fragments continue to bleed and the fundus would *not* de deviated to the right. **Answer 2** is incorrect because overstretched ligaments do *not* cause the uterus to deviate. **Answer 3** is incorrect because a slow rate of involution would be a slow descent of the fundus into the pelvis, *not* a deviation to the right.

TEST-TAKING TIP—Visualize what the uterus looks like after delivery. Would the answer(s) given be a cause of the fundus physically moving to the right side of the body? For example, a slow rate of involution (**Answer 3**) and overstretched ligaments (**Answer 2**) might result in a boggy fundus, but *not* deviation from the midline.
EV, APP, 8, Maternity, PhI, Basic Care and Comfort

85. **(2) The cardiac output is significantly reduced and perfusion will be impaired, leading to almost overwhelming fatigue. Answer 1** is incorrect because the ejection fraction is measuring cardiac *output*, not coronary artery *disease*. Systemic perfusion will be compromised and the client will experience extreme fatigue. **Answer 3** is incorrect because the problem is *not* neurological. **Answer 4** is incorrect because the client's blood pressure will be low, *not* high.

TEST-TAKING TIP—Know the physiological effect of poor perfusion (e.g., significant fatigue).
PL, ANL, 6, M/S: CV, PhI, Physiological Adaptation

86. **(2) It is the antidote for an overdose or toxic level of aspirin, which is the mainstay medication in the treatment of Kawasaki disease. Phytonadione is the generic name for vitamin K.** Answer 1 is incorrect because it is the antidote for an overdose of *heparin.* Heparin is not usually indicated in the treatment of Kawasaki disease. If additional anticoagulant therapy is indicated (such as in the event of aneurysms secondary to Kawasaki disease), warfarin is usually the drug of choice. **Answer 3** is incorrect because it is the antidote for an overdose of iron. Deferoxamine mesylate is the generic name for Desferal. **Answer 4** is incorrect because 80% of all cases of Kawasaki disease occur in children younger than 5 years of age. A diet high in vitamin K would be rich in leafy green vegetables, tomatoes, fish, pork, or beef liver. A child in this age group would probably *resist* eating these food items due to both oral discomfort and general likes and dislikes. Bland foods might be better accepted by the child. An *increase* or decrease in foods high in vitamin K could affect therapy.

TEST-TAKING TIP—Know the antidotes for common childhood overdoses and associated therapies.
IMP, COM, 1, PEDS, PhI, Pharmacological and Parenteral Therapies

87. **(2) The client is scheduled for surgery; and because all of the other clients are stable, completing preoperative orders for this client is the priority.** Answer 1 is incorrect because the client is stable and the pain is not requiring immediate attention. **Answer 3** is incorrect because the Hct, while slightly lower than normal, has *not* dropped *significantly* since the previous test. The level is *not* life-threatening. **Answer 4** is incorrect because the WBC level is *not* elevated significantly to require immediate action by the nurse. It will require *monitoring.*

TEST-TAKING TIP—This is a priority question—think preop assessment as the priority over a client who is stable.
AS, ANL, 1, M/S: Establishing Priorities, SECE, Management of Care

88. **(3) General anesthesia puts the client to sleep. A full recovery will be wakefulness and orientation.** Answer 1 is incorrect because the blood oxygen level is generally *maintained by oxygen* and *ventilatory support* even when the client is asleep for the procedure. **Answer 2** is incorrect because the ability to lift the legs would be an indication of recovery from *spinal* anesthesia. The client may move extremities before being fully awake and oriented. **Answer 4** is incorrect because even during general anesthesia the blood pressure and pulse are *maintained by fluids and drugs.*

TEST-TAKING TIP—Three of the choices are desirable outcomes—the question asks for an indication of "fully" recovered.
EV, ANL, 1, M/S: Postop, PhI, Reduction of Risk Potential

89. **(2) The nurse who is caring for the child would have the most knowledge about how the IV has been functioning and what interventions she may have already taken in regard to the IV. In addition, the nurse caring for the child has the responsibility for the total care of the child.** Answer 1 is incorrect because the charge nurse has not been taking direct physical care of the child and does not know how the IV has been functioning, or what interventions the nurse caring for the child may have already taken. The charge nurse has no way of anticipating how long she may be involved in correct-

ing the situation once she enters the child's room, and the nurse's station should not be left unattended. **Answer 3** is incorrect because pediatric IVs are difficult to start and maintain, and there might be a delay in the call light being answered, which could further jeopardize the IV. This action on the charge nurse's part might also be misinterpreted by the mother. The mother might feel that her child's needs are not being taken seriously. **Answer 4** is incorrect because a nursing student might not have sufficient experience to correctly assess the IV. The ultimate responsibility for the assessment of this IV rests with the nurse caring for the child.

TEST-TAKING TIP—Assessment is the domain and responsibility of the registered nurse who is caring for the child.
IMP, ANL, 7, PEDS, SECE, Management of Care

90. **(4) It is a fall-prevention measure that does not require the use of restraints. Clients who are elderly have difficulty getting out of recliners and deep-seated chairs. Observing a client attempting to get out of the chair would alert the staff to assist the client to ambulate without falling. The nurse can observe the client while performing work at the nurse's station.** Answer 1 is incorrect because restraints can be used only in an *emergency,* and should *not* be in a plan of care. A client's behavior would have to indicate an immediate danger to self or others at the time in order to warrant the use of restraints. **Answer 2** is incorrect because a client with dementia can get easily confused and disoriented. Providing *enclosed* areas free of environmental hazards would be an appropriate fall-prevention nursing action. **Answer 3** is incorrect because having the client sit in the dayroom is a good answer, but it is not the best answer. It places responsibility on other clients to watch the client with dementia.

TEST-TAKING TIP—Prevention is the key concept. Choose the answer that is the least restrictive and the most supportive to the client.
PL, APP, 1, Psych, SECE, Safety

91. **(2) The schedule as described by the client appears to be incorrect and needs to be reviewed by the nurse. The desired goal is regular administration to achieve a therapeutic level.** Answer 1 is incorrect because administration of antibiotics is supposed to be consistent—not increasing daily. Side effects are not a desired outcome. **Answer 3** is incorrect because the first concern should be the dosage schedule. Client teaching before starting the drug should have included the need to immediately report any signs of allergy. **Answer 4** is incorrect because the dosage schedule is usually a consistent number of tablets each day—*not* an increasing dosage. Altering the dosage is *not* the decision of the client.

TEST-TAKING TIP—Three of the choices support the dosage schedule—only one questions it.
IMP, ANL, 1, M/S: Meds, PhI, Pharmacological and Parenteral Therapies

92. **(2) Pain and the stress of labor can cause cardiac decompensation. Providing pain relief for labor is critical for a client with cardiac disease.** Answer 1 is incorrect because the additional stress of surgery and anesthetic agents *can* result in greater morbidity and mortality than a vaginal delivery. **Answer 3** incorrect because pushing in the second stage of labor can lead to cardiac failure. **Answer 4** is incorrect because Valsalva pushing can cause cardiac failure.

TEST-TAKING TIP—Answers 3 and 4 state the same information ("pushing") in different ways; therefore eliminate both.
PL, ANL, 6, Maternity, PhI, Reduction of Risk Potential

93. **(4) It would not be appropriate to give ceftriaxone unless there was no other choice and the reaction to penicillin had been very mild. There is a small chance of cross-reactivity, and the risk of anaphylaxis should be avoided if possible.** Answer 1 is incorrect because acetaminophen (Tylenol) is *not* contraindicated in clients with allergies to penicillin. **Answer 2** is incorrect because diphenhydramine (Benadryl) would actually be *used* to treat an allergic reaction. **Answer 3** is incorrect because there is no known crossover allergy between penicillin and vitamin C. Vitamin C is an essential vitamin for general health.

    TEST-TAKING TIP—Know possible crossover effects. Hint: only one of the choices is an antibiotic.
    PL, COM, 1, M/S: Allergy, PhI, Pharmacological and Parenteral Therapies

94. **(1) During prolonged bedrest the school-age child will become bored. A child in the stage of industry is likely to turn to food for diversion and comfort. Placing additional weight on the femur could delay the healing process and make the return to an ambulatory status more difficult. For this reason, a child with this condition is frequently placed on a low calorie, high protein diet.** Answer 2 is incorrect because constipation is easily prevented with medications, for example docusate sodium (Colace), and increasing fluids and fiber in the diet. **Answer 3** is incorrect because social isolation is easily prevented with cards, telephone contact, and visits from the child's peers. Enlisting the services of the child life specialist would also be beneficial. **Answer 4** is incorrect because pressure ulcers are easily prevented with meticulous skin care and hygiene, and a special pressure-reducing mattress.

    TEST-TAKING TIP—Look for the worst-case scenario in the responses when asked to identify what is "most detrimental" to the child.
    EV, ANL, 4, PEDS, PhI, Basic Care and Comfort

95. **(1, 3, 7)** Answer 1 is a correct answer and should be questioned. Atenolol is a beta-blocker and will further slow the heart rate. Generally the drug is held when the pulse is between 50–60 bpm. Answer 3 is a correct answer and should be questioned. The risk of blood clots from birth control pills is greatly increased when added to other risks such as smoking and increasing age. Answer 7 is a correct answer and should be questioned. Levothyroxine (Synthroid) speeds metabolism and oxygen consumption and would be contraindicated in a recent heart attack. Answer 2 is an incorrect answer because furosemide (Lasix) is a diuretic that would potentially lower the potassium level. The intent would be to increase the amount of K$^+$ lost through the kidneys. **Answer 4** is an incorrect answer because albuterol relaxes airway muscles and *is* a useful treatment in asthma. **Answer 5** is an incorrect answer because insulin carries potassium into the cell and *can* be used to treat high serum K$^+$ levels. **Answer 6** is an incorrect answer because low-dose aspirin *is* used in the prevention of brain attacks (strokes). **Answer 8** is an incorrect answer because a stool softener, such as docusate sodium, *is* often coprescribed because of the great risk for constipation with morphine.

    TEST-TAKING TIP—Know desired drug effects.
    IMP, ANL, 1, M/S: Meds, PhI, Pharmacological and Parenteral Therapies

96. **(1) Heparin given IV initially will reach a therapeutic anti-coagulation level faster. Warfarin (Coumadin) requires generally 72 hours to achieve a therapeutic level. Once the desired level is reached, the heparin will be discontinued and the warfarin will be taken PO to maintain the blood** level. Answer 2 is incorrect because warfarin takes longer to reach the therapeutic level. Heparin is used IV initially to achieve the desired level. **Answer 3** is incorrect because both warfarin and heparin are anticoagulants and can cause bleeding. The antidote for heparin is protamine sulfate. **Answer 4** is incorrect because both heparin and warfarin are anticoagulants and can cause bleeding. The antidote for warfarin is vitamin K.

    TEST-TAKING TIP—Know route of administration and effect time.
    IMP, COM, 6, M/S: Blood, PhI, Pharmacological and Parenteral Therapies

97. **(3) Myelomeningocele is a chronic disease that would involve repeated, prolonged exposure to latex products such as catheters, wheelchair cushions and tires, crutches with axillary and hand pads, etc.** Answer 1 is incorrect because a key concept in the development of latex allergy is repeated exposure. Acute gastroenteritis is an acute, self-limiting disease that would not involve repeated, prolonged exposure to latex products. **Answer 2** is incorrect because a urinary tract infection is an acute, self-limiting disease that would not involve repeated, prolonged exposure to latex products. **Answer 4** is incorrect because bronchiolitis is an acute, self-limiting disease that would not involve repeated, prolonged exposure to latex products.

    TEST-TAKING TIP— "Latex gloves" is found in each answer. Think of the problems associated with the use of latex gloves and identify the situation/disease that would involve repeated, prolonged use of latex gloves.
    EV, APP, 1, PEDS, SECE, Management of Care

98. **(1) Insulin requirements increase with the increasing size of the placenta and the release of human placental lactogen (HPL). The client becomes more insulin resistant later in pregnancy, resulting in an increased need for additional insulin.** Answer 2 is incorrect because the insulin requirements decrease *during* (not after) the first trimester and then gradually increase as the pregnancy progresses until delivery. **Answer 3** is incorrect because the insulin dosage *decreases* dramatically after delivery (usually by about half the dose). **Answer 4** is incorrect because the insulin dosage gradually *increases* as the pregnancy progresses.

    TEST-TAKING TIP—Read the options carefully when you have answers that have "increase" and "decrease." It is easy to jump ahead if the answer "looks right." Take your time and think about the whole answer, not just the word *increase* or *decrease*.
    EV, APP, 4, Maternity, PhI, Pharmacological and Parenteral Therapy

99. **(3) Respiratory status is of *primary importance* in a client with Guillain-Barré syndrome, as it is with most clients.** Answer 1 is incorrect because, while pain is an important assessment for this client, it is *not the most important*. **Answer 2** is incorrect because, while cranial nerve assessment and the client's ability to protect the eyes can be impaired with Guillain-Barré, this is *not the most important* assessment. **Answer 4** is incorrect because, even though arterial blood gases may provide useful information about the client's respiratory status, observing the rate, depth, and quality of respirations provides immediate information.

    TEST-TAKING TIP—While all of the options are potentially correct, the question asks for the option that is of *primary* importance; in other words, *most* important.
    AS, APP, 3, M/S: NM, PhI, Basic Care and Comfort

100. **(1) It is not safe to apply restraints to side rails. Bedrails are not securely attached to the bed and clients would have access to the restraint and could try to release themselves.** Answer 2 is incorrect because padding bony prominences and skin *is* the nursing staffs' responsibility when applying restraints. **Answer 3** is incorrect because it *is* appropriate to use knots with hitches that allow for easy removal. If the client aspirates or there is another emergency, the restraints need to be removed quickly. **Answer 4** is incorrect because it *is* correct to apply the restraints in a fashion that allows the client to have maximum movement.

> **TEST-TAKING TIP**—Choose the answer that focuses on the client, and provides the client with the most comfort. Visualize the situation. Reword the question when the stem asks for further teaching; the best answer is the *incorrect* response.
> **IMP, ANL, 1, Psych, SECE, Safety**

101. **(4) Itching under a Boston brace is not an acute or life-endangering situation. The child is able to independently remove the brace at home for hygiene and other purposes. Thus, removal of the brace by the school health office aide would be permitted. If the itching persists, the school nurse would then see this child, but as a "last priority" client.** Answer 1 is incorrect because a reddened elbow could indicate that the child with hemophilia is experiencing a bleed into the joint (hemarthrosis). This would require a nursing assessment at a level that could only be provided by a registered nurse. **Answer 2** is incorrect because a persistent cough can irritate the child's throat and initiate tissue sloughing, which can lead to hemorrhage that can occur up to 10 days following the surgery. This would require a nursing assessment at a level that could only be provided by a registered nurse. **Answer 3** is incorrect because wheezing in a child with asthma must be assessed immediately to prevent a full-blown asthmatic attack. This would require a nursing assessment at a level that could only be provided by a registered nurse.

> **TEST-TAKING TIP**—Three of the options would require assessment by the registered nurse. Select the one option that is potentially least serious, and does not require nursing judgment.
> **EV, ANL, 1, PEDS, SECE, Management of Care: Delegation**

102. **(4)** *Autonomic dysreflexia* is a complication of spinal cord injury and is considered an *emergency*. A key symptom is complaint of a *headache*, accompanied by *severe hypertension*. Answer 1 is incorrect at this time because *autonomic dysreflexia* is considered an *emergency* for this client, and a key symptom is *headache*. Acetaminophen may be administered *later*, but the emergency needs to be assessed and managed first. **Answer 2** is incorrect at this time because the nurse should *first assess* the client's blood pressure to determine if an emergency exists. Although a distended bladder is often a cause of autonomic dysreflexia and catheterizing the client will reverse the problem, the nurse needs to assess the client's *blood pressure* first to determine if an emergency exists. **Answer 3** is incorrect at this time because the nurse needs to first gather more data to determine if autonomic dysreflexia is the cause of the headache; and if it is, to institute measures to reverse it. A call to the physician may be in order, but the nurse needs to first assess and institute appropriate protocols.

> **TEST-TAKING TIP**—Note that assessment is usually the first correct response before an action is taken, as in **Answers 1, 2,** and **3**. Recall that *autonomic dysreflexia* is considered an *emergency* for clients with spinal cord injury; therefore, immediate assessment and intervention is called

for. While all of the options are correct, **Answer 4** represents the step that should be accomplished *first*.
AN, ANL, 3, M/S: Neuro, PhI, Physiological Adaptation

103. **(1) A raised toilet seat helps the client with a total hip replacement avoid *hyperflexion* of the hip joint.** Answer 2 is incorrect because, although enoxaparin is an anticoagulant intended to prevent thrombus formation, *daily* monitoring of coagulation studies is *not required* with this drug. **Answer 3** is incorrect because jogging would be *too much impact and stress* on the new hip joint; quadriceps strengthening can be accomplished with other exercises that are not contraindicated. **Answer 4** is incorrect because the client with a new hip joint should *avoid hip flexion* to, or beyond 90°. *Adduction*, or crossing the affected limb over the center of the body, is also *contraindicated* and can result in dislocation of the new joint.

> **TEST-TAKING TIP**—Answer 1 is the only option that is theoretically correct. **Answers 2** and **3** include concepts that are correct (use of enoxaparin and quadriceps strengthening), but the implementations are incorrect.
> **IMP, APP, 3, M/S: Ortho, PhI, Basic Care and Comfort**

104. **(4) The child's action does require intervention on the part of the registered nurse. The child is not in any immediate danger, but the situation should be dealt with as soon as possible.** Answer 1 is incorrect because, although this is a frequently encountered postoperative behavior on the part of a child who has just had a tonsillectomy, it can aggravate the operative site and should, thus, *not* be ignored or considered normal. **Answer 2** is incorrect because the child will require teaching or reinstruction as to why this behavior could be dangerous. Only the registered nurse could provide this and the rationale for teaching at a level that a 5-year-old child could comprehend. **Answer 3** is incorrect because the child is not in any immediate danger. Instead, the registered nurse needs to stop the child's at-risk behavior before it is necessary to call the pediatrician for medical treatment/intervention.

> **TEST-TAKING TIP**—Know the difference between immediate danger signals associated with a tonsillectomy (e.g., restlessness, excessive clearing of the throat or swallowing) and at-risk behaviors (e.g., blowing the nose or coughing).
> **IMP, APP, 1, PEDS, SECE, Management of Care**

105. **(1) The client's symptoms may indicate placental abruption which can cause fetal distress. By placing the client on the fetal monitor, the nurse can determine if the fetus is in distress.** Answer 2 is incorrect because the client may have a *placenta previa* and a vaginal exam may result in *increased* vaginal bleeding. **Answer 3** is incorrect because tocolytics can be administered by *other routes* than intravenous. An IV access may be necessary, but it would *not* be the *first* action taken by the nurse. **Answer 4** is incorrect because the physician needs to have *additional* information about the fetus and uterine contraction pattern *before* ordering pain medication.

> **TEST-TAKING TIP**—This question asks for priority of nursing actions. Other actions *may* be performed in this case, but the question asked for first priority.
> **IMP, ANL, 1, Maternity, PhI, Reduction of Risk Potential**

106. **(2)** *Maximum heart rate decreases* as people age. In contrast, the maximum exercise heart rate of a 25-year-old may be up to 200 bpm. Answer 1 is incorrect because a normal consequence of aging is an *increase* in *respiratory rate* of up to 12–24 breaths per minute. **Answer 3** is incorrect because as people age, hardening and decreased elasticity of the arteries results in a moderate increase in blood pressure; 110/60 would generally be considered *low or normal for a young or* *middle-aged adult.* **Answer 4** is incorrect because the rib cage becomes more rigid as a normal consequence of aging; therefore *vital capacity* and *chest excursion decrease* with age.

> **TEST-TAKING TIP**—This question involves the expected assessment findings of an *older* adult. All but one of the options provided, **Answer 2**, describe characteristics of a *younger* adult.
> **AS, ANL, 5, M/S: Geriatrics, HPM, Health Promotion and Maintenance**

107. **(3) The elderly client experiencing normal forgetfulness can successfully use memory aids such as calendars and marked pillboxes to remember important tasks. Answer 1** is incorrect because not knowing the day and month indicates impaired orientation, which suggests *dementia*, rather than simple forgetfulness. **Answer 2** is incorrect because it indicates impaired recognition of people important to the client, and is a characteristic of *dementia*. **Answer 4** is incorrect because repeating the same question only moments later is characteristic of *dementia*.

> **TEST-TAKING TIP**—Look for the option that is different from the rest. **Answer 3** involves a method of coping with normal forgetfulness. The other 3 options describe types of cognitive or memory impairment.
> **AS, ANL, 2, M/S: Geriatrics, HPM, Health Promotion and Maintenance**

108. **(1) Magnesium sulfate acts to reduce the chance of seizures in pregnancy-induced hypertension. Answer 2** is incorrect because magnesium sulfate does *not* have a direct effect on the lungs of the fetus. *Steroids* are used to enhance the production of surfactant in fetal lungs. **Answer 3** is incorrect because magnesium sulfate is a smooth muscle relaxant, *not* an antihypertensive. **Answer 4** is incorrect because magnesium sulfate does *not* have an effect on maternal blood flow to the liver and uterus. *Lying on either side* will enhance maternal perfusion.

> **TEST-TAKING TIP**—Look at the main purpose of magnesium sulfate in a client with pregnancy-induced hypertension. Magnesium is also used for preterm labor; but in this case, the client has a diagnosis of HELLP syndrome. Prevention of the complication of seizures is the main objective for administering magnesium sulfate to this client. Don't be fooled by the decrease in blood pressure (**Answer 3**). Magnesium sulfate is *not* an antihypertensive drug.
> **PL, COM, 1, Maternity, PhI, Pharmacological and Parenteral Therapies**

109. **(3) The focus of care for a child with sickle cell anemia is pain control. The registered nurse will want to assess the child's pain status and reload the medication cassette as soon as possible. This action will be the registered nurse's first priority. Answer 1** is incorrect because the registered nurse would *expect* that the dressing on a new tracheostomy would require frequent changes. The registered nurse will want to assess the tracheostomy and change the dressing as soon as possible, but this is *not* the first priority. **Answer 2** is incorrect because the registered nurse would *expect* that the urine produced by a child with acute glomerulonephritis would be bloody (hematuria). The registered nurse will want to assess the urine and compare it to other voided specimens, but this is *not* the first priority. **Answer 4** is incorrect because the registered nurse would *expect* that vomiting will occur in a child with pyloric stenosis. The registered nurse will want to assess and record the amount of the emesis, but this is *not* the first priority.

> **TEST-TAKING TIP**—Three of the responses involve expected symptoms of the child's disease process. Select the one answer that is different.
> **EV, ANL, 6, PEDS, SECE, Management of Care: Priority**

110. **(3) The nurse has just met this family and needs to further assess the infant's attachment behaviors. Stranger anxiety can begin as early as 6 months of age. Not experiencing anxiety when exposed to strangers can indicate insecure attachment in the infant. Answer 1** is incorrect because it is premature to offer reassurance; this can stop the conversation, and does not encourage elaboration or expression of feelings. **Answer 2** is incorrect because the nurse needs to assess the parent-infant relationship *before* referring the client. Parenting classes may not be an appropriate referral. **Answer 4** is incorrect because showing concern may increase guilt or anxiety in the parent. Reassuring the client to "not worry" is false reassurance, and is not a therapeutic response.

> **TEST-TAKING TIP**—Note the time frame. The nurse is in the initial phase of the therapeutic relationship, which calls for more *assessment*. This is the *first* step in the nursing process. Avoid answers that stop conversation or offer false reassurance (**Answers 1** and **4**).
> **AS, APP, 5, Psych, HPM, Health Promotion and Maintenance**

111. **(4) An unexpected admission to the hospital is stressful for ethnic elders: they are removed from their familiar ethnic community and support system. Allowing a familiar object in the client's room provides a source of comfort and reassurance. Answer 1** is incorrect because relatives and friends often provide emotional and spiritual support for the ethnic elder who is hospitalized. **Answer 2** is incorrect because allowing the client to speak a native language provides emotional support. Family members or professional translators can be used as needed. **Answer 3** is incorrect because familiar foods provide comfort and support for the ethnic elder, unless the foods are contraindicated for the client's condition

> **TEST-TAKING TIP**—Look for the option that *acknowledges* and *supports* the client's ethnicity and culture (**Answer 1**). The other three options *discourage* important aspects of the client's culture: language, food, family, and friends.
> **IMP, APP, 7, M/S: Geriatrics, HPM, Health Promotion and Maintenance**

112. **(4) Clients who are elderly may take longer to process new information. Simple instructions, repeated often, is a useful teaching strategy. Answer** 1 is incorrect because it takes a dictatorial approach rather than a collaborative approach. **Answer 2** is incorrect because not all clients who are elderly have shorter attention spans, and the teaching session should not be rushed. **Answer 3** is incorrect because distractions, such as other people in the room, may interfere with the client's learning

> **TEST-TAKING TIP**—**Answer 4** is the only theoretically correct option that addresses learning characteristics of clients who are elderly.
> **IMP, APP, 7, M/S: Geriatrics, HPM, Health Promotion and Maintenance**

113. **(1) The onset of a headache in a child with epilepsy could precipitate a seizure or indicate a closed head injury. The registered nurse will want to assess this child first. Answer 2** is incorrect because feeling scared and shaky is most probably a reaction to the stress of the accident in a child with diabetes mellitus. It is 7:30 A.M. and this child would have tested the blood glucose level, taken the prescribed amount of insulin, and eaten breakfast at home prior to leaving for

school. The registered nurse will want to assess this child as priority number 2. **Answer 3** is incorrect because feeling stiff and sore in the morning is a common complaint in a child with rheumatoid arthritis. However, this child could have sustained a musculoskeletal injury and should be assessed as priority number 4. **Answer 4** is incorrect because shoulder level pain is a common complaint in a child with scoliosis. The Milwaukee brace is used almost exclusively in a child with kyphosis so the registered nurse would expect the pain to be centered in the neck and shoulders. However, this child could have sustained a musculoskeletal injury despite the protection that the brace would have offered, and should be assessed as priority number 3.

> **TEST-TAKING TIP**—Neurological clients and injuries (**Answer 1**) would always take priority over other types of clients and injuries.
> **AN, ANL, 1, PEDS, SECE, Management of Care: Priority**

114. **(2) Herpes can be directly transmitted to the infant during a vaginal birth. Answer 1** is incorrect because pelvic inflammatory disease does *not* have a direct influence on the method of delivery. **Answer 3** is incorrect because herpes on the lip *cannot* be transmitted during a *vaginal* birth via the birth canal. **Answer 4** is incorrect because group B beta strep can be treated *during labor*, to decrease the possibility of transmission to the infant during the birth process.

> **TEST-TAKING TIP**—This question uses the key word "always", meaning there is no time when a vaginal delivery is appropriate. A cesarean section *must* be performed in the incidence of *genital* herpes.
> **AN, COM, 1, Maternity, SECE, Safety and Infection Control**

115. **(2) The client who is elderly may test as false negative because of diminished hypersensitivity-type immune response. It is best to do the 2-step TB skin test and have client repeat the test 1–3 weeks after the first test. If the second skin test is still negative, then the client can be informed that he or she does not have TB. If the second test is positive, then the client should receive a follow up chest x-ray and prophylactic treatment. Answer 1** is incorrect because hypersensitivity-type immune response diminishes as a normal consequence of aging, so the client who is elderly may test false negative. **Answer 3** is incorrect because it is not necessary to subject the client to the cost and risk of a chest x-ray after 1 skin test. A better response would be to have the client repeat the skin test in 1–3 weeks and base any follow-up on the results of the second skin test. **Answer 4** is incorrect because, even though the client who is elderly may be at increased risk for TB, the client should not be started on medications until a second skin test or chest x-ray indicates a need.

> **TEST-TAKING TIP**—**Answer 2** provides the most reasonable and cost-effective response. **Answers 3** and **4** may be instituted, but involve significant cost and risk to the client, and should not be instituted unless needed.
> **EV, ANL, 1, M/S: Geriatrics, SECE, Safety and Infection Control**

116. **(1) The foundation of traditional Chinese medicine is herbal therapy, and it is important to know which herbal medicines the client has been taking because they can interact with allopathic medications. Answer 2** is incorrect because the client's health beliefs *can* be incorporated into Western medicine practices. **Answer 3** is incorrect because herbal medicines are not necessarily benign; they can react negatively with allopathic medications. **Answer 4** is incorrect because it is not necessary to position the client in Fowler's to maintain the flow of *qi*. The client may find Chinese therapies, for example acupuncture, useful in addition to hospital treatment regimen.

> **TEST-TAKING TIP**—Look for the option that recognizes the effect that the client's health practices may have on Western treatment regimen.
> **PL, APP, 7, M/S: Geriatrics, PsI, Psychosocial Integrity**

117. **(3) A calm, well-lit environment reduces stimuli that may exacerbate withdrawal symptoms. Answer 1** is incorrect because the client who is chemically dependent postoperatively may need *higher* doses of pain medicine to achieve relief. The nurse will also frequently assess the client for excess sedation and respiratory depression. This answer represents a common misconception about the client who is drug and alcohol dependent, that is, administering pain medications will make the client's addiction "worse." **Answer 2** is incorrect because it is inappropriate to apply restraints until assessment indicates a need. In addition, restraints may make the client more agitated. **Answer 4** is incorrect at this time. The immediate postoperative period is not the time to address long-term goals for this client.

> **TEST-TAKING TIP**—Of the 2 possible correct options (**Answers 3** and **4**), **Answer 3** addresses immediate postoperative concerns and is most appropriate at this time.
> **IMP, APP, 3, M/S: Postop, PsI, Psychosocial Integrity**

118. **(1, 3, 5) Answer 1 is correct because infection usually causes an increase in respiratory rate. Answer 3 is correct because an infected uterus will begin to exhibit contractions. Answer 5 is correct because tachycardia is a common symptom of an infection. Answer 2** is incorrect because an infection in the mother would cause tachycardia in the fetus, *not* bradycardia. **Answer 4** is incorrect because hyperglycemia is *not* generally found in infections, unless the client has undiagnosed diabetes.

> **TEST-TAKING TIP**—In this type of question, each option should be considered as a separate true-false question. With each possible answer, ask: Is it true of the condition described? If true, choose the answer; if false, discard the option.
> **AS, APP, 1, Maternity, PhI, Reduction of Risk Potential**

119. **(1) This child is at greatest risk of becoming more hypoxic during the evacuation once being removed from the wall-operated oxygen delivery system. The charge nurse should request backup assistance from the respiratory therapy department to assist in monitoring the child during the evacuation and deliver the needed oxygen via portable tanks. Answer 2** is incorrect because this child is receiving intermittent decompression. The nasogastric tube could be safely disconnected from the wall-operated suction delivery system for a brief period of time during the evacuation and then reconnected to a portable suction machine. The pediatric nursing staff can perform this task without additional assistance. **Answer 3** is incorrect because this child can safely be removed from the enteral feeding pump delivery system during the evacuation and placed on a hand-held gravity drip delivery system. The pediatric nursing staff can perform this task without additional assistance. **Answer 4** is incorrect because this child can remain on the PCA pump during the evacuation. The PCA pump has a backup battery system that will continue to deliver the required medication even when it is disconnected from the electrical outlet in the wall. The pediatric nursing staff can perform this task without additional assistance.

TEST-TAKING TIP Three of the responses require knowing how a specific type of client care system works. The correct response involves critical thinking regarding how to continue delivering lifesaving oxygen to a child who is hypoxic when the delivery system must be temporarily discontinued.
IMP, APP, 1, PEDS, SECE, Management of Care: Priority

120. **(1) Children at this age are beginning to develop** *autonomy,* **according to Erikson's theory of personality development. Short periods of separation will help the child to accomplish this developmental task, but prolonged separation should be avoided until the child has successfully completed the task.** **Answer 2** is incorrect because the parent should be encouraged to *ignore* and not reinforce temper tantrums. **Answer 3** is incorrect because saying "no" is common in the toddler period, but it is *not an important* communication. Many toddlers will say "no" when they really mean "yes." **Answer 4** is incorrect because when toddlers play with other toddlers, they *need* good adult supervision. Playing with other children gives the parent an opportunity to teach the child how to share and play appropriately.

TEST-TAKING TIP—Focus on age-appropriate behavior. Note that the children are age 1–3 years and ask yourself if the answer is reasonable for the situation.
IMP, APP, 5, Psych, HPM, Health Promotion and Maintenance

121. **(4) An advance directive documents the client's wishes if and when the client becomes incapacitated and unable to make decisions. It is the health-care team's responsibility to adhere to those wishes to the extent allowed by the law and hospital policy.** **Answer 1** is incorrect because this response dismisses the client's concerns. **Answer 2** is incorrect because the nurse should not "take sides." The nurse is an objective party whose primary responsibility is for the client's welfare. **Answer 3** is incorrect because a "no code" order before a diagnosis is made is premature.

TEST-TAKING TIP—Focus on the option that directly and most objectively addresses the client's concerns (Answer 4).
IMP, ANL, 7, M/S: Legal, SECE, Management of Care

122. **(3) It gives the child specific information as to when to expect to see the mother. While a 4-year-old child would not yet be able to tell time, the child would comprehend when dinner time is and thus be reassured about seeing the mother later in the day.** **Answer 1** is incorrect because it does not address the child's concern. It offers both an implication that the child is wrong for crying, and that the child can be bribed into acceptable behavior by a visit to the playroom. **Answer 2** is incorrect because it is too vague and does not offer the child the needed information as to when the child may expect to see the mother. **Answer 4** is incorrect because it does not address the child's concern. It informs the child about the mother's present whereabouts, but does not address the issue of when to expect to see the mother.

TEST-TAKING TIP—Look for the response that offers the most age-appropriate information.
IMP, APP, 5, PEDS, PsI, Psychosocial Integrity

123. **(1) The nurse is accountable for evaluating the information, even though she delegated the task to licensed, assistive personnel.** **Answer 2** is incorrect because the person delegating the task still retains accountability, even though the licensed vocational/practical nurse (LVN/LPN) agreed to perform the task. **Answer 3** is incorrect because the physi-

cian is not responsible for this particular aspect of the client's care. **Answer 4** is incorrect because the person delegating is ultimately responsible for the *task*, although the hospital is ultimately responsible for the client's *welfare*.

TEST-TAKING TIP—Notice how this question is worded: who is accountable for this *task*? Although all of the parties involved are accountable for various aspects of the client's *welfare*, the nurse-delegator remains accountable for the specific task.
IMP, APP, 1, M/S: Legal, SECE, Management of Care

124. **(1) It identifies a baseline of knowledge for the nurse and client to build upon, and opens the door to new learning on the client's part.** **Answer 2** is incorrect because it is inappropriate to change the client's medication dosage until the reasons for the elevated glucose levels are determined. **Answer 3** is incorrect because the reasons for the client's poor glucose control may not be lack of knowledge. It would be better to assess the knowledge level, and then tailor an educational program to meet the needs. **Answer 4** incorrect because it blames the client for the elevated glucose levels, and sounds somewhat threatening.

TEST-TAKING TIP—*Assessment* is always the best place to start when planning care for clients.
AS, APP, 4, M/S: Endocrine, PhI, Basic Care and Comfort

125. **(1) Late decelerations are indicators of fetal distress caused by decreased blood flow to the placenta. High blood pressure and abruption are associated with cocaine use and fetal distress.** **Answer 2** is incorrect because polyhydramnios is related to *fetal renal* defects or *maternal diabetes*. **Answer 3** is incorrect because macrosomia is associated with *maternal diabetes*. **Answer 4** is incorrect because hyperbilirubinemia is found in infants with *blood incompatibility* or *liver immaturity*, not cocaine use by the mother.

TEST-TAKING TIP—There are common complications of pregnancy listed in this question. Think about each complication and the causes of each condition. Macrosomia (**Answer 3**) and polyhydramnios (**Answer 2**) can be eliminated, because these are both common complications of *maternal diabetes*. Hyperbilirubinemia is associated with prematurity and could be a complication of this pregnancy. This question asks for the *complication* of cocaine use in pregnancy; high blood pressure and abruption leading to fetal distress are commonly associated with the use of cocaine.
AS, APP, 5, Newborn, HPM, Health Promotion and Maintenance

126. **(3) The client's perception of her need to learn a particular skill influences the success of any teaching session.** *Before* **surgery, many clients do not understand that use of an incentive spirometer prevents atelectasis and pneumonia** *after* **surgery.** **Answer 1** is incorrect because the client's occupation as a high school teacher indicates that she is a woman who is well-educated and who would have little difficulty in learning how to use an incentive spirometer. **Answer 2** is incorrect because the client's occupation as a high school teacher would most likely not hinder her ability to learn to use an incentive spirometer. **Answer 4** is incorrect because the client's social situation has little bearing in this instance.

TEST-TAKING TIP—Recall several of the factors that influence client teaching: intelligence, educational level, environment, social support, occupation, perceived need, relevance, and immediacy. Look for the factor that is *pertinent to this case*.
AN, APP, 7, M/S: Preop, PhI, Reduction of Risk Potential

127. **(1) Girls *do* begin puberty before boys and thus are more developed at an earlier age. Girls usually begin to show signs of puberty about 2 years before boys show similar signs. Answer 2** is incorrect because girls do begin puberty first. There is no reason for the school nurse to pay a visit to the classroom to assess the growth and development of these students. **Answer 3** is incorrect because the school nurse fails to take responsibility for answering a question that is within the scope of the nurse's knowledge base and practice. This is an example of "passing the buck." In this instance, the school nurse shifts responsibility to the school physician. **Answer 4** is incorrect because the ethnic mix of the students in the classroom does not factor into why the girls are more developed than the boys. It is true that ethnicity has a role in the ultimate size of a child, but girls of most ethnic groups develop earlier than do boys of the same ethnic group.

> **TEST-TAKING TIP**—There are two contradictory responses: *normal* or *abnormal*. Decide which it is and select the option that is different (i.e., "normal").
> IMP, APP, 5, PEDS, HPM, Health Promotion and Maintenance

128. **(3) The nurse should gather more information, such as the client's wishes, the client's prognosis for regaining consciousness, the effect that the herbs are likely to have on the medical regimen, and the family dynamics to determine the ethically correct action. Answer 1** is incorrect because the herbs may interfere with the medical treatment regimen. It would be better to gather more data first. **Answer 2** is incorrect because the family may view administration of the herbs as an important care measure. It would be best to gather more data first. **Answer 4** is incorrect because staff input is only a part of the information that should be collected before deciding whether or not to comply with the family's wishes.

> **TEST-TAKING TIP**—The question is whether the nurse should, or should not, give medicinal herbs as the family has requested, when insufficient information is presented to determine the correct action. Collecting more data is the correct thing to do.
> IMP, ANL, 7, M/S: Herbal Meds, SECE, Management of Care

129. **(4) Sore nipples are usually caused by a poor latch. Making sure the infant has a good latch will help the client avoid sore nipples. Answer 1** is incorrect because this will not help the client's sore nipples. **Answer 2** is incorrect because this is a treatment for engorgement, *not* sore nipples. **Answer 3** is incorrect because this is the treatment for engorgement when the client is not breastfeeding.

> **TEST-TAKING TIP**—Focus on the *infant* here, not the breasts (**Answers 2** and **3**). When there are options that look familiar, carefully read the options and don't jump at the first answer that seems recognizable.
> IMP, APP, 4, Maternity, HPM, Health Promotion and Maintenance

130. **(2) The client has redefined aspects of life based on physical limitations and has found an alternative exercise program. Answer 1** is incorrect because recent memory loss is a sign of dementia and is *not a normal* characteristic of aging. **Answer 3** is incorrect because reducing contact with friends can lead to loneliness, and can be a sign that the client who is elderly may be depressed. **Answer 4** is incorrect because recognizing and accepting the aging process is a normal characteristic of aging and will help the client be successful.

> **TEST-TAKING TIP**—Find the answer that is different from the others. The correct answer is a positive action taken by the client and the incorrect answers are signs that the client's condition is diminishing.
> AN, ANL, 5, Psych, HPM, Health Promotion and Maintenance

131. **(4) Nurses are answerable for their actions. Accountability does not mean that the nurse acted correctly or incorrectly, competently or incompetently, but that the nurse is answerable. Answer 1** is incorrect because there is insufficient information in the scenario to determine the nurse's competence; the nurse could be viewed as incompetent because the error was made; however, the circumstances of the error are unknown. **Answer 2** is incorrect because "professionalism" is a broad term that encompasses many values essential to nursing. **Answer 3** is incorrect because reliability refers to the degree to which the nurse can be counted upon to act correctly. If this nurse reliably follows agency protocol for medication errors, the question must be asked: how often does this nurse commit medication errors?

> **TEST-TAKING TIP**—Consider the values that constitute a professional nurse: altruism, equality, esthetics, freedom, human dignity, justice, and truth. Focus on the option that falls within these values.
> IMP, APP, 1, M/S: Legal, SECE, Management of Care

132. **(2) Respect for the client self-determination is at the core of any nursing code of ethics. Answer 1** is incorrect because the nurse should remain as objective as possible when caring for clients. **Answer 3** is incorrect because an ethically correct action is not always the same as a legally correct action. **Answer 4** is incorrect because the physician's orders specify medical treatments, but do not address ethical issues.

> **TEST-TAKING TIP**—Choose the option that is client-focused. **Answers 1, 3,** and **4** all involve the nurse's perspective or the physician's. In contrast, **Answer 2** addresses the client as an individual.
> AN, ANL, 7, M/S: Legal/Ethics, SECE, Management of Care

133. **(3) Urinary tract infections are more common during pregnancy and bladder infections may irritate the uterus and cause preterm contractions. Answer 1** is incorrect because chorioamnionitis is related to prolonged rupture of membranes, multiple intrapartum vaginal exams, and internal fetal monitoring. **Answer 2** is incorrect because pelvic inflammatory disease is a chronic infection caused by a microbe which is sexually transmitted. **Answer 4** is incorrect because kidney stones are unrelated to urinary tract infections and are relatively *uncommon* in pregnancy.

> **TEST-TAKING TIP**—Consider the risk factor of frequent urinary tract infections; then consider the effect of pregnancy on the genitourinary system. Chorioamnionitis and pelvic inflammatory disease are infections, but are *not* related to frequent urinary tract infections.
> AN, APP, 8, Maternity, PhI, Physiological Adaptation

134. **(3) Clients have the right to refuse treatment, even if they are confused and disoriented. Also remember that it is important to document the medications as "not given" and the reason. Answer 1** is incorrect because, although the physician should be notified that the client is confused and agitated, the physician cannot order the client to take the medications. It is the nurse's responsibility to administer the medications. **Answer 2** is incorrect because, although clients should be informed about their medications, a client who is confused may have difficulty understanding the information. **Answer 4** is incorrect because using force ("restrain the

client") to get the client to take medications is called assault and battery, and is illegal, even with a client who is confused.

> **TEST-TAKING TIP**—Look for the answer that provides the most positive outcome for the client. **Answers 1** and **4** involve *others*, not the client.
> **IMP, ANL, 7, M/S: Legal, SECE, Management of Care**

135. **(4) Assessment is always the first step in the nursing process. The nurse must obtain information (subjective as well as objective) that will provide data about what the child is and is not eating before a plan of action and care can be devised.** Answer 1 is incorrect because, while the action in itself is not incorrect, it does not provide the nurse with an individualized picture of this specific child and the child's specific eating patterns. **Answer 2** is incorrect because, while the action in itself is not incorrect, it does not provide the nurse with an individualized picture of this specific child and the child's specific eating patterns. **Answer 3** is incorrect because 4-year-old children still have food habits such as food fads and strong taste preferences. Also, 4-year-olds also tend to be rebellious. Thus, it is unlikely that the child would self select appropriate, acceptable foods.

> **TEST-TAKING TIP**—Assessment provides the foundation for all subsequent nursing actions. It is always the first step taken by the nurse and is the correct response here.
> **IMP, APP, 4, PEDS, PhI, Basic Care and Comfort**

136. **(2) Harm occurred to the client.** Answer 1 is incorrect because the client was not harmed or put in danger by incorrect care. **Answer 3** is incorrect because the client was not harmed or put in danger by incorrect care. **Answer 4** is incorrect because the client was not harmed by incorrect care.

> **TEST-TAKING TIP**—Look for the answer that places the client in *danger of being harmed* by incorrect care.
> **IMP, ANL, 7, M/S: Legal, SECE, Management of Care**

137. **(3) The client with pregnancy-induced hypertension is the least stable of the clients, and IV magnesium sulfate requires additional observation by an RN.** Answer 1 is incorrect because a LVN/LPN *could* care for a client with a stable wound infection, and the supervising RN could administer the IV antibiotics. **Answer 2** is incorrect because a client with a third degree laceration *could* be assigned to a LVN/LPN. **Answer 4** is incorrect because an LVN/LPN *could* care for a pregnant client whose condition is stable, with a diagnosis of hyperemesis. The supervising RN could manage the IV medications.

> **TEST-TAKING TIP**—When determining appropriate assignments, the clients who are most stable are the best choices for an LVN/LPN. A client who is critical or unstable, or a client with risk factors that may lead to a changing condition, should not be assigned to an LVN/LPN.
> **PL, APP, 1, Maternity, SECE, Management of Care: Delegation**

138. **(1) The purpose of unusual occurrence, or incident, reports are to identify recurrent client-care problems so that they may be prevented in the future.** Answer 2 is incorrect because the purpose of unusual occurrence reports is to *prevent lawsuits*. **Answer 3** is incorrect because, although the nurse is obligated to continually evaluate own performance, unusual occurrence reports are *intended to prevent* problems, *not punish* the nurse. **Answer 4** is incorrect because the intent of an unusual occurrence report is to solve problems; it is not intended to be punitive. Keep in mind, however, that unusual occurrence reports document specific client-care problems, and would be reviewed in the event of a lawsuit.

> **TEST-TAKING TIP**—Look for the answer that positively addresses *client* problems, rather than hospital or nurse problems.
> **PL, COM, 7, M/S: Legal, SECE, Management of Care**

139. **(3) It states simply, yet correctly, what the DDST does and thus answers the mother's question.** Answer 1 is incorrect because the DDST assesses children from 0–6 years of age in 4 categories: personal-social, fine motor-adaptive, language, and gross motor. Screening tests, such as the DDST, should *not* be used for diagnostic purposes (example: to determine if the child is "normal") but rather to determine if further assessment is needed. The DDST does not supply the "whole picture" regarding development. **Answer 2** is incorrect because it is vague and does not supply the mother with sufficient information about what exactly the DDST does test. It is the nurse's responsibility to supply the mother with information prior to any screening procedure as to exactly what is the purpose and intent of the screening procedure. **Answer 4** is incorrect because the DDST does not test for intelligence. A test such as the Kaufman Brief Intelligence. Test would supply information regarding the child's intelligence quotient.

> **TEST-TAKING TIP**—Look for the most simple, yet comprehensive, answer that a parent could comprehend.
> **IMP, COM, 7, PEDS, PhI, Reduction of Risk Potential**

140. **(4) This response is age-typical and provides health teaching about normal relationship changes that occur after the children leave home.** Answer 1 is incorrect because it stops the conversation and may not be true. **Answer 2** is incorrect because it is false reassurance and may not be true. **Answer 3** is incorrect because experiencing loss in life will come in the *later* years of life.

> **TEST-TAKING TIP**—Eliminate trite clichés (**Answers 1** and **2**) and a response that is too definitive (e.g., **Answer 3**: "You will …").
> **IMP, APP, 5, Psych, HPM, Health Promotion and Maintenance**

141. **(3) Since this client is dilated at 29 weeks gestation, tocolytics are ordered to decrease contractions, IV hydration is used to prevent maternal dehydration, and bedrest is to decrease pressure on the cervix.** Answer 1 is incorrect because strict bedrest can lead to the development of thrombophlebitis. **Answer 2** is incorrect because strict bedrest in pregnancy can lead to thrombophlebitis. **Answer 4** is incorrect because a cervical cerclage is placed earlier than 29 weeks gestation to prevent spontaneous abortion caused by cervical incompetence.

> **TEST-TAKING TIP**—First, break down the answers into individual options. If one option can be easily eliminated, all the answers with that same option can also be eliminated (e.g., **Answers 1** and **2**).
> **PL, APP, 5, Maternity, PhI, Pharmacological and Parenteral Therapies**

142. **(1) G is the designation for total number of pregnancies, in this case 5; *P* is preterm deliveries, the number of deliveries more than 20 weeks, but less than 37 weeks; *T* is term deliveries, greater than 37 weeks gestation, in this case 0. *AB* is the total number of abortions including spontaneous and induced, in this case 3.** Answer 2 is incorrect because the calculation for total pregnancies is incorrect. It should be a total of five. The *P* is incorrect; the two spontaneous abortions are counted incorrectly. **Answer 3** is incorrect because the 27-week-gestation pregnancy is counted as

a full-term delivery. **Answer 4** is incorrect because the *G* is incorrectly calculated as 6, rather than 5.

> **TEST-TAKING TIP**—Calculate the answer before looking at the options. Then compare the answers with your calculation.
> **AN, COM, 5, Maternity, HPM, Health Promotion and Maintenance**

143. **(1, 4, 6) Answer 1 is correct because an ileostomy produces liquid stool. The client's daily fluid intake should be 2–3 liters to prevent dehydration from loss of fluid via stool. Answer 4 is correct because fecal drainage, or a poorly fitting ostomy appliance can irritate and erode the stoma and surrounding skin. Answer 6 is correct because the client with an ileostomy is often concerned about loss of sexual appeal or leakage of fecal material during sexual activity. Answer 2** is incorrect because an ileostomy produces liquid stool; therefore, the client is at risk for fluid volume deficit, not excess. **Answer 3** is incorrect because an ileostomy produces liquid stool; therefore, constipation is not a typical problem. However, the client should be counseled to avoid foods that can cause blockages in the intestine, such as whole grains, nuts, and some raw vegetables. **Answer 5** is incorrect because a client with an ileostomy is more likely at risk for *nutrition less than body requirements*.

> **TEST-TAKING TIP**—Remember that an ileostomy produces liquid stool. Therefore, many of the potential risks for this client involve *the loss* of liquid stool: fluid volume deficit, nutrition less than body requirements, and irritation of the stoma and surrounding skin. In addition, altered sexuality is a concern for any client with a bowel or urinary diversion.
> **EV, ANL, 8, M/S: GI, PhI, Physiological Adaptation**

144. **(1, 4, 5) Answer 1 is correct because the client's right to confidentiality was violated when the nurse left the computer screen showing the client's medications. Answer 4 is correct because the client's rights to privacy and confidentiality were violated when the physician and nurse talked about client information across the nurse's station. Answer 5 is correct because the client's right to confidentiality was violated when the nursing students discussed their clients in a public place. Answer 2** is incorrect because clients have the right to refuse treatment. **Answer 3** is incorrect because the client's rights were not violated in this case. The client, however, did not fulfill the responsibility to inform the health-care team about allergy to penicillin. **Answer 6** is incorrect because the client does not have the right to have an unlimited number of visitors, particularly if it is disruptive to other clients. While the hospital's goal is to promote the client's welfare, the hospital does have a responsibility to provide equitable care for all clients. In addition, the client and family have a responsibility to make reasonable accommodations that allow the hospital to fulfill this obligation.

> **TEST-TAKING TIP**—Notice that **Answers 2, 3,** and **6** refer to the client; it would be difficult for clients to violate their own rights. Instead, focus on the options that involve actions by the hospital or staff.
> **EV, ANL, 7: Legal, SECE, Management of Care**

145. **75–125.** The first step is to convert 165 lb to 75 kg (165/2.2). The next step is to determine the dose range per *day* by multiplying 75 kg by 3 mg and 5 mg, respectively (225–375 mg/day). The final step is to divide the dose range by 3, which is the number of doses given per day (q8h).

> **TEST-TAKING TIP**—There are several steps to completing this problem. The essential part is remembering

that "q8h" means 3 doses will be given per day; therefore the dose range of 225–375 must be divided by 3 to get the final answer.
PL, ANL, 1, M/S: Calculation, PhI, Pharmacological and Parenteral Therapies

146. **(3) The best way to help preschoolers overcome fear is to actively involve them in finding ways of dealing with frightening experiences. Turning on a night light at bedtime could supply the preschooler with both the necessary assurance and sense of control needed to face the fear. Answer 1** is incorrect because preschoolers tend to have fears of the dark, being left alone (especially at bedtime), fears about animals and monsters. This is a *normal* part of a preschooler's development and does not require a psychiatric evaluation. **Answer 2** is incorrect because preschoolers have vivid imaginations on their own and viewing television before bedtime is probably not the stimulus of choice for the behavior. **Answer 4** is incorrect because pet therapy programs are generally used in pediatrics to bolster a child's self-esteem and increase the child's abilities to relate to others rather than overcoming normal childhood fears.

> **TEST-TAKING TIP**—Look for the simple, positive intervention that might remedy the situation before selecting more complex responses to the question.
> **IMP, APP, 7, PEDS, PsI, Psychosocial Integrity**

147. **(3) It allows the child to have a say in what happens and thus assists the child to maintain a sense of control. Obviously, the choices offered to the child would be assessed for appropriateness by the nurse and the parents. Answer 1** is incorrect because, while the response in itself is a good idea, it will provide needed socialization for the child rather than assisting the child to maintain a sense of control. **Answer 2** is incorrect because, while the response in itself is a good idea, it will provide needed emotional release and diversion for the child rather than assisting the child to maintain a sense of control. **Answer 4** is incorrect because it implies that the child will not have limits set. This could be detrimental to the child's recovery.

> **TEST-TAKING TIP**—The key to the correct response in this question is the phrase "as possible." It sets a limit on what will and what will not be acceptable.
> **IMP, APP, 5, PEDS, PsI, Psychosocial Integrity**

148. <u>**23.**</u> The physician's order directs the nurse to replace the client's potassium, 2-for-1, to 5.5 mEq/L. The first, and most crucial, step is to determine how many tenths below 5.5 mEq/L the client's K$^+$ is. Subtract 3.2 from 5.5 and the answer is 2.3, or *23 tenths*. The next step is to double 23 because the order says to give *2 mEq* of potassium for each tenth; the nurse needs to give 46 mEq of potassium. Finally, figure out how many milliliters of potassium should be taken from the vial on hand. This can be done with a simple ratio:
2 mEq/1 mL = 46 mEq/x mL. Solve for x and the answer is 23 mL.

> **TEST-TAKING TIP**—The most difficult part of this question is figuring out how many *tenths* below 5.5 mEq/L is the client's potassium level. In this case, the answer is *23 tenths, not 2.3.*
> **IMP, APP, 1, M/S: Cardiac, PhI, Pharmacological and Parenteral Therapies**

149. **(3, 4, 6) Answer 3 is correct because calcium levels decrease in chronic renal failure. The milk would provide a source of calcium as well as protein that is of high biological value. Four ounces of fluid would fit into the client's fluid

restriction, **Answer 4 is correct because lettuce and cucumber are not contraindicated for the client with chronic renal failure, and would be considered 1 vegetable exchange. Answer 6 is correct because clients with chronic renal failure increase the fat and carbohydrate calories in their diets. The bread would *not* be contraindicated.** Answer 1 is incorrect because the client with chronic renal failure on hemodialysis should restrict protein intake to 1.0–1.5 g/kg to help reduce nitrogenous wastes. Two chicken breasts would exceed the protein restriction. **Answer 2** is incorrect because the client with chronic renal failure on hemodialysis should restrict potassium intake to 2–3 grams per day. Eight ounces of tomato juice, along with the rest of the client's diet for the day, would most likely exceed the client's potassium allowance. In addition, fluids are restricted for clients with chronic renal failure, and 8 ounces of fluid would be too much. **Answer 5** is incorrect because, although clients in chronic renal failure derive most of their calories from carbohydrate and fat, they should restrict sodium. Mayonnaise is generally high in sodium.

TEST-TAKING TIP—Recall dietary guidelines for clients with chronic renal failure: restricted protein, restricted fluids, restricted sodium and potassium, increased carbohydrates and fat. Choose the food items that fit these guidelines (**Answers 3, 4,** and **6**).
EV, ANL, 4, M/S: Renal, PhI, Basic Care and Comfort

150. **(1) These are normal behavior changes seen in adolescents.** Answer 2 is incorrect because it is during the *latency* age period that the child is concerned with accomplishing tasks. **Answer 3** is incorrect because the adolescent's relationship with parents is usually *strained*. **Answer 4** is incorrect because crying frequently for no reason *is* a sign of moodiness, and is covered in **Answer 1**, the correct answer.

TEST-TAKING TIP—Focus on *normal* behavior and eliminate **Answer 3**. Choose the umbrella answer, the answer that is the most inclusive. Note the age-appropriate answer and eliminate **Answer 2**.
AS, ANL, 5, Psych, HPM, Health Promotion and Maintenance

151. **(3) No tolerance to constipation will occur. The client needs instruction on the importance of diet, fluids, and possibly stool softeners to manage the long-term problem.** Answer 1 is incorrect because tolerance will develop to most adverse effects of narcotics except constipation. If confusion occurred, the drug would likely have been changed and not continued on a long-term basis. **Answer 2** is incorrect because tolerance will develop to most adverse effects of narcotics except constipation. If the blood pressure was dangerously low, the narcotic would have been changed. **Answer 4** is incorrect because tolerance will develop to most adverse effects of narcotics except constipation. If respiratory depression, an adverse effect, was present, the narcotic would likely have been changed because of the risk to the client.

TEST-TAKING TIP—The key is "long-term" effect. If the other three side effects occurred, the drug would be stopped or the dosage changed.
PL, COM, 8, M/S: Substance Use, PhI, Pharmacological and Parenteral Therapies

152. **(1, 4) Answer 1 is correct because swelling of the face, feet, and hands can be symptoms of pregnancy-induced hypertension which requires immediate evaluation. Answer 4 is correct because headaches that are unrelieved by acetaminophen need to be evaluated immediately because this can be an indicator of pregnancy-induced hypertension.** Answer 2 is incorrect because uterine contractions during

position changes are a *normal* part of pregnancy. **Answer 3** is incorrect because decreased vaginal discharge does *not* require medical intervention. **Answer 5** is incorrect because increased fetal movement is an indicator of a *healthy* fetus.

TEST-TAKING TIP—The key word in this question is "immediate." Examine each of the options individually; decide if the symptom needs immediate medical attention. If not, eliminate that option.
IMP, APP, 1, Maternity, HPM, Health Promotion and Maintenance

153. **(1) Foot drop, which is plantar flexion, can be prevented by dorsiflexing the feet in rigid boots or high-top shoes.** Answer 2 is incorrect because the feet will still plantar-flex. While keeping the sheets off the feet minimizes the pressure on the feet, boots or shoes are the only thing that will prevent foot drop. **Answer 3** is incorrect because turning will prevent pressure sores, but while on the back, the foot will tend to drop. **Answer 4** is incorrect because raising the heels off the bed will prevent pressure sores, but will *not* prevent plantar flexion.

TEST-TAKING TIP—Asks for the "best action." Consider which choice keeps foot in normal position.
PL, COM, 3, M/S: Ortho, PhI, Basic Care and Comfort

154. **(4) Endometritis is an infection of the endometrial lining that is characterized by a temperature greater than 100.4°F, tender uterus, and foul-smelling lochia.** Answer 1 is incorrect because a urinary tract infection is not associated with foul smelling *lochia*. **Answer 2** is incorrect because endometriosis is a condition in which endometrial tissue, the tissue that lines the inside of the uterus, grows outside the uterus and attaches to other organs in the abdominal cavity, such as the ovaries and fallopian tubes. It is *not* an infection. **Answer 3** is incorrect because bacterial vaginosis is an infection of the vagina. It is usually caused by an overgrowth of bacteria normally present in the vagina.

TEST-TAKING TIP—Be aware that terms seem similar, that is, they may be only slightly different, but they have *very different meanings* (e.g., **Answer 2** and **Answer 4**).
AN, APP, 1, Women's Health, SECE, Safety and Infection Control

155. **(4) This is an immediate, age-appropriate intervention that the nurse can take to correct the situation. The child life specialist could play a game about drinking (e.g., a tea party) with the toddler and persuade the toddler to drink the desired fluids. If this intervention fails, then the nurse should document the I&O, ask for the mother's assistance, and report the situation to the pediatrician.** Answer 1 is incorrect because there has been no weight loss and thus the toddler is not becoming dehydrated. There is no need to notify the pediatrician at the present time. **Answer 2** is incorrect because it is not known when the mother might be coming back to visit with the child and it might not be soon enough. The toddler *does* need to start drinking as soon as possible. **Answer 3** is incorrect because, while documenting the toddler's I&O is a correct action on the nurse's part, it is not the best action for the nurse to take at the present time because a direct intervention is needed rather than an intervention on paper (i.e., "Document …").

TEST-TAKING TIP—Always select the simplest, fastest intervention first in a noncritical or life-threatening situation.
IMP, ANL, 6, PEDS, PhI, Basic Care and Comfort

156. **(1) It is an inappropriate nursing action. The client will breathe more easily in a semi-Fowler's position. The legs**

are elevated in a modified-Trendelenburg, and the trunk is flat. Ankle edema will lessen when the client is supine. **Answer 2** is incorrect. Adequate nutrition with modification in sodium intake *is* appropriate. **Answer 3** is incorrect because teaching about indications of increasing failure *is* appropriate. **Answer 4** is incorrect because it *is* appropriate to provide time for the client to voice concerns.

> **TEST-TAKING TIP**—Look for the choice that would potentially result in client discomfort or distress. Question asks about what is *not* ok.
> **PL, COM, 6, M/S: CV, PhI, Basic Care and Comfort**

157. **(4) The Hct is very low. It would be important to check the vital signs to determine if the client is experiencing signs of poor perfusion. The physician should be notified immediately of the lab results and vital signs.** Answer 1 is incorrect because hemoconcentration results in an *increase* in the Hct. The normal range for the Hct is 35%–45%; 23% is very low. **Answer 2** is incorrect because 23% is *very low* and would indicate the client has been bleeding. **Answer 3** is incorrect because 23% would not be considered a slight drop. The normal range is 35%–45%.

> **TEST-TAKING TIP**—Know the acceptable ranges for common lab tests. Ask if a specific value is "OK" or "not OK." Two of the answer choices focus on "not OK." Choose the one that requires immediate attention.
> **AN, ANL, 6, M/S: GI, PhI, Reduction of Risk Potential**

158. **(2) The peritoneum is filled with carbon dioxide during the procedure and the pressure on the diaphragm can cause not only shoulder pain but more complaints of nausea and vomiting than the open cholecystectomy.** Answer 1 is incorrect because pneumonia is *unlikely* with the laparoscopic approach. It is a greater risk with the conventional open cholecystectomy. **Answer 3** is incorrect because the procedure is done using general anesthesia, *not* spinal anesthesia. **Answer 4** is incorrect because a T tube would be inserted during an *open* cholecystectomy with exploration of the common bile duct.

> **TEST-TAKING TIP**—Two possible choices—only one would occur with general anesthesia.
> **IMP, COM, 4, M/S:GI, PhI, Reduction of Risk Potential**

159. **(2) Procedures of any type should not be continued when the child is crying, protesting, upset, or frightened. The nurse should stop and reassure the child. The nurse may need to do this several times during the procedure. This is to be expected in this age group despite having prepared the child for the procedure before actually beginning the procedure. A 3-year-old child is very concerned about being hurt and has many body mutilation fears and issues.** Answer 1 is incorrect because, while it is a correct action in itself, it is *not the first* action that the nurse should take. **Answer 3** is incorrect because, while it is a correct action in itself, it is *not the first* action that the nurse should take. **Answer 4** is incorrect because the pediatrician expects that the nurse will accomplish the removal of the nasogastric tube, and sedation is not used in pediatrics for simple procedures such as the removal of a nasogastric tube. Sedation is used in more painful and complex procedures such as a bone marrow aspiration (BMA).

> **TEST-TAKING TIP**—A primary goal in nursing is to "do no harm." Select the answer that would accomplish this goal.
> **IMP, ANL, 7, PEDS, PsI, Psychosocial Integrity**

160. **(4) This answers the client's question truthfully and directly. Answer 1** is incorrect because research does

indicate that the influenza virus in utero can cause schizophrenia in the infant. **Answer 2** is incorrect because it offers false reassurance and does not address the client's question. **Answer 3** is incorrect because the nurse should avoid "why" questions, and it belittles the client for asking the question.

> **TEST-TAKING TIP**—Eliminate the trite cliché and incorrect answer (**Answer 2**). **Answers 1** and **4** are both causes of schizophrenia; however, long answers with technical language are usually not the best answer, so **Answer 1** can be eliminated.
> **IMP, APP, 5, Psych, HPM, Health Promotion and Maintenance**

161. **(3) The Pap smear checks for changes in the cells of the cervix that may indicate an infection, abnormal cells, or cancer. Answer 1** is incorrect because the Pap smear *does not* detect the presence of *chlamydia trachomatis*. **Answer 2** is incorrect because the test for neural tube defects is an *alpha-fetoprotein (AFP) test*. **Answer 4** is incorrect because an *amniocentesis* is the test to obtain fetal cells for genetic testing.

> **TEST-TAKING TIP**—Select the option that is different: **Answers 1, 2, and 4** relate to the fetus. Only **Answer 3** relates to the woman.
> **PL, APP, 1, Women's Health, HPM, Health Promotion and Maintenance**

162. **(2) Exercise will *increase* the HDL level and lower the LDL level, thus slowing or delaying the progression of the coronary heart disease. Answer 1** is incorrect because exercise *will* improve stamina and strength, and is an expected outcome. **Answer 3** is incorrect because exercise *will* improve peripheral blood flow and perfusion to the extremities. **Answer 4** is incorrect because exercise is an important activity to reduce all types of stress.

> **TEST-TAKING TIP**—Read the stem carefully. Looking for something that is undesirable. **Answers 1, 3,** and **4** *are* desirable.
> **IMP, APP, 6, M/S:CV, HPM, Health Promotion and Maintenance**

163. **(2) Treatment will often be a combination of clarithromycin (Biacin), metronidazole (Flagyl), and omeprazole (Prilosec) or ranitidine (Zantac) for one week. A second week might be given for 10% of the clients. Answer 1** is incorrect because 90% of all peptic ulcers are caused by *H. pylori* inflammation. While antacids are still used to increase gastric pH and strengthen the gastric mucosal barrier, antibiotics are the most important component of treatment for PUD. **Answer 3** is incorrect because stress is *not* the cause of PUD in 90% of clients. *Gastritis*, an inflammation of the gastric mucosa, *is* linked to prolonged emotional tension. **Answer 4** is incorrect because the priority for treatment is *prevention* of bleeding. A nasogastric tube would likely be inserted to assess bleeding if present. The Minnesota or Blakemore tubes are used in the treatment of esophageal varices.

> **TEST-TAKING TIP**—The "most effective" action is *eliminating* the cause. All other choices merely *manage* symptoms.
> **PL, ANL, 4, M/S:GI, PhI, Reduction of Risk Potential**

164. **(4) Constipation should be avoided in clients with a fourth-degree episiotomy. Stool softeners and increased fluid intake will assist in preventing constipation. Answer 1** is incorrect because increasing roughage alone will not prevent constipation. **Answer 2** is incorrect because hot packs will not act to assist healing in a fourth-degree episiotomy. **Answer 3** is incorrect because ice packs are used to decrease swelling for the *first 24 hours* after delivery.

TEST-TAKING TIP—Visualize what a fourth-degree episiotomy looks like. It is important to know the complications of an extensive episiotomy.
PL, APP, 8, Maternity, PhI, Basic Care and Comfort

165. **(2) Acidosis will occur from fat metabolism. Fluids are essential to prevent damage to the kidneys. The nurse should determine if the client's physician is aware of this dietary change because a diet without carbohydrates is not considered healthy. Some complex carbohydrates are recommended so that fat burning can occur without acidosis.** Answer 1 is incorrect because a diet with no carbohydrates is generally not recommended. Some carbohydrates are needed to prevent acidosis from occurring as a result of fat metabolism. Extremes in dietary modification should not be recommended without consultation with a client's physician. **Answer 3** is incorrect because the nurse has the responsibility to ensure that the client is not at risk for adverse effects from an unhealthy or extreme weight loss program. **Answer 4** is incorrect because the nurse should not reinforce a diet that is not balanced and has the potential for adverse consequences.

TEST-TAKING TIP—Choose the only choice that addresses concern with eliminating one major dietary component (CHO).
IMP, APP, 4, M/S: Diet, PhI, Basic Care and Comfort

166. **(3) Racemic epinephrine has a rapid onset, but the peak effect is observed in 2 hours. Additional doses may need to be administered every 20–30 minutes in the pediatric intensive care unit or every 3–4 hours on the pediatric unit. The nurse needs to focus on the child's respiratory status in order to identify the return of airway obstruction and treat it promptly while waiting for a pediatric bed to become available.** Answer 1 is incorrect because the child will be coughing and may have laryngeal spasms. Oral fluids could potentially be aspirated. The child's hydration needs will be handled via the intravenous route. In a child with mild croup, which can be managed at home, oral fluids are essential. In a child with severe croup, intravenous fluids are essential. **Answer 2** is incorrect because, while oxygen may be needed, it is *not* the priority nursing intervention. **Answer 4** is incorrect because respiratory monitoring equipment supplements, but *does not replace,* visual observations of the child. Racemic epinephrine, not oxygen, will cause mucosal vasoconstriction, which will decrease the subglottic edema accompanying laryngotracheobronchitis.

TEST-TAKING TIP—See the word "assessing" in **Answer 3,** which is the key to answering this question correctly, as well as knowing the action of racemic epinephrine. "Assessing" *before* "administering" or "measuring."
IMP, APP, 6, PEDS, PhI, Pharmacological and Parenteral Therapies

167. **(1) A low carbohydrate diet will be high in protein and fats.** Answer 2 is incorrect because the diet is extremely high in carbohydrates. Breads that are 100% whole grain, and identified as complete protein breads, may be included in the diet. **Answer 3** is incorrect because cereals, creamed soups, and canned fruits are all high in carbohydrates. **Answer 4** is incorrect because the candied fruits in fruitcake and the sugar in applesauce would not be on the diet. Fruits are generally restricted, although some are lower in carbohydrate and may be included.

TEST-TAKING TIP—Know food choices for basic food groups.
IMP, KNOW, 4, M/S: Diet, PhI, Basic Care and Comfort

168. **(2) The pyloric muscle, rather than the stomach, is entered during the surgical correction. Absence or a decrease in bowel sounds following a pyloromyotomy is normally not a problem, and feeding can usually be resumed as soon as the infant is fully awake.** Answer 1 is incorrect because beginning incremental glucose (and/or electrolyte) water feedings when the infant is fully awake is a *standardized* procedure following a pyloromyotomy. **Answer 3** is incorrect because routine vital signs are a *standardized* procedure following a pyloromyotomy. **Answer 4** is incorrect because strict I&O is a *standardized* procedure following a pyloromyotomy.

TEST-TAKING TIP—The key to answering this question is to know that a pyloromyotomy is usually done via laparoscope which results in a shorter surgical time, and does not enter the stomach. Thus peristalsis (i.e., bowel sounds) is not usually affected.
AN, ANL, 1, PEDS, SECE, Management of Care

169. **(1) Obstruction of the cystic duct from gall stones causes distention of the gallbladder and a characteristic sudden steady pain in the epigastric, subscapular or right upper quadrant of the abdomen that peaks in 30 minutes.** Answer 2 is incorrect because pain with endometriosis is *not* located consistently in one place and would *not* begin *suddenly.* **Answer 3** is incorrect because the pain of irritable bowel syndrome (IBS) is typically in the lower left quadrant of the abdomen. **Answer 4** is incorrect because Crohn's, an inflammatory bowel disease, will have a "colicky" type of pain in the lower abdominal quadrants, associated with diarrhea.

TEST-TAKING TIP—Know typical causes of pain in abdominal quadrants. Think about location of organ or structure causing pain.
AN, COM, 3, M/S: GI, PhI, Basic Care and Comfort

170. **(1, 2, 5, 6) Answer 1 is correct because social isolation with other prodromal symptoms is an early sign that the client may have a psychotic episode. Answer 2 is correct because magical thinking is an early indicator that the client is beginning to have a psychotic episode. Answer 5 is correct because sensing the presence of a force is a prodromal sign. Answer 6 is correct because a change in cognitive functioning, such as a drop in school grades, is an early warning of an approaching psychotic break.** Answer 3 is incorrect because hallucinations and delusions are symptoms of psychosis and are *not prodromal* signs. **Answer 4** is incorrect because hallucinations and delusions are symptoms of psychosis and are *not prodromal* signs.

TEST-TAKING TIP—The correct answers involve changes in perception *without* full psychosis. If you do not know what prodromal symptoms are, look at clues in the stem. The question asks for symptoms *before* psychosis. It does *not* ask for signs of psychosis.
AS, ANL, 2, Psych, HPM, Health Promotion and Maintenance

171. **(4) Treatment of the eyes of a newborn infant prevents the complication of permanent eye damage.** Answer 1 is incorrect because many people do *not know* they have gonorrhea, because although they are infected, they do not have any symptoms. **Answer 2** is incorrect because the infection transmitted at birth affects the *eyes* of the newborn infant causing permanent damage. It does not affect the genitals of the newborn. **Answer 3** is incorrect because the antibiotics used to treat gonorrhea infections *are safe* to use during pregnancy.

TEST-TAKING TIP—Read the answers carefully; sometimes the answer can appear to be correct when it is not correct due to one word in the sentence.
IMP, COM, 1, Maternity, SECE, Safety and Infection Control

172. **(3) The laparoscopic procedure involves usually 4 small incisions. There are no drains and the client is able to go home in less than 24 hours.** Answer 1 is incorrect because there are *no drains* with a laparoscopic cholecystectomy. A T tube is used if exploration of the common bile duct occurred with the *conventional* surgical approach. **Answer 2** is incorrect because there are *no drains* with the laparoscopic approach. If a drain is needed to drain bile, the client would not have a laparoscopic cholecystectomy. **Answer 4** is incorrect because a midline incision describes the *conventional* surgical approach used for gallbladder removal.

TEST-TAKING TIP—Know the advantages of selected surgical techniques (e.g., no drains). Eliminate two options that focus on "drains".
IMP, KNOW, 8, M/S:GI, PhI, Reduction of Risk Potential

173. **(3) The contrast agent used is iodine-based. In severe allergic reactions anaphylactic shock could result. The contrast may still be given to clients who report allergies. The client will be pretreated with an antihistamine or corticosteroid.** Answer 1 is incorrect because *no tube* is inserted with the test. A contrast dye is either injected or a dilute oral barium may be given. **Answer 2** is incorrect because the client is *NPO* for 6–12 hours before an abdominal CT. A high fat diet is consumed during an oral cholecystogram (gallbladder series), which is rarely used. **Answer 4** is incorrect because the lead apron would *obscure* the area to be visualized during the test.

TEST-TAKING TIP—The key word is "contrast." Think potential allergy.
IMP, COM, 8, M/S: GI, PhI, Reduction of Risk Potential

174. **(1) A barium enema (lower GI series) is indicated for clients experiencing altered bowel habits. The intestines must be free of feces for the test to be accurate. A low residue or clear liquid diet is taken for 2 days before the test. A potent laxative and an oral agent to clean the bowel is given the day before. A suppository or enema may be given the morning of the test.** Answer 2 is incorrect because the barium is instilled rectally, *not* orally as with a barium swallow or upper GI series. **Answer 3** is incorrect because the barium is instilled rectally, *not* orally as with a barium swallow or upper GI series. **Answer 4** is incorrect because the client needs to be on a low residue or clear liquid diet for several days to reduce fecal volume. A full meal would *not* be indicated before the test.

TEST-TAKING TIP—Look for patterns. Three of the choices involve taking something orally but the test is an enema!
PL, COM, 8, M/S: GI, PhI, Reduction of Risk Potential

175. **(3) In Hirschsprung's disease a lack of peristalsis in the lower colon causes an accumulation of intestinal contents and distention. The abdominal circumference will provide the nurse will both baseline and ongoing data regarding the progression of the accumulation of intestinal contents.** Answer 1 is incorrect because, while weight is in itself an important assessment to determine the newborn's hydration status, it is not the most important nursing assessment. **Answer 2** is incorrect because, while hydration is in itself an important assessment to determine the newborn's perfusion status, it is not the most important nursing assessment.

Answer 4 is incorrect because, while laboratory values such as hemoglobin/hematocrit, sodium and potassium are in themselves important assessments to determine the newborn's metabolic status, they are not the most important nursing assessment.

TEST-TAKING TIP—Knowing the pathophysiology associated with Hirschsprung's disease is the key to answering this question correctly.
AS, APP, 8, PEDS, PhI, Reduction of Risk Potential

176. **(3) Most women with a diagnosis of breast cancer do not have *any* identified pattern of risk factors.** Answer 1 is incorrect because while it is the most common risk factor, most women with breast cancer do *not* have any identified risk factors. **Answer 2** is incorrect because although "not breastfeeding" *is* a risk factor, it is not so for most women with breast cancer. **Answer 4** is incorrect because breast self examination is *no longer recommended* as a screening tool for breast cancer. A recent study showed that breast self-exam did not prevent mortality. It is recommended to have a yearly clinical breast exam by a medical professional as well as a mammogram.

TEST-TAKING TIP—The question asks about women with a confirmed diagnosis of breast cancer and what these women have in common. Do not confuse this with the identification of risk factors for the development of breast cancer.
AN, APP, 5, Women's Health, HPM, Health Promotion and Maintenance

177. **(3) Successful post-exposure prophylaxis has been seen with the use of 2 drugs (zidovudine and lamivudine) for 4 weeks.** Answer 1 is incorrect because post-exposure prophylaxis is recommended for *4 weeks*, and 1 of the drugs should be zidovudine. **Answer 2** is incorrect because two *drugs* are recommended for post-exposure prophylaxis, including zidivudine. **Answer 4** is incorrect because the likelihood is high that something in the sharps container contains HIV. Treatment needs to begin *immediately*.

TEST-TAKING TIP—Use a process of elimination—remember combination therapy and repeated doses. Only 1 answer lists two drugs.
PL, APP, 1, M/S: Infectious Disease, PhI, Pharmacological Therapy

178. **(4) The client is very cold. The normal range for the temperature in centigrade is 36°– 37.5°C with an average of 37°C. Hypothermia will disrupt normal physiology and needs to be corrected quickly.** Answer 1 is incorrect because the vital signs do *not* indicate the need for rapid infusing of fluids or in large volume. Shock is a complication of hypothyroidism; however, the pulse and blood pressure are within *normal* ranges. **Answer 2** is incorrect because the immediate concern is severe hypothermia. Warming the client can be done easily and quickly, followed by administration of medications. **Answer 3** is incorrect because warming needs to be done regardless of the results of the thyroid levels.

TEST-TAKING TIP—A priority question—where all choices are correct, select the one that directly improves the client's comfort level. Eliminate two invasive actions (**Answers 1** and **3**) and one medication action.
IMP, ANL, 3, M/S: Endocrine, PhI, Reduction of Risk Potential

179. **(1) In infants with hydrocephalus, the head grows at an abnormal rate.** Answer 2 is incorrect because the site of the shunt malfunction is in the ventricles rather than the

abdomen. The shunt provides drainage of the cerebral spinal fluid (CSF) from the ventricles into an extracranial compartment (usually the peritoneum). The abdominal circumference would not be increasing. **Answer 3** is incorrect because difficulty in sucking and feeding will be present only if hydrocephalus is allowed to progress and no intervention is taken. This infant *is* being admitted to the pediatric unit for a surgical intervention. **Answer 4** is incorrect because in an infant with hydrocephalus, lethargy, rather than hyperactivity, is usually noted.

> **TEST-TAKING TIP**—Note the term "cephalus," meaning *head*, which corresponds with **Answer 1**, the best option.
> **AS, APP, 2, PEDS, PhI, Basic Care and Comfort**

180. **(1) Preoccupation with appearance and inflated ideas about the body and beauty is a sign of a disturbance in the body image, which is central to the diagnosis of anorexia nervosa and bulimia. Answer 2** is incorrect because adolescents use their body to attract the opposite sex. This is a *normal* part of developing a sound body image. **Answer 3** is incorrect because it is *normal* for adolescent girls to compare their body to peers and to feel anxious over the changes. **Answer 4** is incorrect because this statement indicates that the client is experiencing *normal* thoughts associated with developing a body image.

> **TEST-TAKING TIP**—When two of the answers say the same thing, they both cannot be the answer. **Answers 3** and **4** both say that the client is comparing her body to peers and that she is nervous about the changes. Look at emotive terms: "makes me nervous" (**Answer 3**); "kind of *scary*" (**Answer 4**); "I *hate* my body" (**Answer 1**). Choose the most negative and strongest emotion here as the best answer.
> **AS, ANL, 5, Psych, HPM, Health Promotion and Maintenance**

181. **(3) Radioactive iodine is excreted in the urine. Radiation precautions for body secretions are instituted for 3 days after ingestion. Answer 1** is incorrect because the therapy is usually done on an outpatient basis. The client receives the dosage and usually goes home unless the dose is extremely large. The restriction is close contact, *not* no contact. The client should avoid close contact, and sleep alone for 1 week. **Answer 2** is incorrect because acetaminophen or aspirin *can* be given if local irritation results from the irradiation concentration in the neck. Radioactive iodine is taken orally on an empty stomach. **Answer 4** is incorrect because the radiation is taken orally. There is *no topical skin irritation.* If there is any irritation it would be in the throat.

> **TEST-TAKING TIP**—A key word is *radioactive*—choose an option that relates to excretion of radioactive waste.
> **PL, APP, 3, M/S: Radiation, SECE, Safety and Infection Control**

182. **(4) A negative CST is contractions without late decelerations, and reactive means accelerations, indicating good oxygenation. Answer 1** is incorrect because a negative contraction stress test (CST) demonstrates the absence of late decelerations with contractions; nonreactive indicates the lack of accelerations. It does demonstrate adequate *placental perfusion*, but does *not* indicate *good oxygenation*. **Answer 2** is incorrect because a positive CST shows the presence of late decelerations in two of three contractions. It shows some problems with oxygen transport through the placenta. Reactivity is the presence of baseline variability and accelerations, an indicator of good oxygenation; therefore, this answer is *not possible. You cannot have good oxygenation and late decelerations.* **Answer 3** is incorrect because a posi-

tive CST shows the presence of late decelerations in two of three contractions. It shows some problems with oxygen transport through the placenta. Nonreactive is the lack of accelerations. This is an indicator of probable uteroplacental insufficiency and *poor oxygenation.*

> **TEST-TAKING TIP**—Review the meanings of antenatal testing terms. In this case, *a positive* CST is *not a good outcome.* A *negative* CST is an indicator of *good* fetal oxygenation.
> **EV, ANL, 6, Maternity, PhI, Reduction of Risk Potential**

183. **(4) Late decelerations are indicators of uteroplacental insufficiency and poor fetal oxygenation, requiring immediate intervention and notification of the physician responsible for the care of the client. Answer 1** is incorrect because early decelerations are caused by compressions of the fetal head; and increased baseline variability *can* be an indicator of fetal distress, but this pattern does *not* require immediate intervention. **Answer 2** is incorrect because variable decelerations are umbilical cord compression. Average baseline variability is an indicator of *good* fetal oxygenation. **Answer 3** is incorrect because variable decelerations in the presence of increased baseline variability *may* be an indicator of developing fetal distress, requiring intervention, but *not* immediate intervention.

> **TEST-TAKING TIP**—The key words in this question are "immediate intervention." While some of the options require increased observation, *late* decelerations require immediate intervention to prevent a poor fetal outcome.
> **EV, ANL, 6, Maternity, PhI, Physiological Adaptation**

184. **(1) The morphine ordered prn for pain can be given very quickly with IV push; whereas, the other medications must infuse over 30 minutes. Comfort and pain management is also a priority. The decision about the order of the remaining drugs is more difficult. The frequency of the drug is an indication of the half-life—more frequent, shorter half-life. However, if the client is having seizures and the phenytoin level was low, the second choice would be phenytoin. Answer 2** is incorrect because the drug would need to be given over more than 30 minutes, whereas morphine can be rapidly given by IV to relieve the client's pain. The half-life of vancomycin is longer than the other drugs, so it might be given *last.* **Answer 3** is incorrect because the drug would need to given over more than 30 minutes, whereas morphine can be rapidly given by IV to relieve the client's pain. If the phenytoin level is low and the client has been having seizures, phenytoin would likely be the second drug to give. **Answer 4** is incorrect because morphine can be given more rapidly to relieve the client's pain. Metronidazole (Flagyl) if ordered IV will take 30 minutes to administer.

> **TEST-TAKING TIP**—Priority question—three of the drugs need to be given in a "timely" manner. Choose the one option that is not a specific time and is an analgesic.
> **IMP, APP, 3, M/S: Meds, PhI, Pharmacological and Parenteral Therapies**

185. **(3) This is the only choice where the possible roommate is not severely immunocompromised. A client with a history of MRSA often has a small number of organisms still present even though previously treated. Being isolated may also be an appropriate decision. The closeness in the ages of the clients would also more likely increase social interaction. Answer 1** is incorrect because clients with HIV are immunocompromised and would be susceptible to MRSA. **Answer 2** is incorrect because chemotherapy reduces the WBC production in the bone marrow. Ten days after therapy

is often the time when the WBC are the lowest; the client would be vulnerable to infection. **Answer 4 is incorrect because any client with a surgical incision is at risk for an infection.**

> **TEST-TAKING TIP**—While no roommate might be preferred, consider which client would have the greatest resistance to infection.
> **PL, ANL, 1, M/S: Infection, SECE, Safety and Infection Control**

186. **(3) It is _not_ desirable to place the infant in a slightly head-down position, because this interferes with the flow of cerebral spinal fluid (CSF), which needs to flow freely following the revision of the shunt. Answer 1** is incorrect because it _is_ desirable to place the infant on the nonopera-tive side to prevent mechanical pressure and obstruction to the shunt. **Answer 2** is incorrect because it _is_ desirable to maintain the infant flat in bed for the first 24 postoperative hours to prevent the formation of a subdural hematoma. **Answer 4** is incorrect because it _is_ desirable to gradually increase the angle of the head of the bed with each postop-erative day, as this promotes venous drainage and reduces cerebral swelling postoperatively.

> **TEST-TAKING TIP**—Three of these responses _are_ posi-tive postoperative interventions that assist in the flow of cerebral spinal fluid (CSF). Select the one response that could impede the flow of CSF.
> **AS, APP, 1, PEDS, SECE, Management of Care**

187. **(1) The first line of defense for infection is the skin. Skin breakdown from decubiti will increase the risk of infec-tion. Nosocomial infections (hospital-acquired) are the leading cause of death in the United States. Answer 2** is incorrect because there are _no_ immunizations for the type of organisms that are likely to invade an open sore on the skin (e.g., _Staphylococcus aureus)._ **Answer 3** is incorrect because heat is _not preventive,_ but would be therapeutic. Often cold is applied initially after an injury to reduce swelling. Heat after 24 hours is used to improve blood flow to an area of injury. **Answer 4** is incorrect because the desired outcome is _prevention_ of infection by maintaining skin integrity. Infectious agents are _not allergens._

> **TEST-TAKING TIP**—Know the normal defenses against infection (i.e., skin).
> **IMP, APP, 1, M/S: Infection Control, PhI, Reduction of Risk Potential**

188. **(2) A reduction or cessation of pain should alert the nurse to the possibility of a rupture of the appendix. The reduc-tion or cessation of pain may be due to a decrease in the sensation of pressure after the appendix bursts. The child's statement warrants further investigation and should be reported immediately by the nurse to the pediatrician. Answer 1** is incorrect because pain _is_ expected on the right side of the abdomen at McBurney's point with appendicitis. A school-age child would probably describe the location of the pain in general rather than specific terms and locations. **Answer 3** is incorrect because thirst _is_ to be expected in this child. The child would have been placed on NPO status in anticipation of possible surgery (appendectomy). **Answer 4** is incorrect because the child is probably running a fever due to the inflamed appendix, and _would_ complain of feeling hot.

> **TEST-TAKING TIP**—Three of the responses are all expected reactions, one is not. The question calls for select-ing a potentially _serious,_ not expected reaction.
> **AN, ANL, 3, PEDS, PhI, Reduction of Risk Potential**

189. **(3) The spleen has an important role in phagocytosis of circulating organisms. Clients are at increased risk for infection for up to 3 years following removal of the spleen. Answer 1** is incorrect because the spleen has no effect on reducing the risk of cancer of the lung from smoking. **Answer 2** is incorrect because the spleen has no effect on reducing hypersensitivity to allergens. **Answer 4** is incorrect because the role of the spleen is phagocytosis of organisms in the blood, _not_ topical irritants.

> **TEST-TAKING TIP**—Know the function of major organs. Consider the consequence of each choice—septicemia (bloodstream infection) is often fatal.
> **IMP, APP, 1, M/S: GI, PhI, Reduction of Risk Potential**

190. **(2) Promoting a sense of accomplishment in children at latency age will increase the child's self-esteem, and there-fore could prevent depression in adolescence. Chronic low self-esteem is a symptom of depression. Answer 1** is incor-rect because advocating for a teen suicide crisis line _will not prevent_ the development of depression. Suicide is a symptom of depression and if the teens are calling a crisis line they _already_ have depression. **Answer 3** is incorrect because offer-ing parental education to recognize the signs and symptoms of depression will _not prevent_ depression, but will assist with _early detection_ of depression. **Answer 4** is incorrect because a depression screening tool will help the adolescent _identify_ depression, but will _not help_ prevent its development.

> **TEST-TAKING TIP**—Look for key words in the stem. Preventing depression indicates that the condition cannot be present. Also, the three incorrect answers address inter-ventions in adolescences. The correct answer is the only answer addressing _latency_ age. This makes this answer different from the others.
> **IMP, APP, 5, Psych, HPM, Health Promotion and Maintenance**

191. **(1) Amoxicillin is an antibiotic and a common sign of an infection is an elevated temperature. A normal tempera-ture (37°C) would indicate the treatment was effective. Answer 2** is incorrect because the blood level of the drug does _not_ tell you if the drug has been effective. **Answer 3** is incorrect because itching would be a possible indication of a drug _allergy, not_ drug effectiveness. **Answer 4** is incorrect because completing the prescribed length of therapy does _not_ indicate if the signs or symptoms of infection are gone.

> **TEST-TAKING TIP**—The stem asks for an indication of effectiveness.
> **EV, ANL, 1, M/S: Meds, PhI, Pharmacological and Parenteral Therapies**

192. **(2) The risk of infection is very high. Neutrophils are part of the granulocyte component of the WBCs. A deficiency occurs with levels below 1000/mm³ and infection with levels at 500/mm³ or below. The client should avoid crowds and people with infection. Preventing inhalation of airborne contaminants with use of a mask and good hand-washing are important. Answer 1** is incorrect because the client is at high risk for infection and should be placed in a _private_ room. **Answer 3** is incorrect because raw or uncooked foods should be avoided during periods of neutropenia (low absolute neutrophil count) because bacte-ria are present. **Answer 4** is incorrect because the concern is infection, _not_ an allergy.

> **TEST-TAKING TIP**—A priority—keep the client safe (mask promotes safety).
> **PL, APP, 1, M/S: Blood, PhI, Reduction of Risk Potential**

193. (1, 2, 3) Answer 1 is correct because jaw control is often compromised in a child with cerebral palsy. Stabilizing the jaw provides more control when feeding the child and reduces the risk of aspiration. Answer 2 is correct because chewing and swallowing are often compromised in a child with cerebral palsy. Feeding the child slowly allows additional time for these activities and reduces the risk of aspiration. Answer 3 is correct because fine and gross motor skills are often compromised in a child with cerebral palsy. The toddler is in the stage of autonomy and will want to self-feed. Specialized utensils will assist the toddler and the parents in the feeding process, and may also reduce the risk of aspiration. Answer 4 is incorrect because while a gastrostomy tube provides a quick, efficient means of providing the toddler with a sufficient amount of food and fluid, it should not be the primary means of sustenance. The goal in feeding a toddler with cerebral palsy is to promote normal, independent feeding techniques which minimize the risk for aspiration but prevent dependency on mechanical means of feeding, such as a gastrostomy tube.

> **TEST-TAKING TIP**—Think "what this toddler *can* do" rather than "what this toddler *cannot* do," and then select all of the answers that would apply.
> **IMP, APP, 4, PEDS, PhI, Basic Care and Comfort**

194. (4) A child who is immunosuppressed should be placed in a private room. Steroids are the prime therapeutic agents in the management of a child with nephrotic syndrome. Answer 1 is incorrect because the child with nephrotic syndrome will be placed on high-dose steroids. While the child waiting for a hypospadias repair is not a potential source of infection, the child with nephrotic syndrome will be immunosuppressed and should be in a private room. Answer 2 is incorrect because the child with pneumonia *is* a potential source of infection to the child who is immunosuppressed and has nephrotic syndrome. Answer 3 is incorrect because the child with tonsillitis *is* a potential source of infection to the child who is immunosuppressed and has nephrotic syndrome.

> **TEST-TAKING TIP**—Choose the option that is different from the others: three options include a roommate; one option has no roommate.
> **IMP, APP, 1, PEDS, SECE, Management of Care**

195. (1) Strengthening the pelvic floor muscles (Kegel exercises) will decrease the incidence of stress incontinence. Answer 2 is incorrect because it is not the best approach. The drug combination is a common regimen for urge incontinence and other conditions where the bladder is *overactive*. Answer 3 is incorrect because these devices were not popular in the United States and are no longer readily found. Answer 4 is incorrect because the health benefits of exercise outweigh the annoyance of stress incontinence. If pelvic floor exercises do not improve the problem, alternatives to exercise are available (e.g., biofeedback or pseudoephedrine).

> **TEST-TAKING TIP**—A priority question—think which choice gives the client the greatest control over the situation.
> **PL, APP, 8, M/S: GU, PhI, Basic Care and Comfort**

196. (4) If the infant is Rh positive, the mother could develop antibodies to the fetal blood cell antigens. RhoGAM acts to block the formation of maternal antibodies. Answer 1 is incorrect because she *will* need a RhoGAM injection during the third trimester and after delivery, if the fetus is Rh positive. Answer 2 is incorrect because the client will *not* need to receive RhoGAM if the infant is Rh negative. Answer 3 is incorrect because the third trimester injection is given to protect the *current* pregnancy from possible Rh sensitization *during* the last trimester.

> **TEST-TAKING TIP**—Two options (Answers 2 and 4) state that she will need RhoGAM "if" the *mother* is *negative* and the *infant* is *positive* (Answer 4), there could be a problem that calls for RhoGAM.
> **IMP, ANL, 5, Maternity, PhI, Pharmacological and Parenteral Therapies**

197. (3) The first line of therapy for urge incontinence caused by detrusor instability is nonpharmacological: timed toileting or bladder retraining. Pelvic floor exercises, electrical stimulation and, if necessary, drugs such as tolterodine or oxybutynin may be used. Answer 1 is incorrect because catheterization increases the risk of infection and detrusor irritability. Answer 2 is incorrect because repeated catheterization would increase the risk of infection and does not address the overactivity of the detrusor muscle. Answer 4 is incorrect because fluids are important in preventing bladder infection that could contribute to the detrusor irritability.

> **TEST-TAKING TIP**—The "best" choice gives the client control and has "return to normal" as the goal. Eliminate the options that involve catheters and "restriction."
> **PL, APP, 8, M/S: GU, PhI, Basic Care and Comfort**

198. (1) Maintaining the IV access is the priority. The new bag of solution would be started at a rate that keeps the vein open while determining if the 1000 mL bag was ever hung or had rapidly infused. Answer 2 is incorrect because checking the records further delays maintaining patency of the IV site. After the vein is kept open, *then* the nurse can determine what has occurred. Answer 3 is incorrect as there are *no observable signs of distress.* A keep-open rate with a new bag of solution will not put the client at risk if the 1000 mL had been infused too rapidly. Answer 4 is incorrect because it would not be the first priority. If the unit was never hung, an incident report would not be completed.

> **TEST-TAKING TIP**—Priority questions will likely have more than one correct answer—think of what is best (safest) for the client, that is, "keep open." Eliminate two choices that focus on paperwork (Answers 2 and 4).
> **IMP, ANL, 6, M/S: Fluids, PhI, Pharmacological and Parenteral Therapies**

199. (2) Severe facial edema and 4+ protein are indicators of severe pregnancy-induced hypertension. Answer 1 is incorrect because weight gain can be caused by something other than severe pregnancy-induced hypertension. Answer 3 is incorrect because *trace* proteinuria is *not* an indicator of severe pregnancy-induced hypertension. The findings could be gestational or chronic hypertension. Answer 4 is incorrect because *slight* pedal edema is not an indicator of pregnancy-induced hypertension.

> **TEST-TAKING TIP**—Examine each of the symptoms and determine if it is consistent with the diagnosis of pregnancy-induced hypertension. If one of the symptoms is not found in severe pregnancy-induced hypertension, eliminate that answer.
> **AS, APP, 5, Maternity, PhI, Physiological Adaptation**

200. (3) It encourages the expression of feelings and allows an assessment of the danger for the mother. If the nurse can

relieve the daughter's frustration and make an appropriate referral, abuse could be prevented. Answer 1 is incorrect because the daughter has not hit the client, but is asking for help in dealing with the frustration of taking care of her mother. It is important to inform the daughter of the law, but *not as the first* response. It does *not* acknowledge the daughter's feelings and it *stops the flow* of conversation. **Answer 2** is incorrect because it offers false reassurance and is not truthful. Clients with Alzheimer's do *not* improve. **Answer 4** is incorrect because it gives an opinion (one that is not therapeutic) and stops the flow of the conversation.

> **TEST-TAKING TIP**—Choose the response that is most open-ended in encouraging the expression of feelings, and does not "talk down" to the client.
> **IMP, APP, 5, Psych, HPM, Health Promotion and Maintenance**

201. **(4) It is stated in a positive manner, and informs the parents that an infant's status can change rapidly and constant assessment is required to prevent any such changes from posing a threat to the infant. Answer 1** is incorrect because, while the infant is stable, changes can happen rapidly in an infant. Continuous assessment is necessary to detect such changes. **Answer 2** is incorrect because, while this may be the policy on the pediatric unit, it does not supply the parents with information and a rationale for the nurse's actions. **Answer 3** is incorrect because, while the parents should discuss their concerns with the pediatrician, it passes the buck to the pediatrician. It is within the scope of the nurse's practice to answer the question posed by the parents.

> **TEST-TAKING TIP**—Avoid responses in which the nurse does not fully function within the scope of nursing practice.
> **IMP, APP, 3, PEDS, PhI, Basic Care and Comfort**

202. **(2) The definition of HELLP includes hemolysis of RBCs, elevated liver enzymes, and decreased platelet count. Answer 1** is incorrect because *increased* platelets are *not* a part of HELLP syndrome. **Answer 3** is incorrect because hemoconcentration is *not* a specific symptom of HELLP syndrome. **Answer 4** is incorrect because *increased* liver enzymes are found in HELLP syndrome.

> **TEST-TAKING TIP**—Remember the definition of HELLP: H is hemolysis, EL is elevated liver enzymes, and LP is decreased or lowered platelets.
> **AN, COM, 5, Maternity, PhI, Reduction of Risk Potential**

203. **(2) The answer involves the removal of microorganisms prior to entering sterile tissue. Answer 1** is incorrect because using clean gloves is part of standard precautions used for every client, but is not surgical aseptic technique. **Answer 3** is incorrect because the HEPA mask prevents the transmission of microorganisms from the client to the nurse. **Answer 4** is incorrect because disposing of a used syringe in a sharps container is part of standard precautions, not surgical aseptic technique.

> **TEST-TAKING TIP**—Remember that surgical aseptic technique, or sterile technique, encompasses practices that prevent microorganisms from entering sterile tissue or the vascular space.
> **IMP, APP, 1, M/S: Infect. Control, SECE, Safety and Infection Control**

204. **(4) The dressing acts as a reservoir for the infectious agent. Changing the dressing disrupts the reservoir. Answer 1** is incorrect because the dressing is a reservoir. **Answer 2** is incorrect because the dressing is a reservoir. **Answer 3** is incorrect because the dressing is a reservoir.

> **TEST-TAKING TIP**—Elements of the chain of infection overlap. In this case, the dressing is a relatively stable place for the infectious agent to survive. The dressing was not transported (**Answer 1**), the survival conditions of the infections were not disrupted (**Answer 2**), and the host defenses were not addressed (**Answer 3**).
> **AN, APP, 1, M/S: Infect. Control, SECE, Safety and Infection Control**

205. **(3) Delivery of the fetus is the only cure for pregnancy-induced hypertension. The termination of pregnancy reverses the pregnancy-induced hypertension. Answer 1** is incorrect because magnesium sulfate is *not* a cure for pregnancy-induced hypertension. It *prevents the complication* of seizures in pregnancy-induced hypertension. **Answer 2** is incorrect because antihypertensive agents (e.g., Aldomet) are not a cure for pregnancy-induced hypertension. The agents act to *lower* the blood pressure, *not* to cure pregnancy-induced hypertension. **Answer 4** is incorrect because a change in diet has *no effect* on pregnancy-induced hypertension.

> **TEST-TAKING TIP**—The key word in this question is "cure." Look for the option that is a cure for pregnancy-induced hypertension, *not* a treatment for the complications.
> **IMP, APP, 5, Maternity, PhI, Reduction of Risk Potential**

206. **(1) The mask prevents the transmission of microorganisms from the nurse to the client's central line. Answer 2** is incorrect because rinsing the suction catheter serves to keep the suction tubing patent, and is not an action associated with infection control. **Answer 3** is incorrect because wearing clean gloves to remove the lunch tray prevents transmission of microorganisms from the client to the nurse, who could act as a carrier. **Answer 4** is incorrect because wearing clean gloves prevents transmission of microorganisms from the client to the nurse.

> **TEST-TAKING TIP**—Consider the direction of transmission of microorganisms. **Answers 3** and **4** prevent the transmission of microorganisms from *client to nurse*, while the correct answer prevents transmission for *nurse to client*.
> **IMP, APP, 1, M/S: Infect. Control, SECE, Safety and Infection Control**

207. **(4) Skin thins as the client ages, predisposing the client to skin tears and pressure ulcers, which dramatically reduce the skin's ability to act as a barrier to infection. Answer 1** is incorrect because saliva production *decreases* with age, not *increases*. **Answer 2** is incorrect because cough effort *decreases* with age, not *increases*. **Answer 3** is incorrect because cell-mediated immunity *decreases* with age, not *increases*.

> **TEST-TAKING TIP**—**Answer 4** is the only answer that is consistent with the physiology of aging, and is the only option that does not contain the word "increased."
> **AS, ANL, 1, M/S: Geriatrics, SECE, Safety and Infection Control**

208. **(4) The nurse's first action should be to assess the IV insertion site completely. This can only be done by removing the central line dressing and noting the appearance of the insertion site. Then the nurse will have sufficient information with which to decide to withhold further IV fluids and notify the pediatrician. Answer 1** is incorrect because severe damage can occur if even a very small amount of chemotherapy infiltrates surrounding tissue. The integrity of the central line must be established first *before* the nurse

proceeds with any other interventions. **Answer 2** is incorrect because damage can occur if agents such as heparin and/or normal saline infiltrate surrounding tissue. The integrity of the central line must be established first before the nurse proceeds with any other interventions. **Answer 3** is incorrect because, while not administering any IV fluids and notifying the pediatrician is a sound idea, the nurse needs *more* information before notifying the pediatrician.

> **TEST-TAKING TIP**—Assessment is always the first step that the nurse should take when investigating any questionable situation involving client care.
> **IMP, APP, 6, PEDS, PhI, Pharmacological and Parenteral Therapies**

209. **(4) This client has three risk factors: age, the stress of an injury, and immobility with the broken hip. Answer 1** is incorrect because this client has one risk factor: surgical repair which involves an incision into sterile tissues. **Answer 2** is incorrect because this client has one risk factor: surgical repair which involves an incision into sterile tissues. **Answer 3** is incorrect because this client has one risk factor: diabetes, a chronic disease.

> **TEST-TAKING TIP**—Count the number of risk factors for each client.
> **AN, ANL, 1, M/S: Infect. Control, SECE, Safety and Infection Control**

210. **(3) The family is providing for the need of the 16-year-old to be with friends while reducing the stimulation for the client. Answer 1** is incorrect because with proper education, the 16-year-old son should be able to stay with the client. This is inappropriate division of labor within the family. **Answer 2** is incorrect because if there is a financial need for the daughter to work, alternative care for the client during the day should be explored. **Answer 4** is incorrect because silence may be an indication that the son *is* having trouble with the living arrangement, and is having difficulty getting his needs met within the family.

> **TEST-TAKING TIP**—Look for the answer that promotes the developmental needs of the family members and is an age-appropriate answer. Look for the answer that is different; the correct answer is a *positive* action taken by the family, *not* "afraid" (**Answer 1**), *not* "worried (**Answer 2**), *not* "very silent" (**Answer 4**).
> **AS, ANL, 7, Psych, PsI, Psychosocial Integrity**

211. **(3) Chickenpox falls into the category of airborne diseases, and requires a *private room with negative airflow* to prevent microorganisms from *escaping* the room. Answer 1** is incorrect because, while MRSA does call for a private room, negative airflow is *not necessary*. **Answer 2** is incorrect because a client with neutropenia should be in a room with *positive* airflow to prevent microorganisms from *entering* the room. **Answer 4** is incorrect because a private room is *not essential* for this client, although it may be desirable. The client with an infected, draining wound, however, should *not* be assigned a room with a client who is newly postoperative.

> **TEST-TAKING TIP**—Notice that the question specifies a private room with *negative airflow*. This means that microorganisms are prevented from escaping the room.
> **IMP, ANL, 1, M/S: Infect. Control, SECE, Safety and Infection Control**

212. **(3) These are both primary causes of third trimester bleeding. Answer 1** is incorrect because these are causes of *first* trimester bleeding. **Answer 2** is incorrect because a retained placenta is a cause of *postpartum* bleeding, not third

trimester bleeding. **Answer 4** is incorrect because ectopic pregnancy is a *first* trimester complication.

> **TEST-TAKING TIP**—*Third trimester* is the key concept in this question. This is the last part of pregnancy before delivery. Consider the options with the third trimester as the overall concept. Does this condition exist in the third trimester? If not, eliminate the option
> **AN, COM, 5, Maternity, HPM, Health Promotion and Maintenance**

213. **(3) It provides the child with factual information that a school-age child could comprehend. The reason for hair loss is different from the grandfather's, and when the child's hair comes back it might be a different color. Answer 1** is incorrect because it offers a solution but fails to provide the child with needed information regarding hair loss and its return. **Answer 2** is incorrect because it offers a solution but fails to provide the child with needed information regarding hair loss and its return. **Answer 4** is incorrect because although it acknowledges the child's feelings regarding hair loss, it fails to provide the child with needed information regarding hair loss and its return.

> **TEST-TAKING TIP**—All of the responses are psychosocial in nature. Select the response that *best* answers the child's need for information.
> **IMP, APP, 7, PEDS, PsI, Psychosocial Integrity**

214. **(3) A preschool-age child with persistent vomiting and diarrhea is at risk for dehydration and must receive prompt evaluation and treatment. It could safely be assumed that this child may have already lost weight and had been dehydrated during the course of hospitalization due to the chemotherapy that was undoubtedly given. Extra attention must be paid so that this situation does not occur again and necessitate re-hospitalization. Answer 1** is incorrect because a preschool-age child can *often* be fussy or irritable without a medical reason and even when back in own home environment. **Answer 2** is incorrect because a preschool-age child *often* has difficulty getting to sleep at nighttime even when back in own home environment. **Answer 4** is incorrect because a preschool-age child *often* has many food likes and dislikes and tends to be a fussy eater even when back in own home environment.

> **TEST-TAKING TIP**—Three of these responses (**Answers 1, 2, and 4**) involve pre-school growth and development. Select the one response that is physiological and could place the child in real jeopardy.
> **IMP, APP, 6, PEDS, PhI, Reduction of Risk Potential**

215. **(3) The Glasgow Coma Scale is the preferred tool to evaluate clients with head injuries in an acute setting. Answer 1** is incorrect because it evaluates mental status, *not neurological* status, and should be performed on a client who is *conscious*. **Answer 2** is incorrect because this evaluates part of mental status, *not neurological* status, and should be performed on a client who is *conscious*. **Answer 4** is incorrect because this evaluates *only part* of neurological status.

> **TEST-TAKING TIP**—Distinguish between evaluation of mental status (**Answers 1** and **2**) and evaluation of neurological status (**Answer 3**)
> **IMP, APP, 2, M/S: Neuro, PsI, Psychosocial Integrity**

216. **(2) Insufficient data are presented to arrive at a specific diagnosis; the nurse must be objective when observing the client's mode of dress. Answer 1** is incorrect because the nurse should be objective in evaluating appearance, realizing that the client's mode of dress may be driven by peer group influences and personal taste. **Answer 3** is incorrect because the nurse needs to collect more data before arriving at a

conclusion. **Answer 4** is incorrect because the nurse needs to collect more data to determine *if a deficit exists* in personal hygiene.

> TEST-TAKING TIP—Beware of options that lead the nurse to a conclusion or plan of action based on insufficient data.
> AN, ANL, 7, Psych, PsI, Psychosocial Integrity

217. **(1) Interpretation of this phrase requires abstract thought.** Answer 2 is incorrect because this evaluates the client's *judgment.* **Answer 3** is incorrect because this evaluates the client's *recent memory.* **Answer 4** is incorrect because this evaluates the client's *language ability.*

> TEST-TAKING TIP—Focus on the option that requires an interpretation, rather than simply describing (**Answer 2**), or stating words (**Answers 3** and **4**).
> IMP, APP, 2, Psych, PsI, Psychosocial Integrity

218. **(3) Constant vigilance required of the family fits a defining characteristic for this diagnosis. Answer 1** is incorrect because there are no data to support a nursing diagnosis of *neglect.* **Answer 2** is incorrect because there are no data to support a nursing diagnosis of *hopelessness.* **Answer 4** is incorrect because there are no data to support a nursing diagnosis of *ineffective family coping.*

> TEST-TAKING TIP—The data in the stem of the question provide defining characteristics for only one nursing diagnosis: **Answer 3.**
> AN, ANL, 1, M/S: Geriatrics, PsI, Psychosocial Integrity

219. **(4) The client's symptoms are a result of dehydration and developing diabetic ketoacidosis. Answer 1** is incorrect because an overdose of insulin would result in *hypoglycemia.* This client has hyperglycemia. **Answer 2** is incorrect because heroin drug use would probably *not* result in the symptoms listed. **Answer 3** is incorrect because pregnancy-induced hypertension would manifest in an increased blood pressure. This client has a low blood pressure.

> TEST-TAKING TIP—Diabetic complications include hypoglycemia and hyperglycemia. Determine which symptoms are associated with each of the complications. Recall that this client has hyperglycemia.
> AN, ANL, 4, Maternity, PhI, Physiological Adaptation

220. **(1, 2, 3, 5, 6)** Answer 1 is a normal unconscious defense mechanism mobilized by clients to protect the integrity of the self. Clients use the mechanism to deal with the perceived threat over time. Answer 2 is a normal unconscious defense mechanism mobilized by clients to protect the integrity of the self. Clients use the mechanism to deal with the perceived threat over time. Answer 3 is a normal unconscious defense mechanism mobilized by clients to protect the integrity of the self. Clients use the mechanism to deal with the perceived threat over time. Answer 5 is a normal defense mechanism mobilized by clients to protect the integrity of the self. Clients use the mechanism to deal with the perceived threat over time. Answer 6 is a normal defense mechanism mobilized by clients to protect the integrity of the self. Clients use the mechanism to deal with the perceived threat over time. Answer 4 is incorrect because suicide is *not a normal* defense mechanism, but is a dysfunctional coping mechanism or strategy.

> TEST-TAKING TIP—Look for the answer that is different from the others. Suicide can be a symptom of depression and/or an ineffective coping mechanism. Recall definitions of the ego defense mechanisms.
> AS, COM, 7, Psych, PsI, Psychosocial Integrity

221. **(3) This behavior conveys to the client that the nurse understands and accepts some of his feelings about the new ostomy. Answer 1** is incorrect because, although this is an essential activity, it does not directly address the client's self-image. **Answer 2** is incorrect because providing privacy is appropriate, unless the client gives permission for the family to observe and they will be participating in the care of the stoma. **Answer 4** is incorrect because the client will take his cues from the nurse's reaction to the stoma. If the nurse expresses distaste, verbally or nonverbally, this reinforces the distastefulness of the ostomy to the client.

> TEST-TAKING TIP—**Answers 1** and **2** do not address self-concept, while **Answer 4** supports a negative self concept.
> IMP, APP, 8, M/S: GI, PsI, Psychosocial Integrity

222. **(3) Chorioamnionitis is a common complication of frequent vaginal exams. Answer 1** is incorrect because pelvic inflammatory disease is a serious infection in the upper genital tract/reproductive organs (uterus, fallopian tubes and ovaries) of a woman. PID can be sexually transmitted or naturally occurring. It is not caused by frequent pelvic exams. **Answer 2** is incorrect because endometriosis is a condition in which tissue like the endometrium is found outside the uterus, causing pelvic pain. Frequent vaginal exams do not place the client at risk for endometriosis. **Answer 4** is incorrect because frequent vaginal exams *do not* cause a premature rupture of membranes.

> TEST-TAKING TIP—The key concept is the relationship between infection and frequent vaginal exams, after the rupture of membranes. Think about which of the conditions is an infection during the labor process.
> AN, APP, 1, Maternity, SECE, Safety and Infection Control

223. **(1) Anaphylaxis is a life-threatening event. This is the priority item that the parents must obtain.** Answer 2 is incorrect because, while it is an excellent idea in itself, it would *not* take *priority* over obtaining the anaphylaxis kit. **Answer 3** is incorrect because, while it is an excellent idea in itself, it would *not* take *priority* over obtaining the anaphylaxis kit. **Answer 4** is incorrect because, while it is an excellent idea in itself, it would *not* take *priority* over obtaining the anaphylaxis kit.

> TEST-TAKING TIP—Think of Maslow's hierarchy of needs when attempting to answer this question. Physiological needs and safety and security are always priorities.
> IMP, APP, 1, PEDS, PhI, Reduction of Risk Potential

224. **(2) Requiring progressively larger doses is consistent with physical *dependence*. Answer 1** is incorrect because *repeated* behavior of driving under the influence indicates drug *abuse.* **Answer 3** is incorrect because *repeated* failure to fulfill work obligations is suggestive of drug *abuse.* **Answer 4** is incorrect because a single incident of intoxication does not necessarily constitute drug dependence or abuse.

> TEST-TAKING TIP—Although there is often a very fine line between drug abuse and drug dependence, *repeated* problems in the client's work, social, or personal life indicates *abuse.* Regardless of the specific classification, the client needs better pain management.
> AS, ANL, 7, M/S: Substance Abuse, PsI, Psychosocial Integrity

225. **(4) The elderly population has a higher use of over-the-counter drugs such as analgesics, laxatives, antacids, and vitamins than younger populations.** Answer 1 is incorrect because, at present, illegal drug use among the elderly is minimal. **Answer 2** is incorrect because adverse effects of the

interaction of drugs and alcohol increases with age. **Answer 3 is incorrect because the effects of aging alter the client's** response to drug abuse.

> **TEST-TAKING TIP**—Body processes change as clients age; therefore, it makes sense that the elderly client will have more and different reactions to alcohol and drugs than younger populations (**Answers 2** and **3**).
> AN, ANL, 7, M/S: Geriatrics, PsI, Psychosocial Integrity

226. (1) **Withdrawal from narcotics includes these symptoms as well as anxiety and restlessness. Answer 2** is incorrect because symptoms of alcohol withdrawal include insomnia, delirium, and seizures. **Answer 3** is incorrect because withdrawal from benzodiazepines include insomnia, delirium, and seizures. **Answer 4** is incorrect because symptoms of cocaine withdrawal include severe depression, prolonged sleep, and apathy.

> **TEST-TAKING TIP**—Picture flu-like symptoms for narcotic withdrawal. **Answers 2** and **3** call for *neurological* symptoms. **Answer 4** calls for remembering *behavioral* symptoms.
> AS, COM, 7, M/S: Substance Abuse, PsI, Psychosocial Integrity

227. (2) **The Pavlik harness is to be worn at least 23 hours a day. It can usually be removed just for skin checks and bathing purposes. It is designed so that diaper changes do not necessitate removing the harness. Answer 1** is incorrect because it *is* an appropriate action on the mother's part and *does not* warrant additional evaluation or teaching on the part of the nurse. A shirt and socks serve as a barrier to prevent skin irritation from the harness. **Answer 3** is incorrect because it *is* an appropriate action on the mother's part and *does not* warrant additional evaluation or teaching on the part of the nurse. Frequent position changes decrease the risk of developing pressure sores or circulatory compromise. **Answer 4** is incorrect because it *is* an appropriate action on the mother's part and *does not* warrant additional evaluation or teaching on the part of the nurse. Keeping the hips abducted relocates the femoral head into the acetabulum while gently stretching the restrictive soft tissue.

> **TEST-TAKING TIP**—Note that the question calls for a *problem* response, not what is OK. Knowing the purpose of and care required for a Pavlik harness is essential in answering this question correctly.
> EV, ANL, 3, PEDS, PhI, Basic Care and Comfort

228. (2) **The client would have first had an abnormal 1 hour glucola test and then the 3 hour glucola test, usually during the third trimester, because the increasing level of human placental lactogen leads to increasing insulin resistance. Answer 1** is incorrect because the 1 hour glucola test is used as a screening tool to determine *if further testing* is needed, *not* a *basis* for diagnosis. **Answer 3** is incorrect because a 1 hour glucola is the *screening tool* used for *further* testing. **Answer 4** is incorrect because family history is a risk factor for gestational diabetes but does *not* make the *definitive* diagnosis of gestational diabetes.

> **TEST-TAKING TIP**—Think about the glucose levels of women who are pregnant in each trimester. In the first trimester, the glucose levels are low, then the levels increase each trimester, with the third trimester exhibiting increasing insulin resistance.
> AN, COM, 4, Maternity, PhI, Reduction of Risk Potential

229. (2) **A prolonged interval between an injury and the treatment is a signal of elder abuse. Observing the client's interactions with the daughter provides valuable information about this potential problem. Answer 1** is incorrect because, although grooming provides information about the level of care the client receives, it does not provide direct information about the injury or the possibility of elder abuse. **Answer 3** is incorrect because, although this presents information about the client's mental status, it does not provide direct information about the injury or the possibility of elder abuse. **Answer 4** is incorrect because this provides information about the level of care the client receives, but it does not provide direct information about the injury or the possibility of elder abuse.

> **TEST-TAKING TIP**—The first priority is to treat the wrist injury. The nurse should also key in on the delay in treatment, which is suggestive of elder abuse or neglect. Observing the interaction between the client and daughter provides the *most direct* insight into a potential problem.
> AS, ANL, 1, Geriatrics: Substance Abuse, PsI, Psychosocial Integrity

230. (1) **The nurse is respecting the client's privacy and maintaining a calm and nonjudgmental stance to the behavior. The nurse is setting limits on the behavior. Answer 2** is incorrect because the nurse is violating the client's right to confidentiality and is placing the responsibility of the behavior solely on the visitor. **Answer 3** is incorrect because the nurse would belittle the adult client and his visitor by interrupting the sexual activity, and "telling" is a form of scolding the behavior. **Answer 4** is incorrect because hypersexuality is a symptom commonly seen in clients with mania. The client is most likely acting on impulse and needs firm limits and simple directions. Once the client's mania is under control, the nurse can discuss any underlying issues.

> **TEST-TAKING TIP**—Visualize clients experiencing mania. Choose a response that is most accepting and nonjudgmental of the options available. Do not accuse or belittle the client (**Answers 2** and **3**). **Answer 4** encourages the expression of feelings, but this would not be effective in limiting inappropriate behavior until the mania is under better control.
> IMP, APP, 7, Psych, PsI, Psychosocial Integrity

231. (3) **Immediate intervention is needed in a crisis. Answer 1** is incorrect because immediate intervention is needed in a crisis—*long-term* goals can be addressed when the crisis is over. **Answer 2** is incorrect because immediate intervention is needed in a crisis. An extensive evaluation of life stressors can be undertaken *after* the immediate crisis is passed. **Answer 4** is incorrect because the nurse is a valuable *support* for the client in a crisis.

> **TEST-TAKING TIP**—Crisis means that the problem the client is experiencing is *urgent* and requires *immediate intervention*. **Answers 2** and **3** involve long-term activities that are useful for preventing future crises, while **Answer 4** leaves the client to manage alone.
> IMP, APP, 7, Psych, PsI, Psychosocial Integrity

232. (3) **Clients do have the right to be informed about treatment and to refuse treatment, even if it will result in their death. Answer 1** is incorrect because, legally, passive euthanasia is a gray area and laws vary by state. **Answer 2** is incorrect because active euthanasia is *not* a constitutional right, but is treated as a *crime* in most states. **Answer 4** is incorrect because *active* euthanasia involves a *deliberate action* that results in the death of the client.

> **TEST-TAKING TIP**—Focus on the words "passive" and "active," then choose the answer that is consistent with the meanings of these terms.
> AN, COM, 7, M/S: End of Life, PsI, Psychosocial Integrity

233. **(4) Thrill and bruit, which indicate viability of the access, should be assessed every shift. Answer** 1 is incorrect because *no blood* should be drawn from the AV fistula, nor should any constricting bands or pressure dressings be applied. **Answer 2** is incorrect because *no medications* or injections should be administered via the AV fistula, other than what is administered during a dialysis session. **Answer 3** is incorrect because the AV fistula is a surgically constructed hemodialysis access beneath the skin. There is *no tubing*, except for dialysis sessions.

> **TEST-TAKING TIP**—The rule is that any hemodialysis access device, be it long-term or short-term, is used only for dialysis, and nothing else. The second rule is that a long-term hemodialysis access such as an AV fistula, should not be used for injections, blood draws, IVs, or blood pressures.
> **IMP, APP, 6, M/S: Renal, PhI, Basic Care and Comfort**

234. **(4) A newborn infant is producing insulin based on the mother's blood sugar and continues to produce insulin after the umbilical cord is cut, which ends the blood sugar supply. The infant *can* suffer profound hypoglycemia as a result. Answer** 1 is incorrect because hypothermia is a *complication of prematurity* due to a decrease in brown fat deposits. **Answer 2** is incorrect because hypotension in a newborn is *not* a complication of diabetes. **Answer 3** is incorrect because infants of mothers who are diabetic produce insulin based on the mother's blood sugar, and *rarely* demonstrate hyperglycemia after birth.

> **TEST-TAKING TIP**—Focus on the "hypo" reactions. The key is to determine which of the "hypos" is caused by diabetes.
> **AN, APP, 4, Newborn, HPM, Health Promotion and Maintenance**

235. **(4) The proper position of the fingertips for palpation of a contraction is over the fundus of the uterus, and palpating the duration of the contraction by palpating the contraction from beginning to the end. Answer** 1 is incorrect because the contraction begins *at* the fundus, *not below* the umbilicus. **Answer 2** is incorrect because the duration of a contraction is the amount of time the uterus is contracting, measured from the beginning of the contraction to the *end of the same* contraction. **Answer 3** is incorrect because the *frequency* is determined by the number of contractions during a specified length of time, i.e., 3 contractions in a 10-minute period.

> **TEST-TAKING TIP**—The key word in this question is "palpation." Determine which of the options is specifically about palpation and read the options carefully.
> **IMP, APP, 5, Maternity, HPM, Health Promotion and Maintenance**

236. **(1) Conservative management for a client with cholelithiasis includes a low fat diet. Answer 2** is incorrect because morphine tends to cause more spasm of the ducts than Demerol (meperidine). **Answer 3** is incorrect because a cholecystectomy is not necessarily inevitable, although it is a treatment option for recurrent or severe cases of cholelithiasis. Other treatment options also exist, such as diet, gallstone-dissolving medications given orally or injected directly into the gallbladder, and the use of sound waves to break up gallstones and make them easier to pass. **Answer 4** is incorrect because the high fat content of dairy products can precipitate an attack.

> **TEST-TAKING TIP**—Focus on the options that are opposites: **Answers 1** and **4**; and pick the one that fits with the pathophysiology of cholelithiasis.
> **IMP, APP, 4, M/S: GI, PhI, Basic Care and Comfort**

237. **(3) A client with Ménière's disease should follow a low sodium diet to reduce fluid retention in the inner ear. Answer** 1 is incorrect because clients with Ménière's disease should follow a low sodium diet; fat content is not pertinent to Ménière's disease. **Answer 2** is incorrect because there is no indication that megavitamin therapy benefits a client with Ménière's disease. **Answer 4** is incorrect because alcohol should be restricted in the diet of a client with Ménière's disease, along with caffeine and nicotine.

> **TEST-TAKING TIP**—Focus on the option that is consistent with the pathophysiology of Ménière's disease: excess fluid in the inner ear.
> **IMP, APP, 4, M/S: Ear, PhI, Basic Care and Comfort**

238. **(4) The effects of the medication used to treat attention deficit-hyperactivity disorder are decreasing at this time of day whether the frequency of administration is once or twice a day. The child would more likely be hungry at this time of day and willing to consider eating a nutritious snack to provide needed calories to prevent additional weight loss. Answer** 1 is incorrect because the medication used to treat attention deficit-hyperactivity disorder is taken in the morning, if the medication is prescribed to be taken once a day. The child would not be hungry at this time of day because of the medication and would not need to have a snack. **Answer 2** is incorrect because the medication used to treat attention deficit-hyperactivity disorder is still fully effective in the mid-morning. The child would not be hungry at this time of day due to the medication, and unlikely to want a snack. **Answer 3** is incorrect because the medication used to treat attention deficit-hyperactivity disorder is still fully effective in the mid-afternoon, or a second dose is given at this time of day. The child would not be hungry at this time of day due to the medication, and unlikely to have a snack.

> **TEST-TAKING TIP**—Knowing the duration of the effects of the medications (psychostimulants) used to treat attention deficit-hyperactivity disorder is essential in answering this question correctly.
> **IMP, ANL, 4, PEDS, PhI, Pharmacological and Parenteral Therapies**

239. **(4) The grandmother is widowed and raising the child alone. The management of such a child's unpredictable moods and high energy could lead to caregiver role strain. The nurse realizes that if the grandmother becomes overly stressed and strained in caring for her grandson, the other nursing diagnoses (*risk for injury, impaired social interaction, non-compliance*) could quickly become reality. The nurse will focus the plan of care on assisting the grandmother to prevent this from happening. Answer** 1 is incorrect because, while it is a valid concern due to the child's high level of impulsiveness and excitability, it is not the nurse's primary concern. **Answer 2** is incorrect because, while it is a valid concern due to the child's chronic episodes of impulsive behavior which tend to interfere with normal, age-appropriate social development and interaction, it is not the nurse's primary concern. **Answer 3** is incorrect because, while it is a valid concern due to the complexity of caring for such a child (behavioral modification program, medication, special education, etc.), it is not the nurse's primary concern.

> **TEST-TAKING TIP**—Focus on the role of the grandmother in caring for and coping with the child when answering this question.
> **AN, ANL, 7, PEDS, PsI, Psychosocial Integrity**

240. **(2) A client in the middle phase of Alzheimer's does not always recognize family members. This action indicates to

the nurse that the adult child does not understand the disease process, and this is a nursing concern. **Answer 1** is incorrect because placing locks high on outside doors *will* protect the client from wandering. **Answer 3** is incorrect because during this phase of Alzheimer's, it *would be unsafe* to drive an automobile. Central to the disease process is denial, so it is unlikely that the client would give permission. **Answer 4** is incorrect because this option demonstrates that the adult child *has* an understanding of the disease process and is seeking solutions to the problem.

> **TEST-TAKING TIP**—The stem calls for what *is* a concern, i.e., requires an intervention. Look for similarities in the answers. **Answers 1** and **3** both do mobilize safety measures for the client. Once these answers are eliminated, **Answer 2** is a *maladaptive* response and is a concern for the nurse.
> **AN, ANL, 7, Psych, PsI, Psychosocial Integrity**

241. **(3) The condition described is caput succedaneum, a collection of fluid in the subcutaneous tissues of scalp, not limited by bony sutures. Answer 1** is incorrect because this is a made-up combination of the two terms cephalohematoma and caput succedaneum It is *not an actual condition.* **Answer 2** is incorrect because hemangiomas are abnormally dense collections of dilated small blood vessels (capillaries) that may occur in the *skin* or *internal* organs. **Answer 4** is incorrect because cephalohematoma is a subperiosteal collection of blood that does *not cross* suture lines.

> **TEST-TAKING TIP**—Visualize the fetal scalp and the bones that make up the fetal skull. Think about what causes a soft bump on the fetal scalp that crosses suture lines.
> **AN, APP, 5, Maternity, HPM, Health Promotion and Maintenance**

242. **(2) Smaller, more frequent meals are less tiring for the client. In addition, clients with Parkinson's disease often have difficulty with chewing and swallowing; and food that is cut into small pieces is more manageable. Answer 1** is incorrect because clients with Parkinson's disease often suffer from constipation, so fluid should be *increased* to 3000 mL per day. **Answer 3** is incorrect because the client with Parkinson's disease may find these difficult to chew and swallow. **Answer 4** is incorrect because *weekly weights* are appropriate to track the client's *nutritional* status. *Daily weight* is for tracking *hydration* status.

> **TEST-TAKING TIP**—Consider the nature of Parkinson's disease, which involves neuromuscular dysfunction resulting in difficulty with voluntary muscle movement, including dysphagia. **Answer 2** is the only option that addresses this concept.
> **IMP, APP, 4, M/S: NM, PhI, Basic Care and Comfort**

243. **(4) Physical dependence may occur with long-term use of valproic acid. Answer 1** is incorrect because valproic acid toxicity increases with use of salicylates. **Answer 2** is incorrect because valproic acid may cause drowsiness. **Answer 3** is incorrect because valproic acid is not a prn medication, and should not be abruptly discontinued.

> **TEST-TAKING TIP**—The primary use for valproic acid is to control seizure activity. **Answer 4** is the only option that is consistent with the pharmacological profile of valproic acid.
> **IMP, APP, 1, M/S: Neuro, PhI, Pharmacological and Parenteral Therapies**

244. **(1, 3, 4) Answer 1** is correct because prioritizing her treatment options may restore some life control for the client. **Answer 3** is correct because, although seemingly inappropriate in these circumstances, the effectiveness of humor to reduce stress is well-known. **Answer 4 is correct because spiritual activities can often help reduce stress and can be a source of strength for the client. Answer 2** is incorrect because, although useful in some circumstances, sedatives will not help the client cope, but will mask symptoms of stress. **Answer 5** is incorrect because the client's social network may be a source of strength and support for the client. She may, however, need to revise her social calendar to preserve energy. **Answer 6** is incorrect because this may be an important source of physical and spiritual activity for the client.

> **TEST-TAKING TIP**—Focus on the options that provide the client with support, a means of reducing stress, or more control over her life.
> **PL, ANL, 3, M/S: Cancer, PsI, Psychosocial Integrity**

245. **(2) A child with attention deficit-hyperactivity disorder will experience a "leveling out" from the medication as opposed to "highs" or "lows." Becoming a "drug abuser" of the medication regime is unlikely. Answer 1** is incorrect because a child with attention deficit-hyperactivity disorder is usually not interested in abusing the medication regime because the effect of the medication on the child is opposite to that which is produced in a normal child. **Answer 3** is incorrect because no documentation exists that "drug holidays" prevent dependency or incorrect usage of the medication. "Drug holidays" are controversial in the treatment of attention deficit-hyperactivity disorder. Many sources recommend that a constant level of medication be maintained to prevent undesirable behavior in the child. **Answer 4** is incorrect because, while this may prevent abuse while the mother is administering the medication, ultimately the child will have to self-administer the medication. The potential for abuse of the medication does increase as the child reaches adolescence and the age of experimentation.

> **TEST-TAKING TIP**—Focus on the option that implies "no problem" and does not need prevention.
> **IMP, ANL, 2, PEDS, PhI, Pharmacological and Parenteral Therapies**

246. **(3, 6) Answer 3 is correct because pain is a subjective experience, and is different for every person. Answer 6 is correct because pain is a signal to modify behavior, e.g., a client with tendonitis in the elbow will refrain from playing tennis for a few days. Answer 1** is incorrect because pain can, and often does, occur in the absence of identifiable tissue injury. **Answer 2** is incorrect because the client is not likely to become addicted. Clients generally stop using analgesics when the need for them is gone. **Answer 4** is incorrect because psychogenic pain involves neurochemical activity in the brain and spinal cord, just as physiological pain does. **Answer 5** is incorrect because clients can doze, even if they are in pain.

> **TEST-TAKING TIP**—The primary rule for assessment and management of pain is that pain occurs whenever the client says it does, and with whatever characteristics the client describes. Therefore, eliminate the options that contradict this principle: **Answers 1, 2, 4,** and **5.**
> **AN, ANL, 3, M/S: Pain, PhI, Basic Care and Comfort**

247. **22.** The infant should weigh approximately 22 pounds or more; 1000 grams = 1 kilogram; 1 kilogram = 2.2. pounds. Therefore, 3400 grams = 3.4 kilograms or 7.48 pounds; 7.48 pounds x 3 = 22.4 pounds.

> **TEST-TAKING TIP**—An infant's birth weight should double by 6 months of age and triple by 1 year of age.
> **AN, APP, 5, PEDS, HPM, Health Promotion and Maintenance**

248. <u>15.</u> The solution contains 2 mg/mL of aminophylline (1000 mg/500 mL). Divide 30 mg/hr by 2 mg/mL to get the answer.

> **TEST-TAKING TIP**—Don't forget to convert 1 gram to 1000 mg before doing the rest of the problem.
> **IMP, APP, 6, M/S: Calculation, PhI, Pharmacological and Parenteral Therapies**

249. **(4) This can be an indicator of congenital hip dysplasia and needs to be reported to the physician.** Answer 1 is incorrect because these are uric crystals, a *normal* finding in a newborn. **Answer 2** is incorrect because these are *normal* in dark skinned infants. **Answer 3** is incorrect because this is a *normal* finding in a newborn.

> **TEST-TAKING TIP**—Think about normal newborn assessment and look for the option that is *not* a normal finding in a newborn.
> **AS, APP, 5, Newborn, HPM, Health Promotion and Maintenance**

250. **(4) A client who is dying should be encouraged to cry. Tears are an important part of the grieving process.** Answer 1 is incorrect because appropriate coping with dying involves *reviewing* life in the past as a way to reconcile with their life. Looking to the future would indicate that the client is *denying* the impending death. **Answer 2** is incorrect because the client who is dying needs to learn how to deal with separation from family and friends. Avoiding discussing feelings with family would be *ineffective* coping. **Answer 3** is incorrect because this statement indicates that the client is *denying* the terminal condition.

> **TEST-TAKING TIP**—Look for similarities in the answers. **Answers 1** and **3** say the same thing (i.e., focus on the future) and they both cannot be correct. Once these answers are eliminated, choose the answer that indicates that the client is expressing feelings.
> **EV, ANL, 7, Psych, PsI, Psychosocial Integrity**

251. **(3) Reflex contraction of the bladder is not coordinated with relaxation of the sphincter in spinal cord injury. Consequently the bladder does not empty with voiding, and retention of urine predisposes to urinary tract infection.** Answer 1 is incorrect because restricting fluids may reduce the urine volume but would *not improve* bladder emptying. **Answer 2** is incorrect because applying bladder pressure particularly when the sphincter is closed could result in *injury*. **Answer 4** is incorrect because these anticholinergic drugs are used with urge incontinence, *not* urinary *retention*.

> **TEST-TAKING TIP**—Know the effect of a spinal cord injury on the bladder (i.e., urinary retention). Think what could occur with prolonged retention.
> **PL, APP, 8, M/S: Neuro, PhI, Reduction of Risk Potential**

252. **(4) The onset of thelarche (changes in nipples and areola and development of a small bud of breast tissue in an adolescent girl) occurs at 11 years of age (average); or between 9 to 13.5 years (range). This is usually the earliest, most visible change associated with puberty and should definitely be assessed.** Answer 1 is incorrect because the development of 32 teeth is *not* expected until the adolescent is approximately 18–21 years of age. A 12-year-old could be expected to have approximately 28 teeth (including permanent teeth and molars). **Answer 2** is incorrect because the development of "adult-like" vital signs is *not* expected until the adolescent is approximately 18 years of age. **Answer 3** is incorrect because the onset of menstruation is *not* expected until 12.8 years (average) or between 10.5–15 years (range).

> **TEST-TAKING TIP**—Review Tanner's Stages of Sexual Development and remember that breast development marks the onset of puberty in an adolescent girl.
> **AS, APP, 5, PEDS, HPM, Health Promotion and Maintenance**

253. **(4) Inability to void can cause bladder distention, uterine atony, and increased postpartum bleeding. This client needs to be assessed first to determine the amount of lochia and her bladder status.** Answer 1 is incorrect because if the client has been stable in the bleeding after delivery, and has been treated throughout her pregnancy with heparin, she does not need to be seen first. **Answer 2** is incorrect because difficulty in having a newborn latch on does not make the client most at-risk for a complication. **Answer 3** is incorrect because pyelonephritis, which is being treated with antibiotics, is not the most unstable condition of the clients presented.

> **TEST-TAKING TIP**—When determining which client needs to be seen first, think about the client whose condition is most unstable, and choose that client.
> **EV, ANL, 8, Maternity, PhI, SECE: Management of Care**

254. **(3) The International Normalized Ratio (INR), the standardization of the prothrombin time, is on the high side of the normal range of 2–3.5. The slower rate of clotting may be a problem particularly during surgery that involves a prosthesis.** Answer 1 is incorrect because the type of surgery requires close assessment of the *potential* for clotting problems. **Answer 2** is incorrect because the hematocrit is within the *low normal* range for women. **Answer 4** is incorrect because the sodium level is within *normal* range.

> **TEST-TAKING TIP**—Know the normal values for routine lab tests. Only one test (i.e., clotting) is abnormal.
> **AN, ANL, 6, M/S: Ortho, PhI, Reduction of Risk Potential**

255. **(2) The client's serum glucose level is dangerously low and will interfere with accurately assessing level of consciousness as the client is waking up from anesthesia. Glucose is needed for normal brain functioning. The lowest normal for serum glucose is 70 mg/dL.** Answer 1 is incorrect because it is *too soon* for any indication of wound infection. The slight elevation in the WBC is most likely related to the reason for the GI surgery. **Answer 3** is incorrect because the blood is *well saturated* with oxygen. If a higher blood oxygen level was desired, red blood cells would have to be given to increase oxygen-carrying capacity. The hematocrit is low for a man and low normal for a woman. **Answer 4** is incorrect because the potassium level is low normal and needs to be *maintained*, if not increased.

> **TEST-TAKING TIP**—Know the normal values for lab test. If more than one test is abnormal, ask which value places the client at the greatest risk.
> **AN, ANL, 1, M/S: Postop, PhI, Reduction of Risk Potential**

256. **(4) The client appears to have an infection and blood loss. Both of these conditions are potentially life-threatening and are the priority for treatment.** Answer 1 is incorrect because the PTT is actually on the high side of *normal*, which is 20–35 seconds. **Answer 2** is incorrect because whole blood or packed red cells do not contain WBC, and do *not need* special filtering. **Answer 3** is incorrect because *no further assessment* of the client's condition is needed. Waiting for a worsening condition could be life-threatening.

> **TEST-TAKING TIP**—Determine which values are *abnormal* and choose a response that addresses blood loss and an infection.
> **IMP, ANL, 6, M/S: Trauma, PhI, Physiological Adaptation**

257. **(2) Clients with complement deficiency typically have either an increased susceptibility to bacterial infections or increased likelihood of an autoimmune disease. Answer 1** is incorrect because the deficiency predisposes the client to infection or an autoimmune disease, *not an allergic* reaction. **Answer 3** is incorrect because *no specific* diet is known to improve complement deficiencies. **Answer 4** is incorrect because it is important to protect from infection or the seriousness of the infection. Vaccinations *would be* one way to minimize the risk of infection.

> **TEST-TAKING TIP**—Look for patterns. Only one choice is assessment: the others are "plans" or "implementation."
> **IMP, APP, 1, M/S: Resp.; PhI, Reduction of Risk Potential**

258. **(3) Diuresis regularly occurs between the 2nd and 5th day postpartum. Answer 1** is incorrect because a urinary tract infection after delivery is *not* the most common cause of increased voiding after delivery. **Answer 2** is incorrect because increased fluid intake does *not* account for the increased diuresis that happens normally after delivery. **Answer 4** is incorrect because there is *decreased* tone of the bladder and dilated ureters and renal pelvis.

> **TEST-TAKING TIP**—Think about the normal postpartum changes that occur during the first few days after delivery. Which of the possible explanations best fits the client's current condition?
> **AN, APP, 8, Maternity, HPM, Health Promotion and Maintenance**

259. **(2) Saying "dada" and "mama" (specific) is expected in a 1-year-old infant. Answer 1** is incorrect because jabbering (rapid, indistinct talk) is associated with a 7–9-month-old infant. **Answer 3** is incorrect because pointing to at least one named body part is associated with a 12–18-month-old toddler. **Answer 4** is incorrect because combining two or three words is associated with a 19–24-month-old toddler.

> **TEST-TAKING TIP**—Speech, like other aspects of growth and development, proceeds from simple to complex. A 1-year-old child must conquer simple, individual words before moving on to combination of words or identification of words.
> **AS, APP, 5, PEDS, HPM, Health Promotion and Maintenance**

260. 8–10.

> **TEST-TAKING TIP**—Disease may begin at ages 40–65; it is progressive with irreversible loss of cerebral function due to cortical atrophy.
> **AS, KNOW, 2, Psych, PsI**

261. **(1) The client is at high risk for infection and the priority would be prevention. The client with neutropenia can quickly develop septicemia. Handwashing is an effective action to prevent cross-contamination. Neutropenia is defined as an absolute neutrophil count of 1000/mm³ and is often due to myelosuppression from chemotherapy. Answer 2** is incorrect because there is *no evidence of a fluid volume deficit.* If the client presented in septic shock, rapid infusion of fluids would be a high priority. **Answer 3** is incorrect because pain is *not* associated with neutropenia specifically. The cause of the neutropenia may be due to cancer where pain management would also be a nursing concern. However, *the risk of infection is the first* concern. **Answer 4** is incorrect because neutropenia is *not* affected by allergens. The client may have related allergies; however, the priority on admission is the *prevention* of infection.

> **TEST-TAKING TIP**—Think client safety—handwashing would be best with any client. Also, choose a KIS (Keep It Simple) response that would be noninvasive.
> **IMP, APP, 1, M/S: Blood, SECE, Safety and Infection Control**

262. **(4) The first action a nurse should take is to control the bleeding. Uterine massage is the first action to control the increased blood flow. Answer 1** is incorrect because the first action should be to control the bleeding, *before* calling the physician. The client could have a very significant blood loss during the time it takes the nurse to call the physician. **Answer 2** is incorrect because getting the client up to void may result in fainting or additional blood loss. **Answer 3** is incorrect because two pads soaked in an hour is *too much* bleeding. More than one pad per hour is an unusual amount of bleeding 6 hours after delivery.

> **TEST-TAKING TIP**—Prioritize the actions the nurse should take. Stopping the bleeding is the most important action the nurse can take in this situation.
> **EV, APP, 6, Maternity, PhI, Physiological Adaptation**

263. **(3) The goal is to promote adequate nutrition through oral intake. Symptom management would be the initial nursing action. Answer 1** is incorrect because the goal is to *resume oral* intake. Parenteral nutrition would not be the initial action following removal of the Salem sump. **Answer 2** is incorrect because the goal is to *support oral* intake. Insertion of a percutaneous endoscopic gastrostomy (PEG) would not be the next step after removal of the Salem sump. **Answer 4** is incorrect because an antacid would not diminish the nausea, anorexia, or the fullness that the client is experiencing.

> **TEST-TAKING TIP**—Look for the choice that promotes "normal" oral intake. See the pattern of choices: 2 tubes, 2 meds. Choose a med that is *before* eating, not *with* the meal.
> **IMP, APP, 4, M/S: Cancer, PhI, Basic Care and Comfort**

264. **(4) The mother "expects" a behavior that the toddler can not deliver. Toddlers do not understand the concept of sharing. Answer 1** is incorrect because toddlers are messy eaters. The mother demonstrates *positive* coping abilities by preventing "messes" through the use of a plastic sheet on the floor under the high chair during mealtimes. **Answer 2** is incorrect because toddlers often say "no" but mean "yes" (and vice versa!). The mother demonstrates *positive* coping abilities by only offering choices that are already acceptable no matter what selection the toddler makes. **Answer 3** is incorrect because toddlers believe everything is "mine." The mother demonstrates *positive* coping abilities by verbalizing her feelings about a normal (but negative) developmental behavior exhibited by the toddler.

> **TEST-TAKING TIP**—Look for similarities in responses. Three of the four responses dealt with *positive* coping mechanisms on the mother's part.
> **EV, ANL, 5, PEDS, HPM, Health Promotion and Maintenance**

265. **(2) Assistive devices allow the client to self-manage the basic activities of daily living. Answer 1** is incorrect because the goal is to promote *client independence.* Rest periods should be planned; however, the client should carry out the basic activities of daily living. **Answer 3** is incorrect because *continuous cold can damage* the skin. Cold does reduce pain; however, application is *intermittent.* **Answer 4** is incorrect because wrapping in a flexed position does not encourage mobility. Range of motion exercises should be reinforced.

266. **(1) The symptoms presented may indicate pregnancy-induced hypertension. The nurse needs additional assessment information, including vital signs and reflexes.** **Answer 2** is incorrect because the client does not have complaints consistent with labor. A vaginal exam is not the most important nursing intervention for this client. **Answer 3** is in correct because the headache can be a symptom of pregnancy-induced hypertension and further evaluation needs to be performed first before pain medication is given. **Answer 4** is incorrect because contractions are a *normal* finding in a client who is at term in the pregnancy and is part of the normal assessment, but is *not the first* action the nurse should take for this client.

267. **(2)** *Discoid* **LE is a more mild form and involves only the skin. Treatment measures are conservative. Systemic LE is more severe and avoiding sun exposure is also important.** **Answer 1** is incorrect because the skin rash is an inflammation, which is aggravated by the sun. Moisture may *increase* the risk of an infection. **Answer 3** is incorrect because the rash is *not* due to an allergen. The rash is also *not* due to dryness. **Answer 4** is incorrect because alcohol and the light treatment will *increase* the dryness and *aggravate* the inflammation.

268. **(3) Infection is the leading cause of death in clients who are immunocompromised. The staff nurse should not take care of these clients to prevent any possibility (however slim) of exposing them to the chickenpox (varicella) virus.** **Answer 1** is incorrect because the incubation period for chickenpox is 2–3 weeks; and the period of communicability is 1 day before eruption of lesions, to 6 days after the first crop of vesicles when crusts have formed. The staff nurse has already been exposed to chickenpox through the child and it is too early to determine if the staff nurse will develop the disease. It might also be assumed that if the staff nurse works in pediatrics, she has been immunized against the chickenpox. Sending the staff nurse home is not justifiable. **Answer 2** is incorrect because while chickenpox is transmitted by droplet (airborne) spread, the staff nurse is not demonstrating any signs or symptoms of the disease. It is not necessary for the staff nurse to wear a face mask. **Answer 4** is incorrect because clients who have previously had chickenpox have naturally acquired, active immunity against the disease and are unlikely to acquire the disease again. The staff nurse would not be limited to caring for just these clients.

269. **(1) An activated PTT of 120 is very high. If the client had been receiving heparin before surgery, it should have been stopped at least 6 hours before surgery to reduce the risk** of bleeding. The blood sample may have been drawn out of a line with heparin in it. If this is a true value, the surgery will be canceled. **Answer 2** is incorrect because this value is *very high*, particularly if the client has not been receiving heparin. **Answer 3** is incorrect because the heparin should have been stopped at least 6 hours before surgery. This would *not* be a therapeutic level for a surgical client. **Answer 4** is incorrect because this test is used to monitor heparin therapy, *not* warfarin.

270. **(4) Restoring a client's sleep cycle is a priority. Lack of sleep can contribute to external stimuli overload and can compound the client's manic symptoms. The restoration of the client's sleep cycle can indicate that the client's condition is improving.** **Answer 1** is incorrect because *psychosocial* needs are *not* a priority of care. **Answer 2** is incorrect because a client's self-care deficit has a less of an impact on the physiological needs of the client than sleep disturbance. **Answer 3** is incorrect because *psychosocial* needs are *not* a priority of care.

271. **(3) Painless vaginal bleeding is associated with placenta previa; and an ultrasound exam would have information about the location of the placenta.** **Answer 1** is incorrect because intercourse may cause spotting, but does *not* cause a *moderate* amount of bleeding. **Answer 2** is incorrect because the client stated she had painless bleeding. This question would be a part of the normal assessment, but *not* the *first* action of the nurse. **Answer 4** is incorrect because a cervical exam can cause a small amount of bleeding, but *not* a *moderate* amount of bleeding.

272. **(3) National statistics about elder abuse demonstrate that family members are the most likely to abuse their loved ones through neglect.** **Answer 1** is incorrect because although these individuals are often abusers, they are not the most frequent. **Answer 2** is incorrect because although strangers could be abusers, they are *not* the most frequent. **Answer 4** is incorrect because being an abuser would be inconsistent with being a professional, although it does occur.

273. **(4) The child** *is* **in imminent danger of airway obstruction and only** *experienced* **personnel should accompany the child to the radiology department. Most emergency departments prefer that the child** *not* **be transported but remain on the parent's lap in the examination area during portable radiology.** **Answer 1** is incorrect because the child *is* in imminent danger of airway obstruction and *must* be kept NPO until an acceptable airway is established. **Answer 2** is

Incorrect because the child *is* in imminent danger of airway obstruction, and a patent IV line *must* be maintained in order to administer life-saving medications. **Answer 3** is incorrect because the child *is* in imminent danger of airway obstruction. Examination of the throat with a tongue blade is contraindicated until properly experienced personnel and equipment are on hand to proceed with immediate intubation or tracheostomy in the event that the examination precipitates further or complete airway obstruction.

> **TEST-TAKING TIP**—Three of the answers are safe; one answer might jeopardize the child due to inexperience on the new graduate's part. Select that answer.
> **EV, ANL, 6, PEDS, PhI, Reduction of Risk Potential**

274. **(1, 2, 3)** Answer 1 is correct because *Haemophilus influenzae* type b is a leading cause of ear infection in infants and young children which, in turn, *can* lead to development of meningitis. The *H. influenzae* type b (Hib) immunization protects against such ear infections and subsequent meningitis. Answer 2 is correct because ear infections *can* lead to development of meningitis. This is due to inability of the immune systems of infants and young children to localize infection and prevent the spread of infection (especially of an ascending nature). Tugging at the ear is a classic sign of infection in preverbal infants or young children. Answer 3 is correct because propped bottles allow the fluid to dribble from the mouth into the ear; and moisture in the ear *can* lead to infection and development of meningitis. It also interferes with human contact during feeding. Answer 4 is incorrect becauses holding an infant or young child in the arms (supine position) encourages the dribbling of fluid and food from the mouth into the ear; the moisture in the ear *can* lead to infection and development of meningitis. The upright feeding position is preferred.

> **TEST-TAKING TIP**—The key to answering this question correctly is to understand the nature of ascending infection and apply it to ear infection and meningitis.
> **EV, APP, 1, PEDS, PhI, Reduction of Risk Potential**

275. **(3)** The client has symptoms of pulmonary embolus. The oxygen saturation level is low, indicating hypoxia. Anxiety and tachypnea are also symptoms of PE. The client has been unable to ambulate because of lower leg fractures, which increases the risk for PE. **Answer 1** is incorrect because the symptoms are consistent with pulmonary embolus and *impaired oxygenation*. **Answer 2** is incorrect because the priority is responding to the low oxygen saturation and tachypnea. **Answer 4** is incorrect because the priority is stabilizing the cardiopulmonary system, and oxygen would be indicated. After the oxygen is in place, a call to the MD for orders would be appropriate.

> **TEST-TAKING TIP**—A priority is something the nurse can do to make the client comfortable—breathe more easily.
> **AN, ANL, 6, M/S: Cardiopulmonary, PhI, Physiological Adaptation**

276. **(1)** The vital signs are on the high side of normal which would be consistent with preoperative anxiety. **Answer 2** is incorrect because the temperature is *below normal*. **Answer 3** is incorrect because the blood pressure and pulse do *not* reflect fluid volume deficit. **Answer 4** is incorrect because the oxygen saturation and pain levels are not indicative of any concern.

> **TEST-TAKING TIP**—Know the normal levels. Also look for patterns—three choices imply there is a possible problem; only one choice states "no increased risk."
> **AN, ANL, 1, M/S: Preop, PhI, Reduction of Risk Potential**

277. **(2)** Maintaining a patent airway is the priority and will be easier with a client who is conscious. Complications from vomiting, such as aspiration, are more likely with a client who is sedated. Answer 1 is incorrect because bowel sounds would *not* be expected to return *immediately* after surgery. Bowel sounds return in 24–36 hours. Answer 3 is incorrect because *sensation* and *movement* cannot be determined *until* the client is awake and can respond to commands. **Answer 4** is incorrect because there should be *no* impairment of bladder function and the ability to void.

> **TEST-TAKING TIP**—Priority questions usually have more than one correct answer. Think of the very first thing you would do. Because the timing is the immediate post-op period, you would eliminate **Answers 1** and **3**.
> **AS, APP, 1, M/S: Postop, PhI, Reduction of Risk Potential**

278. **(1)** Physiological jaundice usually appears on the second to fourth day in normal full-term infants. **Answer 2** is incorrect because liver failure would appear *before* 3 days of age. **Answer 3** is incorrect because neonatal sepsis symptoms include lethargy, *and poor feeding*. **Answer 4** is incorrect because jaundice caused by blood incompatibility appears *before* 24 hours of age.

> **TEST-TAKING TIP**—The key concept in this question is time frame: 3 days old. **Answers 2** and **4** occur in an *earlier* time frame. Normal physiological jaundice is common during this time frame (i.e., 3 days).
> **AN, APP, 1, Newborn, PhI, Physiological Adaptation**

279. **(3)** Excessive use of decongestants may actually result in rebound swelling. Corticosteroid nasal spray may also be used to reduce mucosal inflammation. **Answer 1** is incorrect because headaches are a symptom of sinusitis and may continue to occur *until* the infection is cleared. **Answer 2** is incorrect because humidification is more effective when *warm*. Normal saline irrigations may also be used. **Answer 4** is incorrect because there is *no* restriction of fluids with sinusitis. Instead, drinking sufficient fluids would help to rinse away any postnasal discharge from the back of the throat.

> **TEST-TAKING TIP**—Consider how each choice relates to the diagnosis—would it improve or aggravate the symptoms? Therefore, eliminate **Answer 2**. Choose the option that suggests caution (e.g., "use conservatively").
> **IMP, APP, 1, M/S: ENT, PhI, Reduction of Risk Potential**

280. **(3)** Clients with manic behavior have poor insight into the seriousness of their behaviors and lack judgment. The family's perceptions of the client's behaviors are probably more realistic. Answer 1 is incorrect because a client experiencing mania has an *elevated* mood and is euphoric. **Answer 2** is incorrect because clients who are in a manic phase of bipolar illness do *not* usually experience auditory hallucinations. Delusions of grandeur are common. **Answer 4** is incorrect because clients with mania are socially *hyperactive*.

> **TEST-TAKING TIP**—Eliminate the choices that you know are not correct. Visualize clients who have mania; denial and excessive spending are prominent symptoms of the disorder. Auditory hallucinations are symptoms for *schizophrenia*, and hopelessness and social isolation are prominent symptoms of *depression*.
> **AS, ANL, 7, Psych, PsI, Psychosocial Integrity**

281. **(2)** The bleeding can be excessive and obstruct the airway or pool in the oral cavity. **Answer 1** is incorrect because the purpose of the packing is to act as a tamponade and promote clot formation. Removal of the packing and forcing air through the nose would dislodge the clots. The packing *remains in place* 48–72 hours. **Answer 3** is incorrect because

there is *no* restriction on diet with epistaxis. If a large amount of blood has been swallowed, the client may complain of nausea. **Answer 4** is incorrect because sitting upright is more likely to prevent plugging of the eustachian tube, *not* the *alignment* of the head.

> **TEST-TAKING TIP**—Think client safety—if bleeding is severe enough to require hospitalization, aspiration is a risk.
> **IMP, APP, 6, M/S: ENT, PhI, Reduction of Risk Potential**

282. **(1) The infant who is bottle-fed does not receive the same protection against respiratory viruses and allergy that comes from breast milk. Also, the bottle is likely to be propped, which also contributes to possible infection. In combination, these factors contribute to development of ear infection in the infant who is bottle-fed, which can lead to meningitis.** Answer 2 is incorrect because the infant who is breast-fed receives secretory immunoglobulin A (IgA) which limits the exposure of the eustachian tube and middle ear mucosa to microbial pathogens and foreign proteins. Reflux of milk up the eustachian tube is less likely to occur in infants who are breast-fed because of the semivertical positioning during breast feeding compared with bottle feeding. **Answer 3** is incorrect because a 2-year-old child would have received all of the required *Haemophilus influenzae, type b,* immunizations which would provide protection against ear infection and subsequent meningitis. In addition, such a child would always be fed in the upright position and would probably also have a gastrostomy tube in place for feedings. These measures would also prevent the development of ear infection that could lead to meningitis. **Answer 4** is incorrect because while living with a smoker (passive smoking) is believed to be a risk factor for ear infections and subsequent meningitis, it does not have the direct, established relationship that bottle feeding does. Tobacco smoke inhalation may increase the risk of a blocked eustachian tube by impairing mucociliary function, causing congestion of soft nasopharyngeal tissues, or predisposing clients to upper respiratory infection.

> **TEST-TAKING TIP**—Any child is at risk for ear infection and subsequent meningitis. In order to answer the question correctly, identify the specific *risk factors* associated with the diseases.
> **AN, ANL, 1, PEDS, HPM, Health Promotion and Maintenance**

283. **(3) Chickenpox is transmitted by droplet (airborne) spread and requires *respiratory* isolation. The most important component of this type of isolation is a *face mask*. The new graduate is correct in putting on a gown and gloves prior to entering the room but has overlooked the face mask, the most essential item needed in this type of isolation technique.** Answer 1 is incorrect because the child is in isolation and disposable items, rather than nondisposable items, *should* be used whenever possible. This reduces the possibility of contamination and also reduces cost factors in the sterilization of non-disposable items. **Answer 2** is incorrect because the child is in isolation and disposable items, rather than nondisposable items, *should* be used whenever possible. This reduces the possibility of contamination and also reduces cost factors in the sterilization of nondisposable items. **Answer 4** is incorrect because a covered waste container *should* be placed directly outside of the room. The face mask worn in the room will be placed in the covered waste container when exiting the room.

> **TEST-TAKING TIP**—The transmission of the disease determines the type of isolation and the required items needed to enforce the isolation technique.
> **EV, ANL, 1, PEDS, SECE, Management of Care**

284. **(2) This is the appropriate treatment for engorgement when the client plans to breastfeed. Answer 1** is incorrect because the client is likely engorged, and ice would suppress lactation. **Answer 3** is incorrect because ice is the treatment recommended for *suppression* of lactation. It will do nothing to relieve the engorgement, nor assist the infant to latch-on and feed. **Answer 4** is incorrect because giving the infant formula will *not* relieve the engorgement.

> **TEST-TAKING TIP**—Look at options that group together. **Answers 1 and 3** use ice packs, **Answers 2 and 4** use warm packs. This reduces the choices to two options: ice packs or warm packs. Eliminate the choices with ice packs, which cause suppression of lactation. Then examine the remaining two options (**Answers 2 and 4**); eliminate the option that includes formula (**Answer 4**).
> **IMP, APP, 4, Maternity, PhI, Basic Care and Comfort**

285. **(1) This client is at high risk for developing thrombophlebitis because of the operative delivery, pregnancy and obesity. Early ambulation will help prevent clot formation.** Answer 2 is incorrect because it is a part of the treatment for this client, but it is *not* the most important nursing action. **Answer 3** is incorrect because pain control is important for any hospitalized client; it is the fifth vital sign, but *not* the most important action. **Answer 4** is incorrect because intake and output are *routine* for all surgical clients, but *not* the most important action.

> **TEST-TAKING TIP**—This is a question of priority. The most life-threatening complication is clot formation and risk of embolism. The nursing action that addresses this complication is early ambulation.
> **PL, APP, 1, Maternity, PhI, Reduction of Risk Potential**

286. **(3) Drug therapy is the only effective treatment for TB. Clients often discontinue medications when they begin to feel better. The client may appear to be symptom-free but the organism is still present.** Answer 1 is incorrect because prednisone is *not* a drug of choice for TB and it has *no* effect on urine color. **Answer 2** is incorrect because using the spirometer, if needed, is *not* the most important aspect of TB treatment. **Answer 4** is incorrect because initial treatment is daily doses of combined drug therapy for a minimum of 6–12 months. *Sputum culture*, not a repeat skin test, and the absence of symptoms would be used to determine treatment effectiveness.

> **TEST-TAKING TIP**—Look for similar words in stem and option— "TB skin test" and "anti-TB drugs."
> **IMP, COM, 1, M/S: Infection Control, PhI, Pharmacological and Parenteral Therapies**

287. **100 μg/hr.** 100 mg of MS over 24 hours is about 4 mg/hr. Based on the table, the client would require 100 μg/hr.

> **TEST-TAKING TIP**—This is a basic ratio calculation—dose on hand versus desired dose.
> **PL, APP, 3, M/S: Calculation, PhI, Pharmacological and Parenteral Therapies**

288. **0.** The total amount of acetaminophen that can be safely ingested is 4 g or 4000 mg. The client is taking 1 g or 1000 mg every 6 hours for a total of 4 g or 4000 mg. No additional Tylenol tablets can be safely taken.

> **TEST-TAKING TIP**—Know basic conversions from grams and milligrams.
> **PL, COM, 3, M/S: Calculation, PhI, Pharmacological and Parenteral Therapies**

289. **2.** A dose every 6 minutes equals 10 doses in 1 hour for a total of 2 mg of hydromorphone every hour.

290. (2) Delusions are a symptom that indicates that the client's
thoughts are altered. **Answer 1** is incorrect because in auditory hallucinations the nursing diagnosis is sensory/percep-
tual alterations. **Answer 3** is incorrect because clients who
express anxiety do *not* have altered thought process. **Answer
4** is incorrect because clients with depression do *not* have
altered thought process.

> TEST-TAKING TIP—Eliminate the choices that are not
> theoretically correct. Anxiety and depression (**Answers 3**
> and **4**) are symptoms which do *not* alter the client's
> thought process. Visualize clients who have auditory
> hallucinations and delusions. Hearing voices (**Answer 1**)
> is alteration in the client's *senses*. Clients who are
> delusional are expressing *thoughts* that are not based in
> reality.
> AS, ANL, 7, Psych, PsI, Psychosocial Integrity

291. <u>5</u> To compute the dose, use the dose on hand and the
desired dose ratio:

$$\frac{900 \text{ mg} \times 200 \text{ mg}}{22.5 \times 900} = \frac{4500}{} = 5 \text{ mL}$$

> TEST-TAKING TIP—Set the problem up using the
> basic dose on hand versus desired dose equation.
> PL, COM, 1, M/S: Calculation, PhI, Pharmacological and
> Parenteral Therapies

292. (3) The cause of the muscular weakness can be the result
of over- or undertreatment with anticholinesterase compounds. If the muscle weakness is due to under treatment,
the client will get stronger with Tensilon. Answer 1 is
incorrect because the muscular weakness is *not visible* with a
scan. **Answer 2** is incorrect because the problem is *not*
related to *ventilation and perfusion*. **Answer 4** is incorrect
because urinary catecholamine excretion is done to assess
adrenal medullary function.

> TEST-TAKING TIP—Look for patterns and pick the
> one that is different. Three of the choices are laboratory
> tests; one is a drug.
> IMP, APP, 3, M/S: Endocrine, PhI, Physiological
> Adaptation

293. (2) Glomerulonephritis is an immune-complex disease
(i.e., a reaction that occurs as a by-product of an
antecedent streptococcal infection with certain strains of
the group A β-hemolytic *Streptococcus*). The infection
begins primarily in the throat or skin. Answer 1 is incorrect because it is an emotional response (but typical for a 6-
year-old child) rather than a response that demonstrates
understanding of the cause of glomerulonephritis. Children
in this age group often tend to associate illness with "punishment" for misbehavior. **Answer 3** is incorrect because
glomerulonephritis is an immune-complex disease (i.e., a
reaction that occurs as a byproduct of an antecedent streptococcal infection with certain strains of the group A β-
hemolytic *Streptococcus*). While signs and symptoms of
glomerulonephritis are manifested in the appearance of the
urine (thick; reddish-brown; decreased amounts), the infection begins primarily in the *throat* or skin. **Answer 4** is
incorrect because glomerulonephritis is an immune-
complex disease (i.e., a reaction that occurs as a by-product
of an antecedent streptococcal infection with certain strains
of the group A β-hemolytic *Streptococcus*). The infection is
not transmitted from "person-to-person." The infection
begins primarily in the throat or skin.

294. (2) Evidence has been found that all cultures practice some
form of abuse when all abuse categories are considered—
physical, emotional, financial, and neglect. Answer 1 is
incorrect because elder abuse has been found to be present
in all cultures. It is, however, often defined and executed
differently in various cultures, which makes it hard to
assess. **Answer 3** is incorrect because elder abuse has been
found to be present in all cultures. **Answer 4** is incorrect
because elder abuse has been found to be present in all
cultures

> TEST-TAKING TIP—Look for the choice (**Answer 2**)
> that includes **Answers 1** and **3** (i.e., covers all cultures and
> subgroups).
> AN, KNOW, 7, M/S: Geriatrics, PsI, Psychosocial Integrity

295. (1) The change in dosage is accurate and the activated PTT
is nearing $1\frac{1}{2}$ to 2 times the control, but the desired therapeutic level has not been reached. Answer 2 is incorrect
because the change in rate will not deliver the correct
amount of heparin. **Answer 3** is incorrect because the
change in rate will not deliver the correct amount of
heparin. **Answer 4** is incorrect because there is no indication
that the change in dosage is an unusual order.

> TEST-TAKING TIP—Think about what is being
> asked—key word is "bolus" in the stem and correct answer.
> IMP, APP, 6, M/S: Meds, PhI, Pharmacological and
> Parenteral Therapies

296. (3) This client is a grand multipara delivering her sixth
infant. This places her at a higher risk for uterine atony
and associated hemorrhage. Answer 1 is incorrect because
this client has *no identified risk* factors for postpartum
hemorrhage. **Answer 2** is incorrect because this client does
have increased blood loss associated with surgery, but she
does not have *additional risk factors* associated with postpartum hemorrhage. **Answer 4** is incorrect because, although
this client does have increased risk with vacuum-assisted
delivery and a large infant, these risk factors *are not greater
than the risk* of postpartum hemorrhage in the client who is
a grand multipara.

> TEST-TAKING TIP—Carefully examine all risk factors
> in each option. Each client has some risk factors; however,
> choose the client with the highest risk.
> AN, ANL, 6, Maternity, PhI, Physiological Adaptation

297. (4) The nurse has assumed an active, problem solving role
in the situation. Patient-controlled analgesia (PCA) could
be suggested to the pediatrician by the nurse. This technique has been used successfully for sickle cell–related
pain. The child is old enough to operate the PCA. The PCA
reinforces the child's role and responsibility in managing
the pain and provides flexibility for pain which may vary
in severity over time. Answer 1 is incorrect because warm
compresses are an example of supportive therapy (increase
blood flow and oxygen supply via vasodilation) rather than
pain control. The warm compresses should be continued.
Answer 2 is incorrect because the nurse can not arbitrarily
disregard the pediatrician's order for analgesia without first
discussing the situation with the pediatrician. The nurse
may also be making a promise to the child that will not be
possible to keep. **Answer 3** is incorrect because it implies
that there is no choice in the situation. It also "passes the
buck" to the pediatrician and implies that the nurse is
powerless to intervene in the situation.

TEST-TAKING TIP—Two of the answers involve a violation of the nurse's role in client care; one of the answers implies that the nurse has no input about client care; select the answer that allows the nurse to be actively involved in the management of client care.
IMP, APP, 3, PEDS, PhI, Basic Care and Comfort

298. **(3) Using one eye results in seeing only one image. Answer 1** is incorrect because this does *not* address the double vision. **Answer 2** is incorrect because the problem is double vision, *not* difficulty swallowing. **Answer 4** is incorrect because the problem is *not* acuity, but seeing double.

TEST-TAKING TIP—Narrow the choice. Diplopia involves vision. Only one of the options minimizes the specific double vision problem.
IMP, APP, 2, M/S: Neuro, SECE, Safety and Infection Control

299. **(1) This client is the most at risk for developing complications related to the delay in treatment. The high bilirubin level can lead to kernicterus. Answer 2** is incorrect because this is a *routine* injection that can be done at any time during the scheduled shift. It is a preventative measure, not treatment for an acute condition. **Answer 3** is incorrect because this client's condition is not the most unstable. Her care would *not* be compromised by a delay in treatment. **Answer 4** is incorrect because hyperemesis needs treatment, but a delay will *not* result in a poor client outcome.

TEST-TAKING TIP—This is a question about priority. Think of the client who may have a poor outcome if there is a delay in nursing care. In this case, the infant's bilirubin level continues to increase until phototherapy is started.
IMP, ANL, 1, Maternity, SECE, Management of Care: Priority

300. **(1, 3, 5) Answer 1 is correct because insomnia is a common withdrawal symptom and can be treated with a benzodiazepine. Answer 3 is correct because agitation is treated with benzodiazepines and is a symptom during the detoxification phase. Answer 5 is correct because benzodiazepine medications will prevent withdrawal seizures. Answer 2** is incorrect because benzodiazepines are used for detoxification and will *not prevent* relapse. Relapse prevention occurs in the recovery phase of treatment. **Answer 4** is incorrect because benzodiazepines will *not prevent* weight loss, although establishing proper nutrition is an important part of the detoxification phase. **Answer 6** is incorrect because benzodiazepine medications will *not* treat or prevent suicide.

TEST-TAKING TIP—Read the stem carefully. The question asks for treatment of alcohol withdrawal with benzodiazepine medications. The answers have to be correct for both the detoxification *time frame* and the drug.
IMP, ANL, 7, Psych, PsI, Psychosocial Integrity

301. **(4) The TPN should be maintained at a consistent rate. Slowing it down can precipitate *hypoglycemia*, while increasing the rate, or "catching up," can result in *hyperglycemia*. Answer 1** is incorrect because it is inappropriate to add NPH, an *intermediate-acting insulin*, to the TPN solution. **Answer 2** is incorrect because the client's fingerstick blood glucose should be checked *every 6 hours* for several days after the TPN is initiated. **Answer 3** is incorrect because this is appropriate for *discharge* teaching; but if the client is in an acute care setting, maintaining the correct flow rate is the nurse's responsibility.

TEST-TAKING TIP—Answering this question correctly required careful reading of the question: the incorrect options were *only partially wrong*. Insulin is often added

to TPN solutions (**Answer 1**), but always *regular* insulin, and in *smaller* amounts. Fingerstick blood glucose levels should be performed on a client who has just started TPN (**Answer 2**), but levels should be checked *more often* than once a day. Teaching the client about managing own TPN (**Answer 3**) is appropriate, if the client is going to be *discharged* with TPN.
IMP, APP, 4, M/S: Metab., PhI, Pharmacological and Parenteral Therapies

302. **(2) Beta-adrenergic blockers are contraindicated for the client with asthma using albuterol. Answer 1** is incorrect because there is *no* contraindication for fluoxetine. **Answer 3** is incorrect because there is *no* contraindication for ranitidine. **Answer 4** is incorrect because there is *no* contraindication for ipratropium. This medication is often used in conjunction with albuterol.

TEST-TAKING TIP—Consider the drug classifications: fluoxetine is an *antidepressant*, ranitidine is an *H_2-histamine receptor agonist*, and ipratropium is a *bronchodilator*. In general, these categories are *not* contraindicated with albuterol. Beta-adrenergic blocking medications can cause bronchospasm, and are contraindicated with albuterol.
IMP, APP, 6, M/S: Resp., PhI, Pharmacological and Parenteral Therapies

303. **(1) This statement is part of the teaching for the client about what is a normal process of cord separation. Answer 2** is incorrect because it is *not* recommended to cover the umbilical stump with any dressing or covering. **Answer 3** is incorrect because antibiotic ointment will *not* assist in the separation of the cord. **Answer 4** is incorrect because it is *not necessary* to apply *any* solutions to the umbilical cord.

TEST-TAKING TIP—Three options focus on an action to take; one option is an information-giving statement. Choose the option that is different from the others (**Answer 1**).
IMP, APP, 5, Newborn, HPM, Health Promotion and Maintenance

304. **(1, 5) Answer 1 is correct because an infant who is wet will lose a lot of heat. Answer 5 is correct because the bath should not be performed until the infant's temperature is stable. Answer 2** is incorrect because eye prophylaxis and vitamin K should be given within *one hour* after delivery. **Answer 3** is incorrect because vernix *does not need to be removed* and it does not cause infection. **Answer 4** is incorrect because extensive handling does not facilitate bonding.

TEST-TAKING TIP—Think about the immediate needs of a newborn in transition. Choose the two options that focus on temperature regulation.
IMP, APP, 5, Newborn, HPM, Health Promotion and Maintenance

305. **(2) Over-the-counter lotion may not be applied to the infant's skin. For the infant with eczema, all lubrication must be prescribed. Usually the lubricant is a nonlipid, hydrophilic agent (e.g., *Cetaphil*). Answer 1** is incorrect because tepid baths (up to 4 times a day) *are* recommended for the infant with eczema. The tepid water is comforting to the infant and the bath should be immediately followed by the application of a prescribed lubricant while the skin is still moist. **Answer 3** is incorrect because the infant with eczema has breaks in the skin (first line of defense) and is at *risk for* infection. Standard precautions, such as gloves, *should* be worn when giving direct client care to prevent infection. **Answer 4** is incorrect because covering the infant's hands will prevent scratching at the lesions which are pruritic. 100% cotton mittens or socks *are* frequently used

for this purpose. Elbow restraints are not used because the antecubital space is a common site for eczema.

> **TEST-TAKING TIP**—In the hospital setting, *all* substances administered/applied to a client must be prescribed.
> **EV, ANL, 1, PEDS, SECE, Management of Care**

306. **(1) Verifying the correct information *prevents* transfusion reactions. Answer 2** is incorrect because running the blood slowly at first, which is correct technique, will help *minimize* a transfusion reaction, but won't *prevent* a reaction. **Answer 3** is incorrect because y-type tubing is used to facilitate the administration of normal saline immediately before and after the transfusion, but *does not prevent* a transfusion reaction. **Answer 4** is incorrect because frequent vital signs help detect the presence of a transfusion reaction, and although appropriate, will *not prevent a reaction.*

> **TEST-TAKING TIP**—As the question states, focus on the action that *prevents* the transfusion reaction.
> **IMP, APP, 6, M/S: Blood, PhI, Pharmacological and Parenteral Therapies**

307. **(3) Red spots with a white center on the buccal mucosa describe Koplik spots, which are a defining characteristic of measles. This is a *specific* rather than a *general* response. Answer 1** is incorrect because it is a *general* response rather than a *specific* response. Fever and malaise could be associated with many common, communicable diseases of childhood. **Answer 2** is incorrect because it is a *general* response rather than a *specific* response. A rash on the face, trunk, and limbs could be associated with many common, communicable diseases of childhood. **Answer 4** is incorrect because it is a *general* response rather than a *specific* response. A dry cough could be associated with many common, communicable diseases of childhood.

> **TEST-TAKING TIP**—Three of the responses are general in nature; select the one that is different (specific in nature).
> **AS, APP, 1, PEDS, PhI, Physiological Adaptation**

308. **(2) Increased blood glucose is a characteristic of Cushing's syndrome. Answer 1** is incorrect because Cushing's syndrome is characterized by *increased corticosteroids.* Administering additional corticosteroids would be inappropriate. **Answer 3** is incorrect because decreased resistance to infection is a characteristic of *Addison's* disease. **Answer 4** is incorrect because improving self-esteem is a long-term goal for the client, and is *not* appropriately addressed during an *acute* illness.

> **TEST-TAKING TIP**—Notice that the question specifies a client who is acutely ill. **Answer 4** addresses long-term concerns, while **Answers 1** and **3** are relevant to Addison's disease, rather than Cushing's syndrome.
> **IMP, APP, 6, M/S: Endocrine, PhI, Reduction of Risk Potential**

309. **(3) The client's dose of corticosteroids needs to be *increased during times of physical or emotional stress* to compensate for the increased levels of corticosteroids needed by the body at these times. Answer 1** is incorrect because doses of corticosteroids must be *adjusted periodically* to meet the individual needs of the client. **Answer 2** is incorrect because the dose of corticosteroid will most likely need to be *increased* during times of stress. **Answer 4** is incorrect because the client with Addison's disease will need lifetime replacement of corticosteroids.

> **TEST-TAKING TIP**—Remember the basic pathophysiology of Addison's disease: deficiency of corticosteroids, which requires lifetime replacement therapy.

IMP, APP, 5, M/S: Endocrine, PhI, Reduction of Risk Potential

310. **15 and 27.**

> **TEST-TAKING TIP**—Think: young adulthood (15–27 years of age)
> **AS, KNOW, 3, Psych, PsI, Psychosocial Integrity**

311. **(2) SIADH results in fluid retention and decreased serum osmolality due to the excess secretion of antidiuretic hormone (ADH). Answer 1** is incorrect because SIADH has nothing to do with cellular resistance to insulin. **Answer 3** is incorrect because *body weight* and *fluid volume* both *increase* due to the fluid retention characteristic of SIADH. **Answer 4** is incorrect because *urinary output decreases* in SIADH, and dilutional *hypo*natremia occurs.

> **TEST-TAKING TIP**—Consider the pathophysiology of SIADH: secretion of antidiuretic hormone far above that dictated by plasma osmotic pressure, which, in turn, causes fluid retention.
> **AS, COM, 6, M/S: Renal, PhI, Physiological Adaptation**

312. **(1, 2, 3) Answer 1** is correct because a strawberry-like tongue is a defining characteristic of scarlet fever. A white strawberry-like tongue is usually noted during the first 1–2 days of the disease, while a red strawberry-like tongue is usually noted after 4–5 days of the disease. It is usually noted during the acute exanthema of the disease. **Answer 2** is correct because a sore throat is a defining characteristic of scarlet fever. Group A β-*hemolytic streptococci* is the causative agent for scarlet fever, while the spread of the disease is droplet. The sore throat is due to the tonsillitis that usually accompanies scarlet fever. It is usually noted during the acute exanthema of the disease. **Answer 3** is correct because circumoral pallor is a defining characteristic of scarlet fever. It is usually noted when the face is flushed during the acute exanthema of the disease. **Answer 4** is incorrect because the rash associated with scarlet fever is red, pinhead-size punctuate lesions which rapidly become generalized but are absent on the face. Crusted lesions are associated with chickenpox.

> **TEST-TAKING TIP**—Know all of the characteristics generally associated with common, communicable childhood diseases AND the characteristics associated ONLY with that common, communicable childhood disease.
> **AS, APP, 1, PEDS, PhI, Physiological Adaptation**

313. **(2) Diphtheria is a serious childhood disease. It is characterized by the formation of a membrane over the tonsils, uvula, soft palate and posterior pharynx. The child is at *high risk* for airway obstruction and a tracheostomy tray must be kept by the bedside. The nurse should assess this child first. Answer 1** is incorrect because fifth disease is a relatively benign childhood disease. It is characterized by a "slapped face" appearance and a rash. Hospitalization of the child is usually not necessary unless the child becomes dehydrated or is immunosuppressed. This child is at *no risk* for airway obstruction. The nurse should assess this child last. **Answer 3** is incorrect because while pertussis is a serious childhood disease, it is not as serious as diphtheria. It is characterized by paroxysms of coughing. The child is at *moderate risk* for airway obstruction. The nurse should assess this child *second.* **Answer 4** is incorrect because while measles is a serious childhood disease, it is not as serious as diphtheria (or pertussis). It is characterized by a rash and potential complications such as pneumonia. The child is at *low risk* for airway obstruction. The nurse should assess this child *third.*

> **TEST-TAKING TIP**—Know the most serious consequence of each disease; then rank them in order of impor-

tance. Maintaining a patent airway is always the highest priority.
AN, ANL, 1, PEDS, SECE, Management of Care

314. **(1) These findings are consistent with ARDS. Generally accepted criteria for ARDS include refractory hypoxemia, pulmonary artery wedge pressure <18 mm Hg, and a predisposing condition for ARDS. Answer 2** is incorrect because pulmonary artery wedge pressure does *not increase* with ARDS, unless the client also has congestive heart failure. **Answer 3** is incorrect because the hallmark of ARDS is refractory hypoxemia, therefore a client with ARDS is *not likely* to have a Po$_2$ of 90 mm Hg. In addition, pulmonary artery wedge pressure does *not increase* with ARDS, unless the client also has congestive heart failure. **Answer 4** is incorrect because the hallmark of ARDS is refractory hypoxemia, therefore a client with ARDS is *not likely* to have a Po$_2$ of 96 mm Hg. In addition, pulmonary artery wedge pressure does *not increase* with ARDS, unless the client also has congestive heart failure.

TEST-TAKING TIP—Select the option that is different. **Answers 2, 3,** and **4** all indicate *increased* pulmonary artery wedge pressure, while **Answer 1** indicates a normal wedge pressure. Normal wedge pressure combined with a *low Po$_2$* makes **Answer 1** the correct choice.
AS, APP, 6, M/S: Resp., PhI, Physiological Adaptation

315. **(2) Rubbing the infant's back is a proper method of stimulation. Answer 1** is incorrect because vigorous suctioning of the mouth and nose may cause swelling of the mucous membranes. **Answer 3** is incorrect because shaking an infant is *never* a proper method of infant stimulation. **Answer 4** is incorrect because dilating the anal sphincter can cause *damage* and is not recommended as a method of stimulating an infant to breathe.

TEST-TAKING TIP—Eliminate interventions that may cause injury to the infant ("vigorous," "shaking," and "dilating").
IMP, COM, 6, Newborn, PhI, Physiological Adaptation

316. **(4) Standing away from the bed while a shock is delivered prevents health-care personnel from receiving a shock. Answer 1** is incorrect because alcohol can *ignite* when electric current is passed through it. **Answer 2** is incorrect because it is *inappropriate to further sedate a client who is unconscious.* **Answer 3** is incorrect because *cardioversion* is the first *treatment of choice* for a client who is *unconscious.*

TEST-TAKING TIP—Notice that the question specifies a client who is unconscious. **Answers 2** and **3** are appropriate for a client who is *conscious and hemodynamically stable.* **Answer 1** reflects a dangerous practice.
IMP, APP, 6, M/S: Cardiac, PhI, Physiological Adaptation

317. **(3) Fluids and antibiotics are generally given before surgery to hydrate the client, and treat potential or actual urinary tract infections. Answer 1** is incorrect because restricting fluids will make the client more susceptible to infection and may cause dehydration. **Answer 2** is incorrect because sexual function is not generally lost as a result of TURP. **Answer 4** is incorrect because the purpose for the TURP is to *relieve obstruction* by the prostate. A large catheter such as a 16 Fr most likely cannot be passed through the obstruction of the prostate gland.

TEST-TAKING TIP—Focus on the two options that are almost *opposite*: **Answer 1** indicates *restricting* fluid, while **Answer 3** *gives* the client fluid. In this case, the correct answer is almost counter-intuitive. If the client cannot empty the bladder, it would almost make sense to

withhold additional fluid; however, many clients have already self-restricted fluids and the client is often at risk for dehydration.
IMP, APP, 6, M/S: GU, PhI, Physiological Adaptation

318. **(2) The APGAR score is an indicator of how well the infant is making the transition to extrauterine life. Answer 1** is incorrect because the APGAR score is *not* used to determine whether *resuscitation* is required. **Answer 3** is incorrect because the APGAR score is *not an indicator* of the likelihood of developing *cerebral palsy.* **Answer 4** is incorrect because the APGAR score is *not an indicator of long-term neurological* damage.

TEST-TAKING TIP—Eliminate the three options that imply dire problems (**Answers 1, 3** and **4**). Choose the option that calls for assessment ("additional observation").
AN, COM, 5, Newborn, HPM, Health Promotion and Maintenance

319. **(3) This position facilitates ventilation of the remaining right lung. Answer 1** is incorrect because the client should have the head of the bed *elevated* to facilitate ventilation. **Answer 2** is incorrect because the client should have the head of the bed *elevated* to facilitate ventilation. **Answer 4** is incorrect because the client should not be positioned with the remaining right lung dependent.

TEST-TAKING TIP—When a lung is removed, nursing care is aimed at optimizing function of the remaining lung. In this case, positioning the client on the *right* side impairs ventilation of the *right lung;* therefore, **Answer 4** can be eliminated. In addition, the client should be positioned with the head of the bed *elevated;* therefore, **Answers 1** and **2** ("flat") can be eliminated.
IMP, APP, 6, M/S: Resp., PhI, Basic Care and Comfort

320. **(2) This intervention will help the client's sleep pattern and is a nonpharmacological intervention. Answer 1** is incorrect because administering a hypnotic is *not* a nonpharmacological treatment. **Answer 3** is incorrect because it *includes* a pharmacological intervention, although suggesting that the client lay down to allow the medication to work would enhance its effectiveness. **Answer 4** is incorrect because drinking 2–3 glasses of wine before bedtime *may contribute* to insomnia.

TEST-TAKING TIP—Look for clues in the stem and eliminate the choices that are the pharmacological interventions. Choose the answer that will cause the least harm (i.e., depending on the client's history, suggesting that a client drink alcohol [**Answer 4**] *could have harmful* implications.)
IMP, APP, 3, Psych, PhI, Basic Care and Comfort

321. **(4) Due to the body's inability to resist infection in sickle cell anemia, infection is the leading cause of death. Keeping immunizations updated, staying away from others who are ill, and handwashing are critical interventions for the toddler with sickle cell anemia. Answer 1** is incorrect because, while encouraging the toddler to eat a balanced diet is a good response, toddlers have definite food likes and dislikes. They are also independent and want to feed themselves. The toddler's appetite will decline around 2 years of age because the toddler is not growing as fast as in infancy. It is best to avoid "battles" over eating. The *quality* of the food is more important than the *quantity.* **Answer 2** is incorrect because, while encouraging the toddler to engage in non-strenuous play activities is a good response, toddlers are high energy, vigorous players. They can not pace themselves when playing and tend to play until exhausted. It is best to monitor the toddler's play and prevent it from reaching this level. However, this measure must be tempered with an awareness

of the toddler's need to live a normal life. Overprotection of the toddler should be avoided. **Answer 3** is incorrect because, while protecting the toddler from excess exposure to the sun is a correct response, the toddler needs free, unstructured, outdoor play time. It is best to provide weather-appropriate outdoor clothing and to offer additional fluids to prevent overheating, which can lead to dehydration that can precipitate a sickling episode.

> **TEST-TAKING TIP**—All of the responses are reasonable; select the one response that correlates with the "worst case scenario" should the mother not follow the nurse's advice.
> **PL, APP, 1, PEDS, PhI, Reduction of Risk Potential**

322. **(1, 2) Answer 1 is correct because morning sickness is related to hormone fluctuation that occurs prior to the establishment of the placenta as the source of pregnancy hormones. Answer 2 is correct because fetal movement (quickening) usually is perceived by the pregnant woman by 16–18 weeks of gestation. Answer 3 is incorrect** because urinary frequency is a result of *hormonal* influences of pregnancy, not as a result of increased susceptibility to urinary tract infections. **Answer 4 is incorrect** because easy fatigability is characteristic of *first* trimester, not *third* trimester of pregnancy. **Answer 5 is incorrect** because *moderate* bleeding is *not normal* in any trimester. Spotting may be normal, but not moderate bleeding. It may be a sign of imminent spontaneous abortion.

> **TEST-TAKING TIP**—Think accurate symptoms for a "time frame"—early (i.e., first trimester) *concerns*.
> **IMP, APP, 5, Maternity, HPM, Health Promotion and Maintenance**

323. **(4) Raynaud's phenomenon is often associated with underlying collagen diseases such as rheumatoid arthritis, scleroderma, and systemic lupus erythematosus. Answer 1 is** incorrect because Raynaud's Phenomenon is a vasospastic disorder of *small cutaneous arteries*, therefore ulnar and radial pulses are *not* affected. **Answer 2 is incorrect** because coldness and numbness *occurs* in the affected extremities, followed by throbbing pain and swelling. **Answer 3 is** incorrect because affected tissues first exhibit *pallor* from the vasoconstriction, then *cyanosis*, before becoming *hyperemic* as the episode subsides.

> **TEST-TAKING TIP**—Raynaud's phenomenon is a disorder of *small cutaneous arteries* in which vasospasm *episodically* occurs. Knowing this, **Answer 1** can be eliminated. **Answer 2** can be eliminated because vasospastic pain is likely to be *more severe*, and **Answer 3** is only partially correct.
> **AS, APP, 6, M/S: Vascular, PhI, Physiological Adaptation**

324. **(3) This statement reflects a lack of understanding on the client's part. Answer 1 is incorrect** because exercise *is* strongly recommended in the management of hypertension; therefore, this statement *does* reflect understanding of the treatment. **Answer 2 is incorrect** because restricting salt intake *is* strongly recommended in the management of hypertension; therefore, this statement *does* reflect understanding of the treatment. **Answer 4 is incorrect** because stress reduction *is* strongly recommended in the management of hypertension; therefore, this statement *does* reflect understanding of the treatment.

> **TEST-TAKING TIP**—The question asks which statement indicates *lack of understanding* by the client of the management of hypertension; therefore, the correct answer is the "wrong" one.
> **EV, APP, 6, M/S: CV, PhI, Reduction of Risk Potential**

325. **(1) Elevated serum lipids, hypertension, and smoking are all major, modifiable risk factors, which means that these risk factors are known to significantly increase the risk of coronary artery disease, However, because they are *modifiable* risk factors, risk can be reduced by changes in the client's behaviors. Answer 2 is incorrect because** *gender* is not a modifiable risk factor. Diabetes mellitus is considered a contributing factor: it is associated with coronary artery disease, but the significance and prevalence is not clear. **Answer 3 is incorrect** because family history is not modifiable. **Answer 4 is incorrect** because age is not modifiable, and diabetes mellitus is a contributing factor.

> **TEST-TAKING TIP**—Differentiate between *modifiable* (serum lipids, hypertension, smoking, obesity), *non-modifiable* risk factors (age, gender, family history), and *contributing* factors (diabetes mellitus).
> **AN, APP, 1, M/S: Cardiac, HPM, Health Promotion and Maintenance**

326. **(3) "Spill kits" should be readily accessible and contain all the materials necessary to clean up the spill. Answer 1 is** incorrect because this may delay clean up of the spill. **Answer 2 is incorrect** because the spill should be cleaned up immediately. And, if the nurse exits the room, what about the client? **Answer 4 is incorrect** because calling the fire department is most likely not necessary for a small spill such as this. The nurse can check with risk management in the agency to be certain.

> **TEST-TAKING TIP**—Two of the options (**Answers 1** and **4**) call on others to take action; only 1 option focuses on the nurse *doing something* definitive other than "exiting" the room (**Answer 3**). Chemotherapeutic agents, or any hazardous material, should be neutralized as quickly as possible to prevent toxic effects. Housekeeping *may well be trained* to clean up such a spill; however, the nurse administering the chemotherapy *should* be versed in spill management.
> **IMP, APP, 1, M/S: Hazard, SECE, Safety and Infection Control**

327. **(2) The oxygen saturation in the placenta is about the same as maternal capillary blood. Answer 1 is incorrect** because the oxygen saturation in the placenta *is less* than maternal arterial blood. **Answer 3 is incorrect** because the average oxygen saturation in the intervillous space *is less* than 96%. **Answer 4 is incorrect** because the oxygen saturation in the intervillous space *can not be greater* than maternal capillary blood.

> **TEST-TAKING TIP**—Eliminate **Answers 1 and 4** that say "greater than maternal," because the values of fetal blood can not be greater than the maternal supply. Choose the option that says "about the same as maternal blood."
> **AN, COM, 5, Maternity, HPM, Health Promotion and Maintenance**

328. **(4) The difficulties associated with attention deficit-hyperactivity disorder are most often related to relationships and school. Early identification of the disorder is critical because the characteristics of attention deficit-hyperactivity disorder significantly interfere with the normal course of emotional and psychological development and performance. Answer 1 is incorrect** because while risk factors for the development of attention deficit-hyperactivity disorder include toxins (such as exposure to lead-based paint commonly found in older homes), the exact etiology of this disorder is unknown. **Answer 2 is incorrect** because while risk factors for the development of attention deficit-hyperactivity disorder include sensitivity to foods (such as

chocolate, cow's milk, eggs, and sucrose) or food additives (such as aspartame [*Nutrasweet*]), the exact etiology of this disorder is unknown. Diet as a factor in this disorder continues to generate controversy, but, *some* children do show improvement in behavior when certain foods are eliminated from the diet. **Answer 3** is incorrect because while risk factors for the development of attention deficit-hyperactivity disorder include difficulty in disciplining the child, the exact etiology of this disorder is unknown. The focus is on the prevention of undesired behavior. The family is assisted in developing effective parenting skills such as positive reinforcement, rewarding small increments of desired behaviors and age-appropriate consequences (e.g., time-outs, response-cost) as opposed to discipline based on punishment.

> **TEST-TAKING TIP**—Three of the responses do not directly involve the child; select the one response that *does* involve the child.
> **AS, APP, 2, PEDS, PsI, Psychosocial Integrity**

329. **(2) Smoking cigarettes is a known risk factor for bladder cancer. Answer 1** is incorrect because low fiber diet is *not* a recognized risk factor for bladder cancer. **Answer 3** is incorrect because history of hysterectomy is *not* a recognized risk factor for bladder cancer. **Answer 4** is incorrect because history of *occasional* urinary tract infections is *not* a recognized risk factor for bladder cancer. However, bladder cancer is associated with frequent or chronic bladder infections.

> **TEST-TAKING TIP**—The option that is an important risk factor for many other cancers (**Answer 2**) is a good bet for bladder cancer as well; choose the most common risk factor (smoking).
> **AN, APP, 8, M/S: Renal, HPM, Health Promotion and Maintenance**

330. **(3) It is theorized that children who are obese can become obese later in life as a result of an increased number of cells available for fat storage. Answer 1** is incorrect because this intervention would *not prevent* obesity, but would help the client deal with the feelings associated with being obese. This answer is more appropriate for an *adult* client. **Answer 2** is incorrect because this intervention is *not appropriate for a child*. **Answer 4** is incorrect because nurses should encourage healthy eating of *all* basic food groups.

> **TEST-TAKING TIP**—Look for the age-appropriate answer. Read the stem carefully; the question asks for *prevention* of *childhood* obesity.
> **IMP, APP, 4, Psych, PhI, Basic Care and Comfort**

331. **(4) The client's own report is the best indicator of the pain experience. Answer 1** is incorrect because vital signs are not a reliable indicator of pain. Blood pressure may *increase or decrease* in response to pain. **Answer 2** is incorrect because the experience of pain is individual *regardless* of the client's diagnosis or type of surgery. **Answer 3** is incorrect because the client's body movements do not represent a complete picture of the client's pain.

> **TEST-TAKING TIP**—Answers 1, 2, and 3 are methods of pain assessment often used by nurses to gauge the client's pain; however, none are as accurate or reliable as the client's own report (**Answer 4**).
> **AN, ANL, 3, M/S: Pain, PhI, Basic Care and Comfort**

332. **(1) Tricyclic antidepressants are considered adjuvant drugs and are often used in the management of chronic pain. Answer 2** is incorrect because NSAIDs are nonopioid analgesics, *not* adjuvant drugs. **Answer 3** is incorrect because nonopioids, such as acetaminophen, are considered analgesics, *not* adjuvant drugs. **Answer 4** is incorrect because

narcotic agonist analgesics are considered analgesics, *not* adjuvant drugs.

> **TEST-TAKING TIP**—Adjuvant drugs have some analgesic effects, but not significant effects and are not traditionally used as analgesics. **Answer 1** is the only option consistent with the definition of an adjuvant.
> **AN, COM, 3, M/S: Pain, PhI, Basic Care and Comfort**

333. **(2, 5) Answer 2 is correct because amniotic fluid does provide some protection to the fetus from trauma. Answer 5 is correct because the amniotic fluid provides cushioning to the fetus. Answer 1** is incorrect because amniotic fluid *does not* prevent bacterial infections. **Answer 3** is incorrect because the *placenta* provides oxygen to the fetus. **Answer 4** is incorrect because the amniotic fluid *does not help* dilation of the cervix during labor.

> **TEST-TAKING TIP**—Choose options that apply to functions of the amniotic fluid (**Answers 2** and **5**). Eliminate options that apply to the placenta (**Answer 3**).
> **AN, APP, 5, Maternity, HPM, Health Promotion and Maintenance**

334. **(1) The onset of chest pain in a child with sickle cell anemia could signal the development of acute chest syndrome. This is a serious complication of sickle cell anemia. It is clinically similar to pneumonia. The resulting pulmonary infiltrate can lead to sickling in the small blood vessels of the lungs leading to occlusion and stasis. The staff nurse should assess this child *first*. Answer 2** is incorrect because the toddler has had genitourinary surgery (circumcision for narrowing or stenosis of the preputial opening of the foreskin), incontinence should be *expected*. Also, the toddler may not have been toilet trained prior to the surgery. The added stress of hospitalization could also contribute to regression and incontinence. The staff nurse should assess this child *last*. **Answer 3** is incorrect because the baby who has acute gastroenteritis is *expected* to have green, liquid stools. It would be reasonable to expect that the baby would have an IV and be on strict I & O. The nurse would know this information from the end-of-shift report. The staff nurse should assess this baby *third*. **Answer 4** is incorrect because a child with asthma would be *expected* to have retractions. However, this child could *potentially* have difficulty maintaining a patent airway. The nurse should assess this child *second*.

> **TEST-TAKING TIP**—Assessing for and maintaining a patent airway is *always* the staff nurse's first priority.
> **AN, ANL, 6, PEDS, SECE, Management of Care: Priority**

335. **(3) The client on a cooling blanket is susceptible to "freeze burn" in distal extremities. Answer 1** is incorrect because tepid sponge baths, with or without alcohol, have not been shown to be any more effective than antipyretic medication at reducing fever. **Answer 2** is incorrect because the muscle activity involved with shivering produces heat, which is counterproductive to fever-reducing measures. **Answer 4** is incorrect because fans have not been shown to be any more effective than antipyretic medication at reducing fever.

> **TEST-TAKING TIP**—Answers 1 and 4 represent past nursing practice; these methods are used less today. Knowledge of the heat-producing mechanisms of the body, leads the nurse to **Answer 3**.
> **IMP, APP, 1, M/S: Metab., PhI, Basic Care and Comfort**

336. **(2) The client is 1 centimeter dilated, which is the latent phase of labor. She has not changed her dilation, so she is most likely in a prolonged latent phase. Answer 1** is incorrect because the client *has not established a regular labor*

pattern to determine if she is experiencing a failure-to-progress. **Answer 3** is incorrect because she is *not in the second stage* of labor. **Answer 4** is incorrect because she is *not in active labor*.

> **TEST-TAKING TIP**—Remember there are four stages of labor and three phases of the first stage of labor. Don't confuse labor stages and phases.
> **AN, APP, 5, Maternity, HPM, Health Promotion and Maintenance**

337. (1) **Airway or breathing problems should be treated first.** **Answer 2** is incorrect because airway or breathing problems should be treated first, and this child does not have a problem with airway or breathing. **Answer 3** is incorrect because airway or breathing problems should be treated first, and this client does not have a problem with breathing or airway. **Answer 4** is incorrect because airway or breathing problems should be treated first, and this client does not have a problem with breathing or airway.

> **TEST-TAKING TIP**—According to principles of triage, clients with airway or breathing problems (**Answer 1**) should be treated first, followed by clients with circulation problems (probably **Answer 3**). A child with a laceration, who is awake and alert (**Answer 2**) or a fracture (**Answer 4**) are not the priorities here.
> **AN, ANL, 1, M/S: Trauma, SECE, Management of Care: Triage**

338. (2) **The child with fifth disease (erythema infectiosum) has a communicable but relatively benign, self-limiting disease and could safely be discharged from the hospital.** Hospitalization of the child is usually *not* necessary unless the child was dehydrated or is immunosuppressed. **Answer 1** is incorrect because the child with glomerulonephritis who has an elevated albumin level is still in the acute phase of the disease and cannot be safely discharged from the hospital. **Answer 3** is incorrect because the child with osteomyelitis who is on long-term antibiotic therapy must complete the course of therapy in order to avoid the complications of osteomyelitis (i.e., soft tissue abscess or spread of infection to the joint). This child could *potentially* be discharged for at-home IV antibiotic therapy, but that would take advance planning which could not be accomplished immediately in order to make room for a client being admitted from the scene of the disaster. **Answer 4** is incorrect because the child with asthma who has retractions is still in the acute phase of the disease and cannot be safely discharged from the hospital.

> **TEST-TAKING TIP**—Rank the diseases in order of acuity and discharge the *least* acute client.
> **AN, ANL, 1, PEDS, SECE, Management of Care: Triage**

339. (3) **The fracture should be positioned *above heart level* to promote venous return and reduce swelling.** **Answer 1** is incorrect because a fracture should be positioned *above heart level*, if possible, to promote venous return. **Answer 2** is incorrect because not all fractures require traction weight, such as fractures that are not displaced, or fractures that are casted. **Answer 4** is incorrect because the affected area should be positioned *above heart level*, if possible. Positioning the affected area at heart level is appropriate if the nurse suspects compartment syndrome.

> **TEST-TAKING TIP**—This question boils down to: at what level does the nurse position a fracture? The common-sense answer is above heart level (**Answer 3**). Below heart level is never appropriate (**Answer 1**), and at heart level (**Answer 4**) is helpful if compartment syndrome is suspected.
> **IMP, APP, 3, M/S: Ortho, PhI, Physiological Adaptation**

340. (1) **Maintaining adequate hydration would be the priority nursing goal.** **Answer 2** is incorrect because clients with bulimia usually have a normal weight or are slightly overweight. Weight gain would not be a nursing goal. **Answer 3** is incorrect because insight into maladaptive eating patterns is a *long-term* goal of treatment. **Answer 4** is incorrect because although expressing feelings associated with binging and purging behaviors is an important goal of treatment, it is *not* a priority.

> **TEST-TAKING TIP**—Note the time frame and eliminate the answers that are long-term. Remember Maslow's hierarchy and choose answers that address physiological needs *before* psychosocial needs.
> **EV, APP, 4, Psych, PhI, Basic Care and Comfort**

341. (2) **Pregnancy results in increased iron absorption.** **Answer 1** is incorrect because most women who are pregnant *do require* iron supplementation during pregnancy. **Answer 3** is incorrect because the fetus *will produce* hemoglobin *even if* the mother is anemic. **Answer 4** is incorrect because maternal hemoglobin *does not* rise during the second half of pregnancy with supplementation.

> **TEST-TAKING TIP**—The point to consider is whether or not the client *needs* to take iron as a supplement. Eliminate **Answer 1** that says "not required." Eliminate **Answer 3** because it focuses on the fetus rather than the mother. Eliminate **Answer 4** because it implies that iron supplements are not required.
> **PL, APP, 4, Maternity, PhI, Pharmacological and Parenteral Therapies**

342. (2) **Lactulose is used to treat constipation and hepatic encephalopathy by reducing ammonia levels in clients with hepatic disease. In hepatic encephalopathy it works by binding with ammonia, which is excreted in feces. It also works by pulling water into the colon, which results in diarrhea. Therefore, diarrhea (an expected result of lactulose) indicates that the medication is working.** **Answer 1** is incorrect because lactulose is used to *treat* constipation. **Answer 3** is incorrect because a decreased potassium level is an undesirable side effect of lactulose. **Answer 4** is incorrect because lactulose is not given for pain.

> **TEST-TAKING TIP**—Look at two options that are opposites (constipation vs. diarrhea). Choose diarrhea (an expected result of lactulose).
> **EV, ANL, 8, M/S: GI, PhI, Pharmacological and Parenteral Therapies**

343. (4) **The client is not having a respiratory emergency, and coughing and deep breathing can be tried first.** **Answer 1** is incorrect because the client with COPD should not receive oxygen at more than 2 L/min unless an emergency exists. **Answer 2** is incorrect because suctioning would be traumatic and invasive. More conservative measures can be used first. **Answer 3** is incorrect because a more conservative measure can be used first.

> **TEST-TAKING TIP**—Choose the most conservative measure first, in a nonemergency. Blood gas analysis of this client indicates a move toward respiratory acidosis and is suggestive of hypoventilation. However, there is no emergency here, so the basic nursing measure of coughing and deep breathing should be tried first. A nebulizer treatment (**Answer 3**) can be pursued if coughing and deep breathing are not effective in improving the client's blood gases. Suctioning is not yet indicated in this case (**Answer 2**), and increasing the oxygen flow (**Answer 1**) is inappropriate unless a respiratory emergency exists.
> **IMP, ANL, 6, M/S: Resp., PhI, Reduction of Risk Potential**

344. **(1) The toddler does not have a concept of time. It would be most appropriate to explain the procedure as simply as possible to the toddler *immediately* before giving the preoperative sedation. If the explanation is given to the toddler any earlier than that, it will not be remembered and possibly may not be understood.** Answer 2 is incorrect because the toddler does not have a concept of time. The toddler would enjoy the puppet but the next day would not remember the explanation of the procedure. This intervention would be better for a preschooler who does have a concept (although limited) of time. **Answer 3** is incorrect because the toddler does not have the attention span nor cognitive abilities necessary to understand being read a story about the heart. This intervention would be better for the young school-age child. **Answer 4** is incorrect because the toddler does not have the cognitive abilities necessary to correlate the model of the heart to the procedure that will take place. This intervention would be better for the older school-age child.

> **TEST-TAKING TIP**—To answer this question correctly, correlate the age and developmental stage of the child with the nursing intervention.
> **IMP, APP, 5, PEDS, HPM, Health Promotion and Maintenance**

345. **(3) African-American men are at greatest risk of developing hypertension; and this client is a smoker, which is considered a major risk factor.** Answer 1 is incorrect because, while history of hypertension is a risk factor, there is another client at greater risk. **Answer 2** is incorrect because, while obesity is a risk factor, and African-American women are at greater risk for hypertension than Caucasian women, there is another client at greater risk. **Answer 4** is incorrect because, while diabetes is a contributing factor to hypertension, there is another client who is at greater risk.

> **TEST-TAKING TIP**—Choose the client with the most risk factors. **Answer 1** has age, gender, and family history as risk factors. **Answer 2** has race and obesity as risk factors. **Answer 4** has age, gender, and diabetes as risk factors. **Answer 3**, on the other hand, has age, race, gender, and cigarette smoking as risk factors.
> **AN, ANL, 5, M/S: CV, HPM, Health Promotion and Maintenance**

346. **(2) An EKG monitor is necessary to evaluate the effectiveness of the cardioversion.** Answer 1 is incorrect because chest compressions may *not necessarily* be done during cardioversion. **Answer 3** is incorrect because alcohol is *not used* during a cardioversion. **Answer 4** is incorrect because sodium bicarbonate is *not* used during cardioversion, *unless* the client's arterial blood gases indicated acidosis.

> **TEST-TAKING TIP**—Think cardioversion = cardiac; choose the option directly related to cardiac (EKG). The question refers to *cardioversion*, not *defibrillation*. Defibrillation is done during a cardiac emergency, when a back board would most likely be used for chest compressions (**Answer 1**) and sodium bicarbonate would be on hand in case of acidosis (**Answer 4**).
> **IMP, APP, 6, M/S: Cardiac, PhI, Physiological Adaptation**

347. **(1) The pressure on the fetal head causes the molding and overlapping of the sutures in the fetal head.** Answer 2 is incorrect because the shape of the head is *not trauma-related*. **Answer 3** is incorrect because the normal molding process does *not cause brain damage*. **Answer 4** is incorrect because the molding is *not related to hydrocephalus*.

> **TEST-TAKING TIP**—Visualize the infant's head after delivery. The changes are a normal part of the delivery

process, not a pathological finding. Choose the option that is different from the three options that focus on pathology (**Answers 2, 3** and **4**).
> **IMP, 5, COM, Newborn, HPM, Health Promotion and Maintenance**

348. **28.** The drip rate is determined as follows: $\dfrac{700\ mL}{4\ hr} \times 10$ gtt/mL =28 gtt/min

> **TEST-TAKING TIP**—The calculation is easier if it is reduced to smaller components. First divide 700 mL by 4 hours to get the hourly rate of 175 mL/hr. It is much easier to set the equation up as follows:
> $\dfrac{175\ mL}{60\ min} \times 10$ gtt/mL = 28gtt/min.
> **IMP, APP, 6, M/S: Calculation, PhI, Pharmacological and Parenteral Therapies**

349. **(3) Taking appropriate actions independently is the classic behavior associated with the development of autonomy. Note that this response does not provide for the toddler to take unnecessary risks or engage in inappropriate actions. The parent would select and supervise the type of actions that the toddler would take independently.** Answer 1 is incorrect because learning the difference between right and wrong is part of *moral-ethical* development for the toddler rather than development of autonomy. **Answer 2** is incorrect because providing opportunities for play with another child is part of *social* development for the toddler rather than the development of autonomy. **Answer 4** is incorrect because helping the toddler to complete tasks would *discourage* the development of autonomy. However, the parent would select and supervise the type of tasks that the toddler would engage in to insure that the tasks are age-appropriate and could be accomplished by the toddler.

> **TEST-TAKING TIP**—Autonomy is a synonym for independence; look for the answer that contains the word *independence*.
> **PL, APP, 5, PEDS, HPM, Health Promotion and Maintenance**

350. **(2) A high protein diet would increase the workload on the liver. If the liver is severely damaged, a high protein diet should be avoided.** Answer 1 is incorrect because a high protein diet would *not* affect the Hbg/Hct of the client, although it is an important test to r/o anemia and elevated WBC. **Answer 3** is incorrect because the hemoglobin would be tested in a CBC and would indicate anemia, but not liver function. **Answer 4** is incorrect because a urinalysis would indicate malnutrition, but would *not* give the nurse important information about the *liver function* of the client.

> **TEST-TAKING TIP**—Eliminate choices that give the same answer: CBC and hemoglobin (**Answers 1** and **3**). Choose the answer that relates to the condition: liver damage is a common consequence of chronic alcoholism.
> **AS, APP, 4, Psych, PhI, Basic Care and Comfort**

351. **(1) Swallowing is an effort and requires an unhurried, quiet environment. Start with foods that require no chewing and are easily swallowed and progress as tolerated. Alternate with thickened liquid to ensure that food is not being left in the mouth.** Answer 2 is incorrect because the problem is with swallowing, *not speaking*. **Answer 3** is incorrect because liquids should be *thickened* to aid in swallowing. **Answer 4** is incorrect because the problem is swallowing, *not visual*.

> **TEST-TAKING TIP**—Look for an option that defines the problem—swallowing.
> **PL, APP, 3, M/S: Neuro, PhI, Physiological Adaptation**

352. (3) Quitting smoking or avoiding cigarette smoke reduces the risk of a cardiovascular incident to the same risk as someone who has never smoked. **Answer 1** is incorrect because the risk of cardiovascular disease (hypertension) is already present. The intent is to identify a modifiable risk factor. **Answer 2** is incorrect because a cholesterol under 240 mg/dL would be a positive fact. Current recommended cholesterol levels should be below 200 mg/dL. **Answer 4** is incorrect because age is not a modifiable risk factor.

> **TEST-TAKING TIP**—The question is looking for a *preventable* problem or a problem with the greatest potential for *modification*.
> **AS, APP, 6, M/S: CV, HPM, Health Promotion and Maintenance**

353. (1) Reaching for objects is a fine motor-adaptive skill that the average, normal 4–6-month-old infant should be able to demonstrate. **Answer 2** is incorrect because demonstrating a pincer grasp is a fine motor-adaptive skill that the average, normal *7–9-month*-old infant should be able to demonstrate. **Answer 3** is incorrect because lifting head 45–90 degrees while on stomach is a gross motor skill that the average, normal *birth-3-month*-old infant should be able to demonstrate. **Answer 4** is incorrect because pulling self up into sitting position is a gross motor skill that the average, normal *7–9-month*-old infant should be able to demonstrate.

> **TEST-TAKING TIP**—Remember that growth and development follows a directional pattern: cephalocaudal (head to toe); proximodistal (trunk to extremities); and, differentiation (simple to complex). Correlate the directional pattern with the age of the child when answering the question.
> **AN, APP, 5, PEDS, HPM, Health Promotion and Maintenance**

354. (2, 4) **Answer 2** is correct because fetal kick counts provide reassurance of fetal well-being, and decreased fetal movements can be an indicator of possible problems with placental perfusion and fetal oxygenation. **Answer 4** is correct because rest and work need to be monitored during pregnancy to decrease cardiac complications. **Answer 1** is incorrect because a client with class II cardiac disease usually delivers *without* an increased risk of mortality for the mother. Cardiac disease in pregnancy is based on the New York classifications of heart disease. Clients with class I heart disease have the least complications. Clients with class IV cardiac disease have a high risk of maternal death during delivery. **Answer 3** is incorrect because it is *not necessary* to hospitalize a client with class II heart disease. **Answer 5** is incorrect because cesarean section presents an *increased risk* to the mother with cardiac disease.

> **TEST-TAKING TIP**—Choose the least invasive or least stringent plans of action. Eliminate **Answers 1, 3** and **5,** which have aggressive options.
> **PL, APP, 6, Maternity, PhI, Physiological Adaptation**

355. (1) The client is able to visualize the injection if she administers the insulin in her abdomen. **Answer 2** is incorrect because insulin should be injected *before* breakfast. **Answer 3** is incorrect because exercise does *not* help to utilize the insulin. **Answer 4** is incorrect because the client is likely to need additional insulin as the pregnancy progresses due to increasing insulin resistance.

> **TEST-TAKING TIP**—Eliminate **Answers 3** and **4** because gestational diabetes differs from non-gestational diabetes in that insulin requirements usually increase *in spite of* the client's compliance with the treatment regime.
> **PL, APP, 4, Maternity, PhI, Pharmacological and Parenteral Therapies**

356. (1) The first dose of the measles, mumps, and rubella vaccine (MMR) is routinely given between 12 and 15 months of age. **Answer 1** is incorrect because the second dose of the hepatitis B vaccine (HepB) *is* routinely given between 1 and 4 months of age. **Answer 2** is incorrect because the second dose of the inactivated polio vaccine (IPV) *is* routinely given at 4 month of age. **Answer 3** is incorrect because the second dose of the pneumococcal vaccine (PCV) *is* routinely given at 4 months of age.

> **TEST-TAKING TIP**—Review and memorize the current Recommended Childhood and Adolescent Immunization Schedule (available at www.cdc.gov/nip). Also, think of the order of decreasing maternal-conferred immunity when answering the question.
> **EV, APP, 1, PEDS, SECE, Management of Care**

357. (1, 3, 4) **Answer 1** is correct because death from pneumococcal pneumonia increases with age and the vaccination is usually a one time dose. **Answer 3** is correct because those over 60 or with a chronic illness should receive a flu shot annually. **Answer 4** is correct because people who are elderly are prone to falls and have a weakened immune system. A tetanus shot is preventative. **Answer 2** is incorrect because this vaccination is *not routinely* recommended. **Answer 5** is incorrect because it is recommended for adults who are at high risk for exposure to chickenpox, such as teachers or day care workers. **Answer 6** is incorrect because it is recommended for those at high risk for contact with contaminated blood.

> **TEST-TAKING TIP**—Consider the age group and likely exposure.
> **AS, COM, 1, M/S: Infection Control, HPM, Health Promotion and Maintenance**

358. (3) The head and neck are maintained in an aligned position at all times and supported. The collar is hard and can cause skin breakdown. The collar liner should be changed daily and the underlying skin cleansed. **Answer 1** is incorrect because turning the head from side to side may cause injury to the spine. **Answer 2** is incorrect because the client may be experiencing weakness and there is no support for the neck if the collar is removed. **Answer 4** is incorrect because the collar liner must be changed and the skin cleaned daily to prevent breakdown. The presence or absence of a spinal injury may not be determined in less than 24 hours.

> **TEST-TAKING TIP**—Think of the response that provides the greatest safety from injury. Eliminate **Answer 1** because it involves *movement* of the head; eliminate **Answer 2** because it does not use *alignment* of head with torso.
> **AS, APP, 3, M/S: Neuro, PhI, Reduction of Risk Potential**

359. (1) Spinal precautions mean position restrictions. The spine must be kept in a neutral position—no twisting, flexing, or extending. This can only be done with logrolling and the help of other nurses. **Answer 2** is incorrect because the first priority is preventing further damage to the spine even *before* treatment is determined. **Answer 3** is incorrect because the client should be flat and the spine in a neutral position—*no* flexion. **Answer 4** is incorrect because the first priority is preventing further trauma to the spine. Checking for numbness or weakness would be done, but *not first*.

> **TEST-TAKING TIP**—The priority is *prevention—not treatment or management* of injury.
> **PL, APP, 3, M/S: Neuro, PhI, Reduction of Risk Potential**

360. (2) If the client takes Ativan daily for more than 4 weeks, dependency can occur. Ativan is a short-term treatment for anxiety and should be used only on an as-needed basis to augment other treatments. **Answer 1** is incorrect because the medication does not result in motor coordination but motor *incoordination*. Both parts of this answer have to be correct. **Answer 3** is incorrect because Ativan does *not* always work. **Answer 4** is incorrect because Ativan should be tapered *slowly* and only *if* the client has developed dependency. If the client takes the medication occasionally, then tapering is not necessary.

> **TEST-TAKING TIP**—Make sure all parts of the answer are correct (**Answer 1**). Avoid answers that may imply absolutes like "always" (**Answer 3**).
> **IMP, APP, 7, Psych, PhI, Pharmacological Therapy**

361. **(3) Not voiding for 8 hours may result in infection, as well as more severe problems. A straight catheterization may be done or the Foley reinserted to allow for the bladder reflexes to recover. Answer 1** is incorrect because the potential for *bladder distention will not be relieved* by a prostate evaluation. **Answer 2** is incorrect because waiting can result in severe bladder distention, infection, damage to the kidneys, and even bladder rupture. **Answer 4** is incorrect because increasing oral intake does *not* correct the inability to void.

> **TEST-TAKING TIP**—Eliminate options that further delay voiding—only one choice deals with the problem "now."
> **PL, APP, 8, M/S: GU, PhI, Physiological Adaptation**

362. **(2) Proper disposal of a controlled substance is witnessed destruction. Answer 1** is incorrect because the proper handling of this controlled substance is *witnessed* destruction. **Answer 3** is incorrect because the drug is a narcotic and it needs to be properly destroyed. **Answer 4** is incorrect because the drug remaining in the patch needs to be destroyed and witnessed to prevent abuse potential.

> **TEST-TAKING TIP**—The principles of safe medication disposal apply here. Only one option states that the disposal is witnessed.
> **IMP, APP, 3, M/S: Legal, PhI, Pharmacological and Parenteral Therapies**

363. **(1, 2) Answer 1 is correct because PID is more common with an IUD in place. Signs and symptoms of infection need to be evaluated by a medical professional. Answer 2 is correct because these are common side effects of an IUD. Answer 3** is incorrect because there is a *higher risk with oral* contraceptives. **Answer 4** is incorrect because uterine perforation is a *rare* occurrence. **Answer 5** is incorrect because it is safe for client who smokes to use an IUD.

> **TEST-TAKING TIP**—Choose **Answers 1 and 2,** the options that contain the common side-effects of an IUD and common complications involving infection. Eliminate uncommon occurrences (**Answers 3 and 4**).
> **AN, APP, 1, Women's Health, HPM, Health Promotion and Maintenance**

364. **(4) The changes associated with pregnancy and delivery require a diaphragm to be refitted after delivery. Answer 1** is incorrect because breastfeeding *is not* an effective method of contraception. **Answer 2** is incorrect because an IUD *can* be used by a woman who is breastfeeding without additional complications. **Answer 3** is incorrect because breastfeeding *does not reliably suppress* ovulation.

> **TEST-TAKING TIP**—Read the options carefully to determine if the statement is true. Key words and phrases to eliminate as the incorrect options include "effective," "should not," and "will not."
> **IMP, COM, 5, Women's Health, HPM, Health Promotion and Maintenance**

365. **(3) The first set in client assessment is obtaining vital signs. The client is exhibiting classic symptoms of hypertension, which include frequent early morning headaches, lightheadedness, palpitations, fatigue, forgetfulness, alteration in vision (white spots or blurring), epistaxis (nose bleeds) and shortness of breath on exertion. Answer 1** is incorrect because this is *not the first* action that the nurse should take. The client is not exhibiting signs of poor oxygenation. The nurse should start with vital sign data. **Answer 2** is incorrect because this is not the first action that the nurse should take. The client is not exhibiting symptoms of ketone dumping. This action requires a *physician order*. **Answer 4** is incorrect because neurological assessment is *not the first* action that the nurse should take. The nurse should start with vital sign data.

> **TEST-TAKING TIP**—Ask which option is most likely to explain all of the signs and symptoms.
> **AN, ANL, 6, M/S: CV, PhI, Reduction of Risk Potential**

366. **(2) The first action is to verify placement of the PICC in the superior vena cava via x-ray report. It is unsafe to use the PICC line until appropriate placement has been verified. Insertion of a PICC line can be a difficult process and the catheter can migrate up into the inferior jugular vein or down into the right atrium where it can cause cardiac ectopy. Answer 1** is incorrect because this is *not the first* action the nurse should take. Placement of the PICC in the SVC must be verified first by chest x-ray. **Answer 3** is incorrect because appropriate placement of a PICC is verified by x-ray, *not* ultrasound; and should be in the superior vena cava, *not the right ventricle*. **Answer 4** is incorrect because aspiration of blood *does not indicate* where the distal end of the catheter is placed. Blood can be aspirated when the PICC is inappropriately placed in another blood vessel or the right atrium.

> **TEST-TAKING TIP**—Look at the two options that state "confirm—placement." Eliminate (**Answer 3**), the obviously wrong option.
> **IMP, APP, 6, M/S: CV, PhI, Reduction of Risk Potential**

367. **(2) Blocks in multiple shapes, sizes, and colors are ideal for a toddler *and* appropriate for the hospital setting as well as for the toddler's medical condition. A toddler with meningitis should engage in "quiet" or "non-stimulating" types of activity that is provided by playing with blocks. Answer 1** is incorrect because, while a push-pull type of toy such as a wagon is ideal for a toddler, it would not be appropriate in a hospital setting. **Answer 3** is incorrect because "arts and crafts" type of toys such as crayons and finger paints are too advanced for the toddler. These types of toys are better for the preschooler. **Answer 4** is incorrect because a storybook is too advanced for the toddler. This type of toy is better for the preschooler.

> **TEST-TAKING TIP**—Match the toy to the child's medical condition as well as to the age of the child.
> **IMP, APP, 5, PEDS, HPM, Health Promotion and Maintenance**

368. **(4) Glycosylated hemoglobin (hemoglobin A$_{1c}$) is a method for assessing control of diabetes. Glucose molecules attach to the circulating hemoglobin A molecules and remain there for the lifetime of the red blood cell (approximately 120 days). The attachment is not reversible. Glycosylated hemoglobin reflects the average blood glucose levels that have taken place during the previous 2–3 months and therefore the degree of blood glucose level control. Answer 1** is incorrect because while

self-monitoring of blood glucose (SMBG) has improved diabetes management and has been used successfully by children from the onset of diabetes, its main purpose is to enable the child to change the insulin regimen to maintain blood glucose level in the euglycemic (normal) range. **Answer 2** is incorrect because urine testing for glucose is *no longer* used for diabetic management. There is a poor correlation between simultaneous glycosuria and blood glucose concentrations. Urine testing can be used to detect *ketonuria.* **Answer 3** is incorrect because fasting glucose levels are most useful in confirming the diagnosis of diabetes.

> **TEST-TAKING TIP**—Gluc, gluco, glyc, and glyco come from the Greek language and mean "sweet." Think "control of blood sugar or sweetness" and select the correct answer.
> **IMP, APP, 4, PEDS, PhI, Reduction of Risk Potential**

369. **(3) The right brachial vein is accessed in the area of the right antecubital and is the vein of choice for PICC placement. The right brachial vein provides the *straightest access* to the superior vena cava where the distal end of the PICC should be placed. Answer 1** is incorrect because labs can be drawn from the hand veins. A PICC line *cannot* be placed in hand veins because they are too small and have multiple bifurcations. **Answer 2** is incorrect because labs can be drawn from the left and right lower forearms. A PICC line *cannot* be placed in the lower forearms. **Answer 4** is incorrect because labs can be drawn from the hand veins. A PICC line cannot be placed in hand veins because they are too small and have multiple bifurcations.

> **TEST-TAKING TIP**—Think about the type of line—a central catheter.
> **PL, COM, 6, M/S: Vascular, PhI, Pharmacological and Parenteral Therapies**

370. **(1) Paxil is used for the treatment of depression, and elimination of suicidal ideation is a priority nursing goal for clients who are depressed. Answer 2** is incorrect because improvement in the client's mood is a *lower* priority than the client's *safety.* **Answer 3** is incorrect because reducing insomnia is a *lower* priority than safety. **Answer 4** is incorrect because appetite is a *lower* priority than suicide.

> **TEST-TAKING TIP**—If you do not recognize the medication, look at the answers for clues. All of the answers are symptoms of depression. Focus on the key word in the stem and choose the answer with the *highest* priority: safety.
> **EV, ANL, 7, Psych, PhI, Pharmacological Therapy**

371. **(1) Naegele's rule is based on the first day of the last menstrual period. Answer 2** is incorrect because the day of conception is usually *not absolutely certain.* **Answer 3** is incorrect because the last day of the period *can vary* tremendously from woman to woman and from month to month. It is not a reliable measurement. **Answer 4** is incorrect because the day of ovulation is *variable.*

> **TEST-TAKING TIP**—Eliminate the three options that can have variations (**Answers 2, 3, and 4**); only one option is specific (**Answer 1**). Remember Naegele's rule and the calculation for estimated date of delivery.
> **AN, COM, 5, Maternity, HPM, Health Promotion and Maintenance**

372. **(2) Metoprolol is a β-1 selective inhibitor that will decrease blood pressure and heart rate by competitively blocking the response to beta adrenergic stimulation. Answer 1** is incorrect because famotidine is a histamine H_2 agonist that *inhibits gastric acid secretion.* **Answer 3** is incorrect because

diazepam is a benzodiazepine given for *anxiety disorders* and *skeletal muscle relaxation.* **Answer 4** is incorrect because Lasix is a *diuretic.*

> **TEST-TAKING TIP**—Know the drugs most commonly used in acute MI.
> **PL, KNOW, 6, M/S: CV, PhI, Pharmacological and Parenteral Therapies**

373. **(1) Ortolani's test is only done on infants under 4 months of age. Adduction contractures develop at about 6–10 weeks of age and Ortolani's "click" disappears despite the presence of developmental dysplasia of the hip(s) (DDH). Answer 2** is incorrect because the presence of 4 teeth is a *normal finding* in a 10-month-old infant. This physical finding during the first 2 years of life can be calculated: *age of the child in months − 6 = number of teeth.* Example: 10 months of age − 6 = 4 teeth. **Answer 3** is incorrect because the presence of an open anterior fontanel is a *normal finding* in a 10-month-old infant. *Normally* the *anterior* fontanel fuses between 12–18 months of age. *Normally* the *posterior* fontanel closes by 2 months of age. **Answer 4** is incorrect because the presence of Babinski's sign (the dorsiflexion of the big toe and fanning of the other toes) is a *normal finding* in a 10-month-old infant. The presence of Babinski's sign is *abnormal* after about 1 year of age or when locomotion begins. A positive Babinski's sign after 1 year of age may indicate spinal cord lesions and requires further neurological examination.

> **TEST-TAKING TIP**—Know the critical time periods for the presence *and* absence of key physical assessment findings in an infant.
> **EV, APP, 5, PEDS, SECE, Management of Care**

374. **(1) Beta-blockers competitively block response to beta-adrenergic stimulation. This results in a decrease in heart rate and blood pressure. Discharge medication education on beta-blockers should include teaching the client to take the pulse daily prior to taking the medication, and to hold the medication if the pulse rate is low (the hold rate is ordered by physician). Education must also include signs and symptoms of hypotension (especially postural hypotension), lightheadedness, dizziness, fatigue. An alteration/decrease in sexual function may also occur and should be discussed. Answer 2** is incorrect because beta-blockers can be taken without regard to meals and are *not affected* by dietary intake with the exception of antacids. Beta-blockers should not be taken with antacids. **Answer 3** is incorrect because beta-blockers do *not* cause potassium depletion nor increased urine output. **Answer 4** is incorrect because beta-blockers can be taken without regard to meals and are *not affected* by dietary intake with the exception of antacids. Beta-blockers should not be taken with antacids.

> **TEST-TAKING TIP**—Think about the intended drug effects. Eliminate two options that refer to dietary restrictions, which are not applicable here.
> **PL, APP, 6, M/S: CV, PhI, Pharmacological and Parenteral Therapies**

375. **(4) B-type natriuretic peptide (BNP) is a blood test that helps evaluate heart failure. BNP test measures the level of B-type natriuretic peptide hormone that is produced by the ventricles when they are over stretched and cannot work effectively to pump blood. The higher the BNP level, the worse the heart failure is likely to be. Levels are measured in picograms (pg) per milliliter (mL) and are correlated with classes of cardiac failure I–IV. Answer 1** is incorrect because pancreatic function is evaluated by

amylase and *lipase* levels. **Answer 2** is incorrect because pleural effusions are evaluated by *chest x-ray*. **Answer 3** is incorrect because kidney function is evaluated by *creatinine* and *blood urea nitrogen* (BUN) levels.

> **TEST-TAKING TIP**—Look for an option that causes respiratory distress (e.g., cardiopulmonary). Which one would likely cause acute distress?
> **IMP, COM, 6, M/S: Cardiopulmonary, PhI, Reduction of Risk Potential**

376. **(1)** These are the landmarks used to determine position of the fetal head. **Answer 2** is incorrect because the pelvic inlet is not directly related to the position of the fetal head. **Answer 3** is incorrect because the ischial spines determine the *station* of the fetal head, *not* the position of the head. **Answer 4** is incorrect because there are two temporal bones, there are *no temporal sutures*.

> **TEST-TAKING TIP**—Focus on the options that contain the word "fetal" (**Answers 1 and 4**). In **Answer 4**, two terms were mixed together to create "temporal suture", a structure *that does not exist.*
> **AN, APP, 5, Maternity, HPM, Health Promotion and Maintenance**

377. **(3)** A positive CT of the head indicates hemorrhage. A thrombolytic agent is contraindicated in hemorrhage because it causes bleeding. Clients with acute brain attack symptoms must have a CT scan of the head completed and read by a radiologist to rule out hemorrhage. If hemorrhage is present in the brain as indicated by a positive CT scan, then a thrombolytic agent cannot be given because this will increase the size of the hemorrhagic brain attack and can cause death. **Answer 1** is incorrect because a positive computed tomography (CT) of the head indicates a hemorrhage and shows up as a white mass on CT. A thrombolytic agent is contraindicated in hemorrhage. **Answer 2** is incorrect because a positive CT of the head indicates hemorrhagic brain attack, *not* ischemic brain attack. An ischemic brain attack would not be visualized on CT scan until approximately 12–24 hours after the initial brain injury, when the infarcted and ischemic tissues can be visualized as gray-colored changes on the brain scan. **Answer 4** is incorrect because a positive CT of the head indicates a hemorrhagic brain attack. A thrombolytic agent is only given for an ischemic brain attack with onset of symptoms that are less than 3 hours old. Infusing a thrombolytic agent when the client has a hemorrhagic brain attack diagnosis or an ischemic brain attack that is greater than 3 hours old is contraindicated because of the risk of bleeding.

> **TEST-TAKING TIP**—Know that the positive CT result means hemorrhage; therefore, eliminate **Answers 2 and 4** ("ischemic").
> **AN, COM, 6, M/S: Neuro, PhI, Physiological Adaptation**

378. **>10%–15%.** Knowledge of the infant's weight loss is *critical*. Based on this information, the infant's state of dehydration will be determined (mild, moderate, or severe) and replacement fluids will be ordered. A variety of diseases could be responsible for this finding, but, the *most likely* cause will be pyloric stenosis (an acquired disease of infancy characterized by hypertrophy of the pyloric sphincter and subsequent vomiting after feeding). In the event that pyloric stenosis is the medical diagnosis, the nurse will *also* want to obtain the infant's vital signs, prepare for a venipuncture to obtain baseline blood studies to confirm the presence of metabolic alkalosis, and, set-up for a nasogastric tube insertion. Surgery (pyloromyotomy) will be required for the correction of this condition; *but*, preoperatively the infant must be

rehydrated and *metabolic alkalosis–corrected* with parenteral fluid and electrolyte administration determined by the infant's weight. Replacement fluid therapy *usually* delays surgery for 24–48 hours.

> **TEST-TAKING TIP**—Weight is the basis on which parenteral fluid and electrolyte administration (as well as medication dosage) is calculated and is the foundation for the infant's care.
> **AS, KNOW, 4, PEDS, PhI, Basic Care and Comfort**

379. **(1)** The most important assessment information prior to administering diltiazem is blood pressure. Diltiazem can cause symptomatic hypotension and is to be withheld if SBP <90 mm Hg. **Answer 2** is incorrect because blood pressure is the most important assessment information prior to administering diltiazem. The goal in giving a calcium channel blocker like diltiazem for atrial arrhythmias is to slow SA and AV node conduction, thus slowing heart rate. The therapeutic effect of the drug is a slowed heart rate. Once this is obtained, the drug is given to maintain a slowed heart rate. **Answer 3** is incorrect because the most important assessment information prior to administering Diltiazem is blood pressure. One of the indicators of the strength of peripheral pulses is blood pressure. If the peripheral pulses are weak, the nurse should check the blood pressure. **Answer 4** is incorrect because the most important assessment information prior to administering diltiazem is blood pressure. If the blood pressure is low, the urine output will be low. A low urine output indicates the nurse should check the blood pressure.

> **TEST-TAKING TIP**—Know that the potential side effect is hypertension, which can affect heart rate, peripheral pulses and urine output.
> **AS, APP, 6, M/S: CV, PhI, Pharmacological and Parenteral Therapies**

380. **(3)** Clients with depression who require hospitalization are most likely a suicide risk. Tricyclic antidepressant medications are fatal in an overdose, and the suicide risk is higher when the mood is beginning to improve and the client has more energy. Tricyclic medications begin to take effect in 2–4 weeks, placing this client at highest risk for harm. **Answer 1** is incorrect because the client is being treated appropriately for mania with mood stabilizing medication. Lithium levels should be stable by 3 weeks into treatment. This client needs to be assessed for lithium toxicity on an ongoing basis, but *not* the priority. **Answer 2** is incorrect because although this client is at risk for extrapyramidal symptoms 6 hours after the initiation of Haldol, since the client is also taking an antiparkinsonian agent, the risk is reduced. **Answer 4** is incorrect because this client is at risk for relapse and to an adverse reaction to Antabuse *if* the client begins to drink, but this client would be next priority.

> **TEST-TAKING TIP**—This question is a priority question because it asks who the nurse should see *first*. Visualize each situation to determine the client at the highest risk of harm.
> **PL, APP, 7, Psych, PhI, Pharmacological Therapy**

381. **(4)** Severe pregnancy-induced hypertension would cause intrauterine growth restriction (IUGR) and a small measurement. **Answer 1** is incorrect because macrosomia would likely result in a *larger* measurement. **Answer 2** is incorrect because polyhydramnios would cause overdistention of the uterus and a *larger* measurement. **Answer 3** is incorrect because maternal diabetes is associated with macrosomia and a *larger* measurement.

TEST-TAKING TIP—Remember after 20 weeks gestation, the fundal height measurement should be approximately the same as the weeks of gestation. If the measurement is small, the fetus is small or not growing. If too large a measurement, the fetus could be very large or have too much amniotic fluid.
AN, ANL, 5, Maternity, HPM, Health Promotion and Maintenance

382. **(4) Sanguineous drainage of greater then 100 mL/hr in the client who is in the immediate postoperative period following a thoracotomy indicates hemorrhage. The physician should be notified immediately. Answer 1** is incorrect because sanguineous chest tube drainage in the client who is post operative after a thoracotomy should be *less* than 100mL/hr. **Answer 2** is incorrect because pneumothorax occurs when there is *air* between the visceral and the parietal pleura, which causes compression of the lung and results in acute respiratory distress. **Answer 3** is incorrect because chyle drainage is a milky color that results from disruption of the lymphatic drainage system.

TEST-TAKING TIP—Sanguineous = blood. Is this drainage type and volume normal or not? Hemorrhage involves volume of blood.
AS, COM, 6, M/S: Postop, PhI, Physiological Adaptation

383. **(1) Fetal circulation has high pulmonary vascular resistance. Answer 2** is incorrect because the pulmonary blood flow in a fetus is *low*, not high. **Answer 3** is incorrect because there is a *low* resistance of the ductus arteriosus. **Answer 4** is incorrect because there is *low* umbilicoplacental resistance.

TEST-TAKING TIP—Review the fetal circulation. It is common for the facts to be opposite of the true answer. Read carefully and slowly.
AN, COM, 5, Maternity, HPM, Health Promotion and Maintenance

384. **(2) A normal potassium level is 3.5–5.5 mEq/L and the client has a high potassium level of 5.9 with potassium continuing to infuse in the IV fluid. The RN should stop the IV, maintain the IV site by flushing the IV with normal saline or heparin per agency protocol, and notify the physician immediately for a change in IV fluid order. Answer 1** is incorrect because a normal potassium level is 3.5–5.5mEq/L; and the client has a *high* potassium level of 5.9 with potassium continuing to infuse in the IV fluid at a rate of 40mEq/L. This needs to be addressed *immediately*, *not* in 6 hours with a lab recheck. **Answer 3** is incorrect because a normal potassium level is 3.5–5.5 mEq/L, and the client has a high potassium level of 5.9 with potassium continuing to infuse in the IV fluid. Decreasing the IV rate to 50 mL/hr would still result in the infusion of potassium when the potassium level is elevated. It would also decrease the hourly fluid intake for a client who is admitted for dehydration. The physician should be notified immediately, because decreasing the IV rate requires a physician order. **Answer 4** is incorrect because a normal potassium level is 3.5–5.5mEq/L; the client has a high potassium level of 5.9 with potassium continuing to infuse in the IV fluid. The nurse should notify the physician *immediately* of the lab value and obtain a change in IV fluid orders.

TEST-TAKING TIP—Choose the only option that stops the infusion of potassium.
AN, ANL, 6, M/S: F-E, PhI, Reduction of Risk Potential

385. **(3) Positioning the client to maintain the head and neck alignment will facilitate cerebral spinal fluid drainage and prevent increased intracranial pressure due to impediment** of cerebral spinal fluid drainage. Answer 1 is incorrect because the HOB should be maintained at *greater than* or equal to 30 degrees, unless specifically ordered otherwise by the physician. **Answer 2** is incorrect because grouping multiple nursing activities like turning, bathing, linen change, and suctioning will dramatically *increase* intracranial pressure for an extended amount of time. To minimize increase in intracranial pressure, nursing activities should be planned to give the client 30–60 minute breaks between activities. The intracranial pressure will increase with any activity, but the pressure will have an opportunity to decrease to safer levels if activities are *not* clustered. **Answer 4** is incorrect because positioning to prevent increase in intracranial pressure is focused on alignment of the *head* and *neck* and elevation of the HOB at 30 degrees, *not* the legs.

TEST-TAKING TIP—Think about the effect of each option on the ICP. *Only one will decrease the ICP.*
PL, APP, 2, M/S: Neuro, PhI, Physiological Adaptation

386. **(3) First priority assessment in caring for a client who is postanesthesia is airway and oxygenation assessment. Anesthetic agents affect respiratory rate and quality. Answer 1** is incorrect because the first priority assessment in caring for a client who is postanesthesia is *airway* and *oxygenation* assessment. The *second* priority is blood pressure and heart rate. **Answer 2** is incorrect because the first priority assessment in caring for a client who is postanesthesia is airway and oxygenation assessment. The *third* priority is temperature to evaluate if the client is warm enough or has an escalating temperature associated with an adverse reaction to anesthesia, called *malignant hyperthermia*. **Answer 4** is incorrect because first priority assessment in caring for a client who is post anesthesia is airway and oxygenation assessment. Pain assessment is the *fourth* priority and should be addressed as soon as other vital signs have been taken.

TEST-TAKING TIP—With a priority question, think about the ABCs first (Airway, Breathing, Circulation).
AS, APP, 2, M/S: Postop, PhI, Reduction of Risk Potential

387. **(1, 2, 3, 4) Answer 1 is correct because until the nurse reviews the child's chart for signs and symptoms of previous abuse (suspicious bruises, fractures, etc.), there is no way of knowing if this is an isolated versus a repeated behavior on the mother's part. The chart may not provide all of the needed information. However, this is still an *appropriate* action on the nurse's part. Answer 2 is correct because the nurse has witnessed an inappropriate action taken by the mother against the child. The nurse is using the "chain of command" by notifying the supervisor. The supervisor will interpret and enforce the clinic's policy regarding such matters. This is an *appropriate* action on the nurse's part. Answer 3 is correct because the nurse recognizes that corporal punishment (spanking, hitting, slapping, etc.) should be a "last resort" and never used in public. Both mother and child will benefit from a "cooling off" period. This is an *appropriate* action on the nurse's part. Answer 4 is correct because while corporal punishment *does* cause a dramatic short-term decrease in undesirable behavior, it is a flawed approach to discipline. It focuses on what the child *should not* do rather than what the child *should* do. Other better techniques of discipline such as behavior modification and "time-outs" should be explored with the parent. This is an *appropriate* action on the nurse's part.**

TEST-TAKING TIP—All of the responses to this question are appropriate. In an alternate item question you are allowed to select all the responses that are applicable.
IMP, APP, 7, PEDS, PsI, Psychosocial Integrity

388. **(4) Egg white is a potential allergen for an infant less than 1 year of age. For this reason, egg white (such as in scrambled eggs, soft or hard boiled eggs, etc.) should be avoided during the first year of life. Cooked egg yolk, which is less allergenic in nature, may be safely introduced to the infant between 9 months and 1 year of age.** Answer 1 is incorrect because there is no documentation that this is a true fact. Infants *do* show preferences for certain flavors (especially sweet tasting foods such as applesauce and fruits). For this reason, it is usually suggested that vegetables be introduced prior to fruits. Once infants have tasted "sweetness," they will sometimes reject the relatively bland flavor, of vegetables. Answer 2 is incorrect because the odor, flavor, and texture of the food are what appeal to the infant rather than the "look" or color of the food. Answer 3 is incorrect because the "slippery" consistence of egg white is not the issue. This response would imply that the *only* way the infant would eat the egg white is uncooked (raw). *Raw* egg white should *not* be given to anyone regardless of age because of possible bacterial contamination, rather than the *risk of* choking or aspiration

> **TEST-TAKING TIP**—Foods are introduced to an infant in a specific sequence that is least likely to cause an allergic response (i.e., cereals→vegetables→fruits→proteins).
> **IMP, APP, 4, PEDS, PhI, Basic Care and Comfort**

389. **(1) Fluid in the water-seal chamber *should fluctuate* and move up with inspiration and down with expiration on a newly inserted chest tube. The absence of fluctuations on a newly inserted chest tube must be identified and corrected because it indicates incorrect tube placement, or problems with the chest drainage system. A chest x-ray is always required to determine if the problem is due to incorrect tube placement or if the tube has become dislodged. The chest drainage system should be evaluated for: malfunction due to inappropriate setup, or obstruction of the tubing due to dependent loops filled with fluid, kinked tubing, or the client may be lying on the tubing.** Answer 2 is incorrect because an air leak is present when there is *continuous* or *intermittent bubbling* in the water-seal chamber. **Answer 3** is incorrect because presence of subcutaneous emphysema is *assessed by palpating* the client's chest around the chest tube insertion site for the presence of air under the skin, which indicates an air leak. **Answer 4** is incorrect because the appropriate suction level is assessed on a wet suction unit by confirming that the fluid *level* is at the *desired mark* in the suction control chamber when the suction is turned off.

> **TEST-TAKING TIP**—Ask yourself: Is this OK or not OK? **Answers 2** and **3** say that it is "not OK." Choose the option that is different (**Answer 1**— "expected"). Know normal function of tubes.
> **AS, COM, 6, M/S: Thoracic, PhI, Reduction of Risk Potential**

390. **(1, 2, 3, 5)** Answer 1 is correct because motor restlessness (akathisia) is an extrapyramidal symptom seen in clients taking Haldol. Answer 2 is correct because limb and neck spasms (dystonia) are extrapyramidal symptoms seen in clients taking Haldol. Answer 3 is correct because cogwheeling (parkinsonism) is an extrapyramidal symptom seen in clients taking Haldol. Answer 5 is correct because a shuffling gait (parkinsonism) is an extrapyramidal side effect seen in clients taking Haldol. Answer 4 is incorrect because tardive dyskinesia is seen only after *long-term* antipsychotic therapy. **Answer 6** is incorrect because clients taking anti-psychotic medications do *not* usually experience cardiac changes. This side effect is more common with tricyclic antidepressant medications and monoamine oxidase inhibitors (MAOIs).

> **TEST-TAKING TIP**—Look for the answers that are different from the others. The correct answers involve changes in the *muscular* functions, which are very different from *cardiac* arrhythmias (**Answer 6**). Also, note that the question states that the client *recently* began treatment with Haldol. This would eliminate tardive dyskinesia (**Answer 4**) as a correct answer.
> **AS, ANL, 3, Psych, PhI, Pharmacological Therapy**

391. **(2) The chest tube should be immediately unclamped. The client still has an air leak that is causing a build up of air in the pleural space, collapsing part of the lung, and causing breathing difficulty. The clamp must be removed from the chest tube immediately to allow this air to escape and the lung to re-expand.** Answer 1 is incorrect because the first priority is to remain with the client and address the breathing difficulty by unclamping the chest tube clamp. The physician should be notified as *priority number 4* in this answer sequence. **Answer 3** is incorrect because the first priority is to address the breathing difficulty by unclamping the chest tube clamp. The client should then be assessed for the presence of new or expanded subcutaneous emphysema, which would indicate an air leak. This is *priority number 3* in this answer sequence. **Answer 4** is incorrect because the first priority is to address the breathing difficulty by unclamping the chest tube clamp. The client should be placed on 2L nasal cannula, as *priority number 2* in this answer sequence.

> **TEST-TAKING TIP**—Address the *cause of the problem* first. The chest tube clamp is the probable cause of the breathing difficulty. The oxygen treats a *symptom* (**Answer 4**).
> **AN, ANL, 6, M/S: Resp.; PhI, Physiological Adaptation**

392. **(1) The kinked chest tube tubing does not allow for drainage of air or fluid from the pleural space. This will causes pressure to build up and push against the lung, collapsing the lung and shifting it to the unaffected side. The client will experience respiratory difficulty progressing to respiratory distress and tension pneumothorax. The tension pneumothorax causes a precarious drop in blood pressure as the large blood vessels in the thoracic cavity are compressed and the heart does not receive adequate blood volume to pump out.** Answer 2 is incorrect because the kinked chest tube tubing does not allow for drainage of air or fluid from the pleural space, increasing the risk of *pneumothorax, not air leak* **Answer 3** is incorrect because kinked chest tube tubing does not allow for drainage of air or fluid from the pleural space, thus increasing the risk of pneumothorax, *not* hemorrhage. **Answer 4** is incorrect because kinked chest tube tubing does not allow for drainage of air or fluid from the pleural space, increasing the risk of pneumothorax. Cardiac tamponade occurs when there is a *fluid collection between the pericardial membrane and the heart muscle,* which prevents the heart from pumping effectively.

> **TEST-TAKING TIP**—With *chest tubes*, think *pulmonary* difficulties. When you are deciding between two options, choose the one with the greatest risk.
> **AS, COM, 6, M/S: Thoracic, PhI, Reduction of Risk Potential**

393. **(3) The client is receiving a daily potassium supplement and the nurse should assess the serum potassium level to make sure that it is not elevated, prior to administering additional potassium. The client has undergone coronary angiography and intervention, which requires the use of a dye that can be toxic to the kidneys and cause impaired renal function. Impaired renal function can lead to increased potassium levels.** Answer 1 is incorrect because the potassium level is the most important factor for the nurse to assess. These medications do not *affect blood pressure.* **Answer 2** is incorrect because Troponin is a cardiac biomarker used in diagnosis of an acute myocardial infarction which the nurse would expect to be elevated in the client with an acute MI. **Answer 4** is incorrect because the potassium level is the most important factor for the nurse to assess.At this time there is *no immediate concern for blood clots*; therefore, checking peripheral pulses is not indicated.

> **TEST-TAKING TIP**—Look for the key concept: A low K^+ is life-threatening for a client with a cardiac condition.
> AS, COM, 6, M/S: CV, PhI, **Pharmacological and Parenteral Therapies**

394. **(4) A serum creatinine of greater than 2.5 is indicative of renal impairment. The increase in creatinine from 1.8 mg/dL to 2.8 mg/dL is a significant change because the client has a history of renal insufficiency and has undergone coronary angiography, which required the use of a dye that can be toxic to the kidneys and cause further damage to the glomeruli. Answer 1** is incorrect because the increase in serum creatinine is the most significant value. Troponin is one of the lab values used in the diagnosis of an acute myocardial infarction. The reference range is 0–0.03 ng/mL. The troponin is *expected to be elevated* in the client with an acute MI. The *amount* of increase in this lab value is *insignificant.* **Answer 2** is incorrect because an increase in WBC from 6000/mm³ to 11,000/mm³ indicates an inflammatory response that occurs when there is death of cardiac cells with an acute MI, and with the tissue trauma of heart catheterization. The reference range for an adult is 5000–10,000/mm³. **Answer 3** is incorrect because the increase in serum creatinine is the most significant result. CPK-MB is an isoenzyme specific for the cardiac muscle that indicates damage to the myocardial cells. The reference range for CPK-MB is 0.6 ng/mL–3.5 ng/mL. *It is expected to be elevated* in the client with an acute MI. The amount of increase is *insignificant.*

> **TEST-TAKING TIP**—Three of the options have an *expected* elevation from the MI; the kidneys appear to have sustained further damage.
> AN, ANL, 6, M/S: CV, PhI, **Reduction of Risk Potential**

395. **(2) The blood gases indicate an uncompensated respiratory acidosis. The client is hypoventilating. To increase ventilation, the client should increase deep breathing and activity levels to facilitate better O_2/CO_2 exchange. Instructing the client to use the bedside inspirometer is an excellent tool for encouraging deep breathing and giving the client a specific measured respiratory goal—10 times per hour when awake. Walking should also be advised. Answer 1** is incorrect because the ABGs indicate an uncompensated respiratory acidosis. The client is hypoventilating. Since the CO_2 is already elevated, breathing slowly would increase the CO_2, decrease the pH and worsen the respiratory acidosis. **Answer 3** is incorrect because the ABGs indicate only mild hypoxia with a PaO_2 of 77. Placing the client on 6L nasal cannula O_2 would *overcorrect* the PaO_2 and result in oxygen levels that are too high. High PaO_2 levels can damage the alveoli. **Answer 4** is incorrect because the ABGs indicate an uncompensated respiratory acidosis. Fluids will *not improve* a respiratory blood gas alteration.

> **TEST-TAKING TIP**—Know the normal ranges for arterial blood gases in order to choose the correct intervention.
> IMP, ANL, 6, M/S: ABG, PhI, **Physiological Adaptation**

396. **(1) Late school-aged children need precise and concrete information, such as how the penis becomes erect, before attempting to learn about other more complex sexual** issues. Also, this age group is not yet thinking on an abstract or hypothetical level. They need to "begin at the beginning" when acquiring new information and learn from the simple to the complex. They must learn how their bodies function sexually before they can progress to other topics dealing with sex. **Answer 2** is incorrect because while learning how diseases are sexually transmitted is a correct answer, it is *not* the most basic information with which to begin a sex education program. This information should correctly be incorporated into classes given later in the school semester. **Answer 3** is incorrect because while learning how to be sexually responsible is a correct answer, it is *not* the most basic information with which to begin a sex education program. This information should correctly be incorporated into classes given later in the school semester. **Answer 4** is incorrect because while learning how AIDS is transmitted is a correct answer, it is *not* the most basic information with which to begin a sex education program. This information should correctly be incorporated into classes given later in the school semester.

> **TEST-TAKING TIP**—The responses to this question range from simple to complex. Remember that late-school age children learn in an "easy→hard" sequence, and select the correct answer.
> IMP, APP, 5, PEDS, HPM, **Health Promotion and Maintenance**

397. **(3) Walking along a nature trail *would* promote the development of gross motor and social skills. It would provide a group of active, creative, and imaginative 5-year-old children with the opportunity to select, explore, and share observations and experiences gained while walking on the nature trail. Answer 1** is incorrect because finger painting is a fine motor-adaptive activity as well as an individual activity. It would *not* promote the development of gross motor or social skills. **Answer 2** is incorrect because playing house is a fine motor-adaptive activity. It *would* promote social skills but would *not* promote the development of gross motor skills. **Answer 4** is incorrect because while playing soccer *would* promote the development of gross motor skills, it is too advanced a game (cognitively, socially, and physically) for a group of 5-year-old children. Soccer is a competitive game and better suited for school-age children. It would *not* promote the development of social skills in a group of 5-year-old children as this group enjoys associative play, but *without* rigid organization or rules such as found in playing soccer.

> **TEST-TAKING TIP**—The responses in this question are either fine motor-adaptive or gross motor. Compare the gross motor responses and select the response that *best* incorporates the associative play practices and needs of a group of 5-year-old children.
> IMP, APP, 5, PEDS, HPM, **Health Promotion and Maintenance**

398. **(3) The fetus produces insulin based on the mother's blood sugar. Answer 1** is incorrect because insulin does *not cross the placenta.* **Answer 2** is incorrect because insulin levels of the infant are *not* usually low at birth. **Answer 4** is incorrect because insulin *does not cross the placenta.*

> **TEST-TAKING TIP**—Remember insulin does not cross the placenta; therefore, two of the options can be eliminated.
> AN, COM, 4, Maternity, PhI, **Physiological Adaptation**

399. **(3) Respiratory movements are an indicator of a healthy fetus. Answer 1** is incorrect because a healthy fetus *does*

make respiratory movements. **Answer 2** is incorrect because there is no air in utero to create a crying noise. **Answer 4** is incorrect because asphyxia results in *increased* respiratory efforts, gasping, in utero.

> **TEST-TAKING TIP**—Look at two contradictory options: no respiratory movements (**Answer 1**) versus "demonstrates…respiratory motions" (**Answer 3**). Eliminate most options with an absolute "no."
> **AN, COM, 6, Maternity, HPM, Health Promotion and Maintenance**

400. **(4) The parents should give the child small amounts of fluids to maintain hydration and should continue the medication. The parents should also be giving the child acetaminophen (*Tylenol*) for the fever.** **Answer 1** is incorrect because this medication is a tricyclic antidepressant with withdrawal symptoms of nausea and vomiting. If the medication is stopped suddenly, the client's flu symptoms (e.g., vomiting) could be exacerbated. **Answer 2** is incorrect because the parents should *not* be instructed to hold the medication. The parent should notify the doctor if the fever persists for more than 3 days. **Answer 3** is incorrect because the parents should be giving the child *only clear liquids.* Food would only increase the vomiting.

> **TEST-TAKING TIP**—Look at the pattern: two choices that "hold" the medication and two answers "continue" the medication. It is a choice between "clear liquids" and food. Go with the "safest" answer of *fluids*.
> **IMP, APP, 7, Psych, PhI, Pharmacological Therapy**

401. **(3) Propranolol is a beta-blocker and should be used with *caution* in clients who have COPD because it can cause bronchospasm.** **Answer 1** is incorrect because amitriptyline, along with other tricyclic antidepressants, *is effective* in the management of chronic pain. **Answer 2** is incorrect because enoxaparin is an anticoagulant that *is used* to prevent deep vein thrombosis in clients who have had orthopedic surgery. **Answer 4** is incorrect because lovastatin *is* a drug commonly prescribed for hypercholesterolemia.

> **TEST-TAKING TIP**—Remember the classification of each drug and choose the drug that should *not* be given because it is inappropriate for the condition listed. **Answer 3** *is inappropriate* for the condition listed.
> **AN, ANL, 1, M/S: Meds, PhI, Pharmacological and Parenteral Therapies**

402. **(2) Humidification helps liquefy secretions in the sinus cavities, which reduces the risk for bacterial infection.** **Answer 1** is incorrect because salt water gargles are helpful for *pharyngitis*, but *not* sinusitis. **Answer 3** is incorrect because classic antihistamines make secretions more viscous, and consequently more difficult to get rid of. **Answer 4** is incorrect because corticosteroids in the form of *nasal* sprays are preferred for treating and preventing sinusitis.

> **TEST-TAKING TIP**—Note that two options (**Answers 3** and **4**) are medications, and are not *primary nursing* actions to suggest to the client. One goal of nursing treatment for sinusitis is to facilitate the movement of mucus out of the sinus cavities. **Answer 2** facilitates this goal.
> **PL, APP, 1, M/S: Resp., PhI, Reduction of Risk Potential**

403. **(4) Stretch marks change after delivery and may or may not occur during pregnancy.** **Answer 1** is incorrect because stretch marks *do not* occur in *all* pregnancies. **Answer 2** is incorrect because women who are nulliparous *frequently do develop* stretch marks. **Answer 3** is incorrect because stretch marks *do not completely disappear* after delivery.

> **TEST-TAKING TIP**—The key words "all" (**Answer 1**) and "completely" (**Answer 3**) are clues that the answer is probably incorrect.
> **PL, APP, 5, Maternity, HPM, Health Promotion and Maintenance**

404. **(2) The most likely cause of the problem is that the NG tube is plugged with gastric contents or has adhered to the gastric mucosa and is no longer draining. Irrigating the tube with 30 cc of water should clear any obstructions and free the tube from the gastric mucosa.** **Answer 1** is incorrect because problem-solving should be done first. Inserting a new NG tube would cause the client unnecessary discomfort. **Answer 3** is incorrect because having the client take a few deep breaths will not solve the NG problem. **Answer 4** is incorrect because turning the suction higher may cause additional trauma to the gastric mucosa.

> **TEST-TAKING TIP**—**Answers 1** and **4** involve potential additional trauma to the client and can be eliminated. **Answer 3** does not address gastric decompression; therefore, **Answer 2** is the only correct option.
> **IMP, ANL, 8, M/S: GI, PhI, Reduction of Risk Potential**

405. **(1) High-pitched bowel sounds can be heard *above* the area of obstruction because peristalsis continues to the point of obstruction.** **Answer 2** is incorrect because high-pitched bowel sounds are heard *above* the area of obstruction, *not below*. **Answer 3** is incorrect because bowel sounds are not completely absent with bowel obstruction. Peristalsis continues to the point of obstruction. **Answer 4** is incorrect because a client with bowel obstruction does not have a fever unless peritonitis or strangulation of the bowel has occurred.

> **TEST-TAKING TIP**—Focus on the two options that are opposites: **Answers 1** and **2**. Then, recall that in bowel obstruction, peristalsis continues up to the obstruction; therefore, it makes sense that bowel sounds can be heard *before* the obstruction, but *not after*.
> **AS, ANL, 8, M/S: GI, PhI, Reduction of Risk Potential**

406. **(3) This response describes the Galant reflex (or trunk incurvation reflex). This reflex is present in a newborn and disappears by 4 weeks of age.** **Answer 1** is incorrect because this response describes the *parachute* reflex. This reflex appears at about *7–9 months* of age and persists indefinitely. **Answer 2** is incorrect because this response describes the *Landau* reflex. This reflex appears at about *6–8 months* of age and lasts until approximately 12–24 months of age. **Answer 4** is incorrect because this response describes the *neck-righting* reflex. This reflex appears at about *3 months* of age and lasts until approximately 24–36 months of age.

> **TEST-TAKING TIP**—Know the onset and disappearance of key reflexes in an infant. Think: simple reflexes (responses) in the younger infant and more complex reflexes (responses) in the older infant.
> **AS, APP, 5, PEDS, HPM, Health Promotion and Maintenance**

407. **(3) Severe episodes of hypertension are a hallmark of pheochromocytoma, evidenced by severe headache, profuse sweating, and tachycardia.** **Answer 1** is incorrect because pulse rate, although important, is *not the most important* thing to monitor. **Answer 2** is incorrect because blood sugar, although important, is *not the most important* thing to monitor. **Answer 4** is incorrect because urine output is *not directly related* to pheochromocytoma.

> **TEST-TAKING TIP**—Think "life-threatening!" The question asks for the *most important* (most life-

threatening) thing to monitor. Recall that pheochromocytoma, a rare tumor of the adrenal gland, causes periodic episodes of hypertension. Pulse rate and blood sugar (**Answers 1** and **2**) can rise as a result of this disease; however, neither of these is as *immediately life-threatening* as hypertension. Alteration in urine output (**Answer 4**) is not a significant characteristic of pheochromocytoma.
AS, APP, 6, M/S: Endocrine, PhI, Physiological Adaptation

408. (1, 2, 3, 4) Answer 1 is correct because "baby walkers" allow the infant to independently move about the pediatric unit. This is because the "baby walker" allows the infant's feet to touch the floor. The infant can "walk" and gain access to hazards on the pediatric unit. Answer 2 is correct because unoccupied cribs with the crib rails in the down position pose a hazard. The hospitalized child may be tempted to climb back into the crib but fall in the process. Regardless of the child's ability to get into or out of the crib, unoccupied cribs should have the crib rails in the "up" position at all times. Answer 3 is correct because latex balloons pose a serious threat to children of all ages (hospitalized as well as non-hospitalized). If the balloon bursts, the child may ingest a piece of the balloon. If the piece is aspirated or swallowed, it is extremely difficult to remove and may result in choking. Latex balloons should *never* be permitted in the hospital setting. Substitute Mylar or paper balloons for latex balloons. Answer 4 is correct because the method of transporting hospitalized infants is determined by the infant's age, condition and destination. Transporting an infant in a bassinet or crib would be a safe method of transportation as well as comfortable for the infant. An unsafe method of transportation would be to carry an infant to the destination. The UAP carrying the infant could slip and fall while walking and the infant could be injured during the fall.

> **TEST-TAKING TIP**—All of the responses seem reasonable. In an alternate-item question you are allowed to select all of the responses that are applicable.
> **IMP, APP, 1, PEDS, SECE, Safety and Infection Control**

409. (2) Both the plasma and erythrocytes increase during pregnancy. Answer 1 is incorrect because blood volume increases *until it peaks* at about 32–34 weeks gestation. Answer 3 is incorrect because blood volume increases by *about 50%* over prepregnant values. Answer 4 is incorrect because the volume increase is due to increases in *both plasma and erythrocytes.*

> **TEST-TAKING TIP**—All the options include increase in blood volume. Think about what *causes* the increase. Select the most *inclusive* answer (**Answer 2**).
> **AN, COM, 6, Maternity, HPM, Health Promotion and Maintenance**

410. (1) Lithium is a naturally occurring salt that affects the kidneys. Clients with impaired renal function should use the medication with great caution. The nurse should make sure that the doctor has assessed the renal function before initiating the treatment. Answer 2 is incorrect because the client's alcohol use in the *past* would *not* affect the initiation of treatment. Answer 3 is incorrect because a client's *liver* function will *not* be affected by lithium. Answer 4 is incorrect because a regular diet does not affect lithium treatment. Fluid and sodium intake can change lithium blood levels and the client should avoid changes in fluid and sodium intake. Clients on low sodium diets will need special instructions and monitoring of lithium blood levels.

> **TEST-TAKING TIP**—Eliminate choices that would be less harmful to the client. *History* of alcohol and diet would

cause the least harm. Ask yourself what is true of lithium; does it affect the kidneys or liver?
AN, ANL, 7, Psych, PhI, Reduction of Risk Potential

411. (1) Developing severe weakness within 1 hour of the administration of Tensilon indicates a cholinergic crisis, or overdose of anticholinesterase drugs. The antidote for a cholinergic crisis is atropine. Answer 2 is incorrect because it would be inappropriate to administer an anti-cholinesterase drug, such as pyridostigmine, to a client in cholinergic crisis. Answer 3 is incorrect because checking for constricted pupils does not provide useful information. Pupil constriction does not occur during a cholinergic crisis. Answer 4 is incorrect because intubation is *not* the first action. Atropine should be used first to *counteract* the toxic effects of the anticholinesterase drug.

> **TEST-TAKING TIP**—Focus on the two options that involve a similar action; **Answers 1** and **2** involve administration of drugs. Then recall that a Tensilon test can be used to differentiate underdosing from overdosing of anti-cholinesterase drugs.
> **IMP, APP, 1, M/S: NM, PhI, Pharmacological and Parenteral Therapies**

412. (4) S_1 is best heard at the 5th intercostal space, left mid-clavicular line. The S_1 heart sound represents the closing of the mitral and tricuspid valves and is best heard at the apex. Answer 1 is incorrect because this describes the *aortic* area. Answer 2 is incorrect because this describes the *pulmonic* area. Answer 3 is incorrect because this describes the *tricuspid* area.

> **TEST-TAKING TIP**—Notice that **Answer 4** is the only option that does *not* specify the sternal border. When unsure of the correct answer, choose the option that is different.
> **AS, COM, 6, M/S: Cardiac, PhI, Physiological Adaptation**

413. (4) Cardiac output is increased during the entire duration of pregnancy. Answer 1 is incorrect because cardiac output *remains* increased throughout pregnancy. Answer 2 is incorrect because cardiac output is *decreased in the supine* position. Answer 3 is incorrect because it is *increased* during the stress of the *second stage* of labor.

> **TEST-TAKING TIP**—Three of the options include increased cardiac output; one answer that relates to labor is too limited (**Answer 3**), and can be eliminated. Two options state the cardiac output "increases…decreases" (**Answers 1** and **3**). Choose the option that is different ("increases…and remains elevated").
> **PL, COM, 6, Maternity, PhI, Physiological Adaptation**

414. (4) Research has shown that maintaining recommended dietary levels of potassium and calcium has a beneficial effect on hypertension. Answer 1 is incorrect because goals for physical activity should be realistic. Although the client should aim for 30 minutes/day of moderate intensity activity, setting unrealistic goals (5 miles/day, 6 days/week) does not ensure success. Answer 2 is incorrect because the relationship between stress reduction activities and hypertension is controversial. Answer 3 is incorrect because eliminating caffeine from the diet has not been conclusively shown to have a beneficial effect on hypertension.

> **TEST-TAKING TIP**—Look at the verbs: "increase," "enroll," "eliminate," "maintain." Choose the *dietary* option to *maintain.*
> **IMP, APP, 6, M/S: CV, HPM, Health Promotion and Maintenance**

415. **(2) Wall suction should be set at 120 mm Hg for tracheal suctioning. Answer 1** is incorrect because, while putting sterile saline down the trachea can help liquefy secretions, 10 cc is *too much*. The correct amount should be 2–3 cc. **Answer 3** is incorrect because 20–30 seconds is *too long* to apply suction. Suction should be applied for about 10 seconds. **Answer 4** is incorrect because deflating the cuff *may compromise* the client's airway.

> **TEST-TAKING TIP—Answers 1, 2,** and **3** are all partially correct, but **Answers 1** and **3** involve too much saline or too long to suction.
> **IMP, APP, 6, M/S: Resp., PhI, Reduction of Risk Potential**

416. **(4) The supine position causes arterial hypotension and decreased blood flow to the uterus and the placenta. Answer 1** is incorrect because the supine position causes compression of the vena cava, *decreasing* venous return. **Answer 2** is incorrect because supine position causes a *decreased* cardiac output. **Answer 3** is incorrect because it causes a *decrease* in the blood flow to the lower extremities.

> **TEST-TAKING TIP—**Three options say "increased" (**Answers 1, 2,** and **3**). **Answer 4** implies "decreased." Choose the option that is different.
> **IMP, APP, 6, Maternity, PhI, Physiological Adaptation**

417. **(2) Coughing may indicate pneumothorax from the insertion procedure. Answer 1** is incorrect because it is expected that *venous* blood will flow briskly from the catheter hub just before the tubing is attached. This is an indicator that the catheter *is correctly placed* in a central vein. **Answer 3** is incorrect because mild pain at the insertion site, particularly after the local anesthetic has worn off, is *not unusual*. **Answer 4** is incorrect because sinus rhythm is *normal*.

> **TEST-TAKING TIP—**Choose the option that is different: 3 options are normal; 1 is not. **Answer 2** presents the only abnormal event during the insertion of the central catheter.
> **EV, ANL, 6, M/S: CV, PhI, Reduction of Risk Potential**

418. **(1) An infant who requires an apnea monitor may have difficulty breathing and feeding at the same time. Removing the apnea monitor at feeding time would be especially dangerous. The apnea monitor is effective *only* if it is used. Answer 2** is incorrect because a child with a neurogenic bladder is routinely placed on clean intermittent catheterization (CIC) guidelines. This means that the same catheter *will* be reused but *only* after thorough cleaning between uses. Clean intermittent catheterization (CIC) is effective *only* if the guidelines are followed. **Answer 3** is incorrect because a newborn with developmental hip dysplasia *must* wear the Pavlik harness 23 hours a day to maintain the hips in an abducted position. The Pavlik harness is effective *only* if it is used. **Answer 4** is incorrect because a 12-year-old child with hemophilia could reasonably be expected to self-administer the IV clotting factor. Between 9–12 years of age, children with hemophilia are usually taught to begin self-administration of the IV clotting factor. The IV clotting factor is effective *only* if it is used.

> **TEST-TAKING TIP—**All of these answers contain *at-risk-for* elements. But the danger of respiratory difficulty takes priority over the other situations.
> **EV, ANL, 1, PEDS, SECE, Safety and Infection Control**

419. **(3) The back seat is the safest area of the car, and a rear-facing car seat provides the best protection for the disproportionately heavy head and weak neck of the newborn. This position minimizes the stress on the neck by spreading the forces of a frontal crash over the entire back, neck** and head while the spine is supported by the back of the car seat. If the car seat was facing forward, the head would whip forward because of the force of the crash, and would create enormous stress on the neck. **Answer 1** is incorrect because while a musical mobile is a desirable toy for the newborn and does provide desirable auditory stimulation, it is *not critical* information that the mother must understand prior to going home. This information can be safely delayed until the newborn is seen at a well-baby visit in the pediatrician's office. **Answer 2** is incorrect because, whereas the general rule is that the mattress is too small if two adult fingers can be placed between the mattress and crib frame, the newborn is unlikely to suffocate by becoming wedged in the space between the mattress and the crib frame. This can be prevented by placing large, rolled towels in the space to create a snug fit until a more suitable mattress can be purchased. **Answer 4** is incorrect because, whereas sucking is the newborn's chief pleasure, it is *not critical* information that the mother must understand prior to going home. This information can be safely delayed until the newborn is seen at a well-baby visit in the pediatrician's office. The use of a pacifier is not mandatory for the mother.

> **TEST-TAKING TIP—**This questions provides two "nice to do" responses and two "must do" responses. Of the "must do" responses one is more critical than the other. Select that response.
> **IMP, ANL, 1, PEDS, SECE, Safety and Infection Control**

420. **≥2.0.** The *therapeutic* blood level for lithium is 0.8–1.6 mEq/L. Blood levels *over* 1.6 may place the client at *risk for* lithium toxicity. Clients with blood levels higher than 2.0 mEq/L are at *high risk* and need to be assessed for lithium toxicity.

> **TEST-TAKING TIP—**Memorize therapeutic blood levels for all medications taken by clients that can reach toxic levels!
> **AS, COM, 3, Psych, PhI, Pharmacological Therapy**

421. **(3) Dehydration is a major, potentially life-threatening problem in the early stages of burn treatment. A patent IV is required to prevent dehydration. Answer 1** is incorrect because, although infection is a serious threat to the client, *topical*, not parenteral, antibiotics are often the *first* treatment for burns. **Answer 2** is incorrect because there are *other, more important* issues to address in the *early* stages of caring for a client with burns. **Answer 4** is incorrect because, although pain management is important, there are other more immediate life-threatening problems.

> **TEST-TAKING TIP—**Although **Answers 1, 2,** and **4** are important concerns, the *most important* for a client with serious burns initially is fluid replacement.
> **PL, ANL, 6, M/S: Integ., PhI, Physiological Adaptation**

422. **(1) This indicates hyponatremia. The normal range for sodium is 135–150 mEq/L. Answer 2** is incorrect because, although low, a hematocrit of 31% is still greater than the point at which most clients will be transfused, which is 25%–30%. **Answer 3** is incorrect because treatment for low platelets is not usually started unless the platelet count drops *below* 50,000. **Answer 4** is incorrect because the *normal range* for potassium *is* 3.5–5.0 mEq/L.

> **TEST-TAKING TIP—Answer 4** represents a normal potassium level and is not of concern. **Answers 1, 2,** and **3** all represent abnormal values, but a sodium level of 120 mEq/L is seriously low and will produce symptoms ranging from nausea and malaise to seizures and coma. A sodium level of 120 mEq/L should be attended to immediately.
> **EV, ANL, 1, M/S: F-E, PhI, Reduction of Risk Potential**

423. (3) Knee-chest will facilitate the rotation from occiput posterior to occiput anterior position. **Answer 1** is incorrect because the fetus is likely in an occiput posterior position; and the fetus is not likely to rotate with the client in a semi-Fowler's position. **Answer 2** is incorrect because although the left lateral position is preferred for optimal perfusion to the placenta, the fetus will not easily rotate in this position. **Answer 4** is incorrect because Trendelenburg is not a recommended position for labor. It decreases the positive effects of gravity on the cervix.

> **TEST-TAKING TIP**—The key to this question is the characteristic symptom of back pain. This is usually associated with a fetus in an occiput posterior position. Rotating the fetus will relieve the back pain and facilitate the delivery.
> **IMP, APP, 3, Maternity, PhI, Basic Care and Comfort**

424. (2) Emptying the bag when it is about half full will prevent problems with the bag falling off from the weight of the effluent. **Answer 1** is incorrect because the bag should be emptied *before* it gets "too heavy". **Answer 3** is incorrect because the bag *can* be more than one-third full. Emptying the bag when it is only one-third full could be expensive for the client, who would need to buy supplies more frequently. **Answer 4** is incorrect because a client with an ileostomy will need to wear an ostomy bag *all the time*, because the effluent from an ileostomy is mostly liquid.

> **TEST-TAKING TIP**—Remember that an ileostomy produces liquid stool; therefore, **Answer 4** can be eliminated because the client will need to wear a bag all the time. **Answer 2** is the best compromise of the remaining options.
> **EV, ANL, 8, M/S: GI, PhI, Basic Care and Comfort**

425. (2) This tests *cranial nerve III, the oculomotor nerve.* **Answer 1** is incorrect because this tests *cranial nerve V, the trigeminal nerve.* **Answer 3** is incorrect because this tests *cranial nerve XII, the hypoglossal nerve.* **Answer 4** is incorrect because this tests *cranial nerve I, the olfactory nerve.*

> **TEST-TAKING TIP**—Differentiation of cranial nerves generally requires simple memorization. Cranial nerve III is part of a triad of nerves (III, IV, and VI) which tests direct and consensual light reflexes, which are the cardinal positions of gaze, and movement of the eyeballs.
> **AS, KNOW, 2, M/S: Neuro, PhI, Reduction of Risk Potential**

426. (2) The front-facing position in the middle of the back seat of the car is the best and safest position in which to place a toddler's car seat. The transition point for switching to the forward-facing position is defined by the manufacturer of the car seat, but it is generally at a body weight of 9 kilograms (20 pounds) and at 1 year of age. **Answer 1** is incorrect because the rear-facing position in the middle of the back seat of the car is the best and safest position in which to place an *infant's* car seat. Infants should face the rear from birth to 20 pounds and as close to 1 year of age as possible. **Answer 3** is incorrect because severe injuries and deaths in toddlers (as well as in other age groups) have occurred from air bags deploying on impact. The air bag could strike the head and upper torso of a toddler riding in the front seat of the car, causing neurological and chest injuries. **Answer 4** is incorrect because this position still poses dangers to the toddler. If there is no back seat and a toddler *must* ride in the front, the passenger-side air bag should be switched off (and the seat placed as far back as possible) to reduce the risk; however, the middle of the back seat remains the *safest* position.

> **TEST-TAKING TIP**—Know the ages and weights and positions for car seat safety. The younger and smaller the

child, the greater the need for safety (and protective equipment).
IMP, APP, 1, PEDS, SECE, Safety and Infection Control

427. (4) Flat, pinkish-red macules on the face, neck, and trunk of a 5-year-old child *are* a cause of immediate concern. These lesions would most likely be those associated with rubella (German measles), a highly communicable disease of childhood. These skin lesions *must* be reported immediately to the school pediatrician for confirmation in order to prevent the *potential* spread of the disease to other children in the kindergarten class. **Answer 1** is incorrect because slightly elevated, crusted lesions on the pinna of the ear of a 2-year-old toddler are *not* a cause of immediate concern. These lesions would most likely be those associated with *eczema.* **Answer 2** is incorrect because superficial but elevated pustules on the cheeks of a 16-year-old adolescent are *not* a cause of immediate concern. These lesions would most likely be those associated with *acne.* **Answer 3** is incorrect because elevated vesicles on the palms of the hands of a 7-year-old child are *not* a cause of immediate concern. These lesions would most likely be those associated with *blisters.*

> **TEST-TAKING TIP**—The presence of skin lesions in *several* areas of the body is more likely to be a cause for concern (such as communicability) than if the skin lesions appeared in only one area of the body.
> **AN, ANL, 1, PEDS, SECE, Safety and Infection Control**

428. (4) This client has *multiple* problems—including a chronic disease, acute recovery from the amputation, and rehabilitation—that will require a multidisciplinary approach. **Answer 1** is incorrect because, while this client will need postoperative care, and probably counseling or a support group, this client will not require the most complex care. **Answer 2** is incorrect because, while this client will need nursing care and possible rehabilitation, this client will not require the most complex care. **Answer 3** is incorrect because, unless unforeseen complications occur, this client will only need acute nursing care and discharge teaching.

> **TEST-TAKING TIP**—All the clients will require nursing care for recovery. In addition, all clients may require a physician's or surgeon's care. The clients in **Answers 1, 2,** and **4** will also need posthospital care for counseling or rehabilitation. However, the client in **Answer 4** is very young to have a limb amputated as a result of diabetes and should meet with a diabetes educator.
> **AS, ANL, 3, M/S: Endocrine, SECE, Management of Care: Priority**

429. (3) The postpartum assessment includes fundal location, lochia, and perineum. **Answer 1** is incorrect because since the fourth stage of labor is the *immediate* postpartum period, fetal heart rate would *no longer* be a part of the assessment. **Answer 2** is incorrect because since the delivery *has already occurred*, dilation, effacement, and station are *no longer* assessed. **Answer 4** is incorrect because placental separation is a part of the *third stage* of labor.

> **TEST-TAKING TIP**—Time frame is the key in this question (fourth stage of labor). Do not confuse *stages* and *phases* of labor.
> **AS, APP, 5, Maternity, HPM, Health Promotion and Maintenance**

430. >**0.08%.**
Blood alcohol levels of 0.08% and higher indicate the client is intoxicated.

> **TEST-TAKING TIP**—Memorize this blood alcohol level!
> **AS, KNOW, 7, Psych, PhI, Reduction of Risk Potential**

431. **(3) The nurse should approach the client who is blind from the front, and speak in a normal tone of voice.** **Answer 1** is incorrect because the client is *vision*-impaired, not *hearing*-impaired. Speaking louder than normal *will not help* the client to see better, and may startle the client. **Answer 2** is incorrect because if the nurse speaks *too softly*, the client *may not recognize* that the nurse is speaking. **Answer 4** is incorrect because the client is blind and *will not see* facial expressions.

> **TEST-TAKING TIP**—Use a process of elimination to arrive at the correct answer: **Answers 1** and **2** address *hearing* function, rather than *visual* function, and **Answer 4** is clearly incorrect.
> **AN, ANL, 2, M/S: Sens.-Percep., SECE, Management of Care**

432. **(1) Stage 1 of Lyme disease consists of the tick bite at the time of inoculation, followed by the development of *erythema chronicum migrans* (ECM) at the site of the bite. The lesion begins as a small erythematous papule that enlarges radially over a period of 3–32 days, resulting in a large circumferential ring with a raised, edematous doughnut-like border. The thigh, groin, and axilla are common sites. The lesion is described as "burning," feels warm to the touch, and may be pruritic. Constitutional symptoms such as fever, headache, malaise, and generalized lymphadenopathy may also be observed.** **Answer 2** is incorrect because stage 2 of Lyme disease is the most serious stage and is characterized by systemic involvement of the *neurologic, cardiac* and *musculoskeletal* systems. **Answer 3** is incorrect because stage 3 of Lyme disease is the late stage and is characterized by musculoskeletal pain that involves the tendons, bursae, muscles, and synovia. These symptoms may develop *months or years later* after the initial infection from the tick bite. **Answer 4** is incorrect because Lyme disease just has three stages.

> **TEST-TAKING TIP**—Knowing the signs and symptoms of each stage of the disease assists in selecting the correct answer.
> **AN, ANL, 1, PEDS, SECE, Safety and Infection Control**

433. **(2) Exhaling through pursed lips helps prolong exhalation and prevent bronchiolar collapse.** **Answer 1** is incorrect because it is preferable for clients to inhale through the nose because air is warmed and humidified more effectively via the nose than the mouth. **Answer 3** is incorrect because the exhale should be *approximately 3 times the length of the inhale* to prevent bronchiolar collapse. **Answer 4** is incorrect because, although clients with COPD often use accessory muscles to breathe (neck and upper chest muscles), using these muscles requires more energy and will fatigue the client.

> **TEST-TAKING TIP**—Focus on the two options that involve exhaling, **Answers 2** and **3**.
> **IMP, APP, 6, M/S: Resp., PhI, Reduction of Risk Potential**

434. **(4) The response addresses the client's concerns about her body image and reassures the client that it takes some time for the process.** **Answer 1** is incorrect because it *negates* the client's concerns about body image. **Answer 2** is incorrect because it takes about *four weeks* for the uterus to return to nonpregnant size. **Answer 3** is incorrect because vigorous exercise *is not* recommended for the *immediate* postpartum period.

> **TEST-TAKING TIP**—Choose the option that addresses the client's concerns and gives reassurance.
> **IMP, APP, 7, Maternity, PsI, Psychosocial Integrity**

435. **(3) Colostrum contains important immunoglobulins that protect the infant against infection.** **Answer 1** is incorrect because the colostrum is replaced by mature milk at *3–5 days* postpartum. **Answer 2** is incorrect because colostrum *does* contain vitamins. **Answer 4** is incorrect because antigens do *not provide protection* against infection.

> **TEST-TAKING TIP**—Think about the composition of colostrum and the role of colostrum in the infant's nutrition.
> **IMP, COM, 4, Maternity, HPM, Health Promotion and Maintenance**

436. **(2) Placing a HEPA mask on the client will effectively prevent the transmission of TB while the client moves through the hospital.** **Answer 1** is incorrect because, while HEPA masks are effective at blocking the transmission of TB, the mask should be placed on the client. **Answer 3** is incorrect because TB is transmitted via *airborne droplets* from the respiratory system. A gown and gloves will *not* prevent airborne transmission. **Answer 4** is incorrect because, although it may be courteous to inform the radiology department that the client is coming, the best measure to prevent transmission of TB while in radiology is to place a HEPA mask on the client.

> **TEST-TAKING TIP**—The goal in this situation is to *prevent* the transmission of TB while the client is *mobile*. **Answer 2** provides the most effective option.
> **IMP, APP, 1, M/S: CD, SECE, Safety and Infection Control.**

437. **(1) Ticks that are responsible for Lyme disease lurk in grass, shrubbery, weeds, and heavily wooded areas. Walking in the center of hiking trails helps to avoid tick-infested areas.** **Answer 2** is incorrect because dark colored clothing increases the difficulty in spotting ticks. *Light* colored clothing makes it easier to spot ticks. Other measures, such as tucking pant legs into socks and wearing long-sleeved shirts tucked into long-legged pants, also assist in preventing tick bites. **Answer 3** is incorrect because ticks should *not* be removed with fingers. Ticks should be grasped with tweezers (forceps) as close as possible to the point of attachment. If bare hands touch the tick during removal, the hands should be thoroughly washed with soap and water. **Answer 4** is incorrect because while insect repellents such as those containing diethyltoluamide (DEET) or permethrin can protect against tick bites, parents should be advised to use them cautiously. These repellents are absorbed through the skin and can cause toxicity in infants and children. These preparations should *not* be used on a child younger than 1 year of age. In older children the preparation should be sprayed on the child's clothing rather than directly on the child's skin.

> **TEST-TAKING TIP**—Connect the source of the infection (tick bite) with the answer that *most directly avoids* an encounter with the insect.
> **IMP, APP, 1, PEDS, SECE, Safety and Infection Control**

438. **(1) Clients with arterial occlusive disease should *not* have their feet soaked in water because this may cause *maceration of the skin*.** **Answer 2** is incorrect because placing the client's bed in reverse Trendelenburg at 10 degrees *facilitates* arterial flow to the lower extremities. **Answer 3** is incorrect because the use of sheepskin between overlapped toes helps *prevent* pressure sores. **Answer 4** is incorrect because walking just until pain is experienced, but no further, *helps* the client develop collateral circulation in the extremities.

TEST-TAKING TIP—The question asks to identify an *inappropriate* behavior by the nurse's aide; therefore, the "wrong" action is the *right* answer.
EV, ANL, 3, M/S: Vascular, SECE, Management of Care

439. (3) The activity of walking to the restroom increases heart rate, which in turn, can reveal a new murmur that has occurred as a result of the MI. Answer 1 is incorrect because it is not useful to know if the client has a family history of heart murmur. Heredity is *not a typical risk factor* for heart murmur. Answer 2 is incorrect because, although chest pain is an important assessment in clients who have had an MI, it will *not* provide useful information regarding the *new* heart murmur. Answer 4 is incorrect because heart murmur *is not a side effect* of Inderal.

TEST-TAKING TIP—The question focuses on complications of MI for which the nurse should be alert. Answers 1 and 4 do not involve complications of MI. Answers 2 and 3 refer to complications of MI, but only Answer 3 is directly related to the murmur.
EV, ANL, 6, M/S: Cardiac, PhI, Physiological Adaptation

440. (1) Clients are confused for 30 minutes after the treatment, and family members need to be prepared to help orient the client. Answer 2 is incorrect because the client *should be informed* of all aspects of the treatment and the outcome associated with the treatments. Answer 3 is incorrect because the family should help orient the client *during* the initial confusion. Answer 4 is incorrect because the client may see an improvement in mood anywhere from 6 to 25 treatments. This statement is not accurate.

TEST-TAKING TIP—Eliminate any answer that withholds information from the client (Answer 2). You can also eliminate Answer 4, which is *too* specific (i.e., 6 treatments for *all* clients).
IMP, APP, 7, Psych, PhI, Reduction of Risk Potential

441. (2) Tracheal and mediastinal shifts are hallmarks of tension pneumothorax, a life-threatening condition which requires *immediate treatment* with closed chest drainage. Answer 1 is incorrect because intubating the client is *not yet necessary*. The tracheal and mediastinal shifts should be managed *first*. Answer 3 is incorrect because a paracentesis would be performed to drain the *peritoneal cavity*. Answer 4 is incorrect because the tracheal and mediastinal shifts indicate tension pneumothorax, which is an emergency and should be treated immediately.

TEST-TAKING TIP—Knowing that the question describes an emergency, focus on the two options (Answers 1 and 2) that address the specific problem of tension pneumothorax. Of the two options, Answer 1 may eventually be necessary, but does not directly treat the pneumothorax.
PL, ANL, 6, M/S: Resp., PhI, Reduction of Risk Potential

442. (1) Delivery normally causes the bladder to become edematous with an increased capacity. Answer 2 is incorrect because nerve damage from an epidural is *rare* and is *not the most likely* reason for the client's condition. Answer 3 is incorrect because damage to the urinary tract is *uncommon* even with a forceps assisted delivery. Answer 4 is incorrect because dehydration after delivery is not the most likely of the options to result in inability to void.

TEST-TAKING TIP—The key to this question is the term "most likely" reason. Think of the normal, common changes with delivery of an infant. Three of the options

focus on complications (although they are uncommon). One option is a "normal" result of delivery.
AN, APP, 8, Maternity, HPM, Health Promotion and Maintenance

443. (4) Whereas the management of celiac disease involves the exclusion of grain products such as wheat, rye, barley, and oats, it includes other products (such as corn, rice and millet) as substitute grain products. The idea of "building a special cake" would likely appeal to children who are in the industrious school-age phase and will fulfill the wish for a birthday cake without violating any dietary principles and restrictions. Answer 1 is incorrect because celiac disease is a life-long condition and is managed by the exclusion of glutens from the diet. Compliance with the diet is to be *encouraged* rather than *discouraged* by the nurse. Answer 2 is incorrect because while it acknowledges the child's feelings and frustrations with the diet, it ends in a guilt-inducing manner. This response could serve to make the school-age child, who wants to be just like "all of the other kids in my class," hostile and noncompliant with the dietary restrictions. Answer 3 is incorrect because the child with celiac disease is often also lactose-intolerant; therefore, dairy products, such as ice cream, must be avoided. However, offering another "type" of birthday cake is a good idea as long as it does not violate any dietary principles and restrictions.

TEST-TAKING TIP—When answering a question regarding celiac disease, think: an increase in *grain* causes a decrease in *growth* (i.e., [M] failure to thrive [FTT]) or an increase in *grain* causes *gastrointestinal pain* (abdominal distension, chronic diarrhea, anorexia) or *grain = gone* (from the child's diet).
IMP, APP, 4, PEDS, PhI, Basic Care and Comfort

444. (3) Isordil can cause *dizziness* and the client *should avoid driving* until the effects of the drug are known. Answer 1 is incorrect because the client should *not reduce* the dosage due to headache. Headache is a common side effect of Isordil and can be treated with acetaminophen. Answer 2 is incorrect because Isordil should be taken *continuously* to *prevent* angina. Answer 4 is incorrect because alcohol can *increase* the *hypotensive* effects of Isordil.

TEST-TAKING TIP—It is helpful to remember that Isordil is an *antihypertensive* used for *long-term* treatment of angina. Answers 1 and 2 contradict the *preventative* goal of treatment with Isordil. Answers 3 and 4 address the anti-hypertensive effects of the drug, but Answer 3 presents the *safest* option.
EV, ANL, 6, M/S: CV, PhI, Pharmacological and Parenteral Therapies

445. (4) Osteoarthritis is not a life-threatening disease and hip replacement is generally voluntary. Answer 1 is incorrect because the client has not been hospitalized long enough to achieve a stable blood glucose, and would be discharged to an environment with little support. Answer 2 is incorrect because the CK-MB is elevated, which is indicative of MI, and the client is most vulnerable to complications within the first 48 hours after MI. Answer 3 is incorrect because the client's oxygen saturation is only 90% on 3 L/min. This client is not sufficiently stable to be discharged.

TEST-TAKING TIP—Focus on the option that presents the client who is most stable, Answer 4.
EV, ANL, 1, M/S: Triage, SECE, Management of Care

446. (2) Although it is preferable not to discharge this client, the client exhibits *normal oxygen saturation on room air*.

Answer 1 is incorrect because a fat embolus is a *serious complication* of long bone fracture, and the client should *not* be discharged until the embolus is no longer a danger. **Answer 3** is incorrect because the added risk factors of *advanced age* and *dementia* dictate that this client not be discharged until the heart failure is resolved and the client is stable. **Answer 4** is incorrect because as long as the client requires a nasogastric tube, the client also needs *fluid replacement* and careful *monitoring of hydration status.*

TEST-TAKING TIP—Notice that **Answer 2** is the only option that describes a client with assessment findings within a *normal range.*
EV, ANL, 6, M/S: Triage, SECE, Management of Care

447. **(1) Acid-fast bacilli indicates tuberculosis, which poses a significant public health risk. TB is communicable, requires long-term treatment, is potentially fatal, and can be difficult to detect, treat, and track. Answer 2** is incorrect because scabies, while a nuisance, is easily treated and is not life-threatening, and therefore not considered a significant public health hazard. **Answer 3** is incorrect because rubella is no longer a public health hazard because of the routine immunization of most children. **Answer 4** is incorrect because strep throat is easily detected and treated with antibiotics, and is not considered a significant public health hazard.

TEST-TAKING TIP—Consider threat to life and ease of treating the infection. **Answers 3** and **4** present diseases that, at one time, were potentially fatal, but because of antibiotics and vaccines, are no longer threats. **Answer 2** presents a health problem that is not fatal.
AN, ANL, 1, M/S: CD, SECE, Safety and Infection Control

448. **(2) Lunch away from home is particularly difficult for the school-age child with celiac disease. Bread, luncheon meats, and instant soups are not allowed because of gluten content. For families on a restricted budget, the diet may add an additional financial burden because many inexpensive or convenience foods cannot be used. The standard purchased lunch at school would likely contain glutens, and the child could not eat the foods that are usually offered in the school cafeteria (e.g., pizza, spaghetti). There would be the added temptation to "trade" lunches with a child who is not on the restricted diet, or to purchase a "forbidden" food. Answer 1** is incorrect because breakfast is usually eaten at home and would be prepared and/or supervised by the parents. The child's approval of and satisfaction with the meal might be an issue, but dietary compliance would not present the most difficulty. **Answer 3** is incorrect because dinner is usually eaten at home and would be prepared and/or supervised by the parents. The child's approval of and satisfaction with the meal might be an issue, but dietary compliance would not present the most difficulty. **Answer 4** is incorrect because a bedtime snack is usually eaten at home and would be prepared and/or supervised by the parents. The child's approval of and satisfaction with the snack might be an issue, but dietary compliance would not be an issue.

TEST-TAKING TIP—Three of the responses involve meals/snacks usually eaten at home or with parental supervision; select the one response that is different.
EV, ANL, 4, PEDS, PhI, Basic Care and Comfort

449. **(4) Pain that is unrelieved by medication given an hour ago requires additional assessment. The nurse should first check the episiotomy site. A common complication involving the episiotomy during the first 24 hours postpartum is hematoma formation, which causes additional pain when sitting, with increasing pressure on the area. Answer 1** is incorrect because additional pain medication would *not* be the *first* action taken. **Answer 2** is incorrect because 4 hours is *not enough time* for an infection in the episiotomy to be evident. **Answer 3** is incorrect because the client is having pain at her *episiotomy* site, assessing the bleeding would not be the first action taken.

TEST-TAKING TIP—Note that three options call for assessment. Focus on **Answers 2** and **4** (the perineum). Then consider the time frame since delivery, and ask yourself why pain medication would not be effective (could it be a hematoma or infection?).
IMP, ANL, 5, Maternity, PhI, Basic Care and Comfort

450. **(3) An elevated TSH indicates that the client may have hypothyroidism, which could be the cause of the client's depression. The physician may want to order lab tests for the next morning. If the client needs to be started on thyroid medication, it should occur as soon as possible. Answer 1** is incorrect because there is *not* a contraindication for antidepressant medications and benzodiazepines. The nurse *should discuss* the finding *with the client* and assess for benzodiazepine dependency and observe the client for signs of withdrawal. The physician can be notified of the finding in the morning if the client is not at risk for withdrawal. **Answer 2** is incorrect because *history* of sexual abuse is *not* a current emergency. The physician can be notified the next day. **Answer 4** is incorrect because this information can be given to the physician the *next* day. Also, this information needs to be communicated to the unit *social worker.*

TEST-TAKING TIP—Focus on the key word: "immediately." This indicates that harm would come to the client if an action is not taken. Next, remember Maslow's hierarchy and choose physiological needs *before* psychosocial.
AN, ANL, 7, Psych, PhI, Reduction of Risk Potential

451. **(3) The client has critical, life-threatening arterial blood gas alterations with a pH of 7.19. The immediate treatment should be intubation and mechanical ventilation to support oxygenation. Answer 1** is incorrect because the arterial blood gases indicate a severe hypoxia ($Po_2 = 46$). Increasing the O_2 via nasal cannula will *not be effective in correcting* the PaO_2 for a client who has asthma with bronchoconstriction. **Answer 2** is incorrect because the client has critical, life-threatening arterial blood gas alterations with a pH of 7.19, requiring immediate stabilization of the airway by intubation and mechanical ventilation to support oxygenation. Once this is completed, *then* treatment will include IV Solu-Medrol for inflammation of the bronchioles associated with asthma. **Answer 4** is incorrect because the client has critical, life-threatening arterial blood gas alterations with a pH of 7.19. The immediate priority is to secure the airway by intubating the client and supporting oxygenation via mechanical ventilation. Once the airway is secured, then treatment will also include medications that are bronchodilators.

TEST-TAKING TIP—Remember the ABCs—airway and breathing first. The key word is *immediate* treatment to reverse respiratory failure.
AN, ANL, 6, M/S: ABG, PhI, Physiological Adaptation

452. **(1) The client is exhibiting assessment findings that are consistent with right lung pneumonia including cough, difficulty breathing, crackles, and decreased breath sounds on the affected side, and increased breath sounds on the unaffected side. Diagnostic studies for pneumonia are: chest x-ray, sputum culture, and bronchoscopy if sputum culture is inconclusive. Answer 2** is incorrect because assessment findings that would be consistent with cardiac

tamponade include: decreased/muffled *heart sounds, jugular* vein distention, and hypotension. **Answer 3** is incorrect because assessment findings that would be consistent with pulmonary edema include: bilateral crackles, pink frothy sputum, S_3 gallop. **Answer 4** is incorrect because assessment findings that would be consistent with pleural friction rub include sharp/stabbing pain and a crackling/rubbing sound on inspiration.

> **TEST-TAKING TIP**—Think about the presenting symptoms and the pathophysiology for each option.
> **AN, ANL, 6, M/S: Resp.; PhI, Physiological Adaptation**

453. **(2) Each of these assessments is important in prenatal care to identify high-risk conditions during pregnancy.** Answer **1** is incorrect because cervical dilation is *not* a part of each prenatal visit. **Answer 3** is incorrect because cervical dilation is *not* assessed at each visit. **Answer 4** is incorrect because *measurement of the pelvic* diameter is *not* a part of each visit.

> **TEST-TAKING TIP**—Notice the words "each visit" in the question. Consider which measurements are important in every visit and which assessments are done occasionally during prenatal visits.
> **IMP, COM, 5, Maternity, HPM, Health Promotion and Maintenance**

454. **(2) The first action the nurse should take is to assess the client. A heart rate of 168 will not allow time between beats for adequate filling volume to enter the right and left ventricles. Consequently, the *blood pressure will drop*, which will significantly decrease perfusion to the brain and other organs.** Assessing the client's level of consciousness is also a rapid way to determine perfusion to the vital organs. Then, the physician must be notified STAT for medication orders to control the rapid heart rate, and to give additional assessment information about heart rate, blood pressure, level of consciousness, and lab data. If the blood pressure is dropping rapidly to precarious levels (SBP less then 90), or the client is losing consciousness, a "code blue" must be called. **Answer 1** is incorrect because the first action the nurse should take is to directly assess the *client*, not to monitor the ECG. **Answer 3** is incorrect because the first action the nurse should take is to directly assess the *client*. Then, the physician should be notified STAT not only about the ECG rhythm change, but also to give additional assessment data that may help determine the medical treatment. **Answer 4** is incorrect because the first here-and-now action the nurse should take is to directly assess the client, *not* to check the chart (there-and-then).

> **TEST-TAKING TIP**—Look for an option which includes direct *observation* of the client first (e.g., vital signs and LOC).
> **IMP, APP, 6, M/S: Cardiac, PhI, Physiological Adaptation**

455. **(3) Long-term lead ingestion causes permanent, irreversible neurological damage (i.e., seizures, learning disabilities, mental retardation, etc.). Seizure precautions include an age-appropriate oral airway (as well as suction equipment and oxygen), which is the most important piece of equipment for the staff nurse to place at the toddler's bedside.** Answer **1** is incorrect because, while chelation therapy for lead ingestion is usually administered intravenously and an IV pole will be required, it is *not* the most important piece of equipment for the staff nurse to place at the toddler's bedside. **Answer 2** is incorrect because, while chelation therapy for lead ingestion is nephrotoxic and monitoring intake and output (I & O) on a special form will be required, it is *not* the most important article for the staff nurse to place at the toddler's bedside. **Answer 4** is incorrect

because, while a age appropriate pain (related to lead poisoning and its treatment) assessment scale will be required, it is *not* the most important piece of equipment for the staff nurse to place at the toddler's bedside.

> **TEST-TAKING TIP**—All of the responses are correct; select the most important piece of equipment (an oral airway) for the most serious consequence of long-term lead ingestion (neurological damage such as seizures).
> **IMP, ANL, 1, PEDS, PhI, Reduction of Risk Potential**

456. **(1) Aminoglycoside antibiotics are nephrotoxic and a serum creatinine level is the lab test that best evaluates renal function. Creatinine is a by-product of muscle catabolism that is normally filtered by the glomeruli and excreted in the urine. The adverse/toxic effects of aminoglycosides can result in damage to the glomeruli, affecting their ability to clear waste products, thereby increasing creatinine levels which indicates renal impairment. If nephrotoxic effects occur, the drug dose must be adjusted or discontinued.** Answer **2** is incorrect because a serum amylase level assists in the diagnosis of acute pancreatitis and other *pancreatic* and *liver* problems. **Answer 3** is incorrect because a serum troponin is a cardiac biomarker with specificity and sensitivity to detect myocardial damage. When cardiac injury occurs, troponin is released from the cardiac muscle into the serum circulation. The troponin levels peak 3–6 hours post injury and return to normal levels of 0–0.3 ng/mL after 5–7 days. Troponin levels are one of the primary tests used in the diagnosis of *acute myocardial infarction*. **Answer 4** is incorrect because a serum white blood cell count would be used to evaluate the *effectiveness* of the antibiotic, *not the adverse/toxic* effects. If the infecting organism is susceptible to the antibiotic and infection is being controlled, the WBC count will go down, indicating effective antibiotic treatment. Conversely, if the antibiotic is not effective in fighting the infection, the WBC count will be unchanged or continue to rise.

> **TEST-TAKING TIP**—Think how most medications are metabolized—kidneys or liver. Amylase would not be the test to determine kidney involvement. The question asks about *toxic* effects, not about a diagnostic marker (**Answer 3**) or about effectiveness (**Answer 4**).
> **EV, COM, 1, M/S: Meds, PhI, Reduction of Risk Potential**

457. **(3) A child with nephrotic syndrome is usually placed on a diet with no additional salt (NAS) at the table. In addition, foods with very high sodium content are excluded from the diet. Peanut butter *does* meet this criteria and *must* be removed from the child's tray.** Edema is always one of the characteristics of nephrotic syndrome. Although edema cannot be eliminated by a low sodium diet, the rate of increase of edema may be slowed. **Answer 1** is incorrect because the child with nephrotic syndrome is usually placed on a diet with NAS at the table. In addition, foods with very high sodium content are to be excluded from the diet. A scrambled egg does *not* meet this criterion (high sodium) and need *not* be removed from the child's tray. **Answer 2** is incorrect because the child with nephrotic syndrome is usually placed on a diet with NAS at the table. In addition, foods with very high sodium content are excluded from the diet. A glass of milk does *not* meet this criteria and need *not* be removed from the child's tray. **Answer 4** is incorrect because the child with nephrotic syndrome is usually placed on a diet with NAS at the table. In addition, foods with very high sodium content are to be excluded from the diet. A slice of melon does *not* meet this criterion and need *not* be removed from the child's tray.

TEST-TAKING TIP—Think of the edema that accompanies nephrotic syndrome and the role that sodium plays in fluid retention.
EV, ANL, 4, PEDS, SECE, Basic Care and Comfort

458. **(1) These are the malformations associated with fetal alcohol syndrome. Answer 2** is incorrect because these are complications of *maternal diabetes*. **Answer 3** is incorrect because these are complications of *Rh sensitization*. **Answer 4** is incorrect because these are *neural tube defects*.

TEST-TAKING TIP—These are all malformations, complications of prenatal exposure. When presented with options where all look possible, eliminate options you know are caused by other conditions.
AN, APP, 1, Maternity, PhI, Physiological Adaptation

459. **(3) The client's history and lab data are most consistent with the development of ARDS. One of the major risk factors for development of ARDS is sepsis. A smoking history also increases the risk for ARDS. The cardinal signs of ARDS are: refractory hypoxia (increasing Fio_2 does not significantly increase the client's Pao_2), and bilateral patchy infiltrates ("white out") on chest x-ray. This is a result of noncardiogenic pulmonary infiltrates that flood the alveoli with fluid, impairing gas exchange. Answer 1** is incorrect because the client's history and lab data are most consistent with the development of ARDS, *not* pulmonary embolism. The cardinal signs of pulmonary embolism are: sudden acute dyspnea, sharp chest pain, tachycardia, hypotension, and tachypnea. **Answer 2** is incorrect because the client's history and lab data are most consistent with the development of ARDS, *not* COPD. While the client does have a smoking history, which increases the risk for the development of COPD, chronic obstructive pulmonary disease is a progressive disease involving a diagnosis of emphysema, bronchitis, or asthma. Acute exacerbations are a result of a recent cold or respiratory infection. Assessment findings are consistent with cough, tenacious mucous production, wheezes/crackles, and possible changes in chest structure ("barrel" chest). **Answer 4** incorrect because the client's history and lab data are most consistent with the development of ARDS, *not* pneumothorax. The cardinal signs of pneumothorax are: tracheal deviation, asymmetrical chest motion, diminished breath sounds on the affected side, and dark areas on chest x-ray.

TEST-TAKING TIP— Compare and contrast the cardinal signs for these respiratory conditions; match up the signs in the stem with the correct condition in the options.
AN, ANL, 6, M/S: Resp.; PhI, Physiological Adaptation

460. **(4) All three of the listed electrolytes would be decreased in clients with anorexia. Answer 1** is incorrect because malnutrition, which is central to anorexia nervosa, causes a *decrease* in essential electrolytes. **Answer 2** is incorrect because all three of the listed electrolytes would be *decreased* in the client. **Answer 3** is incorrect because *all three* of the listed electrolytes would be *decreased* in the client.

TEST-TAKING TIP—Narrow the choices between the two opposite actions, hypo-hyper; then focus on the correct choice. Make sure that all choices in the answer are correct.
AS, APP, 4, Psych, PhI, Physiological Adaptation

461. **(2) The type of cesarean section will determine if the client must have another cesarean section or if she can attempt a vaginal delivery. Answer 1** is incorrect because fundal height measurement does not need to be performed first. **Answer 3** is incorrect because these assessments are a part of the initial assessment, but these do not need to be performed first. **Answer 4** is incorrect because these assessments can be delayed without affecting the client outcome.

TEST-TAKING TIP—Notice the word "first." Clients with a previous classical cesarean section are at high risk for uterine rupture and need to be delivered by repeat cesarean section.
AS, APP, 5, Maternity, PhI, Reduction of Risk Potential

462. **(3) Monitoring the child's weight on a weekly basis helps to identify early stages of fluid retention. This helps parents identify signs of a relapse before edema occurs. Early detection and avoidance of relapse is the nurse's priority for at-home-care teaching. Answer 1** is incorrect because while compliance with dietary restrictions is essential in the control of nephrotic syndrome, the child is usually discharged home on a diet with *no* additional salt (NAS) at the table *rather than a low sodium* diet. **Answer 2** is incorrect because, while it is important to anticipate the appetite stimulant effects of the steroids and the subsequent weight gain that steroids can cause, it is *not* the nurse's *priority* for at-home-care teaching. **Answer 4** is incorrect because immunizations should be *withheld* for 6 months until after the completion of steroid therapy. Although immunizations may trigger a relapse, the pneumococcal vaccine and other immunizations are important to protect the child from serious preventable infections.

TEST-TAKING TIP—Edema formation is a critical element of nephrotic syndrome; select the response (weight) that most closely relates to edema formation.
IMP, APP, 1, PEDS, SECE, Management of Care

463. **(2) The subjective and objective assessment data are most consistent with pulmonary emboli. The client's fracture of the lower extremity and immobility are primary risk factors for pulmonary emboli. The cardinal subjective assessment findings of pulmonary emboli include: sudden onset of anxiety, restlessness, feelings of impending doom, difficulty breathing, and sharp chest pain (especially on inspiration). The objective assessment findings include: tachycardia, tachypnea, hypotension, and crackles, with decreased breath sounds, and possible pleural rub on the affected side. Answer 1** is incorrect because the assessment findings that would be consistent with cardiac tamponade would include: decreased/muffled heart sounds, jugular vein distention, and hypotension. **Answer 3** is incorrect because the objective and subjective assessment findings are most consistent with pulmonary emboli, *not* pneumothorax. The objective assessment findings consistent with pneumothorax are: tracheal deviation, asymmetrical chest motion, diminished breath sounds on the affected side, and a possible cough. The subjective assessment findings are similar to pulmonary emboli and include sudden onset of sharp chest pain and difficulty breathing. However, the client's fracture of the lower extremity and immobility are primary risk factors for pulmonary emboli. **Answer 4** is incorrect because assessment findings that would be consistent with pulmonary edema include bilateral crackles, pink frothy sputum, and S_3 gallop.

TEST-TAKING TIP—With three options involving the lungs, select the condition where the risk factors would be fracture of the lower extremity and immobility.
AN, ANL, 6, M/S: Resp.; PhI, Physiological Adaptation

464. **(1) The lab test that is most appropriate to evaluate the client's status after giving furosemide (Lasix) is a serum potassium level. Furosemide is a loop diuretic that causes**

excretion of potassium along with water. A decrease in potassium level can cause PVCs. Critically low levels of potassium can result in lethal arrhythmias such as ventricular fibrillation. Potassium levels must be monitored when giving IV furosemide. Potassium supplements will be administered as needed to keep potassium levels within normal range. **Answer 2** is incorrect because serum creatinine level is the lab test that best evaluates *renal* function, *not* cardiac. **Answer 3** is incorrect because serum troponin assists in the diagnosis of acute myocardial infarction and is not affected by furosemide. **Answer 4** is incorrect because a white blood cell (WBC) test helps evaluate *infection* and is not affected by furosemide.

TEST-TAKING TIP—Remember: diuretics → loss of H₂O + loss of K⁺.
AS, COM, 6, M/S: Fluid/Electrolyte, PhI, Reduction of Risk Potential

465. **(1) The medications for this client are monitored by one pharmacy. This has been proven to decrease the negative effects from polypharmacy—multiple meds, prescribed by multiple MD/NPs; no one is clear about what others are prescribing.** **Answer 2** is incorrect because using another person's medications *could lead to serious* side effects. **Answer 3** is incorrect because confusion *would be a concern* and may signal drug side effects or other health problems. The client needs help to schedule taking medication in manageable time frames. **Answer 4** is incorrect because medication errors are likely when the client is unable to read times, doses, medication names.

TEST-TAKING TIP—Key word is "least."
AS, ANL, 1, M/S: Geriatrics, HPM, Health Promotion and Maintenance

466. **(4) Boys (men) must be informed at some point that they will be unable to produce offspring. This may be caused by blockage of the vas deferens with abnormal secretions or by failure of normal development of the wolffian duct structures. It is important that the distinction be made between sterility and impotence. Normal sexual relationships can be expected. It** *does* **deal with the adolescent's developmental milestone of** *identity versus role confusion* **(adolescents identify themselves as sexual beings when changes in body functions, body image, and identification of gender preferences occur).** **Answer 1** is incorrect because while the onset of diabetes mellitus is a strong possibility due to pancreatic fibrosis, it is *not* applicable to the adolescent's developmental milestone of *identity versus role confusion.* **Answer 2** is incorrect because while quality of life and end-of-life issues are needed topics of discussion, they are not needed at this point in time. Although cystic fibrosis remains an incurable, fatal disease, the median life expectancy for an individual with cystic fibrosis is currently 31 years of age. It is *not* applicable to the adolescent's developmental milestone of *identity versus role confusion.* **Answer 3** is incorrect because while lung transplantation is the final therapeutic option in children with advanced pulmonary vascular disease and hypoxia, it does not describe the adolescent in this question. It is *not* applicable to the adolescent's developmental milestone of *identity versus role confusion.*

TEST-TAKING TIP—Remember the behavioral indicators that relate to the developmental milestone (i.e., central task) of each stage of growth and development.
IMP, APP, 5, PEDS, HPM, Health Promotion and Maintenance

467. **(1) Prolonged rupture of membranes for more than 24 hours is associated with an increased rate of infection.**

Answer 2 is incorrect because prolonged latent phase does *not* put the client at a higher risk for infection. **Answer 3** is incorrect because two vaginal exams *are not frequent enough* to increase the risk of infection. **Answer 4** is incorrect because a first degree tear is *not a high risk factor* for infection.

TEST-TAKING TIP—The key concept is "highest risk". Think about the risk factors of each client. If the client has no high risk factors, eliminate that answer.
AN, ANL , 1, Maternity, SECE, Safety and Infection Control

468. **(3) Research and current practice follow a guide that says "start low and go slow" for all medications for older adults. The dosage may start at ¹/₃ and move up to ¹/₂ of the dose for a younger person.** **Answer 1** is incorrect because research in the past 10 years has shown that older bodies generally require one-half of the dose of a younger body because of changes in metabolism, distribution, and absorption. **Answer 2** is incorrect because the older adult generally needs a *lower* dose because of changes in the ability to metabolize the drug. **Answer 4** is incorrect because the dosage is generally about 50% of the dose for a younger person.

TEST-TAKING TIP—When in doubt, choose the conservative answer.
IMP, APP, 5, M/S: Geriatrics, PhI, Pharmacological and Parenteral Therapies

469. **(1) Lethargy and sedation are the most common side effects of medications in older adults. As a result, many clients have impaired ability to perform self-maintenance, such as ADLs and IADLs.** **Answer 2** is incorrect because side effects are often *different* or the *opposite* of those seen in younger clients because of changes in absorption, distribution, and metabolism. **Answer 3** is incorrect because medications *frequently cause* mental changes in older clients because of changes in absorption, distribution, and metabolism. **Answer 4** is incorrect because therapeutic effects are frequently *less predictable* because of changes in absorption, distribution, and metabolism.

TEST-TAKING TIP—Look for the option that anticipates *problems.*
AN, ANL, 5, M/S: Geriatrics, PhI, Pharmacological and Parenteral Therapies

470. **(3) Stabilizing the physical condition is the priority goal at this time.** **Answer 1** is incorrect because the priority goal is to *stabilize* the client's inflicted *wound* after the crisis. This would be an important *short-term* goal. **Answer 2** is incorrect because it not the priority. Treating the auditory hallucinations would come *after* the blood flow is stopped and the wound is sutured. **Answer 4** is incorrect because the client will identify new coping strategies *after* the hallucinations are under control and the client is not actively suicidal.

TEST-TAKING TIP—Remember "safety first" and Maslow's hierarchy of treating physiological needs *before* psychosocial needs.
EV, ANL, 1, Psych, PhI, Physiological Adaptation

471. **(1) Drop attacks, provoked by head or neck movement resulting in reduced vertebral artery blood flow, occur without warning and therefore cannot be anticipated.** **Answer 2** is incorrect because although postural HTN is a risk factor for falls, medications can be given to *control* it. **Answer 3** is incorrect because although moderate to severe cognitive impairment (CI) is a risk factor for falls, *mild* CI is *not.* **Answer 4** is incorrect because "continues" suggests this is not a new behavior and that tolerance is likely to be present. This amount is usually *manageable* by older adults.

TEST-TAKING TIP—Look for an action that is safety-based and for which there is little preparation by the client or nurse. See the similarity between "falls" in the stem and "drop" in **Answer 1**.
AS, COM, 3, M/S: Geriatrics, SECE, Safety and Infection Control

472. **(3) Because of the decrease in quadriceps strength, elders are more likely to fall getting up or down from the toilet or bed.** Answer 1 is incorrect because the situation, while a risk, is not the greatest risk and could be *prevented* with careful *attention*. **Answer 2** is incorrect because the situation, while a risk, is not the greatest risk and could be *prevented* with handrails and *non-skid strips*. **Answer 4** is incorrect even though it describes a risky situation that can contribute to falls, it does not present the greatest risk because they can be *removed*.

TEST-TAKING TIP—Look for the answer that is due to decrease in muscular strength as a risk factor that cannot be prevented.
IMP, APP, 1, M/S: Geriatrics, SECE, Safety and Infection Control

473. **(1) These are common complications of prolonged (post-dates) pregnancy.** Answer 2 is incorrect because *polyhydramnios is not common* in postdates pregnancy. **Answer 3** is incorrect because *precipitous delivery is not a common* risk factor of postdates pregnancy. **Answer 4** is incorrect because *placenta previa is uncommon* in postdates pregnancy.

TEST-TAKING TIP—In each option, separate the options into individual components, and ask yourself if it is true or false for each choice. When even one component of the answer is false, eliminate that answer.
AN, APP, 5, Maternity, PhI, Reduction of Risk Potential

474. **(3) In the early postpartum period, uterine atony is a common cause of postpartum hemorrhage. Nursing intervention can help avoid unnecessary blood loss.** Answer 1 is incorrect because breastfeeding initiation is essential, but not the most important nursing intervention. **Answer 2** is incorrect because while parental involvement is important, avoiding hemorrhage is the most important nursing intervention. **Answer 4** is incorrect because good hygiene is important, but not the most important intervention in the early postpartum period.

TEST-TAKING TIP—When thinking about the priority, which intervention will prevent the worst complication? In this case, a life-threatening postpartum hemorrhage is the worst outcome
PL, APP, 5, Maternity, PhI, Reduction of Risk Potential

475. **(3) Plotting each student's height and weight on a growth curve form would give the school nurse the most accurate assessment of each student's growth and development.** Measurement of physical growth in children is a key element in evaluating their health status. Physical growth parameters include weight, height, skinfold thickness, arm and head circumference. Values for these growth parameters are plotted on percentile charts and the child's measurements in percentiles are compared with those of the general population. **Answer 1** is incorrect because while obtaining each student's weight is a good idea, the interval between "weigh-ins" is too long. A semester is approximately 18 weeks in length. This does not allow for early intervention by the school nurse in the event that any of the students are lagging behind in age-appropriate weight gain or experiencing inappropriate weight loss. **Answer 2** is incorrect because while asking the parents to submit a weekly food

intake diary is a good idea, it would not represent the accurate, total picture of each student's actual nutritional intake. Elementary school students can and do obtain food from sources (e.g., vending machines, friends) other than the parents. **Answer 4** is incorrect because, while it is a good idea to arrange for a dietitian to evaluate each student, it is not appropriate *until* each student's placement on the growth curve form has been plotted by the school nurse. Students demonstrating a low percentile on the growth curve form should then be evaluated by the dietitian.

TEST-TAKING TIP—Because growth is a continuous but uneven process, the most reliable assessment lies in obtaining and then comparing growth measurements over time.
IMP, APP, 4, PEDS, PhI, Basic Care and Comfort

476. **(4) A toddler will push away an overfilled plate because the toddler is overwhelmed by its size. Many parents do not understand the amount of food the toddler actually requires and tend to serve too much food to the toddler. The nurse should instruct the mother that a general guide to the serving size for a toddler is one tablespoon per year of age for solid food (e.g., vegetables) or one-fourth to one-third the adult portion size (for food such as milk). Too much food is a frequent reason why the toddler does not finish all of the food.** Answer 1 is incorrect because a toddler's appetite and food preferences are usually sporadic. A toddler may typically eat one food for three days in a row and then suddenly refuse to eat it again for days. Such food "jags" do *not* ensure a balanced diet but attempts to alter them are met with resistance by the toddler. The nurse should instruct the mother to include three items from the groups in the Food Guide Pyramid at each meal, in an effort to assist the toddler to develop a variety of taste preferences and well-balanced habits. **Answer 2** is incorrect because a toddler has a decreased nutritional need and decreased appetite in a phenomenon known as *physiological anorexia*. They become picky, fussy eaters with strong taste preferences. There may be no typical eating pattern. They may eat voraciously one day and almost nothing the next. The toddler is increasingly aware of the nonnutritive function of food: the pleasure of eating, the social aspect of mealtime, the control of refusing food. The nurse should instruct the mother to avoid "forcing" food in an effort to achieve an adult-like eating pattern. **Answer 3** is incorrect because a toddler may *not* have the patience or attention span to sit at the table for a meal, especially if mealtime is consistently unpleasant emotionally or is scheduled immediately after active play. Nutritious snacks can, if necessary, replace a meal. The snacks must supply adequate calories, protein, carbohydrate, calcium, and vitamin C.

TEST-TAKING TIP—Three of the responses involve *how* the toddler eats; one response involves *an action taken by the mother*. Select the response that is different.
IMP, APP, 4, PEDS, PhI, Basic Care and Comfort

477. **(2) A normal oral temperature for an older adult is 96.9–98°F. There would only be a slight elevation indicative of infection.** Answer 1 is incorrect because a *decreased or absent* febrile response in infection is most likely. **Answer 3** is incorrect because there is *less* perspiration due to a *decline in* sweat glands. **Answer 4** is incorrect because the thirst response is *decreased* due to age-related changes affecting the hypothalamus.

TEST-TAKING TIP—Review "normals" for older adults. **Answers 1, 3**, and **4** refer to "increase"; select the answer that means "less." Also focus on two contradictory

options: increased fever and decreased temperature and select only a slight temp (**Answer 2**).
AS, COM, 5, M/S: Geriatrics, PhI, Physiological Adaptation

478. (3) While thinking and retelling reasons for deciding to take on the caregiver role, initial positive expectations will be reinforced that can help caregivers refocus from overwhelming tasks back to remembering the "big picture." It puts life back into perspective. Answer 1 is incorrect because although routine is helpful to complete caregiving tasks, the caregiver has to continue to seek out other person-renewing situations. This often doesn't happen when performing specific daily routines. **Answer 2** is incorrect because caregivers, while acknowledging the past, must look toward the future to continue to find meaning in the present. **Answer 4** is incorrect because caregivers need to ask for respite *before* life gets too hard. It is an ongoing need and has been proven to extend the lives of caregivers, as well as have positive effects on the care recipient.

> **TEST-TAKING TIP**—Review caregiver needs and consider ways to return the sense of control to an often uncontrollable situation.
> **IMP, COM, 5, M/S: Geriatrics, PsI, Psychosocial Integrity**

479. (1) The caregiver has recognized that she cannot continue to care for her husband. She needs support with her decision and assistance in letting go and addressing her feelings about her needs and losses from the situation. Answer 2 is incorrect because although respite care is always a good intervention during early and middle caregiving stages, at this time the client has recognized she can no longer manage the required caregiving responsibilities. Respite care would only serve as a *temporary* solution. **Answer 3** is incorrect because the husband's mental deterioration does not allow for relying on him for current decisions. **Answer 4** is incorrect because the client is not asking for cognitive input about the disease. At this point in the caregiving process, the client needs assistance with letting go and taking care of herself.

> **TEST-TAKING TIP**—Key phrase is "final stage of caregiving."
> **IMP, COM, 5, M/S: Geriatrics, PsI, Psychosocial Integrity**

480. (2, 3, 4) Answer 2 is correct because the severe weight loss and the purging associated with the disorder place the client at high risk for electrolyte imbalances. Answer 3 is correct because the purging behavior associated with this condition can lead to dehydration and electrolyte imbalances. Answer 4 is correct because clients with catatonia are frequently unable to eat or drink without assistance, and are at high risk for fluid volume deficit. Answer 1 is incorrect because clients with depression do *not* have fluid volume deficit as a priority diagnosis. Loss of *appetite* is a common symptom of depression, but the clients usually maintain fluid intake. **Answer 5** is incorrect because fluid intake is *not* usually associated with dementia. **Answer 6** is incorrect because clients with a borderline personality disorder are *not* at risk for inadequate fluid intake.

> **TEST-TAKING TIP**—Look for the answers that are similar. Anorexia and bulimia are both eating disorders. Note the key words in the stem, "most likely." This indicates that the conditions would be common in the disorder. Next, visualize the symptoms that are associated with each psychiatric condition and ask yourself if symptoms are

common, and if they would place the client at a high risk for *fluid* volume deficit.
PL, ANL, 4, Psych, PhI, Physiological Adaptation

481. (2) Cerumen is the most reversible common cause of hearing loss. It must be ruled out before continuing with further assessment to determine cause. Answer 1 is incorrect because the ear has difficulty discriminating among loud sounds. Answer 3 is incorrect because it is important to determine the cause first. Answer 4 is incorrect because it does not address the possible cause.

> **TEST-TAKING TIP**—Remember: "assessment" before "intervention."
> **IMP, APP, 2, M/S: Geriatrics, PhI, Physiological Adaptation**

482. (1) Botox has been used to reduce spasticity in targeted muscles. Prime candidates for Botox injections are children with spasticity confined to the lower extremities, because the drug weakens spasticity so that the muscles can be stretched and the child can ambulate with or without assistive devices. The drug is injected into the muscle (commonly the quadriceps, gastrocnemius, or medial hamstrings) and the effect of the drug lasts approximately 3 months. Answer 2 is incorrect because the nurse was not present at the interaction that took place between the pediatrician and the mother. The nurse has no validation that miscommunication has occurred. Answer 3 is incorrect because the *nurse* can correctly assess the parent's knowledge of the drug and supply needed additional information. If, following the nurse's instruction, the mother still requires additional information about the drug, the nurse can notify the pediatrician regarding the mother's questions. Answer 4 is incorrect because oral skeletal muscle relaxants (i.e., Dantrium, Lioresal, Robaxin) have been used with only moderate success to decrease spasticity. In addition, these drugs must be taken several times a day in order to be effective. These drugs may be more readily available, but they do not provide the long-lasting relief obtained by a single injection that is associated with Botox.

> **TEST-TAKING TIP**—A goal in the nursing care of the child with cerebral palsy is to reduce spasticity and improve movement while promoting an optimum developmental course; select the response that is a *teaching* intervention about *this* drug.
> **IMP, APP, 3, PEDS, PhI, Pharmacological and Parenteral Therapies**

483. (1) Difficulty in hearing high pitched sounds and sibilant consonants contributes to a word discrimination problem and difficulty in separating background sounds from the same consonants and sounds that form conversation. Answer 2 is incorrect because the difficulty does *not* center around *low* pitched tones, unless cerumen is a problem. Answer 3 is incorrect because although disinterest may be a response when it is hard to hear conversations, it is not the most correct answer. Answer 4 is incorrect because it does not explain why the client is unable to discriminate words; the answer is incomplete.

> **TEST-TAKING TIP**—Choose the most inclusive and specific answer.
> **AN, COM, 2, M/S: Geriatrics, PhI, Physiological Adaptation**

484. (4) Poor latch is the most common reason for soreness and nipple blisters. Answer 1 is incorrect because nursing *too long is not* the cause of nipple blisters. Answer 2 is incorrect because thrush *does not* cause nipple blisters. **Answer 3** is incorrect because mastitis is a *hard, red spot* on the breast.

TEST-TAKING TIP—All of these interventions may be of some help, but correcting the latch is the most helpful for this client.
IMP, APP, 4, Maternity, HPM, Health Promotion and Maintenance

485. **(3) "Increased muscle tone" would *not* contribute to incontinence. In the elderly, muscle tone is *decreased*. Answer 1** is incorrect because all of the stated reasons *do* contribute to incontinence. **Answer 2** is incorrect because all of the stated reasons *do* contribute to incontinence. **Answer 4** is incorrect because these *are* all factors that contribute to incontinence.

TEST-TAKING TIP—Review physiological causes of incontinence. "Least likely" is a key phrase.
AS, COM, 8, M/S: Geriatrics, PhI, Basic Care and Comfort

486. **(1) During the first trimester fetal development is mainly structural, and exposure to substances can cause congenital malformations. Answer 2** is incorrect because the second trimester is mainly functional development. Congenital malformations occur during the *first* trimester. **Answer 3** is incorrect because the placenta does *not* provide a barrier *to all* substances. **Answer 4** is incorrect because the effects of drug use can be important in *all* trimesters.

TEST-TAKING TIP—The key word "all" is used in one of the answers about the correct trimester (first). "All" is a word that usually indicates that the answer can be eliminated (**Answer 3**). Choose the one option about "first trimester" (**Answer 1**) that does not have the word "all" in the statement.
AN, APP, 5, Maternity, HPM, Health Promotion and Maintenance

487. **(2) The categories of impaired cognition and mobility problems are the most common reasons (forget, put off, or not be able to physically reach the bathroom when needed) that cause incontinence in elders. Answer 1** is incorrect because *family history* is *not* necessarily a common factor, although *age* is. **Answer 3** is incorrect because *family history* is *not* necessarily a cause of incontinence. **Answer 4** is incorrect because of a *vague* reference to medications and diseases in *general* as most common risk factors.

TEST-TAKING TIP—Stem says two MOST common—usually they are also the most obvious reasons (i.e., loss of cognition and mobility), rather than family history (**Answers 1** and **3**).
PL, COM, 8, M/S: Geriatrics, HPM, Health Promotion and Maintenance

488. **(2) Research has shown that when clients have fewer than 6 incontinent instances per day, they are more likely to be able to control their urine and are good candidates for bladder training. Answer 1** is incorrect because this functional disability is an impediment to getting to the bathroom quickly when needed. **Answer 3** is incorrect because urge incontinence is sudden and usually uncontrollable. This client is not a good candidate for bladder training. **Answer 4** is incorrect because this client is not the *most* likely candidate. Surgery may correct the problem for *some* incontinency concerns.

TEST-TAKING TIP—Key phrase is "most likely."
AS, COM, 8, M/S: Geriatrics, PhI, Physiological Adaptation

489. **(1) Outpatient visits to refill the pump and make dosage adjustments are scheduled about every 4–6 weeks depending on the child's response to the treatment. Parents are *not* taught how to refill the pump. Refilling the pump** requires the services of a multidisciplinary team. **Answer 2** is incorrect because the pump's dosage cannot be changed without special equipment (i.e., telemetry wand and a computer). The pump delivers a set dose as opposed to a sliding scale dose. **Answer 3** is incorrect because the intrathecal baclofen delivered by the pump *decreases* the child's spasticity; improves function, gait, and motor control, and generally improves the child's health. It does *not* "cure" cerebral palsy nor allow the child to perform age-appropriate physical activities in a completely normal manner. **Answer 4** is incorrect because it is not the pump that is rejected. The child is *screened before* pump placement by the infusion of a "test dose" of intrathecal baclofen delivered via a lumbar puncture. Close monitoring for side effects (as well as for relief of spasticity) takes place for several hours after the infusion. If a positive effect is noted, the child is considered a candidate for pump placement. If a negative effect is noted, the child is referred to other forms of treatment.

TEST-TAKING TIP—Think: what would best relieve spasticity on a *continuing* basis and select the response that contains "*regular*" and "*scheduled*."
PL, APP, 3, PEDS, PhI, Pharmacological and Parenteral Therapies

490. **(2) Administering Librium, which is an anticonvulsant medication, may prevent a seizure. This is the first nursing action. Answer 1** is incorrect because this is *not the first preventive* nursing action. On day 2 of withdrawal, the client is likely to experience delirium tremors and can have a seizure at any minute. **Answer 3** is incorrect because it not the priority. The client's blood pressure is most likely high; and *after* the medication is given, the blood pressure should be monitored frequently. **Answer 4** is incorrect because this is not a nursing action. The physician needs to order IV fluids before the nurse can begin the treatment. The nurse can push fluids, but this action would occur *after* Librium is given to the client.

TEST-TAKING TIP—This is a priority question and a medical emergency. Look at the answers for clues. Both **Answer 1** and **Answer 2** address an action for seizure control. Choose the direct *action* that is preventive.
IMP, APP, 7, Psych, PhI, Physiological Adaptation

491. **(3) Elders need to stay hydrated throughout the day; but limiting fluids in the evening decreases the body's need to void as the body slows down during sleep. Answer 1** is incorrect because if fluid is limited throughout the day, dehydration will occur. **Answer 2** is incorrect because this should be the LAST incontinence management measure and used only when all else fails. **Answer 4** is incorrect because although it would be helpful to refer the client to try to determine the cause of incontinence, the question asks for a *nursing* intervention that deals with the problem in the *present*.

TEST-TAKING TIP— "Best" and "ongoing nursing intervention" give direction toward the correct answer. Focus on the two options that involve "fluids" and select the time-limited one (i.e., night).
IMP, APP, 8, M/S: Geriatrics, PhI, Basic Care and Comfort

492. **(2) This will help increase the clarity *without* increasing the glare to the point that reading is more difficult. Answer 1** is incorrect because elders should use sunglasses that have *yellow* or *amber* lenses to filter the UV rays and decrease glare. **Answer 3** is incorrect because elders should use warm incandescent, not *bright* lighting to decrease glare. **Answer 4** is incorrect because this level of intensity *increases* glare.

TEST-TAKING TIP— The concern is to reduce glare, at the *lowest* level of light intensity.
IMP, APP, 2, M/S: Geriatrics, HPM, Health Promotion and Maintenance

493. **(4) The nurse's goal is to keep the client awake during the day. If activities are planned in the day when the client usually tries to take a nap, the distraction will assist in decreasing the frequency of daytime naps. Answer 1** is incorrect because clients need to be assisted in sleeping during the *night*. Daytime naps increase the probability of decreased duration of nighttime sleep as well as quality of sleep. **Answer 2** is incorrect because clients with cognitive impairment usually sleep *lightly* and less efficiently. **Answer 3** is incorrect because this will increase daytime napping, as they will be more fatigued.

TEST-TAKING TIP—Remember Maslow's basic needs–uninterrupted sleep is the most restorative.
PL, APP, 3, M/S: Geriatrics, PhI, Basic Care and Comfort

494. **(2) Research describes individuals experiencing periodic waves of grief lasting 20–40 minutes for a year or more after significant loss is experienced. Answer 1** is incorrect because her response is considered an integral and *normal* phase in the grieving process. **Answer 3** is incorrect because this is a *normal* response to loss, and *unless it continues* and becomes chronic grief, psychiatric intervention is not warranted. **Answer 4** is incorrect because the response is a *normal* time frame for the grieving process.

TEST-TAKING TIP—Choose the one option that says this is normal grieving.
AN, COM, 7, Psych: Geriatrics, PsI, Psychosocial Integrity

495. **150 mL** of magnesium sulfate solution at a rate of 300 mL/hr via IV pump.

TEST-TAKING TIP—Calculate 40 g/1000 cm = 4 g/100 mL. The order reads "6 g in 30 min"; calculate 4 g/100 mL (6 g = 150 mL infused over 30 minutes= rate of 300 mL per hour).
IMP, COM, 2, Maternity, PhI, Pharmacological and Parenteral Therapies

496. **(1) Increased agitation often leads to physical injury and falls. Answer 2** is incorrect because this occurs with *long-term* restraint use and immobility. **Answer 3** is incorrect because if agitation is prevented or controlled and restraints are properly applied, physical injury is *less likely* to happen. **Answer 4** is incorrect because if agitation is managed, the risk of falling is decreased.

TEST-TAKING TIP—By selecting **Answer 1**, **Answers 3** and **4** will be included.
AS, COM, 3, Psych: Geriatrics, SECE, Safety and Infection Control

497. **(1) It includes all forms of abuse. Answer 2** is incorrect because clients are often afraid to tell someone how they are treated for fear of subsequent harm. **Answer 3** is incorrect because abuse is often *not observed*. **Answer 4** is incorrect because abuse and neglect can *be emotional as well* as physical. This choice is not the most encompassing answer.

TEST-TAKING TIP—Choose the most inclusive answer.
IMP, COM, 7, M/S: Legal, PsI, Psychosocial Integrity

498. **(3) A certain level of math skills is required to calculate the pump's infusion rate. These math skills are usually evident about 10 years of age. Answer 1** is incorrect because the pump delivers regular and lispro (Humalog) insulin. Both types of insulin *are commonly used* in the control of diabetes mellitus (type 1) in children. **Answer 2** is incorrect because a child with diabetes mellitus (type 1) *cannot* be controlled by oral hypoglycemic agents. Insulin will *always* be required for the control of diabetes mellitus (type 1). **Answer 4** is incorrect because the pump's alarm system *tells* the child (and parents) exactly what the malfunction is (i.e., low battery reserve, an occluded needle or tubing, or an uncontrolled insulin delivery rate).

TEST-TAKING TIP—Remember: all pumps (i.e., IV, enteral, etc.) require some type of calculation in order to operate; select the response that has the word "math" in it.
IMP, APP, 5, PEDS, PhI, Reduction of Risk Potential

499. **(1) Daily weight more rapidly reflects changes in fluid status. Answer 2** is incorrect because effectiveness of any therapy requires that the client be clinically assessed, in addition to reviewing lab values. **Answer 3** is incorrect because swelling *may take some time* to dissipate even after the client's vascular volume is stabilized. **Answer 4** is incorrect because a decreased pulse rate may occur for *several* reasons, *not* necessarily because the heart failure is being managed effectively.

TEST-TAKING TIP—Notice that the question asks for the *best* indicator of treatment effectiveness. The goals of treatment of congestive heart failure include reducing excess intravascular fluid. While **Answers 1** and **3** both relate to fluid status, the best indicator is one that is also the quickest indicator (**Answer 1**).
EV, ANL, 6, M/S: Cardiac, PhI, Pharmacological and Parenteral Therapies

500. **(1) Prolonged starvation associated with anorexia can lead to cardiac changes. Answer 2** is incorrect because the client would have *hypo*glycemia, *not* hyperglycemia (high blood sugar). **Answer 3** is incorrect because it is *not a physiological* symptom. **Answer 4** is incorrect because the client may have metabolic *alkalosis, not* acidosis.

TEST-TAKING TIP—Visualize the symptoms associated with anorexia nervosa (severe weight loss, vomiting, and purging); then, ask yourself if the answer is true for the symptoms. Remember *all parts* of the answer need to be correct.
AS, APP, 4, Psych, PhI, Physiological Adaptation

Guidelines and Tips for International Nurses and Repeat Test-Takers

Sally L. Lagerquist

This unit addresses the special concerns of candidates who have taken the test more than once, as well as international nurses who are graduates of nursing programs outside of the United States.

Since 1977, the authors of this book have had a long history of highest passing results in helping repeat test-takers and international nurses to pass, because we have developed *an approach that works!* We give you guidelines, strategies, and tips that give *you* the skills and confidence to PASS.

This unit will help put you in the frame of mind of an exam question writer and an entry-level nurse (which is what is tested on the exam), so that logic, practice, and a systematic approach can lead you to the best answer(s).

Tips for NCLEX-RN® Candidates Who Must Repeat the Exam

Purpose of This Section

Repeat test-takers have somewhat different needs, different starting points, and a different time frame from those who are first-time NCLEX-RN® candidates: that is, figuring out *why* they did not pass, what the Candidate Performance Report (CPR) *means* that they received, and what to do *next*.

Also refer to **Unit 1—Orientation** in **How to Use This Book as a Study Guide: Where to Begin, While Reviewing, After Reviewing; Key Points to Recall; Memorization Strategies;** information about the structure and format of the computer-adaptive NCLEX-RN®; and **How to Prepare Physically and Mentally.**

What Is the Difference Between Taking This Exam for the First Time and Repeating It?

You are "ahead of the game"! You have already received feedback about your exam-related strengths and weaknesses. You know what the exam is really like and what areas to emphasize. You also know what study methods did *not* work for you. Look at the experience you had in taking the exam as a "dry-run" for helping you to *pass next time.*

What Are Some Risk Factors for Not Passing the First Time?

1. It can readily be *what* you used to study. Often, it is a matter of *what* review materials you used that were not as helpful as other resources could be. Remember, some study aids are better than others. For next time, get a *fresh* start. Use *different* review materials.

2. Using *too many study aids,* from *too many different resources.* You wind up finding that theory and questions in books contradict each other; and there is no one to "referee" as to which books have the right information when books disagree.

3. Reviewing *only with questions and answers in books* will not help you to systematically cover *all* the theory that you need to review.

4. Reviewing *primarily with computer tests* is too time-consuming. You can cover more questions in less time by using a book. In addition, when you get through the thousands of questions on the disk or computer test, you cannot be sure that you have reviewed all that you need to know in each subject area, because the material is both limited and fragmented (i.e., it is not by concepts or systems). Compare this with a book that has *detailed* explanations for wrong and correct answers, where so much *more* helpful information can be seen at a glance on each page.

5. Taking the exam when you are *not ready, just because* you set an exam date.

6. Going into the exam with little or no review because of life circumstances (e.g., illness, moving, vacations, marriage, baby, job).

It Is Not a Matter of How Much You Study for the Test, but *How* You Use the Review Material

At this point in your exam prep, do not start with page 1 and go through page 800+. This is usually overwhelming and not confidence-building. *You* need a *focused* review, starting with your *weakest* area and leaving what you feel most comfortable with toward the end of your reviewing. Discern if you mostly need a review of theory, test-taking strategies, or both. This will determine where you start.

How Do You Know What You Need to Review?

This is based on knowing what the NCLEX-RN® Candidate Performance Report (CPR) means. Look at the eight client subneeds listed in the CPR that came with your NCLEX® results. Look at the areas where the **boldface** print states that your performance was below the passing standard or near the passing standard (which indicates the amount of improvement you need). This means that these are the areas (#1 through #8) that should be the major focus of your content review to **PASS NEXT TIME** (e.g., *Management of Care, Safety and Infection Control, etc.*).

If the computer stopped when you took only 75–100 questions, this probably means that you have significant deficiencies and gaps in certain areas of *nursing content.*

If the computer stopped when you took more than 100 but less than 200 questions, this usually means that you have *some* identifiable areas where you need to review certain content, as well as to improve your test-taking skills. **Appendix C** will show you where to go in this book to *read* in your areas where improvement is needed.

If the computer stopped between 200 and 265 (the maximum number) questions, you were close to passing. Your problem area may very well be a difficulty with or an inconsistency in *answering the questions* when more than one answer could be correct. In this case, help is on the way! Go right to the **Sixty Guidelines and Test-Taking Tips** section in this unit. These test-taking strategies are designed to help you to pull the question apart to show you:

1. How to choose the best answer when all four options could be right.
2. How to narrow your choices down to two possible answers.
3. How to decide between two options.
4. What to do when you haven't a clue!

You *can learn* our *proven* test-taking techniques for success on NCLEX-RN®. By following our guidelines before you repeat the exam, you can get quick feedback on your exam-related problem areas in order to better predict your next NCLEX® results *before* you take it (i.e., whether you are at risk for not passing).

What to Do to Pass Next Time

STEP ONE: ASSESS yourself. In this book, take the **Pre Test, Practice Test,** and **Final Test** all at once (a total of 700 questions).

STEP TWO: Score yourself at the end. Determine what percent correct you had in each of these three integrated tests.

STEP THREE: In any of the tests where you had less than 80% correct, tally the **client need subcategories** that your wrong answers represented. Each question is coded by various categories; *you* need to focus primarily on the *last* category (i.e., the eight client subneeds that are written out). The codes are found after the rationale paragraphs

for each question in the answer section of each test. For example, if most of the questions that you missed in the **Pre Test, Practice Test,** and **Final Test** were represented by the code *Management of Care,* **Appendix C** will list the pages in this book where this content is covered.

STEP FOUR: Go to **Appendix C** and look up where to find *content* in your most problematic area(s). *Read* these pages carefully.

STEP FIVE: Go to **Appendix E** and look up *where* there are all the *questions* in the book that focus on your *most problematic* area(s). Let's say it is *Management of Care; take* each of those questions that are listed, unit by unit, in your problem area(s). *Score* yourself. Go for 80% correct on these *difficult* questions.

How Will You Know That You Are Well Prepared and Ready to Retake the Exam?

When you are getting 80% correct in all of the 2530 questions in this book and on the accompanying disk, you are ready!

Most of all, you are ready when you change the "tape recorder" in your mind that keeps saying "I have failed" to "I haven't **PASSED** yet," and from "I hope I pass" to **"I WILL PASS!"**

A Guide for Graduates of Nursing Schools Outside the United States

International nurses who are educated outside the United States can use this book to serve their special needs.

1. To check their experiences, skills, and knowledge for *equivalency* to those of nursing candidates from U.S. programs, in terms of their ability to deliver effective and safe health care as determined by U.S. standards of practice.
2. To identify cultural differences in perception of client needs and nursing responses and actions (see **Unit 3: Management of Care, Legal and Ethical Aspects in Nursing** and **Cultural Diversity**).
3. To obtain state board of nursing addresses, to find out requirements and procedures to apply to take the RN licensure exam in their state (see **Appendix O**).
4. To learn about the structure and format of the exam (see **Unit 1**).
5. To learn how to prepare for the exam (see **Unit 1**).
6. To practice taking tests made up of multiple-choice and fill-in questions (see questions and test-taking tips in **Units 1, 3, 4, 5, 6, 7, 8, 9, 10, 11, 12,** and **13**).
7. To assess the level of language difficulty in reading the exam.
8. To become skilled in test-taking techniques (see following section).

If you are an international nurse and wish to compare your preparation with that of U.S.-educated nurses, you will find that the practice questions with detailed answers with test-taking tips for each question that are included at the end of each major content unit can serve as an effective **self-assessment** guide. If you find that you need further in-depth study after taking the practice tests and reviewing the essential content presented in outline format throughout the book, you may wish to seek assistance from online or classroom review courses or self-paced review on DVD, CD, videocassette, or audiocassette tapes. In addition, **Unit 10** may help you review **drugs** used in the United States that may be called by other names outside the United States.

Cultural differences may be one cause of incorrect answers stemming from your different perception of clients' needs or nursing action. In addition, **Unit 3** contains the code of ethics and standards of nursing practice and legal aspects that pertain to nursing *in the United States.* We suggest that the international nurse become familiar with these sections to determine what is *emphasized* in this country. **Appendix B** addresses important client needs.

To assist the nurse in making contact with Boards of Registered Nursing, **Appendix O** contains a directory of addresses to write for information about each state's specific requirements for application to take the RN licensing exam.

The **Orientation** unit (see **Unit 1**) is designed to help the international nurse know **what to expect during the exam,** what the **exam structure and format** will be like, **what content will be covered,** and how it will be **scored.** It will also help the exam candidate learn **how to study** for the test, **how to take a multiple-choice test,** and **how to reduce test-taking anxiety.**

If you are concerned about your ability to read and comprehend English as it might be used in the exam, first check yourself by looking at the exam questions in this book. The terms used here are those used in the health care field and are considered to be those a nurse needs to know and use. If the vocabulary is different from yours or is difficult, look at the list of common terms in **Appendix L.** You may also want to consult local colleges for courses in *English as a second language (ESL courses).*

If you are not familiar with or proficient in taking exams with multiple-choice questions when more than one answer looks good, the approximately 2530 sample test questions in this book and the accompanying disk will provide you with sufficient practice for taking such a test. The following section on test-taking tips was specifically included to help you choose the best answer(s) by *narrowing* your choices to *increase* your chances of selecting the best answer(s).

Test-Taking Tips and Guidelines: Sixty Strategies to Use in Answering Questions

In a standard *four-answer multiple-choice* question, if you can systematically eliminate false answers, you can reduce the four-answer question to a two-answer one and thereby make your chances as good as those in the true-false type of question; that is, odds will favor your guessing half of the answers correctly. Other questions will ask you to "select all that apply" from 5–6 options by clicking in the correct boxes to select the answers (*multiple-response* questions).

In the **alternate** items, you may see charts and tables, or you may find pictures and graphs requiring identification of a correct location ("*hot spot*") by either point-and-click or fill-in-the-blank. In the items requiring a *calculation*, determine which numbers are needed to figure out the correct numerical answer and use the drop-down calculator to fill in the blank. Another alternate item is the "drag and drop–ordered" response, in which you are asked to arrange all the correct responses in priority order.

We think that the following pointers will assist you to narrow down your choices systematically and intelligently.

1. *Always, all, everyone, never, none, must.* Answers that include *global* words such as these should be viewed with caution because they imply that there are no exceptions. There are very few instances in which a correct answer is that absolute. Any suggested answer, such as in the following:

   Nurses should exercise caution in interviewing clients who have an alcohol use/dependency problem because:

   1. These clients *always* exaggerate.
   2. These clients are *never* consistent.

   should be looked at with care because any exception will make that a false response. A more reasonable answer to the preceding might be "Clients who have an alcohol use/dependency problem may not be reliable historians."

2. *Broadest, most comprehensive answers.* Choose the answer that includes all the others, which is referred to here as the "*umbrella effect.*" For example, in answering the question:

   A main nursing function in group therapy is to:

   1. Help clients give and receive feedback in the group.
   2. Encourage clients to bring up their concerns.
   3. Facilitate group interaction among the members.
   4. Remind clients to address their comments to the group.

   Number 3 is the best choice because all the other choices fall under it.

3. Test how *reasonable* the answer is by posing a specific situation to yourself. For example, the question might read, "The best approach when interviewing children who have irrational fears is to: (1) Help them analyze why they feel this way." Ask yourself if it is reasonable to use Freudian analysis with 2-year-old children.

4. *Focus on the client.* Usually the reason for doing something with a client is *not* to preserve the good reputation of the *doctor, hospital,* or *nurse,* or to enforce *rules.* Wrong choices would focus on enlisting the client's cooperation for the purpose of fulfilling orders or because it is the rule. On seeing a client out of bed against orders, instead of just saying, "It's against doctor's orders for you to get up," you might better respond by focusing on how the client is reacting to the restriction on his mobility, by saying, for example, "I can see that you want to get up and that it is upsetting to you to be in bed now. Let me help you get back to bed safely and see what I can do for you."

5. *Eliminate any answer that takes for granted that anyone is unworthy or ignorant.* For example, in the question, "The client should not be told the full extent of her condition because … ," a poor response would be, "… she would

not understand." Choose an answer that focuses on the client as a worthy human being.

6. When you do *not* know the best answer, and need to guess, *look for the answer that may be different from the others.* For example, if all choices but one are stated in milligrams and the exception reads "1 g," that choice may be a *distractor* or the *best choice.*

7. Read the question carefully to see if a *negative* modifier is used. If the question asks, "Which of the following is least helpful," be sure to gear your thinking accordingly. Emphasize a key word such as *least* as you read the questions.

8. *Do not look for a pattern* in the correct answers. If you have already selected option 3 for several questions in a row, do not be reluctant to choose option 3 again, if you think that it is the correct response.

9. *Look for the choices that you **know** either **are** correct or **may be** incorrect.* You can save time and narrow your selection by using this strategy. This strategy is also useful when the question requires you to select *all options that apply.* Read each option and determine if it is correct or not; if correct, click on the box to the left of the option. There is no partial credit if you select some but not all that apply.

10. In eliminating potentially wrong psychosocial answers, remember to look for examples of what has been included in the *nontherapeutic response* list in **Unit 6.**

11. Wrong choices tend to be either *very brief* or *very long and involved.*

12. Better psychosocial nursing responses to select are those responses that (a) focus on *feelings* (unless safety is at stake!): "How did that make you feel?" (b) *reflect* the client's comments: "You say that made you angry"; (c) communicate *acceptance* of the client by the nurse rather than criticism or a value judgment; (d) *acknowledge* the client: "I see that you are wincing"; and (e) stay in the *here-and-now*: "What will help now?" Examples of better choices can be found in the *therapeutic responses* list in **Unit 6.**

13. Look for the *average, acceptable, safe, common, typical,* "garden variety" responses, not the "exception to the rule," esoteric, or controversial responses.

14. Eliminate the response that may be the best for a *physician* to make. Look for an *RN role-appropriate psychosocial response;* for example, *psychiatrists* analyze the *past,* and *nurses* in general focus on *present* feelings and situations.

15. *Look for similarities and groupings* in responses and the one-of-a-kind key idea in multiple-choice responses.

Example: *At which activity would it be important to protect the client who is on phenothiazines from the side effects of this drug?*

1. *Sunday church services.*
2. *A twilight concert.*
3. *A midday movie in the theater.*
4. *A luncheon picnic on the hospital grounds.*

Choices 1, 2, and 3 all involve indoor activities. Choice 4 involves outdoor exposure during the height of the sun's rays. Clients need to be protected against photosensitivity and burns when on phenothiazines.

16. Be sure to note whether the question asks for what is the *first* or *initial* response to be made or action to be taken by the nurse. The choices listed may all be correct, but in this situation selecting the response with the *highest priority* is important. If the question asks for an *immediate* action, probably all answers are correct and you need to choose the *priority* answer.

17. When you do not know the specific facts called for in a question, use your *skills of reasoning;* for example, when an answer involves amounts or time (mainly *numbers*) and you do not know the answer and cannot find any basis for reasoning (all else being equal), *avoid the extreme* responses (the highest or lowest numerical values).

18. *Give special attention to questions in which each word counts.* The purpose of this type of question may be not only to test your knowledge but also to see if you can read accurately and find the main point. In such questions, each answer may be a profusion of words, but there may be one or two words that make the critical difference. If the option has several aspects, *all* the parts must be correct for that answer to be correct. If you can eliminate one aspect in an answer, you can eliminate the other options with that aspect.

19. All else being equal, select the response that you best *understand.* Long-winded statements are likely to be included as distractors and may be a lot of words signifying little or nothing, such as "criteria involved in implementing conceptual referents for standardizing protocol." You may want to eliminate *unusual* or *highly technical* language. Relate the situation to something that is *familiar* to you.

20. *Apply skim-reading techniques.* Read the practice questions in this book quickly. Pick out *key* words (write them down, if that is helpful to you). Translate, into *your own* words, the gist of what is asked in the question. You might close your eyes at this point and see if the answer "pops" into mind. *Then,* skim the answer choices, looking for the response that corresponds to what first came into your mind. Key ideas or themes to look for in psychosocial responses have been covered in this section—look for a "feeling" response, acceptance, acknowledgment of the client, and reflection, for example.

21. Look for the *best* answer, not the right answer; for example, *incorrect* action may be the *best* answer *if* the stem asks for an action that is *not appropriate* (e.g., "Which of the following is an inappropriate action?" can be rephrased to say "Which action is wrong?").

22. To narrow down the choices, first find two *contradictory* options; for example, hypo—hyper, flex—extend, give—withhold, dilate—constrict; then focus on which one may be the correct or best choice.

23. Focus on the *age-appropriate* answer (e.g., "When caring for a *toddler,* with what safety issue should the nurse be concerned?").

24. *Time* sequence points to the best choice; e.g., ask yourself *when* is this taking place (e.g., prenatal or postpartum; preoperative or postoperative; before, during, or after; early or late; immediately?).

25. In medication administration questions, apply the *5 rights:*

    - Right Medication
    - Right Route
    - Right Client
    - Right Dosage
    - Right Time

26. When more than one answer looks right, choose the *first step* of the nursing process (*assess* before "implement"). Assessment words and phrases indicate priority:

    - Ascertain
    - Assess
    - Check
    - Collect
    - Detect
    - Determine
    - Find out
    - Identify
    - Look
    - Monitor
    - Observe
    - Obtain information
    - Recognize

27. Isolate the *verbs* from the rest of the question (e.g., *ask* is better than *tell, give,* or *ignore*).

28. Do not overlook the obvious answer: **KIS** (**K**eep **I**t **S**imple); for example, the best answer for what to do when there is a malodor in the room of a client with a colostomy is to "check the stoma for fecal leakage." If it smells like feces, check for feces.

29. As you read what is given for assessment findings (e.g., signs and symptoms) ask yourself: Is this *OK?* or is it *not OK?*

30. When two options are correct, choose the one that covers them *both* (i.e., *incorporates* the other, like a telescope).

    Example: *Two hours after a liver biopsy, the nurse finds the client lying on the left side. What is the best nursing action at this time?*

    1. *Check for bleeding.*
    2. *Turn the client onto the right side.*

    Both options are correct, but choose option 2 because it incorporates option 1; it is possible to *check for bleeding* while *turning* the client over onto the right side (where the liver is), to put pressure on the site (as a *preventive* measure when postbiopsy bleeding is possible).

31. Look at *root* words to give you a clue: for example, hemi = one-half (hemianopsia = "half without vision"). Break down unfamiliar words in the stem.

32. Remember *Maslow*—"soma before psyche"—physiological needs are *before* psychosocial (i.e., physical needs first). Use Maslow's hierarchy to establish *priorities* when more than one answer looks correct.

    Example: *What is the priority nursing care for a client after ECT?*

    1. *Reorient to time and place.*
    2. *Put the side rails up.*
    3. *Explain that memory loss is an expected outcome.*

    When all three options are good (as in this case), select the *physical* aspect of care first (option 2) rather than either of the two psychosocial options.

33. Think *safety* as the best choice when more than one answer could be right. Safety is a *priority.* See the preceding example, where putting side rails up is a "safety" action.

34. *Visualize the condition, behavior, situation,* and the options to help you choose the best answer. Form a *mental image* (e.g., what *flexion* looks like versus *extension*); *visualize and sound out the answers* (e.g., to eliminate trite clichés or "authoritarian"-sounding responses such as "That's not allowed here").

35. "Would that you could that the *ideal* be possible." Choose an answer for the "ideal," not real, world. Do not rely solely on real-world experiences to answer NCLEX® questions (i.e., on the exam, answer as if you *have* all the time, all the staff, and all the equipment).

36. When in doubt as to which answer is best, use the *process of elimination* first (e.g., eliminate what you know is incorrect) to narrow your choice to two options. The best choice will provide an answer to what the question is *asking.*

37. Apply the *ABCS* when the question calls for priorities:

    - **A**irway
    - **B**reathing
    - **C**irculation
    - **S**afety

38. An important goal is to *maximize* client actions. For example, choose options that have indicator words for "encourage":

    - Reinforce
    - Support
    - Facilitate
    - Assist
    - Help
    - Aid
    - Foster

39. Try to turn options into *true-or-false responses* if possible in order to narrow down to two possible options; for example, when a question asks about adjusting insulin dosage, ask yourself, "What is true about adjusting the dose?" "Is it true or false that dosage is increased when the client has an infection?" (True). "Is it true or false that dosage is decreased when blood glucose level increases?" (False). If you find no "true" answers, look at the choices for a "maybe" answer.

40. Use *acronyms* and memory aids to help remember theory in selecting an answer (see **Appendix N**).

SWISS—management of Cushing's:
- Sugar (hyperglycemia)
- Water (fluid retention)
- Infection (prone to …)
- Sodium (retention)
- Sex changes (no menses)

5 Ps of assessing fracture:
- Pain
- Pallor
- Pulselessness
- Paresthesia
- Paralysis

WOUND[2] healing—affected by:
- Wound dimensions
- Overweight
- Undiagnosed infections
- Nutritional deficiencies
- Diabetes, Disabilities (e.g., immunosuppressed)

41. *Reword* the question if the stem says "further teaching is necessary" (e.g., the *best* answer will have an *incorrect* statement).

42. Recognize what is *normal;* for example, the data presented are normal. Or is the sign/symptom presented an "*Oh! Oh!*" (meaning that a problem exists)?

43. Do *not delegate* functions of assessment, evaluation, and nursing judgment to an LVN/LPN or CNA (Certified Nursing Assistant) (e.g., do *not* delegate: admitting a client from the OR to the unit; establishing a plan of care; teaching or giving telephone advice; handling invasive lines).

44. *Do delegate* activities to LVN/LPN or CNA for clients who are *stable* with *predictable* outcomes (e.g., help ambulate a client who is 2 days postsurgery). *Do delegate* to LVN/LPN or CNA activities that involve *standard,* unchanging procedures (e.g., take vital signs after ambulation, *do clean* catheterizations, *simple* dressing changes, suction chronic tracheostomies using *clean* technique).

45. In *positioning* a client, decide what you are trying to *prevent* (e.g., contractures) or *promote* (e.g., venous return).

46. To help decide in which position to place a client, form a mental image of each position in the options (e.g., picture supine, high Fowler, semi-Fowler, Sims, prone, Trendelenburg, lithotomy, dorsal recumbent).

47. When none of the options looks good, identify the nursing *concept* implied in the *options* given (e.g., risk factors for infection).

48. When in doubt, first reread the *question stem* to obtain clues, then reread the options. When you come across a question that is about unfamiliar nursing content (e.g., paracentesis), first ask yourself, "What is the topic of the question?" then "What do the *answer choices mean?*" and then reword the question using the clues from the *options.*

Example: *What is most important for the nurse to ask a client immediately after a paracentesis?*

1. *"Are you in pain?"*
2. *"Do you feel dizzy?"*
3. *"Does your underwear fit better around the belt line?"*
4. *"Do you need to urinate?"*

The first clue is in the question stem: *most important, immediately after.* Then, based on rereading the options, you can reword the question to, "What is an untoward reaction (complication) after this procedure?" The answer choices relate to *expected* outcomes (1, 3), a question that is not relevant to ask *after* the procedure (4), and a *complication* (2), which is the correct option.

49. Recognize *expected* outcomes of drugs and treatments/procedures.

Example: *What will indicate improvement in the condition of the client who has anorexia nervosa?*

1. *The client has gained weight.*
2. *The client weighs herself every day.*
3. *The client eats all the foods served to her.*
4. *The client asks the parents to bring her favorite foods.*

Choose the option that shows progress toward the goal (in this condition, it is weight gain that is expected).

50. When you do *not* know the answer, choose what will cause the *least harm.*

Example: *The nurse suspects abdominal wound dehiscence when lifting the edges of the client's dressings. What should the nurse do next?*

1. *Tell the client to remain quiet and not cough.*
2. *Offer a warm drink to help relax the client.*
3. *Place the client with feet elevated.*
4. *Change the dressing.*

Option 1 is the best answer, because it will not *add* damage that could happen with changing the position or the dressing.

51. Take care of the *client first,* not the equipment or the family (unless a family member is the focus of the question).

52. If one option has *generally, usually, tends to* but other options do not have these qualifiers, use the one option that does have the qualifier as the best answer.

53. Look for a *similar* word or phrase used in the question and in one of the options. For example, if the question states that the client is on an *intermediate*-acting insulin (NPH), and the stem asks for its peak action, look for a *middle* time—between a choice of: 4 hours after the injection, 6–12, 12–14, or 15–18. Choose 6–12 hours (as the midpoint).

54. If two options say the same thing, *neither* can be the answer because both are distractors.

Example: *What might the nurse expect to see when a client with cirrhosis is hospitalized with ascites?*

1. *Client is likely to be anorexic.*
2. *Client's intake will be poor, especially if served large portions.*

You can eliminate both of these options because they are saying the same thing in different words: the client is likely to be not interested in eating.

55. Don't "pass the buck"—think what is a *nursing action* that an RN can do *before* calling the MD.

    Example: *After surgery, a client with diabetes complains of nausea, appears lethargic and flushed, with BP 108/78, P 100, R 24 and deep. What is the next action?*

    1. *Call the MD.*
    2. *Check the client's glucose.*
    3. *Give an antiemetic.*
    4. *Change the IV infusion rate.*

The nurse should *assess* (option 2) *before* calling the MD (who may *then* order an antiemetic, option 3, and alter the IV infusion rate, option 4).

56. Focus on key words in the *stem* of the question as your clue:

    - Best
    - Essential
    - Highest
    - Immediate
    - Least likely
    - Most
    - Most appropriate
    - Most likely
    - Vital

57. "Action" does not always mean choose an "implementation" type of answer. The question may ask: "What is the best nursing action?" However, the answer may be an "assessment" option.

    Example: *What is the best action for the nurse to take when a mother at the clinic reports that her child who has diabetes is hyperglycemic in the morning (215 mg/dL), although the child has been well controlled with NPH and regular insulin before breakfast and dinner?*

    1. *Suggest that the mother give the bedtime snack earlier.*
    2. *Suggest that the insulin be given later in the evening.*
    3. *Suggest that they continue with the same regimen.*
    4. *Check the blood sugar now, and suggest that the mother check it during the night.*

Choose "check," which is an "assessment" response (option 4), although the question (the stem) is phrased as an implementation ("best action" is an implementation).

58. Remember the *nursing hierarchy*. Go to the next line of *nursing* authority (e.g., staff→ charge nurse; LPN/LVN→ staff nurse) when the question asks to whom to report a situation; for example, if the question is about an LVN/LPN, the best answer is to report to the staff nurse.

59. When the question includes lab values, ask yourself whether the given value is "Oh! Oh!" (meaning too high or too low); or "Eh" (meaning not a particular problem). For example, a serum K$^+$ of 8.5 is "Oh! Oh!" (too high).

60. *Prevention* is a key concept (e.g., when the question deals with infection control, and in health teaching).

    Example: *The primary objective in ileostomy teaching with a client during early postoperative period is to:*

    1. *Facilitate maintenance of intake and output records.*
    2. *Control unpleasant odors.*
    3. *Prevent skin excoriation around the stoma.*
    4. *Reduce the risk of postoperative wound infection.*

Choose "prevention" (option 3), which in turn may prevent contamination of abdominal incision (option 4). Options 1 and 2 are *secondary* objectives.

Confidence, Performance, Pass!

This **Unit 2** is aimed at helping you to take NCLEX-RN® with more and improved test-taking skills.
THINK: ↑ confidence
THINK: ↑ performance
THINK: Pass NCLEX-RN®

Guidelines and Tips

Unit 3

Management of Care, Cultural Diversity, Ethical and Legal Aspects, and Nursing Trends

Sally L. Lagerquist and Kathleen Snider

MANAGEMENT OF CARE

I. **Concepts of management**
A. *Definitions*
1. *Case management*—process that involves comprehensive coordination of activities and services provided to the client throughout the continuum of care or episode. *Activities* include: case finding, screening, intake, assessment, problem identification, **prioritization** of client's problems and needs, planning, reassessment, evaluation, documentation, designing and monitoring clinical pathways, and identification of variances.
2. *Continuous quality improvement*—process used to make improvements in client care; indicators of excellence are identified and process involves actively including input from and **collaboration** with the client (whose needs are at the center of the process), the family, and all health-care team members.
3. *Incidents/variance reports*—part of quality improvement, where occurrences take place in a health-care agency that are not typical according to medical orders, may be an accident, or may be a violation of policy and procedures (e.g., wrong medication dose, a client or visitor falls, needle stick by nurse). These are considered unexpected incidents, exceptions that happen during client care.
4. *Quality assurance*—activities that evaluate the quality of care provided to clients to ensure that it meets predetermined standards of excellence.
5. *Resource management*—providing appropriate number and type of resources needed by clients to achieve desired outcomes.
6. *Supervision*—process of guiding, encouraging, and assessing the work of others to whom tasks were delegated.

7. *Delegate responsibility and direct nursing care provided by others*—based on particular client/family needs and on job description, roles, functions, and skills of other nursing personnel: client's condition (stable or medically fragile), *complexity* of required care, *potential risks for harm* to client, degree of needed *problem-solving* expertise, *predictability* of outcome, type and *level of client interaction* required. *Important:* The person who delegated the task has the responsibility and final accountability for effective completion of task.

B. *Management theories*
1. *Microlevel* theories: clarify and predict behavior (e.g., motivation) of the individual, with input on the group/organization (e.g., group dynamics).
2. *Macrolevel* theories: focus on best ways to make changes within an organization, organizing projects, obtaining resources, attaining goals.
3. *Intrapersonal/interpersonal* theories:
a. *Cognitive:* belief—a person's motivation is based on expectations about what will happen as a result of own behavior; involves goal setting, with regular feedback to increase motivation to achieve.
b. *Scientific management:* belief—repetition of task will result in expertise.
c. *Neoclassical management:* based on Maslow (i.e., person continuously strives to meet higher level needs); **ERG** (**E**xistence, **R**elatedness, **G**rowth); job redesign (i.e., ensures that task has validity, significance, autonomy, and feedback).
d. *Social/reinforcement:* belief—motivation comes from learning from those with whom a person identifies; conditioned by reinforcement.
C. *Management behaviors*
1. *Decision maker*

a. Initiator of new projects.

b. Crisis handler (e.g., interpersonal conflicts among staff).

c. Resource allocator (people, physical, financial).

d. Negotiator.

2. *Communicator*

a. Monitor of data collection and processing.

b. Dissemination of collected information.

c. Speaker on behalf of agency.

3. *Representative*

a. Institutional figurehead.

b. Group leader.

c. Liaison between agency and community.

II. Establishing priorities

A. When managing a number of clients at the same time, the nurse needs to set priorities by *assessing types of care* needed:

1. Decide on the *most important nursing activity* (giving a medication? performing a treatment? taking vital signs? providing nutrition? measuring I&O, etc.)

2. Identify the *first* action the nurse needs to take.

3. Select the *best* nursing action.

4. Determine which client needs *immediate* care.

B. Determine priorities with the guidance of:

1. **Maslow's hierarchy of needs** (see **Figure 6.1**).

a. Choose *physiological* needs (survival) as the highest level of priority

b. Followed by *safety* needs

c. Then *psychological* needs (care and belonging).

d. Lastly, *self-actualization* needs.

2. **Steps of the Nursing Process (APIE)**

a. First, is *assessment (data collection)*

b. Then, *plan* (goals)

c. Followed by *implementation* (actions)

d. Finally, *evaluation* (outcome)

3. **ABCS**

a. Airway (e.g., patent airway)

b. Breathing

c. Circulation

d. Safety

4. **RACE** (e.g., in event of fire)

a. *Remove* the client

b. Then sound the *alarm*

c. *Call* the fire department

d. *Extinguish* the fire

III. Disaster planning

A. *Definition:* any man-made (e.g., toxic material spill, riot, explosion, structural collapse) or naturally occurring (e.g., communicable disease epidemic, flood, hurricane, earthquake) event that results in destruction or devastation that causes suffering, creates human needs, and cannot be alleviated without support

B. *Goal:* reduce vulnerability to prevent recurrence

C. *Benefits* of a disaster plan:

1. Decrease in costs of damage control.

2. Decreased extent and duration of injury.

3. Decreased loss of life.

4. Increased ability to respond to unforeseen disasters.

D. *Health-care components*

1. Early warning signals, with *realistic* expectations.

2. Brief and succinct assessment of those at risk.

3. Simple, flexible rescue chains that unfold in organized stages/steps.

E. *Nursing responsibilities*

1. *Nurses at the scene:* assisting with rescue, evacuation, and first aid.

2. *Nurses at the hospital:* triaging victims and providing acute care.

a. *Triage:* a system of client evaluation to set up priorities, assign appropriate staff, and start treatment.

(1) *In emergencies:* greatest risk receives priority.

(2) *In major disasters:* selection is based on doing what can be done to benefit the *largest* number; those needing highly specialized care may be given minimal or no care. First, take care of those needing *minimal* care to save their lives, and who in turn can be available to help others.

3. *Nurses at community shelters or health clinics:* assessing, planning, implementing, and evaluating ongoing health-care needs of victims.

F. *Level of prevention*

1. *Primary prevention:* prevention of disaster and limiting consequences when cannot be prevented.

a. *Nursing activities:* identification of factors that pose actual or potential problem.

2. *Secondary prevention:* responding to the disaster, halting it, and resolving problems caused by it.

a. *Nursing activities:* assessment of extent of injuries; tagging victims for treatments and evaluation; providing first aid; identifying complications; coordinating activities of shelter workers.

3. *Tertiary prevention:* recovery and prevention of recurrence.

a. *Nursing activities:* implementing community's disaster plan; providing continuous assessment, planning, implementation, and evaluation; providing counseling as needed to victims and co-workers; educating the public about disaster preparedness.

IV. Emergency response plan: fire safety and preparedness

A. Know location of:

1. Escape routes, escape doors. Keep fire exits clear.

2. Available equipment.

a. Fire alarms.

b. Fire sprinkler controls.

c. Fire extinguishers.

B. Identify fire hazards.

1. Faulty electrical equipment and wiring.

2. Overloaded circuits.

3. Plugs not properly grounded.

4. Smoking.
5. Combustible substances → spontaneous combustion.

C. Prevention.
1. Report frayed or exposed electrical wires.
2. *Avoid* overloaded circuits.
3. *Don't* use extension cords.
4. Use only three-pronged grounded plugs.
5. *Avoid* clutter.
6. Remove cigarettes and matches from room; control smoking according to institutional policy; limit smoking to designated areas.
7. Immediately report smoke odors and burning.

D. Action to take in event of fire in immediate vicinity:
1. Move clients to safety (triage those who are not ambulatory or are otherwise incapacitated).
2. Sound alarm.
3. Close all windows and doors.
4. Shut off valves for O_2.
5. Follow agency policy about *announcing* fire and location, *notifying* fire company, and evacuation plan.
6. *Avoid* using elevators.

V. Safe use of equipment (see also p. 132)
A. Suspect malfunction in equipment when it:
1. Does not work consistently or correctly.
2. Makes unusual noise.
3. Gives off unusual odor.
4. Produces extreme temperature.
5. Produces sparks.

B. Replace immediately; don't repair it.
C. Call maintenance department to check for safety and repair.
D. When O_2 is in use:
1. Secure the O_2 according to institutional policy.
2. Remove flammable liquids from the area.
3. Put up "oxygen in use" signs.

CULTURAL DIVERSITY IN NURSING PRACTICE*

With increasing ethnocultural diversity among health-care clients and staff, health-care providers must increase their sensitivity to and knowledge of cultural concepts, be aware of both similarities and differences in values and beliefs that exist across cultures, and know how this may affect health-care delivery. Important objectives are to increase respect and sensitivity for diversity in order to minimize potential for transgressing cultural norms, and to provide culturally conscious health-care and working relationships among clients and staff from dissimilar cultures.

The purpose of this section is to provide a framework/structure for assessing, planning, and implementing culturally conscious interventions.

*Sally Lagerquist (was in *Addison-Wesley's Nursing Examination* Review ed. 2, Unit 7, p. 633, oop)

We have selected 10 essential areas as guidelines for assessing cultural characteristics that have implications for health and health care: **communication, family roles, biocultural ecology, high-risk health behaviors, nutrition, pregnancy and childbearing practices, death rituals, spirituality, health-care practices,** and **health-care practitioners.**

I. Communication
A. *Language*
1. What is the usual *volume* and *tone* of speech?
a. *Guidelines:* use interpreters (to provide meaning behind words) rather than translators (who just restate words); *avoid* use of relatives and children; use interpreters of same age and gender when possible. Select the words you use carefully, *avoiding* buzz words and jargon. Speak clearly, pacing yourself to be neither too fast nor too slow. Words that are slurred, have many syllables in them, or are too technical make communication more difficult. Speaking too fast may overload the client and make it difficult for the client to follow. Speaking too slowly may lose the client's attention.
(1) Select the gestures you use with care, using your nonverbal behavior to underscore your words and your actions. The proper use of gestures can clarify a message, and drawings can sometimes be helpful. Be careful, however; not all gestures mean the same thing in all cultures.

B. *Cultural communication patterns (**Table 3.1**)*
1. Willingness to share their *thoughts and feelings.*
2. Use and meaning of *touch* between family, friends, same sex, opposite sex, with health-care provider.
3. *Personal space:* meaning of distance and physical proximity.
4. *Eye contact:* special meaning for staring (rude, "evil eye"); for avoidance of eye contact (e.g., not caring, not listening, not trustworthy); variation of eye contact among family, friends, strangers, and socioeconomic groups.
5. *Facial* expression: how emotions are shown (or not) in facial expressions; use and meaning of smiles.
6. *Standing, greeting* strangers: what is acceptable.

C. *Concept of time:* past, present or future oriented; social time vs. clock time
D. *Names:* expected greetings by health-care providers

II. Family roles
A. *Gender roles:* patriarchal or egalitarian; change in perceived head of household during different life stages; male/female norms (e.g., stoic, modest)
B. *Prescriptive* (*should* do), *restrictive* (should *not* do), *taboo* behaviors for children and adolescents
1. *Prescriptive* (e.g., "Fat children are healthy").
2. *Restrictive* practices (e.g., silence, not anger, at parents).
3. *Taboo* (e.g., discussion of sexuality).

C. *Family roles and priorities*
1. Family goals and priorities (family needs may have priority over individual health needs).
2. Developmental tasks.
3. Aged: status and role.
4. Extended family (biological and nonbiological): role and importance.
5. How social status is gained: through heritage? Educational accomplishments?

D. *Alternative lifestyles*
1. Nontraditional families: single parents, blended families, communal families, same-sex families.

III. Biocultural ecology

A. *Variations in color of skin* and *biological variations*
1. **Skin color:** special problems/concerns: assessment of jaundice, "Mongolian" spots, and blood/oxygenation levels in *dark skin. Considerations for health care:*
   a. Assessment of *anemia*: examine oral mucosa and nailbed capillary refill.
   b. Assessment of *jaundice* (e.g., in Asian people): look at sclera.
   c. Assessment of rashes: palpate.
   d. Get a baseline of skin color from family.
   e. Use direct sunlight.
   f. Look at areas with least amount of pigmentation.
   g. Compare skin in corresponding areas.
2. *Biological* variations in **body, size, shape, and structure:** long bones, width of hips and shoulders, flat nose bridges (relevance for fitting eyeglasses), shorter builds (at variance with normative growth curves); mandibular and palatine dimensions (relevance for fitting dentures); teeth (peg, extra, natal, large size); ears (free, floppy, attached); eyelids (epicanthic folds).
3. *Diseases and health conditions:*
   a. Specific risk factors related to **climate, topography** (e.g., air pollution, mosquito-infested tropical areas).
   b. **At-risk groups for endemic** diseases (those that occur continuously in a specific ethnic group): e.g., malaria, liver and renal impairment, infectious blindness and scleral infections, otitis media, respiratory diseases (e.g., tuberculosis, coccidioidomycosis).
   c. Increased **genetic** *susceptibility* for diseases and health conditions (e.g., diabetes, dwarfism, muscular dystrophy, cystic fibrosis, myopia, keloid formation, gout, cancer of stomach is more prevalent in blood type O, sickle cell anemia, Tay-Sachs).
4. Variations in **drug metabolism** (e.g., cardiovascular effects of propranolol in Chinese; peripheral neuropathy in Native Americans on isoniazid).
5. Variations in **blood groups** (e.g., Native Americans usually are type O and no type B; Rh negative nonexistent in Eskimos, more often in Whites); twinning (dizygote) is highest among African-Americans.

IV. High risk health behaviors

A. Use of alcohol, tobacco, recreational drugs
B. Level of physical activity; increased calorie consumption
C. Use of safety measures (e.g., seat belts and helmets and safe-driving practices)
D. Self-care using folk and magicoreligious practices before seeking professional care

V. Nutrition

See also **Unit 9, Cultural Food Patterns.**

A. *Meaning* of food: symbolic, socialization role; denotes caring and closeness and kinship, and expression of love and anger
B. Common foods and rituals
1. Major ingredients commonly used (high sodium, fat, spices).
2. Preparation practices (e.g., kosher does not mix meat with dairy in cooking, eating, serving).
3. Afternoon tea (British), morning coffee (American).
4. Fasting (e.g., Muslims, Catholics, Jews).
5. Foods not allowed (e.g., no shellfish or pork in kosher diet).
C. Nutritional deficiencies and food limitations
1. Enzyme deficiencies (e.g., in *glucose*-6-phosphate dehydrogenase deficiency, *fava bean* can cause hemolysis and acute anemic crisis).
2. Food intolerances (e.g., *lactose deficiency*).
3. Significant nutritional deficiencies, such as *calcium* (Southeast Asian immigrants).
4. Native food limitations that may cause special health difficulties, such as *poor intake of lysine and other amino acids* (Hindu).
D. Use of food for health promotion, to treat illness, and in disease prevention
1. "Hot and cold" theories.

VI. Pregnancy and childbearing practices

A. *Fertility* and views toward pregnancy, contraception, and abortion
B. *Prescriptive, restrictive, and taboo* practices related to *pregnancy, birthing* practices, and *postpartum period*
1. *Pregnancy:* foods, exercise, intercourse, and avoiding weather-related conditions.
2. *Birthing process:* reactions during labor, presence of men, position for delivery, preferred types of health-care practitioners, place for delivery.
3. *Postpartum* period: bathing, cord care, exercise, foods, role of men.

VII. Death rituals

A. Death rituals and expectations
1. Cultural expectations of response to death and grief.
2. Meaning of death, dying, and afterlife.
   a. Euthanasia.
   b. Autopsies.
B. Purpose of death rituals and mourning practices
C. Specific burial practices (e.g., cremation)

VIII. Spirituality

A. Use of prayer, meditation, or symbols

B. Meaning of life and individual sources of strength

C. Relationship between spiritual beliefs and health practices

IX. Health-care practices

   A. *Health-seeking beliefs and behaviors*

   1. Beliefs that influence health-care practices.

      a. Perception of illness (e.g., punishment for sin, work of malevolent persons).

   2. Health promotion and prevention practices.

      a. Acupuncture.

      b. Yin and yang;

         (1) Increased yin results in nervous, digestive disorders.

         (2) Increased yang results in dehydration, fever, irritability.

   B. *Responsibility* for health care

   1. Acute care: curative or fatalistic.

   2. Who assumes responsibility for health care?

   3. Role of health insurance.

   4. Use of over-the-counter medications.

   C. *Folklore practices*

   1. Combination of folklore, magicoreligious beliefs, and traditional beliefs that influence health-care behaviors.

   D. *Barriers to health care* (e.g., language, economics, geography)

   E. *Cultural responses to health and illness*

   1. Beliefs and responses *to pain* that influence interventions.

      a. Special meaning of pain.

   2. Beliefs and views about *mental illness/mental health care.*

      a. Therapies must include *extended* families as opposed to individuals or nuclear families.

      b. Cultural and racial as well as individual components must be considered when assessing precipitating or predisposing causes of illness (e.g., need to atone for sins).

      c. Values may conflict: for example, individualism versus concern for family or social interactions; self-actualization versus survival needs.

      d. Some ethnic groups *do not value or possess* qualities required for some psychiatric therapies, such as verbal skills, introspection, ability to delay gratification, and ability to discuss personal problems with strangers.

      e. Therapy resources *may not be accessible or considered useful or relevant* for members of some ethnic groups.

      f. Common feelings and behavior patterns may be shared by many "minority" groups:

         (1) Feelings of *inferiority and inadequacy,* often a result of prejudice and racism.

         (2) *Incompetent* behavior as an outcome of feeling inferior and inadequate.

         (3) *Suppressed anger,* resulting in displaced hostility and paranoid ideas.

         (4) *Withholding and withdrawal;* not comfortable with sharing feelings or experiences.

         (5) *Selective inattention;* may block out or deny frustration or insults.

         (6) *Overcompensation* in some areas to make up for denied opportunities in other areas.

   3. Different perception of *mentally and physically* handicapped.

   4. Beliefs and practices related to *chronic* illness and *rehabilitation.*

   5. Cultural perceptions of the *sick role.*

   F. *Acceptance of blood transfusions and organ donation*

X. Health-care practitioners

   A. Traditional vs. biomedical care

   1. Does the *age* of practitioner matter?

   2. Does the *gender* of practitioner matter?

   B. Status of health-care provider

   1. How different members of health-care practice see each other.

XI. Additional cultural considerations—for other cultural influences related to children and families, refer to **Table 3.1.**

RELIGIOUS AND SPIRITUAL INFLUENCES ON HEALTH

Religious and spiritual beliefs can have a major impact on health and illness. Each religion has its own rituals and traditions that must be observed, with the belief that if these are not followed, the outcomes may negatively affect the client's well-being or their family.

I. Definition:

   A. *Religion*—an organized belief system in God or supernatural, using prayer, meditation, or symbols

   B. *Spirituality*—encompasses more than religious beliefs; includes values, meaning, and purpose in life; can provide inspiration and sustain a person or group during crisis

   C. *Values clarification*—aligns values and beliefs so that they are consistent with goals

◆ **II. Assessment *of religious and spiritual beliefs***

   A. Beliefs about birth and what follows death

   B. Code of ethics about right and wrong

   C. View of health, causes of illness, or what may be the cure for the problem

   D. Dietary laws

   E. Relationship of mind, body, and spirit

   F. Importance of work and money as they relate to religion

   G. Pain: purpose of, response to, treatment for

   H. Importance of family

   I. Meaning of life, individual sources of hope and strength

   J. Religious practices that conflict with health practices and use of health services

◆ **III. Analysis/nursing diagnosis**

   A. *Risk for spiritual distress* related to prolonged pain; health-care choices that are in conflict with religious

TABLE 3.1	Cultural Influences on Health-Care Practices with Children and Adults

Cultural Group	Belief	Practice
African Americans (numerous groups from varying locales)	*Health* is viewed as harmony with nature *Illness* may be viewed as "will of God" or a "punishment" (especially in children); illness can be caused by "natural" (polluted food/water) as well as "unnatural" (hex) sources May distrust health-care practitioner who is from the majority group (shown by silence) Reluctant to give permission for organ	Self-care and folk medicine prevalent Try home remedies first or consult with an "old woman" in the community (especially for children) May make use of root doctors, spiritualist, voodoo priests May seek opinion of Black minister, who is highly influential in health-care decisions
Americans (usually of white, European descent)	*Health* is viewed as a combination of physical and emotional well-being *Illness* may be viewed in rational/scientific terms; believe in germ and stress theories Increasing interest in health promotion as reflected in life style May view alternative health care as possibility/valuable, either independently or in conjunction with Western medicine	Believe that infant can "tell" mother its health-care needs Early/routine prenatal and well baby/child care and immunizations Increasing reliance on/demand for "specialists" in child health care
Asian Americans (numerous groups from varying locales)	*Health* is viewed as a balance between energy forces of yin (cold) and yang (hot); harmony with universal order; pleasing good spirits/avoiding evil spirits *Illness* may be viewed as an "imbalance" Child's good health reflects well upon the parent/family Honor and "face" important Suppress emotions	Goal of health-care therapy: restore balance of yin and yang Restoration of health with: tai chi, acupressure/acupuncture, diet, folk healers, herbs, massage, moxibustion (heat applied to skin over specific areas) *Avoid* dairy because of lactose intolerance Trend: use combination of Eastern and Western treatment modalities and prevention Elderly treated with respect Close, extended families Direct eye contact may show disrespect
Hispanic and Mexican Americans (numerous groups from varying locales)	*Health* is viewed as a reward/"good luck" *Illness* may be viewed as punishment or an imbalance between hot and cold Individual is passive recipient of disease, which is caused by external forces (supernatural)	"Curandero" (folk healer) may be consulted before a health-care practitioner from the majority group "Hot" diseases are treated with "cold" remedies (does not refer to temperature) Use: herbs, prayers, religious artifacts/rituals; visits to shrines (strong association between religion and health) Children highly valued/desired and taken everywhere with family, which can lead to interruptions when consulting with health-care practitioner Elderly treated with respect Men make key decisions in matters outside of the home Silence may indicate disapproval of plan of care Very emotionally expressive when grieving
Native Americans (numerous tribes from varying locales)	*Health* is viewed as a state of harmony with nature and the universe *Illness* may be viewed as a price to be paid for past/future deeds All disorders believed to have *supernatural* aspects/influences	Going to the physician/hospital is associated with illness/disease; may delay seeking care as health state is viewed as part of a "natural process" (example: adolescent becomes pregnant) Reliance on: diviners/diagnosticians, herbs, medicine man, rituals, singers; may carry objects to protect self against witchcraft Children who are obstinate are respected, while children who are docile are considered weak; can lead to conflict with health-care practitioner from majority group Elderly treated with respect Blood and organ donation generally not accepted. Handshake, light touch Ok, but maintain respectful distance while interacting

Adapted from Wong, D: Whaley and Wong's Nursing Care of Infants and Children, ed 7. Mosby, St Louis, 2003.

practices; anxiety and guilt due to violating religious beliefs; lashing out against the religion

◆ **IV. Nursing care plan/implementation**
    A. Acknowledge client's beliefs
      1. Provide contact with clergy of choice.
      2. Provide opportunity to carry out practices not detrimental to client's health.
    B. Do *not* impose beliefs and values of health-care system

◆ **V. Evaluation/outcome criteria**
    A. Increased satisfaction related to medical care decision
    B. Decrease in feelings of stress, guilt, depression, anger

NURSING ETHICS

Nursing ethics involves rules and principles to guide right conduct in terms of moral duties and obligations to protect the rights of human beings. In nursing, ethical codes provide professional standards and formal guidelines for nursing activities to protect both the nurse and the client.

  I. Code of ethics—serves as a frame of reference when judging priorities or possible courses of action. *Purposes:*
    A. To provide a basis for regulating relationships between nurse, client, co-workers, society, and profession.
    B. To provide a standard for excluding unscrupulous nursing practitioners and for defending nurses unjustly accused.
    C. To serve as a basis for nursing curricula.
    D. To orient new nurses and the public to ethical professional conduct.
  II. ANA Code of Ethics for Nurses incorporates the following key elements of what the nurse needs to do*:
    A. Demonstrate respect for *human dignity* and *uniqueness* of individual regardless of health problem or socioeconomic level
    B. Maintain client's *right to privacy* and *confidentiality*
    C. Protect the client from *incompetent, unethical,* or *illegal* behavior of others
    D. Accept *responsibility* for informed individual nursing judgment and behavior
    E. Maintain *competence* through ongoing professional development and *consultation*
    F. Maintain responsibility when *delegating* nursing care, based on competence/qualification criteria
    G. Work on maintaining/improving standards of care in employment setting
    H. Protect consumer from misinformation/misrepresentation
  III. Bioethics—a philosophical field that applies ethical reasoning process for achieving clear and convincing

reasons to issues and dilemmas (conflicts between two obligations) in health care.†
    A. Purpose of applying ethical reflection to nursing concerns:
      1. Improve quality of professional nursing decisions.
      2. Increase sensitivity to others.
      3. Offer a sense of moral clarity and enlightenment.
    B. Framework for analyzing an ethical issue:
      1. Who are the relevant participants in the situation?
      2. What is the required action?
      3. What are the probable and possible benefits and consequences of the action?
      4. What is the range of alternative actions or choices?
      5. What is the intent or purpose of the action?
      6. What is the context of the action?
    C. Principles of bioethics:
      1. *Autonomy*—the right to make one's own decisions.
      2. *Nonmalfeasance*—the intention to do no wrong.
      3. *Beneficence*—the principle of attempting to do things that benefit others.
      4. *Justice*—the distribution, as fairly as possible, of benefits, resources, and burdens.
      5. *Veracity*—the intention to tell the truth.
      6. *Confidentiality*—the social contract guaranteeing another's privacy.
  IV. Client bill of rights†
    A. Right to appropriate treatment that is most supportive and least restrictive to personal freedom.
    B. Right to individualized treatment plan, subject to review and reassessment.
    C. Right to active participation in treatment, with the risk, side effects, and benefits of all medication and treatment (and alternatives) to be discussed.
    D. Right to give and withhold consent (exceptions: emergencies and when under conservatorship).
      1. *Advance directives:* legal, written, or oral statements made by a person who is mentally competent about treatment preferences. In the event the person is unable to make these determinations, a designated surrogate decision-maker can do so. Each state has own specific laws with restrictions.
        a. **Living will:** legal document stating person does not wish to have extraordinary lifesaving measures when not able to make decisions about own care.
        b. **Durable power of attorney:** legal document giving designated person authority to make health-care decisions on client's behalf when client is unable to do so.
    E. Right to be free of experimentation unless following recommendations of the National Commission on Protection of Human Subjects (with informed, voluntary, written consent).
    F. Right to be free of restraints and seclusion except in an emergency.
    G. Right to humane environment with reasonable protection from harm and appropriate privacy.

---

*Adapted from recording at JONA and Nurse Educator's Joint Leadership Conference, 1981, A. J. Davis, "Ethical Dilemmas in Nursing."

†Adapted from AAA Code of Ethics on Nurses, Washington, DC.

H. Right to confidentiality of medical records.

I. Right of access to personal treatment record.

J. Right to as much freedom as possible to exercise constitutional rights of association (e.g., use of telephone, personal mail, having visitors) and expression.

K. Right to information about these rights in both written and oral form, presented in an understandable manner at outset and periodically thereafter.

L. Right to assert grievances through a grievance mechanism that includes the power to go to court.

M. Right to obtain *advocacy* assistance.

1. *Definition:* an *advocate* is a person who pleads for a cause or who acts on a client's behalf.

2. *Goals:* help client gain greater self-determination and encourage freedom of choices; increase sensitivity and responsiveness of the health-care, social, political systems to the needs of the client.

3. *Characteristics:* assertiveness; willingness to speak out for or in support of client; ability to negotiate and obtain resources for positive outcomes; willingness to take risks, and take necessary measures in instances of incompetent, unethical, or illegal practice by others that may jeopardize client's rights.

N. Right to criticize or complain about conditions or services without fear of retaliatory punishment or other reprisals.

O. Right to referral to complement the discharge plan.

V. **Conflicts and problems—Ethical dilemmas**

A. *Personal values versus professional duty*—nurses have the right to refuse to participate in those areas of nursing practice that are against their personal values, as long as a client's welfare is not jeopardized. *Example:* therapeutic abortions.

B. *Nurse versus agency*—conflict may arise regarding whether or not to give out needed information to a client or to follow agency policy, which does not allow it. *Example:* a teenager who is emotionally upset asks a nurse about how to get an abortion, a discussion that is against agency policy.

C. *Nurse versus colleagues*—conflict may arise when determining whether to ignore or report others' behavior. *Examples:* you see another nurse steal medications; you know that a peer is giving a false reason when requesting time off; or you observe a colleague who is intoxicated.

D. *Nurse versus client/family*—conflict may stem from knowledge of confidential information. Should you tell? *Example:* client or family member relates a vital secret to the nurse.

E. *Conflicting responsibilities*—to whom is the nurse primarily responsible when needs of the agency and the client differ? *Example:* an MD asks a nurse not to list all supplies used for client care, because the client cannot afford to pay the bill.

F. *Ethical dilemmas*—stigma of diagnostic label (e.g., AIDS, schizophrenia, addict); involuntary psychiatric confinement; right to control individual freedom; right to suicide; right to privacy and confidentiality.

LEGAL ASPECTS OF NURSING

I. **Definition of terms**

A. *Common law:* accumulation of law as a result of judicial court decisions.

B. *Civil law* (private law): law that derives from legislative codes and deals with relations between private parties.

C. *Public law:* concerns relationships between an individual and the state. The thrust of public law is to attain what are deemed valid public goals, such as reporting child abuse.

D. *Criminal law:* concerns actions against the safety and welfare of the public, such as robbery. It is part of the public law.

E. *Informed consent:* implies that significant benefits and risks of any procedure, as well as alternative methods of treatment, have been *explained;* person has had *time* to ask questions and have these answered; person has agreed to the treatment *voluntarily* and is legally competent to give consent; and communication is in a *language known to the client.*

F. *Reasonably prudent nurse:* nurse must react as a reasonably prudent nurse trained in that specialty area would react. For example, if a nurse works with fetal monitors, she must know how to use the monitors, know how to read the strips, and know what actions to take based on the findings.

II. **Nursing licensure**—mandatory licensure required in order to practice nursing.

A. *Nurse Practice Act:* each state has one to protect nurses' professional capacity to set educational requirements, to distinguish between nursing and medical practice, to define scope of nursing practice, to legally control nursing through licensing, and to define standards of professional nursing.

B. *American Nurses Association* (2004): "The practice of nursing means the performance for compensation of professional services requiring substantial specialized knowledge of the biological, physical, behavioral, psychological, and sociological sciences and of nursing theory as the basis for assessment, diagnosis, planning, intervention, and evaluation in the promotion and maintenance of health; the casefinding and management of illness, injury, or infirmity; the restoration of optimum function; or the achievement of a dignified death. Nursing practice includes but is not limited to: administration, teaching, counseling, supervision, delegation, and evaluation of practice and execution of the medical regimen, including the administration of medications and treatments prescribed by any person authorized by state law to prescribe. Each registered nurse is directly accountable and responsible to the consumer for the quality of nursing care rendered" (American Nurses Association: *Nursing: Scope and Standards of Practice.* American Nurses Association, Washington, D.C.).

C. *Revoking a license:* Board of Examiners in each state in the United States and each province in Canada has the power to revoke licenses for just cause, such as incompetence in nursing practice, conviction of crime, drug addiction, obtaining license through fraud, or hiding criminal history (see section **XI A, B, C,** p. 131).

III. Crimes and torts

A. *Crime:* an act committed in violation of societal law and punishable by fine or imprisonment. A crime does not have to be intended (as in giving a client an accidental overdose that proves to be lethal).
   1. *Felonies:* crimes of a serious nature (e.g., murder) punishable by imprisonment of longer than 6 months.
   2. *Misdemeanors:* crimes of a less serious nature (e.g., shoplifting), usually punishable by fines or short prison term or both.

B. *Tort:* a wrong committed by one individual against another or another's property. Fraud, negligence, and malpractice are torts (e.g., losing a client's hearing aid, or bathing the client in water that causes burns).
   1. *Fraud:* misrepresentation of fact with intentions for it to be acted on by another person (e.g., falsifying college transcripts when applying for a graduate nursing program).
   2. *Negligence:* "Omission to do something that a reasonable person, guided by those *ordinary* considerations which ordinarily regulate human affairs would *do;* or doing something which a reasonable and prudent person would *not* do" (Brent N: *Nurses and the Law.* Saunders, Philadelphia, 1997). Types of negligent acts related to:
      a. Sponge counts: incorrect counts or failure to count.
      b. Burns: heating pads, solutions, steam vaporizers.
      c. Falls: side rails left down, infant left unattended.
      d. Failure to observe and take appropriate action—forgetting to take vital signs and check dressing in a client who is newly postoperative.
      e. Wrong medicine, wrong dose and concentration, wrong route, wrong client
      f. Mistaken identity—wrong client for surgery.
      g. Failure to communicate—ignore, forget, fail to report complaints of client or family.
      h. Loss of or damage to client's property—dentures, jewelry, money.
   3. *Malpractice:* part of the law of negligence as applied to the *professional* person; any professional misconduct, unreasonable lack of skill, or lack of fidelity in professional duties, such as accidentally giving wrong medication or forgetting to give correct medication or instilling wrong strength of eyedrops into the client's eyes. Proof of intent to do harm is not required in acts of commission or omission.

IV. **Invasion of privacy**—compromising a person's right to withhold self and own life from public scrutiny. *Implications for nursing—avoid* unnecessary discussion of client's medical condition; client has a right to refuse to participate in clinical teaching; obtain consent before teaching conference.

V. **Libel and slander**—wrongful action of communication that damages person's reputation by print, writing, or pictures (libel), or by spoken word using false words (slander). *Implications for nursing*—make comments about client only to another health team member caring for that client.

VI. **Privileged communications**—information relating to condition and treatment of client requires confidentiality and protection against invasion of privacy. This applies only to court proceedings. Selected person does not have to reveal in court a client's communication to him or her. The purpose of privileged communication is to encourage the client to communicate honestly with the treating practitioner. It is the client's privilege at any time to permit the professional to release information.

   Therefore, if the client asks the nurse to testify, the nurse must truthfully give all information. However, if the nurse is a witness against the client, without the client's permission to release information, the nurse must keep the information confidential by invoking the privileged communication rule if the state law recognizes it and if it applies to the nurse.

VII. **Assault and battery**—violating a person's right to refuse physical contact with another.
   A. Definitions
      1. *Assault*—the attempt to touch another or the threat to do so and person fears and believes harm will result.
      2. *Battery*—physical harm through willful touching of person or clothing, without consent.
   B. *Implications for nursing*—need to obtain consent to treat, with special provisions when clients are underage, unconscious, or mentally ill.

VIII. **Good Samaritan Act**—protects health practitioners against malpractice claims resulting from assistance provided at scene of an emergency (unless there was willful wrongdoing) as long as the level of care provided is the same as any other reasonably prudent person would give under similar circumstances (see also section VII, p. 130).

IX. **Nurses' responsibilities to the law**
   A. A nurse is liable for nursing acts, even if directed to do something by an MD.
   B. A nurse is *not* responsible for the negligence of the employer (hospital).
   C. A nurse is responsible for refusing to carry out an order for an activity believed to be injurious to the client.
   D. A nurse cannot legally diagnose illness or prescribe treatment for a client. (This is the MD's responsibility.)
   E. A nurse is legally responsible when participating in

a criminal act (such as assisting with criminal abortions or taking medications from client's supply for own use).

F. A nurse should reveal client's confidential information only to appropriate health-care team members.

G. A nurse is responsible for explaining nursing activities but not for commenting on medical activities in a way that may distress the client or the MD.

H. A nurse is responsible for recognizing and protecting the rights of clients to refuse treatment or medication, and for reporting their concerns and refusals to the MD or appropriate agency people.

I. A nurse must respect the dignity of each client and family.

X. **Organ donation**
  A. Legal aspects to protect potential donors and to expedite acquisition
    1. Prohibits selling of organs (National Organ Transplant Act).
    2. Guidelines regarding who can donate, how donations are to be made, and who can receive donated organs (Uniform Anatomical Gift Act).
    3. Legal definition of brain death (Uniform Determination of Death Act)—*absence of: breathing movement, cranial nerve reflex, response to any level of painful stimuli, and cerebral blood flow;* and *flat EEG.*
  B. Donor criteria
    1. Contraindications for being organ donor: *HIV-positive* status and *metastatic cancer.*
    2. Prospective donors of both organs and tissues: those with no neurological functions, but have cardiopulmonary functions.
    3. Prospective donors of only tissues: those with no cardiopulmonary function (e.g., can donate corneas, eyes, saphenous veins, cartilage, bones, skin, heart valves).
  C. Management of donor
    1. Maintain body temperature at greater than 96.8°F with room temperature at 70°–80°F, warming blankets, warmer for intravenous fluids.
    2. Maintain greater than 100% PaO_2 and suction/turn and use positive end-expiratory pressure (PEEP) to prevent *hypoxemia* caused by airway obstruction, *pulmonary edema.*
    3. Maintain central venous pressure at 8–10 mm Hg and systolic blood pressure at greater than 90 mm Hg to prevent *hypotension* caused by complete dilation of systemic vasculature due to destruction of brain's vasomotor center, cessation of antidiuretic hormone production, and decreased cardiac output. Give fluid bolus and vasopressors, and monitor sodium levels.
    4. Maintain fluid and electrolyte balance due to volume depletion. Monitor for *hyponatremia, hyperkalemia* and *hypokalemia,* and intake and output.
    5. Prevent infections due to invasive procedures (e.g., tubes, catheters) by using *aseptic* technique.

Questions Most Frequently Asked by Nurses About Nursing and the Law

I. **Taking orders**
  A. *Should I accept verbal phone orders from an MD?* Generally, no. Specifically, follow your hospital's by-laws, regulations, and policies regarding this. Failure to follow the hospital's rules could be considered negligence.
  B. *Should I follow an MD's orders if (a) I know it is wrong, or (b) I disagree with his or her judgment?* Regarding (a)—no, if you think a reasonable, prudent nurse would not follow it; but first inform the MD and record your decision. Report it to your supervisor. Regarding (b)—yes, because the law does not allow you to substitute your nursing judgment for a doctor's medical judgment. Do record that you questioned the order and that the doctor confirmed it before you carried it out.
  C. *What can I do if the MD delegates a task to me for which I am not prepared?* Inform the MD of your lack of education and experience in performing the task. Refuse to do it. If you inform the MD and still carry out the task, both you and the MD could be considered negligent if the client is harmed by it. If you do not tell the MD and carry out the task, you are solely liable.

II. **Obtaining client's consent for medical and surgical procedures:** *Is a nurse responsible for getting a consent for medical/surgical treatment?* Obtaining consent requires explaining the procedure and risks involved, which is the MD's responsibility. A nurse may accept responsibility for *witnessing* a consent. This carries with it little legal liability other than obtaining the correct signature and describing the client's condition at time of signing.

III. **Client's records (documentation)**
  A. *What should be written in the nurse's notes?* All facts and information regarding a person's condition, treatment, care, progress, and response to illness and treatment. Document consent or refusal of treatment. Purpose of record: factual documentation of care given to meet legal standards; used to refute unwarranted claims of negligence or malpractice.
  B. *How should data be recorded?* Entries should:
    1. State date and time given.
    2. Be written, signed, and titled by caregiver or supervisor who observed action.
    3. Follow chronological sequence.
    4. Be accurate, factual, objective, complete, precise, and clear.
    5. Be legible; use black pen.
    6. Use universal abbreviations.
    7. Have all spaces filled in on documentation forms; leave no blank spaces.

IV. **Confidential information**
  A. *If called on the witness stand in court, do I have to reveal confidential information?* It depends on your

state, because each state has its own laws pertaining to this. Consult a lawyer. Inform the judge and ask for specific directions before relating in court information that was given to you within a confidential, professional relationship.

B. *Am I justified in refusing (on the basis of "invasion of privacy") to give information about the client to another health agency to which a client is being transferred?* No. You are responsible for providing continuity of care when the client is moved from one facility to another. Necessary and adequate information should be transferred between professional health-care workers. The client's consent for this exchange of information should be obtained. Circumstances under which confidential information can be released include:

1. By authorization and consent of the client.
2. By order of the court.
3. By statutory mandate, as in reporting cases of child abuse or communicable diseases.

V. **What is the Health Insurance Portability and Accountability Act (HIPAA)?**

A. Importance of this act for nurses: nurses need to be able to answer client questions regarding the national privacy standards. The principles of the law reinforce professional responsibility to avoid unintentional disclosure of information (e.g., in elevators and hallways).

B. Overview of HIPAA: The first-ever federal privacy standards to protect clients' medical records and other health information provided to health plans, doctors, hospitals, clinics, nursing homes, pharmacies, and other health-care providers took effect on April 14, 2003. Developed by the Department of Health and Human Services (HHS), these new standards provide clients with **access** to their medical records and **more control** over how their personal health information is used and disclosed. The standards represent a uniform, federal floor of privacy protections for consumers across the country. State laws providing additional protections to consumers are not affected by this new rule.

C. Client protections: The new privacy regulations ensure a national floor of privacy protections for clients by limiting the ways that health plans, pharmacies, hospitals, and other covered entities can use clients' personal medical information. The regulations protect medical records and other individually identifiable health information, whether it is on paper, in computers, or communicated orally. Key provisions and points related to these new standards include:

1. **Access to medical records**. Clients generally should be able to see and obtain copies of their medical records within 30 days of request, and to request corrections if they identify errors and mistakes. The covered entities must consider the changes, but do not have to agree to the changes, and they may charge clients for the cost of copying and sending the records.

2. **Notice of privacy practices.** Covered entities must provide a notice to their clients stating how they may use personal medical information and their rights under the new privacy regulation. Clients also may ask covered entities to restrict the use or disclosure of their information beyond the practices included in the notice, as long as the restriction does not interfere with activities related to treatment, payment, or operations (e.g., family members may not be given information about a diagnosis without client permission).

3. **Limits on use of personal medical information.** The privacy rule sets limits on how covered entities may use individually identifiable health information. The client has a right to have access to accounting (i.e., the right to know *who* has been given access to their protected health information). The health-care facility must be able to produce a *list* describing people, companies, or agencies who have received protected information. In addition, clients must sign a specific authorization before a covered entity can release their medical information to a life insurer, a bank, or another outside business for purposes not related to their health care.

4. **Prohibition on marketing.** HIPAA sets new restrictions and limits on the use of client information for *marketing* purposes. Covered entities must first obtain an individual's specific authorization before disclosing their client information for marketing. At the same time, the rule permits doctors and other covered entities to communicate freely with clients about treatment options and other health-related information, including disease-management programs.

5. **Stronger state laws may remain in effect.** The new federal privacy standards do not affect state laws that provide additional privacy protections for clients. The privacy rule will set a national "floor" of privacy standards that protect all Americans, but any state law that provides additional protections would continue to apply. When a state law requires a certain disclosure—such as reporting an infectious disease outbreak to the public health authorities—the federal privacy regulations would not preempt the state law.

6. **Confidential communications.** Under the privacy rule, a client can request that covered entities take reasonable steps to ensure that communications with the client are confidential. The client has the right to request that communications about protected health information remain anonymous if mailed.

7. **"Minimum necessary" rule.** It guides the provider to use only the minimum amount of information necessary to meet the client care needs. The actual diagnosis may not be needed. This would relate to the use of e-mail or faxes to communicate client information.

8. **Telephone requests for personal health information.** Inpatient confidentiality must be protected. The nurse may be able to verify whether a client is in the hospital, but only if the caller asks for the client by name; otherwise the caller should be directed to the client or family.

9. **Complaints about violations of privacy.** A health-care facility must identify the privacy officer and state how to contact the officer.

D. There are additional situations where medical information may be disclosed without authorization, such as:

1. For workers' compensation or similar programs.
2. For public health activities (e.g., reporting births or deaths; injury or disability; abuse or neglect of children, elders and dependent adults; or reactions to medications), to prevent or control disease or injury.
3. To a health oversight agency, such as the State Department of Health Services.
4. In response to a court or administrative order, subpoena, warrant or similar process.
5. To law enforcement officials in certain limited circumstances.
6. To a coroner, medical examiner, or funeral director.
7. To organizations that handle organ, eye, or tissue procurement or transplantation.
8. Public health: information may be used or disclosed to avert a serious threat to health or safety of an individual or the public.
9. Food and Drug Administration (FDA): health information relating to adverse events with respect to immunizations and/or health screening tests may be disclosed.
10. For members of the armed forces, health information may be disclosed as required by military command authorities.
11. To notify a person who may have been exposed to a disease or may be at risk for contracting or spreading a disease or condition.

VI. **Liability for mistakes**—yours and others.

A. *Is the hospital or the nurse liable for mistakes made by the nurse while following orders?* Both the hospital and the nurse can be sued for damage if a mistake made by the nurse injures the client. The nurse is responsible for own actions. The hospital would be liable, based on the doctrine of *respondeat superior.*

B. *Who is responsible if a nursing student or another staff nurse makes a mistake? The supervisor? The instructor?* Ordinarily the instructor and/or supervisor would not be responsible unless the court thought the instructor and/or supervisor was negligent in supervising or in assigning a task beyond the capability of the person in question. No one is responsible for another's negligence unless he or she contributed to or participated in that negligence. Each person is personally liable for his or her own

negligent actions and failure to act as a reasonably prudent nurse.

C. *Am I responsible for injury to a client by a staff member who was observed (but not reported) by me to be intoxicated while giving care?* Yes, you may be responsible. You have a duty to take reasonable action to prevent a client's injury.

VII. **Good Samaritan Act:** *For what would I be liable if I voluntarily stopped to give care at the scene of an accident?* You would be protected under the Good Samaritan Act and required to live up to reasonable and prudent nursing standards in those specific circumstances. You would not be treated by the law as if you were performing under professional standards of properly sterile conditions, with proper technical equipment (see also **Section VIII, p. 127**).

VIII. **Leaving against medical advice (AMA):** *Would I or the hospital be liable if a client left "AMA," refusing to sign the appropriate hospital forms?* None of the involved parties would ordinarily be liable in this case as long as (a) the medical risks were explained, recorded, and witnessed, and (b) the client is a competent adult. The law permits clients to make decisions that may not be in their own best health interest. You cannot interfere with the right and exercise of the decision to accept or reject treatment.

IX. **Restraints:** *Can I put restraints on a client who is combative even if there is no order for this?* Only in an emergency, for a limited time (not longer than 24 hours), for the limited purpose of protecting the client from injury—*not* for convenience of personnel. Notify attending MD immediately. Consult with another staff member, obtain client's consent if possible, and get co-worker to witness the record. Check frequently to ensure restraints do not impair circulation, cause pressure sores, or other injury. Remove restraints at the first opportunity, and use them only as a last resort after other reasonable means have not been effective. Restraints of any degree may constitute *false imprisonment.* Freedom from unlawful restraint is a basic human right protected by law. In July 1992, the Food and Drug Administration (FDA) issued a warning that use of restraints "no longer represents responsible, primary management of a client's behavioral problem." It is necessary to advise the client and family of decision to restrain, explain risks and benefits, and obtain informed consent.

In July 1996, the Joint Commission on Accreditation of Healthcare Organizations (JCAHO) recommended standards to minimize injury and complications from the use of restraints:

- Use *alternatives* to physical restraints whenever possible (e.g., offer explanations; ask someone to stay with client; use clocks, calendars, TV, and radio).
- Use only under supervision of *licensed* health-care provider.
- Use according to manufacturer's direction to avoid strangulation or circulation impairment.
- Documentation must include: time applied and

removed; type; medical reason (description of dangerous behavior) and alternatives tried before application of restraints; response.

▶ **A.** *Nursing responsibilities*
1. Provide padding to protect skin, bony prominences, and intravenous lines.
2. Secure restraints to parts of bed or chair that will move with the client and not constrict movement. *Never* secure restraints to bed rails or mattress.
3. Use knots with hitches for easy removal, as required.
4. Maintain proper body alignment when securing restraints.
5. Remove restraints at least every 2 hours to allow for activities of daily living.

X. Wills: *What do I do when a client asks me to be a witness to her or his will?* There is no legal obligation to participate as a witness, but there is a moral and ethical obligation to do so. You should not, however, help draw up a will because this could be considered practicing law without a license. You would be witnessing that (a) the client is signing the document as her or his last will and testament; (b) at that time, to the best of your knowledge, the client (testator) was of sound mind, was lucid, and understood what the client was doing (i.e., the client must not be under the influence of drugs or alcohol or otherwise unable to know what she or he is doing); and (c) the testator was under no overt coercion, as far as you could tell, but was acting freely, willingly, and under own impetus.

XI. Disciplinary action

A. *For what reasons may the RN license be suspended or revoked?*
1. Obtaining license by fraud (omission of information, false information).
2. Negligence and incompetence; assuming duties without adequate preparation.
3. Substance abuse.
4. Conviction of crime (state or federal).
5. Practicing medicine without a license.
6. Practicing nursing without a license (expired, suspended).
7. Allowing unlicensed person to practice nursing or medicine that places the client at risk.
8. Giving client care while under the influence of alcohol or other drugs.
9. Habitually using drugs.
10. Discriminatory and prejudicial practices in giving client care (pertaining to race, skin color, religion, sex, age, or ethnic origin).
11. Falsifying a client's record; failure to maintain a record for each client.
12. Breach in client confidentiality.
13. Physically or verbally abusing a client.
14. Abandoning a client.

B. *What could happen to me if I am proven guilty of professional misconduct?*

1. License may be revoked.
2. License may be suspended.
3. Behavior may be censured and reprimanded.
4. You may be placed on probation.

C. *Who has the authority to carry out any of the aforementioned penalties?* The State Board of Registered Nursing that granted your license.

D. *I am the head nurse. One of my nursing aides has a history of failing to appear to work and not giving notice of or reason for absence. How should I handle this?* An employee has the right to know hospital policies, what is expected of an employee, and what will happen if an employee does not meet the expectations stated in his or her job description or in hospital policies and procedures. As a head nurse, you must document behavior factually, clearly, and concisely, as well as any discussion and decision about future course of action. The employee must have the chance to read and sign this documentation. The head nurse then sends a copy to her or his supervisor.

XII. Floating: *Is a nurse hired to work in psychiatry obligated to cover in the intensive care unit (ICU) when the latter is understaffed?* The issue is the hiring contract (implied or expressed). The contract is a composite of the mutual understanding by involved parties of rights and responsibilities, any written documents, and hospital policies. If the nurse was hired as a psychiatric nurse, he or she could legally refuse to go to the ICU. If the hospital intends to float personnel, such a policy shouldbe clearly stated during the hiring process. Also at this time the employer should determine the employee's education, skills, and experience. On the other hand, if emergency staffing problems exist, a nurse should go to the ICU regardless of personal preference, but should request orientation and not assume responsibility beyond level of experience or education.

XIII. Dispensing medication: *Can a nurse legally remove a drug from a pharmacy when the pharmacy is closed (during the night) if the MD insists that the nurse go to the pharmacy to get the specifically prescribed medication immediately?* Within the legal boundaries of the Pharmacy Act, a nurse may remove one dose of a particular drug from the pharmacy for a particular client during an unanticipated emergency within a limited time and availability of resources. However, the hospital should have a written policy for the nurse to follow and should authorize a specific person to use the services of the pharmacy under certain circumstances.

XIV. Illegible orders: *What should I do if I cannot decipher the MD's handwriting when she or he persists in leaving illegible orders?* Talk to the MD regarding the dangers of your giving the wrong amount of the wrong medication via the wrong route at the wrong time. If that does not help, follow appropriate channels. Do **not** follow an order you cannot read. You will be liable for following orders you thought were written.

Legal Aspects

XV. Heroic measures: *The wife of a client who is terminally ill approaches me with the request that heroic measures not be used on her husband. She has not discussed this with him but knows that he feels the same way. Can I act on this request?* No. The client is the only one who can legally make the decision as long as he or she is mentally competent.

XVI. Medication: *An MD orders pain medication prn for a client. The client asks for the medication, but when I question her she says the pain "isn't so bad." If in my judgment the client's pain is not severe, am I legally covered if I give half of the pain medication dosage ordered by the MD?* A nurse cannot substitute his or her judgment for the MD's judgment. If you alter the amount of medication prescribed by the MD without a specific order to do so, you may be liable for practicing medicine without a license.

XVII. Malfunctioning equipment: *At the end-of-shift report the nurse going off duty tells me that the tracheal suctioning machine is malfunctioning and describes how she got it to work. Should I plan to use the machine in the evening shift and follow her suggestions about how to make it work?* Do not plan to use equipment that you know is not functioning properly. You could be held liable because you could reasonably foresee that proper functioning of equipment would be needed for your client. You have been put on notice that there are defects. Report this to the supervisor or person responsible for maintaining equipment in proper working order. (Also **see p. 121: Safe Use of Equipment**)

Ethical and Legal Considerations in Intensive Care of the *Acutely Ill* Neonate

I. Responsibilities of the health agency
  A. Provide a neonatal intensive care unit (NICU) or transfer to another hospital.
  B. *Personnel—adequate number trained in neonate diseases, special treatment, and equipment.*
  C. Equipment—adequate supply on hand, functioning properly (especially temperature regulator in incubator, oxygen analyzer, blood-gas machine).

II. Infants who are dying
  A. Decision regarding resuscitation in cardiac arrest, with brain damage from cerebral anoxia. It is difficult to predict the effect of anoxia in infancy on the child's later life.
  B. Decision to continue supportive measures.
  C. Issue of euthanasia, such as in severe myelomeningocele at birth.
    1. Active euthanasia (giving overdose).
    2. Passive euthanasia (not placing on respirator).

III. Extended role of nurse in NICU—may raise issues of nursing practice versus medical practice, as when a nurse draws blood samples for blood gas determinations without prior order. To be legally covered:

  A. The nurse must be trained to perform specialized functions.
  B. The functions must be written into the nurse's job description.

IV. Issue of negligence—such as cross-contamination in nursery.

V. Issue of malpractice—such as assigning care of an infant who is critically ill on respirator to a student or aide who is untrained.
  A. May be liable for inaccurate bilirubin studies for neonatal jaundice; may be legally responsible if brain damage occurs in absence of accurate laboratory tests.
  B. May be liable for brain damage in an infant due to respiratory or cardiac distress. Nurse must make sure that there are frequent blood gas determinations to ensure adequate oxygen to prevent brain damage. Nurse also must make sure that the infant is not receiving too high a concentration of oxygen, which may lead to retrolental fibroplasia.

Legal Aspects of Psychiatric Care

I. Four sets of criteria to determine criminal responsibility at time of alleged offense
  A. *M'Naghten Rule* (1832)—a person is not guilty if:
    1. Person did not know the *nature and quality* of the act.
    2. Person could not distinguish right from wrong— if person did not know what he or she was doing, person did not know it was wrong.
  B. *The Irresistible Impulse Test* (used together with M' Naghten Rule)—person knows right from wrong, but:
    1. Driven by *impulse* to commit criminal acts regardless of consequences.
    2. Lacked premeditation in sudden violent behavior.
  C. *American Law Institute's Model Penal Code (1955) Test*
    1. Not responsible for criminal act if person lacks capacity to "appreciate" the wrongfulness of it or to "conform" conduct to requirements of law.
    2. Excludes "an abnormality manifested only by repeated criminal or antisocial conduct"— namely, psychopathology.
    3. Includes "knowledge" and "control" criteria.
  D. *Durham Test* (Product Rule—1954): accused is not criminally responsible if act was a "product of mental disease." Discarded in 1972.

II. Types of admissions
  A. *Voluntary:* person, parent, or legal guardian applies for admission; person agrees to receive treatment and to follow hospital rules; civil rights are retained.
  B. *Involuntary:* process and criteria vary among states **(Figure 3.1).**

III. Legal and civil rights of clients who are hospitalized— the right to:
  A. Wear own clothes, keep and use personal possessions and reasonable sum of money for small purchases.

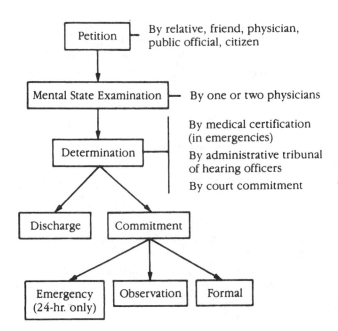

FIGURE 3.1 Typical procedure for involuntary commitment.

B. Have individual storage space for private use.

C. See visitors daily.

D. Have reasonable access to confidential phone conversations.

E. Receive unopened correspondence and have access to stationery, stamps, and a mailbox.

F. Refuse shock treatments, lobotomy.

IV. **Concepts central to community mental health (Community Mental Health Act, 1980)**

A. *Systems* perspective: scope of care moves beyond the individual to the community, with influences from biological, psychological, and sociocultural forces.

B. Emphasis on *prevention: primary* (reduce incidents by preventing harmful social conditions); *secondary* (early identification and treatment of disorders to reduce duration); *tertiary* (early rehabilitation to reduce impairment from disorders).

C. *Interdisciplinary collaboration:* flexible roles based on unique areas of expertise.

D. *Consumer participation and control.*

E. *Comprehensive services:* ambulatory care, partial hospitalization, 24-hour hospitalization and emergency care; consultation and education; screening services.

F. *Continuity of care.*

Legal Aspects of Preparing a Client for Surgery

I. No surgical procedure, however minor, can proceed without the voluntary, informed, and written consent of the client.

A. Surgical permits are witnessed by the physician, nurse, or other authorized person.

B. Surgical permits protect the client against unsanctioned surgery and also protect the surgeon and hospital staff against claims of unauthorized operations.

C. *Informed consent* means that the operation has been fully explained to the client, including possible complications and disfigurements, as well as whether any organ or parts of the body are to be removed.

D. Adults and emancipated minors may sign their own operative permits if they are mentally competent; permission for surgery of minor children and adults who are incompetent or unconscious must be obtained from a responsible family member or guardian.

E. The signed operative permit is placed in a prominent place on the client's chart and accompanies the client to the operating room.

F. *Legal issues in the emergency room: record keeping* plays an essential role in both the prevention and defense of malpractice suits. Detailed documentation not only provides for continuity of care but also perpetuates evidence that care was appropriately given. Records should:

1. Be written legibly.
2. Clearly note events and time of occurrence.
3. Contain all lab slips and results of other tests.
4. Describe events and clients objectively.
5. Clearly note physician's parting instructions to the client.
6. Be signed where appropriate, such as with doctor's orders.
7. Contain descriptions of every event that might lead to a lawsuit, such as fights, injuries, equipment failures.

G. *Consent*—although there is no law requiring written consent before performing medical treatment, all elective procedures can only be performed if the client has been fully informed and voluntarily consents to the procedure.

1. If informed consent cannot be obtained because of the client's condition and immediate treatment is necessary to save life or safeguard health, the emergency rule can be applied. This rule implies consent. However, if time allows, it is advisable to obtain either oral or written informed consent from someone who has authority to act for the client.

2. Verbal consents should be recorded in detail, witnessed and signed by *two* individuals.

3. Written or verbal consent can be given by alert, coherent, or otherwise competent adults, by parents, legal guardian, or person in *loco parentis* (one standing in for the parent with the parent's rights, duties, and responsibilities) of minors or adults who are incompetent.

4. If the minor is 14 years old or older, consent must be acquired from the minor as well as from the parent or legal guardian. *Emancipated minors* can consent for themselves.

TRENDS IN NURSING PRACTICE

I. Overall characteristics
A. Some trends are subtle and slow to emerge; others are obvious and quickly emerge.
B. Trends may conflict; some will prevail, others get modified by social forces.

II. General trends
A. *Broadened focus of care*—from care of ill to care of sick and healthy, from care of individual to care of family. Focus on prevention of illness, promotion of optimum level of health, holism.
B. *Increasing scientific base*—in bio-social-physical sciences, not mere reliance on intuition, experience, and observation.
C. *Increasingly complex technical skills* and use of *technologically advanced equipment,* such as monitors and computers.
D. *Increased independence* in use of judgment, such as teaching nutrition in pregnancy and providing primary prenatal care.
E. *New roles,* such as *nurse-clinician,* require advanced skills in a particular area of practice. *Examples:* psychiatric nurse consults with staff about problems; *primary care* nurse takes medical histories and does physical assessment; one nurse coordinates 24-hour care during hospital stay; *independent nurse practitioner* has her or his own office in community where clients come for care; case management.
F. *Community nursing services* rather than hospital-based; needs of the healthy are served as well as those of the ill.
G. *Development of nursing standards* to reflect specific nursing functions and activities.
   1. Ensure *safe* standard of care to clients and families.
   2. Provide criteria to measure *excellence* and *effectiveness* of care.

III. Trends in care of childbearing family
A. *Consumerism:*
   1. Consumer push for humanization and individualization of health care during the childbearing cycle to reflect client's role in decision making, preferences, and cultural diversity.
   2. Emphasis on family-centered care (including father, siblings, grandparents).
   3. Increase in options available for conduct of birth experience and setting for birth: birthing homes, alternative birth center (ABC) in hospitals; birthing chairs; side-lying position for birth; family-centered cesarean birth; health-care provider (MD, RN, lay midwife); length of postpartum stay.
   4. Increased consumer awareness of legal issues, client's rights.
   5. Major nursing role: client advocate.
B. *Social trends:*
   1. Alternative lifestyles of families—single parenthood, communal living, surrogate motherhood, marriages without children.
   2. Earlier sexual experimentation—availability of assistance to emancipated minors.
   3. Increase in number of older (>38 yr) primiparas.
   4. Legalization of abortion; availability to emancipated minors.
   5. Smaller families.
   6. Rising divorce rates.
C. *Technologies:*
   1. Development of genetic and bioengineering techniques.
   2. Development of prenatal diagnostic techniques, with options for management of each pregnancy.
   3. In vitro fertilization and embryo transplantation.

IV. Trends in community mental health (1960s–1990s)
A. Shift from institutional to community-based care.
B. Preventive services.
C. Consumer participation in planning and delivery of services.
D. Original 12 essential services (1975) reduced to 5 (indicated by asterisk [*]) (1981).
   *1. 24-hour inclient care.
   *2. Ambulatory care.
   *3. Partial hospitalization (day or night).
   4. Emergency care.
   *5. Consultation and education.
   6. Follow-up care.
   7. Transitional services.
   8. Services for children and adolescents.
   9. Services for elderly.
   *10. Screening services (courts).
   11. Alcohol abuse services.
   12. Drug abuse services.
E. Protecting human rights of persons in need of mental health care.
F. Developing an advocacy program for those who are chronically mentally ill.
G. Improving delivery of services to underserved and high-risk populations (e.g., minorities).

V. ANA Standards of Clinical Nursing Practice*
A. Use of *nursing process:* assessment, nursing diagnosis, planning, implementation, evaluation, outcome identification.
B. Performance appraisal review.
C. Continuing education.
D. Collegiality; *peer review.*
E. Ethics.
F. Interdisciplinary collaboration.
G. Research.
H. Resource utilization—utilization of community health systems.

VI. *Four levels* of nursing practice
A. *Promotion of health* to increase level of wellness. *Example:* provide dietary information to reduce risks of coronary artery diseases.

---

*Adapted from the complete description in American Nurses Association: *2004 Nursing: Scope and Standards of Practice.* American Nurses Association, Washington, DC, 2004. Reprinted with permission. (Rationale and assessment factors for the Standards of Clinical Nursing Practice are available from the American Nurses Association.)

B. *Prevention of illness or injury. Example:* immunizations.

C. *Restoration of health. Example:* teach how to change dressing, care for wound.

D. *Consolation of dying*—assist person to attain peaceful death.

VII. *Four components* of nursing care

A. *Nursing care activities*—assist with basic needs, give medications and treatments; observe response and adaptation to illness and treatments; teach self-care; guide rehabilitation activities for daily living.

B. *Case management*—*a process that includes coordination of total client care*—all health team members should work together toward common goals.

C. *Continuity of care*—process of ensuring that ongoing physical, medical, and emotional health-care needs are assessed, planned for, and coordinated with all providers, for desired outcomes, without interruption of service when the location of care is transferred.

D. *Evaluation of care*—flexibility and responsiveness to changing needs: clients' reactions and perceptions of their needs.

VIII. *Three main nursing roles* in relation to care of clients and their families (emphasis of each role varies with the situation, with adaptation of skills and modes of care as necessary)

A. *Therapeutic role* (instrumental). *Function:* work toward "cure" in acute setting.

B. *Caring role* (expressive). *Function:* provide support through human relations, show concern, demonstrate acceptance of differences.

C. *Socializing role. Function:* offer distractions and respite from focus on illness.

NURSING ORGANIZATIONS

I. **International Council of Nurses (ICN)**

A. *Purpose:* to provide a medium through which national nursing associations can work together and share common interests; formed in 1899

B. *Functions*

1. Serves as representatives of and spokespersons for nurses at international level.
2. Promotes organization of national nurses' associations.
3. Assists national organizations to develop and improve services for public health practice of nursing and social/economic welfare of nurses.

II. **World Health Organization (WHO)**—special intergovernmental agency of the United Nations, formed in 1948

A. *Purpose:* to bring all people to the highest possible level of health

B. *Functions:* provides assistance in the form of education, training, improving health standards, fighting disease, and reducing water pollution in member countries

III. **American Nurses Association (ANA)**—national professional association in the United States, composed of the nurses' associations of the 50 states, Guam, Virgin Islands, Puerto Rico, and Washington, DC

A. *Purpose:* to foster high standards of nursing practice and promote the education and welfare of nurses

B. *Functions:* officially represents professional nurses in the United States and internationally; defines practice of nursing; lobbies and promotes legislation affecting nurses' welfare and practice

IV. **National League for Nursing (NLN)**—composed of both individuals and agencies

A. *Purpose:* to foster the development and improvement of all nursing services and nursing education

B. *Functions*

1. Provides educational workshops.
2. Assists in recruitment for nursing programs.
3. Provides testing services for both RN and LPN (LVN) nursing programs.

Questions

Select the one answer that is best for each question, unless otherwise directed.

1. A physician orders the elixir form of a medication. The nurse, familiar only with the injectable form of the medication, believes the order is incorrect. The nurse should:
   1. Ask the two physicians who are currently on the unit whether the medication should be given as the nurse understood the order.
   2. Ask the head nurse if the order is correct.
   3. Call the physician who ordered the medication.
   4. Contact the nursing supervisor about the problem.

2. A client had been receiving a drug by injection over a number of weeks. As the clinical symptoms changed, the physician wrote an order on the client's order sheet changing the mode of administration from injection to oral. When the nurse on the unit, who had been off duty for several days, was preparing to give the medication by injection, the client objected and referred the nurse to the physician's new orders. The nurse should:
   1. Go back to the order sheet and check for the order.
   2. Talk with the nurse who had taken care of this particular client while he or she had been off duty.
   3. Talk with the head nurse about the advisability of using oral rather than injectable medications.
   4. Check the order sheet for the changed order and then speak with the attending physician concerning the changed order.

3. A nurse had been caring for a client whose vital signs had previously been unstable. The nurse had not had a coffee break or a lunch break all day. By 2 P.M. the client had been stable for a number of hours. The physician in charge had seen the client and had told the nurse that the client appeared "much improved." The nurse should:
   1. Leave for lunch break.
   2. Forego lunch break because of the client's previous unstable condition.
   3. Arrange to eat lunch in the client's room.
   4. Discuss the situation with the nurse in charge of the unit and determine who should cover the client while the staff nurse is at lunch.

4. In a certain hospital, whenever there are clients in the recovery room, two nurses are usually present. The hospital policy expects the nurses to take their breaks before clients arrive from surgery. On this particular day, there are two nurses on duty and two clients in the recovery room who have had minor surgeries performed that morning. One nurse had not had a coffee break that morning. That nurse should:
   1. Stay because hospital policy expects there to be two nurses in attendance while there are clients in the recovery room.
   2. Leave for coffee break because there are only two clients in the recovery room and one nurse can handle two clients quite easily.
   3. Talk with the nursing supervisor and secure permission from him or her.
   4. Leave to get coffee and come right back.

5. While driving down a freeway, a nurse spots an overturned car with the driver lying next to the car. The nurse:
   1. May drive on without stopping, or stop and render emergency first aid, without liability.
   2. May stop, start to render aid, and then leave, without liability.
   3. Must stop at the scene of an accident and render first aid.
   4. May stop and render aid, but if he or she performs a medical act, he or she may be charged with illegal practice of medicine.

6. For which reason would a nurse's license be revoked or the nurse be put on probation?
   1. The nurse lost a malpractice suit.
   2. The nurse was found guilty of practicing while under the influence of drugs or alcohol.
   3. The nurse was accused of negligence.
   4. The nurse gave a wrong medication.

7. A nurse who applies restraints on a client *may* be held liable by the client for restraint of freedom of movement (false imprisonment) if the nurse:
   1. Does not immediately obtain an order from the physician.
   2. Does so after other means to subdue the client have failed.
   3. Tries but fails to obtain the client's consent.
   4. Applies restraints for the convenience of the personnel.

8. The nurse has been working with a man who is terminally ill for weeks. The client is lucid. His wife pleads with the nurse not to use heroic measures on her husband but to let him die "with dignity." The nurse should:
   1. Tell the wife that she needs to talk with the attending physician, client (if possible), and other significant people about her concerns.
   2. Act on the wife's request.
   3. Ignore the wife's request and proceed with the client's care.
   4. Tell the wife that to do as she requested would be equivalent to murdering the client.

9. Which statement concerning consent is *false*?
   1. If an informed consent is not obtained from the client, the nurse, doctor, and/or hospital may be liable for assault.
   2. One need only obtain a general consent to treatment.
   3. In an emergency a nurse may do what she or he can do to save life and limb, even in cases in which she or he has no consent.
   4. Consent may be given by conduct as well as expressed words.

10. A nurse gave a client the wrong medication. The client was seriously injured. The client sued. Who will most likely be held liable?
    1. The nurse.
    2. No one, because it was just an accident.
    3. The hospital.
    4. The nurse and the hospital.

11. The supervisor of a cardiovascular unit, responsible for checking staffing patterns, assigned a particular staff nurse to work on the unit because that nurse had many years of experience on that unit. That evening, this staff nurse made a treatment error and a client was injured. Who is liable?
    1. The staff nurse.
    2. The staff nurse and the supervisor.
    3. The staff nurse and the hospital.
    4. The staff nurse, the supervisor, and the hospital.

12. Nurse A noticed that Nurse B was intoxicated while giving care. However, Nurse A did not report this fact to the supervisor. That same day, Nurse B made a medication error and a client was injured. Who *may* be held responsible?
    1. Nurse B (the one who is intoxicated).
    2. Nurse A, Nurse B, and the hospital.
    3. Nurse A (the one who did not report Nurse B).
    4. Nurse B (the one who is intoxicated) and the hospital.

13. A graduate nurse who was new to a unit was caring for an elderly client. The physician on call ordered a treatment that the nurse had not heard of. The nurse should:
    1. Inform the physician of the nurse's lack of education and experience and refuse to do the treatment without supervision.
    2. Inform the physician of the nurse's lack of education and experience and then proceed to perform the treatment.
    3. Refuse to perform the treatment.
    4. Carry out the treatment to the best of the nurse's ability.

14. The day nurse tells the night nurse that the suction equipment in a client's room is not working properly. The night nurse, who will be working with this client, should:
    1. Follow the day nurse's suggestions on how to get the malfunctioning equipment to work.
    2. Continue to use the malfunctioning machine, hoping that it will function for the night shift.
    3. Ask the supervisor how to work with the malfunctioning equipment.
    4. Replace the equipment or report it to whomever is responsible for maintaining equipment in proper working condition.

15. An adult client who is competent has refused treatment and wishes to leave AMA (against medical advice). The client has also refused to sign any of the appropriate AMA forms. Which statement is inaccurate?
    1. The physician and/or hospital is always liable for any injury that might occur as a result of the client's decision to leave AMA.
    2. The law usually permits adult clients who are competent to make decisions that may not be in their own best health interest.
    3. Even if the client is an adult who is competent, the law may interfere with the client's decision to refuse medical treatment if the client has small children who need care.
    4. The physician might be held liable if it can be proven that the client did not receive sufficient information about risks involved with leaving AMA.

16. The only Spanish-speaking nurse in the emergency department admitted a 6-year-old child. The child's mother explained in Spanish that she had removed two ticks from the child the previous day. The child was now running a very high temperature and had a rash on the abdomen. The nurse reported the information to the emergency department physician, who did not speak Spanish. The nurse failed to tell the doctor about the ticks. The physician diagnosed the child as having measles. Over the course of the day, the child's health deteriorated until the child died. Who is liable?
    1. The nurse.
    2. The nurse and the physician.
    3. The nurse and the hospital.
    4. The physician.

17. A nurse was on weekend call for the operating room. Late Saturday night, the nursing supervisor called the nurse to say

that they were expecting a client who needed an emergency appendectomy within the hour. While gowning the surgeon, the nurse smelled alcohol on the doctor's breath. The nurse mentioned this to the anesthesiologist, who also admitted smelling alcohol on the surgeon. Both the nurse and the anesthesiologist felt the surgeon was somewhat unstable on his feet. However, neither the nurse nor the other doctor said anything. If the client had been injured during the surgery, who would have been liable?
1. Nurse, anesthesiologist, surgeon, and hospital.
2. Nurse and surgeon.
3. Surgeon and hospital.
4. Hospital, surgeon, and anesthesiologist.

18. A child about 11 months old was brought by the mother to a hospital for examination, diagnosis, and treatment. The child was seen by a nurse and physician. At the time, the child was suffering from a comminuted spiral fracture of the right tibia and fibula that gave the appearance of having been caused by twisting. The child also had numerous bruises and burns on the body. In addition, there was a nondepressed linear fracture of the skull in the process of healing. When approached, the child demonstrated fear and apprehension. The mother had no explanation for the child's wounds. No further x-rays were taken, and the child was released to the mother without making a report to concerned agencies. One month later the child was brought in again by the mother and was seen by a different physician. The second physician correctly diagnosed the battered-child syndrome and filed the proper reports. The child was placed in a foster home, and the foster home filed suit. Who may be liable?
1. First nurse, first doctor, and hospital.
2. First doctor.
3. No one.
4. First nurse.

19. While getting a client ready for surgery, the nurse removed the client's dentures. The nurse wrapped the dentures in a towel so as not to break them and left them on the bedside stand. While the nurse was out of the room, two nursing aides stripped the bed and threw all the linen, including the towel, in the laundry hamper. Upon returning from surgery, the client requested the dentures. However, the nurse and nursing aides were unable to find them. Who is liable?
1. The nurse.
2. The nurse and the hospital.
3. The nurse and nursing aides.
4. The nurse, nursing aides, and hospital.

20. A teenage girl who had complained of dizziness the previous day wanted to take a shower. The physician gave permission for the client to shower with assistance. The nurse started to get the girl out of bed and over to the shower. The nurse questioned the client about her dizziness. The girl replied that she was not dizzy. The mother then said that she would watch her daughter in the shower and help her back to bed. The nurse then left the room. While the nurse was out, the client fainted getting back into bed. The client injured her head. Who is liable?
1. The nurse.
2. The doctor, nurse, and hospital.
3. The nurse and the hospital.
4. No one.

21. What does voluntary admission require of the individual?
1. The individual must ask to be admitted to a psychiatric hospital and must agree to abide by its rules.
2. The request for hospitalization must originate with the individual to be admitted.
3. The individual must make written application to a hospital, agree to treatment, and agree to abide by the rules.
4. The individual is responsible for the hospital bill.

22. Standards of practice for psychiatric mental health nursing have been developed by:
1. A joint commission of psychiatric nurses and psychiatrists.
2. Psychiatric nurses who are members of the American Nurses Association.
3. A panel of representative psychiatric nurses in the United States.
4. The Division on Psychiatric and Mental Health Nursing Practice of the American Nurses Association.

23. The standards of practice for psychiatric mental health nursing are organized around:
1. Different models of treatment.
2. Rights of the clients.
3. The nursing process.
4. Legal aspects of treatment.

24. The ICN's Code for Nurses, "Ethical Concepts Applied to Nursing," approved by the Council of Nurse Representatives states that:
1. The professional body of nurses of a particular country carries the responsibility for nursing practice and for maintaining competence.
2. The hospital employing the nurse carries the responsibility for nursing practice and for maintaining competence.
3. The laws of the country in which the nurse works carry the responsibility for nursing practice and for maintaining competence.
4. The individual nurse carries personal responsibility for nursing practice and for maintaining competence by continual learning.

25. The National Health Planning and Resource Development Act of 1974 allows:
1. Physicians the largest representation on local and state health-care boards that make decisions about health care.
2. Hospital administrators the largest representation on local and state health-care boards that make decisions about health care.
3. The consumer the largest representation on local and state health-care boards that make health-care decisions.
4. Health professionals as a group the largest representation on local and state health-care boards that make health-care decisions.

26. A client who is terminally ill tells the nurse during a home health-care visit that he does not want CPR when the time comes. What should be the nurse's next action?
1. Document the request in the health-care plan.
2. Talk to the family about this request.
3. Obtain an order from the MD.
4. Share this information with other members of the home health-care team.

27. Which situation would be an example of professional malpractice by a nurse?
1. An infant is injured as a result of incorrect information provided to the parents by the nurse on the use of a child safety restraint in the car.
2. The nurse inadvertently throws away the container holding the client's dentures.
3. A client is ambulating in the hall and slips on a recently mopped floor, causing injury to the leg.
4. A visitor who is sitting by the client's bed is hit by a falling IV pole while the nurse is changing the IV tubing, and requires stitches for a laceration.

28. When checking the IV solution at the beginning of the shift, it was discovered that an incorrect solution was running. After changing the solution to the correct order, an appropriate nursing action would be to:
1. Report the discovery of the error to the supervisor.
2. Document the error and correction in the medical record.
3. Fill out an incident report according to hospital policy.
4. Assure the client that the error had no adverse effects.

Answers/Rationales/Tips

1. **(3)** The nurse would be negligent for any untoward effects of the drug if she or he failed to contact the physician who ordered the drug before the nurse administered it. In *Norton v. Argonaut Insurance Co.* [144 So. 2nd 249 (La. Ct. App. 1962)], the court stated that it was the responsibility of the nurse to clarify the order with the physician *involved,* not with other nurses (**Answers 2** and **4**). **Answer 1** is incorrect because the doctors on the unit are not the ones who wrote the order.

> **TEST-TAKING TIP**—Apply the concept of negligence: omission to do something that a *reasonable* person guided by *ordinary* considerations would *do;* and go directly to the source for clarification.
> **IMP, APP, 1, Legal, SECE, Management of Care**

2. **(4)** Although **Answer 1** is a correct answer, **Answer 4** is the *best* answer because the nurse would validate the changed order and learn the physician's rationale for the change. In *Larrimore v. Homeopathic Hospital Association* [54 Del. 449, 181 A. 2d 573 (1962)], the court found that the nurse who went ahead and gave the medication was negligent. The courts went on to say that the jury could find the nurse negligent by applying ordinary common sense to establish the applicable standard of care. **Answers 2** and **3** are incorrect because talking with nurses is not the direct way to clarify and validate an order.

> **TEST-TAKING TIP**—Eliminate two options related to talking to other nurses. Although the two other choices are good, select the more inclusive option.
> **IMP, APP, 1, Legal, SECE, Management of Care**

3. **(4)** The nurse would come back to the client revitalized after having a lunch break, and the client would be covered the whole time the nurse is away. In deciding that the nurse would not be negligent to leave such a client, the court would emphasize that the question of liability should be determined in light of the circumstances as they existed at the time. When the nurse left the client, it was not foreseeable that an increased risk to the client would result. On the contrary, the client would be looked after, and the nurse's needs would also be met. *Child v. Vancouver General Hospital* [71 W.W.R. 656 (1979)]. **Answer 1** does not provide for client's care. **Answers 2** and **3** are not necessary actions, for the client's condition at the time did not warrant the nurse foregoing lunch or eating in the client's room.

> **TEST-TAKING TIP**—Client's condition (stable) allows for continuity of care (by delegation) while the nurse is at lunch. Choose the option that is different (taking a lunch break).
> **IMP, ANL, 7, Legal, SECE, Management of Care**

4. **(1)** In a court of law, hospital policy may be used to set the standard of care by which the nurses' actions are judged. Because the hospital policy states that two nurses must be in attendance while clients are in the recovery room, both the nurse who left (**Answers 2** and **4**) and the supervisor who authorized the nurse's absence (**Answer 3**) would be held liable

KEY TO CODES FOLLOWING RATIONALES:

Nursing process: **AS**, assessment; **AN**, analysis; **PL**, plan; **IMP**, implementation; **EV**, evaluation; *=code not applicable. *Cognitive level:* **COM**, comprehension; **APP**, application; **ANL**, analysis. *Category of human function:* **1**, protective; **2**, sensory-perceptual; **3**, comfort, rest, activity, and mobility; **4**, nutrition; **5**, growth and development; **6**, fluid-gas transport; **7**, psychosocial-cultural; **8**, elimination. *Client need:* **SECE**, safe, effective care environment; **HPM**, health promotion/maintenance; **PsI**, psychosocial integrity; **PhI**, physiological integrity. (Client subneed appears after Client need code.) See appendices for full explanation.

for any untoward effect on the client. *Laidlaw v. Lions Gate Hospital* [70 W.W.R. 727 (1969)].

> **TEST-TAKING TIP**—In following hospital policy, standards of care are met.
> **IMP, APP, 1, Legal, SECE, Management of Care**

5. **(1)** The court has stated that no one is obliged by law to assist a stranger, even if he or she can do so by a word and without the slightest danger to himself or herself. Hence, **Answer 3** is incorrect. But once one has undertaken to give assistance, the law imposes on him or her a duty of care toward the person assisted. Hence **Answer 2** is incorrect. The court also states that under emergency circumstances, a nurse, like any other person, may perform a medical act to preserve life and limb. Either law or custom exempts such actions from coming within the medical practice acts. This, then, would rule out **Answer 4.**

> **TEST-TAKING TIP**—Apply the *Good Samaritan Act.*
> **PL, APP, 7, Legal, SECE, Management of Care**

6. **(2)** *All State Practice Acts* list "guilty of practicing while under the influence of drugs or alcohol" as a reason for revocation of a license or for putting a nurse on probation. **Answers 1, 3,** and **4** *may* cause revocation of a license; however, *other* circumstances would have to be considered first, such as the frequency with which these had occurred.

> **TEST-TAKING TIP**—Refer to the *State Practice Acts* for reasons for license revocation.
> **EV, APP, 7, Legal, SECE, Management of Care**

7. **(4)** Freedom from unlawful restraint is a basic human right. Restraints of any type may constitute false imprisonment. False imprisonment is an actionable tort for which a nurse may be held liable by a client. The client may have an actionable case of false imprisonment if the restraints were applied for staff convenience only. Most likely the nurse would not be held liable for false imprisonment even if the nurse does not immediately obtain an order from the physician for the restraints. However, **Answer 1** is not the *best* choice. Restraints should be used only in *emergency* situations for a *limited time,* for the *limited purpose* of protecting the client, and not for the convenience of the staff. Even though the client's consent (**Answer 3**) is not usually obtainable under the circumstances, the nurse should try to obtain it in order to avoid being held liable for false imprisonment. However, these restraints should only be applied as a last resort (**Answer 2**).

> **TEST-TAKING TIP**—Select the option that violates client's rights.
> **EV, APP, 7, Legal, SECE, Safety and Infection Control**

8. **(1)** This type of case is an example of the most difficult medical ethical and legal questions today. The answers are ambiguous at best. However, in this case **Answer 1** would be best because neither the nurse (**Answer 3**), the wife (**Answer 2**), nor the doctor can make that decision as long as the client is an adult who is competent. **Answer 4** is incorrect because the nurse's values should not supersede the wife's concerns for her husband's welfare.

> **TEST-TAKING TIP**—The best answer includes the client; the decision is *not* the nurse's to make, and the nurse should not ignore the wife's request.
> **IMP, APP, 7, Legal, SECE, Management of Care**

9. **(2)** *Assault* is the unjustifiable attempt to touch another person or the threat to do so in such circumstances as to cause the other to reasonably believe that it will be carried out. The lack of informed consent is an important part of the meaning of assault. Consent is a defense to an action for assault. However, if the treatment or procedure goes beyond the client's consent (as it probably would if consent was only to "general"

treatment, as in **Answer 2**), the nurse, the doctor, and/or the hospital may be liable. Hence, **Answer 1** is a *true* statement. In an emergency situation in which the nurse is trying to save the client's life, if the client does not or cannot consent to treatment, the nurse usually will not be held to have assaulted the client. Hence, **Answer 3** is also a *true* statement. Consent may be given by conduct as well as by expressed words, as in **Answer 4**. For example, in a case in which a person held up his arm to be vaccinated, the court said he had consented. However, it is best to get the consent in writing, specifically outlining the treatment or procedure to be performed. The consent will most likely be deemed invalid, however, if the client is a child, is mentally incompetent, or is intoxicated.

> **TEST-TAKING TIP**—Eliminate the three *true* statements.
> **EV, APP, 7, Legal, SECE, Management of Care**

10. **(4)** *Both* the nurse and the hospital can be sued for damages if a mistake the nurse makes injures the client. The nurse is always responsible for his or her own actions. The hospital, as the employer, will be vicariously liable under the *respondeat superior doctrine*—the employer is liable for the negligent conduct of its nurses when the act was committed within the scope of employment. **Answers 1** and **3** are incomplete; **Answer 2** is incorrect.

> **TEST-TAKING TIP**—The best answer is based on the *respondeat superior doctrine*, under which the hospital is also liable.
> **EV, APP, 7, Legal, SECE, Management of Care**

11. **(3)** The hospital is *always* initially held liable under the theory of *respondeat superior*—vicarious liability of the employer. **Answers 2** and **4** are incorrect because the supervisor would *not* be responsible unless the court thought that the supervisor was negligent in supervising or assigning a task beyond the capabilities of another. In this case, the staff nurse had had numerous years of experience on the cardiovascular unit. Without further data, the supervisor would not be considered negligent for assigning this nurse to the cardiovascular unit. **Answer 1** is incomplete.

> **TEST-TAKING TIP**—The best answer is based on *respondeat superior*, under which the hospital is also liable.
> **AN, APP, 7, Legal, SECE, Management of Care**

12. **(2)** This answer includes all parties: the hospital, Nurse A, and Nurse B. The hospital, as the employer, might be held liable under the theory of *respondeat superior*—vicarious liability. Nurse B would be held responsible because each nurse is personally liable for his or her own negligent actions. Nurse A might also be held responsible because every nurse is obligated to act so that clients are safe from injury. In this case, Nurse A knew of B's intoxicated state. Nurse A did not act as a *reasonably prudent nurse* in failing to inform a supervisor. **Answers 1, 3,** and **4** are incomplete.

> **TEST-TAKING TIP**—The best answer is based on both the doctrine of *respondeat superior* and *reasonably* prudent behavior.
> **AN, APP, 7, Legal, SECE, Management of Care**

13. **(1)** If the nurse informs the physician and still carries out the treatment (**Answer 2**), both the nurse and the physician could be held liable if the client is negligently harmed. The nurse would be liable for not acting as a reasonably prudent nurse, and the physician would be liable because he or she knew of the nurse's lack of knowledge and did not step in to protect the client. If the nurse does not tell the physician and still carries out the treatment (**Answer 4**), the nurse would be solely liable. The nurse should not refuse to perform the treatment (**Answer 3**) unless she or he has no supervision.

> **TEST-TAKING TIP**—For an educated guess, first eliminate the two options in which the nurse performs the treatment (**Answers 2** and **4**). Then eliminate **Answer 3** because to refuse without notifying the MD is not enough.
> **IMP, APP, 7, Legal, SECE, Management of Care**

14. **(4)** As a nurse, you should *not* plan to use equipment that you know is malfunctioning. You could be held liable because you were on notice and could reasonably foresee that properly functioning equipment would be needed by your client. Hence, **Answers 1, 2,** and **3** are incorrect.

> **TEST-TAKING TIP**—Eliminate the three options that involve working *with* malfunctioning equipment.
> **IMP, APP, 1, Legal, SECE, Safety and Infection Control**

15. **(1)** This is the *only clearly false* option. Neither the physician nor the hospital would ordinarily be liable if (a) the medical risk is explained and a full report concerning the incident is documented and (b) the client is an adult who is competent. The court does not usually interfere with one's right to refuse treatment, as in **Answer 2**. However, the court will closely scrutinize a situation in which the client's refusal to accept treatment results in death or in the client's inability to care for children. If the children might be left as wards of the court, the court may force the client to accept treatment, as in **Answer 3**. Hence, **Answers 2, 3,** and **4** do not apply, because they are true.

> **TEST-TAKING TIP**—Eliminate the three true/correct options pertaining to AMA.
> **EV, APP, 7, Legal, SECE, Management of Care**

16. **(3)** The court in *John Ramsey, Jr. et al. v. Physicians Memorial Hospital, Inc. et al.* stated that "evidence supported finding that the failure of nurse to notify physician of client history involving removal of ticks from one of the children constituted a violation of her duties as a nurse, and failure to relate the information to the physician was the contributing proximate cause of death of the child." The hospital is *also* held liable under the doctrine of *respondeat superior* for the negligent conduct of its nurses when committed within the scope of their employment. Hence, **Answer 1** is incomplete because it does not include the hospital. The physician would most likely *not* be held liable because of the language barrier and the nurse's clear failure to communicate. Hence, **Answers 2** and **4** are incorrect.

> **TEST-TAKING TIP**—Choose the option that involves the hospital under *respondeat superior doctrine*.
> **EV, APP, 1, Legal, SECE, Management of Care**

17. **(1)** Both nurses and doctors are under a duty to protect the safety of their clients. In this case, the client's safety was potentially jeopardized, yet neither the anesthesiologist nor the nurse reported the situation. Therefore, if something had happened to the client during surgery, the court could have made a good argument that all were negligent. Hence, **Answers 2, 3,** and **4** are incomplete. What can a nurse do in a situation as described here? First, for the nurse's own safety, he or she should prepare a summary of the incidents. The nurse might also consult with nurse colleagues who have worked with the physician, because they could confirm or deny the problem and possibly offer support. Second, the nurse should report the incident to the supervisor and director of nursing, who have a liaison with the surgical/medical staff. If the action is not pursued successfully, the nurse can bring the problem to the attention of the hospital administrator. Again, if no action is forthcoming, the nurse may seek out a board member who might be sensitive to the situation. In any case, these are difficult situations that may arise. There is no easy solution.

TEST TAKING TIP—The best answer is the *most inclusive;* failure to report by *both* nurse and doctor can be seen as negligence, and the hospital will also be liable.
AN, APP, 1, Legal, SECE, Management of Care

18. **(1)** Most state statutes provide that every hospital to which any person is brought who is suffering from any injuries inflicted by another must report the fact immediately to the local law enforcement authorities. Most state statutes also impose the same duty on other health-care professionals, school officials and teachers, child care supervisors, and social workers. Hence **Answers 2** and **4** are incomplete; **Answer 3** is incorrect. From *Landeros v. Flood* as well as other cases, it seems clear that the responsibility of professional people—doctors, nurses, and others who must deal with children who are injured—includes the duty to report suspicious evidence to the proper authorities.

TEST-TAKING TIP—Choose the *most inclusive* answer, involving *all* concerned as mandated by state laws regarding reporting suspected abuse.
AN, APP, 7, Legal, SECE, Management of Care

19. **(2)** However, it could be argued that **Answer 1** is correct. The nurse's liability for the negligent loss of or damage to a client's property is based on the nurse's duty as a person, trained or untrained, to act as a reasonable and ordinary, prudent person. In this case, the nurse put the dentures in a towel without a label. The nurse might reasonably expect that aides would be stripping the linen after the client left for surgery. Therefore, this act was not that of an ordinary prudent person. The nurse would be liable. Because the nurse is liable, the hospital, as employer, *might* also be held liable. This would be for court determination. Because the aides had no knowledge of the dentures, and they were acting reasonably, they would not be liable for the lost dentures. Hence, **Answers 3** and **4** are incorrect.

TEST-TAKING TIP—Remember, the hospital may also be liable under *respondeat superior.* Eliminate the two options that include the aides, who were acting as an ordinary prudent person would act.
AN, APP, 7, Legal, SECE, Management of Care

20. **(4)** Although **Answer 4** is best, this is a very close case. When family members help with a client who is hospitalized, liability becomes complicated. Where members of the nursing team offer to assist clients in bathing, feeding, and so on, and an apparently capable family member prefers to assist the client, this is usually acceptable and neither the hospital nor the health-care team is liable. Thus, **Answers 1, 2,** and **3** can be eliminated as correct choices. However, the nurse should never assume that the presence of a family member obviates the nurse helping the client.

TEST-TAKING TIP—Eliminate options **1, 2,** and **3** that include the nurse and the hospital, because they are not liable when family members prefer to assist.
AN, APP, 1, Legal, SECE, Safety and Infection Control

21. **(3)** The request must be in writing. **Answers 1** and **2** are true but incomplete. **Answer 4** has nothing to do with voluntary admission.

TEST-TAKING TIP—Choose the *complete* response (**Answer 3**) and eliminate **Answers 1** and **2** as incomplete. Eliminate **Answer 4** as irrelevant to the question.
EV, COM, 7, Legal, SECE, Management of Care

22. **(4)** This division of the ANA sets the standards; therefore, **Answer 1** cannot be correct. **Answers 2** and **3** are also incorrect, although they may be part of **Answer 4.**

TEST-TAKING TIP—When two or more options are correct (**Answers 2** and **3**), choose the one that encompasses them (**Answer 4**). Eliminate **Answer 1** because it includes an MD.
*****COM, 7, SECE, Management of Care: Ethics**

23. **(3)** **Answers 1, 2,** and **4** may be referred to in the standards, but the standards were organized around the nursing process.

TEST-TAKING TIP—When all four options are right, choose the umbrella option that includes them all.
*****COM, 7, SECE, Management of Care: Ethics**

24. **(4)** This is what the document states. *Other* choices (**1, 2, 3**) do not give the individual nurse primary responsibility.

TEST-TAKING TIP—Eliminate the three options ("body of nurses," "hospital," "laws") that do not focus on the *individual* nurse (**Answer 4**).
*****COM, 7, SECE, Management of Care: Ethics/Legal**

25. **(3)** The Act states that the boards must be composed of 60% *consumers* who are not affiliated with any health professional group; hence, **Answers 1, 2,** and **4** are incorrect.

TEST-TAKING TIP—Choose the option that focuses on the *consumer.*
*****COM, 7, Legal, SECE, Management of Care**

26. **(3)** A *Do Not Resuscitate* (DNR) order is required. **Answers 1, 2,** and **4** are also appropriate, but not as great a priority as notifying the MD, who must provide a written order.

TEST-TAKING TIP—Prioritization is required. Note the key words "next action."
IMP, APP, 7, Legal, SECE, Management of Care

27. **(1)** The definition of *malpractice* is the "incorrect or negligent treatment of a client." Included would be incorrect instructions that resulted in injury. **Answers 2** and **3** are careless and would likely require the *hospital* to compensate the client for the loss or injury. **Answer 4** is an *accident,* not malpractice or negligence.

TEST-TAKING TIP—Think of the meaning of the word *malpractice*—"bad practice." Which situation puts the client at risk because of the nurse's action?
EV, APP, 7, Legal, SECE, Management of Care

28. **(3)** A quality assurance report or incident report should be completed and submitted according to hospital policy. The report would indicate that the MD was notified of the status of the client, and any orders as a result of the error. The supervisor (**Answer 1**) should be notified, but *not before* completing the incident report. It is also most important to notify the MD before completing the report. Incidents are not usually documented in the client (medical) record (**Answer 2**). If unsure of hospital policy, hospital risk management should be consulted. Open communication with clients is important (**Answer 4**); however, *unless* there was an adverse effect that required additional treatment or a change in treatment, it is unlikely that the physician will inform the client.

TEST-TAKING TIP—When two options are correct, select the one that encompasses the other. The incident report (**Answer 3**) also serves to inform the supervisor (**Answer 1**).
IMP, ANL, 7, Legal, SECE, Management of Care

---

* Nursing Process step is **not applicable** to this question.

Nursing Care of the Childbearing Family

Janice McMillin

GROWTH AND DEVELOPMENT

Biological Foundations of Reproduction

General overview: This review of the structures, functions, and important assessment characteristics of the reproductive system provides essential components of the database required for accurate nursing judgments. Comparing normal characteristics and established patterns with nursing assessment findings assists in identifying client needs and in planning, implementing, and evaluating appropriate goal-directed nursing interventions.

Female Reproductive Anatomy and Physiology

I. **Structure of pelvis (Figure 4.1)**
   A. Two hip bones (right and left innominate: sacrum, coccyx).
   B. False pelvis—upper portion above brim, supportive structure for uterus during last half of pregnancy.
   C. True pelvis—below brim; pelvic inlet, midplane, pelvic outlet. Fetus passes through during birth.

II. **Pelvic measurements**
   A. Diagonal conjugate—12.5 cm or greater is adequate size; evaluated by examiner.
   B. Conjugate vera—11 cm is adequate size; can be measured by x-ray (not commonly performed).
   C. Obstetric conjugate—measured by x-ray (not commonly performed).
   D. Tuber-ischial diameter—9–11 cm indicates adequate size; evaluated by examiner.

III. **Female external organs**
   A. Mons veneris—protects symphysis.
   B. Labia majora—covers, protects labia minora.
   C. Labia minora—two located within labia majora.
   D. Clitoris—small erectile tissue.
   E. Hymen—thin membrane at opening of vagina.
   F. Urinary meatus—opening of urethra.

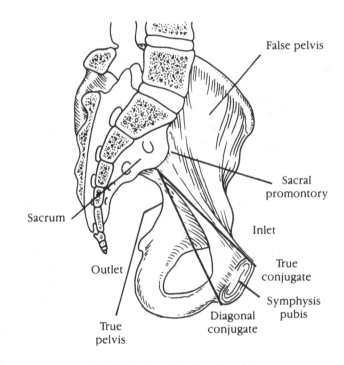

FIGURE 4.1   The female pelvis.

   G. Bartholin glands—producer of alkaline secretions that enhance sperm motility, viability.
IV. **Internal structures (Figure 4.2)**
   A. Vagina—outlet for menstrual flow, depository of semen, lower birth canal.
   B. Cervix—cone-shaped neck of the uterus that protrudes into the vagina.
   C. Uterus—muscular organ that houses fetus during gestation.
   D. Fallopian tubes—two tubes stretching from cornua of uterus to ovaries; transport ovum.
   E. Ovaries—two oval-shaped structures that produce ovum and hormones (estrogen and progesterone).
   F. Breasts—two mammary glands capable of secreting milk for infant nourishment.

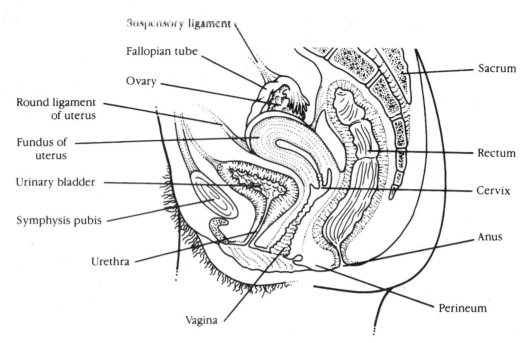

FIGURE 4.2 **Female internal reproductive organs.**

V. Menstrual cycle (Figure 4.3)
A. Reproductive hormones
1. *Follicle-stimulating hormone (FSH)*—secreted during the first half of cycle; stimulates development of graafian follicle; secreted by anterior pituitary.
2. *Interstitial cell-stimulating hormone, luteinizing hormone (ICSH, LH)*—stimulates ovulation and development of corpus luteum; secreted by pituitary.
3. *Estrogen*—assists in ovarian follicle maturation; stimulates endometrial thickening; responsible for development of secondary sex characteristics; maintains endometrium during pregnancy.

Secreted by ovaries and adrenal cortex during cycle and by placenta during pregnancy.
4. *Progesterone*—aids in endometrial thickening; facilitates secretory changes; maintains uterine lining for implantation and early pregnancy; relaxes smooth muscle. Secreted by corpus luteum and placenta.
5. *Prostaglandins*—substances produced by various body organs that act hormonally on the endometrium to influence the onset and continuation of labor. A medication that may be used to facilitate onset of second trimester abortion; also used to efface the cervix before induction of labor in term pregnancies.

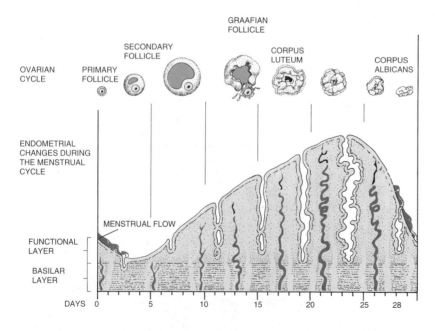

FIGURE 4.3 **The menstrual cycle.**
(From Venes, D [ed]: Taber's Cyclopedic Medical Dictionary, ed. 20. FA Davis, Philadelphia, 2005, p. 1341.)

B. **Ovulation**—maturation and release of egg from ovary; generally occurs 14 days *before* beginning of next menses.

C. **Menstruation**—vaginal discharge of blood and fragments of the endometrium; cyclic; occurs in response to dropping levels of estrogen and progesterone.

D. **Fertilization**—impregnation of ovum by sperm.

E. **Implantation**—fertilized ovum attaches to uterine wall for growth.

F. **Menopause**—normally occurring cessation of menses with gradual decrease in amount of flow and increase in the time between periods at end of fertility cycle; average age, 51–52. Early menopause rare but may be influenced by hypothyroidism, surgical ovarian removal, overexposure to radiation. *Treatments* during menopause for symptom relief: hormonal replacement therapy, isoflavanoids, vitamins B and E for hot flashes, vaginal creams for dyspareunia (painful intercourse), and calcium for osteoporosis. Alternative treatments include herbal supplements and soy.

G. **Spinnbarkeit**—stretchable, thin cervical mucus present at ovulation.

◆ **VI. Assessment of reproductive tract/reproductive health:**
   A. Health history
      1. Menarche: onset and duration.
      2. Menstrual problems.
      3. Contraceptive use.
      4. Pregnancy history.
      5. Fertility problems.
      6. Lifestyle choices that may have an impact on health and reproductive decision making.
   B. Physical examination
      1. External, internal reproductive organs.
      2. Breast examination.
      3. *Mammography*—every 1–2 years for women beginning age 40; annually beginning age 50; more frequently if have **risk factors for breast cancer:**
         a. Mother, daughter, or sister had breast cancer.
         b. Menses before age 11, or menopause before age 45 or after age 55.
         c. Previous benign needle biopsies.
         d. Birth of first child >30 years old.
         e. High-fat diet, obesity.
         f. Obesity after menopause.
         g. Daily alcohol intake of 2–5 drinks per day.
         h. Nulliparous.
         i. Personal history of cancer.
         j. Defects in certain genes (BRCA1, BRCA2, HER, and p53).
      4. Pap smear—First Papanicolaou (Pap) smear at age 18 or earlier if sexually active; then annually until 3 consecutive normal Paps. After 3 consecutive normal Paps, physician discretion is recommended.
      5. Tests for sexually transmitted diseases (STDs).

◆ **VII. Analysis/nursing diagnosis:**

A. *Health-seeking behaviors* related to health promotion.

B. *Health-seeking behaviors* related to menopause.

◆ **VIII. Nursing care plan/implementation:**
   A. Discuss anatomy and physiology of reproductive tract.
   B. Review menstruation, ovulation, fertilization.
   C. Explain need for periodic Pap smears, annual gynecological exams, including mammography.
   D. Discuss lifestyle choices and sexuality issues that might affect health.

◆ **IX. Evaluation/outcome criteria:**
   A. Woman displays basic understanding of anatomy and physiology.
   B. Woman understands cycle and contraception.
   C. Woman regularly seeks preventive care and performs monthly breast self-examination (BSE).

Decision Making Regarding Reproduction

General overview: During the reproductive years, the woman who is sexually active often faces the decision to postpone, prevent, or terminate a pregnancy. The nursing role focuses on assisting her to make an informed decision consistent with individual needs.

   I. Family planning
◆ A. **Assessment:**
      1. Determine interest in and present knowledge of methods of family planning.
      2. Identify factors affecting choice of method: cultural and religious objections, contraindications for individual methods, motivation/ability to follow chosen method successfully, financial considerations, and sexual orientations.
◆ B. **Analysis/nursing diagnosis:** *knowledge deficit* regarding family planning methods/options.
◆ C. **Nursing care plan/implementation**—Goal: *health teaching*—to facilitate informed decision making, selection of option appropriate to individual needs, desires.
      1. Describe, explain, discuss options available and appropriate to the woman. Include information on advantages and disadvantages of each option (**Tables 4.1** and **4.2**).
      2. Demonstrate, as necessary, method selected.
      3. Quick health teaching reminders for missed oral hormone preparations:
         a. Woman should take one pill at the same time every day for 21 (or 28) days.
         b. If woman misses one pill, she should take it as soon as she remembers it; she should then take the next one at the usual time.
         c. If woman misses two or more pills in a row in the first 2 wk of her cycle, she should take 2 pills for 2 days and use a backup method of contraception for the next 7 days.
         d. If woman misses two pills in the third week, or three or more pills anytime:

(1) A *Sunday starter* should keep taking pills until the next Sunday, then start a new pack that Sunday. She should use a backup method of contraception for the next 7 days.

(2) A *day 1 starter* should throw out the rest of the pack and start a new pack that day. She should use a backup method of contraception for the next 7 days.

e. *28-day pill pack:* If woman misses any of the seven pills that do not have any hormones, she should throw out the pills missed and keep taking one pill a day until the pack is empty. She does not need a backup method of contraception.

4. Alert woman to discontinue use of *oral hormone contraceptive* preparations and report any of the following symptoms to the physician **STAT**. Signs of potential problems: "ACHES"*

A—Abdominal pain: possible problem with the liver or gallbladder.

C—Chest pain or shortness of breath: possible clot within lungs or heart.

H—Headaches (sudden or persistent): possibly caused by stroke (brain attack) or hypertension.

E—Eye problems: possible vascular incident or hypertension.

S—Severe leg pain: possible thromboembolic process.

5. Signs of *potential problems* related to IUD use: "PAINS"*

P—Period (menstrual) late, abnormal spotting or bleeding.

A—Abdominal pain, pain during coitus (dyspareunia).

I—Infection, abnormal vaginal discharge.

N—Not feeling well; fever or chills.

S—String missing (nonpalpable on vaginal self-examination, or not seen on speculum examination).

*Source: Hatcher, R, et al: Contraceptive Technology, ed. 16. Irving, New York.

6. **Toxic Shock Syndrome** (TSS)

a. *Signs/symptoms*
(1) Fever of sudden onset—over 102°F (38.9°C).
(2) Hypotension—systolic pressure <90 mm Hg; orthostatic dizziness; disorientation.
(3) Rash—diffuse, macular erythroderma (resembling sunburn).
(4) Sore throat; severe nausea, vomiting.
(5) Copious vaginal discharge.

b. *Instructions for prevention*
(1) General
(a) *Avoid* use of tampons, cervical caps, and diaphragms during the postpartum period (6 wk).
(b) Do *not* use any of the above if you have a history of TSS.
(c) Call physician if you experience sudden onset of a high fever, vomiting, diarrhea, or skin rash.
(d) Insert clean tampons and contraceptive devices with clean hands.
(e) Remove within prescribed time limits.
(2) Tampons
(a) Change tampons every 3–6 hr.
(b) Do *not* use superabsorbent tampons.
(c) For overnight protection, substitute other products such as sanitary napkins or minipads.
(3) Diaphragm or cervical cap
(a) *Avoid* use during your menstrual period.
(b) Remove within 8 hr after intercourse (diaphragm must be removed no later than 24 hr; the cap, no later than 48 hr).

TABLE 4.1	Contraception		
Method	**Action/Effectiveness**	**Advantages**	**Disadvantages and Side Effects**
Hormonal Contraceptives			
Pill—combination of estrogen and progesterone Oral contraceptives (daily)	■ Suppresses ovulation by suppressing production of FSH and LH ■ *Most efficient* form of contraception (99.7%) if used consistently	■ Convenient; easy to take ■ Withdrawal bleeding cycles are predictable ■ Not related to sex act ■ Safe for older nonsmoking women until menopause ■ Many noncontraceptive health benefits (oral)	■ *Absolute contraindications* (e.g., thromboembolic or coronary artery disease; some cancers or liver disease) ■ *Relative contraindications* (e.g., migraines, hypertension, immobility 4 wk or more, abnormal genital bleeding) ■ Some decrease in glucose tolerance ■ Effectiveness decreased if taken during use of barbiturates, phenytoin, antibiotics ■ **No protection against STDs**

(Continued on following page)

Method	Action/Effectiveness	Advantages	Disadvantages and Side Effects
Contraceptive patch—combination of estrogen and progesterone (change q wk)	■ Suppresses ovulation ■ Thickens cervical mucus ■ Decreases sperm penetration ■ 99% effective in women <198 lbs; 92% effective in women >198 lbs	■ Convenient ■ Patch applies to abdomen, buttocks, upper arm, or upper torso ■ Changed 1/week	■ *Absolute contraindications* (e.g., thromboembolic or coronary artery disease, some cancers or liver disease) ■ *Relative contraindications* (e.g., migraines, hypertension, immobility 4 wk or more, allergic reaction to patch) ■ **No protection against STDs**
Mini-pill—Progestin only (PO daily)	■ Impairs fertility ■ Thickens cervical mucus ■ Decreases sperm penetration ■ Alters endometrial maturation ■ *Effectiveness:* undetermined; can reach 100% reliability if used exactly as prescribed	■ Convenient, easy to take	■ Ovulation may occur ■ Irregular bleeding, mood changes, weight gain ■ May change glucose and insulin values ■ **No protection against STDs**
Depo-Provera—synthetic progesterone (IM q 3 months)	■ Suppresses ovulation ■ Thickens cervical mucus ■ Changes the uterine lining, making it harder for sperm to enter or survive in the uterus ■ *Effectiveness:* 99.7%	■ Private ■ Effective after 24 hours ■ Does not require regular attention ■ Does not interrupt sex play ■ Has no estrogen ■ May decrease risk for ovarian and uterine cancers	■ Requires injections every 3 months ■ Delay of return to fertility ■ Possible weight gain and irregular bleeding ■ **No protection against STDs**
Emergency Postcoital Contraception			
Estradiol (100 μg) and levonorgestrel (0.5 mg)	■ Antifertility; taken within 72 hr of unprotected sex ■ Take as soon as possible; repeat 12 hr later ■ *Effectiveness:* 75%–85%	■ Available, prn	■ Nausea, headache, dizziness
Intrauterine Devices (IUDs)			
Small, T-shaped, medicated device inserted into uterine cavity	■ Prevents fertility	■ Can be used by women who cannot use hormonal contraception; no disruption of ovulation pattern	■ *Contraindications:* history of PID, pregnancy, undiagnosed genital bleeding, genital malignancy, abnormal uterine cavity, severe cervicitis, HIV/AIDS, history of ectopic pregnancy, history of toxic shock

(Continued on following page)

Maternal-Infant

TABLE 4.1	Contraception *(Continued)*		

Method	Action/Effectiveness	Advantages	Disadvantages and Side Effects
▪ Copper (Paragard)	▪ Recommended for women who have had at least one child ▪ Damages sperm in transit to fallopian tube	▪ Can be used effectively for 10 yr (Paragard)	▪ *Risks:* uterine perforation, infection (may be followed by PID) in the first 3 mo of insertion; unnoticed expulsion ▪ *Side effects* (especially with Paragard): heavy flow, spotting between periods, and cramping within first few months of insertion
▪ Progesterone (Mirena)	▪ Alters cervical mucus and endometrial maturation ▪ *Effectiveness:* 90%–99%	▪ Change every yr (Mirena) ▪ Less blood loss during menses and decreases primary dysmenorrhea	▪ Must check for string after each menses and before intercourse ▪ **No protection against STDs**
Mechanical Barriers			
Diaphragm: shallow rubber device that fits over cervix	▪ Barrier preventing sperm from entering cervix (**if** it is correct size, undamaged, correctly placed, and is used with spermicide) ▪ *Effectiveness:* 83%–90%; 99% in highly motivated women	▪ Does not interrupt sex act, except to add spermicide just before act* ▪ Insert up to 6 hr before intercourse and leave in place for 6 hr after last intercourse, but not longer than 24 hr† ▪ Safe: no side effects from well-fitted device if woman is not allergic to diaphragm or spermicide ▪ Decreased incidence of vaginitis, cervicitis, PID	▪ Requires careful cleansing with warm water and mild soap; powder with cornstarch, and store away from heat. ▪ Size/fit must be checked after birth, second/third trimester abortion, weight gain or loss of 15–20 lb or more, or every 2 yr ▪ Spermicide must be reinserted for additional acts that may follow after initial intercourse
Cervical cap: $1\frac{1}{4}''$ – $1\frac{1}{4}''$ soft natural rubber dome with a firm but pliable rim	▪ Physical barrier to sperm ▪ Spermicide inside cap adds a chemical barrier ▪ *Effectiveness* depends on its fit. ▪ 80%–91% effective for nulliparas ▪ 60%–74% effective in multiparas	▪ Worn for 8 hr but not longer than 48 hr ▪ No need to add spermicide for repeated acts of intercourse	▪ Need a Pap smear every yr: higher rate of conversion from class I to class III‡ ▪ If in-place over 48 hr, it produces an odor and might be associated with TSS‡ ▪ Cannot be worn during menstrual flow (menses) or up to at least 6 wk postpartum ▪ *Contraindications:* abnormal Pap smear, hard to fit, history of TSS or genital infection, allergy ▪ Change after genital surgery, abortion, or birth, major change in weight ▪ Must be checked each yr ▪ **Does not protect against STDs**
Female condom: vaginal sheath of natural latex rubber with flexible rings at both the closed and the open ends	▪ Barrier preventing sperm from entering vagina	▪ Apply up to 8 hr in advance of intercourse; spermicide added just before intercourse	▪ Cost

(Continued on following page)

Method	Action/Effectiveness	Advantages	Disadvantages and Side Effects
	▪ *Effectiveness* similar to other mechanical methods used with spermicide (79%–95%) *Note:* Male and female condoms should not be used at the same time	▪ Heightens sensation for man ▪ About as satisfying for both woman and man as intercourse without it ▪ **Provides protection from STDs**	▪ A new one must be used for every act of intercourse
Condom: thin, stretchable latex sheath to cover penis	▪ Barrier preventing sperm from entering vagina, applied over erect penis before loss of preejaculatory drops and is held in place as penis is withdrawn ▪ Spermicidal foam, jelly, or cream is also used* ▪ *Effectiveness* rate: 64%–98% when used with spermicide	▪ Safety—no side effects ▪ **Provides protection from spread of STDs** With spermicide (0.5 g of nonoxynol-9) added to interior or exterior surface, provides protection from STDs, including HIV	▪ Check expiration date ▪ Requires high motivation to use correctly/consistently ▪ Must be properly applied and removed ▪ Sheath may tear during intercourse ▪ Can have small undetectable holes
Chemical Barriers			
Spermicide: aerosol foams, foaming tablets, suppositories, creams, and films (VCF)	▪ Physical barrier to sperm penetration ▪ Chemical action on sperm (kills sperm) ▪ Nonoxynol-9 has a bacteriostatic action ▪ *Effectiveness* rate: 70%–98% when used with diaphragm or condoms	▪ Increases effectiveness of mechanical barriers ▪ Ease of application. Aids lubrication of vagina* ▪ Requires no medical examination or prescription ▪ May be used during lactation ▪ Backup for missed oral contraceptive pills	▪ Messy ▪ Some people are allergic to preparations ▪ Tabs or suppositories take 10–15 min to dissolve ▪ If it is only method being used, each intercourse should be preceded (by 30 min) by a fresh application; may be allergenic
Other Methods			
Natural family planning: BBT each morning before any physical activity	▪ Requires sexual abstinence during woman's fertile period (4 d before ovulation), and for 3 or 4 days after ovulation	Physically safe to use—no drugs or appliances are used; meets requirements of most religions	▪ Effectiveness depends on high level of motivation and diligence ▪ Requires fairly predictable menstrual cycle
Symptothermal variation: BBT plus cervical mucus changes	▪ *Effectiveness:* about 80%		
Calendar method			
Predictor test for ovulation			

*Spermicide provides lubrication, but if additional lubrication is needed, use water-based products only (e.g., K-Y Jelly).
†TSS: toxic shock syndrome. Although there is no direct link between TSS and use of the diaphragm or cervical cap, a possible association remains (see **p. 144**).
‡Class I Pap smear: no abnormal cells; III Pap smear: suspicious abnormal cells present.

Maternal-Infant

TABLE 4.2	Sterilization	
Method	**Advantages**	**Disadvantages and Side Effects**
Men		
Vas deferens is occluded (ligated and severed; bands; clips) to prevent passage of sperm	▪ Relatively simple surgical procedure	▪ Sterility is not immediate; sperm are cleared from vas after about 15 ejaculations; need to have follow-up semen analysis to confirm sterility
	▪ Does not affect endocrine function, production of testosterone	▪ Antibody produced to own sperm
	▪ Does not alter volume of ejaculate	▪ Some men become impotent due to psychological response to procedure
	▪ Tubal reconstruction usually possible (90%)	▪ Fertility after tubal reconstruction (30%–85%)
		▪ **Does not protect against STDs**
Women		
Both fallopian tubes are ligated and severed, or occluded with bands or clips to prevent passage of eggs; fulguration of the tubes at the cornu is most effective	▪ Abdominal surgery utilizing 1-inch incision and laparoscopy	▪ Major surgery (if done by laparotomy) with possible complications of anesthesia, infection, hemorrhage, and trauma to other organs; psychological trauma in some
	▪ Greater than 99.5% effective	▪ Success rate for pregnancy after tubal reversal using microsurgical techniques: 40%–75%
Hysterectomy or oophorectomy or both	▪ Abdominal or vaginal surgery	
	▪ Absolute sterility	

◆ D. **Evaluation/outcome criteria:**
1. Woman avoids or achieves a pregnancy as desired.
2. Woman expresses comfort and satisfaction with method selected.

II. **Infertility**
   A. **Definition:** inability to conceive after 1 yr of unprotected intercourse.
   B. **Pathophysiology:** contributing factors—hormonal deficiencies, reproductive system disorders, congenital anomalies, male impotence, sexual knowledge deficit, debilitating disease.
◆ C. **Assessment:**
1. History—general health, reproduction, social history.
2. *Maternal diagnosis*
   a. Basal body temperature (BBT) (**Figure 4.4**).
   b. Endocrine studies.
   c. Huhner (postcoital).
   d. Rubins (tubal patency).
   e. Hysterosalpingogram (tubal patency).
3. *Male diagnosis*—history, physical examination, laboratory studies (e.g., semen analysis).
◆ D. **Analysis/nursing diagnosis:** *altered sexuality, altered family process* related to infertility.

◆ E. **Nursing care plan/implementation:**
1. Provide emotional support.
2. Explain testing procedures for diagnosis.
3. Assist with referral process.
◆ F. **Evaluation/outcome criteria:**
1. The couple conceives, or,
2. If the couple does not conceive, they accept referral for help with adoption, other reproductive alternatives, or childlessness.

III. **Interruption of Pregnancy**—also known as elective, voluntary, or therapeutic abortion. Once the diagnosis of pregnancy and the length of gestation are established, the woman faces the decision to interrupt or to maintain the pregnancy (**Table 4.3**).
   A. **Decision-making stage:**
◆ 1. **Assessment:**
   a. Health history:
      (1) Determine woman's feelings about the pregnancy, reasons for considering abortion, level of maturity; if decision was already made before she came to clinic, how was decision made? Does she have a support system?
      (2) Identify factors influencing/complicating

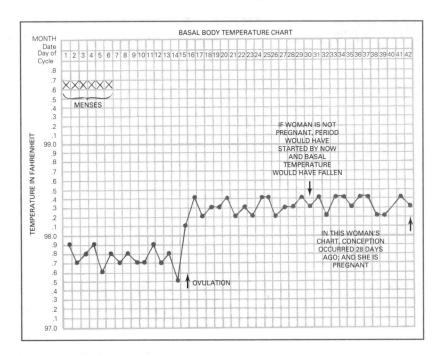

FIGURE 4.4 Basal body temperature chart. (From Venes, D [ed]: Taber's Cyclopedic Medical Dictionary, ed. 20. FA Davis, Philadelphia, 2005.)

TABLE 4.3	Interruption of Pregnancy (Elective/Voluntary Abortion)	
Method	**Advantages**	**Disadvantages and Side Effects**
First-Trimester Procedures		
Early uterine evacuation (EUE)—aspiration of endometrium through undilated cervix	Performed for women who have not yet missed a menstrual period 100% effective if implantation site is not missed	Cervical trauma may occur and may lead to incompetent cervix Hemorrhage
RU 486 (mifepristone)—a progesterone antagonist; taken up to 7 wk gestation (56 days LMP); taken orally	Prevents implantation of fertilized egg Most effective in early gestation, during luteal phase, within 10 days of first missed period	Slight nausea and fatigue during period of bleeding Uterine aspiration may be needed if RU 486 does not work
Misoprostol (Cytotec)—initiates uterine contractions; given intravaginally	Softens cervix and aids in expelling products of conception	
Uterine aspiration (vacuum or suction curettage)—cannula suction under local anesthesia, following cervical dilatation, usually with laminaria tent	Relatively few complications—minimal bleeding, minimal discomfort Outpatient procedure	Performed after one or two missed menstrual periods Cervical or endometrial trauma possible
Surgical dilation and curettage (D & C)—cervix dilated with laminaria tents; endometrium scraped with metal curette or flexible aspiration tip, under local anesthesia (paracervical block)	After cervix is dilated, procedure takes about 15 min	Performed after one or two missed periods

(Continued on following page)

Maternal-Infant

TABLE 4.3	Interruption of Pregnancy (Elective/Voluntary Abortion) *(Continued)*	
Method	**Advantages**	**Disadvantages and Side Effects**
	Outpatient procedure	
	Relatively few complications (≤1%): bleeding like a heavy period, some cramping	Possible but rare; cervical trauma, uterine perforation infection, hemorrhage
Second-Trimester Procedures		
D & E (dilation and evacuation)—extends D & C and vacuum curettage up to 20 wk gestation	Woman does not experience labor	Requires 3 d for laminaria to dilate cervix; procedure done on third day
Second- and Third-Trimester Procedures		
Hysterotomy—cesarean delivery	Available for gestations more than 14–16 wk	*After:* major surgery complications—hemorrhage and infection possible
	Preferred method if woman wishes a tubal ligation or hysterectomy to follow	Fetus may be born alive, causing ethical, moral, religious, and legal problems

her decisions (religious beliefs, cultural mores, peer and family pressures).
(3) Information needs.
b. Physical examination.
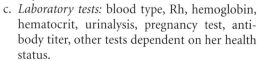
c. *Laboratory tests:* blood type, Rh, hemoglobin, hematocrit, urinalysis, pregnancy test, antibody titer, other tests dependent on her health status.

◆ 2. **Analysis/nursing diagnosis:**
a. *Ineffective coping* related to emotional conflicts associated with need for decision to continue/terminate pregnancy.
b. *Altered family* process related to intrafamily conflict associated with need for/decision to continue/terminate pregnancy.
c. *Anticipatory grieving* related to loss of pregnancy/child.
d. *Altered self-concept, self-esteem disturbance* related to possible guilt feelings associated with pregnancy/termination.
e. *Knowledge deficit* related to available options.

◆ 3. **Nursing care plan/implementation:**
a. Goal: *emotional support* to minimize impact on self-image and self-esteem.
(1) Maintain accepting, nonjudgmental attitude.
(2) Encourage verbalization of feelings, perceptions, and values.
(3) Support woman's decision.
b. Goal: *health teaching* to facilitate informed decision making.
(1) Explain and discuss available options as applicable (see **Table 4.3**).
(2) Describe procedure selected and what to expect after procedure.

c. Goal: *minimize impact on intrafamily relations, family process.* Where applicable, encourage open communication between deciding partners.

◆ 4. **Evaluation/outcome criteria:**
a. Woman states she understands all information necessary to give consent.
b. Woman expresses comfort and satisfaction with the decision.

B. Preoperative period

◆ 1. **Assessment:**
a. Reassess woman's emotional and physical status and current feelings regarding decision.
b. Determine woman's current knowledge/understanding of authorization form, anticipated procedure, and consequences (informed consent).
c. Monitor woman's physiological and (if awake) psychological response to procedure.

◆ 2. **Analysis/nursing diagnosis:**
a. *Anxiety/fear* related to procedure, potential complications
b. *Knowledge deficit* related to ongoing procedure, sights, sounds, and sensations experienced.

◆ 3. **Nursing care plan/implementation:**
a. Goal: *provide opportunity to reconsider decision regarding termination of pregnancy.*
(1) Check to ensure all required permission (informed consent) forms have been signed/filed.
(2) Refer to physician if woman is ambivalent or insecure in decision.
b. Goal: *reduce anxiety/fear related to procedure.*
(1) Explain all anticipated preoperative, operative, and postoperative care.

(2) Assist with procedure; if woman is awake, explain what is happening and what she may be experiencing.

c. Goal: *emotional support* to facilitate effective coping.

(1) Encourage verbalization of feelings, fears, concerns.

(2) Support woman's decision.

◆ 4. **Evaluation/outcome criteria:** woman does not experience physiological or psychological problems during procedure.

C. Postoperative period

◆ 1. **Assessment:**

a. Monitor *physiological* response to procedure (vital signs, blood loss, uterine cramping).

b. Determine *psychological* response (happy, relieved; guilt feelings, lowered self-esteem).

c. Determine desire for family planning information.

◗▭ d. Determine need for Rho(D)immune globulin, *Rubella* vaccination

◆ 2. **Analysis/nursing diagnosis:**

a. *Pain* related to procedure.

b. *High risk for infection* related to lack of knowledge of postabortal self-care.

◆ 3. **Nursing care plan/implementation:**

a. Goal: *provide and explain postoperative care.*

(1) Administer intravenous (IV) fluids.

(2) Administer medications prn for discomfort.

◗▭ (3) Administer oxytocic meds for uterine atony, prn.

(4) If mother is *Rh-negative*, 8 or more weeks of gestation, and laboratory tests indicate no current sensitization (i.e., she is Coombs negative):

(a) Explain rationale for postabortion administration of Rho (D antigen) immune globulin (RhoGAM).

◗▭ (b) Administer RhoGAM, as ordered.

(5) Provide and explain perineal care

b. Goal: *health teaching* to facilitate active participation in own health maintenance, informed decision making, provide predischarge anticipatory guidance (also provide in written form with attention to woman's level of reading skill and understanding, and in her native language whenever possible):

(1) Immediately report any cramping, excessive bleeding, signs of infection.

(2) Provide name and telephone number of person to call if she has questions.

(3) Schedule a postabortal checkup.

(4) Discuss contraception, if woman indicates interest; or give her place and name to call for information later.

(5) Discuss resumption of tampon use (3 days–3 wk as ordered) and sexual intercourse (1 wk–3 wk as ordered).

(6) Discuss need to *avoid* douching.

◆ 4. **Evaluation/outcome criteria:**

a. Woman returns for postabortal appointment.

b. Woman suffers no adverse physical sequelae to the procedure.

c. Woman suffers no adverse psychological sequelae to the procedure.

d. Woman is successful in achieving her goal of either contraception or conception at the time she desires.

5. Postabortion psychological impact:

a. Majority—relieved and happy.

b. Small number (5%–10%)—negative feelings, such as guilt or low self-esteem.

CHILDBEARING: PREGNANCY BY TRIMESTER

General overview: This review of the normal physiological and psychosocial changes occurring during each trimester of pregnancy provides essential components of the database for accurate nursing judgments and anticipatory guidance during the prenatal period. Complications of pregnancy are correlated with the trimester of common occurrence; relationships with other NCLEX® categories of human function are described.

I. General aspects of nursing care

◆ **A. Assessment**—based on nursing knowledge of the following:

1. Biophysical and psychosocial aspects of conception and gestation.

2. Parameters of normal pregnancy.

3. Risk factors, signs, symptoms, and implications of deviations from normal patterns of maternal and fetal health.

◆ **B. Analysis/nursing diagnosis:**

1. *Knowledge deficit* related to normal pregnancy-related alterations (physiological and emotional alterations/trimester).

2. *Pain* related to normal physiological alterations in pregnancy.

3. *Altered elimination* related to normal physiological changes during pregnancy (polyuria, constipation).

4. *Altered nutrition* related to increased metabolic needs due to pregnancy.

5. *Impaired adjustment* related to altered self-image; anticipated role change; resurgence of old, unresolved conflicts.

◆ **C. Nursing care plan/implementation:**

1. Goal: *emotional support.*

a. Encourage verbalization of feelings, fears, concerns.

b. Validate normalcy of behavioral response to pregnancy.

2. Goal: *anticipatory guidance.*

a. Facilitate achievement of developmental tasks.

b. Strengthen coping techniques for pregnancy,

lation, birth. Suggest appropriate resources (preparation for childbirth classes).

3. Goal: *health teaching.* Describe, explain, discuss:
   a. Normal physiological alterations during pregnancy.
   b. Common discomforts of pregnancy, management.

◆ **D. Evaluation/outcome criteria:**
1. Woman takes an active, informed part in her pregnancy-related care.
2. Woman copes effectively with common alterations associated with pregnancy (physiological, psychological, role change).
3. Woman successfully carries an uneventful pregnancy to term.

II. Biological foundations of pregnancy
A. Conception
1. *Egg*—life span, approximately 24 hr after ovulation.
2. *Sperm*—life span, approximately 72 hr after ejaculation into female reproductive tract.
3. *Conception* (fertilization)—usually occurs 12–24 hr after ovulation, within fallopian tube.
4. *Implantation* (nidation)—usually occurs within 7–9 days of conception, or about day 21–23 of a 28-day menstrual cycle.
5. *Ovum*—period of conception until primary villi have appeared; usually about 12–14 days.
6. *Embryo*—period from end of ovum stage until measurement reaches approximately 3 cm; 54–56 days.
7. *Fetus*—period from end of embryo stage until birth.

First Trimester
Susceptible to teratogens
Heart functions at 3–4 wk
Eye formation at 4–5 wk
Arm and leg buds at 4–5 wk
Recognizable face at 8 wk
Brain: rapid growth
External genitalia at 8 wk
Placenta formed at 12 wk
Bone ossification at 12 wk

Second Trimester
Less danger from teratogens after 12 wk
Facial features formed at 16 wk
Fetal heartbeat heard by 18–20 wk; with a fetoscope/Doppler at 10–12 wk
Quickening at 18–20 wk
Length: 10 inches, weight: 8–10 oz
Vernix: present

Third Trimester
Iron stored
Surfactant production begins in increasing amounts
Size: 15 inches, 2–3 lb
Calcium stored at 28–32 wk
Reflexes present at 28–32 wk
Subcutaneous fat deposits at 36 wk

Lanugo shedding at 38–40 wk
Average size: 18–22 inches, 7.5–8.5 lb at 38–40 wk

B. Anatomical and physiological modifications
1. *Bases of functional alterations*
   a. *Hormonal*—**Table 4.4** discusses the effects of estrogen and progesterone during pregnancy. Nursing implications provide the knowledge base for the following:
      (1) Anticipatory guidance regarding normal maternal adaptations.
      (2) Early identification of deviations from normal patterns.
   b. *Mechanical*—enlarging uterus → displacement and pressure; increased weight of uterus and breasts → changes in posture and pressure.
2. *Breasts*—enlarged darkened areola; secrete colostrum.
3. *Reproductive organs*
   a. *Uterus*
      (1) Amenorrhea. Occasional spotting common, especially at time of first missed menstrual period.
      (2) Increased vascularity adds to increase in size and softening of the lower uterine segment (*Hegar's sign*).
      (3) Growth is due to hypertrophy and hyperplasia of existing muscle cells and connective tissue.
      (4) Fundal height measurement landmarks:

Uterus	Nonpregnant	Pregnant (At Term)
Length	6.5 cm	32 cm
Width	4 cm	24 cm
Depth	2.5 cm	22 cm
Weight	50 g	1000 g

   b. *Cervix*
      (1) Increased vascularity → softening (*Goodell's sign*) and deepened blue-purple coloration (*Chadwick's sign*).
      (2) Edema, hyperplasia, thickening of mucous lining, and increased mucus production; formation of mucus plug by end of second month.
      (3) Becomes shorter, thicker, and more elastic.
   c. *Vagina*
      (1) Hyperemia deepens color (*Chadwick's sign*).
      (2) Hypertrophy and hyperplasia thicken vaginal mucosa.
      (3) Relaxation of connective tissue.
      (4) pH acidic (4.0–6.0).
      (5) Leukorrhea—nonirritating.
   d. *Perineum*
      (1) Increases in size—hypertrophy of muscle cells, edema, and relaxation of elastic tissue.
      (2) Deepened color—increased vascularization/hyperemia.

TABLE 4.4	Hormones of Pregnancy

Primary Effects	Clinical Implications for Nursing Actions
Estrogen	
Level rises in serum and urine	Basis of test for maternal/placental/fetal well-being
Uterine enlargement	Probable sign of pregnancy
Breast enlargement	Probable sign of pregnancy; increased tingling, tenderness
Genital enlargement: increased vascularization, hyperplasia	Vaginal growth facilitates vaginal birth
Softens connective tissue	Results in backache and leg ache; relaxes joints to increase size of birth canal and rib cage
Alters nutrient metabolism:	*Gastrointestinal and metabolic changes:*
Decreases HCl and pepsin	Digestive upsets
Antagonist to insulin—makes glucose available to fetus	Anti-insulin effect challenges maternal pancreas to produce more insulin; failure of β-cells to respond leads to "gestational" diabetes. For the woman who is insulin-dependent, insulin requirements increase by an average of 67% during the second half of pregnancy
Supports fat deposition	Protect source of energy for fetus
Sodium and water retention; edema of lower extremities (nonpitting)	Meet increased plasma volume needs and maintain fluid reserve
Hematological changes:	
Increased coagulability	Increased tendency to thrombosis
Increased sedimentation rate (SR)	SR loses diagnostic value for heart disease
Vasodilation: spider nevi; palmar erythema	Resolves spontaneously after birth
Increased production of melanin-stimulating hormone	Resolves spontaneously after birth; causes chloasma and linea nigra
Progesterone	
Development of decidua	High levels result in tiredness, listlessness, and sleepiness
Reduces uterine excitability	Protection against abortion/early birth (i.e. *maintains pregnancy*)
Development of mammary glands	Prepares breasts for lactation
Alters nutrient metabolism:	*Nutritional significance:*
Antagonist to insulin	Diabetogenic
Favors fat deposition	Energy reserve
Decreases gastric motility and relaxes sphincters	Favors heartburn and constipation
Increased sensitivity of respiratory center to CO_2	Increased depth, some dyspnea, increased sighing
Decreased smooth-muscle tone:	*Decreased tone can lead to:*
Colon	Constipation
Bladder, ureters	Stasis of urine with $\uparrow$ chance of infection
Veins	Dependent edema; varicosities
Gallbladder	Gallbladder disease
Increased basal body temperature (BBT) by 0.5°C	Discomfort from hot flashes and perspiration
Human Chorionic Gonadotropin	
Maintains corpus luteum during early pregnancy	Placenta must "take over" after a few weeks
Stimulates male testes	Increased testosterone in male fetuses
May suppress immune response	May inhibit response to foreign protein, for example, fetal portion of placenta

(Continued on following page)

Maternal-Infant

TABLE 4.4	Hormones of Pregnancy *(Continued)*

Primary Effects	Clinical Implications for Nursing Actions
	Diagnostic value:
	Basis for pregnancy test
	Decreased level with threatened abortion
	Increased level with multiple pregnancy
	Very high level with hydatidiform mole
Human Placental Lactogen	
Antagonizes insulin	Diabetogenic; may → gestational diabetes or complicate management of existing diabetes
Mobilizes maternal free fatty acids	Increased tendency of ketoacidosis in pregnant diabetic
Prolactin	
Suppressed by estrogen and progesterone	No milk produced before birth
Increased level after placenta is delivered	**Milk production** (lactation) 2–3 days after birth
Follicle-Stimulating Hormone	
Production suppressed during pregnancy; level returns to prepregnant levels within 3 wk after birth	No ovulation during pregnancy; ovulation usually returns within 6 wk for 15%, within 12 wk for 30%
Oxytocin	
Causes uterus to contract when the oxytocin levels exceed those of estrogen and progesterone	Labor induction or augmentation; treatment for postpartum uterine atony

e. *Ovaries*
  (1) Ovum production ceases.
  (2) Corpus luteum persists; produces hormones to wk 10–12 until placenta "takes over."
C. **Alterations affecting fluid-gas transport**
  1. *Cardiovascular system* (**Table 4.5**)
    a. **Physiological changes**
      (1) Heart displaced upward and to the left.
      (2) Circulation:
        (a) Cardiac volume increases by 20%–30%.
        (b) Labor—cardiac output increases by 20%–30%.

(3) Hemoglobin and hematocrit values remain between 10–14 g and 35%–42%; normal drop is 10% during second trimester.
(4) Hypercoagulability—increased levels of blood factors VII, VIII, IX, and X.
(5) Nonpathologic increased sedimentation rate—due to 50% increase in fibrinogen level.
(6) Blood pressure should remain stable with drop in second trimester.
(7) Heart rate often increases 10–15 beats/min at term.

TABLE 4.5	Blood Values

Component	Prepregnant	Pregnant	Postpartum*
WBC	4,000–11,000	9,000–16,000 (↑); 25,000—labor	20,000–25,000 within 10–12 days of birth, then returns to normal
RBC volume	1600 mL	1900 mL	Prepregnant level of 1600 mL
Plasma volume	2400 mL	3700 mL	Prepregnant level of 2400 mL
Hct (PCV)	37%–47%	32%–42% (↓)	At 72°, returns to prepregnant level of 37%–47%
Hgb (at sea level)	12–16 g/dL	10–14 g/dL	At 72°, returns to prepregnant level of 12–16 g/dL
Fibrinogen	250 mg/dL	400 mg/dL	At 72°, returns to prepregnant level of 250 mg/dL

*Postpartum values depend on factors of amount of blood loss, mobilization, and physiological edema (excretion of extravascular water). Normal blood loss for vaginal birth is 300–400 mL.

(8) Compression of pelvic veins → stasis of blood in lower extremities.

(9) Compression of inferior vena cava when supine → bradycardia → reduced cardiac output, faintness, sweating, nausea (*supine hypotension*). *Fetal response:* marked bradycardia due to hypoxia secondary to decreased placental perfusion.

◆ b. **Assessment:**
(1) Apical systolic murmur.
(2) Exaggerated splitting of first heart sound.
(3) Physiological anemia.
(4) Dependent edema in third trimester (**Table 4.6**).
(5) *Vena cava syndrome* (supine hypotension)—drop in systolic blood pressure may occur due to compression of descending aorta and inferior vena cava when supine.
(6) Varicosities (vulvar, anal, leg).

◆ c. **Nursing care plan/implementation:**
Goal: *health teaching*
(1) *Elevate* lower extremities frequently.
(2) Apply support hose.
(3) *Avoid* excess intake of sodium.
(4) Assume *side-lying* position at rest.
(5) Learn signs and symptoms of pregnancy-induced hypertension.

2. *Respiratory system*
a. **Physiological changes:**
(1) Increased: tidal volume, vital capacity, respiratory reserve, oxygen consumption, production of CO_2.
(2) Diaphragm elevated, increased substernal angle → flaring of rib cage.
(3) Uterine enlargement prevents maximum lung expansion in third trimester.

◆ b. **Assessment:**
(1) Shortness of breath or dyspnea on exertion and when lying flat in third trimester.
(2) Nasal stuffiness due to estrogen-induced edema (see **Table 4.6**).
(3) Deeper respiratory excursion.

◆ c. **Nursing care plan/implementation:** Goal: *health teaching*
(1) Sit and stand with good posture.
(2) When resting assume *semi-Fowler's position.*
(3) *Avoid* overdistention of stomach.

D. **Alterations affecting elimination**
1. *Urinary system*
a. **Physiological changes:**
(1) Relaxation of smooth muscle results in conditions that can persist 4–6 wk after birth:
(a) Dilatation of ureters.
(b) *Decreased* bladder tone.
(c) Increased potential for urinary stasis and *infection* (UTI).
(2) *Increased* glomerular filtration rate (50%) during last two trimesters.

(3) *Increased* renal plasma flow (25%–50%) during first two trimesters; returns to near normal levels by end of last trimester.
(4) *Increased* renal-tubular reabsorption rate—compensates for increased glomerular activity.
(5) Glycosuria—reflects kidney's inability to reabsorb all glucose filtered by glomeruli (may be normal or may indicate gestational diabetes; glycosuria always warrants further testing).
(6) *Increased* renal clearance of urea and creatinine (creatinine clearance used as test of renal function during pregnancy).
(7) Hormone-induced turgescence of bladder and pressure on bladder from gravid uterus (see **Table 4.6**).

◆ b. **Assessment:**
(1) Urinary frequency, first and third trimesters (see **Table 4.6**).
(2) Nocturia.
(3) Stress incontinence in third trimester.

◆ c. **Nursing care plan/implementation:**
Goal: *health teaching*
(1) Void with urge, to prevent bladder distention.
(2) Learn signs and symptoms of UTI.
(3) Decrease fluid intake in late evening.
(4) Perform *Kegel* exercises to reduce incontinence.

2. *Gastrointestinal system* (see **Table 4.6**)
a. **Physiological changes:**
(1) General decrease in smooth-muscle tone and motility due to actions of progesterone.
(2) *Intestines:* slowed peristalsis, increased water reabsorption in bowel.
(3) *Stomach*
(a) Gastric emptying time is delayed (e.g., 3 hr vs. $1^1/_2$ hr).
(b) Gastric secretion of HCl and pepsin decreases.
(c) Decreased motility delays emptying; increased acidity.
(4) *Cardiac sphincter* relaxes.
(5) Increasing size of *uterus* and displacement of *intraabdominal organs.*
(6) *Gallbladder:* decreased emptying.

◆ b. **Assessment:**
(1) Nausea and vomiting in first trimester.
(2) Constipation and flatulence.
(3) Hemorrhoids.
(4) Heartburn, reflux esophagitis, indigestion.
(5) Hiatal hernia.
(6) Epulis—edema and bleeding of gums.
(7) Ptyalism—excessive salivation.
(8) Jaundice.
(9) Gallstones.
(10) Pruritus due to increased retention of bile salts.

TABLE 4.6	Common Discomforts During Pregnancy

Discomfort and Cause		Health Teaching
Morning sickness—first 3 mo; nausea and vomiting; may occur anytime, day or night; *cause:* hormonal, psychological, and empty stomach		Alternate dry carbohydrate and fluids hourly; take dry carbohydrate before rising, stay in bed 15 more minutes; *avoid* empty stomach, offending odors, and food difficult to digest (e.g., food high in fat); *avoid* acidic foods (e.g., citrus)
Fatigue (sleep hunger)—first 3 mo; *cause:* possibly hormones; often returns in late pregnancy when physical load is great		Iron supplement if anemic—foods high in *iron, folic acid,* and *protein;* adequate rest
Fainting (syncope)—early pregnancy; due to slightly decreased arterial blood pressure; late pregnancy, due to venous stasis in lower extremities		*Elevate feet;* sit down when necessary; when standing, do not lock knees; *avoid* prolonged standing, fasting
Urinary frequency—enlarging uterus presses on bladder, turgescence of structures from hormone stimulation; relieved somewhat as uterus rises from pelvis; recurs with lightening		*Kegel exercises; limit fluids* just before bedtime to ensure rest; rule out urinary tract infection
Vaginal discharge—mo 2–9; mucus less acidic, and increases in amount (leukorrhea)		Cleanliness important; treat only if infection sets in; douche contraindicated in pregnancy
Hot flashes—heat intolerance, due to increased metabolism → diaphoresis		Alter clothing, bathing, and environmental temperature prn
Headache—cause unknown; possibly blood pressure change, nutritional, tension (unless associated with preeclampsia)		If pain relief needed, consult physician (*avoid* over-the-counter drugs without prescription); reduce tension
Nasal stuffiness—due to increased vascularization; allergic rhinitis of pregnancy		Antihistamines and nasal sprays by *prescription only*
Heartburn—enlarging uterus and hormones slow digestion; progesterone → reverse peristaltic waves → reflux of stomach contents into esophagus		Physician may prescribe an antacid; *avoid* use of antacids containing sodium; instead of leaning over, bend at the knees, keeping torso straight; sit on firm chairs; *limit fatty and fried* foods; small, frequent meals
Flatulence—altered digestion from enlarging uterus and hormones		Maintain regular bowel habits, *avoid* gas-forming foods; antiflatulent may be prescribed
Insomnia—fetal movements, fears or concerns, and general body discomfort from heavy uterus		Medication by prescription only; exercise; side-lying *positions* with pillow supports; change position often; back rubs, ventilate feelings
Shortness of breath—enlarging uterus limits expansion of diaphragm		Good posture; cut down/stop smoking; *position*—supine and upright
Backache—increased elasticity of connective tissue, increased weight of uterus, and increased lumbar curvature		Correct posture, low-heeled, wide-base shoes, and abdominal support (binders); do pelvic rock often; *avoid* fatigue
Pelvic joint pain—hormones relax connective tissue and joints and allow movement within joints		Rest; good posture; will go away after giving birth, in 6–8 wk; *avoid* prolonged standing/walking
Leg cramps—pressure of enlarging uterus on nerve supplying legs; possible causes: lack of calcium, fatigue, chilling, and tension		Stretch affected muscle and hold until it subsides; *do not rub* (may release a blood clot, if present); ↑ calcium intake
Constipation—decreased motility (hormones, enlarging uterus) and increased reabsorption of water; iron therapy (oral)		*Diet*—prunes, fruits, vegetables, roughage, and fluids; regular habits; exercise; sit on toilet with knees up; *avoid* enemas, mineral oil, laxatives
Hemorrhoids—varicosities around anus; aggravated by pushing with stool and by uterus pressing on blood vessels supplying lower body		As above, *avoid* constipation; pure Vaseline or Desitin is mild and sometimes soothing; use any other preparation with prescription only
Ankle edema—normal and nonpitting; gravity		Rest legs often during day with legs and hips raised
Varicose veins—lower legs, vulva, pelvis; pressure of heavy uterus; relaxation of connective tissue in vein walls; hereditary		Progressively worse with subsequent pregnancies and obesity; *elevate* legs above level of heart; support hose may help
Cramp in side or groin—round ligament pain; stretching of round ligament with cramping		To get out of bed, turn to side, use arm and upper body and push up to sitting position

◆ c. **Nursing care plan/implementation:**
  Goal: *health teaching*
 (1) Nausea and vomiting
    (a) *Avoid* fatty food; increase carbohydrates.
    (b) Eat small, frequent meals.
    (c) Eat dry crackers in morning.
    (d) *Decrease* liquids with meals.
    (e) *Avoid* odors that predispose to nausea.
    (f) *Avoid* acidic foods (e.g. citrus, tomatoes).
 (2) Constipation and flatulence
    (a) *Increase* fluids (6–8 glasses/day).
    (b) Maintain exercise regimen.
    (c) Add *fiber* to diet.
    (d) *Avoid* mineral oil laxatives.
    (e) *Avoid* gas-producing foods (e.g., beans, cabbage).
 (3) Heartburn and indigestion
    (a) *Eliminate* fatty, spicy, or acidic foods.
    (b) Eat small, frequent meals (6/day).
    (c) Eat slowly.
    (d) *Avoid* gastric irritants (e.g., alcohol, coffee).
    (e) *Avoid* lying flat.
    (f) Take antacids without sodium or phosphorus.
    (g) Try chewing gum to increase the secretion of alkaline saliva.
    (h) Wait 2–3 hours after meals before lying down.
    (i) Wear loose-fitting clothes.
  (4) Hemorrhoids
    (a) Increase *fluid and fiber* intake.
    (b) Maintain exercise regimen.
    (c) *Avoid* constipation and straining to defecate.
    (d) Take warm sitz baths.
    (e) Apply witch hazel pads.
    (f) *Elevate* hips and legs frequently.
    (g) Use hemorrhoidal ointments only with advice of health-care provider.

E. **Alterations affecting nutrition**
  1. **Physiological changes:**
    a. *Gastrointestinal system*
      (1) Gingivae soften and enlarge due to increased vascularity.
      (2) Increased saliva production.
    b. *Endocrine system*
      (1) *Increased* size and activity of pituitary, parathyroids, adrenals.
      (2) *Increased* vascularity and hyperplasia of thyroid.
      (3) Pancreas—*increased* insulin production during second half of pregnancy, needed to meet rising maternal needs; human placental lactogen (HPL) and insulinase deactivate maternal insulin; may precipitate *gestational diabetes* in women who are susceptible.
    c. *Metabolism*
      (1) Basal metabolic rate (BMR)—*increases* 25% as pregnancy progresses, due to increasing oxygen consumption; protein-bound iodine (PBI) *increases* to 7–10 µg/dL; metabolism returns to normal by sixth postpartal week.
      (2) Protein—need *increased* for fetal and uterine growth, maternal blood formation.
      (3) Water retention—*increased*.
      (4) Carbohydrates—need *increases* to spare protein stores.
        (a) *First half of pregnancy*—glucose rapidly and continuously siphoned across placenta to meet fetal growth needs; may lead to hypoglycemia and faintness.
        (b) *Second half of pregnancy*—placental production of antiinsulin hormones; normal maternal hyperglycemia; affects coexisting diabetes.
      (5) Fat—*increased* plasma-lipid levels.
      (6) Iron—supplements recommended to meet *increased* need for red blood cells (RBCs) by maternal/placental/fetal unit.

◆ 2. **Assessment:**
  a. Weight gain: 20–35 lb (11.5–16 kg); depends on Body Mass Index (BMI) and prepregnant nutritional status.
  b. Normal pattern: first trimester, 2–5 lb (1–2.3 kg); remainder of gestation, approximately 1 lb/wk (0.4–0.5 kg/wk).

◆ 3. **Nursing care plan/implementation:**
  Goal: *health teaching*
  a. Evaluate diet for adequacy of nutrient and caloric intake.
  b. Evaluate cultural, religious, and economic influences on diet.
  c. Review dietary recommendation for pregnancy with woman.
  d. *Avoid* dieting in pregnancy (even if obese).
  e. Supplement diet with *vitamins, iron,* or *folic acid* on advice of health provider.
  f. *Ptyalism:*
    (1) Suck hard candies.
    (2) Perform frequent oral hygiene.
    (3) Maintain adequate oral intake (6–8 glasses/day).
    (4) Use lip balm to prevent chapping.
  g. *Epulis:*
    (1) Frequent oral hygiene.
    (2) Use soft toothbrush.
    (3) Floss gently.
    (4) See dentist regularly.

F. **Alterations affecting protective functions**—*integumentary system*
  1. **Physiological changes**—estrogen-induced vascular and pigment changes.

◆ 2. **Assessment:**
   a. Increased pigmentation (chloasma and linea nigra).
   b. Striae gravidarum (stretch marks).
   c. Increased sebaceous and sweat gland activity.
   d. Palmar erythema.
   e. Angiomas—vascular "spiders."
◆ 3. **Nursing care plan/implementation:**
   Goal: *health teaching*
   a. Bathe or shower daily.
   b. Reassure woman that skin changes decrease after pregnancy.
G. **Alterations affecting comfort, rest, mobility—** *musculoskeletal system*
   1. **Physiological changes**
      a. Progesterone, estrogen, and relaxin-induced relaxation of joints, cartilage, and ligaments.
      b. Function in childbearing—increases antero-posterior diameter of rib cage and enlarges birth canal.
◆ 2. **Assessment:**
   a. Complaint of pelvic "looseness."
   b. Duck-waddle walk.
   c. Tenderness of symphysis pubis.
   d. Lordosis (exaggerated lumbar curve)— *increased* weight of pelvis tilts pelvis forward; to compensate, woman throws head and shoulders backward; complaint of leg and back strain and fatigue (see **Table 4.6**)
   e. Feet often increase by half a shoe size or more.
◆ 3. **Nursing care plan/implementation:**
   Goal: *health teaching*
   a. Good body alignment—tuck pelvis under; tighten abdominal muscles.
   b. Pelvic-rock exercises.
   c. Squat; bend at knees, *not* at waist.
   d. Wear low-heeled, sturdy shoes.
   e. *Avoid* tight-fitting clothing that interferes with circulatory return in legs.
III. **Psychosocial-cultural alterations**
   A. *Emotional changes*—affected by: age, maturity, support system, amount of current stresses, coping abilities, physical and mental health status.
   Developmental tasks of pregnancy:
   1. Accept the pregnancy as real: "I am pregnant;" progress from symbiotic relationship with the fetus to perceiving the child as an individual.
   2. Seek and ensure acceptance of child by others.
   3. Seek protection for self and fetus through pregnancy and labor ("safe passage").
   4. Prepare realistically for the coming child and for necessary role change: "I am going to be a parent."
   B. *Physical bases of changes*
   1. *Increased* metabolic demands may result in anemia and fatigue.
   2. *Increased* hormone levels (steroids, estrogen, progesterone)—affect mood as well as physiology.
   C. *Characteristic behaviors*—**Table 4.7** describes behaviors commonly exhibited in each trimester.

D. *Sexuality and sexual expression*—feelings and expressions of sexuality may vary during pregnancy due to maternal adaptations and physiological changes.
E. *Intrafamily relationships*
   1. Pregnancy is a maturational crisis for the family.
   2. Requires changes in lifestyle and interactions:
      a. Increased financial demands.
      b. Changing family and social relationships.
      c. Adapting communication patterns.
      d. Adapting sexual patterns.
      e. Anticipating new responsibilities and needs.
      f. Responding to reactions of others.

Prenatal Management

I. **Initial assessment:** Goal: *establish baseline for health supervision, teaching, emotional support, or referral.*
II. **Objectives:**
   A. Determine woman's present health status and validate pregnancy.
   B. Identify factors affecting or affected by pregnancy.
   C. Determine current gravidity and parity.
   D. Identify present length of gestation.
   E. Establish an estimated date of delivery (EDD). Nägele's determination of EDD—*subtract 3 mo, add 7 days* to last menstrual period (LMP).
   F. Determine relevant knowledge deficit.
◆ III. **Assessment:** *history*
   A. *Family*—inheritable diseases, reproductive problems.
   B. *Personal*—medical, surgical, gynecological, past obstetric, average nonpregnant weight.
      1. *Gravida*—a pregnant woman.
         a. *Nulligravida*—woman who has *never* been pregnant.
         b. *Primigravida*—woman with a *first* pregnancy.
         c. *Multigravida*—woman with a *second or later* pregnancy.
      2. *Para*—refers to *past pregnancies* (not number of babies) that reached viability (20–22 wk whether or not born alive).
         a. *Nullipara*—woman who has *not* carried a pregnancy to viability (e.g., may have had one or more abortions).
         b. *Primipara*—woman who has carried *one* pregnancy to viability.
         c. *Multipara*—woman who had *two or more* pregnancies that reached viability.
         d. *Grandmultipara*—woman who has had *six or more* viable pregnancies.
      3. *Examples of gravidity/parity.* Several methods of describing gravidity and parity are in common use. One method (**GTPAL**) describes number of "**G**ravida" (pregnancies), **T**erm (or full-term infants), **P**reterm infants, **A**bortions, and number of **L**iving children.
         a. A woman who is pregnant for the *first* time and is currently *undelivered* is designated as 1-0-0-0-0. *After* giving birth to a full-term living neonate, she becomes 1-1-0-0-1.

TABLE 4.7	Behavioral Changes in Pregnancy

◆ Assessment/Characteristics	◆ Nursing Care Plan/Implementation
First Trimester	
Emotional lability (mood swings)	Encourage verbalization of feelings, concerns
Displeasure with subjective symptoms of early pregnancy (nausea, fatigue, etc.)	*Health teaching:* diet, rest, relaxation, diversion
Feelings of ambivalence	Validate normalcy of feelings, behaviors
Second Trimester	
Accepts pregnancy (usually coincides with awareness of fetal movement [i.e., "quickening"])	Encourage exploration of feelings of dependency, introspection, mood swings
Becomes introspective: resolves old conflicts (feelings toward mother, sexual intimacy, masturbation)	Discuss childbirth preparation and preparation-for-parenthood classes; refer, as necessary
Reevaluates self, lifestyle, marriage	
Daydreams, fantasizes self as "mother"	
Seeks out other women who are pregnant and new mothers	
Third Trimester	
Altered body image	Encourage verbalization of concerns, discomforts of late pregnancy
Fears body mutilation (stretching of body tissues, episiotomy, cesarean birth)	Help meet dependency needs; offer reassurance, as possible
Distress over loss of control over body functions (ptyalism, colostrum leakage, leukorrhea, urinary frequency, constipation, stress incontinence)	*Health teaching:* Kegel exercises; preparation for labor. Anticipatory guidance and planning for needs of self, baby, and family in early postpartum
Anxiety for baby (deformity, death)	
Fears pain, loss of control in labor	
Acceptance of impending labor during last 2 wk (ready to "move on")	

b. If a woman's second pregnancy ends in abortion and she has a living child from a previous pregnancy, born at term, she is designated as 2-1-0-1-1.

c. A woman who is pregnant for the fourth time and whose previous pregnancies yielded one full-term neonate, premature twins, and one abortion (spontaneous or induced), and who now has three living children, may be designated as 4-1-1-1-3.

d. Others record as follows: number gravida/number para. Applying this system to the examples given above, those mothers would be designated as follows: a—G1P1; b—G2P1; c—G4P2.

e. Others include recording of abortions:
G1P1 Ab0
G2P1 Ab1
G4P2 Ab1

◆ **IV. Assessment: *initial physical aspects:***
  A. Height and weight.
  B. Vital signs.
  C. Blood work—hematocrit and hemoglobin for anemia; type and Rh factor; tests for sickle cell trait, syphilis, rubella antibody titer, and hepatitis B screen (see also **Table 4.5**).

 D. Urinalysis—glucose, protein, ketones, signs of infection, and pregnancy test (HCG).
  E. Breast examination.
  F. Pelvic examination.
    1. Signs of pregnancy.
    2. Adequacy of pelvis and pelvic structures.
    3. Size and position of uterus.
    4. Papanicolau smear.
    5. Smears for monilial and trichomonal infections.
    6. Signs of pelvic inflammatory disease.
    7. Tests for STD: Gonorrhea (Gonococcus-GC), chlamydia.
  G. *Validation of pregnancy*—physician or midwife makes differential diagnosis between presumptive/probable signs/symptoms of early pregnancy and other signs.
    1. *Presumptive symptoms*—subjective experiences.
      a. Amenorrhea—more than 10 days past missed menstrual period.
      b. Breast tenderness, enlargement.

c. Nausea and vomiting.

d. Quickening (wk 16–18).

e. Urinary frequency.

f. Fatigue.

g. Constipation (50% of women).

2. *Presumptive signs*

a. Striae gravidarum, linea nigra, chloasma (after wk 16).

b. Increased basal body temperature (BBT)

3. *Probable signs*—examiner's objective findings.

a. Positive pregnancy test.

b. Enlargement of abdomen/uterus.

c. Reproductive organ changes (after sixth week):

(1) *Goodell's sign*—cervical softening.

(2) *Hegar's sign*—softening of lower uterine segment.

(3) Vaginal changes (*Chadwick's sign*): purple hue in vulvar/vaginal area.

d. Ballottement (after 16–20 wk).

e. *Braxton Hicks* contractions.

4. *Positive signs of pregnancy:*

a. Fetal heart tones.

(1) Doptone: wk 10–12.

(2) Fetoscope: wk 20.

b. Examiner visualizes and feels fetal movements (usually after wk 24).

c. Sonographic examination (after wk 14) when fetal head is sufficiently developed for accurate determination of gestational age. Pregnancy may be detected as early as fifth or sixth week after LMP.

◆ **V. Assessment: *nutritional status:***

A. Physical findings suggesting poor nutritional status:

1. Skin: rough, dry, scaly.

2. Lips: lesions in corners.

3. Hair: dull, brittle.

4. Mucous membranes: pale.

5. Dental caries.

B. Height, weight, age—average weight gain approximately 24 lb. Range 24–32 lb is best for mother and neonate.

C. Laboratory values—Hemoglobin: <10.5/100 mg Hct: <32% indicates anemia.

D. Nutrition history.

◆ **E. Analysis/nursing diagnosis:**

1. *Altered nutrition: less than body requirements* related to anemia, vitamin/mineral deficit.

2. *Altered nutrition: more than body requirements* related to obesity.

◆ **F. Nursing care plan/implementation:**

Goal: *health teaching.* Nutritional counseling for diet in pregnancy and/or lactation.

◆ **G. Evaluation/outcome criteria:**

1. If *underweight* at conception: should gain 28–42 lb (12.5–18 kg).

2. If *overweight* at conception: 15–25 lb (7–11.5 kg).

3. If *obese* at conception: 15 lb (7 kg) or more.

◆ **VI. Assessment: *psychosocial aspects:***

A. Pregnancy: planned or not; desired or not.

B. Present plans:

1. Carry pregnancy, keep baby.

2. Carry pregnancy, adoption.

3. Abortion.

C. Cultural, ethnic influences on decisions: will influence range of activities, types of safeguarding actions, diet, and health-promotion behaviors.

D. Parenting potential: actively seeking medical care and information about pregnancy, childbirth, parenthood.

E. Family readiness for childbearing and child rearing:

1. Physical maintenance.

2. Allocation of resources: identify support system.

3. Division of labor.

4. Socialization of family members.

5. Reproduction, recruitment, launching of family members into society.

6. Maintenance of order (relationships within family).

F. Perceptions of present and projected family relationships.

G. Review lifestyle for smoking, drugs, alcohol (ETOH), attitudes about pregnancy, health-care practices, and risks for hepatitis and human immunodeficiency virus (HIV).

◆ **VII. Analysis/nursing diagnosis:**

A. *Altered role performance* related to stress imposed by developmental tasks.

B. *Ineffective coping: individual, family* related to stress caused by developmental tasks/crises.

C. *Altered family process* related to developmental tasks. First baby may precipitate individual or family developmental crisis.

◆ **VIII. Nursing care plan/implementation:**

A. Goal: *anticipatory guidance/support.*

1. Discuss mood swings, ambivalent feelings, negative feelings.

2. Reinforce "normalcy" of such feelings.

B. Goal: *increase individual/family coping skills, reduce intrafamily stress.*

1. Reinforce family strengths (both partners), sense of family identity.

a. Encourage open communication between partners; share feelings and concerns.

b. Increase understanding of mutual needs, encourage mutuality of support.

c. Increase tendency of mother to turn to partner as most significant person (as opposed to physician).

d. Enhance bond, success of childbirth preparation classes.

2. Promote understanding/acceptance of role change.

a. Facilitate/support achievement of developmental tasks.

b. Reduce probability of postpartal psychological problems.

c. Promote family bonding.

C. Goal: *health teaching.*
1. *Siblings:*
   a. Alert parents to sibling needs for security, love.
   b. Include sibling in pregnancy experience.
   c. Provide clear, simple explanations of happenings.
   d. Continue demonstrations of love.
   e. Describe increased status ("big sister/brother").
   f. Discuss possible misbehavior to gain attention.
2. *Relatives:* alert parents to possible negative feelings of in-laws.
3. Referral to childbirth preparation/parenting classes.
4. Appropriate community referrals for financial relief to decrease stress and provide aid.

◆ **IX.** **Evaluation/outcome criteria:**
   A. Actively participates in pregnancy-related decision making.
   B. Expresses satisfaction with decisions made.
   C. Demonstrates growth and development in parenting role.
   D. Prepared for the birth and for early parenthood.

Antepartum

I. **Nursing care and obstetric support**
   A. **General aspects of prenatal management**
   1. *Scheduled visits:*
      a. Once monthly—until wk 28.
      b. Every 2 wk—wk 28–36.
      c. Weekly—wk 36 until labor.
   ◆ 2. **Assessment:**
      a. General well-being, signs of deviations, concerns, questions.
      b. Weight gain pattern.
      c. Blood pressure (sitting).
   ▶ d. Abdominal palpation:
      (1) Fundal height; tenderness, masses, hernia.
      (2) Fetal heart rate (FHR).
   ▶ (3) Leopold's maneuvers for presentation (after wk 32).
      e. Laboratory tests:
      (1) Urinalysis—for protein, sugar, signs of asymptomatic infection; drug screen for high-risk groups.
      (2) Venous blood—Hgb, Hct; blood type and Rh; RPR; rubella titer, antibody titer, sickle cell. HIV and hepatitis antigen recommended for all pregnant clients.
      (3) Cultures (vaginal discharge; cervical scrapings, for *Chlamydia trachomatis, Neisseria gonorrhoeae*).
      (4) Tuberculosis (TB) screening in high-risk areas.
      (5) Maternal alpha-fetoprotein screen, 16–18 wk optimum time.
      (6) Serum-glucose screen, 24–28 wk; 1-hour glucose tolerance test.

   f. Follow-up on medications (vitamins, iron) and nutrition.
   g. If TB positive during pregnancy, isoniazid (INH) and rifampin given daily. INH is associated with increase in fetal malformations, particularly neurotoxicity. Pyridoxine administered simultaneously to prevent their development.

B. **Common minor discomforts during pregnancy** (for **Assessment**, see **Table 4.6**).
   1. **Etiology:** normal maternal physiological/psychological alterations in pregnancy.
   ◆ 2. **Nursing care plan/implementation:**
      a. Goal: *anticipatory guidance.* Discuss the importance of adequate rest, exercise, diet, and hydration in minimizing symptoms.
      b. Goal: *health teaching* (see **Table 4.6**).
   ◆ 3. **Evaluation/outcome criteria:** woman avoids, minimizes, or copes effectively with minor usual discomforts of pregnancy.

C. **Danger signs:**
   1. **Etiology:** Specific disease processes are discussed under **Complications.**
   ◆ 2. **Nursing care plan/implementation:**
      Goal: *health teaching*—to safeguard status. Signs to report *immediately:*

   a. **Persistent vomiting** beyond first trimester or severe vomiting at any time. *Possible cause:* Hyperemesis gravidarum.
   b. Fluid discharge from vagina—**bleeding or amniotic fluid** (anything other than leukorrhea). *Possible causes:* Placental problem, rupture of membranes (ROM).
   c. Severe or unusual **pain:** abdominal. *Possible cause:* Abruptio placentae.
   d. Chills or **fever** (if lasts over 24 hours, or over 102°F). *Possible cause:* Infection.
   e. Urinary frequency or **burning on urination.** *Possible cause:* UTI.
   f. **Absence of fetal movements** after quickening, lasting more than 24 hours. *Possible cause:* Intrauterine fetal death.
   g. Visual disturbances—**blurring, double vision,** "spots before eyes." *Possible cause:* Preeclampsia.
   h. **Swelling** of fingers, ankles, hands, feet, or face. *Possible cause:* Preeclampsia.
   i. Severe, frequent, or continual **headache.** *Possible cause:* Preeclampsia.
   j. Muscle irritability or **convulsions.** *Possible cause:* Preeclampsia.
   k. **Rapid weight gain** not associated with eating. *Possible cause:* Preeclampsia.
   l. **More than 4 uterine contractions** per hour (before 38 weeks). *Possible cause:* Preterm labor.

   ◆ 3. **Evaluation/outcome criteria:**
      a. Actively participates in own health maintenance/pregnancy management.
      b. Identifies early signs of potentially serious complications during the antepartal period.
      c. Promptly reports and seeks medical attention.

II. Complications during the antepartum

A. **General aspects:**

1. **Etiology:**

a. Normal alterations and increasing physiological stress of pregnancy affect status of coexisting medical disorders.

b. Conditions affecting mother's general health also affect ability to adapt successfully to normal physiological stress of pregnancy.

c. Aberrations of normal pregnancy.

2. Goal: *reduce incidence of health problems affecting maternal/fetal health and pregnancy outcome.*

a. Identify presence of risk factors and signs and symptoms of complications early.

b. Treat emerging complications promptly and effectively.

c. Minimize effects of complications on pregnancy outcome.

◆ 3. **Assessment:** risk factors:

a. Age:

(1) Adolescent.

(2) Primigravida, age 35 or older.

(3) Multigravida, age 40 or older.

b. Socioeconomic level: lower.

c. Ethnic group

d. Previous pregnancy history:

(1) Habitual abortion.

(2) Multiparity greater than 5.

(3) Previous stillbirths.

(4) Previous cesarean birth.

(5) Previous preterm labor or delivery.

e. Multifetal pregnancy.

f. Prenatal care:

(1) Enters health-care system late in pregnancy.

(2) Irregular/episodic prenatal care visits.

(3) Noncompliance with medical/nursing recommendations.

g. Preexisting or coexisting medical disorders:

(1) Cardiovascular: hypertension, heart disease.

(2) Diabetes.

(3) Other: renal, respiratory, infections, acquired immunodeficiency syndrome (AIDS).

h. Substance abuse.

◆ 4. **Nursing care plan/implementation:**

a. Goal: *health teaching* (discussed under specific health problem).

b. Goal: *early identification/treatment of emerging health problems* (if any).

(1) Monitor status and progress of pregnancy.

(2) Refer for medical management, as necessary.

c. Goal: *emotional support.*

◆ 5. **Evaluation/outcome criteria:**

a. Understands present health status, interactions of coexisting disorder and pregnancy.

b. Accepts responsibility for own health maintenance.

c. Makes informed decisions regarding pregnancy.

d. Minimizes potential for complications of coexisting disorder/pregnancy.

(1) Avoids factors predisposing to health problems.

(2) Understands and implements therapeutic management of coexisting disorder/pregnancy.

(3) Increases compliance with medical/nursing recommendations.

e. Carries uneventful pregnancy to term.

B. **Disorders affecting fluid-gas transport: cardiac disease**

1. **Pathophysiology:** cardiac overload → cardiac decompensation → right-sided failure → pulmonary edema.

2. **Etiology:**

a. Congenital heart defects.

b. Valvular damage—due to rheumatic fever (most common lesion is mitral stenosis, which can lead to pulmonary edema and emboli).

c. Increased circulating-blood volume and cardiac output—exceeds cardiac reserve. Greatest risk: *after 28 weeks of gestation*—reaches maximum (30%–50%) volume increase; *postpartum*—due to diuresis.

d. Secondary to treatment (tx) (e.g., tocolysis and steroids).

e. Pregnancy after valve replacement.

3. Normal physiological alterations during pregnancy that *mimic cardiac disorders:*

a. Systolic murmurs, palpitations, tachycardia, and hyperventilation with some dyspnea on normal moderate exertion.

b. Edema of lower extremities.

c. Cardiac enlargement.

d. Elevated sedimentation rate near term.

◆ 4. **Assessment:**

a. Medical evaluation of cardiac status. Classification of severity of cardiac involvement:

(1) *Class I*—least affected; asymptomatic with ordinary activity.

(2) *Class II*—activities somewhat limited; ordinary activities cause fatigue, dyspnea, angina.

(3) *Class III*—moderate/marked limitation of activity; common activities result in severe symptoms of fatigue, etc.

(4) *Class IV*—most affected; symptomatic (dyspnea, angina) at rest; should avoid pregnancy.

b. **Cardiac decompensation:**

(1) *Subjective symptoms*

Palpitations; feeling that the heart is "racing"

Increasing fatigue or difficulty breathing, or both, with the usual activities

Feeling of smothering and/or frequent cough

Periorbital edema; edema of face, fingers (e.g., rings do not fit anymore), feet, legs

(2) *Objective signs*

Irregular weak, rapid pulse (≥ 100 beats/min)

Rapid respirations (≥ 25 breaths/min)

Progressive, generalized edema

Crackles (rales) at base of lungs, after two inspirations and exhalations

Orthopnea; increasing dyspnea on minimal physical activity

Moist, frequent cough

Cyanosis of lips and nailbeds

◆ 5. **Analysis/nursing diagnosis:**

a. *Fluid volume excess* related to inability of compromised heart to handle increased workload (decreased cardiac reserve → congestive heart failure).

b. *Impaired gas exchange* related to pulmonary edema secondary to congestive heart failure.

◆ 6. **Nursing care plan/implementation:**

a. *Medical management:*

▬▭ (1) Diuretics, electrolyte supplements.

▬▭ (2) Digitalis (dose may need to be higher because of dilution in the increased blood volume of pregnancy).

▬▭ (3) Antibiotics—prophylaxis against rheumatic fever; treatment of bacterial infections during pregnancy.

▬▭ (4) Anticoagulants. Heparin is preferred because its large molecule cannot easily cross placenta. Occasionally, sequelae may include maternal hemorrhage, preterm birth, stillbirth.

(5) Oxygen, as needed.

(6) Mitral valvotomy for mitral stenosis often brings dramatic relief.

b. Goal: *health teaching.*

(1) Need for compliance with therapeutic regimen, medical/nursing recommendations.

(2) Drug actions, dosage, necessary actions (how to take own pulse, reportable signs/-symptoms).

(3) Methods for *decreasing work of heart:*

(a) Adequate *rest*—minimum 10 hr sleep each night; 30 min nap after each meal.

(b) *Avoid* heavy physical *activity* (including housework), fatigue, excessive weight gain, emotional stress, infection.

(c) *Avoid situations* of reduced ambient O$_2$, such as smoking, exposure to pollutants, flight in unpressurized small planes.

c. Goal: *nutritional counseling.*

(1) Well-balanced *diet*; adequate protein, fresh fruits and vegetables, water.

🍽 (2) *Avoid* "junk food," stimulants (caffeine), excessive salt intake.

d. Goal: *anticipatory planning:* management of **labor.**

(1) Goal: *minimize physiological and psychological stress.*

(2) *Medical management:*

(a) Reevaluation of cardiac status before EDD and labor.

(b) Regional anesthesia for labor/birth.

(c) Low-outlet forceps or vacuum extraction birth; episiotomy.

(d) Continuous hemodynamic monitoring.

◆ (3) **Assessment:** continuous.

(a) Physiological response to labor stimuli—*frequent vital signs* (pulse rate most sensitive and reliable indicator of impending congestive heart failure).

(b) Color, respiratory effort, diaphoresis.

(c) Contractions, etc.—same as for any mother in labor.

◆ (4) **Nursing care plan/implementation:** *labor.*

(a) Goal: *safeguard status.*

(1) Report *promptly:* pulse rate over 100; respirations more than 24 between contractions.

(2) Oxygen at 6 liters, as needed.

(b) Goal: *emotional support*—to reduce anxiety, facilitate cooperation.

(1) Encourage verbalization of feelings, fears, concerns.

(2) Explain all procedures.

(c) Goal: *promote cardiac function.* *Position*—semirecumbent; support arms and legs.

(d) Goal: *promote relaxation/control over labor discomfort.* Encourage Lamaze (or other) breathing/relaxation techniques.

(e) Goal: *reduce stress on cardiopulmonary system.* Discourage bearing-down efforts.

(f) Goal: *relieve stress of pain, eliminate bearing-down.* Prepare for regional anesthesia.

▬▭ (g) Goal: *maintain effective cardiac function.* Administer medications, as ordered (e.g., digitalis, diuretics, antibiotics).

e. Goal: *anticipatory planning:* **postpartal** management.

(1) Factors increasing risk of cardiac decompensation:

(a) Delivery → rapid, decreased intraabdominal pressure → vasocongestion and rapid rise in cardiac output.

(b) Loss of placental circulation.

(c) Normal diuresis increases circulating blood volume.

◆ (2) **Assessment:**

(a) Observe for tachycardia or respiratory distress.

(b) Monitor blood loss, I&O—potential hypovolemic shock, cardiac overload due to diuresis.

(c) Pain level—potential neurogenic shock.

(d) Same as for any woman who is post-partum (fundus, signs of infection, etc.).

◆ (3) **Nursing care plan/implementation:** *post-partum.*

(a) Goal: *minimize stress on cardiopulmonary system.*

(i) Rest, dangle, ambulate with assistance.

(ii) Gradual increase in activity—as tolerated without symptoms.

 (iii) *Position:* semi-Fowler's if needed.

(iv) Extra help with newborn care.

◆ 7. **Evaluation/outcome criteria:**

a. Successfully carries uneventful pregnancy to term.

b. Experiences no cardiopulmonary decompensation during labor, birth, or postpartum.

C. **Disorders affecting fluid-gas transport in fetus: Rh incompatibility**

1. **Pathophysiology**—in a mother who is Rh-negative: Rh-positive fetal red blood cells enter the maternal circulation → maternal antibody formation → antibodies cross placenta and enter fetal bloodstream → attack fetal red blood cells → hemolysis → anemia, hypoxia.

a. The mother who is pregnant and Rh-positive carries her infant (Rh negative *or* positive) without incident.

b. The mother who is pregnant and Rh-positive carries an Rh-negative infant without incident.

c. The mother who is pregnant and Rh-positive *usually* carries her first Rh-positive child without problems *unless* she has been sensitized by inadvertent transfusion with Rh-positive blood. *Note:* Fetal cells do not usually enter the maternal bloodstream until placental separation (at abortion, abruptio placentae, amniocentesis, or birth).

2. **Etiology:**

a. The Rh factor is an antigen on the red blood cells of some people (these people are Rh positive); the Rh factor is dominant; a person may be homozygous or heterozygous for Rh factor.

b. A person who is Rh-negative is homozygous for this recessive trait—does *not* carry the antigen; develops antibodies when exposed to Rh-positive red blood cells (isoimmunization) through transplacental (or other) transfusion.

c. Following birth of an infant who is Rh-positive, if fetal cells enter the mother's bloodstream, maternal antibody formation begins; antibodies remain in the maternal circulation.

d. At time of next pregnancy with fetus who is Rh-positive, antibodies cross placenta →

hemolysis. *Note: Degree* of hemolysis depends on amount (titer) of maternal antibodies present.

3. Possible serious complication (fetal)—rare today. Hydrops fetalis—most severe hemolytic reaction: severe anemia, cardiac decompensation, hypoxia, edema, ascites, hydrothorax; may be stillborn.

◆ 4. **Assessment:**

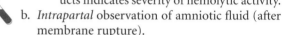 a. *Prenatal*—diagnostic procedures:

(1) Maternal blood type and Rh factor.

(2) Indirect Coombs' test—to determine presence of Rh sensitization (titer indicates amount of maternal antibodies).

(3) Amniocentesis—as early as 26 weeks of gestation—amount of bilirubin byproducts indicates severity of hemolytic activity.

 b. *Intrapartal* observation of amniotic fluid (after membrane rupture).

(1) Straw-colored fluid—mild disease.

(2) Golden fluid—severe fetal disease.

c. *Postnatal* (see **III. A. Rh Incompatibility, p. 242**).

◆ 5. **Nursing care plan/implementation:**

a. Goal: *prevent isoimmunization in women who are Coombs-negative*

(1) *Postabortion*—if no evidence of Rh sensitization (antibody formation) in the mother who is Rh-negative, administer RhoGAM.

(2) *Prenatal*—if no evidence of sensitization, administer RhoGAM at 28 weeks of gestation, as ordered, to all women who are Rh-negative.

(3) *Postpartum*—if no evidence of sensitization, administer RhoGAM within 72 hr of birth to women who are Rh-negative and who gave birth to a baby who is Rh-positive.

Give RhoGAM to:

1. Mother who is Rh-negative who gives birth to neonate who is Rh-positive.

2. Mother who is Rh-negative after spontaneous or induced abortion (>8 wk).

3. Mother who is Rh-negative after amniocentesis or chorionic villus sampling (CVS).

4. Mother who is Rh-negative between 28 and 32 weeks of gestation.

b. Goal: *health teaching.*

(1) Explain, discuss that RhoGAM suppresses antibody formation in susceptible woman who is Rh-negative carrying fetus that is Rh-positive. *Note:* Cannot reverse sensitization if already present.

(2) Required during and after each pregnancy with fetus who is Rh-positive.

◆ 6. **Evaluation/outcome criteria:**

a. Successfully carries pregnancy to term.

b. No evidence of Rh isoimmunization.

c. Birth of viable infant.

D. Disorders affecting fluid-gas transport in fetus: tuberculosis

1. **Pathophysiology:** *M. tuberculosis* primarily is spread as an airborne aerosol from infected → noninfected individuals, through the lung. Initial TB infection usually → latent or dormant infection in hosts with normally functioning immune systems. *M. tuberculosis* is a slow-growing obligate aerobe and a facultative intracellular parasite.

2. **Etiology:**

   a. Symptoms of tuberculosis in pregnancy are vague and nonspecific. Fatigue, shortness of breath, sweating and tiredness can all be attributed to the pregnancy.

   b. Reluctance of health-care professionals to perform a chest x-ray on a woman who is pregnant due to fear of harming the fetus → delay in diagnosis.

3. **Assessment:**

   a. Heaf and Mantoux skin tests (as reliable as in women who are nonpregnant).

   b. Same as for women who are nonpregnant: sputum examination, and culture and scans.

4. **Nursing care plan/implementation:**

   a. Goal: *prevent spread of disease.*

   (1) Initial treatment regimen: isoniazid (INH), rifampin (RIF), and ethambutol (EMB).

   (2) Pyridoxine (vitamin B6) recommended for women who are pregnant and taking INH.

   (3) Routine use of pyrazinamide (PZA) should be *avoided* because of inadequate teratogenicity data.

   (4) *Avoid:* streptomycin (which interferes with development of the ear; may cause congenital deafness).

   b. Goal: *health teaching.*

   (1) Explain, discuss transmission of disease, importance of completion of medication regime.

   (2) Because small concentration of antituberculosis drugs in breast milk do not produce toxicity in the newborn who is nursing, breastfeeding should *not* be discouraged for a woman who is HIV-seronegative and is planning to take (or is taking) INH or other anti-TB medications.

   c. Goal: *TB treatment for women who are HIV-infected and pregnant.*

   (1) If have a positive *M. tuberculosis* culture or suspected TB disease, treat *without delay.*

   (2) Rifamycin.

   (3) Although routine use of pyrazinamide not recommended if pregnant (due to inadequate teratogenicity data), benefits for women who are HIV-infected and pregnant outweigh potential pyrazinamide-related risks to fetus.

E. Disorders affecting fluid-gas transport in fetus: hepatitis B (HBV)

1. **Pathophysiology:** Hepatitis B is one of the most highly transmitted forms of hepatitis from mother to child around the world, especially in developing countries. Virus is highly contagious; the risk that newborn infant will develop hepatitis B is 10%–20% if the mother is positive for the hepatitis B surface antigen; and as high as 90% if she is also positive for the HBeAg (hepatitis Be antigen).

2. **Etiology:** Usually, hepatitis B is passed on during delivery with exposure to the blood and fluids during the birth process.

3. **Assessment:**

   a. Blood: highest concentration.

   b. Semen, vaginal secretions, wound exudates: lower concentration.

   c. Hepatitis B surface antigen = active infection.

4. **Nursing care plan/implementation:**

   a. Goal: *prevent spread of disease.*

   (1) Hepatitis B immune globulin to infant at birth.

   (2) Hepatitis B vaccine at 1 wk, 1 month, 6 months after birth.

   b. Goal: *health teaching.*

   (1) Explain, discuss transmission of disease, importance of completion of vaccination regimen.

   (2) Centers for Disease Control and Prevention (CDC) has recommended that all newborn infants be vaccinated for hepatitis B.

   (3) The risk of HBV infection in children is not only from perinatal transmission from mothers who are HBV-infected, but also from close contact with household members and caregivers who have acute or chronic HBV infection.

   (4) Ensure that all infants born to mothers who are HBsAg-positive (hepatitis B surface antigen) receive timely and appropriate immunoprophylaxis with HBIG (hepatitis B immunoglobulin) and hepatitis B vaccine.

   (5) Discontinue interferon therapy during pregnancy (effect on fetus is unknown).

F. Disorders affecting nutrition: diabetes mellitus

1. **Pathophysiology:** increased demand for insulin exceeds pancreatic reserve → inadequate insulin production; enzyme (insulinase) activity breaks down circulating insulin → further reduction in available insulin; increased tissue resistance to insulin; glycogenolysis/gluconeogenesis → ketosis.

2. **Etiology:** increased metabolic rate; action of placental hormones (see following), enzyme (insulinase) activity.

3. *Normal physiological* alterations during pregnancy that may *affect* management of the woman who is *diabetic*, or *precipitate gestational diabetes* in women who are susceptible:

a. *Hormone production:*
(1) Human placental lactogen (HPL).
(2) Progesterone.
(3) Estrogen.
(4) Cortisol.
b. *Effects of hormones:*
(1) Decreased glucose tolerance.
(2) Increased metabolic rate.
(3) Increased production of adrenocortical and pituitary hormones.
(4) Decreased effectiveness of insulin (increased resistance to insulin by peripheral tissues).
(5) Increased gluconeogenesis.
(6) Increased size and number of islets of Langerhans to meet increased maternal needs.
(7) Increased mobilization of free fatty acids.
(8) Decreased renal threshold, increased glomerular filtration rate; glycosuria common.
(9) Decreased CO_2-combining power of blood; higher metabolic rate increases tendency to acidosis.
c. *Effect of pregnancy on diabetes:*
(1) Nausea and vomiting—predispose to ketoacidosis.
(2) Insulin requirements—relatively stable or may decrease in first trimester; rapid *increase* during second and third trimesters; rapid *decrease* after birth to prepregnant level.
(3) Pathophysiological progression (nephropathy, retinopathy, and arteriosclerotic changes) may appear; existing pathology may worsen.
4. *Effect of poorly controlled diabetes on pregnancy—* increased incidence of:
a. Infertility.
b. UTI.
c. Vaginal infections (moniliasis).
d. Spontaneous abortion.
e. Congenital anomalies (three times as prevalent).
f. Preeclampsia/eclampsia.
g. Polyhydramnios.
h. Preterm labor and birth.
i. Fetal macrosomia—cephalopelvic disproportion (CPD).
j. Stillbirth.
◆ 5. **Assessment:** *gestational diabetes (mellitus)*
a. History:
(1) Family history.
(2) Previous infant 9 lb or more.
(3) Unexplained fetal wastage—abortion, stillbirth, or early neonatal death.
(4) Obesity with very rapid weight gain.
(5) Polyhydramnios (excessive amniotic fluid).
(6) Previous infant with congenital anomalies.

(7) Increased tendency for intense vaginal or urinary tract infections.
(8) Previous history of gestational diabetes
b. Symptoms: **3 "Ps"**—**p**olydipsia, **p**olyphagia, **p**olyuria—and weight loss.
c. *Abdominal assessment:*
(1) Fetal heart rate.
(2) Excessive fundal height.
(a) Polyhydramnios.
(b) Large-for-gestational-age (LGA) fetus. *Note:* With vascular pathology, small-for-gestational-age (SGA) fetus.
d. *Medical diagnosis*—procedures:
(1) 50 g oral glucose tolerance test (GTT): woman ingests 50 g oral glucose solution; 1 hr later plasma glucose obtained. If 140 mg/dL, 3 hr oral GTT ordered.
(2) Abnormal 3-hour GTT: two or more of the following findings are diagnostic of gestational diabetes.

(a) Fasting blood sugar (FBS) ≥ 95 mg/dL.
(b) One hour ≥ 180 mg/dL.
(c) Two hours 155 mg/dL.
(d) Three hours ≥140mg/dL.

(3) *Diabetic classification criteria:*
(a) *Type 1*—autoimmune disease in which the body's immune system destroys pancreatic beta cells; ↓ production of insulin; need additional insulin. About 10% with diabetes are type 1.

(b) *Type 2*— ↑ insulin resistance despite adequate insulin production; *treatment* may include: diet, exercise, weight loss, oral drugs to stimulate release of insulin; or insulin injections. About 90% with diabetes are type 2.
(c) *Gestational*—occurs in about 3% of all pregnancies. GTT administered at 24–28 weeks' gestation; 2 abnormal values indicate diagnosis of gestational diabetes. About 40% of women with gestational diabetes will develop type 2 diabetes within 5 years.
e. Woman with known diabetes—all classes.
(1) Knowledge and acceptance of disease and its management:
(a) Signs and symptoms of hyperglycemia/hypoglycemia (see **Table 7.31**).
(b) Appropriate behaviors (e.g., skim milk for symptoms of hypoglycemia).
(2) Skill and accuracy in monitoring serum glucose (dextrometer use).
(3) Skill and accuracy in preparing and administering insulin dosage; site rotation; subcutaneous injection in abdomen.
(4) Close monitoring—prenatal status assessment every 2 wk until 30 wk, then weekly

until birth. Alert to signs of emerging problems (need for insulin adjustment, polyhydramnios, macrosomia).

(5) Other—as for any woman who is pregnant.

◆ 6. **Analysis/nursing diagnosis:**

a. *Knowledge deficit* related to pathophysiology, interactions with pregnancy, management (e.g., insulin administration).

b. *Altered nutrition, more or less than body requirements,* related to weight gain.

c. High-risk pregnancy: high risk for infection, ketosis, fetal demise, fetal macrosomia, cephalopelvic disproportion, polyhydramnios, preterm labor and birth, congenital anomalies.

◆ 7. **Nursing care plan/implementation:**

a. Goal: *health teaching.*

(1) Pathophysiology of diabetes, as necessary; effect of pregnancy on management.

(2) Signs and symptoms of hyperglycemia, hypoglycemia; appropriate management of symptoms.

(3) Hygiene—to reduce probability of infection.

(4) Exercise—needed to control serum-glucose levels, to regulate weight gain, and for feeling of well-being.

(5) Need for close monitoring during pregnancy.

(6) Insulin regulation:

(a) Requirements vary through pregnancy: *first trimester*—may decrease with some periods of hypoglycemia due to fetal drain; *second trimester*—increased need for insulin; *third trimester*—needs may be triple prepregnant dose; acidosis more common in late pregnancy (precipitated by emotional stress, infection).

(b) Serum-glucose testing—dextrometer, Acucheck, or other.

(c) Preparation and self-administration of insulin injection, as necessary.

(d) Prompt reporting of fluctuating serum-glucose levels.

(7) Diagnostic testing/hospitalization:

(a) Nonstress test.

(b) Sonography.

(c) Amniocentesis.

b. Goal: *dietary counseling.*

(1) Optimal weight gain—about 24 lb.

(2) Needs 25–35 calories/kg of ideal body weight (1800–2600 calories).

(3) Protein—18%–25% (2 g/kg, or about 70 g daily).

(4) Carbohydrates: 50%–60% in complex form (milk, bread).

(5) Fats—25%–30% unsaturated.

(6) *No* fruit juice; no cold cereal; carbohydrate limited.

c. *Medical management:* hospitalize woman for:

(1) Regulation of insulin (oral hypoglycemics **contraindicated** in early pregnancy, due to teratogenicity; crosses placental barrier).

(2) Control of infection.

(3) Determination of fetal jeopardy or indications for early termination of pregnancy.

◆ 8. **Evaluation/outcome criteria:**

a. Understands and accepts diagnosis of diabetes.

b. Actively participates in effective management of diabetes and pregnancy.

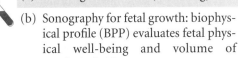

c. Maintains serum-glucose levels within acceptable parameters (e.g., 70–120 mg/dL).

(1) Monitors serum-glucose levels accurately (dextrometer, Acucheck).

(2) Prepares and self-administers insulin appropriately.

(3) Complies with dietary regimen.

9. **Antepartal** *hospitalization*

◆ a. **Assessment:**

(1) *Medical evaluation*—procedures:

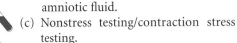

(a) Serum-glucose levels (↓ 120 mg).

(b) Sonography for fetal growth: biophysical profile (BPP) evaluates fetal physical well-being and volume of amniotic fluid.

(c) Nonstress testing/contraction stress testing.

(d) Amniocentesis for fetal maturity. *Note:* L/S ratio may be elevated in women who are diabetic; *phosphatidylglycerol [PG]* more accurate for women who are diabetic.

(2) **Nursing assessment:**

(a) Daily weight, vital signs, FHR q4h, I&O.

▶ (b) Fundal height and Leopold's maneuvers on admission.

◆ b. **Nursing care plan/implementation.**

Goal: *emotional support*—to reduce anxiety and tension, which contribute to insulin imbalance.

(1) Explain all procedures.

(2) Assist with tests for fetal status.

(3) Prepare for possibility of preterm or cesarean birth.

10. *Anticipatory planning*—management of **labor**

◆ a. **Assessment:** continuous.

(1) Signs and symptoms of hyperglycemia, hypoglycemia (see **Table 7.31**). Hourly blood sugar measurements.

(2) Electronic fetal monitoring—to identify signs of fetal distress.

(3) Other—as for any woman in labor.

◆ b. **Nursing care plan/implementation:**

Goal: *safeguard maternal/fetal status.*

 Position: lateral Sims'—to reduce compression of inferior vena cava and aorta due to polyhydhamnios or LGA baby. (Supine hypotensive syndrome results from compression; reduced placental perfusion increases incidence of fetal hypoxia/anoxia.)

c. *Medical management*—varies widely.

  (1) Timing—amniocentesis to determine PG and *phosphatidylinositol* levels (estimate fetal pulmonary surfactant).

  (2) Insulin added to intravenous infusion of 0.9 NaCl and titrated to maintain serum glucose approximately 100 mg/dL. 5%–10% D/W IV needed to prevent hypoglycemia that may lead to maternal ketoacidosis; hyperglycemia may result in newborn hypoglycemia.

  (3) Ultrasound to identify macrosomia >4050 g.

11. *Anticipatory planning*—management of **postpartum**

a. Factors influencing serum-glucose levels:

  (1) Loss of placental hormones that degrade insulin.

  (2) Lower metabolic rate. Woman requiring large doses of insulin may need to triple caloric intake and decrease insulin by one-half.

b. **Assessment:**

  (1) Observe for:

    (a) Hypoglycemia.

    (b) Infection.

    (c) Preeclampsia/eclampsia (higher incidence in women who are diabetic).

    (d) Hemorrhage (associated with polyhydramnios, macrosomia, induction of labor, forceps birth, or cesarean birth).

  (2) Monitor healing of episiotomy/abdominal incision.

c. **Nursing care plan/implementation:**

  (1) *Medical management:* insulin calibration—requirement may drop to one-half or two-thirds pregnant dosage on first postpartum day if woman is on full diet (due to loss of human placental lactogen and conversion of serum glucose to lactose).

  (2) *Nursing management*

    (a) Goal: *euglycemia.* Acucheck, insulin as ordered.

    (b) Goal: *avoid trauma, reduce risk of UTI. Avoid* catheterization, where possible.

    (c) Goal: *health teaching.* Nipple care—to prevent fissures and possible mastitis.

    (d) Goal: *reduce serum-glucose and insulin needs.* Encourage/support breastfeeding → antidiabetogenic effect. *Note:* If *acetonuria* occurs, stop breastfeeding while physician readjusts diet/insulin balance; may pump breasts to maintain lactation. If *hypoglycemic*, adrenalin level rises → decreased milk supply and let-down reflex.

12. *Anticipatory guidance*—**discharge plan/implementation**

a. Goal: *counseling.* Reinforce recommendations of physicians/genetic counselors.

  (1) Risk of infant inheriting gene for diabetes is greater if mother has early-onset, insulin-dependent disease.

  (2) Increased risk of congenital disorders.

b. Goal: *family planning*

  (1) Oral contraceptives are controversial because they decrease carbohydrate tolerance; may be cautiously prescribed for women with no vascular disease and who are nonsmokers. IUD **contraindicated** because of impaired response to infection. Barrier contraceptives (diaphragm or condoms with spermicides) recommended.

  (2) Tubal ligation: if mother has vascular involvement (i.e., retinopathy or nephropathy) increased risk with later pregnancies (see **Table 4.2**).

c. Goal: *health teaching.*

  (1) Self-care measures.

  (2) Importance of eating on time, even if infant must wait to breastfeed or bottle feed.

  (3) Importance of adequate rest and exercise to maintain insulin/glucose balance.

  (4) Organize schedule to care for infant, other children, and her diabetes. Allow time for self.

d. **Evaluation/outcome criteria:**

  (1) Successfully completes an uneventful pregnancy, labor, and birth of a newborn who is normal and healthy.

  (2) Makes informed judgments regarding parenting, family planning, management of her diabetes.

G. Disorders affecting psychosocio-cultural behaviors: substance abuse

1. **Assessment:** woman who is pregnant and abuses substances

a. *Medical history*

  (1) Infections: HIV-positive status, AIDS, STDs, hepatitis, cirrhosis, cellulitis, endocarditis, pancreatitis, pneumonia.

  (2) Psychiatric illness: depression, paranoia, irritability.

  (3) Trauma related to violence.

b. *Obstetric history*

  (1) Spontaneous abortions.

  (2) History of abruptio placentae.

  (3) Preterm labor.

  (4) Preterm rupture of membranes.

  (5) Fetal death.

  (6) Low-birth-weight (LBW) infants.

  (7) Tremors/seizures.

c. *Current pregnancy*

  (1) Preterm labor contractions.

  (2) Hypoactivity or hyperactivity in fetus.

  (3) Poor or decreased weight gain.

(4) STD.

(5) Undiagnosed vaginal bleeding.

(6) Drugs being used and methods of self-administration.

d. *Psychosocial history*

(1) Attitudes re: pregnancy.

(2) Current support system: lacking.

(3) Current living arrangements; lifestyle.

(4) History of psychiatric illness.

(5) History of physical, sexual abuse.

(6) Involvement with legal system.

e. *Physical examination*

f. *Commonly abused substances*

(1) Nicotine.

(2) Alcohol (fetal alcohol syndrome [FAS] or fetal alcohol effects [FAE]).

(3) Marijuana.

(4) Stimulants—cocaine, crack, ice, methamphetamine

(5) Opiates—heroin, methadone, Darvon, codeine, Vicodin, OxyContin.

(6) Sedatives, hypnotics.

(7) Caffeine.

(8) Ecstasy.

g. *Neonatal outcomes*

(1) LBW, small heads.

(2) Irritable, difficult to console.

(3) Disorganized suck-swallow reflex.

(4) Impaired motor development.

(5) Congenital anomalies: genitourinary, gastrointestinal, limb anomalies.

(6) Cerebral infarctions.

(7) Breastfeeding allowed; thought to ease infant withdrawal.

(8) Poor, slow weight gain; failure to thrive.

◆ 2. **Analysis/nursing diagnosis:**

a. *Altered nutrition: less than body requirements—*poor weight gain related to poor nutrition.

b. *Altered nutrition: less than body requirements—*slow fetal growth related to slow gain in weight.

c. *Altered placental function* related to high risk for abruptio placentae.

d. *Noncompliance* with health-care protocols related to persistent drug use.

e. *Altered parenting* related to psychological illness (substance dependence).

◆ 3. **Nursing care plan/implementation:**

a. Early identification of substance abuse.

b. Stabilize physiological status.

c. Fetal surveillance.

d. Urge consistent obstetric care.

e. Refer for social services.

◆ 4. **Evaluation/outcome criteria:**

a. Seeks out and uses social services and drug treatment program.

b. Abstains from illicit substances during pregnancy.

c. Successfully completes an uneventful pregnancy, labor, and birth of normal healthy infant.

Lifestyle Choices and Influences That Impact Health in Pregnancy, Intrapartum, Postpartum, and Newborn (See also STDs, pp. 171–172, 177–180 and substance abuse, pp. 168–169)

I. **Other high-risk women**

A. **An adolescent who is pregnant**

1. **General aspects:**

a. Pregnancy in women between 12 and 17 years old.

b. Incidence has started to ↓; approximately one-third of all births are to adolescents.

c. *Predisposing factors:* early menarche, early experimentation with sex, poor family relationships, poverty, late or no prenatal care, cultural influence.

d. *Associated health problems:* preeclampsia, preterm labor, SGA infants, anemia, bleeding disorders, infections, CPD.

e. *Social problems:* mothers who are poorly educated, child abuse, single-parent families, mothers who are unemployed or working at minimum wage or who lack support system.

◆ 2. **Assessment:**

a. Present physical/health status.

b. Feelings toward pregnancy.

c. Plans for the future.

d. Factors influencing decisions related to self, pregnancy, baby.

e. Signs and symptoms of complications of pregnancy (see **A.1.d.** *Associated health problems*).

f. Need/desire for health maintenance information (family planning).

◆ 3. **Analysis/nursing diagnosis:**

a. *Ineffective coping, individual/family,* related to need to alter lifestyle, plans, expectations.

b. *Altered family processes* related to unexpected/unwanted pregnancy.

c. *Altered parenting* related to intrafamily stress secondary to unexpected pregnancy, developmental tasks.

d. *Self-esteem disturbance* related to altered self-concept, body image, role performance, personal identity.

e. *Knowledge deficit* related to family planning, health maintenance, risk factors, pregnancy options.

f. *Altered nutrition* related to lifestyle

◆ 4. **Nursing care plan/implementation:**

a. Goal: *emotional support.*

(1) Ensure confidentiality.

(2) Establish acceptant, supportive environment.

(3) Encourage verbalization of feelings, concerns, fears, desires, etc.

Maternal-Infant

(1) Maintain continuity of care—consistency of nursing approach, to establish trust, confidentiality.

b. Goal: *facilitate informed decision making.* Discuss available options; aid in exploring implications of possible decisions.

c. Goal: *nutritional counseling* (anemia).
 (1) Needs for own growth and that of fetus.
 (2) High-quality diet—value for character of skin, return to prepregnant figure.
 (3) Include pizza, hamburgers, milkshakes as acceptable—to minimize anger at being "different."

d. Goal: *health teaching.*
 (1) Rest, exercise, hygiene—as for other women.
 (2) Prevention of infection—STD, UTI, etc.
 (3) Breast self-exam; Pap smear.
 (4) Future family planning options (see **Table 4.1**).

e. Goal: *assist in achievement of normal developmental tasks.* Encourage exploration of new role and responsibilities.

f. Goal: *referral to appropriate resources.*
 (1) Abortion; adoption resources.
 (2) Preparation for childbirth and parenting classes.
 (3) Family counseling.
 (4) Social services.

g. Goal: *assist in facilitating/continuing/completing basic education.*
 (1) Communicate with school nurse.
 (2) Explore other options available in community.

◆ 5. **Evaluation/outcome criteria:**
a. Makes informed decisions appropriate to individual and family needs, desires.
b. Actively participates in own health maintenance.
 (1) Complies with medical/nursing recommendations.
 (2) Minimizes potential for complications of pregnancy.
c. Copes effectively with normal physiological and psychosocial alterations of pregnancy.
d. Both woman and baby's father express satisfaction with decision and management of this pregnancy. If parenthood is chosen and pregnancy is successful, accepts parenting role.

B. **Older mother: primigravida over age 35**
 1. **General aspects**—higher incidence of congenital anomalies (e.g., Down syndrome), increased possibility of complications of pregnancy. However, generally it is a conscious decision to have postponed childbearing. Individuals are usually used to making own decisions regarding career and health care.

◆ 2. **Assessment:**
a. Same as for other women who are pregnant.
b. Reaction to reality of pregnancy.
c. Family response to pregnancy.

◆ 3. **Analysis/nursing diagnosis:**
a. *Fear* related to threat to pregnancy.
b. *Knowledge deficit* related to aspects of pregnancy care.

◆ 4. **Nursing care plan/implementation:**
a. Goal: *anticipatory guidance.* Preparation for parenthood, altered lifestyle, potential change of career. Assist with realistic expectations. Refer to "over 30" parents' support group.
b. Goal: *health teaching.* Explain, discuss special diagnostic procedures (**Figure 4.5**) (**Amniocentesis**).
c. Other—same as for other women who are pregnant.

◆ 5. **Evaluation/outcome criteria:**
a. Experiences normal, uncomplicated pregnancy, labor, and birth of a newborn who is normal and healthy.
b. Expresses satisfaction with decision and outcome of this pregnancy.

C. **Older mother: multipara over age 40**
 1. **General aspects**
a. Increased incidence of preexisting and coexisting medical disorders (hypertension, diabetes, arthritis).
b. Increased incidence of complications of pregnancy (preeclampsia/eclampsia, hemorrhage).
c. Smoking is major risk factor.

◆ 2. **Assessment:**
a. Same as for other women who are pregnant.
b. Reaction to pregnancy (varies from pleasure at still being "young enough," to despair, if facing decision to abort).
c. History, signs and symptoms of coexisting disorders.
d. Indications of reduced physical ability to cope with normal physiological alterations of pregnancy.
e. Family constellation: stage of family developmental cycle, responses to this pregnancy (especially adolescents' reaction to parents' pregnancy).

◆ 3. **Analysis/nursing diagnosis:** same as for over-35 age group.

◆ 4. **Nursing care plan/implementation:**
a. Goal: *emotional support.* Encourage verbalization of feelings, fears, concerns.
b. Goal: *referral to appropriate resource.*
 (1) Genetic counseling.
 (2) Abortion/support groups.
 (3) Preparation for childbirth and parenthood classes.
c. Goal: *facilitate/support effective family process.* Involve family in preparation for birth and integration of newborn into family unit.
d. Other—same as for other women who are pregnant.

◆ 5. **Evaluation/outcome criteria:**
a. Makes informed decisions related to pregnancy.

AMNIOCENTESIS

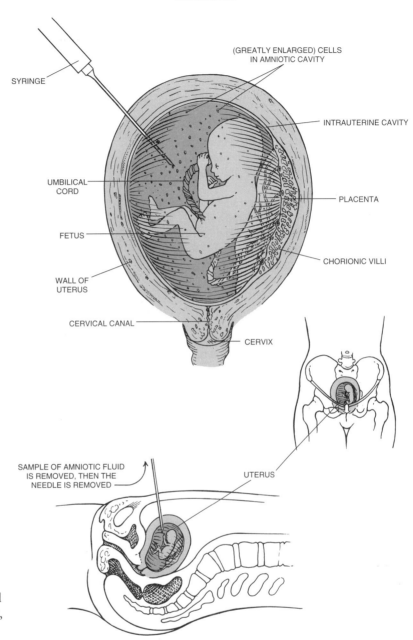

FIGURE 4.5 **Amniocentesis.** (From Venes, D [ed]: Taber's Cyclopedic Medical Dictionary, ed. 20. FA Davis, Philadelphia, 2005.)

b. Expresses satisfaction with decision and outcome of this pregnancy.

c. Experiences uncomplicated pregnancy, labor, and birth of a newborn who is normal and healthy.

D. AIDS

1. **General aspects**—AIDS is a serious condition affecting the immune system. Heterosexual women are considered at risk if they or their sexual partners:

   a. Are HIV-positive.
   b. Use IV drugs (50%).
   c. Received blood between 1977 and 1985 (9%).
   d. Are homosexual or bisexual men (39%).
   e. Have hemophilia.

◆ 2. **Assessment**—general symptoms:

   a. Malaise.
   b. Chronic cough; possible tuberculosis.
   c. Chronic diarrhea.

   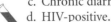 d. HIV-positive.

   e. Weight loss: 10 lb in 2 mo.
   f. Night sweats; lymphadenopathy.
   g. Skin lesions; thrush.
   h. PID; STDs; vulvovaginitis (usually, yeast [*Candidiasis*]), often refractory and severe.

   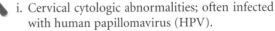 i. Cervical cytologic abnormalities; often infected with human papillomavirus (HPV).

◆ 3. **Analysis/nursing diagnosis:**

   a. *Altered nutrition, less than body requirements,* related to general malaise.

b. *Fatigue,* related to altered health status, weight loss.

c. *Fear* related to progressively debilitating disease.

d. *Knowledge deficit* related to disease progression, treatment, life expectancy.

e. *Ineffective individual coping* related to disease progression.

◆ 4. **Nursing care plan/implementation:**
 a. Identify women at risk.
 b. Protect confidentiality.
 c. Implement standard precautions.
 d. Use proper gloves, gown, handwashing.
 e. Use protective eyewear and mask during labor, birth.

◆ 5. **Evaluation/outcome criteria:**
 a. No further transmission of virus.
 b. Woman's confidentiality maintained.
 c. Standard precautions implemented.
 d. Emotional support implemented.
 e. Supportive groups contacted.

6. **Women who are HIV-positive**—*pregnancy management:*
 a. *Antepartum*
  (1) Increased incidence of other STD (gonorrhea, syphilis, herpes, HPV).
  (2) Increased incidence of cytomegalovirus (CMV).
  (3) Differential diagnosis for all pregnancy-induced complaints.
  (4) Counsel regarding nutrition.
  (5) Advise about risk to infant.
  (6) Counsel regarding safer sex.
 b. *Intrapartum*
  (1) Focus on prevention of transmission.
  (2) Mode of birth not based on disease.
  ▶ (3) External electronic fetal monitoring (EFM) preferred.
  (4) *Avoid* use of fetal scalp electrodes or fetal scalp sampling.
 c. *Postpartum*
  (1) No remarkable alteration in disease progression.
  (2) Breastfeeding **contraindicated.**
  (3) Implement standard precautions for mother and infant.
  (4) Refer to specialists in AIDS care and treatment.

7. **Newborn or neonate:**
 a. **General aspects:** Neonatal AIDS—transmission may be transplacental, contact with maternal blood at birth, or postnatal exposure to parent who is infected (i.e., breastfeeding). Classic signs evident in adult often not present. Common signs: lymphadenopathy, hepatosplenomegaly, oral *candidiasis,* bacterial infections, failure to thrive.
 b. Implement standard precautions for all invasive procedures. Bathe infant immediately after birth to decrease contact with mother's blood. Wear gloves for all contact before first bath.

c. Provide supportive nursing care (thermoregulation, respiratory).
 d. Encourage parent-infant contact.
 e. Provide opportunities for sensory stimuli and touch.
 f. Monitor intake and weight gain.
 g. Observe for signs of infection.
 h. Initiate social service consultation.
 i. Counsel family about vaccinations (should receive all *except* oral polio).
 j. Administer medications as ordered (AZT).

Emergency Conditions by Trimester

See **Table 4.8**

Common Complications of Pregnancy

First Trimester Complications

I. **Complications affecting fluid-gas transport: hemorrhagic disorders**
 A. **General aspects** (review **Table 4.8**)
 ◆ 1. **Assessment:**
  a. Vital signs, output, general status.
  b. Evidence of internal/external bleeding.
  c. Pain.
  d. Emotional response.
  e. Perineal pads saturated and number (pad count).
  f. Speculum examination.
 ◆ 2. **Analysis/nursing diagnosis:**
  a. *Knowledge deficit* related to diagnosis, prognosis, treatment, sequelae.
  b. *Anxiety/fear* related to loss of pregnancy, surgery.
  c. *Fluid volume deficit, potential/actual,* related to excessive blood loss.
  d. *Pain.*
  e. *Ineffective coping, individual/family,* related to knowledge deficit and fear.
  f. *Anticipatory/dysfunctional grieving,* related to loss of pregnancy.
  g. *Disturbance in self-esteem, body image, role performance,* related to threat to self-image as woman and childbearer.
 ◆ 3. **Nursing care plan/implementation:**
  a. Goal: *minimize blood loss, stabilize physiological status.*
   (1) Facilitate prompt medical management.
   (2) Administer IV fluids, blood, as ordered.
   (3) Administer analgesics, as needed.
  b. Goal: *prevent infection.* Strict aseptic technique.
  c. Goal: *emotional support.*
   (1) Encourage verbalization of anxiety, fears, concerns.
   (2) Supportive care for grief reaction (**pp. 369–371**).
 ◆ 4. **Evaluation/outcome criteria:**
  a. Blood loss minimized; physiological status stable.
  b. Copes effectively with loss of pregnancy.

TABLE 4.8	Emergency Conditions

First Trimester

◆ Assessment/Observations	Possible Problem	◆ Nursing Care Plan/Implementation
Fluid-Gas Transport		
a. *Cramping*—with or without bleeding or passage of tissue	Abortion (before 24 wk) Threatened Imminent, Incomplete, Septic	Bedrest, sedation, *avoid* coitus—if threatened; bedrest, start IV fluids and draw blood for laboratory work: CBC, type/crossmatch, electrolytes, platelets, HCG levels
b. *Passage of tissue* (products of conception; grapelike vesicles) or *brown spotting;* fundus too high for gestational age; *blood pressure* elevated. Often associated with hyperemesis gravidarum and preeclampsia	Hydatidiform mole (trophoblastic disease)	Vital signs q5–15 min, prn
c. Severe *pain, shock* out of proportion to amount of overt blood; shoulder-strap pain (*Kehr's sign*), a "referred pain" that indicates intraabdominal bleeding (or rupture of ovarian cyst); amenorrhea of 6–12 wk	Ectopic pregnancy	Save all pads or tissue passed through vagina for physician evaluation **No** rectal or vaginal examination until physician is present
d. Malodorous *discharge; hyperthermia and chills;* tender abdomen	Septic abortion (self-induced or "criminal")	Take complete history, if possible Convulsion precautions if hypertensive
e. *Ecchymosis or bleeding*—with a history that includes any or all of the following: had symptoms of pregnancy, but they subsided; pregnancy test negative; uterine size diminishing; no FHR	Missed abortion with possible DIC (retained dead fetus syndrome)	Emotional support for loss of pregnancy (through nurse's manner, tone of voice, touch, use of woman's name; keep her informed of what is happening); oxygen, prn

Second Trimester

◆ Assessment/Observations	Possible Problem	◆ Nursing Care Plan/Implementation
Fluid-Gas Transport		
a. Cramping; passage of products of conception	Late abortion	Same as for first trimester
b. Labor—cervical changes, "show"	Incompetent cervical os	See physician immediately for possible cerclage
c. *Prolonged* nausea and vomiting; unexplained *hypertension* or *preeclampsia;* passage of dark blood or grapelike vesicles; *absent FHRs;* excessive fundal height for gestation	Hydatidiform mole	Maintain hydration; assess for dehydration; refer to physician
Sensory-Perceptual		
a. *Preeclampsia/eclampsia*	With increased severity: renal failure, circulatory collapse, stroke, coagulation defects (DIC); abruptio placentae; convulsions	Pharmacological management of hypertension (see **Unit 7**)

(*Continued on following page*)

Maternal-Infant

TABLE 4.8	Emergency Conditions *(Continued)*

◆ Assessment/Observations	Possible Problem	◆ Nursing Care Plan/Implementation
Assessment: hypertension first noted after 24 wk; followed by increased proteinuria		**Convulsion precautions:**
Symptoms: blurred or double vision; pain: headache, epigastric (late sign)		1. Emergency tray at bedside
		2. Oxygen/suction
		3. Start IV
Signs: BP 160/110; 3⁺ proteinuria		4. Padded siderails
Edema: facial, digital; pulmonary		5. Limit environmental stimulation
Oliguria		6. Constant observation
Hyperreflexia		7. Deep-tendon reflexes
		8. Daily weight
		9. I&O—strict
		10. Note any complaints and changes
		11. Prepare for lab work (type and crossmatch, CBC, platelets, BUN, and creatinine, uric acid, SGOT, SGPT)
b. *Convulsions* in absence of hypertension, proteinuria, or facial edema	Stroke, epilepsy, drug toxicity; intracranial injury; diabetic complications; encephalopathy	**Convulsion care:**
		1. Oxygen/mask; drugs (Valium, magnesium sulfate IV)
		2. Observe:
		a. Uterine tone, FHR, fetal activity
		b. Signs of labor
		3. Emotional support for woman and family

Signs: BP 160/110; 3^+ proteinuria

Third Trimester

◆ Assessment/Observations	Possible Problem	◆ Nursing Care Plan/Implementation
Fluid-Gas Transport		
a. *Bleeding: painless, bright red,* vaginal	Placenta previa	**No vaginal exam**
		Apply fetal monitor; assess for labor
Contractions or uterine tone normal		*Position:* semi to high-Fowler's
		Ultrasound to verify placental location
b. *Pain:* abdomen rigid and tender to touch	Abruptio placentae	As for placenta previa; *position:* Sims'
Increased uterine tone; signs of shock disproportionate to visible blood loss; may have loss of FHTs; associated with: preeclampsia, multiparity, precipitous labor, oxytocin induction, trauma, cocaine use		Prepare for possible emergency cesarean delivery

B. **Spontaneous abortion:** *before viable age of 20–22 wk*
   1. **Etiology:**
      a. Defective products of conception.
      b. Insufficient production of progesterone.
      c. Acute infections.
      d. Reproductive system abnormalities (e.g., incompetent cervical os).
      e. Trauma (physical or emotional).
      f. Rh incompatibility.
   ◆ 2. **Assessment:** types
      a. *Threatened*—mild bleeding, spotting, cramping; cervix closed.
      b. *Inevitable*—moderate bleeding, painful cramping; cervix dilated, positive Nitrazine test (membranes ruptured).
      c. *Imminent*—profuse bleeding, severe cramping, urge to bear down.
      d. *Incomplete*—fetal parts or fetus expelled; placenta and membranes retained.
      e. *Complete*—all products of conception expelled; minimal vaginal bleeding.
      f. *Habitual/recurrent*—history of spontaneous loss of three or more successive pregnancies.
      g. *Missed*—fetal death with no spontaneous expulsion within 4 weeks.
         (1) Anorexia, malaise, headache.
         (2) Fundal height—inconsistent with gestational estimate.
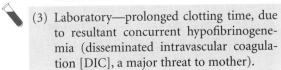
         (3) Laboratory—prolonged clotting time, due to resultant concurrent hypofibrinogenemia (disseminated intravascular coagulation [DIC], a major threat to mother).
      h. *Elective abortions* (intentionally introduced loss of pregnancy).
   ◆ 3. **Analysis/nursing diagnosis:**
      a. *Altered family processes* related to pregnancy, circumstances surrounding abortion.
      b. *Sexual dysfunction* related to compromised self-image, altered interpersonal relationship, guilt feelings.
   ◆ 4. **Nursing care plan/implementation:**
      a. *Threatened*—Goal: *health teaching.* Suggest: *avoid* coitus and orgasm, especially around normal time for menstrual period.
      b. *Incomplete, inevitable, imminent.*
         (1) Goal: *safeguard status.*
            (a) Save all pads, clots, tissue for expert diagnosis.
            (b) Report immediately any change in status, excessive bleeding, signs of infection, shock.
            (c) Prepare for surgery.
         (2) Goal: *comfort measures.*
            (a) Administer analgesics, as necessary.
            (b) Bedrest, quiet diversional activities.
         (3) Goal: *emotional support.*
            (a) Encourage verbalization of fear, concerns.
            (b) Reduce anxiety, as possible.
            (c) If pregnancy terminates, facilitate grieving process; assist in working through guilt feelings (**pp. 205–206**).
            (d) Supportive care for grief reaction (**p. 205**).
         (4) Goal: *prevent isoimmunization* (see **II. C. 5. Rh incompatibility, p. 164**).
         (5) *Medical management:*
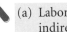
            (a) Laboratory—blood type and Rh factor, indirect Coombs, platelets, serum fibrinogen, clotting time.
            (b) Replace blood loss; maintain fluid levels with IV.
            (c) Dilation and curettage or dilation and evacuation.
            (d) *Habitual*—determine etiology.
   ◆ 5. **Evaluation/outcome criteria:**
      a. *Threatened*—responds to medical/nursing regimen; abortion avoided, successfully carries pregnancy to term.
      b. *Spontaneous abortion*—after uterus emptied.
         (1) Her bleeding is controlled.
         (2) Her vital signs are stable.
         (3) Copes effectively with loss of pregnancy.
         (4) Expresses satisfaction with care.
      c. *Habitual abortion*—cause identified and corrected; carries subsequent pregnancy to successful termination.

C. **Hydatidiform mole** (complete)
   1. **Pathophysiology**—chorionic villi degenerate into grapelike cluster of vesicles; may be antecedent to choriocarcinoma.
   2. **Etiology**—genetic base of complete mole (sperm enters empty egg and its chromosomes replicate; 23 pairs of chromosomes are all paternal); rare complication; more common in women over 45 years of age and women who are Asian.
   ◆ 3. **Assessment:**
      a. Uterus—rapid enlargement; fundal height inconsistent with gestational estimate.
      b. Brownish discharge—beginning about wk 12; may contain vesicles.
      c. Signs and symptoms of preeclampsia/eclampsia (before third trimester), increased incidence of hyperemesis gravidarum.
      d. *Medical evaluation*—procedures:
         (1) Sonography, x-ray, amniography—no fetal parts present; "snowstorm."
         (2) Laboratory test—for elevated human chorionic gonadotropin (HCG) levels.
         (3) Follow-up surveillance of HCG levels for at least 1 yr; persistent HCG level is consistent with choriocarcinoma; x-ray.
   ◆ 4. **Analysis/nursing diagnosis:**
      a. *Anxiety/fear* related to treatment, possible sequelae of hydatidiform mole (choriocarcinoma).
      b. *Potential for injury* related to hemorrhage, perforation of uterine wall, preeclampsia/ eclampsia.
      c. *Fluid volume deficit* related to hemorrhage.

5. **Nursing care plan/implementation:**
   a. *Medical management*
      (1) Monitor for preeclampsia.
      (2) Evacuate the uterus—hysterectomy may be necessary.
      (3) Strict contraception for at least 1 yr to enable accurate assessment of status.
      (4) Choriocarcinoma—chemotherapy (methotrexate plus dactinomycin) or radiation therapy, or both.
   b. *Nursing management*
      (1) Goal: *safeguard status.* Observe for hemorrhage, passage of retained vesicles and abdominal pain, or signs of infection (because woman is at risk for perforation of uterine wall).
      (2) Goal: *health teaching.*
         (a) Explain, discuss diagnostic tests; prepare for tests.
         (b) Discuss contraceptive options.
         (c) Importance of follow-up.
      (3) Goal: *preoperative and postoperative care.*
      (4) Goal: *emotional support.* Facilitate grieving **(p. 205).**
6. **Evaluation/outcome criteria:**
   a. Verbalizes understanding of diagnosis, tests, and treatment.
   b. Complies with medical/nursing recommendations.
   c. Tolerates surgical procedure well.
      (1) Bleeding controlled.
      (2) Vital signs stable.
      (3) Urinary output adequate.
   d. Copes effectively with loss of pregnancy.
   e. Returns for follow-up care/surveillance.
   f. Selects and effectively implements method of contraception; avoids pregnancy for 1 yr or more.

g. Tests for HCG remain negative for 1 yr; no evidence of malignancy.
h. Achieves a pregnancy when desired.
i. Successfully carries pregnancy to term; normal, uncomplicated birth of viable infant.

D. **Ectopic pregnancy (Figure 4.6)**
   1. **Pathophysiology**—implantation outside of uterine cavity.
   2. Types:
      a. Tubal (most common).
      b. Cervical.
      c. Abdominal.
      d. Ovarian.
   3. **Etiology:**
      a. PID—pelvic salpingitis and endometritis.
      b. 43% caused by STD-related factors: 25%, chlamydial; 20%, previous STD.
      c. Tubal or uterine anomalies, tubal spasm.
      d. Adhesions from PID or past surgeries.
      e. Presence of IUD.
   4. **Assessment:** dependent on implantation site.
      a. *Early signs*—abnormal menstrual period (usually following a missed menstrual period), spotting, some symptoms of pregnancy; possible dull pain on affected side.
      b. *Impending or posttubal rupture*—sudden, acute, lower abdominal pain; nausea and vomiting; signs of shock; referred shoulder pain (*Kehr's sign*) or neck pain—due to blood in peritoneal cavity; blood in cul-de-sac may → rectal pressure.
      c. Sharp, localized pain when cervix is touched during vaginal exam; shock and circulatory collapse in some, usually following vaginal examination.
      d. Positive pregnancy test in many women.
   5. **Analysis/nursing diagnosis:**
      a. *Fear* related to abdominal pain and pregnancy status.
      b. *Grief* related to pregnancy loss.

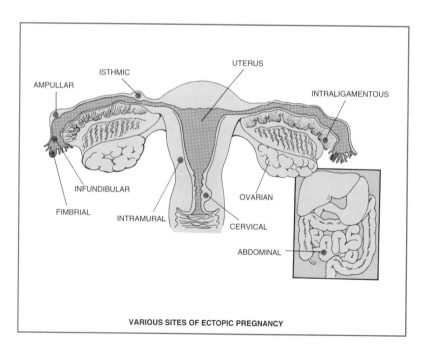

VARIOUS SITES OF ECTOPIC PREGNANCY

FIGURE 4.6   Ectopic pregnancy.
(From Venes, D [ed]: Taber's Cyclopedic Medical Dictionary, ed. 19. FA Davis, Philadelphia, 2001.)

◆ 6. **Nursing care plan/implementation:**
   ◗ a. *Medical management:* Surgical removal/repair. Methotrexate, a folic acid antagonist, which acts by inhibiting cell division (may be used in early ectopic pregnancy).
   b. *Nursing management:*
      (1) Goal: *preoperative and postoperative care, health teaching.*
      (2) Goal: *supportive care for grief reaction;* encourage verbalization of anxiety and concerns of further pregnancies.

◆ 7. **Evaluation/outcome criteria:**
   a. Woman experiences uncomplicated postoperative course.
   b. Woman copes effectively with loss of pregnancy.

II. Complications affecting nutrition/elimination: hyperemesis gravidarum

   A. **Pathophysiology**—pernicious vomiting during first 14–16 wk (peak incidence around 10 weeks of gestation); excessive vomiting at any time during pregnancy. Potential hazards include the following:
      1. Dehydration with fluid and electrolyte imbalance.
      2. Starvation, with loss of 5% or more of body weight; protein and vitamin deficiencies.
      3. Metabolic acidosis—due to breakdown of fat stores to meet metabolic needs.
      4. Hypovolemia and hemoconcentration; *increased* blood urea nitrogen (BUN); *decreased* urinary output.
      5. Embryonic or fetal death may result, and the woman may suffer irreversible metabolic changes or death.

   B. **Etiology:**
      1. Physiological—secretion of HCG, decrease in free gastric HCl, decreased gastrointestinal motility. Increased incidence in hydatidiform mole and multifetal pregnancy (due to high levels of HCG).
      2. Psychological—thought to be related to rejection of pregnancy or sexual relations.

◆ C. **Assessment:**
      1. Intractable vomiting.
      2. Abdominal pain.
      3. Hiccups.
      4. Marked weight loss.
      5. Dehydration—thirst, tachycardia, skin turgor.
      6. Increased respiratory rate (metabolic acidosis).
      7. Laboratory—*elevated* BUN.
      8. *Medical evaluation:* rule out other causes (infection, tumors).

◆ D. **Analysis/nursing diagnosis:**
      1. *Altered nutrition, less than body requirements,* related to inability to retain oral feedings.
      2. *Fluid volume deficit* related to dehydration.
      3. *Ineffective individual coping* related to symptoms, insecurity in role, psychological stress of unwanted pregnancy.
      4. *Personal identity disturbance* related to symptoms or perception of self as inadequate in role, sick, socially unpresentable.

◆ E. **Nursing care plan/implementation:**
      1. Goal: *physiological stability*
         a. Rest GI tract (keep NPO) (e.g., maintain IV fluids, parenteral nutrition).
         ▮◗ b. Progress diet, as ordered; present small feedings attractively; ↑CHO, ↓ fat, ↓ acidic foods.
         c. Weigh daily, assess hydration; note weight gain.
         ◗ d. Antiemetics (IV, suppository).
      2. Goal: *minimize environmental stimuli.*
         a. Limit visitors and phone calls.
         b. Bedrest with bathroom privileges.
      3. Goal: *emotional support.*
         a. Establish accepting, supportive environment.
         b. Encourage verbalization of anxiety, fears, concerns.
         c. Support positive self-image.

◆ F. **Evaluation/outcome criteria:**
      1. Woman's signs and symptoms subside; she takes oral nourishment and gains weight.
      2. Woman's pregnancy continues to term without recurrence of hyperemesis.

III. Complications affecting protective function: STDs. This NCLEX-RN® category measures applications of knowledge about conditions related to client's capacity to maintain defenses and prevent physical and chemical trauma, injury, *infection*, and threats to health status.

   A. **Vaginitis**—inflammation of vagina.
      1. **Pathophysiology**—local inflammatory reaction (redness, heat, irritation/tenderness, pain). May cause preterm labor in pregnancy.
      2. **Etiology:**
         a. Common causative organisms:
            (1) Bacteria—streptococci, *Escherichia coli,* gonococci, Chlamydia, bacterial vaginosis.
            (2) *Viruses*—herpes type II, CMV, HPV
            (3) Protozoa—*Trichomonas vaginalis.*
            (4) Fungi—*Candida albicans.*
         b. Atrophic changes—due to declining hormone level (women who are postmenopausal).
   ◆ 3. **Assessment:** differentiate among common vaginal infections:
         a. Vulvovaginal erythema.
         b. Pruritus, dysuria, dyspareunia.
         c. Vaginal discharge—color, consistency.
   ◆ 4. **Analysis/nursing diagnosis:** *pain* related to inflammation, discharge.
   ◆ 5. **Nursing care plan/implementation:**
         a. Goal: *emotional support.*
         b. Goal: *health teaching.* Instruct woman in self- care measures to promote comfort and healing:
            (1) Perineal care.
            (2) Sitz baths.
            (3) Douching (as ordered). *Not* recommended during pregnancy.
            (4) Exposing vulva to air.
            (5) Cotton briefs.
            (6) Proper insertion of vaginal suppository.
         ◗ (7) Instruct client on antibiotic use, as ordered.

c. Goal: *prevent reinfection*
  (1) Suggest sexual partner use condom until infection is eliminated—or abstain from intercourse.
  (2) Recommend sexual partner seek examination and treatment.
  d. Goal: *medical consultation/treatment.*
    Refer for diagnosis and treatment.
◆ 6. **Evaluation/outcome criteria:**
  a. Woman is asymptomatic; unable to recover organism from body fluids or tissue.
  b. Woman avoids reinfection.
  c. Woman carries pregnancy to term without complications.

B. **Gonorrhea**
  1. **Pathophysiology:**
    a. *Men*—early infection usually confined to urethra, vestibular glands, anus, or pharynx. Untreated: ascending infection may involve testes, causing sterility.
    b. *Women*—early infection usually confined to vestibular glands, endocervix, urethra, anus (vagina is resistant). May ascend to involve pelvic structures (e.g., PID: fallopian tubes, ovaries); scarring may cause sterility.
    c. *Women who are pregnant*—may result in preterm rupture of membranes, amnionitis, preterm labor, postpartum salpingitis.
    d. Sequelae (untreated):
      (1) May develop carrier state (asymptomatic; organism resident in vestibular glands).
      (2) Systemic spread may result in gonococcal:
        (a) Arthritis.
        (b) Endocarditis.
        (c) Meningitis.
        (d) Septicemia.
      e. Newborn—ophthalmia neonatorum (gonococcal conjunctivitis). Untreated sequela: blindness.
  2. **Etiology:** gram-negative diplococcus (*Neisseria gonorrhoeae*).
  3. **Epidemiology:**
    a. Portal of entry—oral or genitourinary mucous membranes.
    b. Mode of transmission—usually sexual contact.
    c. Incubation period: 2–5 days; may be asymptomatic.
    d. Communicable period—as long as organisms are present; to 4 days after antibiotic therapy begun.
◆ 4. **Assessment:**
    a. History of known (or suspected) contact.
    b. *Men:*
      (1) Complaint of mucoid or mucopurulent discharge.
      (2) Medical diagnosis—procedure: urethral discharge Gram stain.
    c. *Women:*
      (1) Often asymptomatic; acute infection: severe vulvovaginal inflammation, venereal warts, greenish-yellow vaginal discharge.
      (2) *Medical diagnosis*—procedure: endocervical culture.
    d. Gonococcal urethritis (men and women)—sudden severe dysuria, frequency, burning, edema.
    e. Salpingitis/oophoritis—severe, sudden abdominal pain, fever (with or without vaginal discharge).
◆ 5. **Analysis/nursing diagnosis:** *impaired tissue integrity* related to tissue inflammation.
◆ 6. **Nursing care plan/implementation:**
    a. Goal: *emotional support.*
    b. Goal: *health teaching* to prevent transmission, sequelae, reinfection.
      (1) Need for accurate diagnosis and effective treatment, follow-up examination in 7–14 days, and culture.
      (2) All sexual partners need examination, treatment.
      (3) Possible sequelae/complications (sterility, carrier state).
    c. Goal: *medical consultation/treatment.*
      (1) Determine allergy to antibiotics.
      (2) Refer for diagnosis and treatment.
        (a) Diagnosis: culture.
        (b) Treatment—ceftriaxone IM, plus doxycycline PO. May use erythromycin or spectinomycin in pregnancy.
        (c) Follow-up culture before birth.
        (d) Notification of sexual partners.
◆ 7. **Evaluation/outcome criteria:**
    a. Verbalizes understanding of mode of transmission, prevention, importance of examination, treatment of sexual contacts.
    b. Informs sexual contacts of need for examination.
    c. Returns for follow-up examinations.
    d. Successfully treated; weekly follow-up cultures: negative on two successive visits.
    e. Avoids reinfection.

C. *Chlamydia trachomatis*
  1. **Pathophysiology:**
    a. Most common sexually transmitted disease in United States.
    b. Initial infection mild in women; inflammation of cervix with discharge.
    c. If untreated, may lead to urethritis, dysuria, PID, tubal occlusion, infertility.
  2. **Etiology:**
    a. *Chlamydia trachomatis* has maternal-fetal effects.
    b. Bacteria can exist only within living cells.
    c. Transmission is by direct contact from one person to another.
◆ 3. **Assessment—maternal:**
    a. Inflamed cervix (may be asymptomatic).

b. Cervical congestion, edema.

c. Mucopurulent discharge.

◆ 4. **Assessment—fetal-neonatal:**

a. Increased incidence of stillbirth.

b. Preterm birth may result.

c. Contact with infected mucus occurs during birth.

d. Newborn may be asymptomatic.

e. Conjunctivitis; may lead to scarring.

f. *Chlamydial* pneumonia.

◆ 5. **Analysis/nursing diagnosis:**

a. *Pain* related to inflamed reproductive organs.

b. *Fatigue* related to inflammation.

c. *Knowledge deficit* related to mode of treatment, disease transmission.

◆ 6. **Nursing care plan/implementation:**

a. Treatment with antibiotics, generally doxycycline or azithromycin. Erythromycin in pregnancy.

b. Provide pain relief, analgesics.

c. Counsel regarding use of condoms, spermicidal agents (containing nonoxynol-9) to prevent reinfection.

◆ 7. **Evaluation/outcome criteria:**

a. Woman understands treatment and shows compliance.

b. Woman understands portal of entry and risk for reinfection.

D. Herpes genitalis

1. **Pathophysiology**—initial infection: varies in severity of symptoms, may be local or systemic; duration: prolonged; morbidity: severe.

2. **Etiology**—Herpes virus type II.

3. **Epidemiology:**

a. Portal of entry—skin, mucous membranes.

b. Mode of transmission—usually sexual.

c. Incubation: 3–14 days.

d. Communicable period—while organisms are present.

◆ 4. **Assessment:**

a. Lesions—painful, red papules; pustular vesicles that break and form wet ulcers that later crust; self-limiting (3 wk).

b. Severe itching, tingling, or pain.

c. Discharge—copious; foul-smelling.

d. Dysuria.

e. Lymph nodes—enlarged, inflammatory, inguinal.

f. Woman who is pregnant—vaginal bleeding, spontaneous abortion, fetal death.

g. May shed virus for 7 wk.

h. *Medical diagnosis*: multinucleated giant cells in microscopic examination of lesion exudate; culture for herpes simplex virus (HSV).

◆ 5. **Analysis/nursing diagnosis:**

a. *Pain* related to inflammation process.

b. *Fear* related to longevity of disease.

c. *Fear* related to no cure for disease.

d. *Knowledge deficit* related to transmission to future partners, suppressive treatment.

◆ 6. **Nursing care plan/implementation:**

a. Goal: *emotional support.*

b. Goal: *health teaching.*

(1) Virus remains in body for life (dormant, noninfectious) in 25%–30% of population; small percentage have symptoms.

(2) Recurrence probable; usually shorter and milder.

(3) Need for close surveillance during pregnancy; cesarean birth may be indicated if woman has active genital lesions or positive culture.

c. Goal: *promote comfort.*

d. Goal: *accurate definitive treatment.* Refer for diagnosis and treatment.

(1) Diagnosis—cervical smears, labial and vaginal smears.

(2) Treatment—acyclovir; used for suppressive treatment only.

◆ 7. **Evaluation/outcome criteria:**

a. Woman remains asymptomatic.

b. Pregnancy continues to term with no newborn effects.

E. Syphilis

1. **Pathophysiology:**

a. *Primary stage:* nonreactive RPR.

(1) *Men:* 3–4 wk after contact, painless, localized penile/anal ulcer (chancre); lymph nodes—enlarged, regional.

(2) *Women:* often asymptomatic; labial, vaginal, or cervical chancre.

(3) Medical diagnosis—procedure: dark-field microscopic examination of lesion exudate.

b. *Secondary stage:* reactive VDRL.

(1) 6–8 wk after infection.

(2) Rash—macular, papular; on trunk, palms, soles.

(3) Malaise, headache, sore throat, weight loss, low-grade temperature.

c. *Latent stage:* reactive serologic test for syphilis (STS). Asymptomatic; noninfectious.

d. *Tertiary stage:*

(1) Gumma formation in skin, cardiovascular system, or central nervous system.

(2) Psychosis.

2. **Etiology:** *Treponema pallidum* (spirochete).

3. **Epidemiology:**

a. Portal of entry—skin, mucous membranes.

b. Mode of transmission—usually sexual.

c. Incubation period—9 days–3 mo.

d. Communicable period—primary and secondary stages.

◆ 4. **Assessment:**

a. *Primary*—chancre, when detectable. *Medical diagnosis*—procedure: dark-field examination of lesion exudate.

b. *Secondary:*
   (1) Malaise, lymphadenopathy, headache, elevated temperature.
   (2) Macular, papular rash on palms and soles; may be disseminated.
   (3) Medical diagnosis—(see **d.**, following).
c. *Tertiary:*
   (1) Subcutaneous nodules (gumma).
   (2) *Note:* Gumma formation may affect any body system; symptoms associated with area of involvement.
d. *Medical diagnosis*—procedures: stages other than primary—STS: VDRL, rapid plasma reagin (RPR), *T. pallidum* immobilization (TPI), fluorescent treponemal antibody absorption (FTA). *False-positive STS* in: collagen diseases, infectious mononucleosis, malaria, systemic tuberculosis.

◆ 5. **Analysis/nursing diagnosis:**
   a. *Pain* related to inflammation process.
   b. *Knowledge deficit* related to treatment and transmission of the disease.

◆ 6. **Nursing care plan/implementation:**
   a. Goal: *emotional support*
      (1) Nonjudgmental.
      (2) Caring, supportive manner.
   b. Goal: *health teaching.*
      (1) Need for accurate diagnosis and treatment, follow-up examinations.
      (2) All sexual partners need examination and treatment.
   c. Goal: *medical consultation/treatment.*
      (1) Refer for diagnosis and treatment.
         Note: In pregnancy—treatment by 18th gestational week prevents congenital syphilis in neonate; however, treat at time of diagnosis.
      (2) Treatment:
         (a) Primary, secondary—benzathine penicillin G, 2.4 million U.
         (b) Other stages—7.2 million U over 3 wk period.
         (c) Erythromycin or doxycycline for clients who are allergic to penicillin.

◆ 7. **Evaluation/outcome criteria:**
   a. If treated by 18th wk of pregnancy, congenital syphilis is prevented.
   b. Appropriate treatment after 18th wk cures both mother and fetus; however, any fetal damage occurring before treatment is irreversible.
   c. Follow-up VDRL: nonreactive at 1, 3, 6, 9, and 12 mo.
   d. *Tertiary*—cerebrospinal fluid examination negative at 6 mo and 1 yr following treatment.
   e. Verbalizes understanding of mode of transmission, potential sequelae without treatment, importance of examination/treatment of sexual contacts, preventive techniques.
   f. Informs contacts of need for examination.

g. Returns for follow-up visit.
h. Avoids reinfection.

F. **PID**
   1. **Pathophysiology**—ascending pelvic infection; may involve fallopian tubes (salpingitis), ovaries (oophoritis); may develop pelvic abscess (most common complication), pelvic cellulitis, pelvic thrombophlebitis, peritonitis.
   2. **Etiology:**
      a. *C. trachomatis.*
      b. Gonococci.
      c. Streptococci.
      d. Staphylococci.
   ◆ 3. **Assessment:**
      a. Pain: acute, abdominal.
      b. Vaginal discharge: foul smelling.
      c. Fever, chills, malaise.
      d. *Elevated* white blood cell (WBC) count.
   ◆ 4. **Analysis/nursing diagnosis:**
      a. *Pain* related to occluded tubules.
      b. *Infertility* related to permanent block of tubes.
      c. *Knowledge deficit* related to transmission of disease.
      d. *Altered urinary elimination* related to dysuria.
   ◆ 5. **Nursing care plan/implementation—for woman who is hospitalized:**
      a. Goal: *emotional support.*
      b. Goal: limit extension of infection.
         (1) Bedrest—*position:* semi-Fowler's, to promote drainage.
         (2) *Force fluids* to 3000 mL/day.
         (3) Administer antibiotics, as ordered.
      c. Goal: *prevent autoinocculation/transmission.*
         (1) Strict aseptic technique (handwashing, perineal care).
         (2) Contact-item isolation.
         (3) *Health teaching:* if untreated: high risk of tubal scarring, sterility, or ectopic pregnancy; pelvic adhesions; transmission of disease.
      d. Goal: *promote comfort.*
         (1) Analgesics, as ordered.
         (2) External heat, as ordered.
   ◆ 6. **Evaluation/outcome criteria:**
      a. Woman responds to therapy; uneventful recovery.
      b. Woman avoids reinfection.

Second Trimester Complications

See **Table 4.8.**

I. **Complications affecting comfort, rest, mobility: Incompetent cervix**
   A. **Pathophysiology**—inability of cervix to support growing weight of pregnancy; associated with repeated spontaneous second trimester abortion.
   B. **Etiology:**
      1. Unknown.
      2. Congenital defect in cervical musculature (exposure to DES).
      3. Cervical trauma during previous birth, abor-

tion; aggressive, deep, or repeated dilation and curettage.

◆ **C. Assessment:**
1. History of habitual, second trimester abortions.
2. Painless, progressive cervical effacement and dilation during second trimester.
3. Signs of threatened abortion or (early third trimester) preterm labor.

◆ **D. Analysis/nursing diagnosis:**
1. *Pain* related to early dilation.
2. *Fear* related to possible pregnancy loss.

◆ **E. Nursing care plan/implementation:**
1. *Medical management*
   a. Cerclage surgical procedure (*Shirodkar, McDonald*).
2. *Preoperative nursing management*
   a. Goal: *reduce physical stress on incompetent cervix.* Bedrest, supportive care.
   b. Goal: *emotional support.* Encourage verbalization of anxiety, fear, concerns.
   c. Goal: *health (preoperative) teaching.* Explain procedure—purse-string suture encircles cervix and reinforces musculature.
   d. Goal: *preparation for surgery.*
3. *Postoperative nursing management*
   a. Goal: *maximize surgical result.* Bedrest, supportive care.
   b. Goal: *health teaching.*
      (1) *Avoid:* strenuous physical activity; straining, infection.
      (2) Report promptly: signs of labor (vaginal bleeding, cramping).
      (3) Need for continued, close health surveillance.

◆ 4. **Evaluation/outcome criterion:** woman carries pregnancy to successful termination.

II. Complications affecting sensory/perceptual functions: pregnancy-induced hypertension (PIH); preeclampsia/eclampsia

A. Pathophysiology:
1. Generalized arteriospasm → increased peripheral resistance, decreased tissue perfusion, and hypertension.
2. *Kidney:*
   a. Reduced renal perfusion and vasospasm → glomerular lesions.
   b. Damage to membrane → loss of serum protein (albuminuria). *Note:* Reduced serum albumin/globulin (A/G) ratio alters blood osmolarity → edema.
   c. Increased tubular reabsorption of sodium → increased water retention (edema).
   d. Release of angiotensin contributes to vasospasm and hypertension.
3. *Brain:* decreased oxygenation, cerebral edema, and vasospasm → visual disturbances and hyperirritability, convulsions, and coma.
4. *Uterus:* decreased placental perfusion → increased risk of SGA baby, abruptio placentae, oligohydramnios.

B. Etiology: unknown. *Risk factors:*
1. Pregnancy—occurs only when a functioning trophoblast is present; more common in *first* pregnancies. Onset: develops after wk 20 of gestation, through labor, and up to 48 hours postpartum.
2. Coexisting conditions—diabetes, multifetal gestation, polyhydramnios, renal disease.
3. Angiotensin gene T235.

◆ **C. Assessment**—types:
1. *Preeclampsia—mild*
   a. **Hypertension**—systolic increase of 30 mm Hg or more over baseline; diastolic rise of 15 mm Hg or more.
   b. **Proteinuria**—1 g/day.
   c. Edema—digital and periorbital; **weight gain** over 0.45 kg (1 lb)/wk.
2. *Preeclampsia—severe*
   a. Increasing hypertension—systolic at or above 160 mm Hg or more than 50 mm Hg over baseline; diastolic, 110 mm Hg or more.
   b. Urine: *proteinuria* (5 g or more in 24 hr); *oliguria* (400 mL or less in 24 hr).
   c. Hemoconcentration, hypoproteinemia, hypernatremia, hypovolemic condition.
   d. Nausea and vomiting.
   e. Epigastric pain—due to edema of liver capsule.
   f. Cerebral or visual disturbances (before convulsive state):
      (1) Disorientation and somnolence.
      (2) Severe frontal **headache**.
      (3) Increased irritability; **hyperreflexia**.
      (4) **Visual disturbance:** blurred vision, halo vision, dimness, blind spots.
   g. **HELLP** Syndrome (Hemolysis, Elevated Liver enzymes, and Low Platelets).
3. *Eclampsia*
   a. Tonic and clonic convulsions; coma.
   b. Renal shutdown—oliguria, anuria.

◆ **D. Assessment—woman who is hospitalized:**
1. Vital signs (blood pressure in side-lying position, pulse, respirations)—q2–4hr, while awake (if mild to moderate preeclampsia) or as necessary. *Note:* Record, report persistent *hypertension.*
2. Fetal heart tones at time of vital signs.
3. Deep-tendon reflexes (DTR) and clonus—to identify/monitor CNS hyperirritability.
4. I&O—to identify diuresis. (*Note:* oliguria indicates pathologic progression.)
5. Urinalysis (clean-catch) for protein, daily or after each voiding, as necessary.
6. Signs of pathologic progression (see above **C. Assessment**—types).
7. Signs of labor, abruptio placentae (*Note:* high blood pressure, or a rapid drop, may initiate abruptio), DIC.
8. Emotional status.

9. Daily weight, amount/distribution of *edema* (pitting; pedal, digital, periorbital)—to identify signs of mobilization of tissue fluid, diuresis.

◆ **E. Analysis/nursing diagnosis:**
1. *Fluid volume excess:* hemoconcentration, edema related to altered blood osmolarity and sodium/water retention.
2. *Altered nutrition, less than body requirements:* protein deficiency related to loss through damaged renal membrane.
3. *Altered tissue perfusion* related to increased peripheral resistance and vasospasm in renal, cardiovascular system.
4. *Altered urinary elimination:* oliguria, anuria related to hypovolemia, vasospasm.
5. *Sensory/perceptual alterations:* visual disturbances, hyperirritability related to cerebral edema, decreased oxygenation to brain.
6. *Anxiety* related to symptoms, implications of pathophysiology.
7. *Diversional activity deficit* related to need for reduced environmental stimuli, bedrest.
8. *Risk for injury* related to seizure.

F. Prognosis:
1. *Good*—symptoms mild, respond to treatment.
2. *Poor*—convulsions (number and duration); persistent coma; hyperthermia, tachycardia (120 beats/min); cyanosis, and liver damage.
3. *Terminal*—pulmonary edema, congestive heart failure, acute renal failure, cerebral hemorrhage. The earlier the symptoms appear, the poorer the outcome for the pregnancy.

◆ **G. Nursing care plan/implementation:** Goal: *health teaching.*
1. *Rest*—frequent naps in *lateral Sims' position.*

2. Immediate report of **danger signs:**
   a. Digital and periorbital edema.
   b. Severe headache, irritability.
   c. Visual disturbances.
   d. Epigastric pain.

▶ 3. *Do roll-over* test (blood pressure while on back and lateral positions).
4. Importance of regular prenatal visits.
5. Monitoring own blood pressure between prenatal visits.

◆ **H. Nursing care plan/implementation—woman who is hospitalized:**
1. Goal: *reduce environmental stimuli,* to minimize stimulation of hyperirritable CNS. Limit visitors and phone calls.
2. Goal: *emotional support.*
   a. Encourage verbalization of anxiety, fears, concerns.
   b. Explain all procedures, seizure precautions.
3. Goal: *supportive care.*
   a. Encourage bedrest—to increase tissue perfusion, promote diuresis.

b. *Position:* lateral Sims'—to reduce risk of supine hypotensive syndrome.
4. Goal: *health teaching.* Rest with reduced stimuli.
5. Goal: *monitor and administer drugs as ordered.*
   a. Anticonvulsants (especially magnesium sulfate).
   b. Antihypertensives.
   c. Diuretics (used rarely, and only in presence of congestive heart failure [CHF]).
   d. Blood volume expanders.
6. Goal: *seizure precautions.* To safeguard maternal/fetal status:
   a. Observe for signs and symptoms of *impending* convulsion:

   (1) Frontal headache.
   (2) Epigastric pain.
   (3) Sharp cry.
   (4) Eyes: fixed, unresponsive.
   (5) Facial twitching.

   b. Emergency items (suction equipment, airway, drugs, IV fluids) immediately available.
▶ 7. Goal: *convulsion care* (woman with eclampsia).

   a. Maintain patent *airway;* administer oxygen.
   b. *Safety*—padded bed rails.
   c. Reduce environmental stimuli: dim lights, quiet.
   d. Observe, report, and record:
      (1) Onset and progression of convulsion.
      (2) If followed by coma or incontinence.
   e. Prepare for immediate cesarean delivery; check FHR. Close observation for 48 hr postpartum, even if no further convulsions.

◆ **I. Evaluation/outcome criteria:**
1. Woman complies with medical/nursing plan of care.
2. Woman's symptoms respond to treatment; progression halted.
3. Woman carries uneventful pregnancy to successful termination.

Third Trimester Complications

See **Table 4.8.**

I. Complications affecting fluid-gas transport
   A. Placenta previa—abnormal implantation; near or over internal cervical os. Increased incidence with multiparas, multiple gestation, previous uterine surgery.
   ◆ 1. **Assessment:**
      a. *Painless, bright red vaginal bleeding* (may be intermittent); absence of contractions, abdomen soft.
      b. If in labor, contractions usually normal.
      c. Boggy lower uterine segment—palpated on vaginal exam. (*Note:* If placenta previa is suspected, internal examinations are **contraindicated.**)

d. *Medical diagnosis—procedure:* sonography—to determine placental site.

◆ 2. **Analysis/nursing diagnosis:**
   a. *Anxiety* related to bleeding, outcome.
   b. *Fluid volume deficit* related to excessive blood loss.
   c. *Altered tissue perfusion* related to blood loss.
   d. *Altered urinary elimination* related to hypovolemia.
   e. *Fear* related to fetal injury or loss.

◆ 3. **Nursing care plan/implementation:**
   a. *Medical management*
      (1) Sterile vaginal examination under double setup.
      (2) Vaginal birth possible if bleeding minimal, marginal implantation; if fetal vertex is presenting so that presenting part acts as tamponade.
      (3) Cesarean birth for complete previa.
   b. *Nursing management.* Goal: *safeguard status.*

◆ 4. **Evaluation/outcome criteria: (Table 4.9)** (see following section on abruptio placentae).

B. **Abruptio placentae**—premature separation of normally implanted placenta from uterine wall.

◆ 1. **Assessment:**
   a. Sudden onset, *severe* abdominal pain.
   b. Increased uterine tone—may contract unevenly, fails to relax between contractions; very tender.
   c. Shock usually more profound than expected on basis of external bleeding or internal bleeding.
   d. *Medical evaluation—procedures:* DIC screening (bleeding time, platelet count, prothrombin time, activated partial thromboplastin time, fibrinogen); sonogram to see placental hemoseparation.

◆ 2. **Analysis/nursing diagnosis:**
   a. *Fluid volume deficit* related to bleeding.
   b. *Potential for fetal injury* related to uteroplacental insufficiency.
   c. *Fear* related to unknown outcome.

3. **Potential complications:**
   a. Afibrinogenemia and DIC.
   b. Couvelaire uterus—bleeding into uterine muscle.
   c. Amniotic fluid embolus.
   d. Hypovolemic shock.

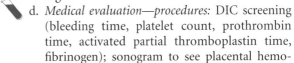

Pathology	Etiology	◆ Assessment	◆ Nursing Care Plan/Implementation
Placenta Previa			
Types:	More common with multiparity, advanced maternal age	**Painless,** *bright red* vaginal bleeding	**No** vaginal or rectal examinations or enemas
Marginal—low-lying	Fibroid tumors	Usually manifests in 8th mo	Bedrest (*high-Fowler's* if marginal previa)
Partial—partly covers internal cervical os	Endometriosis	*Postpartum:* signs of hemorrhage, infection	■ Continuous fetal monitor
Complete—covers internal cervical os	Old uterine scars		■ Maternal vital signs q4h, or prn
	Multiple gestation		■ Note character and amount of bleeding
			Emotional support
Abruptio Placentae			
Types:	Preeclampsia/eclampsia	**Pain: sudden, severe**	*Position:* supine; elevate (right) hip
Partial—small part separates from uterine wall	Before birth of second twin	Abdomen: rigid	■ Monitor: vital signs, blood loss, fetus
Complete—total placenta separates from uterine wall	Traction on cord	Uterus: very tender to touch	■ I&O (anuria, oliguria; hematuria)
Retroplacental—bleeding (concealed)	Rupture of membranes	Fetal hyperactivity; bradycardia, death	
	High parity	Shock: rapid, profound	Prepare for surgery
Marginal—occurs at edges; external bleeding	Chronic renal hypertension	Port-wine amniotic fluid	Emotional support
	Oxytocin induction/augmentation of labor	Signs of DIC	■ Fluid, blood replacement
	Cocaine use	*Postpartum:* signs of atony, infection, pulmonary emboli	
	Trauma		

TABLE 4.9 Comparison of Placenta Previa and Abruptio Placentae

Maternal-Infant

e. Renal failure.

f. Uterine atony, hemorrhage, infection in post-partum.

◆ 4. **Nursing care plan/implementation:**

a. *Medical management*

(1) Control: hemorrhage, hypovolemic shock; replace blood loss.

(2) Cesarean birth.

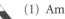 (3) Fibrinogen, crystalloids, blood replacement.

(4) IV heparin—by infusion pump—to reduce coagulation and fibrinolysis.

b. *Nursing management.* Goal: *safeguard status.*

◆ 5. **Evaluation/outcome criteria:**

a. Experiences successful termination of pregnancy.

(1) Woman gives birth to viable newborn (by vaginal or cesarean method).

(2) Woman has minimal blood loss.

(3) Woman's assessment findings within normal limits.

(4) Woman retains capacity for further child-bearing.

b. No evidence of complications (anemia, hypotonia, DIC) during postpartal period.

II. **Complications affecting comfort, rest, mobility**

A. **Polyhydramnios**—amniotic fluid over 2000 mL (normal volume: 500–1200 mL).

1. **Etiology:** unknown. *Risk factors:*

a. Maternal diabetes.

b. Multifetal gestation.

c. Erythroblastosis fetalis.

d. Preeclampsia/eclampsia.

e. Congenital anomalies (e.g., anencephaly, upper-GI anomalies, such as esophageal atresia).

◆ 2. **Assessment:**

a. Fundal height: excessive for gestational estimate.

b. Fetal parts: difficult to palpate, small in proportion to uterine size.

c. Increased discomfort—due to large, heavy uterus.

d. Increased edema in vulva and legs.

e. Shortness of breath.

f. GI discomfort—heartburn, constipation.

g. Susceptibility to *supine hypotensive syndrome*—due to compression of inferior vena cava and descending aorta while in supine position.

h. *Medical diagnosis—procedures:*

(1) Sonography—to diagnose multifetal pregnancy, gross fetal anomaly, locate placental site.

(2) Amniocentesis—to diagnose anomalies, erythroblastosis.

3. **Potential complications:**

a. Maternal respiratory impairment.

b. Premature rupture of membranes (PROM) with prolapsed cord or amnionitis.

c. Preterm labor.

d. Postpartum hemorrhage—due to overdistention and uterine atony.

◆ 4. **Analysis/nursing diagnosis:**

a. *Pain* related to excessive size of uterus impinging on diaphragm, stomach, bladder.

b. *Impaired physical mobility* related to increased lordotic curvature of back, increased weight on legs.

c. *Altered tissue perfusion* related to decreased venous return from lower extremities, compression of body structures by overdistended uterus.

d. *Potential fluid volume deficit* related to potential uterine atony in immediate postpartum, secondary to loss of contractility due to overdistention.

e. *Sleep pattern disturbance* related to respiratory impairment and discomfort in side-lying position.

f. *Anxiety* related to discomfort, potential for complications associated with congenital anomalies.

g. *Altered urinary elimination* (frequency) related to pressure of overdistended uterus on bladder.

◆ 5. **Nursing care plan/implementation:**

a. *Medical management*

(1) Amniocentesis—remove excess fluid very slowly, to prevent abruptio placentae.

(2) Termination of pregnancy—if fetal abnormality present *and* woman desires.

b. *Nursing management*

(1) Goal: *health teaching.*

(a) Need for *lateral Sims' position* during resting; semi-Fowler's may alleviate respiratory embarrassment.

(b) Explain diagnostic or treatment procedures.

(c) Signs and symptoms to be **reported immediately:** bleeding, loss of fluid through vagina, cramping.

(2) Goal: *prepare for diagnostic and/or treatment procedures.*

(a) Permit for amniocentesis.

(3) Goal: *emotional support for loss of pregnancy* (if applicable).

(a) Encourage verbalization of feelings.

(b) Facilitate grieving: permit parents to see, hold infant; if desired, take photograph, footprints for them.

◆ 6. **Evaluation/outcome criteria:**

a. Woman complies with medical/nursing management.

b. Woman's symptoms of respiratory impairment, etc., reduced; comfort promoted.

c. Woman experiences normal, uncomplicated pregnancy, labor, birth, and postpartum.

III. **Diagnostic tests to evaluate fetal growth and well-being**

A. **Daily fetal movement count (DFMC)**

1. Assesses fetal activity.
2. Noninvasive test done by woman who is pregnant.
3. Five to 10 movements per hour: normal activity.
4. Five movements or less per hour may indicate fetal jeopardy or sudden change in movement pattern.
5. Assess for fetal sleep patterns.

B. Nonstress test (NST)
1. Correlates fetal movement with FHR. Requires electronic monitoring.
2. *Reactive test*—three accelerations of FHR 15 beats/min above baseline FHR, lasting for 15 sec or more, over 20 min time period.
3. *Nonreactive test*—no accelerations or acceleration less than 15 beats/min above baseline FHR. May indicate fetal jeopardy. Vibroacoustic simulator (VAS) to differentiate hypoxia from fetal sleep.
4. Unsatisfactory test—data that cannot be interpreted or inadequate fetal activity; repeat.

C. Contraction stress test (CST); oxytocin challenge test (OCT)
1. Correlates fetal heart rate response to spontaneous or induced uterine contractions.
2. Requires electronic monitoring.
3. Indicator of uteroplacental sufficiency.
4. Identifies pregnancies at risk for fetal compromise from uteroplacental insufficiency.
5. Increasing doses of oxytocin are administered to stimulate uterine contractions until 3 in 10-minute period.
6. Interpretation: *negative* results indicate absence of late decelerations with all contractions.
7. *Positive* results indicate late FHR decelerations with contractions.
8. Nipple stimulation (breast self-stimulation test) may also release enough systemic oxytocin to contract uterus to obtain CST. Instruct *not* to do at home.

D. Biophysical profile (BPP)
1. Observation by ultrasound of four variables for 30 min and results of nonstress testing:
   a. Fetal body movements.
   b. Fetal tone.
   c. Amniotic fluid volume.
   d. Fetal breathing movements.
2. Variables are scored at 2 for each variable if present; score of 0 if not present; score of less than 6 is associated with perinatal mortality.

E. Ultrasound
1. Noninvasive procedure involving passage of high-frequency sound waves through uterus to obtain data regarding fetal growth, placental positioning, and the uterine cavity.
2. Purpose may include:
   a. Pregnancy confirmation.
   b. Fetal viability.
   c. Estimation of fetal age.
   d. BPD measurement (biparietal diameter).

   e. Placenta location.
   f. Detection of fetal abnormalities.
   g. Confirmation of fetal death.
   h. Identification of multifetal gestations.
   i. Amniotic fluid index.
3. No risk to mother with infrequent use. Fetal risk not determined on long-term basis.

F. Amniocentesis (see **Figure 4.5**)
1. Invasive procedure for amniotic fluid analysis to assess fetal lung maturity or disease; done after 14 weeks of gestation.
2. Needle placed through abdominal-uterine wall; designated amount of fluid is withdrawn for examination.
3. Empty bladder if gestation greater than 20 wk.
4. Risk of complications less than 1%. Ultrasound *always* precedes this procedure.
5. *Possible complications:* onset of contractions; infections (probably amnionitis); placental punctures; cord puncture; bladder or fetal puncture.

6. Advise women to observe and report the following to physician: fetal hypoactivity or hyperactivity, vaginal bleeding, vaginal discharge (clear or colored), signs of labor, signs of infection.

G. Analysis of amniotic fluid
1. Chromosomal studies to detect genetic aberrations.
2. Biochemical analysis of fetal cells to detect inborn errors of metabolism.
3. Determination of fetal lung maturity by assessing *lecithin-sphingomyelin* ratios.
4. Evaluation of *phospholipids*; aids in determining lung maturity.
5. Determination of *creatinine* levels, aids in determining fetal age. (*Greater than 1.8* mg/dL indicates fetal maturity and the fetal age.)
6. Assesses isoimmune disease.
7. Presence of meconium may indicate fetal hypoxia.

H. Chorionic villus sampling (CVS)
1. Cervically invasive procedure.
2. Advantage—results can be obtained after 10 weeks of gestation due to fast-growing fetal cells.
3. Procedure—removal of small piece of tissue (chorionic villus) from fetal portion of placenta. Tissue reflects genetic makeup of fetus.
4. Determines some genetic aberrations and allows for earlier decision for induced abortion (if desired) from abnormal results. Does not diagnose neural tube defects; clients who have CVS need further diagnoses with ultrasound.
5. Protects "pregnancy privacy" because results can be obtained before the pregnancy is apparent and decisions can be made regarding abortion or continuation of gestation.
6. Risks involve: spontaneous abortion, infection, hematoma, intrauterine death, Rh isoimmunization, and fetal limb defects, if done before 9 weeks of gestation.

Maternal-Infant

THE INTRAPARTAL EXPERIENCE

General overview: This review of the anatomical and phys-iological determinants of successful labor provides baseline data against which the nurse compares findings of an ongo-ing assessment of the woman in labor. Nursing actions are planned and implemented to meet the present and emerging needs of the woman in labor.

I. **Biological foundations of labor**
   A. **Premonitory signs**
      1. *Lightening*—process in which the fetus "drops" into the pelvic inlet.
         a. *Characteristics*
            (1) Nullipara—usually occurs 2–3 wk before onset of labor.
            (2) Multipara—commonly occurs with onset of labor.
         b. *Effects*
            (1) Relieves pressure on diaphragm—breathing is easier.
            (2) Increases pelvic pressure.
               (a) Urinary frequency returns.
               (b) Increased pressure on thighs.
               (c) Increased tendency to vulvar, vaginal, perianal, and leg varicosities.
      2. *Braxton Hicks contractions*—may become more uncomfortable.
   B. **Etiology:** unknown. *Theories* include:
      1. Uterine overdistention.
      2. Placental aging—*declining* estrogen/progesterone levels.
      3. *Rising* prostaglandin level.
      4. Fetal cortisol secretion.
      5. Maternal/fetal oxytocin secretion.
   C. **Overview of labor process**—forces of labor (involun-tary uterine contractions) overcome cervical resist-ance; cervix thins *(effacement)* and opens (0–10 cm *dilation)* (**Table 4.10**). Voluntary contraction of secondary abdominal muscles during the second stage (e.g., pushing, bearing-down) forces fetal descent. Changing pelvic dimensions force fetal head to accommodate to the birth canal by molding (cranial bones overlap to decrease head size).

TABLE 4.10. First Stage of Labor		
Phases of First Stage	◆ **Assessment: Expected Maternal Behaviors**	◆ **Nursing Care Plan/Implementation**
0–4 cm: Latent Phase and Early Active Phase		
1. *Time:* multipara 5–6 hr; nullipara 8–10 hr, average	1. Usually comfortable, euphoric, excited, talkative, and energetic, but may be fear-ful and withdrawn	1. Provide encouragement, feedback for relax-ation, companionship, hydration, nutrition
2. *Contractions:* regular, mild, 5–10 min apart, 20–30 seconds duration	2. Relieved or apprehensive that labor has begun	2. Coach during contractions: signal beginning of contraction, mark the seconds, signal end of contraction; "Follow my breathing," "Watch my lips," etc.
3. Low-back pain and abdominal discomfort with contractions	3. Alert, usually receptive to teaching, coach-ing, diversion, and anticipatory guidance	3. Comfort measures: position change for comfort; praise; keep aware of progress; maintain hydration
4. Cervix thins: some bloody show		
5. *Station:* Multipara −2 to +1; nullipara 0.		
4–8 cm: Midactive Phase, Phase of Most Rapid Dilation		
1. Average *time:* nullipara 1–2 hr; multipara 1½–2 hr	1. Tired, less talkative, and less energetic	1. Coach during contractions; partner (coach) may need some relief
2. *Contractions:* 2–5 min apart, 30–40 seconds' duration, intensity increasing	2. More serious, malar flush between 5 and 6 cm, tendency to hyperventilate, may need analgesia, needs constant coaching	2. *Comfort measures* (to partner too—as needed): position for comfort while prevent-ing hypotensive syndrome; encourage relax-ation, focusing her on areas of tension; provide counterpressure to sacrococcygeal area, prn; praise; keep aware of progress; minimize distractions from surrounding environment (loud talking, other noises); offer analgesics and anesthetics, as appropri-ate; provide hygiene: mouth care, ice chips, clean perineum; warmth, as needed

(Continued on following page)

Phases of First Stage	◆ Assessment: Expected Maternal Behaviors	◆ Nursing Care Plan/Implementation
3. Membranes may rupture now		3. Monitor progress of labor and maternal/fetal response, color of fluid, time of rupture of membranes (ROM)
4. Increased bloody show		4. If monitors are in use, attention on mother; periodically check accuracy of monitor read-outs
5. *Station:* −1 to 0		

8–10 cm: Transition, Deceleration Period of Active Phase

1. Average *time:* nullipara 40 min–1 hr; multipara 20 min	1. If not under regional anesthesia, more introverted; may be amnesic between contractions	1. Stay with woman (couple) and provide constant support
2. *Contractions:* $1^1/_2$–2 min apart, 60–90 seconds duration, strong intensity	2. Feeling she cannot make it; increased irritability, crying, nausea, vomiting, and belching; increased perspiration over upper lip and between breasts; leg tremors; and shaking	2. Continue to coach with contractions: may need to remind, reassure, and encourage her to reestablish breathing techniques and concentration with each contraction; coach panting or "he-he" respirations to prevent pushing
3. Increased vaginal show; rectal pressure with beginning urge to bear down	3. May have uncontrollable urge to push at this time	3. Comfort measures; remind her and partner her behavior is normal and "OK"; coach breathing to quell nausea; offer ice chips
4. *Station:* +13 to +14		4. Assist with countertension techniques woman requested
		5. Monitor contractions, FHR (after each contraction), vaginal discharge, perineal bulging, maternal vital signs; record every 15 min
		6. Assess for bladder filling
		7. Keep mother (couple) aware of progress
		8. Prepare partner for birth (scrub, gown, etc.)

Stages of labor:
1. *First*—begins with establishment of regular, rhythmic contractions; ends with complete effacement and dilation (10 cm); divided into three phases:
   a. Latent and early active.
   b. Active.
   c. Transitional.
2. *Second*—begins with complete dilation and ends with birth of infant.
3. *Third*—begins with birth of infant and ends with expulsion of placenta.
4. *Fourth*—begins with expulsion of placenta; ends when maternal status is stable (usually 1–2 hr postpartum).

D. **Anatomical/physiological determinants**
   1. **Maternal**
      a. *Uterine contractions*—involuntary; birth; begin process of involution.
         (1) *Characteristics:* rhythmic; increasing tone (*increment*), peak (*acme*), relaxation (*decrement*).
         (2) *Effects:*
            (a) Decreases blood flow to uterus and placenta.
            (b) Dilates cervix during first stage of labor.
            (c) Raises maternal blood pressure during contractions.
            (d) With voluntary bearing-down efforts (abdominal muscles), expels fetus (second stage) and placenta (third stage).
            (e) Begins involution.
      ◆ (3) **Assessment:**
            (a) Frequency—time from beginning of one contraction to beginning of the next.
            (b) Duration—time from beginning of contraction to its relaxation
            (c) Strength (intensity)—resistance to indentation.
            (d) False/true labor—differentiation (**Table 4.11**)
            (e) Signs of dystocia (dysfunctional labor) (see **pp. 203, 206**).
      b. *Pelvic structures and configuration:*
         (1) *False positive*—above linea terminalis (line travels across top of symphysis pubis around to sacral promontory); supports gravid uterus during pregnancy.

TABLE 4.11	Assessment: Differentiation of False/True Labor

False Labor	True Labor
Contractions: Braxton Hicks intensify (more noticeable at night); short, *irregular*, little change	*Contractions:* begin in lower back, radiate to abdomen ("girdling"), become *regular*, rhythmic; *frequency, duration, intensity increase*
Discomfort: mostly abdominal and groin	*Discomfort:* mostly low back
Relieved by change of position or activity (e.g., walking)	*Unaffected* by change of position, activity, drinking two glasses of water, or moderate analgesia
Cervical changes—none; *no* effacement or dilation progress	*Cervical changes*—*progressive* effacement and dilation

(2) *True pelvis*—below linea terminalis; divided into:
  (a) Inlet— "brim," demarcated by linea terminalis.
    (i) Widest diameter: transverse.
    (ii) Narrowest diameter: anterior-posterior (true conjugate).
  (b) Midplane—pelvic cavity.
  (c) Outlet.
    (i) Widest diameter: anterior-posterior (requires internal rotation of fetal head for entry).
    (ii) Narrowest diameter: transverse (intertuberous); facilitates birth in occiput anterior (OA) position.
(3) *Classifications*
  (a) Gynecoid—normal female pelvis; rounded oval.
  (b) Android—normal male pelvis; funnel shaped.
  (c) Anthropoid—oval.
  (d) Platypelloid—flattened, transverse oval.

2. **Fetal**
  a. *Fetal head* (**Figure 4.7**).

(1) Bones—one occipital, two frontal, two parietals, two temporals.
(2) Suture—line of junction or closure between bones; sagittal (longitudinal), coronal (anterior), and lambdoidal (posterior, frontal); permit molding to accommodate head to birth canal.
(3) Fontanels—membranous space between cranial bones during fetal life and infancy.
  (a) *Anterior* "soft spot"—diamond shaped; junction of coronal and sagittal sutures; closes (ossifies) by *18 mo.*
  (b) *Posterior*—triangular; junction of sagittal and lambdoidal sutures; closes by *4 mo of age.*
b. *Fetal lie*—relationship of fetal long axis to maternal long axis (spine).
  (1) Transverse—shoulder presents.
  (2) Longitudinal—vertex or breech presents.
c. *Presentation*—fetal part entering inlet first (**Figure 4.8**).
  (1) *Cephalic*—vertex (most common); face, brow.
  (2) *Breech*

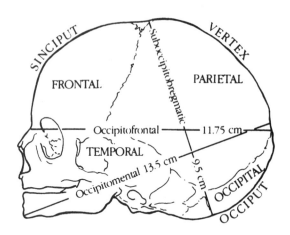
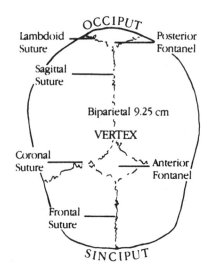

FIGURE 4.7 **The fetal head.** *Bones:* two frontal, two temporal, one occipital. *Sutures:* sagittal, frontal, coronal, lambdoid. *Fontanels:* anterior, posterior. (Used with permission of Ross Products Division, Abbott Laboratories, Inc., Columbus, OH 43216, Clinical Education Aid No. 13.)

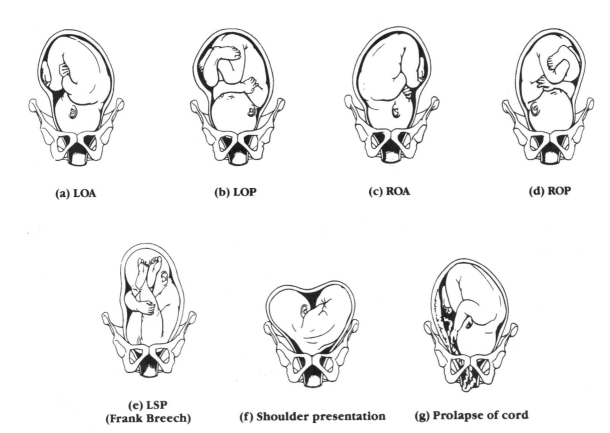

(a) LOA   **(b) LOP**   **(c) ROA**   **(d) ROP**

(e) LSP
(Frank Breech)   **(f) Shoulder presentation**   **(g) Prolapse of cord**

FIGURE 4.8   Categories of fetal presentation. (a) **LOA:** fetal occiput is in left anterior quadrant of maternal pelvis. (b) **LOP:** fetal occiput is in left posterior quadrant of maternal pelvis. (c) **ROA:** fetal occiput is in right anterior quadrant of maternal pelvis. (d) **ROP:** fetal occiput is in right posterior quadrant of maternal pelvis. (e) **LSP:** fetal sacrum is in left posterior quadrant of maternal pelvis. (f) **Shoulder presentation with fetus in transverse lie.** (g) **Prolapse of umbilical cord** with fetus in LOA position. (Used with permission of Ross Products Division, Abbott Laboratories, Inc., Columbus, OH 43216, Clinical Education Aid No. 18.)

(a) *Complete*—feet and legs flexed on thighs; buttocks and feet presenting
(b) *Frank*—legs extended on torso, feet up by shoulders; buttocks presenting.
(c) *Footling*—single (one foot), double (both feet) presenting.
d. *Attitude*—relationship of fetal parts to one another (e.g., head flexed on chest).
e. *Position*—relationship of presenting fetal part to quadrants of maternal pelvis; vertex most common, occiput anterior on maternal left side (LOA) (see **Figure 4.8**).
◆ 3. **Assessment:** determine presentation and position.
▶ a. *Leopold's maneuvers*—abdominal palpation.
(1) *First*—palms over fundus, breech feels softer, not as round as head would be.
(2) *Second*—palms on either side of abdomen, locates fetal back and small parts.
(3) *Third*—fingers just above pubic symphysis, grasp lower abdomen; if unengaged, presenting part is mobile.
(4) *Fourth*—facing mother's feet, run palms down sides of abdomen to symphysis; check for cephalic prominence (usually on

right side), and if head is floating or engaged.
▶ b. *Location of fetal heart tones*—heard best through fetal back or chest.
(1) *Breech* presentation—usually most audible *above* maternal umbilicus.
(2) *Vertex* presentation—usually most audible *below* maternal umbilicus.
(3) Changing location of most audible FHTs (fetal heart tones)—useful indicator of fetal descent.
(4) Factors affecting audibility:
(a) Obesity.
(b) Maternal position.
(c) Polyhydramnios.
(d) Maternal gastrointestinal activity.
(e) Loud uterine bruit—origin: hissing of blood through maternal uterine arteries; synchronous with maternal pulse
(f) Loud funic souffle—origin: hissing of blood through umbilical arteries; synchronous with fetal heart rate (FHR).
(g) External noise, faulty equipment.

Maternal-Infant

c. *Vaginal examination:* palpable sutures, fontanels (triangular-shaped superior, diamond-shaped inferior = vertex presentation, OA position).

4. *Cardinal movements of the* **mechanisms of normal labor**—vertex presentation, positional changes of fetal head accommodate to changing diameters of maternal pelvis (**Figure 4.9**).

   a. *Descent*—head engages and proceeds down birth canal.

   b. *Flexion*—head bent to chest; presents smallest diameter of vertex (suboccipital-bregmatic).

   c. *Internal rotation*—during second stage of labor, transverse diameter of fetal head enters pelvis; occiput rotates 90 degrees to bring back of neck under symphysis (e.g., LOT to LOA to OA); presents smallest diameter (biparietal) to smallest diameter of outlet (intertuberous).

   d. *Extension*—back of neck pivots under symphysis, allows head to be born by extension.

   e. *Restitution*—head returns to normal alignment with shoulders (with LOA, results in head facing right thigh), presents smallest diameter of shoulders to outlet.

   f. *Delivery of head*—shoulders in anterior-posterior position.

   g. *Expulsion*—birth of neonate completed.

◆ 5. **Assessment:** relationship of fetal head to ischial spines (**degree of descent**).

   a. *Engagement*—widest diameter of presenting part has passed through pelvic inlet (e.g., biparietal diameter of fetal head).

   b. *Station*—relationship of presenting part to ischial spines (IS).

      (1) *Floating*—presenting part above inlet, in false pelvis.

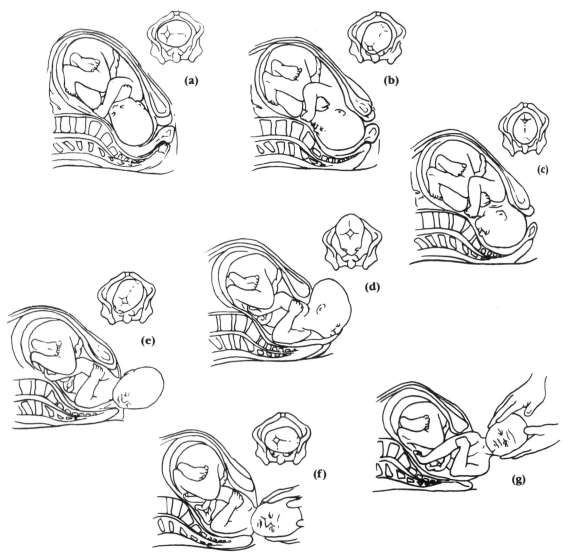

FIGURE 4.9 **Cardinal movements in the mechanism of labor with the fetus in vertex presentation.** (a) Engagement, descent, flexion. (b) Internal rotation. (c) Extension beginning (rotation complete). (d) Extension complete. (e) External rotation (restitution). (f) External rotation (shoulder rotation). (g) Expulsion. (Used with permission of Ross Products Division, Abbott Laboratories, Inc., Columbus, OH 43216, Clinical Education Aid No. 13.)

(2) Station–5 is at inlet (presenting part well above IS).

(3) Station 0—presenting part at IS (engaged).

(4) Station +4—presenting part at the outlet.

E. Warning signs during labor

1. *Contraction*—hypertonic, poor relaxation, or tetanic (greater than 90 sec long and ≤2 min apart).
2. *Abdominal pain*—sharp, rigid abdomen
3. *Vaginal bleeding*—profuse.
4. *FHR*—late decelerations, prolonged variable decelerations, bradycardia, tachycardia (**Figure 4.10**), decreased variability.
5. *Maternal hypertension.*
6. *Meconium-stained amniotic fluid (MSAF).*
7. *Prolonged ROM.*

II. Participatory childbirth techniques

A. Psychoprophylaxis—Lamaze method

1. Premise—conditioned responses to stimuli occupy nerve pathways, reducing perception of pain. Emphasis is on childbirth as a natural event, with a woman who is informed as the active participant. The ability to relax effectively reduces the perception of pain, and the involvement of the coach fosters the family concept.
2. Childbirth partners are taught:
   a. Anatomy and physiology of labor.
   b. Psychology of man and woman.
   c. What to expect in the birthing setting.
   d. Conditioned responses to labor stimuli.
      (1) Concentration on focal point.
      (2) Breathing techniques.
      (3) Need for active coaching to enable woman to:
         (a) Use techniques appropriate to present stage of labor.
         (b) Avoid hyperventilation.
   e. Specific stage—appropriate techniques:
      (1) *First stage of labor—early:* slow, deep chest breathing; *active:* patterned breathing.
      (2) *Transition* (8–10 cm)—rapid, shallow breathing pattern, to prevent pushing prematurely.
         (a) Panting.
         (b) Pant-blow.
         (c) "He-he" pattern.
      (3) *Second stage of labor*
         (a) Pushing (or bearing-down)—aids fetal descent through birth canal.
         (b) Panting—aids relaxation between contractions; prevents explosive birth of head.
   f. Effects on labor behaviors/coping:
      (1) Help mother cope with and assist contractions.
      (2) Prevent premature bearing-down efforts; reduce possibility of cervical lacerations, edema due to pushing on incompletely dilated cervix.
      (3) When appropriate, improve efficiency of bearing-down efforts.

B. Other methods—include parent classes, classes for siblings, multiparas, and those who plan cesarean birth.

III. Nursing actions during first stage of labor

◆ **A. Assessment:** careful evaluation of:

1. *Antepartal history*
   a. EDD
   b. Genetic and familial problems.
   c. Preexisting and coexisting medical disorders, allergies.
   d. Pregnancy-related health problems (hyperemesis, bleeding, etc.).
   e. Infectious diseases (past and present herpes, etc.).
   f. Past obstetric history, if any.
   g. Pelvic size estimation.
   h. Height.
   i. Weight gain.
   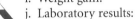 j. Laboratory results:
      (1) Blood type and Rh factor.
      (2) Serology.
      (3) Urinalysis.
      (4) Hepatitis.
      (5) Rubella.
   k. Prenatal care history.
   l. Use of medications.
2. *Admission findings*
   a. Emotional status.
   b. Vital signs.
   c. Present weight.
   d. Fundal height.
   e. Estimated fetal weight.
   f. Edema.
   g. Urinalysis (for protein and glucose).
▶ 3. *FHR*—normal, 110–160 beats/min (see **Figure 4.10**).
   a. Check and record every 15–30 min—monitor fetal response to physiological stress of labor.
   b. *Bradycardia* (mild, 100–110 beats/min, or 30 beats/min lower than baseline reading).
   c. *Tachycardia* (moderate, 160–179 beats/min, or 30 beats/min above baseline reading lasting 5 or more minutes).
▶ 4. *Contractions*—every 15–30 min.
   a. Place fingertips over fundus, use gentle pressure; contraction felt as hardening or tensing.
   b. Time: frequency and duration.
   c. Intensity/strength at acme:
      (1) Weak—easily indent fundus with fingers.
      (2) Moderate—some tension felt, fundus indents slightly with finger pressure.
      (3) Strong—unable to indent fundus.
5. *Maternal response to labor*—assess for effective coping, cooperation, and using effective breathing techniques.
6. *Maternal vital signs*—between contractions.
   a. Response to pain or use of special breathing techniques alters pulse and respirations.

Maternal-Infant

Pattern	Description	Nursing Intervention

Early Decelerations

No intervention required.
Continue observation.
Sterile vaginal examination (SVE) to check for dilation, station.

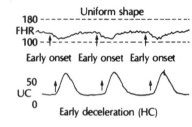

1. FHR begins to slow with the onset of the uterine contraction (UC) and returns to baseline when contraction is over.
2. Fetal head compression occurs.
3. Vagal nerve stimulation.
4. Transient slowing of FHR.

A

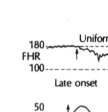

Head compression
(HC)

Late Decelerations

Change maternal position.
Turn off Pitocin; increase rate of maintenance IV.
Begin oxygen by face mask
Notify physician.
Check blood pressure and pulse rate.
Possible candidate for cesarean birth.

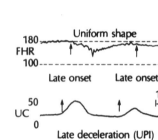

1. FHR begins to fall at height of the UC and returns to baseline after contraction has ceased.
2. FHR usually remains within normal range.
3. Indicates some degree of uteroplacental insufficiency.
4. Baseline variability.

B

Compression of vessels

Uteroplacental insufficiency
(UPI)

Variable Decelerations

Change maternal position to alleviate cord pressure.
Turn off Pitocin; increase rate of maintenance IV.
Begin oxygen by face mask.
Notify physician.
Check blood pressure and pulse rate.
Possible candidate for cesarean birth.
Possible candidate for amnio infusion.

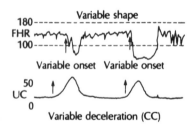

1. Slowing of FHR either with a contraction or in between contractions. Unrelated pattern of FHR and uterine contraction.
2. Pattern may be U shaped or V shaped. Transitory acceleration may precede or follow the deceleration.
3. FHR may fall below 100 beats/min; then returns immediately to baseline.
4. Usually indicates cord compression.

C

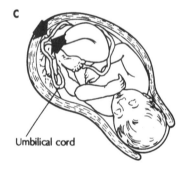

Umbilical cord

**Umbilical cord compression
(CC)**

FIGURE 4.10   Fetal heart rate (FHR) decelerations and nursing interventions.

b. B/P, P, RR—if normotensive: on admission, and then every hour and prn; after regional anesthesia: every 30 min (every 5 min first 20 min).

c. Temp—if within normal range: on admission, and then every 4 hr and prn. Every 2 hr after rupture of membranes.

d. Before and after analgesia/anesthesia.

e. After rupture of membranes (see **Amniotic fluid embolism, p. 208**).

7. Character and amount of *bloody show.*

8. *Bladder* status: encourage voiding every 1–2 hr, monitor output.

a. Determine bladder distention—palpate just above symphysis (full bladder may impede labor progress or result in trauma to bladder).

b. Admission urinalysis—check for protein and glucose.

9. Signs of deviations from normal patterns.

10. *Status of membranes:*

a. Intact.

b. Ruptured (Nitrazine paper turns blue on contact with alkaline amniotic fluid). Fluid may be placed on a glass slide to dry; a fernlike crystallization of sodium chloride will appear. Note, record, and report:

(1) Time—danger of *infection* if ruptured more than 24 hr.

(2) FHR stat and 10 min later—to check for *prolapsed cord.*

(3) Character and color of fluid (see **11.b.** and **c.**).

11. Amniotic fluid.

a. Amount—polyhydramnios (>2000 mL)—associated with *congenital anomalies/ poorly controlled diabetes.*

b. Character—thick consistency or odor associated with *infection.*

c. Color—normally clear with white specks.

(1) Yellow—presence of bilirubin; *Rh or ABO incompatibility.*

(2) Green or meconium stained; if fetus in vertex position, indicates recent *fetal hypoxia* secondary to respiratory distress in fetus.

(3) Port wine—may indicate *abruptio placentae.*

12. *Labor progress:*

a. Effacement.

b. Dilatation.

c. Station.

d. Bulging membranes.

e. Molding of fetal head.

13. *Perineum*—observe for bulging.

◆ **B. Analysis/nursing diagnosis:**

1. *Anxiety, fear* related to uncertain outcome, pain.

2. *Ineffective individual coping* related to lack of preparation for childbirth or poor support from coach.

3. *Altered nutrition: less than body requirements* related to physiological stress of labor.

4. *Altered urinary elimination* related to pressure of presenting part.

5. *Altered thought processes* related to sleep deprivation, transition, analgesia.

6. *Fluid volume deficit* related to anemia, excessive blood loss.

7. *Impaired (fetal) gas exchange* related to impaired placental perfusion.

◆ **C. Nursing care plan/implementation:**

1. Goal: *comfort measures.*

a. Maintain hydration of oral mucosa. Encourage sucking on cool washcloth, ice chips, lollipops, clear liquids (if ordered).

b. Reduce dryness of lips. Apply lip balm.

c. Relieve backache. Apply sacral counterpressure (particularly with occiput posterior [OP] presentation).

d. Encourage significant other to participate.

e. Encourage ambulation when presenting part engaged.

2. Goal: *management of physical needs.*

a. Encourage frequent voiding to prevent full bladder from impeding oncoming head.

b. Encourage ambulation throughout labor; *lateral Sims' position with head elevated to:*

(1) Encourage relaxation.

(2) Allow gravity to assist in anterior rotation of fetal head.

(3) Prevent compression of inferior vena cava and descending aorta *(supine hypotensive syndrome).*

(4) Promote placental perfusion.

c. Perineal prep, if ordered to promote cleanliness.

d. Fleet's enema, if ordered—to stimulate peristalsis, evacuate lower bowel. *Note:* **contraindicated** if:

(1) Cervical dilation (4 cm or more) with unengaged head—due to possibility of cord prolapse.

(2) Fetal malpresentation/malposition—due to possible fetal distress.

(3) Preterm labor—may stimulate contractions.

(4) Painless vaginal bleeding—due to possible placenta previa.

3. Goal: *management of psychosocial needs. Emotional support:*

a. Encourage verbalization of feelings, fears, concerns.

b. Explain all procedures.

c. Reinforce self-concept ("You're doing well!").

4. Goal: *management of discomfort.*

a. Analgesia or anesthesia—may be required or desired—to facilitate safe, comfortable birth.

b. Support/enhance/teach childbirth techniques.

▶ (1) Reinforce appropriate *breathing techniques* for current labor status.

    (a) If woman is **hyperventilating,** to increase Paco$_2$, minimize fetal acidosis, and relieve symptoms of vertigo and syncope, suggest:

        (i) Breathe into paper bag.

        (ii) Breathe into cupped hands.

    (b) Demonstrate appropriate breathing for several contractions—to reestablish rate and rhythm.

5. Goal: *sustain motivation.*

    a. Offer support, encouragement, and praise, as appropriate.

    b. Keep informed of status and progress.

    c. Reassure that irritability is normal.

    d. Serve as surrogate coach when necessary (if no partner, before partner arrives, while partner changes clothes, during needed breaks); assist with effleurage, breathing, focusing.

    e. Discourage bearing-down efforts by pant-blow until complete (10 cm) dilation to avoid cervical edema/laceration.

    f. Facilitate informed decision making regarding medication for relaxation or pain relief.

    g. Minimize distractions: quiet, relaxed environment; privacy.

◆ **D. Evaluation/outcome criteria:**

1. Woman manages own labor discomfort effectively.

2. Woman maintains control over own behavior.

3. Woman successfully completes first stage of labor without incident.

IV. Nursing actions during second stage of labor

◆ **A. Assessment:**

1. Maternal (or couple's) response to labor.

▶ 2. FHR—continuous electronic monitoring, or after each contraction with fetoscope, Doppler.

3. Vital signs.

4. Time elapsed—average: 2 min–1 hr; prolonged second stage increases risk of: fetal distress, maternal exhaustion, psychological stress, intrauterine infection.

5. Contraction pattern—average every $1\frac{1}{2}$–3 min, lasting 60–90 sec.

6. Vaginal discharge—increases.

7. Nausea, vomiting, disorientation, tremors, amnesia between contractions, panic.

8. Response to regional anesthesia, if administered.

    a. Signs of hypotension—reduces placental perfusion, increases risk of fetal hypoxia.

    b. Effect on contractions—note and report any slowing of labor progress.

9. Efforts to bear down—increase expulsive effects of uterine contractions.

10. Perineal bulging with contractions—fetal head distends perineum, crowns; head born by extension.

◆ **B. Analysis/nursing diagnosis:**

1. *Pain* related to strong uterine contractions, pressure of fetal descent, stretching of perineum.

2. *High risk for injury:*

    a. Infection related to ruptured membranes, repeated vaginal examinations.

    b. Laceration related to pressure of fetal head exceeding perineal elasticity.

3. *Impaired skin integrity* related to laceration, episiotomy.

4. *Fluid volume deficit* related to hypotension secondary to regional anesthesia.

5. *Anxiety* related to imminent birth of fetus.

6. *Ineffective individual coping* related to prolonged sensory stimulation (contractions) and anxiety.

7. *Altered urinary elimination* related to anesthesia and contractions, descent of fetal head.

8. *Sleep pattern disturbance.*

◆ **C. Nursing care plan/implementation:**

1. Goal: *emotional support.*

    a. To sustain motivation/control:

        (1) Never leave mother and significant other alone during second stage.

        (2) Keep informed of progress.

▶   (3) Direct bearing-down efforts (pushing) without holding breath* while pushing. Encourage pushing "out through vagina" and encourage mother to touch crowning head; position mirror so woman can see perineal bulging with effective efforts; minimize distractions.

    b. To allay significant other's anxiety: reassure regarding mother's behavior if she is not anesthetized.

    c. Support family choices.

2. Goal: *safeguard status.*

    a. Precautions when putting legs in stirrups:

        (1) If varicosities, **do not put legs in stirrups.**

        (2) *Avoid* pressure to popliteal veins; pad stirrups.

        (3) Ensure proper, even alignment by adjusting stirrups.

        (4) Move legs simultaneously into or out of stirrups—to *avoid* nerve, ligament, and muscle strain.

        (5) Provide proper support to woman not using stirrups. Do **not** hold legs (can cause back injury).

    b. Support woman in whatever position selected for birth (e.g., side-lying position).

▶   c. Cleanse perineum, thighs as ordered.

---

*The woman must be discouraged from using the **Valsalva maneuver** (holding one's breath and tightening abdominal muscles) for pushing during the second stage. This activity increases intrathoracic pressure, reduces venous return, and increases venous pressure. Cardiac output and blood pressure increase, and pulse slows temporarily. During the Valsalva maneuver, fetal hypoxia may occur. The process is reversed when the woman takes a breath.

3. Goal: *maintain a comfortable environment.*
   a. Free of unnecessary noise, light.
   b. Comfortable temperature (warm).
4. *Medical management:*
   a. Episiotomy may be performed to facilitate birth.
   b. Forceps may be applied to exert traction and expedite birth.
   c. Vacuum extraction also used to assist birth.
5. Birthing room birth with alternative positions (squat).

D. Evaluation/outcome criteria:
1. Cooperative, actively participates in birth; maintains control over own behavior.
2. Successful, uncomplicated birth of viable infant.
3. All assessment findings within normal limits (vital signs, emotional status, response to birth).
4. Presence of significant other.

V. Nursing actions during third stage of labor

A. Assessment:
1. Time elapsed—average: 5 min; prolonged third stage (greater than 25 min) may indicate complications (placenta accreta).
2. Signs of *placental separation:*
   a. Increase in bleeding from the vagina.
   b. Cord lengthens.
   c. Uterus rises in abdomen, assumes globular shape.
3. Assess mother's level of consciousness.
4. Examine placenta for intactness and number of vessels in umbilical cord (normal: three. *Note:* two vessels only—associated with increased incidence of congenital anomalies); condition of placenta for calcification, infarcts, etc.

B. Analysis/nursing diagnosis:
1. *Family coping: potential for growth* related to bonding, beginning achievement of developmental tasks.
2. *Fluid volume deficit* related to blood loss during third stage.

C. Nursing care plan/implementation:
1. Goal: *prevent uterine atony.* Administer oxytocin, as ordered.
2. Goal: *facilitate parent-child bonding.*
   a. While protecting neonate from cold stress, encourage parents to see, hold, touch neonate.
   b. Comment about neonate's individuality, characteristics, and behaviors.
   c. After neonate is assessed for congenital anomalies (e.g., cleft palate, esophageal atresia), encourage breastfeeding, if desired.
3. Goal: *health teaching.*
   a. Describe, discuss common neonatal behavior in transitional period (periods of reactivity, sleep, hyperactivity).
   b. Demonstrate removal of mucus by aspiration with bulb syringe.
   c. Demonstrate ways of facilitating breastfeeding.

D. Evaluation/outcome criteria:
1. Woman has a successful, uneventful completion of labor.

   a. Minimal blood loss.
   b. Vital signs within normal limits.
   c. Fundus well contracted at level of umbilicus.
2. Parents express satisfaction with outcome, demonstrate infant attachment.

VI. Nursing actions during the fourth stage of labor—1–2 hr postpartum.

A. Assessment—every 15 min four times; then, every 30 min two times—or until stable—to monitor response to physiological stress of labor/birth.
1. Vital signs:
   a. *Temperature* taken once; if elevated, requires follow-up—may indicate infection, dehydration, excessive blood loss. Note, record, report temperature of 100.4°F (38°C).
   b. *Blood pressure*—every 15 min × 4.
     (1) Returns to prelabor level—due to loss of placental circulation and increased circulating blood volume.
     (2) Elevation may be in response to use of oxytocic drugs or preeclampsia (first 48 hr).
     (3) Lowered blood pressure—may reflect significant blood loss during labor/ birth, or occult bleeding.
   c. Pulse—every 15 min × 4.
     (1) Physiological bradycardia—due to normal vagal response.
     (2) Tachycardia—may indicate excessive blood loss during labor/birth, dehydration, exhaustion, maternal fever, or occult bleeding.
2. Location and tone of fundus—every 15 min × 4 to ensure continuing contraction; prevent blood loss due to uterine relaxation.
   a. Fundus—firm; at or slightly lower than the umbilicus; in midline.
   b. May be displaced by distended bladder—due to normal diuresis; common cause of bleeding in immediate postpartum, uterine atony.
3. Character and amount of vaginal flow.
   a. Moderate lochia rubra.
   b. Excessive loss: if perineal pad saturated in 15 min, or blood pools under buttocks.
   c. Bright red bleeding may indicate cervical or vaginal laceration.
4. Perineum.
   a. Edema.
   b. Bruising—due to trauma.
   c. Distention/hematoma, rectal pain.
5. Bladder fullness/voiding—to prevent distention.
6. Rate of IV, if present; response to added medication, if any.
7. Intake and output—to evaluate hydration.
8. Recovery from analgesia/anesthesia.
9. Energy level.
10. Verbal, nonverbal interaction between woman and significant other.
   a. Dialogue.

Maternal-Infant

b. Posture.
c. Facial expressions.
d. Touching.

11. Interactions between parent(s) and newborn; signs of bonding (culturally appropriate).
    a. Eye contact with newborn.
    b. Calls by name.
    c. Explores with fingertips, strokes, cuddles.

12. Signs of **postpartal emergencies**:
    a. Uterine atony, hemorrhage.
    b. Vaginal hematoma.

◆ **B. Analysis/nursing diagnosis:**
1. *Fluid volume deficit* related to excessive intrapartal blood loss, dehydration.
2. *Altered urinary elimination* related to intrapartal bladder trauma, dehydration, blood loss.
3. *Impaired skin integrity* related to episiotomy, lacerations, cesarean birth.
4. *Altered family processes* related to role change.
5. *Altered parenting* related to interruption in bonding secondary to:
    a. Compromised maternal status.
    b. Compromised neonatal status.
6. *Knowledge deficit* related to self-care procedures, infant care.
7. *Fatigue* related to sleep disturbances and anxiety.
8. *Anxiety* regarding status of self and infant.
9. *Altered nutrition, less than body requirements,* related to decreased food and fluid intake during labor.

◆ **C. Nursing care plan/implementation:**
1. Goal: *comfort measures.*
    a. Position, pad change.
  ▶ b. Perineal care—to promote healing; to reduce possibility of infection.
    c. Ice pack to perineum; as ordered—to reduce edema, discomfort, and pain related to hemorrhoids.
2. Goal: *nutrition/hydration.* Offer fluids, foods as tolerated.
3. Goal: *urinary elimination.*
    a. Encourage voiding—to avoid bladder distention.
    b. Record: time, amount, character.
    c. Anticipatory guidance related to nocturnal diuresis and increased output.
4. Goal: *promote bonding.*
    a. Provide privacy, quiet; encourage sustained contact with newborn.

b. Encourage: touching, holding baby; breastfeeding (also promotes involution).
5. Goal: *health teaching.*
    a. Perineal care—front to back, labia closed (after *each* void/bowel movement).
    b. Handwashing—before and after each pad change; after voiding, defecating; before and after baby care.
    c. Signs to report:
       (1) Uterine cramping/ ↑ pain.
       (2) Increased vaginal bleeding, passage of large clots.
       (3) Nausea, dizziness.

◆ **D. Evaluation/outcome criteria:**
1. Expresses comfort, satisfaction in fourth stage.
2. Vital signs stable, fundus contracted, moderate lochia rubra, perineum undistended.
3. Tolerates food and fluids well.
4. Voids an adequate amount.
5. Demonstrates culturally appropriate contact with infant.
6. Verbalizes abnormal signs to report to physician.
7. Returns demonstration of appropriate perineal care.
8. Ambulates without pain, dizziness, numbness of legs.

VII. Nursing management of the newborn immediately after birth

◆ **A. Assessment:**
1. Mucus in nasophyarynx, oropharynx.
2. *Apgar score:* note and record—at 1 and 5 min of age (**Table 4.12**).
    a. Score of 7–10: *good* condition.
    b. Score of 4–6: *fair* condition; assess for CNS depression.
    c. Score of 0–3: *poor* condition; requires immediate intervention. *Asphyxia neonatorum*—fails to breathe spontaneously within 30–60 sec after birth; HR <100.
3. Number of vessels in umbilical stump.
4. Passage of meconium stool, urine.
5. General physical appearance/status.
    a. Signs of respiratory distress (nasal flaring, grunting, sternal retraction, cyanosis, tachypnea).
    b. Skin condition (meconium-stained, cyanosis, jaundice, lesions).
    c. Cry—presence, pitch, quality.

TABLE 4.12	**Apgar Score**		
Sign	**0**	**1**	**2**
Heart rate	Absent	<100	>100
Respiratory effort	Absent	Slow and irregular	Good and strong, loud crying
Activity: muscle tone	Flaccid	Some flexion or extremities	Active motions, general flexion
Reflex irritability	No response to stimuli	Weak cry or grimace	Cry: vigorous
Appearance: color	Blue, pale	Body pink, extremities blue	Completely pink

d. Signs of birth trauma (lacerations, dislocations, fractures).

e. Symmetry (absent parts, extra digits, gross malformations, ears, palm creases, sacral dimples).

f. Moulding, caput succedaneum, cephalohematoma.

g. Assess gestational age.

6. Identify high-risk infant.

◆ **B. Analysis/nursing diagnosis:**

1. *Ineffective airway clearance* related to excessive nasopharyngeal mucus.

2. *Ineffective breathing pattern* related to CNS depression secondary to intrauterine hypoxia narcosis, prematurity, and lack of pulmonary surfactant.

3. *Impaired gas exchange* related to respiratory distress.

4. *Fluid volume deficit* related to birth trauma; hemolytic jaundice.

5. *Impaired skin integrity* related to cord stump.

6. *High risk for injury* (biochemical, metabolic) related to impaired thermoregulation.

7. *Ineffective thermoregulation* related to environmental conditions/prematurity.

◆ **C. Nursing care plan/implementation:**

1. Goal: *ensure patent airway.*

▶ a. Suction mouth first, then nose; when stimulated, sensitive receptors around entrance to nares initiate gasp, causing aspiration of mucus present in mouth.

▶ b. Suction with bulb syringe.

(1) If deeper suctioning necessary, use DeLee mucus trap attached to suction. Oral use of DeLee is contraindicated due to risk of contact with baby's secretions (new Delee now available that has no such risk).

(2) *Avoid* prolonged, vigorous suctioning.

(a) Reduces oxygenation.

(b) May traumatize tissue, cause edema, bleeding, laryngospasm, and cardiac arrhythmia.

◪ c. Assist gravity drainage of fluids. *Position:* head dependent (Trendelenburg) and side-lying position.

2. Goal: *maintain body temperature*—to conserve energy, preserve store of brown fat, decrease oxygen needs; prevent acidosis. Prevent chilling:

a. Minimize exposure; dry quickly.

b. Keep warm; apply hat.

c. Take temperature hourly until stable.

3. Goal: *identify infant:*

a. Apply Identiband.

b. Take infant's footprints and maternal fingerprints.

4. Goal: *prevent eye infection* (gonorrheal and *chlamydial ophthalmia neonatorum*).

▬● Within 1 hr of birth apply antibiotic ointment in each eye.

5. Goal: *facilitate prompt identification/vigilance for potential neonatal complications.*

a. Record significant data from mother's chart:

(1) History of: pregnancy, diabetes, hypertension, current drug abuse, excessive caffeine, medications, alcohol, malnutrition.

(2) Course of labor, evidence of fetal distress, medications received in labor.

(3) Birth history of anesthesia.

(4) Apgar; resuscitative efforts.

6. Goal: *facilitate prompt identification/intervention in hemolytic problems of the newborn.*

 a. Collect and send cord blood for appropriate tests:

(1) Blood type and Rh factor.

(2) Coombs' test.

▬● b. Give vitamin K to facilitate clotting.

◆ **D. Evaluation/outcome criteria:** successful transition to extrauterine life.

1. Status satisfactory; all assessment findings within normal limits.

2. Responsive in bonding process with parents.

VIII. Nurse-attended emergency birth (precipitate birth). When woman presents without prenatal care (to emergency department), may represent drug abuse. **IMMINENT BIRTH**

◆ **A. Assessment:** identify signs of *imminent birth:*

1. Strong contractions.

2. Bearing-down efforts.

3. Perineal bulging; crowning.

4. Mother states, "It's coming."

◆ **B. Analysis/nursing diagnosis:**

1. *Pain* related to:

a. Strong, sustained contractions.

b. Descent of fetal head.

c. Stretching of perineum.

2. *Anxiety/fear* related to imminent birth.

3. *Ineffective individual coping* related to circumstances surrounding birth; anxiety, fear for self and infant.

4. *Injury* (mother) related to lacerations (vaginal, perineal).

5. *Fluid volume deficit* related to:

a. Lacerations.

b. Uterine atony.

c. Retained placental fragments.

6. *Impaired gas exchange* (infant) related to intact membranes after birth.

7. *Risk for injury* (infant) related to:

a. Precipitate birth.

b. Trauma.

c. Hypoxia.

◆ **C. Nursing care plan/implementation:**

1. Goal: *reduce anxiety/fear*—reassure mother.

2. Goal: *delay birth,* as possible.

a. Discourage bearing-down efforts.

b. Encourage panting.

◪ c. *Side-lying position* to slow descent and allow for more controlled birth.

Maternal-Infant

▶ 3. Goal: *prevent infection.*
    a. Provide clean field for birth.
    b. *Avoid* touching birth canal without gloved hands.
    c. Support perineum (and advancing head) with sterile (or clean) towel.

▶ 4. Goal: *prevent, or minimize, infant hypoxia and perineal lacerations.*
    a. If membranes intact as head emerges, tear at neck to facilitate first breath.
    b. Feel for cord around neck (if present, and if possible, slip cord over head; if tight, *and* sterile equipment at hand, clamp cord in two places, cut between clamps, unwrap cord). If unsterile environment, keep fetus and placenta attached—do not cut cord.

▶ 5. Goal: *facilitate/assist birth.*
    a. Hold head in both hands.
    b. Apply gentle downward pressure to bring anterior shoulder under pubic symphysis.
    c. Gently lift head to ease birth of posterior shoulder.
    d. Support infant as body slips free of mother's body.

▶ 6. Goal: *facilitate drainage of mucus and fluid →* patent airway.
    ▰ a. Hold infant in head-dependent *position.*
    b. Clear mucus with bulb syringe (if available), or use fingertip, wipe with towel.

▶ 7. Goal: *prevent placental transfusion*—hold infant level with placenta until cord stops pulsating; clamp and cut.

▶ 8. Goal: *prevent chilling.*
    a. Wrap infant in towel or other clean material.
    ▰ b. Place infant on *side, head dependent,* on mother's abdomen.
    c. Dry head, cover with cap or material.

9. Goal: *stimulate respiration.* If neonate *fails to breathe* spontaneously:
    a. Maintain body temperature—dry and cover.
    ▶ b. Clear airway
       ▰ (1) *Position:* head *down.*
       (2) Turn head to *side.*
    c. Stimulate.
       (1) Rub back gently.
       (2) Flick soles of feet.
    d. If no response to stimulation:
       ▰ (1) Slightly extend neck to "sniffing" *position* (head tilt–chin lift method).
       (2) Place mouth over newborn's nose and mouth and exhale air in cheeks, saying "ho" (prevents excessive pressure).

▶ 10. Goal: begin *cardiopulmonary resuscitation (CPR)* if no heart rate:
    a. Place infant on firm, flat surface.
    b. With two fingers on sternum depress $1/2$–$3/4$ inch 100 times/min.
    c. Assist ventilation on upstroke of every fifth compression (5:1 ratio).
    d. Go immediately to emergency department.

11. Goal: *maintain infant's body temperature*
    a. Wrap placenta with baby, if cord intact.
    b. Place infant in mother's arms.

PLACENTAL SEPARATION

◆ **A. Assessment**—*third stage:* identify signs of *placental separation.*

◆ **B. Nursing care plan/implementation:**
    1. Goal: *avoid/minimize potential for complications* (everted uterus, tearing of placenta with fragments remaining, separation of cord from placenta).
       a. *Avoid* traction (pulling) on cord.
       b. *Avoid* vigorous fundal massage.
       c. Discourage maternal bearing-down efforts unless placenta visible at introitus.
       d. With fundus well contracted, and placenta visible at introitus, encourage mother to bear down to expel placenta.
    2. Goal: *prevent maternal hemorrhage* (uterine atony).
       a. Encourage breastfeeding, or stimulate nipple.
       b. Gently massage fundus, support lower part of uterus, and express clots when uterus is contracted.
       c. Encourage voiding if bladder is full.
       d. Get to a medical facility.
    3. Goal: *encourage bonding/stimulate uterine contractions.* Encourage breastfeeding.
    4. Goal: *legal accountability* as birth attendant. Record date, time, birth events, maternal and fetal status.

◆ **C. Evaluation/outcome criteria:**
    1. Experiences normal spontaneous birth of viable infant over intact perineum.
    2. Uncomplicated fourth stage—status satisfactory for both mother and infant.
    3. Expresses satisfaction in management and result.

IX. Alterations affecting protective function
    A. Induction of labor—deliberate initiation of uterine contractions.
       1. Indications for:
          a. History of rapid or silent labors, precipitate birth.
          b. Woman resides some distance from hospital (controversial).
          c. Coexisting medical disorders:
             (1) Uncontrolled diabetes.
             (2) Progressive preeclampsia.
             (3) Severe renal disease.
             (4) Cardiac disease.
          d. PROM—spontaneous rupture of membranes before onset of labor and less than 37 wk from last menstrual period.
          Hazards:
             (1) Maternal—intrauterine infection (chorioamnionitis, endometritis).
             (2) Fetal—sepsis; prolapsed cord.
          e. Rh or ABO incompatibility, fetal hemolytic disease.
          f. Congenital anomaly (e.g., anencephaly).

g. Postterm pregnancy with nonreactive non-stress test (NST), or oligohydramnios.

h. Intrauterine fetal demise.

2. *Criteria for induction:*

a. Absence of CPD, malpresentation, or malposition.

b. Engaged vertex of single gestation.

c. Nearing, or at term.

d. Fetal lung maturity.

(1) Survival rate—better at 32 wk or more.

(2) *Lecithin/sphingomyelin* ratio greater than 2:1.

(3) Mother who is diabetic—PG is present in amniotic fluid.

e. "Ripe" cervix—softening, partially effaced, or ready for effacement/dilation (if not already present). *Note:* Intravaginal or paracervical application of prostaglandin gel, or misoprostol may be used to prepare cervix for labor.

3. *Methods:*

a. Amniotomy—artificial rupture of membranes with fetal head engaged and dilation of cervix.

b. Intravenous oxytocin infusion.

4. *Potential complications:*

a. *Amniotomy*—irrevocably committed to birth. **Hazards:**

(1) Prolapsed cord.

(2) Infection.

b. *IV oxytocin infusion:*

(1) Overstimulation of uterus.

(2) Decreased placental perfusion/fetal distress, neonatal jaundice.

(3) Precipitate labor and birth.

(4) Cervical/perineal lacerations.

(5) Uterine rupture.

(6) Postpartum hemorrhage.

(7) Water intoxication—if large doses given in D/W over prolonged period (antidiuretic effect increases water reabsorption).

(8) Hypertensive crisis.

BEFORE INDUCTION

5. **Assessment**—*before induction:*

a. Estimate of gestation (EDD, fundal height, cervical status).

b. *Bishop's score:* evaluation of cervical inducibility.

c. General health status:

(1) Weight, vital signs, FHR, edema.

(2) Status of membranes.

(3) Vaginal bleeding.

(4) Coexisting disorders.

d. History of previous labors, if any.

e. Emotional status.

f. Knowledge/understanding of anticipated procedures:

(1) Amniotomy (artificial rupture of membranes).

(2) Cervical ripening (prostaglandin gel, Cervidil, Cytotec).

(3) IV oxytocin infusion.

(4) Fetal monitoring

g. Preparation for childbirth (Lamaze, etc.); coping strategies. Identify support person.

6. **Analysis/nursing diagnosis:**

a. *Knowledge deficit* related to process of induction.

b. *Anxiety/fear* related to need for induction of labor.

c. *Ineffective individual coping* related to psychological stress.

d. *Pain* related to uterine contractions.

7. **Nursing care plan/implementation:**

a. Goal: *health teaching.*

(1) Explain rationale for procedures:

(a) *Amniotomy.*

(i) Induces labor.

(ii) Relieves uterine overdistention.

(iii) Increases efficiency of contractions, shortening labor.

(b) *Oxytocin infusion.*

(i) Induces labor.

(ii) Stimulates uterine contractions.

(c) *Internal fetal monitor.*

(i) Provides continuous assessment of uterine response to oxytocin stimulation.

(ii) Provides continuous assessment of fetal response to physiological stress of labor.

(2) *Describe procedure*—to reduce anxiety and increase cooperation.

(3) *Explain advantages/disadvantages*—to ensure "informed consent."

b. Goal: *emotional support*—encourage verbalization of concerns; reassure, as possible.

8. **Evaluation/outcome criterion:** woman verbalizes understanding of process, rationale, procedures, and alternatives.

DURING INDUCTION AND LABOR

9. **Assessment**—*during induction and labor:*

a. *Amniotomy*—same as for spontaneous rupture of membranes:

(1) Observe fluid—note color, amount.

(2) Monitor FHR; assess for fetal distress.

(3) Observe for signs of prolapsed cord.

(4) Assess fetal activity.

(a) *Excessive* activity may indicate distress.

(b) *Absence* of activity may indicate distress or demise.

b. *IV oxytocin infusion:*

(1) Continually assess response to oxytocin stimulation/flow rate; always given by controlled infusion.

(a) Uterine contractions.

(b) Maternal vital signs, FHR.

(2) Identify signs of:

(a) *Deviation* from normal patterns:

(i) Lack of response to increasing flow rate.

(ii) Uterine hyperstimulation (contractions—less than 2 min apart).

(iii) Lack of adequate uterine relaxation between contractions.

(b) *Side effects* of oxytocin: diminished output—potential water intoxication.

(c) **Hazards** to mother or fetus:

(i) Sustained (over 90 sec) or tetanic (strong, spasmlike) contractions—potential abruptio placentae, uterine rupture, fetal hypoxia/anoxia/death.

(ii) *Fetal* arrhythmias, decelerations.

(iii) *Maternal* hypertension—potential for hypertensive crisis, cerebral hemorrhage.

◆ 10. **Nursing care plan/implementation:**

a. Same as for other women in labor.

b. If indications of deviations from normal patterns:

(1) Change maternal position.

▬ (2) Stop oxytocin infusion, maintain IV with Ringer's lactate, etc.

▶ (3) Begin oxygen per mask; up to 8–10 L/min.

(4) Notify physician promptly.

(5) Check maternal blood pressure and pulse rate.

c. Anticipatory guidance: may or may not have strong contractions soon after induction starts.

◆ 11. **Evaluation/outcome criteria:**

a. Demonstrates response to oxytocin stimulation.

(1) Establishes desired contraction pattern, not hyperstimulated.

(2) Progresses through labor—within normal limits:

(a) Normotensive.

(b) Voids in adequate amounts.

(c) No evidence of deviation from normal contraction patterns.

b. No evidence of fetal distress.

c. Experiences normal vaginal birth of viable infant.

B. **Operative obstetrics**—procedures used to prevent trauma/reduce hazard to mother or infant during the birth process.

1. **Episiotomy**—incision of perineum to facilitate infant's birth.

a. Rationale:

(1) Surgical incision reduces possibility of laceration.

(2) Protects infant's head from pressure exerted by resistant perineum.

(3) Shortens second stage of labor.

b. Types:

(1) Midline—chance of extension into anal sphincter greater than with mediolateral.

(2) Mediolateral—healing is more painful than midline.

◆ c. **Assessment:**

 (1) **REEDA:**

(a) **R**edness

(b) **E**dema

(c) **E**cchymosis

(d) **D**ischarge

(e) **A**pproximation (suture line intact, separated)

(2) Healing.

(3) Bruised; hematoma.

(4) Tenderness; pain. *Note:* Evaluate complaints of pain carefully. If intense, and unrelieved by usual measures, report promptly. May indicate vulvar, paravaginal, or ischiorectal abscess or hematoma.

◆ d. **Analysis/nursing diagnosis:**

(1) *Pain* related to labor process.

(2) *Impaired skin integrity* related to surgical incision.

(3) *Fluid volume deficit* related to hematoma.

(4) *Sexual dysfunction* related to discomfort.

◆ e. **Nursing care plan/implementation:**

(1) Goal: *prevent/reduce edema, promote comfort and healing.*

(a) Place covered ice pack during immediate postpartum

▬ (b) Administer analgesics, topical sprays, ointments, witch hazel pads, hydrocortisone.

(c) Encourage use of sitz bath or rubber ring.

(d) Encourage Kegel exercises.

(e) Do *health teaching:*

(i) Instruct in tightening gluteal muscles before sitting.

(ii) Instruct to *avoid* sitting on one hip.

(2) Goal: *minimize potential for infection.*

(a) Teach/provide perineal care during fourth stage of labor.

(b) *Health teaching:* instruct in self-perineal care after voiding, defecation, and with each pad change.

◆ f. **Evaluation/outcome criteria:**

(1) Woman's incision heals by primary intention.

(2) Woman demonstrates appropriate self-perineal care.

(3) Woman evidences no signs of hematoma, infection, or separation of suture line.

(4) Woman experiences minimal discomfort.

2. **Forceps-assisted birth**—use of instruments to assist birth of infant.

a. Indications:

(1) Fetal distress.

(2) Maternal need:

(a) Exhaustion.

(b) Coexisting disease, such as cardiac disorder.

(c) Poor progress in second stage.

(d) Persistent fetal OT or OP position.

b. *Criteria* for forceps application:

(1) Engaged fetal head.

(2) Ruptured membranes.

(3) Full dilatation.

(4) Absence of CPD.

(5) Some anesthesia has been given; usually, episiotomy has been performed.

(6) Empty bladder.

c. *Types:*

(1) Low—outlet forceps.

(2) Mid—applied after head is engaged (rarely used).

(3) Pipers—applied to after-coming head in selected breech births (rarely done).

d. *Potential complications:*

(1) *Maternal:*

(a) Lacerations of birth canal, rectum, bladder.

(b) Uterine rupture/hemorrhage.

(2) *Neonatal:*

(a) Cephalohematoma.

(b) Skull fracture.

(c) Intracranial hemorrhage, brain damage.

(d) Facial paralysis.

(e) Direct tissue trauma (abrasions, ecchymosis).

(f) Umbilical cord compression.

◆ e. **Assessment:**

▶ (1) FHR immediately before—and after—forceps application (forceps blade may compress umbilical cord).

(2) Observe mother/newborn for injury or signs of complications.

◆ f. **Analysis/nursing diagnosis:**

(1) *Self-esteem disturbance* related to inability to give birth without surgical assistance.

(2) *Anxiety/fear* related to infant's appearance (forceps marks) or awareness of potential complications.

◆ g. **Nursing care plan/implementation:**

(1) Goal: *minimize feelings of failure due to inability to give birth "naturally."*

(a) Explain, discuss reasons/indications for forceps-assisted birth.

(b) Emphasize no maternal control over circumstances.

(2) Goal: *reduce parental anxiety, maternal guilt over infant bruising/forceps marks.* Explain condition is temporary and has no lasting effects on child's appearance.

◆ h. **Evaluation/outcome criteria:**

(1) Woman verbalizes understanding of reasons for forceps-assisted birth.

(2) Woman evidences no interruption in bonding with infant.

(3) Woman experiences uncomplicated recovery.

3. Vacuum extraction (soft plastic cup with vacuum from a handheld suction pump). Used to assist in rotation or delivery of the fetal head.

a. Risks may include caput succedaneum and cephalohematoma.

b. Causes neonatal jaundice, IVH can result in death.

4. **Cesarean birth**—incision through abdominal wall and uterus to give birth.

a. Indications for *elective* cesarean birth:

(1) Known CPD.

(2) Previous uterine surgery (e.g., myomectomy), repeated cesarean births (depends on type of incision done).

(3) Active maternal genital herpes II infection; human papilloma virus (HPV).

(4) Breech presentation. *Note:* To reduce infant morbidity/mortality, elective cesarean birth is common method of choice.

(5) Neoplasms of cervix, uterus, or birth canal.

(6) Maternal diabetes with placental aging; fetal macrosomia (CPD); >4050 g.

b. *Criteria* for elective cesarean birth:

L/S ratio greater than 2:1—indicates presence of pulmonary surfactant; less risk of respiratory distress syndrome.

c. *Indications for emergency cesarean birth:*

(1) **Fetal:**

(a) *Fetal distress:* prolapsed cord, repetitive late decelerations, prolonged bradycardia.

(b) *Fetal jeopardy:* Rh or ABO incompatibility.

(c) *Fetal malposition*/malpresentation.

(2) **Maternal:**

(a) *Uterine* dysfunction; rupture.

(b) *Placental* disorders:

(i) Placenta previa.

(ii) Abruptio placentae, with Couvelaire uterus.

(c) Severe maternal preeclampsia/eclampsia.

(d) Fetopelvic disproportion.

(e) Sudden maternal death.

(f) Carcinoma.

(g) Failed induction.

d. *Types:*

(1) Low segment—method of choice:

(a) Transverse incision through abdominal wall and lower uterine segment.

(b) Transverse incision through abdominal wall, with vertical incision of lower uterine segment.

(c) Advantages—fewer complications:

(i) Less blood loss.

Maternal-Infant

(ii) More comfortable convalescence.
(iii) Less adhesion formation.
(iv) Lower risk of uterine rupture in subsequent pregnancy/labor and birth.
(v) Cosmetically more acceptable.
(2) Classical—vertical incision through abdominal wall and uterus. May be necessary for anterior placenta previa and transverse lie, <28 weeks' prematurity.
(3) Porro's—hysterotomy followed by hysterectomy. Necessary in presence of:
(a) Hemorrhage from uterine atony.
(b) Placenta accreta/percreta.
(c) Large uterine myomas.
(d) Ruptured uterus.
(e) Cancer of uterus or ovary.
◆ e. **Assessment:**
(1) Maternal physical status.
(a) Vital signs.
(b) Labor status, if any.
(c) Contractions (if any).
(d) Membranes (intact; ruptured).
(e) Bleeding.
(2) Fetal status.
(a) FHR pattern.
(b) Color and amount of amniotic fluid.
(c) Biophysical profile (BPP), if performed.
(3) Maternal emotional status.
(4) Understanding of procedure, indications for, implications.
(5) Other—as for any abdominal surgery (see **Unit 7**).
◆ f. **Analysis/nursing diagnosis:**
(1) *Self-esteem disturbance* related to perceived failure to give birth vaginally.
(2) *Anxiety/fear* related to impending surgery and/or reasons for cesarean birth.
(3) *Ineffective individual coping* related to anxiety and fear for self, infant.
(4) *Fluid volume deficit* related to abdominal surgery or reason for cesarean birth.
(5) *Pain* related to abdominal surgery.
(6) *Constipation* related to decreased bowel activity.
(7) *Altered urinary elimination* related to fluid volume deficit.
◆ g. **Nursing care plan/implementation:**
(1) *Preoperative:*
(a) Goal: *safeguard fetal status.*
(i) Monitor fetal heart rate continually.
(ii) Notify neonatology and neonatal intensive care unit (NICU) of scheduled surgical birth, if suspect complications.
(b) Goal: *health teaching.*
(i) Describe, discuss anticipated anesthesia.

(ii) Explain rationale for preoperative antacids to minimize effects of aspiration: cimetidine, Bicitra, histamine blocker to decrease production of gastric acid. Reglan (metoclopramide), to hasten gastric emptying.
(iii) Describe, explain anticipated procedures—abdominal shave, indwelling catheter, intravenous fluids—to woman and support person.
(c) Other—as for any abdominal surgery.
(d) Prepare for cesarean birth.
(2) *Postoperative:*
(a) Same as for other clients having abdominal surgery (see **Unit 7**).
(b) Same as for other women who are postpartum.
◆ h. **Evaluation/outcome criteria:**
(1) Verbalizes understanding of reasons for cesarean birth.
(2) Successful birth of viable infant.
(3) Evidences no surgical/birth complications.
(4) Evidences no interference with bonding.
(5) Expresses satisfaction with procedure and result.
5. **Trial of labor after cesarean (TOLAC)**
a. Candidates for TOLAC.
(1) Previous low transverse cesarean birth.
(2) Head well-engaged in pelvis (vertex presentation).
(3) Soft, anterior cervix.
(4) Preexisting reason for repeat cesarean birth not apparent.
◆ b. **Assessment:**
(1) Monitor FHR carefully during trial of labor.
(2) Monitor contractions carefully for adequate progress of labor.
(3) Observe mother for signs of complications/uterine rupture.
◆ c. **Analysis/nursing diagnosis:**
(1) *Knowledge deficit* related to trial of labor.
(2) *Fear* related to outcome for fetus.
(3) *Ineffective individual coping* related to labor progress and outcome.

Complications During the Intrapartal Period

I. **General aspects**
   A. **Pathophysiology**—interference with normal processes and patterns of labor/birth result in maternal or fetal jeopardy (e.g., **preterm** labor, **dysfunctional** labor patterns; **prolonged** [over 24 hours] labor; **hemorrhage: uterine rupture**/inversion, **amniotic-fluid embolus**).
   B. **Etiology:**
      1. **Preterm labor**—unknown.
      2. **Dysfunctional labor (dystocia:** see **p. 206**):

a. Physiological response to anxiety/fear/pain—results in release of catecholamines, increasing physical/psychological stress → myometrial dysfunction; painful and ineffectual labor.

b. Iatrogenic factors: premature or excessive analgesia, particularly during latent phase.

c. *Maternal factors:*
   (1) Pelvic contractures.
   (2) Uterine tumors (e.g., myomas, carcinoma).
   (3) Congenital uterine anomalies (e.g., bicornate uterus).
   (4) Pathological contraction ring (*Bandl's* ring).
   (5) Rigid cervix, cervical stenosis/stricture.
   (6) Hypertonic/hypotonic contractions.
   (7) Prolonged rupture of membranes. *Note:* Intrauterine infection may have caused rupture of membranes or may follow rupture.
   (8) Prolonged first or second stage.
   (9) Medical conditions: diabetes, hypertension.

d. *Fetal factors:*
   (1) Macrosomia (LGA).
   (2) Malposition/malpresentation.
   (3) Congenital anomaly (e.g., hydrocephalus, anencephaly).
   (4) Multifetal gestation (e.g., interlocking twins).
   (5) Prolapsed cord.
   (6) Postterm.

e. *Placental factors:*
   (1) Placenta previa.
   (2) Inadequate placental function with contractions.
   (3) Abruptio placentae.
   (4) Placenta accreta.

f. Physical restrictions: when confined to bed, *flat position*, etc.

◆ **C. Assessment:**
1. Antepartal history.
2. Emotional status.
3. Vital signs, FHR.
4. Contraction pattern (frequency, duration, intensity).
5. Vaginal discharge.

◆ **D. Analysis/nursing diagnosis:**
1. *Anxiety/fear* for self and infant related to implications of prolonged or complicated labor/birth.
2. *Pain* related to hypertonic contractions/dysfunctional labor.
3. *Ineffective individual coping* related to physical/psychological stress of complicated labor/birth, lowered pain threshold secondary to fatigue.
4. *High risk for injury* related to prolonged rupture of membranes, infection.
5. *Fluid volume deficit* related to excessive blood loss secondary to placenta previa, abruptio placentae, Couvelaire uterus, DIC.

◆ **E. Nursing care plan/implementation:**
1. Goal: *minimize physical/psychological stress during labor/birth.* Assist woman in coping effectively:
   a. Reinforce relaxation techniques.

b. Support couple's effective coping techniques/mechanisms.

2. Goal: *emotional support.*
   a. Encourage verbalization of anxiety/fear/concerns.
   b. Explain all procedures—to minimize anxiety/fear, encourage cooperation/participation in care.
   c. Provide quiet environment conducive to rest.

3. Goal: *continuous monitoring of maternal/fetal status and progress through labor*—to identify early signs of dysfunctional labor, fetal distress; facilitate prompt, effective treatment of emerging complications.

4. Goal: *minimize effects of complicated labor on mother, fetus.*
   a. *Position* change: lateral Sims'—to reduce compression of inferior vena cava.
   b. Oxygen per mask, as indicated.
   c. Institute interventions appropriate to emerging problems (see specific disorder).

◆ **F. Evaluation/outcome criteria:**
1. Woman has successful birth of viable infant.
2. Maternal/infant status stable, satisfactory.

II. Disorders affecting protective functions. Preterm labor—occurs after 20 weeks of gestation and before beginning of wk 38.

A. Pathophysiology—physiological events of labor (i.e., contractions, spontaneous rupture of membranes, cervical effacement/dilation) occur before completion of normal, term gestation.

B. Etiology—causes may be from maternal, fetal, or placental factors.

C. *Coexisting disorders:*
1. Infections that may cause PROM.
2. PROM of unknown etiology.
3. PIH (preeclampsia/eclampsia).
4. Uterine overdistention.
   a. Polyhydramnios.
   b. Multifetal gestation.
5. Maternal diabetes, renal or cardiovascular disorder, UTI.
6. Severe maternal illness (e.g., pneumonia, acute pyelonephritis).
7. Abnormal placentation.
   a. Placenta previa.
   b. Abruptio placentae.
8. Iatrogenic: miscalculated EDD for repeat cesarean birth (rare).
9. Fetal death.
10. Incompetent cervical os (small percentage).
11. Uterine anomalies (rare).
    a. Intrauterine septum.
    b. Bicornate uterus.
12. Uterine fibroids.
13. Positive fetal fibronectin assay (protein found in fetal tissue, membranes, amniotic fluid, and the decidua) found in cervical/vaginal fluid first half of pregnancy and normally absent through mid to late pregnancy (↑ risk of PTL by 20%).

Maternal-Infant

Maternal-Infant

D. *Prevention:*
1. *Primary*—close obstetric supervision; education in signs/symptoms of labor.
2. *Secondary*—prompt, effective treatment of associated disorders (see **II. C., p. 203**).
3. *Tertiary*—suppression of preterm labor.
   a. Bedrest.
   b. *Position:* side-lying—to promote placental perfusion.
   c. Hydration.
   d. Pharmacological (may require "informed consent"; follow hospital protocol). Beta-adrenergic agents, $MgSO_4$ (recent studies show poor results with $MgSO_4$), Procardia to reduce sensitivity of uterine myometrium to oxytocic and prostaglandin stimulation; increase blood flow to uterus.
   e. May be maintained at home with adequate follow-up and health teaching.

E. **Contraindications for suppression:** Labor is not suppressed in presence of:
1. Placenta previa or abruptio placentae with hemorrhage.
2. Chorioamnionitis.
3. Erythroblastosis fetalis.
4. Severe preeclampsia.
5. Severe diabetes (e.g., "brittle").
6. Increasing placental insufficiency.
7. Progressive cervical dilatation of 4 cm or more.
8. Ruptured membranes (with maternal fever).

F. **Assessment:**
1. Maternal vital signs. Response to medication:
   a. Hypotension.
   b. Tachycardia, arrhythmia.
   c. Dyspnea, chest pain.
   d. Nausea and vomiting.
2. Signs of infection:
   a. Increased temperature.
   b. Tachycardia.
   c. Diaphoresis.
   d. Malaise.
   e. Increased baseline fetal heart rate; ↓ variability
3. Contractions: frequency, duration, strength.
4. Emotional status—signs of denial, guilt, anxiety, exhaustion.
5. Signs of continuing and progressing labor. *Note:* Vaginal examination *only* if indicated by other signs of continuing labor progress:
   a. Effacement.
   b. Dilation.
   c. Station.
6. Status of membranes.
7. Fetal heart rate, activity (continuous monitoring).

G. **Analysis/nursing diagnosis:**
1. *Anxiety/fear* related to possible outcome.
2. *Self-esteem disturbance* related to feelings of guilt, failure.
3. *Impaired physical mobility* related to imposed bedrest.

4. *Knowledge deficit* related to medication side effects
5. *Ineffective individual coping* related to possible outcome.
6. *Impaired gas exchange* related to side effects of medication (circulatory overload; pulmonary edema).
7. *Diversional activity deficit* related to imposed bedrest, decreased environmental stimuli.
8. *Altered urinary elimination* related to bedrest.
9. *Constipation* related to bedrest.

H. **Nursing care plan/implementation:**
1. Goal: *inhibit uterine activity.* Administer medications as ordered—terbutaline, magnesium sulfate, Procardia, Indocin.
2. Goal: *safeguard status.*
   a. Continuous maternal/fetal monitoring.
   b. I&O—to identify early signs of possible circulatory overload.
   c. *Position:* side-lying—to increase placental perfusion, prevent supine hypotension.
   d. Report **promptly** to physician:

   (1) Maternal pulse of 110 or more.
   (2) Diastolic pressure of 60 mm Hg or less.
   (3) Respirations of 24 or more; crackles (rales).
   (4) Complaint of dyspnea.
   (5) Contractions: increasing frequency, strength, duration, or cessation of contractions.
   (6) Intermittent back and thigh pain.
   (7) Rupture of membranes.
   (8) Vaginal bleeding.
   (9) Fetal distress.

3. Goal: *comfort measures.*
   a. Basic hygienic care—bath, mouth care, cold washcloth to face, perineal care.
   b. Back rub, linen change—to promote relaxation.
4. Goal: *emotional support.*
   a. Encourage verbalization of guilt feelings, anxiety, fear, concerns; provide factual information.
   b. Support positive self-concept.
   c. Keep informed of progress.
5. Goal: *provide quiet diversion.* Television, reading materials, handicrafts (may not be able to focus well if on magnesium therapy).
6. Goal: *health teaching*
   a. Explain, discuss proposed management to suppress preterm labor.
   b. Describe, discuss side effects of medication.
   c. Explain rationale for bedrest, position.

I. **If labor continues to progress:**
1. Goal: *facilitate infant survival.*
   a. Administer betamethasone, as ordered, 24–48 hr before birth—to increase/stimulate production of pulmonary surfactant.
   b. Give antibiotic to mother to ↓ chance of neonatal sepsis.
   c. Notify neonatal ICU (NICU)—to increase chances for fetal survival, ensure prompt, expert management of neonate, and provide information and support to parents.

d. Monitor progress of labor to identify signs of impending birth *Note:* May give birth before complete (10 cm) dilation.

e. Consider transfer to high-risk facility.

f. Prepare for birth, or cesarean birth if infant less than 34–36 weeks of gestation.

2. Goal: *emotional support.*

a. Do *not* leave woman (or couple) alone.

b. Encourage verbalization of anxiety, fear, concern.

c. Explain all procedures.

3. Goal: *comfort measures. Note:* Analgesics used conservatively—to prevent depression of fetus/neonate.

4. Goal: *support effective coping techniques.* Encourage support Lamaze (or other) techniques—coach, as necessary; discourage hyperventilation.

5. Goal: *health teaching*—for severe preterm birth.

a. Discuss need for episiotomy, possibility of outlet forceps-assisted birth—to reduce stress on fetal head, or

b. Prepare for cesarean birth—to reduce possibility of fetal intraventricular hemorrhage.

c. Give rationale for avoiding use of medications to reduce contraction pain.

J. Immediate care of neonate:

1. Goal: *safeguard status.*

a. Stabilize environmental temperature—to prevent chilling (isolette or other controlled-temperature bed).

▶ b. Suction, oxygen, as needed; may need intubation.

▬ c. Parenteral fluids, as ordered—to support normal acid-base balance, pH; administer antibiotics, as necessary.

d. Arrange transport to high-risk facility, as necessary.

2. Goal: *continuous monitoring of status.*

▶ a. Electronic monitors—to observe respiratory and cardiac functions.

b. Blood samples—to monitor blood gases, pH, hypoglycemia.

K. Postpartum care: Goal: *emotional support.*

1. Facilitate attachment—photos, if baby transferred or mother unable to visit.

2. If couple, foster sense of mutual experience and closeness.

3. Help her/them maintain a positive self-image.

4. Encourage touching of infant before transport to nursery or high-risk facility; father/partner may accompany infant and report back to mother.

5. Encourage early contact—to facilitate mother's need to ventilate her feelings.

6. Assist parent(s) with grieving process, if necessary.

7. Refer to support group if necessary.

L. *Other*—as for any woman who is postpartum.

◆ **M. Evaluation/outcome criteria:**

1. Woman verbalizes understanding of medical/nursing recommendations and treatments.

2. Woman complies with medical/nursing regimen.

3. Woman experiences no discomfort from side effects of therapy.

4. Woman experiences successful outcome—labor inhibited.

5. Woman carries pregnancy to successful termination.

6. If preterm birth occurs, woman copes effectively with outcome (physiologically compromised neonate, neonatal death).

III. Grief and childbearing experience. The loss of a pregnancy or a newborn, or the birth of a child who is physiologically compromised (preterm, congenital disorder) is a crisis situation. The unexpected outcome can cause the parent(s) to suffer a sense of loss of self-esteem, self-concept, positive body image, feelings of worth (see **p. 225**).

◆ **A. Assessment:**

1. Response to loss of the "fantasy child"/real child.

a. Behavioral—anger, hostility, depression, disinterest in activities of daily living, withdrawal.

b. Biophysical—somatic complaints (stomach pain, malaise, anorexia, nausea).

c. Cognitive—feelings of guilt.

2. Knowledge/understanding/perception of situation.

3. Coping abilities, mechanisms.

4. Support system.

◆ **B. Analysis/nursing diagnosis:**

1. *Ineffective family coping: compromised* related to psychological stress due to fear for infant, guilt feelings, impact on self-image.

2. *Ineffective individual coping* related to anxiety, stress.

3. *Ineffective family coping: disabling* related to disturbance in intrafamily relations secondary to individual coping deficits, recriminations.

4. *Altered parenting* related to lack of effective bonding secondary to emotional separation from infant, feelings of guilt.

5. *Dysfunctional grieving* related to guilt feelings, impact of loss on self-concept.

6. *Disturbance in body image, self-esteem, role performance* related to perceived failure to complete gestational task, produce perfect, healthy infant; associated with sleep deprivation.

7. *Social isolation* related to severe coping deficit, dysfunctional grieving, disturbance in self-esteem.

◆ **C. Nursing care plan/implementation:**

1. Goal: *emotional support.*

a. Provide privacy; encourage open expression/verbalization of feelings, fears, concerns, perceptions.

b. Crisis intervention techniques.

2. Goal: *facilitate bonding, effective coping, or anticipatory grieving processes.*

a. Encourage contact and participation in care of premature or compromised infant.

b. Keep informed of infant's status.

c. Provide realistic data.

3. Goal: *health teaching.*

a. Clarify misperceptions, as appropriate.

b. Discuss, demonstrate infant care techniques (e.g., feeding infant who has cleft lip or palate).

c. Refer to appropriate community resources.

◆ **D. Evaluation/outcome criteria:**

1. Woman verbalizes recognition and acceptance of diagnosis.

2. Woman verbalizes understanding of relevant information regarding treatment, prognosis.

3. Woman makes informed decision regarding infant care.

4. Woman demonstrates comfort and increasing participation in care of neonate.

5. Woman shows evidence of culturally appropriate bonding (eye contact, cuddles, calls infant by name).

IV. Disorders affecting comfort, rest, mobility: dystocia

A. Definition—difficult labor.

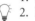 **B.** *General aspects* (*MOTHER,* "**3 Ps**": *P*sych, *P*lacenta, *P*osition):

1. **Pathophysiology**—see specific disorders.

2. **Etiology**—due to effects of factors that affect the FETUS (see also "**3 Ps**"):

a. *POWER:* forces of labor (uterine contractions, use of abdominal muscles).

(1) Premature analgesia/anesthesia.

(2) Uterine overdistention (multifetal pregnancy, fetal macrosomia).

(3) Uterine myomas.

(4) Grand multiparity.

b. *PASSAGEWAY:* resistance of cervix, pelvic structures.

(1) Rigid cervix.

(2) Distended bladder.

(3) Distended rectum

(4) Dimensions of the bony pelvis: pelvic contractures.

c. *PASSENGER:* accommodation of the presenting part to pelvic diameters.

(1) Fetal malposition/malpresentation.

(a) Transverse lie.

(b) Face, brow presentation.

(c) Breech presentation.

(d) Persistent occiput posterior position.

(e) CPD.

(2) Fetal anomalies.

(a) Hydrocephalus.

(b) Conjoined ("Siamese") twins.

(c) Meningomyelocele

(3) Fetal size: macrosomia.

3. **Hazards:**

a. *Maternal:*

(1) Fatigue, exhaustion, dehydration—due to prolonged labor.

(2) Lowered pain threshold, loss of control—due to prolonged labor, continued uterine contractions, anxiety, fatigue, lack of sleep.

(3) Intrauterine infection—due to prolonged rupture of membranes and frequent vaginal examinations.

(4) Uterine rupture—due to obstructed labor, hyperstimulation of uterus.

(5) Cervical, vaginal, perineal lacerations—due to obstetric interventions.

(6) Postpartum hemorrhage—due to uterine atony or trauma.

b. *Fetal:*

(1) Hypoxia, anoxia, demise—due to decreased O_2 concentration in cord blood.

(2) Intracranial hemorrhage—due to changing intracranial pressure.

C. Hypertonic dysfunction

1. **Pathophysiology**—increased resting tone of uterine myometrium; diminished refractory period; prolonged latent phase:

a. *Nullipara*—more than 20 hr.

b. *Multipara*—more than 14 hr.

2. **Etiology**—unknown. Theory—ectopic initiation of incoordinate uterine contractions.

◆ 3. **Assessment:**

a. Onset—early labor (latent phase).

b. Contractions:

(1) Continuous fundal tension, incomplete relaxation.

(2) Painful.

(3) Ineffectual—no effacement or dilation.

c. Signs of fetal distress

(1) Meconium-stained amniotic fluid.

(2) FHR irregularities.

d. Maternal vital signs.

e. Emotional status.

f. *Medical evaluation:* vaginal examination, x-ray pelvimetry, ultrasonography—to rule out CPD (rarely used).

◆ 4. **Analysis/nursing diagnosis:**

a. *Pain* related to hypertonic contractions, incomplete uterine relaxation.

b. *Anxiety/fear* for self and infant related to strong, painful contractions without evidence of progress.

c. *Ineffective individual coping* related to fatigue, exhaustion, anxiety, tension, fear.

d. *Impaired gas exchange (fetal)* related to incomplete relaxation of uterus.

e. *Sleep pattern disturbance* related to prolonged ineffectual labor.

◆ 5. **Nursing care plan/implementation:**

a. *Medical management:*

(1) Short-acting barbiturates (see **Unit 10**)—to encourage rest, relaxation.

(2) Intravenous fluids—to restore/maintain hydration and fluid-electrolyte balance.

(3) If CPD, cesarean birth.

b. *Nursing management:*

(1) Goal: *emotional support*—assist coping with fear, pain, discouragement.

(a) Encourage verbalization of anxiety, fear, concerns.

(b) Explain all procedures.

(c) Reassure. Keep couple informed of progress.

(2) Goal: *comfort measures.*

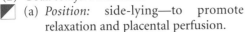 (a) *Position:* side-lying—to promote relaxation and placental perfusion.

(b) Bath, back rub, linen change, clean environment.

(c) Environment: quiet, darkened room— to minimize stimuli and encourage relaxation, warmth.

(d) Encourage voiding—to relieve bladder distention; to test urine for ketones.

(3) Goal: *prevent infection.* Strict aseptic technique.

(4) Goal: *prepare for cesarean birth* if necessary.

◆ 6. **Evaluation/outcome criteria:**

a. Relaxes, sleeps, establishes normal labor pattern.

b. Demonstrates no signs of fetal distress.

c. Successfully completes uneventful labor.

D. Hypotonic dysfunction during labor

1. **Pathophysiology**—after normal labor at onset, contractions diminish in frequency, duration and strength; lowered uterine resting tone; cervical effacement and dilation slow/cease.

2. **Etiology:**

a. Premature or excessive analgesia/anesthesia (epidural block or spinal block).

b. CPD.

c. Overdistention (polyhydramnios, fetal macrosomia, multifetal pregnancy).

d. Fetal malposition/malpresentation.

e. Maternal fear/anxiety.

◆ 3. **Assessment:**

a. Onset—may occur in latent phase; most common during active phase.

b. Contractions: normal previously, demonstrate:

(1) Decreased frequency.

(2) Shorter duration.

(3) Diminished intensity (mild to moderate).

(4) Less uncomfortable.

c. Cervical changes—slow or cease.

d. Signs of fetal distress—rare.

(1) Usually occur late in labor due to infection secondary to prolonged rupture of membranes.

(2) Tachycardia.

e. Maternal vital signs may indicate infection (↑temperature).

f. *Medical diagnosis*—procedures: vaginal examination.

◆ 4. **Analysis/nursing diagnosis:**

a. *Knowledge deficit* related to limited exposure to information.

b. *Anxiety/fear* related to failure to progress as anticipated; fear for fetus.

c. *High risk for injury* (infection) related to prolonged labor or ruptured membranes.

◆ 5. **Nursing care plan/implementation:**

a. *Medical management:*

(1) Amniotomy—artificial rupture of membranes.

(2) Oxytocin augmentation of labor—intravenous infusion of oxytocin to increase frequency, duration, strength, and efficiency of uterine contractions (see **Induction of labor, p. 198**).

(3) If CPD, cesarean birth.

b. *Nursing management:*

(1) Goals: *emotional support, comfort measures, prevent infection*—same as for **Hypertonic dysfunction** (see **p. 206**).

(2) Other (see **Induction of labor, p. 198**).

◆ 6. **Evaluation/outcome criteria:**

a. Reestablishes normal labor pattern.

b. Experiences successful birth of viable infant.

V. Disorders affecting fluid-gas transport: *maternal*

A. Uterine rupture

1. **Pathophysiology**—stress on uterine muscle exceeds its ability to stretch.

2. **Etiology:**

a. Overdistention—due to large baby, multifetal gestation.

b. Old scars—due to previous cesarean births or uterine surgery.

c. Contractions against CPD, fetal malpresentation, pathological retraction ring *(Bandl's).*

d. Injudicious obstetrics-malapplication of forceps (or application without full effacement/ dilation).

e. Tetanic contraction—due to hypersensitivity to oxytocin (or excessive dosage) during induction/augmentation of labor.

◆ 3. **Assessment:**

a. Identify predisposing factors early.

b. *Complete rupture*

(1) Pain: sudden, sharp, abdominal; followed by cessation of contractions; tender abdomen.

(2) Signs of shock; vaginal bleeding.

(3) Fetal heart tones—absent.

(4) Presenting part—not palpable on vaginal examination.

c. *Incomplete rupture*

(1) Contractions: continue, accompanied by abdominal pain and failure to dilate; may become dystonic.

(2) Signs of shock.

(3) May demonstrate vaginal bleeding.

(4) Fetal heart tones—absent/bradycardia.

4. **Prognosis**

a. Maternal—guarded.

b. Fetal—grave.

◆ 5. **Analysis/nursing diagnosis:**

a. *Pain* related to rupture of uterine muscle.

b. *Fluid volume deficit* related to massive blood loss secondary to uterine rupture.

c. *Anxiety/fear* related to concern for self, fetus.

d. *Altered tissue perfusion* related to blood loss secondary to uterine rupture.

e. *Altered urinary elimination* related to necessary conservation of intravascular fluid secondary to blood loss.

f. *Anticipatory grieving* related to expected loss of fetus; inability to have more children.

◆ 6. **Nursing care plan/implementation:**
   a. *Medical management:*
      (1) Surgical—laparotomy, hysterectomy.
      (2) Replace blood loss—transfusion, packed cells.
      (3) Reduce possibility of infection—antibiotics.
   b. *Nursing management:*
      (1) Goal: *safeguard status.*
         (a) Report *immediately;* mobilize staff.
         (b) Prepare for immediate laparotomy.
      ▶ (c) Oxygen per mask—to increase circulating oxygen level.
         (d) Order STAT type and crossmatch for blood—to replace blood loss.
      ▶ (e) Establish IV line—to infuse fluids, blood, medications.
      ▶ (f) Insert indwelling catheter—to deflate bladder.
         (g) Abdominal prep—to remove hair, bacteria.
         (h) Surgical permit (informed consent) for hysterectomy.
      (2) Goal: *emotional support*—to allay anxiety (woman and family).
         (a) Encourage verbalization of fears, anxiety, concerns.
         (b) Explain all procedures.
         (c) Keep family informed of progress.

◆ 7. **Evaluation/outcome criteria:**
   a. Experiences successful termination of emergency; minimal blood loss.
   b. Postoperative status stable.

B. **Amniotic fluid embolus (anaphylactoid syndrome)**
   1. **Pathophysiology:** acute cor pulmonale—due to embolus blocking vessels in pulmonary circulation; massive hemorrhage—due to DIC resulting from entrance of thromboplastin-like material into bloodstream.
   2. **Etiology**—amniotic fluid (with any meconium, lanugo, or vernix) enters maternal circulation through open venous sinuses at placental site; travels to pulmonary arterioles. Triggers cardiogenic shock and anaphylactoid reaction.
      a. Rare.
      b. Associated with: tumultuous labor, abruptio placentae, AROM, placement of intrauterine catheter.
   3. **Prognosis**—poor; often fatal to mother.
◆ 4. **Assessment:**
      a. May occur during labor, at time of rupture of membranes, or immediately postpartum.

b. Sudden dyspnea and cyanosis.
c. Chest pain.
d. Hypotension, tachycardia.
e. Frothy sputum.
f. **Signs of DIC:**
   (1) Purpura—local hemorrhage.
   (2) Increased vaginal bleeding—massive.
   (3) Rapid onset of shock.

◆ 5. **Analysis/nursing diagnosis:**
   a. *Impaired gas exchange* related to pulmonary edema.
   b. *Risk for fluid volume deficit* related to DIC.
   c. *Anxiety/fear* for self and fetus related to severity of symptoms, perception of jeopardy.

◆ 6. **Nursing care plan/implementation:**
   a. *Medical management:*
      (1) IV heparin, whole blood.
      (2) Birth: immediate, by forceps, if possible; or cesarean birth.
      (3) Digitalize, as necessary.
   b. *Nursing management:*
      (1) Goal: *assist ventilation.*
         (a) *Position:* semi-Fowler's.
      ▶ (b) Oxygen under positive pressure.
      ▶ (c) Suction prn.
      (2) Goal: *facilitate/expedite administration of fluids, medications, blood.*
      ▶ (a) Establish intravenous line with large-bore needle.
         (b) Administer heparin, fluids, as ordered.
      (3) Goal: *restore cardiopulmonary functions, if*
      ▶ *needed.* Cardiopulmonary resuscitation techniques.
      (4) Goal: *emotional support* of woman, family.
         (a) Allay anxiety, as possible.
         (b) Explain all procedures.
         (c) Keep informed of status.

◆ 7. **Evaluation/outcome criteria:**
   a. Dyspnea relieved.
   b. Bleeding controlled.
   c. Successful birth of viable infant.
   d. Uneventful postpartum course.

VI. **Disorders affecting fluid-gas transport:** *fetal*
   A. **Fetus in jeopardy**—general aspects:
      1. **Pathophysiology**—maternal hypoxemia, anemia, ketoacidosis, Rh isoimmunization, or decreased uteroplacental perfusion.
      2. **Etiology**—*maternal:*
         a. Preeclampsia/eclampsia, PIH.
         b. Heart disease.
         c. Diabetes.
         d. Rh or ABO incompatibility.
         e. Insufficient uteroplacental/cord circulation due to:
            (1) Maternal hypotension/hypertension.
            (2) Cord compression:
               (a) Prolapsed.
               (b) Knotted.
               (c) Nuchal.
            (3) Hemorrhage; anemia.

(4) Placental problem:
    (a) Malformation of the placenta/cord.
    (b) Premature "aging" of placenta.
    (c) Placental infarcts.
    (d) Abruptio placentae.
    (e) Placenta previa.
(5) Postterm gestation.
(6) Maternal infection.
(7) Polyhydramnios.
(8) Hypertonic uterine contractions.
f. Premature rupture of membranes (PROM) with chorioamnionitis.
g. Dystocia (e.g., from CPD).

◆ 3. **Assessment**—intrapartal:
a. Amniotic fluid examination—at or after rupture of membranes. *Signs of fetal distress:* meconium stained, vertex presentation—due to relaxation of fetal anal sphincter secondary to hypoxia/anoxia. *Note:* Fetus "gasps" in utero—may aspirate meconium and amniotic fluid.
b. Fetal activity:
    (1) Hyperactivity—due to hypoxemia, elevated CO_2.
    (2) Cessation—possible fetal death.
▶ c. Methods of monitoring FHR:
    (1) Fetoscope.
    (2) Phonocardiography with microphone application.
    (3) Internal fetal electrode—attached directly to fetus through dilated cervix after membranes ruptured.
    (4) Doppler probe using ultrasound flow.
    (5) Cardiotocograph—transducer on maternal abdomen transmits sound.
d. Abnormal FHR patterns (see **Figure 4.10, p. 192**).

> (1) Persistent arrhythmia.
> (2) Persistent tachycardia of 160 or more beats/min.
> (3) Persistent bradycardia of 100 or fewer beats/min.
> (4) *Early deceleration*—due to vagal response to head compression.
> (5) *Late deceleration*—due to uteroplacental insufficiency.
> (6) *Variable deceleration*—due to cord compression.
> (7) Decreased or loss of variability in FHR pattern.

e. *Medical evaluation*—procedures: fetal blood gases, pH (rarely performed).
    (1) Purpose—to identify fetal acid-base status.
    (2) Requirements for:
        (a) Ruptured membranes.
        (b) Cervical dilation.
        (c) Engaged head.
    (3) Procedure—under sterile condition, sample of fetal scalp blood obtained for analysis.

(4) Signs of fetal distress:

> (a) pH <7.20 (normal range is 7.3–7.4).
> (b) *Increased* CO_2
> (c) *Decreased* PO_2

◆ 4. **Analysis/nursing diagnosis:**
a. *Impaired gas exchange, fetal,* related to decreased placental perfusion/insufficient cord circulation.
b. *Altered tissue perfusion* related to hemolytic anemia.
c. *High risk for fetal injury* related to hypoxia.

B. Prolapsed umbilical cord
1. **Pathophysiology**—cord descent in advance of presenting part; compression interrupts blood flow, exchange of fetal/maternal gases → fetal hypoxia, anoxia, death (if unrelieved).
2. **Etiology:**
a. Spontaneous or artificial rupture of membranes before presenting part is engaged.
b. Excessive force of escaping fluid, as in polyhydramnios.
c. Malposition—breech, compound presentation, transverse lie.
d. Preterm or fetus who is SGA—allows space for cord descent.
◆ 3. **Assessment:**
a. Visualization of cord outside (or inside) vagina.
b. Palpation of pulsating mass on vaginal examination.
c. Fetal distress—variable deceleration and persistent bradycardia.
◆ 4. **Analysis/nursing diagnosis:**
a. *Impaired gas exchange, fetal,* related to interruption of blood flow from placenta/fetus.
b. *Anxiety/fear, maternal,* related to knowledge of fetal jeopardy.
◆ 5. **Nursing care plan/implementation:**
a. Goal: *reduce pressure on cord.*
    (1) *Position:* knee to chest; lateral modified Sims' with hips elevated; modified Trendelenburg.
    (2) With gloved hand, support fetal presenting part.
▶ b. Goal: *increase maternal/fetal oxygenation:* oxygen per mask (8–10 L/min).
▶ c. Goal: *protect exposed cord:* continuous pressure on the presenting part to keep pressure off cord.
d. Goal: *identify fetal response* to above measures, reduce threat to fetal survival: monitor FHR continuously.
e. Goal: *expedite termination of threat to fetus:* prepare for immediate cesarean birth.
f. Goal: *support mother and significant other* by staying with them and explaining.
◆ 6. **Evaluation/outcome criteria:**
a. FHR returns to normal rate and pattern.
b. Uncomplicated birth of viable infant.

VII. Summary of danger signs during labor (also see Clinical Pathway for Intrapartal Stages that follows this discussion.)

A. Contractions—strong, every 2 min or less, lasting 90 sec or more; poor relaxation between contractions.

B. Sudden sharp abdominal pain followed by board-like abdomen and shock—abruptio placentae or uterine rupture.

C. Marked vaginal bleeding.

D. **FHR** periodic pattern decelerations—late; variable; absent variability (see **Figure 4.10**).

E. Baseline.
  1. Bradycardia (<100 beats/min).
  2. Tachycardia (>160 beats/min).

F. Amniotic fluid.
  1. Amount: excessive; diminished
  2. Odor.
  3. Color: meconium stained; port-wine; yellow.
  4. 24 hr or more since rupture of membranes.

G. Maternal hypotension, or hypertension.

THE POSTPARTAL PERIOD

General overview: This review of the normal physiological and psychological changes occurring during the postpartal period (birth to 6 weeks after) provides the database necessary for assessing the woman's progress through involution, planning and implementing care, anticipatory guidance, health teaching, and evaluating the results. Emerging problems are identified by comparing the woman's status against established standards.

I. **Biological foundations of the postpartal period**
  A. **Uterine involution**—integrated processes by which the uterus returns to nonpregnant size, shape, and consistency.
    ◆ 1. **Assessment:**
      a. Contractions ("afterpains")—shorten muscles, close venous sinuses, restore normal tone.
        (1) Frequency, intensity, and discomfort decrease after first 24 hr.

CLINICAL PATHWAY 4.1: Intrapartal Stages

Category	First Stage	Second and Third Stage	Fourth Stage: Birth to 1 Hour Past Birth
Referral	Review prenatal record Advise CNM/physician of admission	Labor record for first stage	Report to recovery room nurse
◆ Assessments	**Admission Assessments:** Ask about problems since last prenatal visit; labor status (contraction frequency and duration), membrane status (intact or ruptured); coping level; support; woman's desires during labor and birth; ability to verbalize needs; laboratory testing (blood and UA) **Intrapartal Assessments:** Cervical assessment: from 1–10 cm dilation; nullipara (1.2 cm/hr), multipara (1.5 cm/hr) Cervical effacement: from 0%–100% Fetal descent: progressive descent from −4 to +4 Membrane assessment: intact or ruptured; when ruptured, Nitrazine and fern positive, fluid clear, no foul odor *Comfort level:* woman states is able to cope with contractions *Behavioral characteristics:* facial expressions, tone of voice and verbal expressions are consistent with comfort level and ability to cope **Latent Phase:** ▪ BP, P, R q1h if in normal range (BP 90–140/60–90 or not >30 mm Hg systolic or 15 mm Hg diastolic over baseline; pulse 60–90; respirations 12–20/min, quiet, easy) ▪ Temp q4hr; if >37.6°C (99.6°F); or if membranes ruptured, q2hr	**Second Stage Assessments:** ▪ BP, P, R q5–15min ▪ Uterine contraction palpated continuously ▪ FHR q15min (for low-risk women) and q5min (for high-risk women) if reassuring; if nonreassuring, monitor continuously Fetal descent: descent continues to birth *Comfort level:* woman states is able to cope with contractions and pushing *Behavioral characteristics:* response to pushing, facial expressions, verbalization **Third Stage Assessments:** ▪ BP, P, R q5min ▪ Uterine contractions, palpate occasionally until placenta is delivered, fundus maintains tone and contraction pattern continues to birth of placenta **Newborn Assessments:** ▪ Assess *Apgar* score of newborn	**Expected Outcomes:** Appropriate resources identified and used **Immediate postbirth assessments of mother** q15min for 1 hr: ▪ *BP:* 90–140/60–90; should return to prelabor level ▪ *Pulse:* slightly lower than in labor; range is 60–90 ▪ *Respirations:* 12–20/min; easy; quiet ▪ *Temperature:* 36.2°–37.6°C (98°–99.6°F) ▪ *Fundus:* firm, in midline, at the umbilicus ▪ *Lochia:* rubra; moderate amount; <1 pad/hr; no free flow or passage of clots with massage ▪ *Perineum:* sutures intact; no bulging or marked swelling; minimal bruising may be present; no c/o severe pain or rectal pain ▪ *Bladder:* nondistended; spontaneous void of >100 mL clear, straw-colored urine or blood-tinged with lochia; bladder nondistended following voiding ▪ If hemorrhoids present, no tenseness or marked engorgement; <2 cm diameter *Comfort* level: <3 on scale of 1 to 10 *Energy* level: awake and able to hold newborn **Newborn assessments if newborn remains with parents:** ▪ *Respirations:* 30–60; irregular ▪ *Apical pulse:* 120–160 and somewhat irregular

(Continued on following page)

Category	First Stage	Second and Third Stage	Fourth Stage: Birth to 1 Hour Past Birth
	■ Uterine contractions q30min (contractions q5–10min, 15–40sec, mild intensity) ■ FHR q60min (for low-risk women) and q30min (for high-risk women) if reassuring (reassuring FHR has baseline 110–160, LTV average, accelerations with fetal movement, no late or variable decelerations); if nonreassuring, position on side, start O$_2$, assess for hypotension, monitor continuously, notify CNM/physician **Active Phase:** ■ BP, P, R q1hr if WNL ■ Temp as above ■ Uterine contractions q30min: contractions q2–3min, 60 sec, moderate to strong ■ FHR q30min (for low-risk women) and q15min (for high-risk women) if reassuring; if nonreassuring, institute interventions **Transition:** ■ BP, P, R, q30min ■ Uterine contractions q15–30min: contractions q2min, 60–75 sec, strong ■ FHR q30min (for low-risk women) and q15min (for high-risk women) if reassuring; if nonreassuring, see above	■ *Respirations* 30–60, irregular ■ *Apical pulse:* 120–160 and somewhat irregular ■ *Temperature:* skin temp above 36.5°C (97.8°F) ■ *Umbilical cord:* two arteries, one vein (if one artery, assess for anomalies and urine output) ■ *Gestational age:* 38–42 wk	■ *Temperature:* skin temp above 36.5°C (97.8°F); skin feels warm to touch ■ *Skin color:* noncyanotic ■ *Mucus:* small amount, clear, easily suctioned with bulb syringe without skin color change ■ *Behavioral:* newborn opens eyes widely if room is slightly darkened ■ *Movements:* rhythmic; no hand tremors present **Expected Outcomes:** Findings indicate normal progression with absence of complications
Teaching/ psychosocial	Establish rapport Orient to environment, expected assessments, and procedures Answer questions and provide information Orient to EFM if used Teach relaxation, visualization, and breathing pattern if needed Explain comfort measures available Assume advocacy role for woman/ family during labor and birth	Orient to expected assessments and procedures Answer questions and provide information Explain comfort measures available Continue advocacy role	Explain immediate assessments and care after this first hour Teach self-massage of fundus and expected findings Instruct to call for assistance if mother desires to get OOB Begin newborn teaching; bulb syringe, positioning; maintaining warmth Assist parents in exploring their newborn Assist with first breastfeeding experience **Expected Outcomes:** Client and partner verbalize/demonstrate understanding of teaching
▶ **Nursing care management and report**	Straight cath prn if bladder distended If regional block administered monitor BP, FHR, sensation per protocol Provide continuing status reports to CNM/physician Perineal hair clip per woman's request Small enema per woman's request Perform sterile vaginal examination as indicated	Straight cath prn if bladder distended Continue monitoring VS, FHR and sensation if regional block has been given	Straight cath if bladder distended Monitor return of motor ability and sensation if regional block has been given Weigh perineal pads if lochia flow >1 saturated pad in 15 min, presence of boggy uterus and clots; ↓BP, ↑P **Expected Outcomes:** ■ Maternal/fetal well-being maintained and supported ■ Mother and newborn experience safe labor and birth ■ Family participates in process as desired
Activity	Encourage ambulation unless contraindicated Maintain bedrest immediately after administration of IV pain medication, or following regional block Woman rests comfortably between contractions	Position comfortably for birth Woman rests comfortably between pushing efforts and while awaiting birth of placenta	Position of comfort **Expected Outcomes:** ■ Activity maintained as desired unless contraindicated ■ Comfort enhanced by positioning/ movement

(Continued on following page)

Maternal-Infant

CLINICAL PATHWAY 4.1: Intrapartal Stages *(Continued)*

Category	First Stage	Second and Third Stage	Fourth Stage: Birth to 1 Hour Past Birth
▶ Comfort	Institute comfort measures: ambulation, frequent position change, effleurage, focal point, patterned paced breathing, visualization, therapeutic touch, back rub, moist cloths to face, holding hand, words of encouragement, changing underpad, shower, whirlpool, staying with the woman/family, warmed blanket at back, sacral pressure Offer pain medication or administer if requested Assist with administration of regional block	Institute comfort measures ■ *Second stage:* cool cloth to forehead, encouragement, coaching, position of comfort for pushing and birth ■ *Third stage:* cool cloth to forehead, assist parents to see newborn, position mother to hold newborn, provide encouragement	Institute comfort measures: ■ *Perineal* discomfort: gently cleanse and apply ice pack; position to decrease pressure on perineum ■ *Uterine* discomfort: palpate fundus gently ■ *Hemorrhoids:* ice pack ■ *General fatigue:* position of comfort, encourage rest ■ Administer pain medication **Expected Outcomes:** ■ Optimal comfort level maintained ■ Active reduction of pain/discomfort achieved
Nutrition	Ice chips and clear fluids (as ordered) Evaluate for signs of dehydration	Ice chips and clear fluids (as ordered)	Regular diet if assessments are WNL Encourage fluids **Expected Outcomes:** Nutritional needs met
Elimination	Voids at least q2hr; urine: clear, straw-colored, negative or trace for protein Bladder nondistended May have bowel movement Monitor I&O with IVs	May void spontaneously with pushing May pass stool with pushing	Voids spontaneously **Expected Outcomes:** Urinary bladder and bowel function unimpaired
Medications	Administer pain medication per woman's request	Local infiltration of anesthetic agent for birth by CNM/physician Pitocin 10 units IM, IVP per IV tubing, or added to IV fluids	Continue Pitocin infusion Administer pain medication **Expected Outcomes:** Comfort enhanced by pain relieving techniques, administration of analgesia agent or an analgesic or anesthetic block
Discharge planning	Evaluate knowledge of labor and birth process Evaluate support system and need for referral after birth		Provide information if mother to be moved from LDR room Provide opportunity for parents to ask questions regarding newborn Evaluate knowledge of normal postpartum, newborn care **Expected Outcomes:** Mother and newborn transferred to low-risk postpartal and newborn care
Family involvement	Identify available support person(s) Recognize possible impact of culture on responses Observe interaction between woman and partner Create moment alone with woman to identify possible abuse Assess current parenting skills	Provide opportunities for woman and support person(s) to watch newborn assessments Perform newborn assessment on mother's abdomen/ chest if possible	Provide opportunity for parents to be with baby Encourage skin-to-skin contact Darken room to encourage eye-to-eye contact Provide quiet time for new family Parenting: demonstrates early culturally expected parenting behaviors **Expected Outcomes:** ■ Incorporation of newborn into family ■ Family verbalizes comfort with newborn care

Source: Maternal-Newborn Nursing (6th ed), by Olds, London, Ladewig © 2000. Pp. 548–550. Reprinted by permission of Prentice Hall, Inc., Upper Saddle River, NJ.

Maternal-Infant

(2) More common in multiparas and after birth of a large baby; primiparous uterus remains contracted.

(3) Increased by breastfeeding.

b. Autolysis—breakdown and excretion of muscle protein (decreasing size of myometrial cells). Lochia—sloughing of decidua and blood.

c. Formation of *new endometrium*—4–6 wk until placental site healed.

d. *Cervix*

(1) *Immediately following* birth—bruised, small tears; admits one hand.

(2) *Eighteen hours* after birth—becomes shorter, firmer; regains normal shape.

(3) *One week* postpartum—admits two fingers.

(4) Never returns fully to prepregnant state.

(a) Parous os is wider and not perfectly round.

(b) Lacerations heal as scars radiating out from the os.

e. *Fundal height and consistency*

(1) After birth—at umbilicus; size and consistency of firm grapefruit.

(2) Day 1 (first 12 hr)—one finger above umbilicus.

(3) Descends by one finger-breadth daily until day 10.

(4) Day 10—behind symphysis pubis, nonpalpable.

f. *Lochia*

(1) Character:

(a) Days 1–3: rubra (red).

(b) Days 3–7: serosa (pink to brown).

(c) Day 10: alba (creamy white).

(2) Amount:

(a) Moderate: 4–8 pads/day (average 6 pads/day).

(b) Following cesarean birth: less lochia—due to manipulation during surgery.

(3) Odor: normal lochia has characteristic "fleshy" odor; foul odor is characteristic of infection.

(4) Clots: normal: a few small clots, most commonly on arising—due to pooling. *Note:* Large clots and *heavy* bleeding are associated with uterine atony, retained placental fragments.

B. Birth canal

1. *Vagina*—never returns fully to prepregnant state.

a. First few weeks postpartum—thin walled, due to lack of estrogen; few rugae.

b. Week 3: rugae may reappear.

2. *Pelvic floor*

a. Immediately after birth—infiltrated with blood, stretched, torn.

b. Month 6: considerable tone regained.

3. *Perineum*

a. Immediately following birth—edematous; may

have episiotomy (or repaired lacerations); hemorrhoids.

b. Healing, incisional line clean; no separation.

c. Hematoma—blood in connective tissue beneath skin; complains of pain, unrelieved by mild analgesia or heat; perineal distention; painful, tense, fluctuant mass.

C. Abdominal wall

1. Overdistention during pregnancy may → rupture of elastic fibers, persistent striae, and diastasis of the rectus muscles.

2. Usually takes 6–8 wk to retrogress, depending on previous muscle tone, obesity, and amount of distention during pregnancy.

3. Strenuous exercises discouraged until 8 wk postpartum.

D. Cardiovascular system—characteristic changes:

1. Immediately after birth—*increased* cardiac load, due to:

a. Return of uterine blood flow to general circulation.

b. Diuresis of excess interstitial fluid.

2. Volume—returns to prepregnant state (4 L) in about 3 wk. Major reduction—during first week, due to diuresis and diaphoresis.

3. Blood values (see **Table 4.5**).

a. High WBC during labor (25,000–30,000/mm^3), drops to normal level in first few days.

b. Week 1—Hgb, RBC, Hct, elevated fibrinogen return to normal.

4. Blood coagulation

a. During labor: rapid consumption of clotting factors.

b. During postpartum: increased consumption of clotting factors. Hypercoagulability maintained during first few days postpartum; predisposes to thrombophlebitis, pulmonary embolism.

◆ 5. **Assessment: potential complications**—vital signs:

a. *Temperature*—elevated in:

(1) Excessive blood loss, dehydration, exhaustion, infection.

(2) Elevation: 100.4°F (38°C) after first day postpartum suggests puerperal infection.

b. *Pulse*—physiological bradycardia (50–70) common through second day postpartum; may persist 7–10 days; etiology: unknown. *Tachycardia*—associated with: excessive blood loss, dehydration, exhaustion, infection.

c. *Blood pressure*—generally unchanged. *Elevation*—associated with: preeclampsia, essential hypertension.

E. Urinary tract—characteristic changes:

1. Output—increased due to: diuresis (12 hr–5 days postpartum); daily output to 3000 mL.

2. Urine constituents:

a. Sugar—primarily lactose, usually not detected by conventional dipstick.

b. Acetonuria—after prolonged labor; dehydration.

c. Proteinuria—first 2 days in response to the catalytic process of involution ≤1⁺.
3. Dilation of ureters—subsides in first few weeks.
◆ 4. **Assessment: potential complications**—measure first few voidings, palpate bladder to determine emptying.
　　a. Edema, trauma, or anesthesia may → retention with overflow.
　　b. Overdistended bladder—common cause of excessive bleeding in immediate postpartum.

F. **Integument (skin)**—characteristic changes:
　1. Striae—persist as silvery or brownish lines.
　2. Diastasis recti abdominis—some midline separation may persist.
　3. Diaphoresis—excessive perspiration for first few (approximately 5) days.
　4. Breast changes (see **II.A.3. Breasts,** below).
　5. Linea nigra and darkened areola fade.

G. **Legs**
　1. Should have no redness, tenderness, local areas of increased skin temperature, or edema.
　2. May have some soreness from birth position.
　3. *Homans' sign* should be negative (no calf pain when knee is extended and gentle pressure applied to dorsiflex the foot).

H. **Weight**—characteristic changes:
　1. Initial weight loss—fetus, placenta, amniotic fluid, excess tissue fluid.
　2. Weighs more than in prepregnant state (weight maintained in breasts).
　3. Week 6—weight loss is individualized.

I. **Menstruation and ovarian function**—first menstrual cycle may be anovulatory.
　1. *Nonnursing*—ovulation at 4–6 wk; menstruation at 6–8 wk.
　2. *Nursing*—anovulatory period varies (39 days to 6 mo or more); some for duration of lactation; contraceptive value: *very unreliable.*

II. **Nursing management during the postpartal period**
◆ A. **Assessment**—minimum of twice daily.
　1. Vital signs.
　2. Emotional status, response to baby.
　3. *Breasts*
　　a. Observe: size, symmetry, placement and condition of nipples, leakage of colostrum. Normal: although one breast is usually larger than the other, breasts are essentially symmetrical in shape; nipples: in breast midline, erectile, intact (no signs of fissure); bilateral leakage of colostrum is common.
　　b. *Note:* reddened areas, elevations, supernumerary nipples, inverted nipples, cracks.
　　c. Observe for signs of (normal) engorgement (i.e., tenderness, distention, prominent veins). Transient; normally occurs shortly before lactation is established—due to venous and lymphatic stasis.
　　d. Palpate for: local heat, edema, tenderness, swelling (signs of localized infection).

4. Fundus, lochia, perineum.
5. Voiding and bowel function.
6. Legs (see **I.G.**).
7. Signs of complications.
◆ B. **Analysis/nursing diagnosis** (see **VI, Nursing actions during the fourth stage of labor, pp. 195–196**).
◆ C. **Nursing care plan/implementation:**
　1. Goal: *comfort measures.*
　▶ a. Perineal care—to promote healing, prevent infection.
　　b. Sitz baths—to promote healing.
　◖ c. Apply topical anesthetics, witch hazel to episiotomy area, hemorrhoids.
　◖ d. Administer mild analgesia, as ordered.
　　e. Instruct in tensing buttocks on position change —to reduce stress on suture line, discomfort.
　　f. Breast care: mother who *is bottle-feeding*
　　　(1) Wash daily with clear water and mild soap.
　　　(2) Support with well-fitting brassiere.
　　　(3) For engorgement:
　　　　(a) Prevent with tight binder.
　　　　(b) Treat with ice pack and mild analgesic.
　　　　(c) *Avoid* nipple stimulation.
　　　(4) (see also **Breastfeeding and lactation, p. 216**).
　2. Goal: *encourage normal bowel function.* (Normal to take 1–3 days for function to resume.)
　◖ a. Administer stool softeners, as ordered.
　　b. Encourage ambulation.
　🍽 c. Increase *dietary fiber* (salads, fresh fruit, vegetables, bran cereals).
　　d. Provide adequate fluid intake.
　3. Goal: *health teaching and discharge planning.*
　　a. Reinforce appropriate perineal self-care.
　　b. Reinforce hand washing (see **VI. Nursing actions during the fourth stage of labor, pp. 195–196**).
　▶ c. *Infant care*
　　　(1) Bathing, cord care, circumcision care, diapering.
　　　(2) Feeding, burping, scheduling.
　　　(3) Assessment—temperature, skin color, newborn rash, jaundice.
　　　(4) Normal stool cycle and voiding pattern.
　　　(5) Common sleep/activity patterns.
　　　(6) Signs to report **immediately:**

　　　　(a) Fever, vomiting, diarrhea.
　　　　(b) Signs of inflammation or infection at cord stump.
　　　　(c) Bleeding from circumcision site.
　　　　(d) Lethargy, irritability.

　　d. *Self-care*
　　　(1) Adequate rest, nutrition, hydration.
　　　(2) Breast self-examination; wear bra to support breasts and promote comfort.
　　　(3) Normal process of involution; lochial patterns.
　　e. Resumption of intercourse approximately 4 wk postpartum (wait until lochia stops).

(1) Explain that time interval varies as to first postpartal ovulation.

(2) Family planning options may resume if desired:

    (a) If not breastfeeding, oral contraceptives (estrogen and progesterone); low-dose progesterone given to mothers who are breastfeeding (see **Table 4.1**).

    (b) Long-acting progestins (subcutaneous implants or injectable). Safe to use during lactation.

    (c) Use of IUD or diaphragm decided at postpartal checkup.

    (d) Emphasize need to recheck size and fit of diaphragm.

    (e) Other options: condom plus spermicides.

f. Exercises—to restore muscle tone, relieve tension.

    (1) Mild exercise during first few weeks.

        (a) Deep abdominal breathing.

        (b) Supine head-raising.

        (c) Stretching from head to toe.

        (d) Pelvic tilt.

        (e) Kegel—to regain perineal muscle tone.

    (2) Strenuous exercises (sit-ups, leg lifts)—deferred until later in postpartum.

g. Maternal signs to report **immediately:**

> (1) Prolonged lochia rubra.
> (2) Cramping.
> (3) Signs of infection.
> (4) Excessive fatigue, depression.
> (5) Dysuria.

4. Goal: *anticipatory guidance*—discharge planning: mothers are discharged earlier in their postpartum recovery today—(6–48 hr after birth if asymptomatic).

a. Discuss, assist in organizing time schedule. Nap, when possible, when infant asleep—to minimize fatigue.

b. Common maternal emotional/behavior changes, feelings:

    (1) Jealous of infant; guilt feelings.

    (2) "Baby blues"—due to hormonal fluctuations, fatigue, change of lifestyle.

    (3) Feelings of inadequacy.

c. Discuss support groups, aid in identifying supportive people.

◆ **D. Evaluation/outcome criteria:**

1. Woman experiences normal, uncomplicated postpartal period All assessment findings within normal limits.

2. Woman returns demonstrations of appropriate self-care measures/techniques:

    a. Perineal care, pad change, handwashing.

    b. Breast care, breast self-examination.

3. Woman verbalizes understanding of:

    a. Need for adequate rest and diversion.

b. Appropriate time for resumption of intercourse and exercise.

c. Appropriate nutritional intake to meet needs (own and, if breastfeeding, infant's).

d. Signs to be reported immediately.

e. Returns demonstration of appropriate infant care measures.

f. Evidences beginning comfort and increasing confidence in parenting role.

◆ **E. Postpartal assessment—6 or less wk after birth:**

1. Weight, vital signs, urine for protein, complete blood count (CBC).

2. Breast examination lactating or not.

3. Pelvic examination—involution and position of uterus; perineal healing; tone of pelvic floor.

4. Desire for selection of method of contraception.

III. Psychological/behavioral changes. *Achievement of developmental tasks*—progress in assuming maternal role.

◆ **A. Assessment:**

1. *Taking-in* phase—1–3 days following birth.

    a. Talkative; verbally relives labor/birth experience.

    b. Passive, dependent, concerned with own needs (eating, sleeping, elimination).

2. *Taking-hold*—day 3 to 2 wk.

    a. Impatient to control own bodily functions, care for self.

    b. Expresses interest/concern in learning how to care for baby (desire to assume "mothering" role).

    c. Responds to positive reinforcement.

3. *Letting-go*—mother "lets go" of former self-concept, role, lifestyle; begins to integrate new role and self-concept as "mother."

    a. Feelings of insecurity, inadequacy.

    b. Hesitancy in approaching infant care tasks.

4. "Baby blues"—may appear on day 4 or 5. *Note:* Often, father/partner experiences same feelings.

    a. Thought to result from fatigue (sleep deprivation), realization of need for role change, recognition of new responsibilities, hormonal change.

    b. Mild depression, cries without provocation.

    c. Frightened—intimidated by own perceptions of responsibilities, hormonal changes.

5. Lag in experiencing "maternal feelings"—usually resolved within 6 wk.

    a. May contribute to "baby blues."

    b. Guilt regarding lack of "maternal feelings."

    c. Diminished by prompt bonding experience.

◆ **B. Analysis/nursing diagnosis:**

1. *Ineffective family coping: compromised,* related to achieving developmental tasks.

2. *Situational low self-esteem* related to perceived inadequacy in acceptance of maternal role.

3. *Ineffective individual coping* related to "baby blues," lag in experiencing maternal feelings.

◆ C. **Nursing care plan/Implementation:**
1. *Taking-in.* Goal: *emotional support.*
    a. Encourage verbalization of labor/birth experiences; compliment parents on "how well" they did.
    b. Explore feelings of disappointment, if any.
    c. Meet dependency needs; comment on appearance, hair, personal gowns.
    d. Encourage rooming in.
2. *Taking-hold.* Goal: *health teaching.*
    a. Discuss self-care, postpartal physiological/psychological changes.
    b. Demonstrate infant care; mother returns demonstration.

◆ D. **Evaluation/outcome criteria:**
1. Woman demonstrates beginning comfort in maternal role.
2. Woman develops confidence and competence in infant care.
3. Woman expresses satisfaction with self, infant; eager to return home.
4. Woman succeeds in breastfeeding. (Tension inhibits let-down reflex; baby nurses poorly.)

IV. **Breastfeeding and lactation**
    A. **Biological foundations:**
    1. *Antepartal* alterations:
        a. High estrogen/progesterone levels—stimulate proliferation and development of breast ducts.
        b. High progesterone levels—also → development of mammary lobules and alveoli.
    2. *Postpartum* alterations:
        a. Rapid drop in estrogen/progesterone levels.
        b. Increased secretion of prolactin—stimulates alveolar cells → milk.
        c. Suckling—stimulates release of oxytocin →contraction of ducts → milk ejection (let-down reflex).
        d. Engorgement—due to venous and lymphatic stasis.
            (1) Immediately precedes lactation.
            (2) Lasts about 24 hr.
            (3) Frequent feeding reduces engorgement.

◆ B. **Assessment:**
1. Colostrum (yellowish fluid)—continues for first 2–3 days; has some antibiotic, immunologic, and nutritive value.
2. Milk (bluish-white, thin)—secreted on about third day.

◆ C. **Analysis/nursing diagnosis:**
1. *Knowledge deficit* related to breastfeeding techniques.
2. *Pain* related to engorgement.
3. *Personal identity disturbance* related to problems in breastfeeding.
4. *Sleep pattern disturbance* related to discomfort or infant care needs.

◆ D. **Nursing care plan/implementation:**
1. Goal: *promote successful breastfeeding.*

a. Encourage first feeding within 1 hr after giving birth.
b. Encourage emptying both breasts at each feeding and before engorgement to stimulate milk production, prevent mastitis.
c. Encourage rest, relaxation, fluids.
d. *Nutritional* counseling (see **Unit 9**).
    (1) Additional 500 calories daily—may be supplied by one extra pint of milk, one extra egg, and one extra serving of meat, citrus fruit, and vegetable.
    (2) Increase fluid intake to 3000 mL daily.
2. Goal: *prevent or relieve engorgement.*
    ▶ a. Pain: relieved by warm packs, emptying breasts.
    b. Wear good, supportive bra.
    c. Administer analgesics, as ordered/necessary.
3. Goal: *health teaching.*
    ▶ a. Instruct, demonstrate *rooting reflex* and putting infant to breast. Infant must grasp nipple and areola over location of milk sinuses.
    ▶ b. Demonstrate burping techniques, what to do if infant chokes; removing infant from breast.
    ▶ c. Instruct in *basic nipple care.*
        (1) Teach good handwashing.
        (2) Nurse on each breast, making sure areola is in mouth, alternating position of infant.
        (3) Alternate "beginning" breast.
        (4) Break suction before removing infant from breast.
        (5) Air-dry nipples after each feeding and apply lanolin if abraded. *Note:* Creams, lotions, or ointments block secretion of a natural bacteriostatic oil by Montgomery glands—and infant may refuse breast until it is washed. Instead: expressed milk may be massaged gently around nipple.
        (6) Teach daily hygiene of breasts.
    d. Instruct in care of cracked or *fissured nipples.*
        (1) Encourage and support mothers.
        (2) Air-dry nipples after each feeding.
        (3) Use nipple shield if nipples extremely sore.
        (4) Discontinue nursing for 48 hr; maintain milk supply by expressing milk with pump.
    e. Discuss avoiding use of any drugs except under medical supervision—may affect infant or suppress lactation.
    f. Discuss possibility of sexual stimulation during breastfeeding.
        (1) Validate normalcy and acceptability.
        (2) *Note:* During orgasm, milk may squirt from nipples.
    g. Explain that contraceptive value of nursing is unpredictable; the time that ovulation is inhibited varies widely.
    h. Explain *contraindications to breastfeeding:*

(1) Active tuberculosis.

(2) Severe chronic maternal disease.

(3) Mastitis (temporary interruption may be necessary).

(4) Some therapeutic drugs.

(5) Severe cleft lip or palate in newborn (may pump and give in special bottles).

(6) HIV-positive status; AIDS.

◆ **E. Evaluation/outcome criteria:**

1. Woman verbalizes understanding of breastfeeding techniques, nutritional requirements for successful lactation.

2. Woman successfully demonstrates breastfeeding; infant nurses well.

3. Woman demonstrates appropriate burping techniques; clears excessive mucus from infant's mouth without incident.

4. Woman verbalizes understanding of basic breast care techniques:

   a. Self-examination.

   b. Clear water bath.

   c. Drying nipples after bathing, feeding.

   d. Care of cracked or irritated nipples.

   e. Correct infant positioning for feeding.

CLINICAL PATHWAY FOR THE POSTPARTAL PERIOD
(see pp. 218–220)

Complications During the Postpartal Period

I. Disorders affecting fluid-gas transport

A. Postpartum hemorrhage

1. Definition—loss of 500 mL of blood or more during first 24 hr postpartum in vaginal birth; 1000 mL in cesarean birth.

2. **Pathophysiology**—excessive loss of blood secondary to trauma, decreased uterine contractility; results in hypovolemia.

3. **Etiology** (in order of frequency):

   a. Uterine atony

     (1) Uterine overdistention (multipregnancy, polyhydramnios, fetal macrosomia).

     (2) Multiparity.

     (3) Prolonged or precipitous labor.

     (4) Anesthesia—deep inhalation or regional (particularly saddle block).

     (5) Myomata (fibroids).

     (6) Oxytocin induction of labor.

     (7) Overmassage of uterus in postpartum.

     (8) Distended bladder.

   b. Lacerations—cervix, vagina, perineum.

   c. Retained placental fragments—usually delayed postpartum hemorrhage.

d. Hematoma—deep pelvic, vaginal, or episiotomy site.

◆ **4. Assessment:**

   a. Uterus—boggy, flaccid; excessive vaginal bleeding (dark; seepage, large clots) —due to uterine atony, retained placental fragments.

   b. Late signs of shock—air hunger; anxiety/apprehension, tachycardia, tachypnea, hypotension.

   c. Blood values (admission and postpartal)—hemoglobin (Hgb), hematocrit (Hct), clotting time.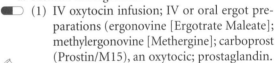

   d. Estimated blood loss: during labor/birth; in early postpartum.

   e. Pain: vulvar, vaginal, perineal.

   f. Perineum: distended—due to edema; discoloration—due to hematoma. May complain of rectal pressure.

   g. Lacerations—bright red vaginal bleeding with firm fundus.

◆ **5. Analysis/nursing diagnosis:**

   a. *Fluid volume deficit* related to excessive blood loss secondary to uterine atony, retained placental fragments.

   b. *Anxiety/fear* related to unexpected complication.

   c. *Altered tissue perfusion* related to decreased oxygenation secondary to blood loss.

   d. *Activity intolerance* related to fatigue.

◆ **6. Nursing care plan/implementation:**

   a. *Medical management:*

     (1) IV oxytocin infusion; IV or oral ergot preparations (ergonovine [Ergotrate Maleate]; methylergonovine [Methergine]; carboprost (Prostin/M15), an oxytocic; prostaglandin.

     (2) Order blood work: clotting time, platelet count, fibrinogen level, Hgb, Hct, CBC.

     (3) Type and crossmatch for blood replacement.

     (4) Surgical:

       (a) Repair of lacerations.

       (b) Evacuation, ligation of hematoma.

       (c) Curettage—retained placental fragments.

   b. *Nursing management:*

     (1) Goal: *minimize blood loss.*

       (a) Notify physician promptly of abnormal assessment findings.

       (b) Order lab work STAT, as directed—to determine blood loss and etiology.

       (c) Fundal massage.

       (d) Administer medications to stimulate uterine tone. For ergot products and carboplast, monitor blood pressure (**contraindicated** in PIH).

     (2) Goal: *stabilize status.*

       (a) Establish IV line—to enable administration of medications and rapid absorption/action. Administer whole blood (with larger catheter).

CLINICAL PATHWAY 4.2: The Postpartal Period

Category	First 4 Hours	4–8 Hours Past Birth	8–24 Hours Past Birth
Referral	Report from labor nurse if not continuing in an LDR room	Lactation consultation as needed	Home nursing, WIC referral if indicated **Expected Outcomes:** Referrals made
◆ **Assessments**	Postpartum assessments q 30min × 2, q1h × 2, then q4hr. Includes: ■ *Fundus:* firm, midline, at or below umbilicus ■ *Lochia rubra* <1 pad/hr; no free flow or passage of clots with massage ■ *Bladder:* voids large amounts of urine spontaneously; bladder not palpable following voiding ■ *Perineum:* sutures intact; no bulging or marked swelling; no c/o severe pain. Minimal bruising may be present. If hemorrhoids present, no tenseness or marked engorgement; <2 cm diameter ■ *Breasts:* soft, colostrum present *Vital signs:* ■ BP: WNL; no hypotension; not > 30 mm systolic or 15 mm diastolic over baseline ■ *Temperature:* <38°C (100.4°F) ■ *Pulse:* bradycardia normal, consistent with baseline ■ *Respirations:* 12–20/min; quiet, easy *Comfort level:* <3 on scale of 1–10	Continue postpartum assessment q4hr × 2, then q8h *Breasts:* evaluate nipple status; should be no evidence of cracks or bruising Observe *feeding* technique with newborn *Vital signs:* assessment q8h; all WNL; report temperature >38°C (100.4°F) Assess *Homan's sign* q8h Continue assessment of *comfort* level	Continue postpartum assessment q8h *Breasts:* nipples should remain free of cracks, fissures, bruising *Feeding* technique with newborn: should be good or improving *Vital signs:* assessment q8h; all WNL; report temperature >38°C (100.4°F) Continue assessment of *comfort* level **Expected Outcomes:** Vital signs medically acceptable, voids qs, postpartum assessment WNL; *comfort level* <3 on 1–10 scale, involution of uterus in process, demonstrates and verbalizes appropriate newborn feeding techniques
Teaching/ psychosocial	Explain postpartum assessments Teach self-massage of fundus and expected findings; rationale for fundal massage Instruct to call for assistance first time OOB and PRN Demonstrate peri-care, surgigator, sitz bath prn Explain comfort measures Begin newborn teaching; bulb suctioning, positioning, feeding, diaper change, cord care Orient to room if transferred from LDR room Provide information on early postpartal period Assess mother/infant attachment	Discuss psychological changes of postpartum period; facilitate transition through tasks of taking on maternal role Discuss peri-care/hygiene; encourage use of supportive brassiere for breast- or bottle-feeding Stress need for frequent rest periods Continue newborn teaching: soothing/comforting techniques, swaddling; return demonstrations indicate woman's understanding Provide opportunities for questions and review; reinforce previous teaching Breastfeeding: nipple care: air-drying, lanolin; proper latch-on technique; tea bags Bottle-feeding: supportive bra, ice bags, breast binder Assess mother/infant attachment	Reinforce previous teaching, complete teaching Discuss involution; anticipated physical changes in first 2 weeks postpartum; postpartal exercises; need to limit visitors Discuss postpartal nutrition; balanced diet **Breastfeeding:** ■ Increase calories by 500 kcal over nonpregnant state (200 kcal over pregnant intake) ■ Explain milk production, let-down reflex, use of supplements, breast pumping, and milk storage **Bottle-feeding:** ■ Return to nonpregnant caloric intake ■ Explain formula preparation and storage Discuss birth control options, sexuality Discuss sibling rivalry and plan for supporting siblings at home Discuss pets; suggestions for improving acceptance of infant by pets **Expected Outcomes:** Mother verbalizes teaching comprehension Positive bonding and emotional behaviors observed

(Continued on following page)

Category	First 4 Hours	4–8 Hours Past Birth	8–24 Hours Past Birth
◆ **Nursing care management and reports**	Ice pack to perineum to decrease swelling and increase comfort Straight catheter prn × 1 if distended or voiding small amounts If continues to be unable to void or voiding small amounts, insert Foley catheter and notify CNM/physician	Sitz baths prn If woman is Rh− and infant Rh+, RhoGAM workup; obtain consent; complete teaching Determine rubella status Obtain consent for rubella vaccine if indicated; explain purpose, procedure, implications of vaccine Obtain hematocrit	Continue sitz baths prn May shower if ambulating without difficulty DC saline lock if present Administer rubella vaccine as indicated **Expected Outcomes:** Using sitz bath; voids qs; lab work WNL; performs ADL without assistance
Activity	Assistance when OOB first time, then prn Ambulate ad lib Rests comfortably between assessments	Encourage rest periods Ambulate ad lib; may leave birthing unit after notifying staff of plan to ambulate off unit	Up ad lib **Expected Outcomes:** Ambulates ad lib
▶ **Comfort**	Institute comfort measures: ■ *Perineal* discomfort: peri-care; sitz baths, topical analgesics ■ *Hemorrhoids:* sitz baths, topical analgesics, digital replacement of external hemorrhoids; side-lying or prone position *Afterpains:* prone with small pillow under abdomen; warm shower or sitz baths; ambulation ■ Administer pain medication	Continue with pain management techniques *Offer alternative pain management options:* distraction with music, television, visitors; massage; warmed blankets or towels to affected area; using breathing techniques when infant latches on to breast and/or during cramping until medication's action is felt	Continue with pain management techniques **Expected Outcomes:** *Comfort* level <3 on 1–10 scale Verbalizes alternative pain management options
Nutrition	Regular diet Fluid ≥2000 mL/day	Continue diet and fluids	Continue diet and fluids **Expected Outcomes:** Regular diet/fluids tolerated
Elimination	Voiding large amounts straw-colored urine	Voiding large quantities May have bowel movement	Same **Expected Outcomes:** Voiding qs; passing flatus or bowel movement
Medications	Pain medications as ordered Methergine 0.2 mg q4th PO if ordered Stool softener Tucks pad prn, perineal analgesic spray	Continue meds Lanolin to nipples PRN; tea bags to nipples if tender; saline flush to Luer local adaptor (if present) q8hr or as ordered May take own prenatal vitamins	Continue medications RhoGAM and rubella vaccine administered as indicated **Expected Outcomes:** Vaccines administered; pain controlled
Discharge planning/ home care	Evaluate knowledge of normal postpartum and newborn care Evaluate support systems	Discuss typical newborn schedule; plan for periods of rest Birth certificate paperwork completed Evaluate plans for transporting newborn; car seat available	Review discharge instruction sheet/checklist Describe postpartum warning signs and when to call CNM/physician Provide prescriptions. Gift packs given appropriate for bottle- or breastfeeding Arrangements for baby pictures as desired Postpartum and newborn visits scheduled **Expected Outcomes:** Discharged home; mother verbalizes postpartum warning s/sx, follow-up appointment times/dates

Maternal-Infant

(Continued on following page)

CLINICAL PATHWAY 4.2: The Postpartal Period *(Continued)*

Category	First 4 Hours	4–8 Hours Past Birth	8–24 Hours Past Birth
Family involvement	Identify available support persons Assess family perceptions of birth experience Parenting: demonstrates culturally expected early parenting behaviors	Involve support persons in care, teaching; answer questions Evidence of parental bonding behaviors present	Continue to involve support persons in teaching, involve siblings as appropriate Plans made for providing support to mother following discharge **Expected Outcomes:** Evidence of parental bonding behavior; support persons verbalize understanding of woman's need for: rest, good nutrition, fluids and emotional support

Source: Maternal-Newborn Nursing (6th ed), by Olds, London, Ladewig © 2000. Pp. 933–934. Reprinted by permission of Prentice Hall, Inc., Upper Saddle River, NJ.

(b) Administer medications, as ordered to control bleeding, combat shock.

(c) Prepare for surgery, as ordered.

(3) Goal: *prevent infection.* Strict aseptic technique.

(4) Goal: *continual monitoring.* Vital signs, bleeding (do pad count or weigh pads), fundal status.

(5) Goal: *prevent sequelae* (*Sheehan's* syndrome).

(6) Goal: *health teaching*—after episode: Reinforce appropriate perineal care and handwashing techniques.

◆ 7. **Evaluation/outcome criteria:**
   a. Maternal vital signs stable.
   b. Bleeding diminished or absent.
   c. Assessment findings within normal limits.

B. **Subinvolution**—delayed return of uterus to normal size, shape, position.
   1. **Pathophysiology**—inability of inflamed uterus (endometritis) to contract effectively → incomplete uterine involution; failure of contractions to effect closure of vessels in site of placental attachment → bleeding.
   2. **Etiology:**
      a. PROM with secondary amnionitis, endometritis.
      b. Retained placental fragments.
      c. Oxytocin stimulation or augmentation of labor of overdistended uterine muscle may interfere with involution.
   ◆ 3. **Assessment:**
      a. Uterus: large, boggy; lack of uterine tone; failure to shrink progressively.
      b. Discharge: persistent lochia; painless fresh bleeding, hemorrhagic episodes.
   ◆ 4. **Analysis/nursing diagnosis:**
      a. *Pain* related to tender, inflamed uterus secondary to endometritis.

   b. *Anxiety/fear* related to change in physical status.
   c. *Knowledge deficit* related to diagnosis, treatment, prognosis.
   d. *High risk for injury* related to infection.
   e. *Fluid volume deficit* related to excessive bleeding.

◆ 5. **Nursing care plan/implementation:**
   a. *Medical management:*
      (1) Have woman void or catheterize; massage fundus.
      (2) Surgical (curettage) —to remove placental fragments.
      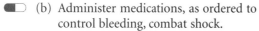(3) Antibiotic therapy—to treat intrauterine infection.
      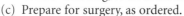(4) Oxytocics—to stimulate/enhance uterine contractions.
   b. *Nursing management:*
      (1) Goal: *health teaching.*
         (a) Explain condition and treatment.
         (b) Describe, demonstrate perineal care, pad change, handwashing.
      (2) Goal: *emotional support.* Encourage verbalization of anxiety regarding recovery, separation from newborn.
      (3) Goal: *promote healing.*
         (a) Encourage rest, compliance with medical/nursing regimen.
         (b) Administer oxytocics, antibiotics, as ordered.

◆ 6. **Evaluation/outcome criteria:**
   a. Verbalizes understanding of condition and treatment.
   b. Complies with medical/nursing regimen.
   c. Demonstrates normal involutional progress.
   d. All assessment findings (vital signs, fundal height, consistency, lochial discharge) within normal limits.
   e. Expresses satisfaction with care.

C. **Hypofibrinogenemia**

1. **Pathophysiology**—decreased clotting factors, fibrinogen; may be accompanied by DIC.

2. **Etiology:**
   a. Missed abortion (retained dead fetus syndrome).
   b. Fetal death, delayed emptying of uterine contents.
   c. Abruptio placentae; Couvelaire uterus.
   d. Amniotic fluid embolism.
   e. Hypertension.

◆ 3. **Assessment:**
   a. Observe for bleeding from injection sites, epistaxis, purpura.
   b. See **DIC assessment, p. 506** in **Unit 7.**
   c. Maternal vital signs, color.
   d. I&O.
   e. *Medical evaluation*—procedures.

> (1) Thrombin clot test—important: size and persistence of clot.
> (2) Prothrombin time—*prolonged.*
> (3) Bleeding time—*prolonged.*
> (4) Platelet count—*decreased.*
> (5) Activated partial thromboplastin time—*prolonged.*
> (6) Fibrinogen (factor I concentration)—*decreased.*
> (7) Fibrin degradation products—*present.*

◆ 4. **Analysis/nursing diagnosis:**
   a. *Fluid volume deficit* related to uncontrolled bleeding secondary to coagulopathy.
   b. *Anxiety/fear* related to unexpected critical emergency.
   c. *Altered tissue perfusion* related to decreased oxygenation secondary to blood loss.

◆ 5. **Nursing care plan/implementation:**
   a. *Medical management:*
      (1) Replace platelets.
      (2) Replace blood loss.
      (3) IV heparin—to inhibit conversion of fibrinogen to fibrin.
   b. *Nursing management:*
      (1) Goal: *continuous monitoring.*
      ▶ (a) Vital signs.
         (b) I&O hourly.
         (c) Skin: color, emergence of petechiae.
         (d) Note, measure (as possible), record, and report blood loss.
      (2) Goal: *control blood loss.*
         (a) Establish IV line, administer fluids or blood products as ordered.
         (b) *Position:* side-lying—to maintain blood supply to vital organs.
      (3) Goal: *emotional support.*
         (a) Encourage verbalization of anxiety, fear, concerns.
         (b) Explain all procedures.
         (c) Remain with woman continuously.
         (d) Keep woman and family informed.

◆ 6. **Evaluation/outcome criteria:**
   a. Bleeding controlled.
   b. Laboratory studies—returning to normal values.
   c. Status stable.

II. **Disorders affecting protective functions:** postpartal infection (**Table 4.13**).

A. **General aspects**

1. Definition—reproductive system infection occurring during the postpartal period.

2. **Pathophysiology**—bacterial invasion of birth canal; most common: localized infection of the lining of the uterus (endometritis).

3. **Etiology:**
   a. Anaerobic nonhemolytic streptococci.
   b. *E. coli.*
   c. *C. trachomatis* (bacteroides).
   d. Staphylococci.

4. Predisposing conditions:
   a. Anemia.
   b. PROM.
   c. Prolonged labor.
   d. Repeated vaginal examinations during labor.
   e. Intrauterine manipulation—e.g., manual extraction of placenta.
   f. Retained placental fragments.
   g. Postpartum hemorrhage.

◆ 5. **Assessment:**
   a. Fever 38°C (100.4°F) or more on two or more occasions, after first 24 hr postpartum.
   b. Other signs of infection: pain, malaise, dysuria, subinvolution, foul lochial odor.

◆ 6. **Analysis/nursing diagnosis:**
   a. *Fluid volume deficit* related to excessive blood loss, anemia.
   b. *Knowledge deficit* related to danger signs of postpartum period.
   c. *High risk for injury* related to infection.

◆ 7. **Nursing care plan/implementation:** prevention
   a. Goal: *prevent anemia.*
      (1) Minimize blood loss—accurate post-partal assessment and management of bleeding.
    (2) *Diet: high protein, high vitamin.*
      (3) Vitamins, iron—suggest continuing prenatal pattern until postpartum checkup.
   b. Goal: *prevent entrance/transport of microorganisms.*
      (1) *Strict aseptic technique* during labor, birth, and postpartum (standard precautions).
      (2) Minimize vaginal examinations during labor.
      (3) Perineal care.
   c. Goal: *health teaching.*
      (1) Handwashing—before and after each pad change, after voiding or defecating.
      ▶ (2) Perineal care—from front to back; use clear, warm water or mild antiseptic solution as a cascade; do *not* separate labia.
      (3) Maintain sterility of pads; apply from front to back.

Maternal-Infant

Maternal-Infant

TABLE 4.13	Postpartum Infections		
Condition/Etiology	◆ **Assessment: Signs/Symptoms**	◆	**Nursing Interventions**

Postpartum Infection

Traumatic labor and birth and postpartum hemorrhage make woman more vulnerable to infection by such bacteria as nonhemolytic streptococci, *Escherichia coli,* and *Staphylococcus species*	Depends on location and severity of infection; usually include fever, pain, swelling, and tenderness Temperature of 100.4°F (38°C) or more after first 24 hr after birth on two or more occasions indicates puerperal infection ("childbed fever")	1. Monitor: Signs and symptoms, drainage (e.g., uterine) 2. Obtain culture and sensitivity 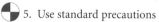 3. Administer *antimicrobial* agents and *analgesic* agents 4. Ensure comfort; encourage rest 5. Use standard precautions 6. *Force fluids* and provide *high* calorie diet 7. Keep family informed of mother's and newborn's progress 8. Promote maternal-infant contact as soon as possible 9. Plan and implement discharge and follow-up care

Endometritis

Microorganisms invade placental site and may spread to entire endometrium	Temperature, chills, anorexia, malaise, boggy uterus, foul-smelling lochia, and cramps	1. Administer *antimicrobial* agents and *analgesic* agents 2. Encourage *Fowler's position* to promote drainage 3. *Force fluids* 4. Take standard precautions

Pelvic Cellulitis or Parametritis

Microorganisms spread through lymphatics and invade tissues surrounding uterus	Fever, chills, lower-abdominal pain, and tenderness	1. Administer *antimicrobial* agents and *analgesic* agents 2. Encourage bedrest 3. *Force fluids*

Perineal Infection

Trauma to perineum makes woman more vulnerable to infection	Localized pain, fever, swelling, redness, and seropurulent drainage	1. Administer *antimicrobial* agents and *analgesic* agents 2. Provide sitz baths or heat/cold applications 3. Take standard precautions

Mastitis

Lesions or fissure on nipples allow entry of microorganisms (e.g., *Staphylococcus aureus*) from infant's nose/mouth or mother's unwashed hands (Breastmilk is a good medium for growth of organism)	Marked engorgement, pain, chills, fever, tachycardia If untreated, single or multiple breast abscesses may form	1. Order culture and sensitivity studies of mother's milk 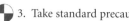 2. Administer *antimicrobial* agents and *analgesic* agents 3. Apply heat or cold therapy 4. Assist with incising and draining abscesses 5. Use standard precautions and perform meticulous handwashing

(Continued on following page)

Condition/Etiology	◆ Assessment: Signs/Symptoms	◆ Nursing Interventions
Thrombophlebitis		*Femoral:*
Infected pelvic or femoral thrombi	Pain, chills, and fever	1. Rest and *elevate* leg
Increased tendency to clot formation during pregnancy, trauma to tissues, and hemorrhage decrease new mother's resistance to infection	*Femoral:* stiffness of affected area or part and positive *Homans'* sign *Pelvic:* severe chills and wide fluctuations in temperature	2. Administer *antimicrobial* agents, *analgesic* agents, and *anticoagulants* *Pelvic:* 1. Encourage bedrest 2. Force fluids 3. Administer *antimicrobial* agents, and *anticoagulants*

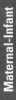

    (4) *Avoid* use of tampons until normal menstrual cycle resumes.

◆ 8. **Evaluation/outcome criteria:**
   a. Woman has assessment findings within normal limits:
     (1) Vital signs.
     (2) Rate of involution (fundal height, consistency).
     (3) Lochia: character, amount, odor.
   b. Woman avoids infection.

B. Endometritis—infection of lining of uterus.
  1. **Pathophysiology** (see **II. A. General aspects**, p. 221).
  2. **Etiology**—most common: invasion by normal body flora (e.g., anaerobic streptococci).
  3. Characteristics:
   a. Mild, localized—asymptomatic, or low-grade fever.
   b. Severe—may lead to ascending infection, parametritis, pelvic abscess, pelvic thrombophlebitis.
   c. If remains localized, self-limiting; usually resolves within 10 days.
◆ 4. **Assessment:**
   a. Signs of infection: fever, chills, malaise, anorexia, headache, backache.
   b. Uterus: large, boggy, extremely tender.
     (1) Subinvolution.
     (2) Lochia: dark brown; foul odor.
◆ 5. **Analysis/nursing diagnosis:**
   a. *Anxiety/fear* related to effects on self and newborn.
   b. *Self-esteem disturbance and altered role performance* related to inability to meet own expectations regarding parenting, secondary to unexpected hospitalization.
   c. *Pain* related to inflammation/infection.
   d. *Ineffective individual coping* related to physical discomfort and psychological stress associated with self-concept disturbance; worry, guilt, concern regarding newborn at home.
   e. *Altered family processes*—interruption of

adjustment to altered life pattern related to postpartal infection/hospitalization.

◆ 6. **Nursing care plan/implementation:**
   a. Goal: *prevent cross-contamination.* Contact-item isolation.
   b. Goal: *facilitate drainage. Position:* semi-Fowler's.
   c. Goal: *nutrition/hydration.*
     (1) *Diet:* high calorie, high protein, high vitamin.
     (2) Push *fluids* to 4000 mL/day (oral or IV, or both, as ordered).
     (3) I&O.
   d. Goal: *increase uterine tone/facilitate involution.* Administer medications, as ordered (e.g., oxytocics, antibiotics).
   e. Goal: *minimize energy expenditure,* as possible.
     (1) Bedrest.
     (2) Maximize rest, comfort.
   f. Goal: *emotional support.*
     (1) Encourage verbalization of anxiety, concerns.
     (2) Keep informed of progress.
◆ 7. **Evaluation/outcome criteria:**
   a. Vital signs stable, within normal limits.
   b. All assessment findings within normal limits.
   c. Unable to recover organism from discharge.

C. Urinary tract infections
  1. **Pathophysiology**—normal physiological changes associated with pregnancy (e.g., ureteral dilation) and the postpartal period (e.g., diuresis, increased bladder capacity with diminished sensitivity of stretch receptors)→ increased susceptibility to bacterial invasion and growth→ ascending infections (cystitis, pyelonephritis).
  2. **Etiology:** usually bacterial.
  3. Predisposing factors:
   a. Birth trauma to bladder, urethra, or meatus.
   b. Bladder hypotonia with retention (due to intrapartal anesthesia or trauma).
   c. Repeated or prolonged catheterization, or poor technique.

d. Weakening of immune response secondary to anemia, hemorrhage.

◆ 4. **Assessment:**
   a. Maternal vital signs (fever, tachycardia).
   b. Dysuria, frequency (flank pain—with pyelonephritis).
   c. Feeling of "not emptying" bladder.
   d. Cloudy urine; frank pus.

◆ 5. **Analysis/nursing diagnosis:**
   a. *Altered urinary elimination* related to diuresis, dysuria, inflammation/infection.
   b. *Pain* related to dysuria secondary to cystitis.
   c. *Knowledge deficit* related to self-care (perineal care).

◆ 6. **Nursing care plan/implementation:**
   a. Goal: *minimize perineal edema.* Perineal ice pack in fourth stage—to limit swelling secondary to trauma, facilitate voiding.
   b. Goal: *prevent overdistention of bladder.*
      (1) Monitor level of fundus, lochia, bladder distention. (*Note:* Distended bladder displaces uterus, limits its ability to contract → boggy fundus, increases its vaginal bleeding.)
      (2) Encourage *fluids* and voiding; I&O.
      (3) Aseptic technique for catheterization.
      (4) Slow emptying of bladder on catheterization—to maintain tone.
   c. Goal: *identification of causative organism*—to facilitate appropriate medication (antibiotics). Obtain clean-catch (or catheterized) specimen for culture and sensitivity.
   d. Goal: *health teaching.* See previous discussion of fluids, general hygiene, diet, and medications.

◆ 7. **Evaluation/outcome criteria:**
   a. Voiding: quantity sufficient (although small, frequent output may mean overflow with retention).
   b. Urine character: clear, amber, or straw colored.
   c. Vital signs: within normal limits.
   d. No complaints of frequency, urgency, burning on urination, flank pain.

D. **Mastitis**—inflammation of breast tissue:
   1. **Pathophysiology**—local inflammatory response to bacterial invasion; suppuration may occur; organism can be recovered from breast milk.
   2. **Etiology**—most common: *Staphylococcus aureus*; source—most common: infant's nose, throat.

◆ 3. **Assessment:**
   a. Signs of infection (may occur several weeks in postpartum).
      (1) Fever.
      (2) Chills.
      (3) Tachycardia.
      (4) Malaise.
      (5) Abdominal pain.
   b. Breast
      (1) Reddened area(s).
      (2) Localized/generalized swelling.
      (3) Heat, tenderness, palpable mass.

◆ 4. **Analysis/nursing diagnosis:**
   a. *Impaired skin integrity* related to nipple fissures, cracks.
   b. *Pain* related to tender, inflamed tissue secondary to infection.
   c. *Disturbance in body image, self-esteem* related to association of breastfeeding with female identity and role.
   d. *Anxiety/fear* related to sexuality; impact on breastfeeding, if any.

◆ 5. **Nursing care plan/implementation:**
   a. Goal: *prevent infection.* Health teaching in early postpartum:
      (1) Handwashing.
      (2) Breast care—wash with warm water only (*no* soap) —to prevent removing protective body oils.
      (3) Let breast milk dry on nipples to prevent drying of tissue.
      (4) Clean bra (with no plastic pads or liners) to support breasts, reduce friction, minimize exposure to microorganisms.
      (5) Good breastfeeding techniques (see **p. 216**).
      (6) Alternate position of infant for nursing to change pressure areas.
   b. Goal: *comfort measures.*
      (1) Encourage bra or binder—to support breasts, reduce pain from motion.
      ▶ (2) Local heat or ice packs as ordered—to reduce engorgement, pain.
      (3) Administer analgesics, as necessary.
   c. Goal: *emotional support.*
      (1) Encourage verbalization of feelings, concerns.
      (2) If breastfeeding is discontinued, reassure woman she will be able to resume breastfeeding.
   d. Goal: *promote healing.*
      (1) Maintain lactation (if desired) by manual expression or breast pump, q4hr.
      (2) Administer antibiotics as ordered.

◆ 6. **Evaluation/outcome criteria:**
   a. Woman promptly responds to medical/nursing regimen.
      (1) Symptoms subside.
      (2) Assessment findings within normal limits.
   b. Woman successfully returns to breastfeeding.

E. **Thrombophlebitis**
   1. **Pathophysiology**—inflammation of a vein secondary to lodging of a clot.
   2. **Etiology:**
      a. Extension of endometritis with involvement of pelvic and femoral veins.
      b. Clot formation in pelvic veins following cesarean birth.
      c. Clot formation in femoral (or other) veins

secondary to poor circulation, compression, and venous stasis.

3. **Assessment:**
   a. Pelvic—pain: abdominal or pelvic tenderness.
   b. Calf—pain: positive *Homans'* sign (pain elicited by flexion of foot with knee extended).
   c. Femoral
      (1) Pain.
      (2) Malaise, fever, chills.
      (3) Swelling— "milk leg."

4. **Analysis/nursing diagnosis:**
   a. *Pain* in affected region related to local inflammatory response.
   b. *Anxiety/fear* related to outcome.
   c. *Ineffective individual coping* related to unexpected postpartum complications, hospitalization, separation from newborn.
   d. *Impaired physical mobility* related to imposed bedrest to prevent emboli formation and dislodging clot (embolus).

5. **Nursing care plan/implementation:**
   a. Goal: *prevent clot formation.*
      (1) Encourage early ambulation.
      (2) *Position: avoid* prolonged compression of popliteal space, use of knee gatch.
      (3) Apply thromboembolic disease (TED) hose, as ordered, preoperatively or postoperatively, or both, for cesarean birth.
   b. Goal: *reduce threat of emboli.*
      (1) Bedrest, with cradle to support bedding.
      (2) Discourage massaging "leg cramps."
   c. Goal: *prevent further clot formation.* Administer anticoagulants, as ordered.
   d. Goal: *prevent infection.*
      (1) Administer antibiotics, as ordered.
      (2) Push *fluids.*
   e. Goal: *facilitate clot resolution.* Heat therapy, as ordered.

6. **Evaluation/outcome criteria:**
   a. Symptoms subside; all assessment findings within normal limits.
   b. No evidence of further clot formation.

III. **Disorders affecting psychosocial-cultural functions—**postpartum depression/psychosis
   A. **General aspects**
      1. Can occur in both new parents and experienced parents.
      2. Usually occur within 2 wk of birth.
      3. Increased incidence among single parents
      4. Increased incidence among women with history of clinical depression.
      5. Most common symptomatology: affective disorders.
      6. Psychiatric intervention required if prolonged or severe; if underlying cause unresolved; increased risk in subsequent pregnancies.
   B. **Etiology**—theory: birth of child may emphasize:
      1. Unresolved role conflicts.
      2. Unachieved normal development tasks.

C. **Assessment:**
   1. Withdrawal.
   2. Paranoia.
   3. Anorexia, sleep disturbance, mood swings.
   4. Depression—may alternate with manic behavior.
   5. Potential for self-injury or child abuse/neglect.

D. **Analysis/nursing diagnosis:**
   1. *Ineffective individual coping* related to perceived inability to meet role expectations ("mother") and ambivalence related to dependence/independence.
   2. *Self-esteem disturbance and altered role performance* related to "femaleness" and reaction to responsibility for care of newborn.
   3. *High risk for violence,* self-directed or directed at newborn, related to anger or depression.
   4. *Ineffective family coping* related to lack of support system in early postpartum.
   5. *Altered family processes* related to psychological stress, interruption of bonding.
   6. *Altered parenting* related to hormonal changes and stress.

E. **Nursing care plan/implementation:**
   1. Goal: *emotional support.*
      a. Encourage verbalization of feelings, fears, anxiety, concerns.
      b. Support positive self-image, feelings of adequacy, self-worth.
         (1) Reinforce appropriate comments and behaviors.
         (2) Encourage active participation in self-care, comment on accomplishments.
         (3) Reduce threat to self-image, fear of failure. Maintain support, gradually increase tasks.
   2. Goal: *safeguard status of mother/newborn.*
      a. Unobtrusive, protective environment.
      b. Stay with woman when she is with infant.
   3. Goal: *nutrition/hydration.*
      a. Encourage selection of favorite foods—to aid security in decision making; counteract anorexia (refusal to eat) by tempting appetite.
      b. Push *fluids* (juices, soft drinks, milkshakes) — to maintain hydration.
   4. Goal: *minimize stress, facilitate effective coping.* Administer therapeutic medications, as ordered.
      a. Schizophrenia—phenothiazines.
      b. Depression—mood elevators.
      c. Manic behaviors—sedatives, tranquilizers.

F. **Evaluation/outcome criteria:**
   1. Woman increases interaction with infant.
   2. Woman expresses interest in learning how to care for infant.
   3. Woman evidences no agitation, depression.
   4. Woman actively participates in caring for self and infant.
   5. Woman demonstrates increasing comfort in mothering role.
   6. Woman has positive family interactions.

THE NEWBORN INFANT

General overview: Effective nursing care of the newborn infant is based on: (1) knowledge of the conditions present during fetal life; (2) requirements for independent extrauterine life; and (3) alterations needed for successful transition. *The first 24 hours are the most hazardous.*

I. **Biological foundations of neonatal adaptation**—*general aspects:*

  A. *Fetal anatomy and physiology*

    1. *Fetal circulation*—four intrauterine structures that differ from extrauterine structures (**Figure 4.11**):

      a. *Umbilical vein*—carries oxygen and nutrient-enriched blood from placenta to ductus venosus and liver.

      b. *Ductus venosus*—connects to inferior vena cava; allows most blood to bypass liver.

      c. *Foramen ovale*—allows fetal blood to bypass fetal lungs by shunting it from right atrium into left atrium.

      d. *Ductus arteriosus*—allows fetal blood to bypass fetal lungs by shunting it from pulmonary artery into aorta.

      e. *Umbilical arteries* (two)—allow return of deoxygenated blood to the placenta.

    2. *Umbilical cord*—extends from fetus to center of placenta: usually 50 cm (18–22 inches) long and 1–2 cm ($\frac{1}{2}$–1 inch) in diameter. Contains:

      a. *Wharton's jelly*—protects umbilical vessels from pressure, cord "kinking," and interference with fetal-placental circulation.

      b. *Umbilical vein*—carries oxygen and nutrients from placenta to fetus.

      c. *Two umbilical arteries*—carry deoxygenated blood and fetal wastes from fetus to placenta. *Note:* Absence of one artery indicates need to rule out intraabdominal anomalies.

    3. *Characteristics of fetal blood*

      a. *Fetal hemoglobin (HbF)*

        (1) Higher oxygen-carrying capacity than adult hemoglobin.

        (2) Releases oxygen easily to fetal tissues.

        (3) Ensures high fetal oxygenation.

        (4) Normal range at term: 12–22 g/dL; average: 15–20 g/dL.

      b. Total blood volume at term: 85 mL/kg body weight; Hct: 38%–62%, average 53%; RBC 3–7 million, average 4.9 million/U.

  B. *Extrauterine adaptation: tasks*

    1. Establish and maintain ventilation, successful gas transfer—requires patent airway and adequate pulmonary surfactant.

    2. Modify circulatory patterns—requires closure of fetal structures.

    3. Absorb and utilize fluids and nutrients.

    4. Excrete body wastes.

    5. Establish and maintain thermal stability.

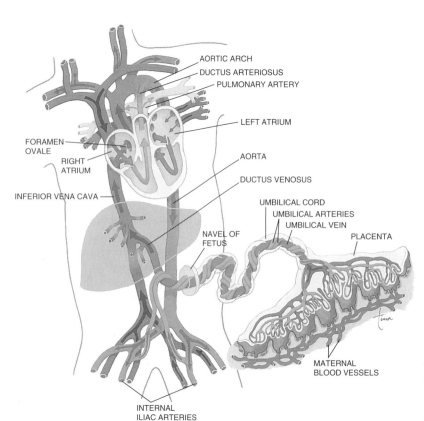

FIGURE 4.11 Fetal circulation. (From Venes, D [ed]: Taber's Cyclopedic Medical Dictionary, ed. 20. FA Davis, Philadelphia, 2005.)

◆ **C. Nursing care plan/implementation**
1. Facilitate successful transition to independent life.
2. Protect infant from physiological stress and environmental hazards.
3. Encourage development of a strong family unit.

II. Admission/assessment: 1–4 hours after birth (see also **Clinical Pathway for Newborn Care**)
   A. Admission assessment of normal, term neonate
   1. Color and reactivity.
   2. General appearance, symmetry.
   3. Length and weight.
   4. Head and chest circumferences.
   5. Vital signs:
      a. Axillary temperature.
      b. Respirations (check rate, character, rhythm).
      c. Apical pulse.
   6. General physical assessment (**Table 4.14**) and reflexes (**Table 4.15**).
   7. Estimate of gestational age (**Table 4.16**).

TABLE 4.14 ◆ Physical Assessment of the Term Neonate		
Criterion	**Average Values and Normal Variations**	**Deviations from Normal**
Vital Signs		
Heart rate	120–140/min, irregular, especially when crying, and functional murmur	Faint sound—pneumomediastinum; and heart rate <100 beats/min or >180 beats/min
Respiratory	30–60/min with short periods of apnea, irregular; vigorous and loud cry	Distress—flaring of nares, retractions, tachypnea, grunting, excessive mucus, <30 respirations/min or >60 respirations/min; cyanosis
Temperature	Stabilizes about 8–10 hr after birth; 36.5–37°C (97.7–98.6°F) axillary	Unreliable indicator of infection due to environmental influences
Blood pressure	60–80/40–50; varies with change in activity level	Hypotension: with RDS Hypertension: coarctation of aorta
Measurements		
Weight	3400 g ($7^1/_2$ lbs); range: 5 lb 8 oz–8 lb 13 oz	Birthweight <2500 g; preterm or SGA infant; >4000 g; LGA infant, evaluate mother for gestational diabetes
Length	50 cm (20 inches); range: 18–22 inches	
Chest circumference	2 cm ($^3/_4$ inch) less than head circumference	If relationship varies, check for reason
Head circumference	33–35 cm (13–14 inches)	Check for microcephalus and macrocephalus
General Assessment		
Muscle tone	Good tone and generalized flexion; full range of motion; spontaneous movement	Flaccid, and persistent tremor or twitching; movement limited; asymmetrical
Skin color	Mottling, acrocyanosis, and physiological jaundice; petechiae (over presenting part), milia, mongolian spotting, lanugo, and vernix caseosa	Pallor, cyanosis, or jaundice within 24 hr of birth Petechiae or ecchymoses elsewhere; all rashes, except erythema toxicum; pigmented nevi; hemangioma; and yellow vernix
Head	Moulding of fontanels and suture spaces; one-fourth of body length	Cephalohematoma, caput succedaneum, sunken or bulging fontanels, closed sutures; excessively wide sutures
Hair	Silky, single strands, lies flat; grows toward face and neck	Fine, wooly; unusual swirls, patterns, hair line; coarse
Eyes	Edematous eyelids, conjunctival hemorrhage; grayish-blue to grayish-brown; blink reflex, usually no tears; uncoordinated movements may focus for a few seconds; good placement on face; cornea is bright and shiny; pupillary reflex equal and reactive to light; eyebrows distinct	Epicanthal folds (in non-Asians); discharges; agenesis; opaque lenses; lesions; strabismus; "doll's eyes" beyond 10 days; absence of reflexes
Nose	Appears to have no bridge; should have no discharge; preferential nose breathers; sneezes to clear nose	Discharge and choanal atresia; malformed; flaring of nares beyond first few moments of life

(Continued on following page)

Maternal-Infant

TABLE 4.14	Physical Assessment of the Term Neonate *(Continued)*	
Criterion	**Average Values and Normal Variations**	**Deviations from Normal**
Mouth	*Epstein's pearls* on gum ridges; tongue does not protrude and moves freely, symmetrically; uvula in midline; reflexes present; sucking, rooting, gag, extrusion	*Cleft lip or palate;* teeth, cyanosis, circumoral pallor; asymmetrical lip movement; excessive saliva; thrush; incomplete or absent reflexes
Ears	Well formed, firm; notch of ear should be on straight line with outer canthus	Low placement, clefts; tags; malformed; lack of cartilage
Face	Symmetrical movements and contours	*Facial palsy* (7th cranial nerve); looks "funny"
Neck	Short, freely movable; some head control	Wry neck, webbed neck; restricted movement; masses; distended veins; absence of head control
Chest	Enlarged breasts, "*witch's milk*"; barrel shaped; both sides move synchronously; nipples symmetrical	Flattened, funnel-chested, asynchronous movement; lack of breast tissue; fracture of clavicle(s); supernumerary or widely spaced nipples; bowel sounds
Abdomen	Dome shaped, abdominal respirations, soft; may have small umbilical hernia; umbilical cord well formed, containing three vessels; dry around base; bowel sounds within 2 hr of birth; voiding; passage of meconium	Scaphoid shaped, omphalocele, diastasis recti, and distention; umbilical cord containing two vessels; redness or drainage around base of cord
Genitalia		
Girl	Large labia; may have pseudomenstruation, smegma; vaginal orifice open; increased pigmentation; ecchymosis and edema following breech birth; pink-stained urine (uric acid crystals)	Agenesis and imperforate hymen; ambiguous labia widely separated, fecal discharge per vagina; *epispadias or hypospadias*
Boy	Pendulous scrotum covered with rugae, and testes usually descended; voids with adequate stream; increased pigmentation; edema and ecchymosis following breech birth	*Phimosis, epispadias,* or *hypospadias;* ambiguous; scrotum smooth and testes undescended *Hydrocele:* collection of fluid in the sac surrounding the testes
Extremities	Synchronized movements, freely movable through full range of motion; legs appear bowed, and feet appear flat; attitude of general flexion; arms longer than legs; grasp reflex; palmar and sole creases; normal contour	Fractures, brachial nerve palsy, *clubbed foot,* phocomelia or amelia, unusual number or webbing of digits, and abnormal palmar creases; poor muscle tone; asymmetry; hypertonicity; unusual hip contour and click sign (*hip dysplasia*); hypermobility of joints
Back	Spine straight, easily movable, and flexible; may have small pilonidal dimple at base of spine; may raise head when prone	Fusion of vertebrae: pilonidal dimple with tuft of hair; *spina bifida,* agenesis of part of vertebral bodies; limitation of movement; weak or absent reflexes
Anus	Patent, well placed; "wink" reflex	Imperforate, and absence of "wink" (absence of sphincter muscle); fistula
Stools	Meconium within first 24 hr; transitional—days 2–5; *breastfed:* loose, golden yellow; *bottle-fed:* formed, light yellow (see **Table 4.17**)	Light-colored meconium (dry, hard), or absent with distended abdomen (*cyctic fibrosis* or *Hirschsprung's disease*); diarrhetic
Laboratory Values		
Hemoglobin (cord)	13.6–19.6 g/dL	Evaluate for anemia and persistent polycythemia
Serum bilirubin	2–6 mg/dL	Hyperbilirubinemia (*term:* 15 mg or more; *preterm:* 10 mg or more)
Blood glucose	40 mg/dL for *term;* >30 mg/dL for *preterm*	Identify hypoglycemia before overt or asymptomatic hypoglycemia—do Dextrostix on all suspected infants (LGA or SGA neonates, or neonates of mothers who are diabetic)

Neurological Examination Specific to gestational age and state of wakefulness

1. Behavioral patterns

a. Feeding	Variations in interest, hunger; usually feeds well within 48 hr	Lethargic. Poor suck, poor coordination with swallow, choking, cyanosis

(Continued on following page)

Criterion	Average Values and Normal Variations	Deviations from Normal
b. Social	Crying is lusty, strong, and soon indicative of hunger, pain, attention seeking. Responds to cuddling, voice by quietness and increased alertness	Absent; no focusing on person holding him/her; unconsolable
c. Sleep-wakefulness	Two periods of reactivity: at birth, and 6–8 hr later. Stabilization, with wakeful periods about every 3–4 hr	Lethargy, drowsiness Disorganized pattern
d. Elimination	Stooling: see Stools	See Stools
	Urination	Diminished number: dehydration
	First few days: 3–4 qd	
	End of first week: 5–6 qd	
	Later: 6–10 qd, with adequate hydration	
2. Reflex response	Bilateral, symmetrical response (see **Table 4–15**)	Absent, hyperactive, incomplete, asynchronous
3. Sensory capabilities		
a. Vision	Limited accommodation, with clearest vision within 7–8 inches. Focuses and follows by 15 min of age. Prefers patterns to plain.	Absence of these responses may be due to absence of or diminished acuity or to sensory deprivation
b. Hearing	By 2 min of age, can move in direction of sound: responds to high pitch by "freezing," followed by agitation; to low pitch (crooning) by relaxing	Absence of response: deafness
c. Touch	Soothed by massaging, warmth, weightlessness (as in water bath)	Unable to be comforted: possible drug dependence
d. Smell	By fifth day, can distinguish between mother's breasts and those of another woman	Newborns who are cocaine-addicted avoid eye contact
e. Taste	Can distinguish between sweet and sour	
f. Motor	Coordinates body movement to parent's voice and body movement	Absence

*Based on Brazelton's method.

TABLE 4.15	◆ Assessment: Normal Newborn Reflexes*	
Reflex	**Description**	**Implications of Deviations from Normal Patterns**
Moro (startle)	Symmetrical *abduction* and *extension* of arms with fingers extended in response to sudden movement or loud noise	Asymmetrical reflex may indicate brachial (Erb's) palsy or fractured clavicle
Tonic neck (fencing)	When head turned to one side, arm and leg on *that* side *extend,* and *opposite* arm and leg *flex*	Asymmetry may indicate cerebral lesion, if persistent
Rooting and sucking	With stimulus to cheek, turns *toward* stimulus, opens mouth, sucks	Absence of response may indicate prematurity, neurological problem, or depressed infant (or not hungry)
Palmar grasp	If palm stimulated, fingers *curl;* holds adult finger briefly	Asymmetry may indicate neurological involvement
Plantar grasp	Pressure on sole will elicit *curling* of toes	Absence/asymmetry associated with defects of lower spinal column
Stepping/dancing	If held in upright position with feet in contact with hard surface, alternately raises feet	Asymmetry may indicate neurological problem
Babinski	Stroking the sole in a upward fashion elicits *hyperextension* of toes	Same as for plantar grasp
Crawling	When placed in prone position, attempts to crawl	Absence may indicate prematurity or depressed infant

*Reflexes are good indicators of the neurological system in infants who are well, but not in neonates who are sick. Infants with infections may not show normal reflexes yet have an intact neurological system.

Maternal-Infant

TABLE 4.16 Estimation of Gestational Age: Common Clinical Parameters

Characteristic	Preterm	Term
Head	Oval—narrow biparietal; large in proportion to body; face looks like "old man"	Square-shaped biparietal prominences; $1/4$ body length
Ears: form, cartilage	Soft, flat, shapeless	Pinna firm; erect from head
Hair: texture, distribution	Fine, fuzzy, or wooly; clumped; appears at 20 wk	Silk; single strands apparent
Sole creases	Starting at ball of foot: $1/3$ covered with creases by 36 wk, $2/3$ by 38 wk	Entire sole heavily creased
Breast nodules	0 mm at 36 wk; 4 mm at 37 wk	10 mm or more
Nipples	No areolae	Formed; raised above skin level
Genitalia		
Girl	Clitoris large, labia gaping	Labia larger, meet in midline
Boy	Small scrotum, rugae on inferior surface only, and testes undescended	Scrotum pendulous, covered with rugae; testes usually descended
Skin: texture, opacity	Visible abdominal veins; thin, shiny	Few indistinct larger veins; thick, dry, cracked, peeling
Vernix	Cover body by 31–33 wk	Small amount in creases or absent at term; postterm: dry, wrinkled
Lanugo	Apparent at 20 wk; by 33–36 wk, covers shoulders	Minimal or no lanugo (depends on parental ethnicity)
Muscle tone	Hypotonia; extension of arms and legs	Hypertonia; well flexed
Posture	Froglike	Attitude of general flexion
Head lag	Head lags; arms have little or no flexion	Head follows trunk; strong arm flexion
Scarf sign	Elbow can extend to opposite axilla	Elbow to midline only; infant resists
Square window	90 degrees	0 degrees
Ankle dorsiflexion	90 degrees	0 degrees
Popliteal angle	180 degrees	<90 degrees
Heel-to-ear maneuver	Touches ear easily	90 degrees
Ventral suspension	Hypotonia; "rag-doll"	Good caudal and cephalic tone
Reflexes		
Moro	Apparent at 28 wk; good, but no adduction	Complete reflex with adduction; disappears 4 mo postterm
Grasp	Fair at 28 wk; arm is involved at 32 wk	Strong enough to sustain weight for a few seconds when pulled up; hand, arm, shoulder involved
Cry	24 wk: weak; 28 wk: high-pitched; 32 wk: good	Lusty; can persist for some time
Length	Under 47 cm (18 $1/2$ inches), usually	50 cm (20 in); range: 18–22 inches
Weight	Under 2500 g (5 lb 5 oz)	3400 g (7 $1/2$ lb); range: 5 lb 8 oz–8 lb 13 oz

◆ **B. Analysis/nursing diagnosis:**
1. *Altered health maintenance* related to separation from maternal support system.
2. *Impaired skin integrity* related to umbilical stump; incontinence of urine and meconium stool; skin penetration by scalp electrode, injections, heel stick, scalpel during cesarean birth; abrasion from obstetric forceps.
3. *Ineffective airway clearance* related to excessive mucus.
4. *Pain* related to environmental stimuli.
5. *Ineffective thermoregulation* related to immature temperature regulation mechanism.

◆ **C. Nursing care plan/implementation:**
1. Goal: *promote effective gas transport.*
   a. Maintain patent airway—to promote effective gas exchange and respiratory function.
   b. *Position:* right side-lying, head dependent (gravity drainage of fluid, mucus).
   c. Suction prn with bulb syringe for mucus.
2. Goal: *establish/maintain thermal stability.*
   a. *Avoid* chilling—to prevent metabolic acidosis.

b. Dry, wrap, and apply hat.
c. Place in heated crib.
d. Monitor vital signs hourly until stable.
3. *Goal: reduce possibility of blood loss.*
   a. Check cord clamp for security.
   b. Administer vitamin K injection, as ordered, in anterior or lateral thigh muscle—to stimulate blood coagulability.
4. *Goal: prevent infection.*
   a. Administer antibiotic treatment to eyes (if not performed in birth room)—to prevent ophthalmia neonatorum.
   b. Treat cord stump (alcohol), as ordered.
   c. Use standard precautions.
5. *Goal: promote comfort and cleanliness.* Admission bath when temperature stable.
6. *Goal: promote nutrition, hydration, elimination.*
   a. Encourage breastfeeding within 1 hr after birth.
   b. Check blood sugar (Dextrostix or Chem-strip) at 30 min, 1, 2, and 4 hr for infants at risk for hypoglycemia (e.g., SGA, LGA, IDM).
   c. First feeding at 1–4 hr of age with sterile water (or formula) if permissible and if not breastfeeding.
   d. Note voiding or meconium stool; report if failure to void or defecate within 24 hr.
7. *Goal: promote bonding.*
   a. Encourage parent-infant interaction (holding, touching, eye contact, talking to infant).
   b. Encourage breastfeeding within 1 hr of birth, if applicable.
   c. Encourage parent participation in infant care—to develop confidence and competence in caring for newborn.
     (1) Assist with initial efforts at feeding.
     (2) Discuss and demonstrate positioning and burping techniques.
     (3) Demonstrate/assist with basic care procedures, as necessary:
       (a) Bath.
       (b) Cord care.
       (c) Diapering.
       (d) Aid parents in distinguishing normal vs. abnormal newborn characteristics.
8. *Goal: health teaching*—to provide anticipatory guidance for discharge.

a. Facilitate sibling bonding.
b. Describe/discuss normal newborn behavior:

> (1) *Sleeping*—almost continual (wakes only to feed) or 12–16 hr daily.
> (2) *Feeding*—from every 2–3 hr to longer intervals; establish own pattern; babies who are breastfed feed more often.
> (3) *Weight loss*—5%–10% in first few days; regained in 7–14 days.
> (4) *Stools*—(**Table 4.17**).
> (5) *Cord care*—drops off in 7–10 days
>   (a) Keep clean and dry.
>   (b) Alcohol may be applied to stump, or it may be allowed to dry naturally.
>   (c) HIV precautions.
> (6) *Circumcision care*
>   (a) Keep clean and dry; heals rapidly.
>   (b) Watch for bleeding.
>   (c) Petroleum jelly, gauze prn, if ordered.
>   (d) Do *not* remove yellowish exudate.

(7) *Physiological jaundice*—occurs 24–72 hr after birth.
  (a) Nonpathologic.
  (b) Need for hydration.
(8) Identify need for newborn screen test after ingestion of milk (done routinely at 24 hr of age and later). Includes screen for congenital hypothyroidism and galactosemia. (See **Table 11.2, Unit 11,** for other newborn screening procedures.)
(9) Describe suggested sensory *stimulation* modalities (mobiles, color, music).
(10) Discuss *safety* precautions:
  (a) Position on back for sleep.
  (b) Infant seat for travel and home safety.
  (c) Maintaining contact/control over infant to prevent falls, drowning in bath.
  (d) Instruct parents in infant cardiopulmonary resuscitation (CPR).
  (e) *Hepatitis B vaccination*—first dose can be given 24–48 hr of life; second dose 1 mo; third dose 6 mo. If infant born to mother who is infected, hepatitis B vaccine and hepatitis B immune globulin should be administered within 12 hr of birth.

Maternal-Infant

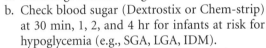

TABLE 4.17	Infant Stool Characteristics		
Age	**Bottle-fed**	**Breastfed**	**Implications of Abnormal Patterns**
1 day	Meconium	Meconium	Absence may indicate obstruction, atresia
2–5 days (transitional)	Greenish yellow, loose	Greenish yellow, loose, frequent	*Note*—At any time:
>5 days	Yellow to brown, firm, 2–4 daily, foul odor	Bright golden yellow, loose, 6–10 daily	*Diarrhea*—greenish, mucus or blood tinged, or forceful expulsion, may indicate infection *Constipation*—dry, hard stools or infrequent or absent stools may indicate obstruction

(11) Describe signs of common health problems to be reported promptly:
  (a) Diarrhea, constipation.
  (b) Colic, vomiting.
  (c) Rash, jaundice.
  (d) Differentiation from normal patterns.

◆ **D. Evaluation/outcome criteria:**
1. Infant demonstrates successful transition to independent life:
   a. Breastfeeds well.
   b. Normal feeding, sleeping, elimination patterns.
   c. No evidence of infection or abnormality.

2. Mother/family evidences bonding.
   a. Eye contact.
   b. Stroking, cuddling.
   c. Crooning, calling baby by name, talking to infant.
3. Mother demonstrates comfort and skill in basic newborn care.
4. Mother verbalizes understanding of subjects discussed:
   a. Safety precautions.
   b. Health maintenance actions.
   c. Signs of normal infant behavior and health.

CLINICAL PATHWAY 4.3: Newborn Care

Category	First 4 Hours	4–8 Hours Past Birth	8–24 Hours Past Birth
Referral	Review labor/birth record Review transitional nursing record Check ID bands Prn consults: orthopedics, genetics, infectious disease	Check ID bands Transfer to mother/baby care at 4–6 hours of age if stable As parents desire, obtain circumcision permit after their discussion with physician Lactation consult prn	Check ID bands every shift **Expected Outcomes:** Mother/baby ID bands correlate at time of discharge; consults completed prn
◆ **Assessments**	Continue assessments begun first hour after birth. *Vital signs:* TPR (q1h × 4), *BP* prn (skin temp 97.8–98.6°F, resp. may be irregular but within 30–60 per min) **Newborn Assessments:** ■ *Respiratory status* with resp. distress scale × 1 then prn. If resp. distress, assess q5–15min ■ *Cord*—bluish white color, clamp in place ■ *Color:* skin, mucous membranes, extremities; trunk pink with slight acrocyanosis of hands and feet ■ Wt (5 lb 8 oz–8 lb 13 oz), length (18–22 inches), HC (12.5–14.5 inches), CC (32.5 cm, 1–2 cm less than head) ■ Extremity movement—may be jerky or brief twitches ■ Gestational age classification—preterm, term, postmature, AGA, SGA, LGA, IUGR ■ Anomalies (cong. anomalies can interfere with normal extrauterine adaptation)	Assess newborn's progress through periods of reactivity *Vital signs:* TPR q8hr and prn, BP prn **Newborn Assessments:** ■ *Skin color* q4h prn (circulatory system stabilizing, acrocyanosis decreased) ■ *Eyes* for drainage, redness, hemorrhage ■ Ausculate *lungs* q4h (noisy, wet resp. normal) ■ Increased mucus production (normal in second period of reactivity) ■ Check *apical pulse* q4h ■ Umbilical cord base for redness, drainage, foul odor, drying, clamp in place ■ Extremity movement q4h ■ Check for expected reflexes (suck, rooting, Moro, grasp, blink, yawn, sneeze, tonic neck, Babinski) ■ Note common normal variations ■ Assess suck and swallow during feeding ■ Note behavioral characteristics ■ Temp before and after admission bath	*VS* q8hr Normal ranges: T, 97.5–99°F; P, 120–160; R, 30–60; BP, 60–80/40–45 mm Hg **Continue Newborn Assessments:** ■ *Skin color* q4h ■ Signs of drying or infection in cord area ■ Check cord clamp in place until removed before discharge ■ Check circ. for bleeding after procedure, then q30min × 2, then q4hr and prn **Expected Outcomes:** Vital signs medically acceptable, color pink, assessments WNL, circ site without s/sx infection, cord site without s/sx infection and clamp removed; newborn behavior WNL
Teaching/ psychosocial	Admission activities performed at mother's bedside if possible; orient to nursery prn, handwashing, assess teaching needs Teach parents use of bulb syringe, signs of choking, positioning, and when to call for assistance	Reinforce teaching about choking, bulb syringe use, positioning, temperature maintenance with clothing and blankets Teach infant positioning to facilitate breathing and digestion	**Final discharge teaching:** diapering, normal void and stool patterns, bathing, nail and cord care, circumcision/uncircumcised penis/genital care and normal characteristics, rashes, jaundice, sleep/wake cycles, soothing activities, taking temperatures, thermometer reading

(Continued on following page)

Category	First 4 Hours	4–8 Hours Past Birth	8–24 Hours Past Birth
	Teach reasons for use of radiant warmer, infant hat, and warmed blankets when out of warmer Discuss/teach infant security, identification	Teach new parents holding and feeding skills Teach parents soothing and calming techniques	Explain s/sx of illness and when to call health care provider Infant safety: car seats, immunizations, metabolic screening; on back for sleep **Expected Outcomes:** Mother/family verbalize comprehension of teaching; demonstrates care capabilities
Nursing care management and reports	Place under radiant warmer Suction nares/mouth with bulb syringe prn Keep bulb syringe with infant Attach security sensor Obtain lab tests: blood glucose; as needed obtain blood type, Rh, Coombs on cord blood Notify physician's office to exchange info about infant's birth and status Maintain standard precautions	Wean from radiant warmer (T 98°F axillary) Place hat on newborn (decreases convection heat loss); hat off when under warmer Chem-strips prn; BP prn Oxygen saturation prn Bathe infant if temp >97.8°F Position on side Suction nares prn (esp. during second period of reactivity) Obtain peripheral Hct per protocol Cord care per protocol (alcohol or natural drying) Fold diaper below cord (for plastic diapers, turn plastic layer away from skin)	Check for hearing test results Weigh before discharge Cord care every shift DC cord clamp before discharge Perform newborn metabolic screening blood tests before discharge Circumcision if indicated. Circumcision care: change diaper prn noting ability to void; follow policy for Gomco or Plastibell care **Expected Outcomes:** Newborn maintains temp, lab test WNL, cord dry without s/sx infection and clamp removed; screening tests accomplished; circ. site without s/sx infection or bleeding
Activity and comfort	Place under radiant warmer or wrap in prewarmed blankets until stable Soothe baby as needed with voice, touch, cuddling, nesting in warmer	Leave in warmer until stable, then swaddle Position on side after each feeding	Place in open crib Swaddle to allow movement of extremities in blanket, including hands to face **Expected Outcomes:** Infant maintains temp WNL in open crib; infant attempts self-calming
Nutrition	Assist newborn to breastfeed as soon as mother/baby condition allows Supplement breast only when medically indicated or per agency policy Initiate bottle-feeding within first hour Gavage feed, SNS, or finger feed, if necessary to prevent hypoglycemia	Breastfeed on demand, at least q3–4hr Teach positions, observe/assist with feeding, breast/nipple care, establishing milk supply, breaking suction, feeding cues, latching on techniques, nutritive suck, burping Bottle-feed on demand, at least q3–6hr Determine readiness to feed and feeding tolerance	Continue breast/bottle-feeding pattern Assess feeding tolerance q4hr Discuss normal feeding requirements, signs of hunger and satiation, handling feeding problems, and when to seek help **Expected Outcomes:** Mother verbalizes knowledge of feeding information; breastfeeds on demand without supplement; bottle—tolerates formula feeding, nipples without problems
Elimination	Note first void and stool if not noted at birth	Note all voids, amount and color of stools q4hr	Evaluate all voids and stools color q8hr **Expected Outcomes:** Voids qs; stools qs without difficulty; stool character WNL; diaper area without s/s skin breakdown or rashes
Medications	Prophylactic ophthalmic ointment OU after baby makes eye contact with parents within 1 hr after birth Administer Aquamephyton IM, dosage according to infant weight per MD/NP order	Hepatitis B injection as ordered by physician after consent signed by parents	Hepatitis B vaccine before discharge **Expected Outcomes:** Baby has received ophthalmic ointment and vitamin K injection; baby has received first hepatitis B vaccine if ordered and parental permission received

(Continued on following page)

Maternal-Infant

CLINICAL PATHWAY 4.3: **Newborn Care** *(Continued)*

Category	First 4 Hours	4–8 Hours Past Birth	8–24 Hours Past Birth
Discharge planning/home care	Hepatitis B consent signed Hearing screen consent signed (if needed) Plan discharge call with parent or guardian in 24 hr to 2 days Assess parents' discharge plans, needs, and support systems	Review/reinforce teaching with mother and significant other Review home preparedness Obtain birth certificate information	Initial newborn screening tests (hearing, blood tests, NBS) before discharge Bath and feeding classes, videos, or written information given Give written copy of discharge instructions Newborn photographs Have car seat available before discharge All discharge referrals made, follow-up appt. scheduled **Expected Outcomes:** Infant discharged home with family; mother verbalizes follow-up appt. time/date
Family involvement	Facilitate early investigation of baby's physical characteristics (maintain temp during unwrapping), hold infant en face Dim lights to help infant keep eyes open	Assess parents' knowledge of newborn behaviors, such as alertness, suck and rooting, attention to human voice, response to calming techniques	Assess mother-baby bonding/interaction Incorporate father and siblings in care Enhance parent-infant interaction by sharing characteristics and behavioral assessment Support positive parenting behaviors Identify community referral needs and refer to community agencies **Expected Outcomes:** Demonstrates caring and family incorporation of infant

Source: Maternal-Newborn Nursing (6th ed), by Olds, London, Ladewig © 2000. Pp. 754–755. Reprinted by permission of Prentice Hall, Inc., Upper Saddle River, NJ.

Complications During the Neonatal Period: The High-Risk Newborn

I. **General overview**—successful newborn adaptation to the demands of independent extrauterine life may be complicated by environmental insults during the *prenatal* period or those arising in the period immediately surrounding birth. The nursing role focuses on minimizing the effect of present and emerging health problems and on facilitating and supporting a successful transition to extrauterine life.

II. **General aspects**—common neonatal risk factors:
  A. Gestational age profile (see **Tables 4.14** and **4.16**):
    1. Prematurity.
    2. Dysmaturity.
    3. Postmaturity.
  B. Congenital disorders.
  C. Birth trauma.
  D. Infections.

III. **Disorders affecting protective functions: neonatal infections**
  A. **Assess for intrauterine infections.**
  B. **Oral thrush (mycotic stomatitis).**
    1. **Pathophysiology**—local inflammation of oral mucosa due to fungal infection.
    2. **Etiology:**
      a. Organism—*Candida albicans.*
      b. More common in newborn who is vulnerable (i.e., sick, debilitated; those receiving antibiotic therapy).
    3. Mode of transmission—direct contact with:
      a. Maternal birth canal, hands, and linens.
      b. Contaminated feeding equipment, staff's hands.
  ◆ 4. **Assessment:**
      a. White patches on oral mucosa, gums, and tongue that bleed when touched.
      b. Occasional difficulty swallowing.
  ◆ 5. **Analysis/nursing diagnosis:**
      a. *Pain* related to irritation of oral mucous membrane secondary to oral moniliasis.
      b. *Altered nutrition, less than body requirements* related to irritability and poor feeding.
  ◆ 6. **Nursing care plan/implementation:**
      Goal: *prevent cross-contamination.*
       a. Aseptic technique; good handwashing.
      b. Give medications as ordered:
        (1) Aqueous gentian violet, 1%–2%: apply to infected area with swab.
        (2) Nystatin (Mycostatin)—instill into mouth with medicine dropper, or apply to lesions with swab, *after* feedings. *Note:* Before medicating, feed sterile water to rinse out milk.
  ◆ 7. **Evaluation/outcome criteria:**
      a. Oral mucosa intact, lesions healed, no evidence of infection.

b. Feeds well; maintains weight or regains weight lost, if any.

C. **Neonatal sepsis**

1. **Pathophysiology**—generalized infection; may overwhelm infant's immature immune system.

2. **Etiology:**

   a. Prolonged rupture of membranes.

   b. Long, difficult labor.

   c. Resuscitation procedures.

   d. Maternal infection (e.g., beta-hemolytic streptococcus vaginosis).

   e. Aspiration—amniotic fluid, formula, mucus.

   f. Iatrogenic (nosocomial)—caused by infected health personnel or equipment.

3. **Assessment:**

   a. Respirations—irregular, periods of apnea.

   b. Irritability or lethargy.

4. **Analysis/nursing diagnosis:**

   a. *Fatigue* related to increased oxygen needs.

   b. *High risk for infection* related to septic condition.

5. **Nursing care plan/implementation:**

    a. Cultures (spinal, urine, blood).

   b. Check vitals.

   c. Monitor respirations.

   d. Give medications, as ordered.

6. **Evaluation/outcome criteria:**

   a. Responds to medical/nursing regimen (all assessment findings within normal limits).

   b. Parent(s) verbalize understanding of diagnosis, treatment; demonstrate appropriate techniques in participating in care (as possible).

   c. Parent(s) demonstrate effective coping with situation; express satisfaction with care.

IV. **Disorders affecting nutrition: infant of the diabetic mother (IDM)**

A. **Pathophysiology**—hyperplasia of pancreatic beta cells → increased insulin production → excessive deposition of glycogen in muscles, subcutaneous fat, and tissue growth. Results in fetal:

1. *Macrosomia*—LGA infant.

2. *Enlarged internal organs*—common.

   a. Cardiomegaly.

   b. Hepatomegaly.

   c. Splenomegaly.

3. Neonatal—inadequate carbohydrate reserve to meet energy needs.

4. Associated with *increased incidence of:*

   a. Congenital anomalies (five times average incidence with pregestational diabetes) includes cardiac, pelvic, and spinal anomalies.

   b. Preterm birth: respiratory distress syndrome (RDS); increased insulin needs prenatally lead to decreased surfactant production.

   c. Fetal dystocia—due to CPD.

   d. Neonatal metabolic problems:

      (1) Hypoglycemia.

      (2) Hypocalcemic tetany.

      (3) Metabolic acidosis.

      (4) Hyperbilirubinemia.

B. **Etiology**—high circulating maternal glucose levels during fetal growth and development; loss of maternal glucose supply following birth; decreased hepatic gluconeogenesis.

C. **Assessment:**

1. Characteristics of IDM.

    2. Hypoglycemia—Dextrostix or Chem-strip to heelstick at:

   a. 30 min × 2.

   b. 1, 2, and 4 hr of age; before meals × 4 or until stable.

   c. Chem-strip: if <20 mg/dL, must draw glucose STAT.

   d. Hypoglycemia laboratory values for preterm and term infants: under 45 mg/dL.

   e. Behavioral signs—tremors; twitching, hypotonia, seizures.

3. Gestational age, since macrosomia may mask prematurity.

4. Hypocalcemia—usually within first 24 hr

   a. Irritability.

   b. Coarse tremors, twitching, convulsions.

5. Birth injuries:

   a. Fractures: clavicle, humerus, skull.

   b. Brachial palsy.

   c. Intracranial hemorrhage/signs of increased intracranial pressure.

   d. Cephalohematoma.

6. Respiratory distress:

   a. Nasal flaring.

   b. Expiratory grunt.

   c. Sternal retraction.

   d. Intercostal retractions.

   e. Cyanosis—central.

7. Jaundice.

D. **Analysis/nursing diagnosis:**

1. *High risk for injury* related to CPD, dystocia.

2. *Altered cardiopulmonary tissue perfusion* related to placental insufficiency, RDS.

3. *Impaired gas exchange* related to RDS.

4. *Altered nutrition, less than body requirements,* related to hypoglycemia, hypocalcemia.

5. *Risk for altered endocrine/metabolic processes* related to hyperbilirubinemia and kernicterus.

E. **Nursing care plan/implementation:**

1. Hypoglycemia—administer formula or IV glucose, as ordered (may cause rebound effect).

2. Preterm/immature—institute preterm care prn.

3. Hypocalcemia—administer oral or IV calcium gluconate, as ordered.

4. Inform pediatrician **immediately** of signs of:

   a. Jaundice.

   b. Hyperirritability.

   c. Birth injury.

   d. Increased intracranial pressure/hemorrhage

F. **Evaluation/outcome criteria:**

1. Infant makes successful transition to extrauterine life.

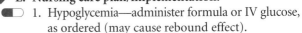

2. Infant responds to medical/nursing regimen. Experiences minimal or no metabolic disturbances (hypoglycemia, hypocalcemia, hyperbilirubinemia).

3. Infant exhibits normal respiratory function and gas exchange.

V. **Hypoglycemia**

A. **Pathophysiology**—low serum-glucose level → altered cellular metabolism → cerebral irritability, cardiopulmonary problems.

B. **Etiology:**

1. Loss of maternal glucose supply.

2. Normal physiological activities of respiration, thermoregulation, muscular activity exceed carbohydrate reserve.

3. Decreased hepatic ability to convert amino acids into glucose.

4. More common in:

  a. Infants of diabetic mothers.

  b. Preterm, postterm infants.

  c. SGA infants.

  d. Smaller twin.

  e. Infant of mother with preeclampsia.

  f. Birth asphyxia.

◆ C. **Assessment:**

1. Jitteriness, tremors, convulsions; lethargy and hypotonia.

2. Sweating; unstable temperature.

3. Tachypnea; apneic episodes; cyanosis.

4. High-pitched, shrill cry.

5. Difficulty feeding.

◆ D. **Analysis/nursing diagnosis:**

1. *Altered tissue perfusion (fetal)* related to placental insufficiency associated with maternal diabetes, preeclampsia, renal or cardiac disorders; erythroblastosis.

2. *Risk for altered endocrine metabolic processes* related to high incidence of morbidity associated with birth asphyxia.

3. *Impaired gas exchange* related to coexisting RDS.

4. *Altered nutrition, less than body requirements,* related to hypoglycemia.

5. *High risk for injury* related to coexisting infection, metabolic acidosis.

◆ E. **Nursing care plan/implementation** (see **IV. infant of the diabetic mother, p. 235**).

◆ F. **Evaluation/outcome criteria** (see **IV. infant of the diabetic mother, p. 235**).

VI. **Disorders affecting psychosocial-cultural functions: neonate who is drug-dependent (heroin)**

A. **General aspects**

1. Maternal drug addiction has been associated with:

  a. Prenatal malnutrition and vitamin deficiencies.

  b. Increased risk of antepartal infections.

  c. Higher incidence of antepartal and intrapartal complications.

2. Infant at risk for:

  a. Intrauterine growth retardation (IUGR).

  b. Prematurity.

  c. Fetal distress.

  d. Perinatal death.

  e. Child abuse.

  f. Sudden infant death syndrome (SIDS) (5–10 times higher than normal).

  g. Learning and behavior disorders.

  h. Poor social adjustment.

B. **Pathophysiology**—withdrawal of accustomed drug levels → physiological deprivation response.

C. **Etiology**—repeated intrauterine absorption of heroin/cocaine/methadone from maternal bloodstream → fetal drug dependency.

◆ D. **Assessment**—degree of withdrawal depends on type and duration of addiction and maternal drug levels at birth.

1. Irritability, hyperactivity, hypertonicity, exaggerated reflexes, tremors, high-pitched cry, difficult to comfort:

  a. *"Step" reflex* (dancing)—infant places both feet on surface; assumes rigid stance—does not "step" or dance.

  b. *"Head-righting" reflex*—holds head rigid; fails to demonstrate head-lag.

2. Nasal stuffiness and sneezing; respiratory distress, tachypnea, cyanosis, or apnea.

3. Exaggerated acrocyanosis or mottling in the infant who is warm.

4. Sweating.

5. Hunger—sucks on fists; feeding problems—regurgitation, vomiting, poor feeding, diarrhea, and increased mucus production.

6. Convulsions with abnormal eye-rolling and chewing motions.

7. Developmental lags/mental retardation.

◆ E. **Analysis/nursing diagnosis:**

1. *High risk for injury* related to convulsions secondary to physiological response to withdrawal, CNS hyperirritability.

2. *Impaired gas exchange* related to respiratory distress secondary to inhibition of reflex clearing of fluid by the lungs.

3. *Altered nutrition, less than body requirements,* related to feeding problems secondary to respiratory distress and GI hypermotility.

4. *High risk for impaired skin integrity* related to scratching secondary to withdrawal symptoms.

◆ F. **Nursing care plan/implementation:**

1. Goal: *prevent/minimize respiratory distress.*

  a. *Position:* side-lying, head dependent—to facilitate mucus drainage.

  b. Suction prn with bulb syringe for excess mucus—to maintain patent airway.

  c. Monitor respirations and apical pulse.

2. Goal: *minimize possibility of convulsions.*

  a. Decrease environmental stimuli—quiet, touch only when necessary, offer pacifier.

  b. Keep warm, swaddle for comfort.

3. Goal: *maintain nutrition/hydration.*

a. Food/fluids—oral or IV, as ordered.

b. I&O.

c. Daily weight.

4. Goal: *assist in diagnosis of drug and drug level.* Collect all urine and meconium during first 24 hr for toxicologic studies.

5. Goal: *maintain/promote skin integrity.*

a. Mitts over hands—to minimize scratching.

b. Keep clean and dry.

c. Medicated ointment/powder, as ordered, q2–4hr, to excoriated areas.

d. Expose excoriated areas to air.

6. Goal: *minimize withdrawal symptoms.* Administer medications, as ordered.

a. Paregoric elixir—to wean from drug.

b. Phenobarbital—to reduce CNS hyperirritability, hyperbilirubinemia.

c. Chlorpromazine (Thorazine), diazepam (Valium)—to tranquilize, reduce hyperirritability. *Note:* Valium is **contraindicated** for the neonate who is jaundiced because it predisposes to hyperbilirubinemia.

d. Methadone.

7. Goal: *emotional support to mother.*

a. Encourage verbalization of feelings of guilt, anxiety, fear, concerns.

b. Refer to social service.

◆ **G. Evaluation/outcome criteria:**

1. Infant responds to medical/nursing regimen.

a. Maintains adequate respirations.

b. Feeds well, gains weight.

c. No evidence of CNS hyperirritability, convulsions; demonstrates normal newborn reflexes.

2. Infant evidences bonding with parent(s). Responsive to mother's voice.

VII. Disorders affecting psychosocial-cultural function: fetal alcohol syndrome (FAS). *General aspects:*

A. Maternal alcohol abuse has been associated with:

1. Malnutrition, vitamin deficiencies.

2. Bone marrow suppression.

3. Liver disease.

4. Child abuse.

B. Infant at risk for:

1. Congenital anomalies (FAS).

2. Mental deficiency; learning disabilities.

3. IUGR.

C. Pathophysiology—permanent damage to developing embryonic/fetal structures; cardiovascular anomalies (ventricular septal defects).

D. Etiology—high circulating alcohol levels are lethal to the embryo; lower levels cause permanent cell damage.

◆ **E. Assessment:**

1. Characteristic craniofacial abnormalities:

a. Short, palpebral fissure.

b. Epicanthal folds.

c. Maxillary hypoplasia.

d. Micrognathia.

e. Long, thin upper lip.

2. Short stature.

3. Irritable, hyperactive, poor feeding.

4. High-pitched cry, difficult to comfort.

◆ **F. Nursing care plan/implementation:**

1. Goal: *reduce irritability.*

a. Reduce environmental stimuli.

b. Wrap, cuddle.

c. Administer sedatives, as ordered.

2. Goal: *maintain nutrition/hydration.*

3. Goal: *emotional support to mother.*

◆ **G. Evaluation/outcome criteria:** (see **VI. neonate who is drug-dependent (heroin), p. 236**).

1. No respiratory distress.

2. Infant feeding properly.

3. Maternal bonding apparent.

4. Social service—home involvement.

VIII. Classification of infants by weight and gestational age

A. Terminology

1. *Preterm, or premature*—37 wk gestation or less (usually 2500 g [5 lb] or less).

2. *Term*—38–42 wk gestation.

3. *Postterm*—over 42 wk.

4. *Postmature*—gestation greater than 42 wk.

5. *Appropriate for gestational age (AGA)*—for each week of gestation, there is a normal range of expected weight (between 10th and 90th percentile).

a. Term infants weighing 2500 g or more are usually mature in physiological functions.

b. If respiratory distress occurs, it is usually related to meconium aspiration syndrome.

6. *SGA or dysmature*—weight falls *below* normal range for age (<10th percentile).

a. Preeclampsia.

b. Malnutrition.

c. Smoking.

d. Placental insufficiency.

e. Alcohol syndrome.

f. Rubella.

g. Syphilis.

h. Multifetal gestation (twins, etc.).

i. Genetic.

j. Cocaine abuse.

7. *LGA*—*above* expected weight for age (>90th percentile). *Note:* If **preterm,** at risk for **RDS.** If **postterm,** at risk for **aspiration** and **sudden intrauterine death.**

a. **Etiology:**

(1) Maternal diabetes or prediabetes.

(2) Maternal weight gain over 35 lb.

(3) Maternal obesity.

(4) Genetic.

b. *Associated problems:*

(1) Hypoglycemia.

(2) Hypocalcemia.

(3) Hyperbilirubinemia.

(4) Birth injury (e.g., fractures, Erb-Duchenne paralysis).

B. *Estimation of gestational age*—planning appropriate care for the newborn requires accurate assessment to differentiate between preterm and term infants.

PRETERM INFANT — Born at 37 weeks of gestation or less.

A. **Pathophysiology**—anatomical and physiological immaturity of body systems compromises ability to adapt to extrauterine environment and independent life.
  1. *Interference with* **protective** *functions*
     a. *Temperature regulation*—unstable, due to:
        (1) Lack of subcutaneous fat.
        (2) Large body surface area in proportion to body weight.
        (3) Small muscle mass.
        (4) Absent sweat or shiver responses.
        (5) Poor capillary response to changes in environmental temperature.
     b. *Resistance to infection*—low, due to:
        (1) Lack of immune bodies from mother (these cross placenta *late* in pregnancy).
        (2) Inability to produce own immune bodies (immature liver).
        (3) Poor WBC response to infection.
     c. *Immature liver*
        (1) Inability to conjugate bilirubin liberated by normal breakdown of RBCs→ increased susceptibility to hyperbilirubinemia and kernicterus.
        (2) Immature production of clotting factors and immune globulins.
        (3) Inadequate glucose stores→increased susceptibility to hypoglycemia.
  2. *Interference with* **elimination:** immature *renal* function—unable to concentrate urine → precarious fluid/electrolyte balance.
  3. *Interference with* **sensory-perceptual functions:** CNS—immature → weak or absent reflexes and fluctuating primitive control of vital functions.
B. **Etiology:** often unknown; preterm labor.
  1. *Iatrogenic*—EDD miscalculated for repeat cesarean birth (rare).
  2. *Placental factors*
     a. Placenta previa.
     b. Abruptio placentae.
     c. Placental insufficiency.
  3. *Uterine factors*
     a. Incompetent cervix.
     b. Overdistention (multifetal gestation, polyhydramnios).
     c. Anomalies (e.g., myomas).
  4. *Fetal factors*
     a. Malformations.
     b. Infections (rubella, toxoplasmosis, HIV-positive status, AIDS, cytomegalic inclusion disease).
     c. Multifetal gestations (twins, triplets).
  5. *Maternal factors*
     a. Severe physical or emotional trauma.
     b. Coexisting disorders (preeclampsia, hypertension, heart disease, diabetes, malnutrition).
     c. Infections (streptococcus, syphilis, bacterial vaginosis, pyelonephritis, pneumonia, influenza, leukemia, UTI).
  6. *Miscellaneous factors*
     a. Close frequency of pregnancies.
     b. Advanced maternal age.
     c. Heavy smoking.
     d. High-altitude environment.
     e. Cocaine use.
C. Factors influencing survival:
  1. Gestational age.
  2. Lung maturity.
  3. Anomalies.
  4. Size.
D. Causes of mortality (in order of frequency):
  1. Abnormal pulmonary ventilation.
  2. Infection.
     a. Pneumonia.
     b. Septicemia.
     c. Diarrhea.
     d. Meningitis.
  3. Intracranial hemorrhage.
  4. Congenital defects.
E. **Disorders affecting fluid-gas transport: RDS**
  1. **Pathophysiology**—insufficient pulmonary surfactant (lecithin) and insufficient number/maturity of alveoli predispose to atelectasis; alveolar ducts and terminal bronchi become lined with fibrous, glossy membrane.
  2. **Etiology:**
     a. Primarily associated with prematurity.
     b. Other *predisposing* factors:
        (1) Fetal hypoxia—due to decreased placental perfusion secondary to maternal bleeding (e.g., abruptio) or hypotension.
        (2) Birth asphyxia.
        (3) Postnatal hypothermia, metabolic acidosis, or hypotension.
  3. Factors *protecting* neonate from RDS:
     a. Chronic fetal stress—due to maternal hypertension, preeclampsia, or heroin addiction.
     b. PROM.
     c. Maternal steroid ingestion (e.g., betamethasone).
     d. Low-grade chorioamnionitis.
  ◆ 4. **Assessment:**
     a. Usually appears during first or second day after birth.
     b. Signs of *respiratory distress:*
        (1) Nasal flaring.
        (2) Expiratory grunt.
        (3) Sternal retractions.
        (4) Tachypnea (60 beats/min or more).
        (5) Cyanosis—central.
        (6) Increasing number and length of apneic episodes.
        (7) Increasing exhaustion.

c. *Respiratory acidosis*—due to hypercapnea and rising CO_2 level.

d. *Metabolic acidosis*—due to increased lactic acid levels and falling pH.

◆ 5. **Analysis/nursing diagnosis:**

a. *Impaired gas exchange* related to lack of pulmonary surfactant secondary to preterm birth, intrapartal stress and hypoxia, infection, postnatal hypothermia, metabolic acidosis, or hypotension.

b. *Altered nutrition, less than body requirements*, related to poor feeding secondary to respiratory distress, ↑ caloric demand.

◆ 6. **Nursing care plan/implementation:**

a. Goal: *reduce metabolic acidosis, increase oxygenation, support respiratory efforts.*

(1) Ensure warmth (isolette at 97.6°F).

▶ (2) Warmed, humidified O_2 at lowest concentration required to relieve cyanosis, through hood, nasal prongs, or endotracheal tube.

▶ (3) Monitor *continuous positive airway pressure (CPAP)*—oxygen–air mixture administered under pressure during inhalation *and* exhalation to maintain alveolar patency.

◪ (4) *Position:* side-lying or supine with neck slightly extended ("sniffing" position); arms at sides.

▶ (5) Suction prn with bulb syringe—for excessive mucus.

▶ b. Goal: *modify care for infant with endotracheal tube.*

(1) Disconnect tubing at adapter.

(2) Inject 0.5 mL sterile normal saline (may be omitted).

(3) Insert sterile suction tube, start suction, rotate tube, withdraw.

(4) Suction up to 5 sec.

(5) Ventilate with bag and mask during procedure.

(6) Reconnect tubing securely to adapter.

(7) Auscultate for breath sounds and pulse.

c. Goal: *maintain nutrition/hydration.*

(1) Administer fluids, electrolytes, calories, vitamins, minerals PO or IV, as ordered.

(2) I&O.

d. Goal: *prevent secondary infections.*

(1) Strict aseptic technique.

(2) Handwashing.

e. Goal: *emotional support of infant.*

(1) Gentle touching.

(2) Soft voices.

(3) Eye contact.

(4) Rocking.

f. Goal: *emotional support of parents.*

(1) Keep informed of status and progess.

(2) Encourage contact with infant—to promote bonding, understanding of treatment.

g. Goal: *minimize possibility of iatrogenic disorders associated with oxygen therapy* (see **F.** and **G.**).

◆ 7. **Evaluation/outcome criteria:**

a. Respiratory distress treated successfully; infant breathes without assistance.

b. Infant completes successful transition to extrauterine life.

F. **Iatrogenic (oxygen toxicity) disorders: retinopathy of prematurity**

1. **Pathophysiology**—intraretinal hemorrhage → fibrosis → retinal detachment → loss of vision.

2. **Etiology**—prolonged exposure to high concentrations of oxygen.

3. **Assessment**—only perceptible retinal change is vasoconstriction.

Note: Arterial blood (PaO_2) gas readings less than 50 or more than 80 mm Hg.

◆ 4. **Nursing care plan/implementation:** Goal: *prevent disorder.* Maintain PaO_2 of 50–70 mm Hg.

◆ 5. **Evaluation/outcome criteria:**

a. Successful recovery from respiratory distress.

b. No evidence of retinopathy.

G. **Iatrogenic (oxygen toxicity) disorders: bronchopulmonary dysplasia (BPD)**

1. **Pathophysiology**—damage to alveolar cells result in focal emphysema.

2. **Etiology**—positive pressure ventilation (CPAP and PEEP) and prolonged administration of high concentrations of oxygen.

◆ 3. **Assessment**—monitor for signs of:

a. Tachypnea.

b. Increased respiratory effort.

c. Respiratory distress.

◆ 4. **Nursing care plan/implementation:**
Goal: *prevent disorder*

▶ a. Use of *positive* pressure devices.

▶ b. Maintain oxygen concentration *below 80%*.

c. Supportive care.

d. Wean off ventilator, as possible.

◆ 5. **Evaluation/outcome criteria:**

a. Successful recovery from respiratory distress.

b. No evidence of disorder.

H. **Intraventricular hemorrhage**

1. **Pathophysiology**—rupture of thin, fragile capillary walls within ventricles of the brain (more common in preterm).

2. **Etiology:**

a. Hypoxia.

b. Respiratory distress.

c. Birth trauma.

d. Birth asphyxia.

e. Hypercapnia.

◆ 3. **Assessment:**

a. Hypotonia.

b. Lethargy.

c. Hypothermia.

Maternal-Infant

d. Bradycardia.

e. Bulging fontanels.

f. Respiratory distress or apnea.

g. Seizures.

h. Cry: high-pitched whining.

◆ 4. **Nursing care plan/implementation:** Goal: *supportive care*—to promote healing.

a. Monitor vital signs.

b. Maintain thermal stability.

▶ c. Ensure adequate oxygenation (may be placed on CPAP).

◆ 5. **Evaluation/outcome criteria:**

a. Condition stable, all assessment findings within normal limits.

b. No evidence of residual damage.

I. Disorders affecting nutrition

1. **Pathophysiology**—underdeveloped feeding abilities, small stomach capacity, immature enzyme system, fat intolerance.

2. **Etiology**—immature body systems associated with preterm birth.

◆ 3. **Assessment:**

a. Weak suck, swallow, gag reflexes—tendency to aspiration.

b. Signs of malabsorption and fat intolerance (abdominal distention, diarrhea, weight loss, or failure to gain weight).

c. Signs of vitamin E deficiency (edema, anemia).

◆ 4. **Analysis/nursing diagnosis:**

a. *Altered nutrition, less than body requirements,* related to poor feeding reflexes, reduced stomach capacity, inability to absorb needed nutrients.

b. *Impaired gas exchange* related to aspiration.

◆ 5. **Nursing care plan/implementation:** Goal: *maintain/increase nutrition.*

🍽 a. Frequent, small feedings—to *avoid* exceeding stomach capacity, facilitate digestion.

b. Frequent "burping" during feeding—to *avoid* regurgitation/aspiration.

💊 c. Supplement vitamin E (alpha-tocopherol) intake, as ordered, in infants who are formula-fed (*Note:* intake adequate in infants who are breastfed.) *Vitamin E actions:*

(1) Antioxidant.

(2) Maintains structure and function of smooth, skeletal, and cardiac muscle.

(3) Maintains structure and function of vascular tissue, liver, and RBC integrity.

(4) Coenzyme in tissue respiration.

(5) Treatment for malnutrition with macrocytic anemia.

d. Encourage parent/family participation.

◆ 6. **Evaluation/outcome criteria:**

a. Feeds well without regurgitation/aspiration.

b. Maintains/gains weight.

c. No evidence of malabsorption, vitamin deficiency.

J. Disorders affecting nutrition/elimination: necrotizing enterocolitis (NEC)

1. **Pathophysiology**—intestinal thrombosis, infarction, autodigestion of mucosal lining, and necrotic lesions; incidence *increased in preterm.*

2. **Etiology**—intestinal ischemia, due to blood shunt to brain and heart in response to:

a. Fetal distress.

b. Fetal/neonatal asphyxia.

c. Neonatal shock.

d. After birth, may result from:

(1) Low cardiac output.

(2) Infusion of hyperosmolar solutions.

e. Complicated by action of enteric bacteria on damaged intestine.

◆ 3. **Assessment**—early identification is **vital.**

a. Abdominal distention or erythema, or both.

b. Poor feeding, vomiting.

🧪 c. Blood in stool.

d. Systemic signs associated with sepsis that may need temporary colostomy or iliostomy:

(1) Lethargy or irritability.

(2) Hypothermia.

(3) Labored respirations or apnea.

(4) Cardiovascular collapse.

e. *Medical diagnosis:*

(1) Increased gastric residual.

🧪 (2) X-ray shows ileus, air in bowel wall.

4. **Analysis/nursing diagnosis:**

a. *Altered nutrition, less than body requirements,* related to inability to tolerate oral feedings, and gastrointestinal dysfunction secondary to ischemia, thrombosis, or necrosis.

b. *Constipation* related to paralytic ileus with stasis; diarrhea related to water loss.

c. *High risk for injury* related to infection, thrombosis, metabolic alterations (acidosis, osmotic diuresis, dehydration, hyperglycemia) due to parenteral nutrition.

d. *Altered parenting* related to physiological compromise and prolonged hospitalization.

e. *Impaired skin integrity* when colostomy is necessary.

◆ 5. **Nursing care plan/implementation:**

a. Goal: *supportive care.*

(1) Rest GI tract: *no oral intake*—to achieve gastric decompression.

💊 (2) IV fluids, as ordered—to maintain hydration.

💊 b. Goal: *prevent infection.* Administer antibiotics, as ordered.

c. Goal: *prevent trauma to skin surrounding stoma.*

◆ 6. **Evaluation/outcome criteria:**

a. Tolerates oral feedings.

b. Demonstrates weight gain.

c. Normal stool pattern.

d. Parents are accepting and knowledgeable about care of infant.

POSTTERM INFANT — Over 42 weeks of gestation.

A. **General aspects**
  1. Labor may be hazardous for mother and fetus because:

    a. Large size of infant contributes to cephalopelvic disproportion; obtain estimate of fetal weight (EFW) by ultrasound.
    b. Placental insufficiency → fetal hypoxia; diagnosis by:
      (1) Contraction stress test.
      (2) Nonstress test.
      (3) Amniotic fluid index (AFI).
    c. Meconium passage (common physiological response) increases chance of meconium aspiration.

◆ B. **Assessment:**
  1. If postmature skin: dry, wrinkled—due to metabolism of fat and glycogen reserves to meet in utero energy needs.
  2. Long limbs, fingernails, and toenails—due to continued growth in utero.
  3. Lanugo and vernix—absent.
  4. Expression: wide-eyed, alert—probably due to chronic hypoxia (oxygen hunger).
  5. Placenta—signs of aging.

◆ C. **Analysis/nursing diagnosis:** *High risk for injury* related to high incidence of morbidity and mortality due to dystocia or hypoxia.

◆ D. **Nursing care plan/implementation:**
  1. **During labor:**
    a. Goal: *emotional support of mother*—may require cesarean birth due to CPD or fetal distress.
    ▶ b. Goal: *continuous electronic monitoring of FHR.* Report *late* decelerations **immediately** (indicate fetal distress).
  2. **After birth:**
    a. Goal: *if born vaginally, prompt identification of birth injuries, respiratory distress.* Continual observation.
    b. Goal: *early identification/treatment of emerging signs of complications.*

      (1) *Hypoglycemia*—Dextrostix readings and behavior.
      (2) Administer oral or intravenous glucose, as ordered.

▶ E. **Evaluation/outcome criterion:** successful transition to extrauterine life (all assessment findings within normal limits).

Congenital Disorders

I. **General overview:** Genetic abnormalities and environmental insults often lead to congenital disorders of the newborn. Successful transition to independent extrauterine life may pose a major challenge to infants compromised by anatomical or physiological disorders. Knowledge regarding the implications of the neonate's structural or metabolic problems enables the nurse to identify early signs of health problems and to plan, provide, and evaluate appropriate outcome-directed care to safeguard the status of the infant with a congenital disorder.

II. **Disorders affecting fluid-gas transport:** *congenital heart disease*

A. **Pathophysiology**—altered hemodynamics, due to persistent fetal circulation or structural abnormalities.
  1. *Acyanotic defects*—no mixing of blood in the systemic circulation.
    a. *Patent ductus arteriosus.*
    b. *Atrial septal defect.*
    c. *Ventriclar septal defect.*
    d. *Coarctation of the aorta.*
  2. *Cyanotic defects*—unoxygenated blood enters systemic circulation.
    a. *Tetralogy of Fallot.*
    b. *Transposition of the great vessels.*

B. **Etiology**—unknown. Associated with maternal:
  1. Prenatal viral disease (e.g., rubella, Coxsackie).
  2. Malnutrition; alcoholism.
  3. Diabetes (poorly controlled).
  4. Ingestion of lithium salts.

◆ C. **Assessment:**
  1. *Patent ductus arteriosus* (see **Figure 5.3, p. 282**).
    a. Characteristic machine murmur, mid to upper left sternal border (cardiomegaly); persists throughout systole and most of diastole; associated with a "thrill."
    b. Widened pulse pressure.
    c. Bounding pulse, tachycardia, "gallop" rhythm.
  2. *Atrial septal defect* (see **Figure 5.1, p. 282**).
    a. Characteristic crescendo/decrescendo systolic ejection murmur.
    b. Fixed S_2 splitting.
    c. Dyspnea, fatigue on normal activity.
    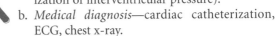
    d. *Medical diagnosis*—cardiac catheterization, x-ray.
  3. *Ventricular septal defect* (see **Figure 5.2, p. 282**).
    a. Loud, harsh, pansystolic murmur; heard best at left lower sternal border; radiates throughout precordium. (*Note:* may be absent—due to high pulmonary vascular resistance → equalization of interventricular pressure).
    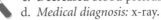
    b. *Medical diagnosis*—cardiac catheterization, ECG, chest x-ray.
  4. *Coarctation of the aorta* (see **p. 284**).
    a. Absent femoral pulse.
    b. Late systolic murmur.
    c. Decreased blood pressure in *lower* extremities.
    d. *Medical diagnosis:* x-ray.
  5. *Tetralogy of Fallot* ("blue" baby) (see **Figure 5.4, p. 282**).
    a. Acute hypoxic/cyanotic episodes.
    b. Limp, sleepy, exhausted; hypotonic extended position—postepisode.

    c. *Medical diagnosis*—cardiac catheterization.

6. Transposition of the great arteries (see **Figure 5.5, p. 283**).
   a. Cyanotic after crying or feeding.
   b. Progressive tachypnea—attempt to compensate for decreased Pao_2, metabolic acidosis.
   c. Heart sounds vary; consistent with defect.
   d. Signs of CHF.
   e. *Medical diagnosis*—cardiac catheterization, x-ray, ECG.
D. Analysis/nursing diagnosis:
   1. *Fluid volume excess* related to persistent fetal circulation, structural abnormalities.
   2. *Impaired gas exchange* related to abnormal circulation, secondary to pathology.
   3. *Altered nutrition, less than body requirements,* related to exhaustion, dyspnea.
E. Nursing care plan/implementation:
   1. Goal: *minimize cardiac workload.*
      a. Minimize crying—snuggle; pacifier—to meet psychological needs.
      b. Keep clean and dry.
   2. Goal: *maintain thermal stability*—to reduce body need for oxygen.
   3. Goal: *prevent infection.*
      a. Strict aseptic technique; standard precautions.
      b. Handwashing.
   4. Goal: *parental emotional support.*
      a. Encourage verbalization of anxiety, fears, concerns.
      b. Keep informed of status.
   5. Goal: *health teaching*—explain, discuss:
      a. Diagnostic procedures.
      b. Treatment procedures.
      c. Basic care modalities.
   6. Goal: *promote bonding.* Encourage to participate in infant care, as possible.
   7. Medical/surgical management: surgical intervention/repair of congenital cardiac abnormality.
F. Evaluation/outcome criteria:
   1. Experiences no respiratory distress in immediate postnatal period.
   2. Completes transfer to high-risk center without incident, if applicable.
   3. Surgical intervention successful, where applicable.
III. Disorders affecting fluid-gas transport: *hemolytic disease of the newborn*
   A. Rh incompatibility
      1. **Pathophysiology** (see **p. 164**).
      2. **Etiology** (see **Rh isoimmunization, p. 164**).
      3. **Assessment:**
         a. *Prenatal*—maternal Rh titers, amniocentesis.
         b. *Intrapartal*—amniotic fluid color:
            (1) Straw-colored: *mild* disease.
            (2) Golden: *severe* fetal disease.
         c. Direct *Coombs' blood;* positive test demonstrates Rh antibodies in fetal blood.
      4. **Nursing care plan/implementation—exchange transfusion:**

a. Goal: *health teaching.*
   (1) Explain purpose and process to parents:
      (a) Removes anti-Rh antibodies and fetal cells that are coated with antibodies.
      (b) Reduces bilirubin levels—indicated when 20 mg/dL in term neonate and 15 mg/dL in preterm.
      (c) Corrects anemia—supplies RBCs that will not be destroyed by maternal antibodies.
      (d) Rh-negative type O blood elicits no reaction; maximum exchange is 500 mL; duration of exchange: 45–60 min.
b. Goal: *minimize transfusion hazards.*
   (1) Warm blood to room temperature, since cold blood may precipitate cardiac arrest.
   (2) Use only fresh blood—to reduce possibility of hypocalcemia, tetany, convulsions.
   (3) Give calcium gluconate, as ordered, after each 100 mL of transfusion.
c. Goal: *prepare for transfusion procedure.* Ready necessary equipment—monitor, resuscitation equipment, radiant heater, light.
d. Goal: *assist with exchange transfusion.*
   (1) Continuous monitoring of vital signs; record baseline, and every 15 min during procedure.
   (2) Record: time, amount of blood withdrawn; time and amount injected; medications given.
   (3) Observe for: dyspnea, listlessness, bleeding from transfusion site, cyanosis, cardiovascular irregularity or arrest; coolness of lower extremities.
e. Goal: *posttransfusion care.*
   (1) **Assessment:**
      (a) Observe for: dyspnea, cyanosis, cardiac arrest or irregularities, jaundice, hypoglycemia; frequent vital signs.
      (b) *Signs of sepsis*—fever, tachycardia, dyspnea, chills, tremors.
   (2) **Nursing care plan/implementation:**
      (a) Maintain thermal stability—to reduce physiological stress, possibility of metabolic acidosis.
      (b) Give oxygen—to relieve cyanosis.
      (c) Keep cord moist—to facilitate repeat transfusion, if necessary.
      (d) Maintain nutrition/hydration—feed per schedule.
5. **Evaluation/outcome criteria:**
   a. Infant's hemolytic process ceases; bilirubin level drops.
   b. Infant makes successful transition to extrauterine life.
   c. Infant experiences no complications of therapeutic regimen.
   d. Infant shows evidence of bonding.

B. **ABO incompatibility**
1. **Pathophysiology**—fetal blood carrying antigens A/B enters maternal type O bloodstream → antibody formation → antibodies cross placenta → hemolyze fetal RBCs. *Note:* less severe than Rh reaction.
2. **Etiology:**
   a. Type O mother carries anti-A and anti-B antibodies.
   b. Even first pregnancy is jeopardized if fetal blood enters maternal system.
   c. Reaction possible if fetus is type A, type B, or type AB and mother is type O.
◆ 3. **Assessment:**
   a. Jaundice within first 24 hr.
   b. Rising bilirubin levels.
   c. Enlarged liver and spleen.
◆ 4. **Nursing care plan/implementation:** Goal: *reduce hazard to newborn.*
   ▶ a. Prepare for exchange transfusion with O negative blood.
   ▶ b. Phototherapy may be ordered if bilirubin is 10 mg/dL, and anemia is mild or absent.
   c. Close monitoring of status.
   d. Supportive care.
◆ 5. **Evaluation/outcome criteria:**
   a. Infant responds to medical/nursing regimen.
   b. Infant's assessment findings within normal limits.

C. **Hyperbilirubinemia**
1. **Pathophysiology**—bilirubin, a breakdown product of hemolyzed RBCs, appears at increased levels; exceeds 13–15 mg/dL. Bilirubin is safe when bound with albumin and conjugated by user for body excretion; danger is when unconjugated and deposits in CNS.
   a. **WARNING:** There is no "safe" serum-bilirubin level; kernicterus is a function of the bilirubin level *and* neonatal age and condition; poor fluid-and-caloric balance subjects the infant (especially the preterm infant) to kernicterus at low serum-bilirubin levels.
   b. *Kernicterus*—high bilirubin levels result in deposition of yellow pigment in basal ganglia of brain → irreversible retardation.
2. **Etiology:**
   a. Rh or ABO incompatibility, during first 48 hr.
   b. Resolution of an enclosed hemorrhage (e.g., cephalohematoma).
   c. Infection.
   d. Drug induced—vitamin K injection, maternal ingestion of sulfisoxazole (Gantrisin).
   e. Bile duct blockage.
   f. Albumin-binding capacity is exceeded.
   g. "Breastfeeding jaundice" (e.g., pregnandiol in milk). Breastfeeding is *not* dangerous and not a cause of physiological jaundice.
   h. Dehydration.
   i. Immature liver (interferes with conjugation).

◆ 3. **Assessment:**
   a. Jaundice noted after blanching skin to suppress hemoglobin color; noted in sclera or mucosa in dark-skinned neonates; make sure light is adequate; spreads from head down, with increasing severity.
   b. Pallor.
   c. Concentrated, dark urine.
   d. Blood level determination—hemoglobin or indirect bilirubin (unconjugated, unbound bilirubin deposits in CNS).
   e. *Kernicterus*—similar to intracranial hemorrhage.
      (1) Poor feeding or sucking.
      (2) Regurgitation, vomiting.
      (3) High-pitched cry.
      (4) Temperature instability.
      (5) Hypertonicity/hypotonicity.
      (6) Progressive lethargy; diminished Moro reflex.
      (7) Respiratory distress.
      (8) Cerebral palsy, mental retardation.
      (9) Death.
◆ 4. **Analysis/nursing diagnosis:**
   a. *Fluid volume (RBC) deficit* related to hemolysis secondary to blood incompatibility.
   b. *High risk for injury* (brain damage) related to kernicterus.
   c. *Altered thought processes* (mental retardation) related to brain damage secondary to kernicterus.
   d. *Knowledge deficit (parental)* related to infant condition.
◆ 5. **Nursing care plan/implementation:**
   a. *Medical management:*
      (1) *Prenatal*—amniocentesis.
      (2) *Postnatal*—exchange transfusion, phototherapy.
   ▶ b. Goal: *assist bilirubin conjugation through phototherapy.*
      (1) Cover closed eyelids while under light to protect eyes. (If biliblanket is used, no need to cover eyes.) Remove eyepads when not under light (feeding, cuddling, during parental visits).
      (2) Expose as much skin as possible—to maximize exposure of circulating blood to light. Remove for only brief periods.
      (3) *Change position* qlhr—to maximize exposure of circulating blood to light.
      (4) *Note:* any loose green stools as bile is cleared through gut; watch for skin breakdown on buttocks.
      (5) Monitor temperature—to identify hyperthermia. (not necessary if using biliblanket.)
      (6) *Push fluids* (to 25% more than average) between feedings—to counteract dehydration. Breastmilk has natural laxative effects that help clear bile.

c. Goal: *health teaching.* Explain, discuss photo-therapy, bilirubin levels, implications.

d. Goal: *emotional support.*
   (1) Encourage verbalization of anxiety, fears, concerns.
   (2) Encourage contact with infant.
   (3) Reassure, as possible.

◆ 6. **Evaluation/outcome criteria:**
   a. Infant's hemolytic process ceases; bilirubin level drops.
   b. Infant makes successful transition to extrauterine life.
   c. Infant experiences no complications of therapeutic regimen.
   d. Infant shows evidence of effective bonding.

Emotional Support of the High-Risk Infant

I. **General aspects**
   A. The high-risk infant has the same *developmental needs* as the healthy term infant:
      1. Social and tactile stimulation.
      2. Comfort and removal of discomfort (hunger, soiling).
      3. Continuous contact with a consistent, parenting person.
   B. Treatment for serious physiological compromise may result in:
      1. Isolation.
      2. Sensory deprivation or noxious stimuli.
      3. Emotional stress.

◆ II. **Assessment**—signs of neonatal emotional stress:
   A. Does not look at person performing care.
   B. Does not cry or protest.
   C. Poor weight gain; failure to thrive.

◆ III. **Analysis/nursing diagnosis:** *sensory/perceptual alterations* related to isolation in isolette, oxygen hood.

◆ IV. **Nursing care plan/implementation:**
   A. Goal: *provide consistent parenting contact.* Assign same nurses whenever possible.
   B. Goal: *emotional support.*
      1. Comfort when crying.
      2. Provide positive sensory stimulation. Arrange time to:
      a. Stroke skin.
      b. Hold hand.
      c. Hum, sing, talk.
      d. Hold in en-face position (nurse looking into infant's eyes).
      e. Hold when feeding, if possible.
   C. Goal: *encourage parents to participate in care*—to:
      1. Reduce their psychological stress, anxiety, fear.
      2. Promote bonding.
      3. Reduce possibility of later child abuse (higher incidence of child abuse against children who have been high-risk infants).

◆ V. **Evaluation/outcome criteria:**
   A. Infant demonstrates successful resolution of physiological problems.
   B. Parents and infant evidence bonding.
   C. Parents express satisfaction with care and result.

General Aspects: Nursing Care of the High-Risk Infant and Family

I. **General overview:** The birth of a physiologically compromised neonate is psychologically stressful for both infant and family and physiologically stressful for the neonate. Effective, goal-directed nursing care is directed toward:
   A. Minimizing physiological and psychological stress.
   B. Facilitating/supporting successful coping or adaptation.
   C. Encouraging parental attachment/separation/grieving, as appropriate.

◆ II. **Assessment**—directed toward determining neonate's present and projected status:
   A. Determine neonate's current physical status.
   B. Identify specific status and diagnosis-related problems and needs.
   C. Describe family psychological status, strengths, and coping mechanisms/skills.
   D. Determine medical/surgical/nursing approach to problems—and prognosis.

◆ III. **Analysis/nursing diagnosis:**
   A. Parental *anxiety/fear* related to physiological compromise of neonate.
   B. *Self-esteem disturbance* related to feelings of guilt or anger.
   C. *Ineffective individual coping* related to severe psychological stress.
   D. *Knowledge deficit* related to diagnosis, treatment, prognosis of infant.
   E. *High risk for altered parenting* related to concern about infant.

◆ IV. **Nursing care plan/implementation:**
   A. Goal: *preoperative and postoperative care.*
      1. Maintain/improve physiological stability.
      a. Temperature stabilization—keep warm.
      b. Oxygenation:
         (1) Position.
      ▶ (2) Administer oxygen, as ordered or necessary.
      c. Nutrition/hydration:
      ◗ (1) Administer/monitor IV fluids.
         (2) Oral fluids, as ordered.
         (3) Feed, as status permits.
      2. Assist with diagnostic testing.
   B. Goal: *emotional support of parents.*
      1. Encourage exploring and ventilating feelings.
      2. Involve parents in decision-making process.
   C. Goal: *health teaching.*
      1. Determine knowledge/understanding of problem.

2. Explain/simplify/clarify, as needed, physician's discussions with parents.
3. Describe/explain/discuss neonate's present status and any auxiliary equipment; teach CPR to family.
4. Refer, as needed, to hospital/community resources.
D. Goal: *promote bonding.* Encourage parental participation in care of the neonate.

◆ V. **Evaluation/outcome criteria:**
A. Parents verbalize understanding of relevant information; make informed decisions regarding infant care.
B. Parents demonstrate comfort and increasing participation in care of neonate.
C. Infant maintains/increases adequacy of adaptation to extrauterine life.
D. If relevant, parents demonstrate progress in grieving process.

Questions

Select the one answer that is best for each question, unless otherwise directed.

1. Which of the following identifies the basal body temperature (BBT) change characteristic of ovulation?
   1. Falls slightly, then increases by about 0.5°C.
   2. Rises slightly, then falls by about 0.5°C.
   3. Is affected by a surge of FSH.
   4. Is due to an estrogen surge.
2. When calculating the 1-minute Apgar, the nurse adds the following assessment findings: heart rate—over 100; respiratory effort—slow and irregular; muscle tone—poor response to slap on soles of feet; weak cry; color—body pink, extremities blue. In view of these assessment findings, which Apgar score should the nurse record?
   1. 5.
   2. 6.
   3. 7.
   4. 8.
3. A pregnant woman's last menstrual period began on April 3. Calculate an accurate estimate of her EDD.
   Fill in the blank: _____ (month and day).
4. A newborn who weighed 7 lb at birth now weighs 6 lb 8 oz. Implementing health teaching, the nurse tells the mother the percentage of birth weight usually lost by normal, healthy babies. Which represents the maximum amount of normal weight loss for this newborn?
   1. 6 oz (170 g).
   2. 8 oz (227 g).
   3. 11 oz (317 g).
   4. 16 oz (454 g).
5. The woman who is pregnant who would likely be given a "trial of labor" for vaginal birth after cesarean (VBAC) is one who had a first:
   1. Cesarean through a classical uterine incision because of severe fetal distress.
   2. Low transverse cesarean for breech presentation; this pregnancy is in vertex presentation.
   3. Cesarean for fetopelvic disproportion.
   4. Low transverse cesarean for active vaginal/perineal herpes infection; culture at 39 weeks, this pregnancy was positive for herpes.
6. A woman who is pregnant is told to increase her intake of foods high in iron. Which food should the nurse suggest as being the best source of iron?

   1. Lean red meat.
   2. Nuts.
   3. Shellfish.
   4. Dairy products.
7. For which complication of pregnancy is a woman who is Rh-negative at risk?
   1. Spontaneous abortion.
   2. Preeclampsia.
   3. Maternal anemia.
   4. Erythroblastosis fetalis.
8. The nurse manager on a maternity unit is informed that a woman who is 36 weeks pregnant with severe preeclampsia is to be admitted to the unit. Which bed assignment is the best choice?
   1. Bed in a double room 50 feet from the nurse's station with a roommate who has rheumatic heart disease.
   2. Bed in a double room next to the nurse's station with a roommate who is a drug addict with withdrawal symptoms.
   3. Bed in a four-bed unit with all other women who are postpartum.
   4. Bed in a four-bed unit with other women who have pyelonephritis, diabetes, and premature rupture of membranes.
9. The nurse analyzes the following data: A woman in labor has remained at 6 cm dilation, +1 station (vertex presentation), with moulding of the baby's head at +2 station for 3 hours. The baby's FHR has increased from a baseline of 140 to 170. The physician orders Pitocin augmentation of labor. The nurse's correct action would be to:
   1. Add Pitocin to the IV and label it correctly.
   2. Start the Pitocin drip using an IV pump.
   3. Accurately chart the Pitocin infusion.
   4. Refuse to carry out the order for Pitocin augmentation.
10. Of the following findings in a full-term newborn, which is not an expected outcome of maternal hormone influence, and therefore should be reported?
    1. "Witch's milk."
    2. Slight vaginal bleeding.
    3. Undescended testicles.
    4. Linea nigra.
11. The nurse is to assign a nurse's aide on the postpartum unit to care for clients. The aide has a cold that day, but no other problems. Which client would the nurse not want to assign to this nurse's aide?
    1. Woman in renal failure.
    2. Woman who has hypertension.
    3. Woman who had a prolonged labor.
    4. Woman who has AIDS.
12. The hematocrit decreases an average of 7%–10% during pregnancy. This is referred to as physiological anemia of pregnancy. Which mechanism best explains this decrease?
    1. The total erythrocyte count increases about 30%; the plasma volume increases about 50%.
    2. The total erythrocyte count increases about 50%; the plasma volume decreases 30%.
    3. The total erythrocyte count decreases 30%; the plasma volume increases about 50%.
    4. The erythrocyte count remains the same; the plasma volume increases 50%.
13. Assessment data indicate an abnormality at 20 weeks of gestation when:
    1. The fundal height measurement is at 4 fingers below the umbilicus.
    2. Fetal movements are felt faintly on the right side of the abdomen.

3. The woman complains of backache and fatigue.
4. The fetal heart rate is 140 and sometimes is difficult to count.

14. When responding to a question from a new mother about producing enough milk for the baby as the baby grows and needs more milk at each feeding, the nurse should explain that:
    1. The mother's milk supply will increase as the infant demands more at each feeding.
    2. The breast milk will gradually become richer to supply additional calories.
    3. Early addition of solid baby foods will ensure an infant's nutritional needs.
    4. As the infant requires more milk, feedings should be supplemented with cow's milk.

15. Which woman would be at highest risk for preterm labor?
    1. The woman who is pregnant and working full-time at a sedentary job.
    2. The woman who is pregnant with twins.
    3. The woman who has gained 35 lb by 36 weeks of gestation.
    4. The woman who is pregnant with her first baby.

16. The nurse considers information regarding smoking cigarettes and marijuana essential for women who are pregnant because it is well established that these activities may lead to:
    1. Infants with mental retardation.
    2. Low-birth-weight infants.
    3. Infants with deformities.
    4. Malnourished infants.

17. Several weeks after the funeral of one of her twin infants, a mother tells the community health nurse that she is experiencing difficulty producing enough breast milk to satisfy the other infant. The most appropriate response for the nurse to make would be:
    1. "You probably have a virus and should see a doctor right away."
    2. "Your baby is probably reacting to the loss of a sibling and not sucking long enough to stimulate an adequate supply."
    3. "Milk production may decrease with an increase in stress."
    4. "The lactation ducts may be occluded."

18. If a woman is pregnant for the second time, but her first pregnancy did not reach viability, what would be her parity using the four-digit scoring system?
    1. 1-0-0-1.
    2. 0-0-1-0.
    3. 0-1-0-0.
    4. 0-1-0-1.

19. In providing health teaching for an expectant couple, what should the nurse tell them is a *probable* sign of pregnancy?
    1. Fetal heart sounds.
    2. Positive pregnancy test.
    3. Fetal movements felt by examiner.
    4. Outline of fetus on sonogram.

20. A woman who is pregnant is hospitalized for preeclampsia. She and her husband express anxiety about having limited insurance, which may not cover this hospitalization. The *most* appropriate nursing intervention would be to:
    1. Refer the couple to social services for possible assistance.
    2. Initiate a family-counseling referral.
    3. Provide supportive counseling.
    4. Assess the couple's needs through discussion.

21. A young woman describes experiencing a heavy vaginal discharge and severe itching for the past 3 days. She is diagnosed as having *Trichomonas vaginalis* infection. Health teaching for this woman should include dosage, administration, and signs and symptoms of side effects of which medication as treatment for this condition?
    1. Tetracycline.
    2. Erythromycin.

3. Nystatin.
    4. Metronidazole.

22. A woman in labor has a history of undiagnosed vaginal bleeding. Which procedure may be *contraindicated* on her arrival in the labor room?
    1. Initiating intravenous therapy.
    2. Taking her blood pressure.
    3. Examining her vaginal canal.
    4. Monitoring FHR.

23. The nurse explains to the client and family that because of excessive bleeding, an emergency hysterectomy will need to be performed:
    1. Upon completion of the necessary surgical preparation.
    2. Immediately.
    3. Within 24 hours.
    4. At the start of the next surgical day.

24. The nurse explains to a client's family that the surgical treatment *most* often implemented for excessive vaginal bleeding due to uterine fibroids is:
    1. Panabdominal hysterectomy.
    2. Vaginal hysterectomy.
    3. Dilation and curettage.
    4. Abdominal hysterectomy.

25. Which precaution would the nurse implement when caring for a neonate born to a woman who is HIV-positive?
    1. The nurse should wear gloves until all blood and amniotic fluid have been removed.
    2. The woman should be encouraged to breastfeed.
    3. The father who is HIV-positive should have limited contact with the child.
    4. The parents should be encouraged to place the infant for adoption since the outlook for the mother is poor.

26. The labor room nurse decides to intervene when the fetal heart rate (FHR) pattern indicates:
    1. A baseline range of 110 to 160 bpm.
    2. Absence of variability.
    3. Early decelerations.
    4. Mild variable decelerations.

27. Which postoperative instruction for a client who had an abdominal hysterectomy includes *inaccurate* information?
    1. Monitor vaginal drainage and report any color changes.
    2. Expect that vaginal discharge will diminish and cease gradually.
    3. Plan on contraception, considering that her ovaries are still intact.
    4. Expect that menses will no longer occur.

28. On the third postoperative day after a mastectomy, the client voiced concern about her husband's reaction to her surgery. Which approach by the nurse is most likely to help minimize this client's concern?
    1. Emphasizing the lifesaving aspects of her surgery.
    2. Explaining that depression and anxiety are common behaviors following radical surgery.
    3. Interviewing the husband to learn about his real reaction to his wife's surgery.
    4. Encouraging her to identify the strengths in her relationship with her husband.

29. Emergency cesarean section is ordered for a woman in active labor due to fetal distress. Which of the following would be part of the nursing interventions at this time?
    Select all that apply.
    1. Obtain an informed consent from the client.
    2. Give reassurance to the woman to alleviate her anxiety about the fetal outcome.
    3. Monitor the fetal heart rate closely.
    4. Place Foley catheter in the client.
    5. Shave client's abdomen.

30. The mother of the newborn on an apnea monitor tells the nurse that her baby looks so frail and sick. The most appropriate response for the nurse to make is:
    1. "Your baby has a life-threatening illness."
    2. "The baby looks fine; you haven't seen many really sick babies."
    3. "I know how you feel. My baby was sick at birth and now he's fine."
    4. "It must be difficult to see your baby look this way."

31. A client, 38 weeks' gestation, is admitted to the labor unit for a scheduled cesarean section under regional anesthesia. During admission process, the client expresses anxiety about pain during the surgical procedure. The most appropriate response to her concerns would be:
    1. "You won't feel anything at all during the surgery."
    2. "The regional block completely eliminates sensation during the surgery."
    3. "You may feel some pressure during surgery."
    4. "You may feel some pain when the incision is made."

32. A client who is pregnant has been instructed to report signs and symptoms of preterm labor immediately. The nurse knows that the client has failed to follow instructions when the client phones after:
    1. Determining that her contractions are occurring every 10 minutes.
    2. Determining that her contractions are continuing after she has emptied her bladder.
    3. Resting in bed on her side for one hour.
    4. Drinking half a cup of water.

33. A client, 36 weeks' gestation, is admitted to the labor and delivery unit with premature rupture of membranes. The fetus is in a transverse lie and the client is prepared for an emergency cesarean section. The client asks what type of incision the physician will use in her surgery. The nurse should realize that the client's primary concern involves the possibility of:
    1. Scarring.
    2. Bleeding.
    3. Infection.
    4 Uterine rupture.

34. At her first prenatal visit, a newly diagnosed pregnant client informs the nurse that she has a family history of cystic fibrosis and questions whether her unborn child is at risk for this disease. The nurse's response is based on the knowledge that most inborn errors of metabolism are:
    1. Caused by exposure to teratogens during the first trimester.
    2. Autosomal recessive inherited disorders.
    3. Caused by the use of illicit drugs during pregnancy.
    4. Random mutations of X-linked genes.

35. A client, newly diagnosed with active tuberculosis infection, is 12 weeks pregnant. In providing anticipatory guidance for this client, the nurse knows the physician will most likely recommend that:
    1. The client should have an abortion as soon as possible.
    2. The client should start NIH and rifampin after giving birth.
    3. The client should start NIH and rifampin now.
    4. The client should start NIH and pyrazinamide after the first trimester.

36. A 19-year-old client is 34 weeks' gestation and has symptoms of yellowish vaginal discharge and burning with urination. Her genital culture reveals gonorrhea. In providing health teaching for the client, the nurse explains that:
    1. Gonorrhea is the most common sexually transmitted disease in the United States and is easily treated with antibiotics.
    2. The client will have to have a cesarean section to avoid transmission of gonorrhea to the fetus during delivery.
    3. The client may need cryotherapy on her cervix if the antibiotics do not cure the infection.
    4. Immunity does not develop after exposure to gonorrhea, and re-infection can occur if sexual partners are not treated.

37. The client is a 42-year-old gravida 4, para 3003, at term, who has been admitted in early labor with a twin gestation. Her admission vital signs: oral temperature was 99.1°F; pulse was 92; respirations were 24; blood pressure was 140/88; fetal heart rate of twin 1 was 138; fetal heart rate of twin 2 was 156. One hour later her blood pressure was 156/92; fetal heart rate of twin 1 was 140; fetal heart rate of twin 2 was 154. The nurse should:
    1. Record the vital signs as normal.
    2. Encourage the client to ambulate to stimulate her labor.
    3. Notify the physician of the change in the blood pressure.
    4. Apply the internal fetal scalp electrode at the next vaginal exam.

38. Which physical sign or test finding is an inconclusive sign of rupture of membranes?
    1. Vaginal discharge with strongly positive nitrazine reaction.
    2. Ferning pattern on a microscope slide of dried fluid from the vagina.
    3. Direct observation of watery fluid coming from the cervix.
    4. Complaint of thin, watery discharge from the vagina for the last 8 hours.

39. The nurse in the prenatal clinic is taking a history from a client who is 26 weeks pregnant. The client states that she has not felt the baby move yet. On physical exam, the nurse notes that the fundus is below the umbilicus. The nurse should:
    1. Record the findings as normal.
    2. Reassure the client that she will feel the baby move in the next week.
    3. Notify the physician that there is a discrepancy between the gestational age of the pregnancy and the findings from this prenatal visit.
    4. Tell the client that the baby has been moving for the past several weeks but that the movements are too weak to be felt.

40. The client expresses a fear that her fetus is getting "too large" for her "to deliver naturally." The nurse knows that cephalopelvic disproportion:
    1. Can always be determined before labor by a manual exam.
    2. Is usually a problem when the fetus is large for gestational age.
    3. Is determined by the size and position of the fetal head and the shape and size of the pelvic bone.
    4. Can be avoided by inducing labor before the estimated date of delivery.

41. In labor and delivery, *engagement* means that the widest diameter of the fetal head has passed the pelvic inlet. Which is an accurate statement about engagement?
    1. Active labor occurs before engagement for most women.
    2. After engagement, the risk of cephalopelvic disproportion is reduced.
    3. Engagement generally occurs late in second stage.
    4. Severe back pain is a sign of engagement.

42. Which menstrual history would suggest that calculating the due date by the date of the last menstrual period might be erroneous?
    1. Interval every 28 days, length 5 days, flow heavy on first 2 days.
    2. Interval 24–26 days, length 3 to 5 days, flow moderate.
    3. Interval 15–45 days, length 2 to 3 days, flow light.
    4. Interval every 28 to 32 days, length 3 days, flow heavy.

43. The nurse is taking a prenatal history and asks the client about contraceptive use before pregnancy. Which response by the client should alert the nurse to a possible error in calculating the due date?
    1. The client states that she only used condoms and foam.
    2. The client states that she finished her package of birth control pills but did not have a period.
    3. The client states that she had her intrauterine device removed and had two periods.
    4. The client states that she was not using contraception.

44. The client has been using oral contraceptive pills for 2 months. Which statement by the client would alert the nurse that the client should stop taking the pills?
    1. "I have had a bad headache constantly for the past week. I can't get rid of it."
    2. "I have a thick yellow discharge from 'down below' with a bad odor."
    3. "My mother has diabetes and takes insulin."
    4. "My boyfriend was just treated for gonorrhea."

45. The nurse is teaching a class on "safe" sex to high school students. Which statement about the use of condoms should the nurse avoid making?
    1. "Condoms should be used every time you have sex because condoms prevent all forms of sexually transmitted diseases."
    2. "Condoms should be used every time you have sex even if you are taking the pill because condoms can prevent the spread of HIV and gonorrhea."
    3. "Condoms should be used even if you have recently tested negative for HIV."
    4. "Condoms should be used because they can prevent infection and because they may prevent pregnancy."

46. The client has just had an intrauterine device (IUD) inserted. Which set of symptoms suggesting a problem with the contraceptive device should the nurse include in health teaching?
    1. Nausea, vomiting, fever, joint pains.
    2. Abdominal pain, late period, fever, and chills.
    3. Headache, heartburn, backache, fatigue.
    4. Clear vaginal discharge, urinary frequency, flank pain.

47. Which statement by the client who is breastfeeding should alert the nurse that her instruction about breastfeeding and family planning was misunderstood?
    1. "I understand that the hormones for breastfeeding may affect when my periods come."
    2. "I may not have periods while I am breastfeeding, so I don't need family planning."
    3. "I can get pregnant as early as one month after my baby was born."
    4. "Breastfeeding causes my womb to tighten and bleed less after birth."

48. The nurse is teaching a class about toxic shock syndrome. Which practice should the nurse strongly discourage in order to prevent toxic shock?
    1. Wash diaphragm after each use.
    2. Remove and wash cervical cap at least every 48 hours.
    3. Change tampons every 2–4 hours.
    4. Use only superabsorbent tampons for overnight protection.

49. The nurse is counseling a couple in their mid-30s who have been trying to get pregnant for about 6 months. They are concerned that one or both of them may be infertile. The best advice the nurse could provide is:
    1. "Start planning adoption. Many couples get pregnant when they are trying to adopt."
    2. "Consult a fertility specialist and start testing now."
    3. "It is not unusual to take 6 to 12 months to get pregnant, especially when the partners are in their mid-30s. Eat well, exercise, and avoid stress."
    4. "Have sex as often as you can, especially around the time of ovulation, to increase your chances of pregnancy."

50. The nurse, who has strong personal anti-abortion values, is interviewing a client who is pregnant and is requesting an abortion. The ethical obligation of the nurse requires that:
    1. The nurse will inform the client of the pro-life viewpoint.
    2. The nurse will discuss the risks of abortion with the client.
    3. The nurse will validate that the client has made an informed decision.
    4. The nurse will refer the client to someone else who can provide counseling.

51. In which situation is it inappropriate to administer RhoGAM?
    1. After abortion in a 10-week gestation, mother is Rh-negative.
    2. Woman who is Rh-negative at 28 weeks of gestation.
    3. Spontaneous abortion at 6 weeks of gestation, mother is Rh-positive.
    4. Abdominal trauma in a mother who is Rh-negative at 16 weeks of gestation.

52. A woman who is multiparous is admitted to labor and delivery at 39 weeks' gestation with orders for Pitocin induction of labor. The nurse performs Leopold's maneuver and feels that the fetal parts are ballotable. The nurse locates the fetal heart rate in the upper right quadrant. A sterile vaginal exam by the nurse reveals the cervix is 2 cm dilated and the presenting part is out of the pelvis. Which of the following are appropriate nursing interventions at this time?
    Select all that apply.
    1. Start an IV with a solution of Lactated Ringer's solution.
    2. Order a regular diet for the client, since she is likely to have a prolnged labor.
    3. Obtain a bedside ultrasound to determine fetal presentation.
    4. Begin the Pitocin induction as ordered by the physician.
    5. Prepare the client for a vacuum-assisted vaginal delivery.

53. In teaching a group of women about postabortion care, the nurse should emphasize that:
    1. Tampons may be used as needed.
    2. Contraception should be initiated as soon as the first period begins.
    3. Douching is permitted as soon as the bright-red bleeding ceases.
    4. Sexual intercourse should be delayed for 1–3 weeks.

54. The nurse is providing anticipatory guidance for a woman who wishes to use natural family planning and has a 28-day menstrual cycle. The woman asks the nurse when she is fertile during her cycle. The best answer for the nurse to provide is:
    1. In a 28-day cycle, ovulation occurs at or about day 14. The egg lives for about 24 hours and the sperm live for about 72 hours. The fertile period would be approximately between day 11 and day 15.
    2. In a 28-day cycle, ovulation occurs at or about day 14. The egg lives for about 72 hours and the sperm live for about 24 hours. The fertile period would be approximately between day 13 and day 17.
    3. In a 28-day cycle, ovulation occurs 8 days before the next period or at about day 20. The fertile period is between day 20 and the beginning of the next period.
    4. It is impossible to determine the fertile period reliably, so it is best to assume that a woman is always fertile.

55. A prenatal client tearfully states that she used drugs before she knew she was pregnant. According to her last menstrual period, she was at approximately 1 week of gestational age when she last used drugs. The nurse knows that:
    1. Drug use in the first trimester always causes congenital anomalies.
    2. Drug use before implantation has a smaller incidence of teratogenic effect.
    3. It is only important to avoid drug use during the period of organ formation, weeks 3–10.
    4. Selected drug use is not harmful in pregnancy.

56. A prenatal client tearfully states that she used drugs before she knew she was pregnant. According to her last menstrual period, she was at approximately 2 weeks of gestational age when she last used drugs. The best reply for the nurse to make is:
    1. "Have you considered abortion since your baby is probably affected by the drug use?"
    2. "You have a bad start on your pregnancy and will probably have problems later on."
    3. "There are tests that can be done to determine if the baby is affected by the drug use."
    4. "Tell me about any drug use since you have been pregnant."

57. The nurse is conducting a class about nutrition to a group of prenatal Latina clients who are anemic. The nurse is aware that many Latinas are lactose intolerant. Which foods should the nurse especially encourage during the third trimester?
    1. Cheese, yogurt, and fish for protein and calcium needs plus prenatal vitamins and iron supplements.
    2. Red beans, green leafy vegetables, and fish for iron and calcium needs plus prenatal vitamin and iron supplements.
    3. Red meat, milk, and eggs for iron and calcium needs plus prenatal vitamins and iron supplements.
    4. Prenatal iron and calcium supplements plus a regular adult diet.

58. A woman comes for her first prenatal visit at 16 weeks' pregnancy. The following lab values are observed by the nurse after the client's visit: WBC 10,000; hemoglobin 11 g/dL; hematocrit 33%; platelets 300,000. Based on interpretation of these lab values, the nurse should:
    1. Report to the physician that the client is anemic.
    2. Refer the client to the nutritionist for counseling concerning a diet for pregnancy.
    3. Record that the client has normal lab values for pregnancy and needs no supplementation.
    4. Dispense prenatal iron and vitamins.

59. For women who are pregnant and are employed during the first half of pregnancy, which set of job classifications poses the least threat of exposure to teratogens?
    1. Construction worker, carpenter's assistant.
    2. Daycare worker, bank teller.
    3. Garden supply worker, hotel domestic.
    4. Hospital nurse, medical assistant.

60. The nurse is teaching a class on common discomforts of pregnancy in the first half of pregnancy. The nurse knows that the instruction has been misunderstood when one client states:
    1. "To avoid morning sickness, I should drink all my fluids with meals."
    2. "To decrease my backache, I should practice the pelvic tilt."
    3. "To avoid heartburn, I should avoid eating just before I go to bed."
    4. "To avoid morning sickness, I should eat some dry crackers before I get out of bed in the morning."

61. The client who is 10 weeks pregnant is complaining of repeated nausea and vomiting. She states that she "can't keep anything down." She has the following vital signs and lab values: temperature 99.4°F, pulse 92, respirations 28, urine specific gravity 1.035, urine protein negative, urine glucose negative, urine ketones large or high. The nurse should:
    1. Record the assessment findings and reassure the client that the nausea and vomiting will go away in a couple of weeks.
    2. Instruct the client to keep dry crackers by her bedside; avoid fluids with meals; and eat small, frequent meals.
    3. Report the findings to the physician because they are indicating severe dehydration and carbohydrate starvation.
    4. Give the client a soft drink and a snack to see if she can keep it down.

62. Constipation in pregnancy is a common and uncomfortable discomfort. Which concept should the nurse teach regarding nutrition to reduce discomfort from constipation?

1. Because progesterone causes decreased tone of smooth muscle, adequate fiber intake to stimulate elimination is important.
2. Because estrogen causes sodium and water retention, excessive fluid intake is discouraged.
3. Because progesterone softens the smooth muscle of the gallbladder, excessive intake of fats is discouraged.
4. Because estrogen softens connective tissue, excessive straining at stool should be discouraged.

63. A client is 36 weeks pregnant and is complaining of swollen ankles. The nurse knows that, for this woman, the ankle edema is probably a normal discomfort of pregnancy when the woman states:
    1. "My ankles are more swollen in the evening than in the morning."
    2. "Sitting or lying flat on my back makes my swelling better."
    3. "My ankles are more swollen in the morning than in the evening, and my fingers are always swollen."
    4. "Whenever my ankles swell up, I get a headache."

64. Some women who are pregnant experience hot flashes, shortness of breath, and heart palpitations during pregnancy. Which statement reflects an accurate statement of self-help measures that the woman who is pregnant might use to reduce her discomfort?
    1. Some of these symptoms are caused by hormones of pregnancy and just have to be tolerated.
    2. Start an exercise program that will increase muscle toning, improve respiration, and maintain overall fitness.
    3. Dress in layers, avoid hot and stuffy rooms, and avoid overexertion.
    4. Avoid eating large meals and sleep in the supine position.

65. Persistent constipation in pregnancy is a common discomfort associated with intake of iron supplements and slowed peristalsis. Which statement by the nurse is an effective nutritional way to reduce the discomfort from constipation?
    1. "Take iron supplements at bedtime, not at mealtime."
    2. "Eat small, frequent meals and avoid foods high in roughage."
    3. "Take a mild bulk-forming laxative to maintain a regular elimination habit."
    4. "Eat foods high in roughage, especially dark green vegetables."

66. The nurse is describing exercises for women who are pregnant to increase tone and fitness and decrease lower backache. Which exercise program should be avoided?
    1. Ten minutes of walking per day with an emphasis on good posture.
    2. Pelvic rock exercise and squats three times a day.
    3. Stand with legs apart and touch hands to floor three times per day.
    4. Ten minutes of swimming or leg kicking in pool per day.

67. A lawyer who is pregnant appears distressed at her prenatal visit. She states that she "doesn't understand what is happening" to her. She cries a lot and has trouble making decisions. Sometimes she feels that she does not want the baby. She feels that she is getting too fat. The best reply by the nurse would be:
    1. "Many women who are pregnant feel that way. Wait until you see the baby. It will be OK."
    2. "Many women have confusing feelings during pregnancy. Some of them are related to hormonal changes. Tell me more about what bothers you."
    3. "It is really important to eat a good diet. You must not lose weight in pregnancy."
    4. "These feelings sound like depression. Maybe you should ask the doctor for some medication."

68. The nurse arrives on the labor and delivery unit and is assigned to a client in labor with the following parity: G4, P0120. The nurse anticipates that:

1. Because the woman is pregnant for the fourth time, she might have a rapid labor.
2. Because the woman has had no full-term pregnancies, she might have a slow labor.
3. Because the woman has had a preterm infant, this infant might be preterm as well.
4. This woman may have many questions about sibling rivalry after her labor and birth.

69. The nurse in the prenatal clinic is doing an interview with a woman at 28 weeks of gestation. The woman complains of palpitations, feelings of smothering, difficulty breathing while doing common household tasks, and a persistent cough. Her vital signs are: blood pressure 120/80, pulse 100, respirations 28. She has edema in her fingers and ankles. The skin around her eyes is puffy and pale. The nurse understands that:
    1. The woman has signs of cardiac decompensation and should see a physician immediately.
    2. The woman is experiencing normal discomforts of pregnancy.
    3. The woman is probably not physically fit and should start a mild exercise program.
    4. The woman should see a nutritionist to check her intake of sodium.

70. A client with a past history of rheumatic heart disease is in the third trimester of her first pregnancy. She is asking the nurse what she should expect in labor. The best reply by the nurse would be:
    1. Plan on a natural childbirth because regional anesthesia in labor has significant cardiovascular risks.
    2. Because an episiotomy may cause excessive bleeding, she should prepare for strong pushing efforts.
    3. Excessive anxiety should be avoided in labor; therefore she will be medicated and her family will stay in the waiting room.
    4. To reduce the burden on her cardiovascular system, she should practice breathing and relaxation exercises.

71. The nurse is explaining how RhoGAM works to a Lamaze class of couples who are expecting. The best explanation would be:
    1. RhoGAM prevents the immune system of the mother who is Rh-negative from attacking the red blood cells of the baby who is Rh-positive.
    2. RhoGAM prevents the immune system of the mother who is Rh-negative from attacking the red blood cells of a baby who is Rh-negative.
    3. RhoGAM prevents the immune system of a baby who is RH-positive from attacking the red blood cells of a mother who is Rh-negative.
    4. RhoGAM prevents the immune system of a baby who is Rh-negative from attacking the red blood cells of a mother who is Rh-positive.

72. The nurse is anticipating the insulin needs of a woman with diabetes who has just been informed that she is pregnant. The nurse is correct when he or she states:
    1. "Pregnancy has no effect on insulin requirements because the fetus produces its own insulin."
    2. "During pregnancy, insulin requirements gradually increase to a peak at term."
    3. "Some women who have diabetes experience a decrease in insulin requirements during the first trimester and an increase in the second and third trimesters."
    4. "Most women who have diabetes experience a prolonged increased insulin requirement after pregnancy and birth."

73. A woman who is pregnant and diabetic is concerned about the well-being of her baby. The nurse is correct when she states that the most important factor for the baby in pregnancy is:

1. "To keep your weight under control."
2. "To keep your serum glucose under one hundred twenty milligrams per deciliter."
3. "To maintain regular sleep and exercise habits."
4. "The genetic code for your baby, which has already been established. There is nothing you can do about it now."

74. Which statement(s) about preterm labor and delivery is/are correct?
    Select all that apply.
    1. The more premature the fetus, the greater the chance of malpresentation.
    2. Cord compression is uncommon in clients with premature rupture of membranes.
    3. The head of the fetus who is preterm is fragile and at risk for intracranial hemorrhage.
    4. Antibiotics are commonly ordered to prevent neonatal sepsis.
    5. All preterm labor is caused by an infection.

75. During a home visit to a mother with a baby who is 1-week-old, the nurse observes that the baby appears anxious and distressed and is difficult to console when crying. The fontanels are slightly sunken. The baby has one or two wet diapers per day. The urine in the diaper is yellow. The mother states that the baby has a hard time latching on to the breast nipple, but she has not offered supplements because she is determined to breastfeed. The most appropriate action by the nurse would be to:
    1. Encourage the mother to continue her breastfeeding efforts and avoid supplements.
    2. Encourage the mother to continue her breastfeeding efforts but offer supplements after breastfeeding.
    3. Suggest that she stop breastfeeding immediately and switch to formula.
    4. Take the baby for a medical evaluation today for dehydration.

76. The nurse is taking care of a woman who has just experienced a second-trimester fetal loss. The mother expresses fear that she will never be able to carry a healthy baby to term. The best response by the nurse is:
    1. "I understand your concern. Tell me about what has happened to you."
    2. "Everyone feels that way after the loss of a baby. It is a normal feeling."
    3. "The loss of one baby does not mean you can't ever have children."
    4. "Have you talked to your doctor about this feeling?"

77. The nurse is providing health education to a woman who is at 26 weeks of gestation and had a prior preterm birth at 30 weeks. The nurse is describing signs of preterm labor. The best description by the nurse includes:
    1. Show and perineal pressure.
    2. Leaking amniotic fluid and rectal pressure.
    3. Backache and pelvic pressure not relieved by rest.
    4. Contractions every 10 minutes.

78. The nurse is talking with a woman in the prenatal clinic who is 28 weeks pregnant. The woman has been informed that her *Chlamydia* test is positive and she has been instructed to take antibiotics for 10 days. The woman explains to the nurse that she has trouble swallowing pills and that she does not have any signs of infection. The most accurate response by the nurse would be:
    1. "You should avoid medication in pregnancy, so don't start the pills until you have obvious vaginal odor and itching."
    2. "*Chlamydia* is a minor infection and is likely to reoccur, so wait until you are closer to term to start the antibiotics."
    3. "*Chlamydia* is associated with preterm labor and newborn pneumonia, so start the medication immediately."
    4. "Have your partner tested for *Chlamydia* and start the antibiotics if he tests positive."

79. A woman who is 12 weeks' pregnant has just been informed that her serological test for syphilis is positive. The nurse should state that:
    1. "This infection can cause fetal abnormalities. Have you considered an abortion?"
    2. "The serological test for syphilis is a screening test. There is another test that must be done to determine if you have an active infection."
    3. "You and your partner must be treated immediately. All of your sexual contacts should be reported to the health department."
    4. "This infection can be transmitted to the baby as it passes down the birth canal. You will be treated just before delivery."

80. The nurse is taking the blood pressure of a 15-year-old woman who is primigravida and at 26 weeks of gestation. At her initial prenatal visit, this woman's vital signs were: blood pressure 90/60; pulse 88; respirations 18. Today her vital signs are: blood pressure 124/76; pulse 92; respirations 22. The nurse should:
    1. Record these vital signs as normal and proceed with routine prenatal care.
    2. Encourage the woman to start a mild exercise program to increase activity tolerance and reduce pulse and respirations.
    3. Immediately refer this woman to the physician for evaluation of pregnancy-induced hypertension.
    4. Record these vital signs as normal, recognizing that the changes are appropriate for second trimester of pregnancy.

81. A 15-year-old adolescent at 26 weeks of gestation with a diagnosis of possible preeclampsia is referred to the nurse for nutrition counseling. The nurse suggests an added serving of protein over the recommended minimum for 15-year-olds who are pregnant because:
    1. The adolescent may not have completed her own growth.
    2. Hypertension problems in pregnancy are associated with loss of protein in the urine.
    3. Hypertension problems in pregnancy are caused by a low-protein diet.
    4. The added protein will ensure that the fetus can grow even with reduced placental circulation.

82. The nurse knows that hypertensive disorders in pregnancy are associated with vasospasm and decreased tissue perfusion. Which symptoms are considered danger signs signaling the increase in severity of preeclampsia?
    1. Headache, ankle edema, polyuria.
    2. Headache, edema of the hands and face, dysuria.
    3. Edema of the hands and face, visual disturbances, irritability.
    4. Irritability, edema of the ankles, visual disturbances.

83. A nurse on the postpartum unit is taking care of a woman who delivered 1 hour ago after a labor complicated by severe preeclampsia. The physician's orders include magnesium sulfate, strict intake and output, and restricted oral intake of fluids. The nurse knows that fluid restriction:
    1. Is appropriate for care before delivery, but the order should be canceled now that the client has delivered.
    2. Will continue until it is evident that output is adequate because of the risk of renal failure.
    3. Will continue only as long as magnesium sulfate is administered because this drug is cleared by the kidneys.
    4. Only relates to the intake of sodium and does not include fluids with no sodium ions.

84. The nurse in the emergency department is evaluating a woman at 37 weeks of gestation who has been admitted with complaints of abdominal pain and some bright-red vaginal bleeding. The nurse knows that:
    1. Placenta previa must be the underlying problem because of the presence of pain.

2. Placental abruption must be the problem because of the presence of bright-red vaginal bleeding.
3. Infection is most likely because of the combination of pain and bleeding.
4. These may be signs of normal labor.

85. A woman whose pregnancy is at term is hospitalized on bedrest with placenta previa. She complains of backache and abdominal cramping. The nurse should:
    1. Check for vaginal bleeding at these early signs of labor.
    2. Remind her of breathing and relaxing exercises in labor.
    3. Assist her with the bedpan so that she can have a bowel movement.
    4. Perform a vaginal exam to check for cervical changes.

86. A woman whose pregnancy is at term is admitted to labor and delivery complaining of severe abdominal pain and no fetal movement for the past 8 hours. Her vital signs are: blood pressure 90/60; pulse 104; respirations 22; fetal heart rate 120. Vaginal exam shows that the cervix is closed and there is clear mucus fluid in the vagina. Her abdomen is rigid and tender. The nurse knows that the most important sign to carefully observe for is:
    1. Vaginal bleeding as a sign of placenta previa.
    2. Uterine contractions obscured by signs of placental abruption.
    3. Normal labor progress.
    4. Rupture of membranes.

87. A woman whose pregnancy is at term is admitted to labor and delivery with a large amount of bright-red vaginal bleeding. Having determined that the woman is in stable condition, the nurse should anticipate that which assessment tests will be done first?
    1. Nonstress test of fetal movement.
    2. Stress test of the fetal heart rate.
    3. Ultrasound for placental location.
    4. Contraction monitoring for signs of labor.

88. The nurse is caring for a woman who is pregnant at 32 weeks of gestation who has been hospitalized with polyhydramnios. The client has been ordered on bed rest in the lateral Sims' position. The nurse knows that this position is important because:
    1. It reduces the risk of preterm labor.
    2. It is easier to monitor the fetus in this position.
    3. It reduces respiratory distress and pressure on the vena cava.
    4. It minimizes the discomfort of backache.

89. The nurse is providing daily hygiene to a woman at 32 weeks of gestation who has been admitted with polyhydramnios. During the bath, the amniotic sac ruptures, with 2000 cc of clear amniotic fluid discharged from the vagina. The nurse knows that this is an obstetric emergency because of the risk of:
    1. Shock from excessive fluid loss.
    2. Sudden onset of tumultuous labor.
    3. Prolapsed cord.
    4. Premature separation of the placenta.

90. The nurse is describing a nonstress test to a woman at 36 weeks of gestation. The woman asks, "What do my baby's movements have to do with how healthy he is?" The best response by the nurse would be:
    1. "When the fetus reaches maturity, he moves a lot more, showing that he has good muscle mass."
    2. "When the fetus gets enough blood, he is stimulated to move because blood stimulates brain activity."
    3. "A slow-moving baby probably has an abnormality in the brain that causes poor nervous stimulation to the muscles in the legs and arm."
    4. "Under control of the brain, the heart rate should speed up when the baby moves to deliver enough oxygen to the muscles."

91. The nurse is describing a contraction stress test to a woman at 36 weeks of gestation. The nurse knows that the client understands the difference between the nonstress test and the contraction stress test when the client states:
    1. "I will only have to have a contraction stress test if there is a significant problem with my baby."
    2. "The contraction stress test is used when my baby is asleep and is not moving enough to do the nonstress test."
    3. "A contraction stress test can only be done when I am in labor."
    4. "I would have a contraction stress test if the results from the nonstress test were uncertain, in order to see for sure if there was a problem with the baby."

92. A client who is pregnant is being observed on the labor and delivery unit for a biophysical profile. The nurse anticipates that this client's pregnancy may be postmature, because this test measures:
    1. Heart rate in response to uterine contractions.
    2. Amount of amniotic fluid.
    3. Serial fetal growth patterns.
    4. Gross anatomical abnormalities of the fetus.

93. A woman who is pregnant has a family history of Down syndrome. Which statement by the nurse about amniocentesis and chorionic villus sampling is accurate?
    1. "Only amniocentesis can look directly at fetal cells and chromosomes."
    2. "Chorionic villus sampling must be done after the sixteenth week of gestation when there is sufficient placental tissue."
    3. "Although both tests involve a needle aspiration, there is little or no risk of harm to the baby."
    4. "Chorionic villus sampling may be performed as early as four weeks before an amniocentesis."

94. The nurse is discussing signs of labor with a class of women who are pregnant and their partners. Which statement by the nurse is accurate about signs of labor?
    1. "Second labors are always faster than first labors. You should go to the hospital when the contractions are no closer than 10 minutes apart."
    2. "Women having their first baby will feel the baby drop (lightening) about 2 weeks before labor begins."
    3. "When labor starts, vaginal bleeding is a sign of a problem and you should go to the hospital."
    4. "The membranes should rupture once the baby descends, putting pressure on the cervix."

95. A woman is pregnant with twins. In evaluating her risks, the nurse knows that which of the following statements is/are true about multifetal pregnancies?
    Select all that apply.
    1. The woman's chance of developing preeclampsia is greatly increased.
    2. The woman's chance of developing preeclampsia is less than a woman carrying a singleton pregnancy.
    3. The woman will probably deliver before her EDD.
    4. The best test to ensure that each fetus is growing is a nonstress test.
    5. The woman's chance of postpartum hemorrhage is greater than if she were carrying a singleton pregnancy.

96. A primipara at term has experienced lightening. The nurse should anticipate which sign of discomfort that would normally accompany lightening?
    1. Urinary frequency.
    2. Dyspnea.
    3. Heartburn.
    4. Constipation.

97. A woman at term pregnancy, gravida 5, para 4004, has been examined by the nurse in the triage room of the labor and delivery unit. The nurse finds that her contractions are 5 minutes apart, cervix is 3 cm dilated and 10% effaced, station 0, membranes intact. The nurse anticipates that:
    1. This woman is at the beginning of active phase and will not deliver for at least 8 hours.
    2. At 3 cm with intact membranes, this woman is still in latent phase and should return home.
    3. This woman is experiencing abnormal labor as evidenced by rapid contractions and progress in dilation without progress in effacement. She should be observed carefully.
    4. This woman appears to be experiencing a normal active labor process for a multipara and should be admitted.

98. The forces of labor have voluntary and involuntary components. In providing support during labor, the nurse knows that:
    1. Voluntary forces are most effectively used in second stage.
    2. Women in labor should be encouraged to voluntarily push with every contraction to assist fetal descent.
    3. Involuntary pushing should be eliminated with analgesics.
    4. There is no way to assist the involuntary forces during first stage.

99. The nurse in labor and delivery has just received report from the nurse going off duty. The client to whom the nurse is assigned has just entered the transition phase of labor. The nurse realizes that the husband who is acting as labor coach may need extra support because:
    1. He has been there for many hours and is getting bored and restless.
    2. The woman in labor is having painful contractions and is irritable and withdrawn.
    3. Birth is imminent.
    4. He should be helping her to push.

100. A woman who is a primipara at term is in active labor and is complaining of severe backache with contractions. Which of the following is not an effective comfort measure?
    1. Massage to the lower back between contractions.
    2. External pressure to the sacrum during contractions.
    3. Assistance with ambulation.
    4. Position on side with pillows between legs.

Answers/Rationales/Tips

1. **(1)** Basal body temperature falls slightly immediately before ovulation, then rises approximately 0.5°C. This characteristic finding aids women in identifying the fertile period of their cycle. **Answer 2** is incorrect because the pattern described is reversed. **Answers 3** and **4** are wrong because ovulation is related to an LH surge.

> **TEST-TAKING TIP**—Remember the characteristic pattern: ↓T, ↑T.
> **AS, COM, 5, Women's Health, HPM, Health Promotion and Maintenance**

KEY TO CODES FOLLOWING RATIONALES:

Nursing process: **AS**, assessment; **AN**, analysis; **PL**, plan; **IMP**, implementation; **EV**, evaluation. *Cognitive level:* **COM**, comprehension; **APP**, application; **ANL**, analysis. *Category of human function:* **1**, protective; **2**, sensory-perceptual; **3**, comfort, rest, activity, and mobility; **4**, nutrition; **5**, growth and development; **6**, fluid-gas transport; **7**, psychosocial-cultural; **8**, elimination. *Client need:* **SECE**, safe, effective care environment; **HPM**, health promotion/maintenance; **PsI**, psychosocial integrity; **PhI**, physiological integrity. (Client subneed appears after Client need code.) See appendices for full explanation.

2. **(1)** Heart rate—2; respiratory effort—1; muscle tone—0; reflex response—1; color—1. Total Apgar score is 5. **Answers 2, 3,** and **4** are incorrect because of inaccurate allocation of points for behaviors described.

> 💡 **TEST-TAKING TIP**—Use the acronym APGAR to help remember the five areas for assessment: A—Appearance, P—Pulse, G—Grimace, A—Activity, R—Respiratory effort.
> **AS, COM, 5, Newborn, PhI, Physiological Adaptation**

3. **January 10.** (Accept alternate formats such as January 10th, Jan. 10, 1/10, etc.) To calculate EDD using Nägele's rule of counting back 3 months and adding 7 days to date of LMP: fourth month – 3 months = first month (January); third day plus 7 days = tenth day; January 10 is her EDD.

> **TEST-TAKING TIP**—Mathematical accuracy is the key to the right answer, using Nägele's rule. Use the formula for calculating the EDD.
> **AN, ANL, 5, Maternity, HPM, Health Promotion and Maintenance**

4. **(3)** Term infants may lose 5%–10% of their birth weight. Arithmetic: 7 x 16 oz = 112 oz; 10% of 112 = 11.2 oz (317.5 g). **Answers 1, 2,** and **4** are wrong because of inaccurate computation.

> **TEST-TAKING TIP**—Accurate multiplication (16 oz = 1 pound) is the key. Remember that 5%–10% loss is OK.
> **AN, APP, 5, Newborn, HPM, Health Promotion and Maintenance**

5. **(2)** The reason for the first cesarean was a breech presentation, and that is not present in this pregnancy. Also, a low transverse uterine incision presents only a very slight risk for uterine rupture with subsequent VBAC deliveries. **Answer 1** is incorrect because the classic vertical incision through the uterus (and subsequent scar) is considered to weaken the uterus and compromise its ability to withstand stretching and contracting. **Answer 3** is incorrect because the original cause (fetopelvic disproportion) remains. **Answer 4** is incorrect because an infant may acquire herpes during passage through an infected birth canal.

> **TEST-TAKING TIP**—Visualize the common uterine incision used and why it would pose the greatest risk for uterine rupture. Eliminate **Answer 3** because the same condition exists *again;* and eliminate **Answer 4** because there is maternal infection *now.* Review the risks of cesarean birth, and specifically the risks of a vaginal birth after a previous cesarean.
> **AN, APP, 1, Maternity, PhI, Reduction of Risk Potential**

6. **(1)** Red meats, egg yolks, and organ meats are the best sources of iron. **Answers 2, 3,** and **4** are incorrect because they do not contain as much iron as red meat.

> **TEST-TAKING TIP**—Knowing the best (highest) food sources of iron will help you choose the best answer.
> **IMP, APP, 4, Maternity, PhI, Basic Care and Comfort**

7. **(4)** Even women who are Rh-negative during their first pregnancy are at some risk for Rh incompatibility; erythroblastosis fetalis results from hemolysis of fetal cells by maternal antibodies. **Answers 1** and **2** are incorrect because the woman who is Rh-negative is *not* more prone to spontaneous abortion or preeclampsia. **Answer 3** is incorrect because *fetal, not* maternal, anemia results from Rh incompatibility.

> **TEST-TAKING TIP**—The focus should be on the potential risk for the fetus. Understand the pathophysiology of Rh isoimmunization.
> **AN, APP, 6, Maternity, PhI, Reduction of Risk Potential**

8. **(1)** A quiet room close to the nurse's station provides the best environment for treatment (observation and decreased stimulation). A private room is ideal, but of these choices, **Answer 1** is the best. **Answers 2, 3,** and **4** are incorrect because too much noise or stimulation can precipitate eclamptic seizures. All of these environments could be too noisy and too stimulating.

> **TEST-TAKING TIP**—Because of severe preeclampsia, choose the *least* stimulating environment (i.e., ↓ noise, ↓ number of people).
> **AN, ANL, 6, Maternity, PhI, Reduction of Risk Potential**

9. **(4)** The data indicate that the woman has an arrest of her labor (potentially cephalopelvic disproportion), and the fetus is developing a tachycardia (fetal distress). It would be contraindicated to augment labor under these circumstances. The nurse should emphasize the assessment findings to the physician. **Answers 1, 2,** and **3** are incorrect because augmentation of labor is *contraindicated* with the current situation.

> **TEST-TAKING TIP**—Because of the risk of hyperstimulation of the uterus, choose the *one* answer that does *not* cause it. Think of client safety, and think of the *legal* responsibility of the RN.
> **IMP, ANL, 1, Maternity, PhI, Pharmacological Therapy**

10. **(3)** Undescended testicles are a condition unrelated to maternal hormonal influence. By 36–38 weeks of gestation, they should be descending through the inguinal canal and into the scrotal sac. **Answers 1, 2,** and **4** are incorrect. They are all a result of maternal hormonal influences and are considered *normal* findings in the full-term neonate.

> **TEST-TAKING TIP**—Eliminate the three options that are related to maternal hormone influence. Key concept is *time* related (i.e., at *term,* not at 36 weeks of gestation or earlier).
> **AS, APP, 5, Maternity, HPM, Health Promotion and Maintenance**

11. **(4)** The woman with AIDS has compromised immunity. The nurse should not assign this client to a health-care provider who has a viral or infectious illness. **Answers 1, 2,** and **3** are incorrect. It would not be as great a risk for clients with renal failure, hypertension, or a prolonged labor to have contact with a health-care provider who has a cold.

> **TEST-TAKING TIP**—Consider the nurse's role in *delegation of care,* and think about client safety as the *priority* when there is a risk of exposure to infectious or viral agents for clients with compromised immunity.
> **PL, ANL, 6, Maternity, SECE, Safety and Infection Control**

12. **(1)** Both red blood cells (RBCs) and plasma increase in pregnancy; but because the plasma increase exceeds the increase in RBC production, there is a decrease in both Hct and Hgb due to hemodilution. **Answers 2, 3,** and **4** are incorrect because the increases are not correct. Neither erythrocyte nor plasma volume decreases during pregnancy.

> **TEST-TAKING TIP**—The increases in both are a protective mechanism for both mother and fetus.
> **AN, ANL, 6, Maternity, HPM, Health Promotion and Maintenance**

13. **(1)** The height of the fundus (single pregnancy) should measure about 20 cm at 20 weeks (*at the umbilicus*). A measurement less than that might indicate inadequate fetal growth or an error in calculation of gestational age. **Answers 2, 3,** and **4** are all findings that would be considered *normal* during the second trimester of pregnancy.

> **TEST-TAKING TIP**—The key point is *when*—that is, when prenatal assessment findings are not normal during the second trimester.
> **AS, APP, 5, Maternity, HPM, Health Promotion and Maintenance**

14. **(1)** As milk is removed from the breast, more is produced. **Answers 2, 3,** and **4** are incorrect because as the infant requires more milk with each feeding, the woman's breasts will meet the demands with adequate nutrition and volume if there is adequate maternal nutrition and hydration. Also, early introduction of solids (**Answer 3**) may make the infant more prone to food allergies. Regular feeding of solids may also lead to decreased intake of breastmilk and has been associated with early cessation of breastfeeding.

> **TEST-TAKING TIP**—Remember the concept that milk production during lactation is a supply-demand system.
> **AN, COM, 4, Maternity, PhI, Basic Care and Comfort**

15. **(2)** The considerable uterine distention involved with multiple gestation can place the woman at risk for premature contractions, cervical dilation, and delivery. If there are risk factors for preterm birth, abstinence from orgasm and nipple stimulation, as well as increased rest during the last trimester, may be recommended to avoid preterm labor. **Answers 1, 3,** and **4** do not necessarily place a woman at increased risk for preterm labor. *Inadequate* weight gain is a risk factor, *not* extra weight gain. A history of preterm labor must always be considered a high-risk factor.

> **TEST-TAKING TIP**—Visualize what happens to the uterus with twins and to what that can lead.
> **AS, APP, 1, Maternity, PhI, Reduction of Risk Potential**

16. **(2)** The one factor that has been *highly* correlated to smoking cigarettes and marijuana is low birth weight. **Answers 1, 3,** and **4** are incorrect because retardation, deformation, and malnourishment do *not* have a *high* correlation to smoking cigarettes and marijuana.

> **TEST-TAKING TIP**—Think *low* birth weight = *high* risk (i.e., high correlation). Choose the *least* serious consequence as the *highest* probability for causing the condition. Review teratogenic and high-risk substances women may use during pregnancy. Know the most common effects of these substances on the fetus/newborn.
> **EV, COM, 5, Maternity, HPM, Health Promotion and Maintenance**

17. **(3)** Many times the physiological response to stress may be a decrease in milk production. This may rectify itself over time, provided the anxiety is controlled. However, as long as the system is under prolonged, intense stress, the milk supply will probably remain diminished. **Answers 1** and **4** are incorrect because the nurse does *not* have physiological *evidence* to substantiate the probability of a virus or of occluded lactation ducts. **Answer 2** is incorrect because the surviving infant is probably *too young* to react physiologically to the twin's death. However, it is possible that the infant is experiencing some emotional trauma in response both to the increase in familial tension and to not hearing or seeing the other twin.

> **TEST-TAKING TIP**—Think funeral = increased stress. Note the similarity between the stem ("producing ... milk") and **Answer 3** ("milk producing"). Review factors that might alter normal lactation.
> **IMP, APP, 5, Maternity, PsI, Psychosocial Integrity**

18. **(2)** The "formula" for determining parity is *TPAL: T* is the number of *term* pregnancies (38 weeks); *P* is the number of

preterm pregnancies (20–37 weeks); *A* is the number of *abortions* (pregnancies that do not reach viability, 20–22 weeks of gestation); *L* is the number of *living children*. This woman's first pregnancy ended in abortion and she has no living children. Her parity is T = 0, P = 0, A = 1, L = 0; or 0-0-1-0. **Answers 1, 3,** and **4** are not correct according to this formula.

> **TEST-TAKING TIP**—Use the TPAL system: term, preterm, abortions, living children.
> **AN, COM, 5, Maternity, HPM, Health Promotion and Maintenance**

19. **(2)** Positive pregnancy test results are considered among the *probable* signs of pregnancy (with the exception of the bioassay test for the beta subunit of HCG, which is accurate). **Answers 1, 3,** and **4** are incorrect because hearing fetal heart sounds, feeling fetal movements, and seeing the fetus are all *positive* signs of pregnancy, not probable signs.

> **TEST-TAKING TIP**—The positive pregnancy test is a *probable* sign. Compare presumptive, probable, and positive signs of pregnancy.
> **IMP, APP, 5, Maternity, HPM, Health Promotion and Maintenance**

20. **(4)** An effective assessment of the couple's needs is obtained through discussing the couple's own perceptions of those needs. **Answers 1** and **2** are incorrect because referral to social services or family counseling may be an appropriate action once a thorough assessment is complete, it should *never* precede discussion with the couple. **Answer 3** is incorrect because supportive counseling may be an appropriate action once a thorough assessment is complete, it also should *never* precede discussion with the couple.

> **TEST-TAKING TIP**—Choose "assess" *before* "refer" or "provide." Review the nurse's role as client advocate and guidelines for proper referral.
> **IMP, APP, 7, Maternity, SECE, Management of Care**

21. **(4)** Metronidazole (Flagyl) is the drug of choice in treating *Trichomonas vaginilis.* **Answers 1** and **2** are incorrect because tetracycline and erythromycin are ineffective against *Trichomonas* infection and are more commonly used in treating *bacterial* disease. **Answer 3** is incorrect because nystatin has little effect on *Trichomonas vaginalis,* but is the drug of choice for *Candida* infection.

> **TEST-TAKING TIP**—Choose the pharmacological agent commonly used for STDs and vaginal infections, rather than bacterial diseases (**Answers 1** and **2**).
> **IMP, COM, 1, Women's Health, PhI, Pharmacological and Parenteral Therapies**

22. **(3)** Examining her vaginal canal is contraindicated initially because of her preadmission history of bleeding. **Answer 1** is incorrect because initiating IV therapy *is* imperative in order to have a line available for any ordered medications or fluids. **Answers 2** and **4** are incorrect because taking her blood pressure and monitoring FHR *are* essential to establish baseline data and to monitor the mother's and infant's status.

> **TEST-TAKING TIP**—The problem may be placenta previa or other bleeding abnormalities in pregnancy. Choose the answer that covers what the nurse would *not* do when the question asks for a procedure that is contraindicated. The problem is *vaginal* bleeding, so select the option that relates to the *vaginal* canal.
> **AN, APP, 1, Maternity, PhI, Reduction of Risk Potential**

23. **(1)** Emergency surgery must be performed to save the life of the client, save the function of an organ or limb, remove a

damaged organ or limb, or stop hemorrhage. Few emergency situations are so urgent as to require immediate response (**Answer 2**), which would eliminate the necessary laboratory data to evaluate the client's physiological response to the situation. Surgical preparation would be completed within 24 hours (**Answer 3**), but this is not the *best* answer. True emergency situations cannot be postponed to the following surgical day (**Answer 4**).

> **TEST-TAKING TIP**—*Emergency* means "right away"; *however,* important things need to be done *before* the surgery can begin. There are preliminary measures such as establishing baseline assessment data, establishing IV lines, determining allergies, and having blood on hand for replacement if necessary. Consider what is best for client.
> **IMP, COM, 1, Women's Health, SECE, Management of Care**

24. **(4)** An abdominal hysterectomy is generally the treatment of choice for uterine fibroids with excessive vaginal bleeding. If the ovaries are not pathologic, there is no reason for surgical removal. A *pan*abdominal hysterectomy (**Answer 1**) involves the removal of the uterus, fallopian tubes, and ovaries and is usually performed for *extensive endometriosis or carcinoma.* A vaginal hysterectomy (**Answer 2**) is the treatment of choice for a prolapsed *uterus,* and a D&C (**Answer 3**) is primarily a *diagnostic* tool, *not* a measure to *control excessive* uterine bleeding.

> **TEST-TAKING TIP**—The key word is "fibroids," which do not require extensive removal of tubes, ovaries, and uterus. Thus, eliminate **Answer 1**. The difference between **Answer 2** (vaginal) and **Answer 4** (abdominal) is that **Answer 2** is done for a prolapsed uterus, *not* for excessive vaginal bleeding from fibroids.
> **IMP, COM, 5, Women's Health, SECE, Management of Care**

25. **(1)** Standard precautions specify that all health-care providers should wear gloves until all blood and amniotic fluid have been removed. Because transmission of the virus may occur via breastmilk, breastfeeding is *discouraged* (**Answer 2**). **Answers 3** and **4** are incorrect because the parents are *encouraged to bond* with the child and the nurse needs to support all positive parental feelings.

> **TEST-TAKING TIP**—The priority is *infection control,* that is, standard precautions (gloves when in contact with body fluids). See the word "precaution" in the stem and an example of standard precautions in **Answer 1**.
> **IMP, APP, 1, Maternity, SECE, Safety and Infection Control**

26. **(2)** Absence of variability (a smooth baseline) is an ominous sign of potential fetal distress. It can result from fetal hypoxia and acidosis and certain drugs that depress the central nervous system. A baseline range of 110–160 bpm is within normal limits (**Answer 1**). Early decelerations (from head compression) are of no clinical significance (**Answer 3**). Mild variable decelerations are usually remedied by changing the woman's position (**Answer 4**).

> **TEST-TAKING TIP**—Look at the key words: "baseline," "absence," "early," "mild." An intervention goes with "absence." Understand basic electronic fetal monitoring (EFM) patterns. Compare early, late, and variable decelerations.
> **EV, APP, 6, Maternity, PhI, Physiological Adaptation**

27. **(3)** Once the uterus is removed, the woman is infertile and contraception is *not* necessary. **Answers 1, 2,** and **4** *should* be included in the teaching plan. Following a hysterectomy, the vaginal flow is usually brownish in nature and will gradually diminish and cease. If the flow continues and is obviously red in nature, the physician must be notified. These signs could indicate a bleeding vessel. Menses will be absent following removal of the uterus.

> **TEST-TAKING TIP**—When a question asks for *inaccurate* information, choose the one that is wrong.
> **IMP, APP, 5, Women's Health, HPM, Health Promotion and Maintenance**

28. **(4)** Initial intervention when clients are reacting to the loss of a significant body part is to encourage verbalization of their fears and to assist them in identifying how they see the change in their body image as well as how it may affect their relationships. One of the most important factors in the client's response to mastectomy surgery is the reaction of her husband or the person with whom she is intimately involved. **Answers 1** and **2** tend to cut off communication in this instance. Many partners are very supportive; others are not. It is therefore also important to assist the partners to talk with each other, not just to the nurse, to acknowledge feelings and concerns (**Answer 3**). The client needs the reassurance of the partner's love and support to work through her own emotional reaction and begin the work of recovery.

> **TEST-TAKING TIP**—Focus on the client, *not* the husband (**Answer 3**); focus on feelings, *not* cognitive explanations (**Answers 1** and **2**).
> **IMP, APP, 7, Women's Health, PsI, Psychosocial Integrity**

29. **(3, 4, 5)** Answer 3 is correct because monitoring the fetal status is the most important function of the nurse at this time, since the cesarean section is being ordered for fetal distress. **Answer 4** is correct because a Foley catheter must be placed before surgery can begin. **Answer 5** is correct because the client needs to have a shave prep for surgery. **Answer 1** is incorrect because *informed* consent is the primary responsibility of the physician. **Answer 2** is incorrect because the nurse *cannot* reassure the client about the fetal outcome when the fetus is showing fetal distress. The nurse cannot *alleviate* realistic fears about the fetal outcome.

> **TEST-TAKING TIP**—The key phrase is *informed* consent; this is a physician role, therefore eliminate this option since the question asks for the *nursing* intervention. Eliminate the option that has an implied *guarantee.* The nurse cannot reassure this client of a positive outcome.
> **AS, ANL, 8, Maternity, PhI, Reduction of Risk Potential**

30. **(4)** The nurse should reflect back to the mother her concerns and listen to her fears. False reassurance and cliché answers are not therapeutic. **Answer 1** is incorrect because it may not be the case, and this answer will only frighten the mother at this time. **Answer 2** is incorrect because even if the mother hasn't seen very ill babies, she is extremely worried about the baby. Simply saying that the baby looks fine is not likely to ease her fears. **Answer 3** is incorrect because this answer is false reassurance and not therapeutic for the mother.

> **TEST-TAKING TIP**—The question asks what the most appropriate response is at this time. Eliminate answers that give false hope or are cliché (**Answers 2 and 3**). **Answer 1** is *not* supportive of the mother in dealing with her newborn's illness.
> **IMP, ANL, 7, Newborn, PsI, Psychosocial Integrity**

31. **(3)** Pressure is a *normal* sensation during a cesarean section. The client should be educated about the difference between pressure and pain during a cesarean section. **Answer 1** is incorrect because the client *will* feel pressure during the surgery, even with a regional anesthetic block. **Answer 2** is incorrect because the block does not *completely* eliminate sensations during surgery. **Answer 4** is incorrect because the effect of the anesthetic block will be carefully checked before beginning surgery. Pain would indicate an *incomplete* anesthetic block, not normal expectation during surgery.

TEST-TAKING TIP—There are two options that basically state the same information; therefore, eliminate **Answers 1 and 2**. Both options state that the client will feel nothing during the surgery. The remaining two options are pain or pressure. Think about which is normal. Eliminate **Answer 4** since pain during surgery is not normal.
IMP, ANL, 7, Maternity, PsI, Psychosocial Integrity

32. **(4)** The client should wait to call until she has assessed her symptoms after consuming *several 8-ounce glasses* of water for hydration. Adequate hydration can decrease uterine activity. **Answer 1** is incorrect because the client *should* call if her contractions are every 10 minutes. **Answer 2** is incorrect because she *should* call if contractions occur after she emptied her bladder. **Answer 3** is incorrect because she *should* call after she rested in bed on her side for an hour.

TEST-TAKING TIP—Three of the actions are appropriate before calling; eliminate these options (**Answers 1, 2, and 3**).
EV, ANL, 5, Maternity, HPM, Health Promotion and Maintenance

33. **(1)** The client is concerned about her body image after surgery. Because of the transverse lie, the physician may have to use a classical (vertical) incision, leaving a larger scar. **Answer 2** is incorrect because while this may be a concern of the client, it is not her *primary* concern about the incision. **Answer 3** is incorrect because while this may be a concern of the client, it is not her *primary* concern about the incision. **Answer 4** is incorrect because while this may be a concern of the client, it is not her *primary* concern about the external incision.

TEST-TAKING TIP—There are three options (**Answers 2, 3, and 4**) that concern surgical risk, and one option (**Answer 1**) that concerns external effects. Choose the option that is different.
AN, ANL, 7, Maternity, HPM, Health Promotion and Maintenance

34. **(2)** Most inborn errors of metabolism are caused by two recessive genes. That is, a woman who is a carrier (one dominant gene and one recessive gene) has a child with a man who is a carrier (one dominant gene and one recessive gene); the fetus has a chance of inheriting two recessive genes and, therefore, having the disease. The unborn child also has the chance of being a carrier of the disease (one dominant gene and one recessive gene). The woman and the father of the baby need additional genetic testing and counseling. **Answer 1** is incorrect because exposure to teratogens during first trimester of pregnancy is the cause of birth defects, not inborn errors of metabolism. **Answer 3** is incorrect because the use of illicit drugs does not cause inborn errors of metabolism. Drug use can cause placental abruption and childhood cognitive disorders. **Answer 4** is incorrect because most inborn errors of metabolism are not usually random mutations, but inherited from carriers of the trait for the disease.

TEST-TAKING TIP—The question asks what causes *most* inborn errors of metabolism. Three of the options (**Answers 1, 3, and 4**) are similar; choose the one option that is different (inherited).
AN, COM, 5, Maternity, HPM, Health Promotion and Maintenance

35. **(3)** The client needs to start treatment immediately. These medications are the primary medications recommended for use in pregnancy. **Answer 1** is incorrect because a therapeutic abortion is not indicated for a client with active tuberculosis

infection, **Answer 2** is incorrect because the client should start medication as soon as possible. Waiting for 6 months until birth is too long a time period. **Answer 4** is incorrect because the client needs to begin medication as soon as the diagnosis is made, and pyrazinamide is not recommended in pregnancy.

TEST-TAKING TIP—Three options focus on start medication for the client. Two of the choices are basically the same, i.e. a delay in treatment (**Answers 1 and 4**). One answer begins treatment *immediately* (**Answer 3**). Choose the different answer.
PL, ANL, 5, Maternity, HPM, Health Promotion and Maintenance

36. **(4)** Gonorrhea can be easily reacquired if sexual partners are not treated. **Answer 1** is incorrect because *Chlamydia* is the most common sexually transmitted disease in the U.S. **Answer 2** is incorrect because having a cesarean section will *not prevent* transmission. **Answer 3** is incorrect because cryotherapy is *not used* for gonorrhea infections.

TEST-TAKING TIP—Carefully read each option; both parts of the answer must be true to have the entire answer be correct. Do not quickly pick the first option that looks right; make sure there is no better answer.
IMP, APP, 1, Maternity, SECE, Safety and Infection Control

37. **(3)** Both the systolic and diastolic measurements have exceeded the normal limit of 140/90. **Answer 1** is incorrect because the second blood pressure is *not* normal. **Answer 2** is incorrect because this intervention is not indicated by the change in blood pressure. **Answer 4** is incorrect because this intervention is not indicated by the change in blood pressure.

TEST-TAKING TIP—The only option that deals with an abnormal finding is **Answer 3**. If you know that the blood pressure is potentially abnormal, it is the only option that fits the question.
AN, ANL, 6, Maternity, PhI, Reduction of Risk Potential

38. **(4)** It is a complaint that many women who are pregnant express, especially just before labor begins, when cervical mucus is shed. It is often confused with amniotic fluid and is inconclusive. **Answer 1** is incorrect because it is a positive reaction produced only by the presence of amniotic fluid diagnosing rupture of membranes. **Answer 2** is incorrect because it is a positive reaction produced only by the presence of amniotic fluid diagnosing rupture of membranes. **Answer 3** is incorrect because it is a positive reaction produced only by the presence of amniotic fluid diagnosing rupture of membranes.

TEST-TAKING TIP—Note that the question asks for an *inconclusive* option. The only option that is not directly observed but comes as subjective data from the client is **Answer 4**. The other three options occur only with the presence of amniotic fluid and *are conclusive* signs of rupture of membranes.
AS, APP, 5, Maternity, PhI, Reduction of Risk Potential

39. **(3)** Fetal movement is normally felt for the first time by 22 weeks of gestation, and the height of the fundus at 26 weeks of gestation is *above* the umbilicus. These findings are abnormal for this gestational age and may signal a complication. **Answer 1** is incorrect because the fundal height and lack of fetal movement are *not* normal for this gestational age. **Answer 2** is incorrect because one possible complication might be fetal demise, and it would be *inappropriate* to reassure the client that she will feel fetal movement or that it has been occurring. **Answer 4** is incorrect because one possible complication might be fetal demise, and it would be *inappro-*

priate to reassure the client that she will feel fetal movement or that it has been occurring.

> **TEST-TAKING TIP**—Whenever the question provides history or physical exam data, the first question to ask is, "Are these findings normal?" If they are not, usually the most appropriate answer will be some sort of report or consultation, unless it is an emergency requiring immediate action.
> **IMP, ANL, 5, Maternity, HPM, Health Promotion and Maintenance**

40. **(3)** Cephalopelvic disproportion is a complication involving *both* the fetal head and the pelvic bones. It cannot be determined by assessment of the bones alone. **Answer 1** is incorrect because cephalopelvic disproportion *cannot* be determined by the size of the *pelvis alone*. **Answer 2** is incorrect because cephalopelvic disproportion cannot be determined by the size of the *fetus alone*. **Answer 4** is incorrect because delivering before the due date has *little impact* on pelvic bones (although it may influence fetal size).

> **TEST-TAKING TIP**—Options with "extreme" words such as *always* are usually wrong. By definition cephalopelvic disproportion requires an answer that has *both* the head and the pelvis in it. **Answer 3** is the only one that includes both terms (head, pelvis). The term *cephalopelvic* in the stem is a tip to the best answer.
> **AN, APP, 5, Maternity, HPM, Health Promotion and Maintenance**

41. **(2)** If the pelvic inlet is big enough to accommodate the fetal head, the rest of the pelvis is probably adequate. **Answer 1** is incorrect because active labor can occur *with or without* engagement. However, primiparas generally have engage-ment before active labor. **Answer 3** is incorrect because, for most women, engagement occurs before or during the active phase of labor. **Answer 4** is incorrect because pelvic and back *pressure* may accompany engagement, but *severe* pain is *unusual*.

> **TEST-TAKING TIP**—The question links the diameter of the fetal head with the pelvic inlet. The only option that relates to those two concepts is **Answer 2**.
> **AS, APP, 5, Maternity, HPM, Health Promotion and Maintenance**

42. **(3)** The assumption that ovulation and fertilization would occur at about day 14 of the cycle would not be true for cycles that are 45 days apart. **Answer 1** is incorrect because ovulation and fertilization would occur at or about day 14 or at the midpoint in the cycle. **Answer 2** is incorrect because, although ovulation and fertilization would occur around day 10–12 rather than day 14, the difference of a couple of days would *not* affect the due date significantly. **Answer 4** is incorrect because, although ovulation and fertilization would occur at or about day 14–18 of the cycle, the differ-ence of these days would *not* affect the due date significantly.

> **TEST-TAKING TIP**—**Answer 3** is the only one with a significantly larger interval between menstrual periods. If a large interval would affect the due date, the largest one is the most likely answer.
> **AN, APP, 1, Maternity, HPM, Health Promotion and Maintenance**

43. **(2)** The client may not have resumed ovulation immediately after stopping the pill and may not have gotten pregnant right away. **Answer 1** is incorrect because condoms and foam *do not affect* the interval of the menstrual cycles. **Answer 3** is incorrect because the two periods after the IUD removal indi-cate resumption of the menstrual cycle. **Answer 4** is incorrect because lack of use of contraception does *not* alter the inter-val of the menstrual cycle (other than pregnancy).

> **TEST-TAKING TIP**—The only option that suggests that there was *not* a normal menstrual cycle before pregnancy is **Answer 2**. A normal menstrual cycle is essential for accurate calculation of the due date by the last menstrual period.
> **EV, APP, 1, Maternity, HPM, Health Promotion and Maintenance**

44. **(1)** Sudden severe headaches may be a sign of hypertension or brain attack associated with pill use. **Answer 2** is incorrect because vaginal infection, although it requires treatment, is *not* a life-threatening complication of pill use. **Answer 3** is incorrect because a family history of diabetes is *not* a sign of a life-threatening complication of pill use. **Answer 4** is incor-rect because exposure to gonorrhea, although it requires treatment, is *not* a life-threatening complication of pill use.

> **TEST-TAKING TIP**—Although each answer suggests a serious problem, only one answer suggests a serious problem *directly* related to pill use.
> **AN, APP, 6, Maternity, PhI, Pharmacological/Parenteral Therapies**

45. **(1)** Condoms do *not* prevent *all* forms of sexually transmitted diseases. **Answer 2** is incorrect because *it is true* that condoms should be used with pills to prevent infection. **Answer 3** is incorrect because *it is true* that condoms should be used even if you have tested negative for HIV. **Answer 4** is incorrect because *it is true* that a primary reason for using condoms is to prevent infection.

> **TEST-TAKING TIP**—The use of the word "all" in the first option is a red flag. Usually avoid use of "extreme" words such as *all* or *none* (but not in this case) because this question does ask for a statement that should be *avoided*. All other answers are true.
> **IMP, APP, 1, Women's Health, SECE, Safety/Infection Control**

46. **(2)** These are the *early* warning symptoms of a complication from the use of the intrauterine device. **Answer 1** is incorrect because these symptoms are *not* strongly associated with complications of the intrauterine device. **Answer 3** is incor-rect because these symptoms are *not* strongly associated with complications of the intrauterine device. **Answer 4** is incor-rect because these symptoms are *not* strongly associated with complications of the intrauterine device.

> **TEST-TAKING TIP**—Symptom lists can be confusing. Do *not* be mislead by the most serious symptoms. Look for the ones that directly relate to the problem in the question.
> **IMP, APP, 1, Women's Health, SECE, Safety/Infection Control**

47. **(2)** It is a common misconception that breastfeeding may prevent pregnancy. **Answer 1** is incorrect because the client has a *correct* understanding that breastfeeding may affect her menstrual cycle. **Answer 3** is incorrect because the client has a *correct* understanding about when fertility resumes after birth. **Answer 4** is incorrect because the client has a *correct* under-standing about the effect of breastfeeding on involution.

> **TEST-TAKING TIP**—When you are looking for a false statement, it is helpful to think of each option as "true" or "false," and then go back and read the stem again. Usually the right answer will then be more obvious.
> **EV, APP, 1, Women's Health, HPM, Health Promotion and Maintenance**

48. **(4)** Superabsorbent tampons for long-term use should be strictly *avoided* to prevent toxic shock. **Answer 1** is incorrect because washing barrier method devices *is* effective protection against toxic shock. **Answer 2** is incorrect because the cervical

cap *should* never be left in more than 48 hours. It is advisable to *remove* it and wash it before 48 hours. **Answer 3** is incorrect because tampons *should* be changed more frequently than 2 to 4 hours to prevent infection.

> **TEST-TAKING TIP**—*Time* is the main issue here, and the longest time span is in **Answer 4**. Note that the question asks for a practice that should be *discouraged*. Superabsorbent tampons left in for longer than 4 hours have been associated with toxic shock syndrome.
> **IMP, APP, 1, Women's Health, SECE, Safety/Infection Control**

49. **(3)** Infertility is not diagnosed until at least 12 months of unprotected intercourse has failed to produce a pregnancy. Older couples will experience a longer time to get pregnant. **Answer 1** is incorrect because it is a *myth*; it rarely happens. **Answer 2** is incorrect because infertility is *not* diagnosed until 12 months of unprotected intercourse has failed to produce a pregnancy. **Answer 4** is incorrect because very frequent intercourse (more often than every 24 hours) depletes the sperm count and *decreases* chances of pregnancy.

> **TEST-TAKING TIP**—**Answer 3** is the only sound self-help advice. It is clearly within the nurse's role to provide this advice.
> **IMP, APP, 5, Women's Health, HPM, Health Promotion and Maintenance**

50. **(4)** It respects client autonomy in decision making. The nurse is obligated to provide either unbiased counseling or a referral. **Answer 1** is incorrect because the nurse is *not* obligated to provide a point of view contrary to the client's decision, and to do so might violate client autonomy. **Answer 2** is incorrect because, although it is appropriate to discuss the risks of a procedure with the client, a nurse with an opposing viewpoint may not be able to give unbiased information. **Answer 3** is incorrect because, although it is an appropriate nursing action, the nurse with an opposing value may not be able to validate informed consent fairly.

> **TEST-TAKING TIP**—Ethical questions are troublesome because there are few clear-cut answers. Look for the option that *respects* the position of the *client without compromising the position of the nurse*.
> **IMP, ANL, 5, Maternity, SECE, Management of Care**

51. **(3)** RhoGAM is not indicated for women who are Rh-positive. **Answer 1** is incorrect because RhoGAM *is* indicated for any first trimester abortion of a woman who is Rh-negative. **Answer 2** is incorrect because RhoGAM *is* indicated at the beginning of the third trimester for women who are Rh-negative and who are unsensitized. **Answer 4** is incorrect because RhoGAM *is* indicated for all women who are Rh-negative and experience abdominal trauma.

> **TEST-TAKING TIP**—The key word in the stem is "inappropriate." Because RhoGAM is given only to mothers who are Rh-negative, the mother who should *not* receive it is the only mother who is Rh-positive (**Answer 3**).
> **IMP, COM, 1, Maternity, PhI, Pharmacological/Parenteral Therapies**

52. **(1, 3)** **Answer 1** is correct because the client will need an IV access for labor induction or cesarean section. **Answer 3** is correct because both the sterile vaginal examination and the Leopold's maneuver revealed ballotable presenting fetal parts. The location of the fetal heart tones in the *upper quadrant* is common in *breech* presentation. The fetal presenting part must be determined before starting labor induction. **Answer 2** is incorrect because the client should be NPO until the fetal

presentation is determined. **Answer 4** is incorrect because the fetal presenting part *must* be determined before starting labor induction. **Answer 5** is incorrect because the client is 2 cm dilated, indicating that the client is in the *first* stage of labor. A vacuum-assisted delivery is performed during the *second* stage of labor.

> **TEST-TAKING TIP**—The key to this question is *ballotable*. When the fetus is ballotable, the fetal presentation must be determined *before* beginning an induction of labor. Eliminate the options that are *not* associated with the start of labor (a regular diet and a vacuum extraction).
> **PL, ANL, 6, Maternity, SECE, Management of Care**

53. **(4)** Sexual intercourse, as a potential source of infection, should be delayed until the cervix is healed. **Answer 1** is incorrect because tampons are a potential source of *infection*. **Answer 2** is incorrect because pregnancy may occur *before* the first period. **Answer 3** is incorrect because douching is a potential source of *infection*.

> **TEST-TAKING TIP**—Knowing that nothing should be inserted in the vagina immediately after an abortion should eliminate **Answers 1** and **3** immediately.
> **IMP, APP, 1, Maternity, PhI, Reduction of Risk Potential**

54. **(1)** It is the most accurate statement of physiological facts for a 28-day menstrual cycle: ovulation at day 14, egg life span 24 hours, sperm life span 72 hours. Fertilization could occur from sperm deposited before ovulation. **Answer 2** is incorrect because the life span of the egg is 24 hours, *not* 72 hours, and the life span of the sperm is 72 hours, *not* 24 hours. **Answer 3** is incorrect because, in a reliable 28-day cycle, ovulation occurs at about day 14, *not* day 20. **Answer 4** is incorrect because the fertile period *can* be reliably, but not absolutely, calculated. It is an unreliable basis for contraception.

> **TEST-TAKING TIP**—The question asks for the period of fertility.
> **IMP, APP, 5, Women's Health, HPM, Health Promotion and Maintenance**

55. **(2)** Before implantation, the fertilized egg is not attached to the uteroplacental connection and is less affected by substances in the maternal blood. **Answer 1** is incorrect because not all drug use is associated with congenital anomalies. **Answer 3** is incorrect because drug use later in pregnancy may affect organ function, *even after* the period of organ formation. **Answer 4** is incorrect because all drugs have potential harmful effects in pregnancy, and the benefit of use should be weighed by the risk of the harmful effects.

> **TEST-TAKING TIP**—Options with absolute words such as "always" in **Answer 1** and "only" in **Answer 3** are usually wrong.
> **AN, APP, 1, Maternity, PhI, Pharmacological/Parenteral Therapies**

56. **(4)** It is an open-ended, neutral response to the client that elicits important information about the extent and currency of drug use. **Answer 1** is incorrect because it incorrectly assumes that the drug use will affect the fetus. **Answer 2** is incorrect because it incorrectly assumes that the drug use will cause complications of pregnancy and childbirth. **Answer 3** is incorrect because there are no tests that can provide absolute reassurance that the fetus has not been affected by drug use.

> **TEST-TAKING TIP**—Open-ended, neutral, nonjudgmental responses are preferable to responses that imply a judgment about the client. You want her to feel comfortable and be open and honest about her drug use.
> **IMP, APP, 1, Maternity, PsI, Psychosocial Integrity**

57. (2) It lists culturally appropriate foods that are high in iron and calcium but would not affect lactose intolerance. **Answer 1** is incorrect because *dairy* products would affect lactose intolerance. **Answer 3** is incorrect because *dairy* products would affect lactose intolerance. **Answer 4** is incorrect because the regular adult diet is *insufficient* for the needs of pregnancy.

> **TEST-TAKING TIP**—Note *lactose intolerance* in the stem. Therefore *dairy products* will eliminate two of the options (**Answer 1** and **Answer 3**).
> **IMP, APP, 4, Maternity, PhI, and Basic Care and Comfort**

58. (2) The lab values indicate hemodilutional anemia of pregnancy, for which dietary counseling is indicated. The platelet and WBC values are normal. **Answer 1** is incorrect because the lab values do *not* indicate anemia but are consistent with the hemodilution process in pregnancy. If the hemoglobin drops to 10 g/dL or less, or the hematocrit drops below 33%, the woman is considered anemic. **Answer 3** is incorrect because the lab values indicate that *hemodilution* is occurring and routine supplementation for pregnancy *is* indicated. **Answer 4** is incorrect because *dispensing* medication is *outside of the scope* of practice of the nurse.

> **TEST-TAKING TIP**—Be careful of facts in the stem, such as the WBC and platelet values that are not reflected in the options. They can be confusing. The focus of the question is the hemoglobin and hematocrit values and the implications for the care of the client.
> **AN, ANL, 6, Maternity, PhI, Reduction of Risk Potential**

59. (1) Although there are a number of physical hazards to these jobs, the exposure to toxins, pesticides, and viruses is limited. **Answer 2** is incorrect because day care workers *are* exposed to many childhood viruses that can be teratogenic to the fetus. **Answer 3** is incorrect because in both job categories there *are* pesticides, cleansers, and solvents that can be teratogenic. **Answer 4** is incorrect because both job categories involve *exposure* to chemical, bacterial, and viral teratogens.

> **TEST-TAKING TIP**—The question specifically addresses teratogens *rather* than work-related injuries.
> **AN, ANL, 1, Maternity, SECE, Safety/Infection Control**

60. (1) Drinking fluids with meals enhances *nausea*. **Answer 2** is incorrect because the pelvic tilt *is* effective in reducing low backache. **Answer 3** is incorrect because lying down after eating promotes gastric reflux. **Answer 4** is incorrect because dry crackers *are* a good source of carbohydrates and help prevent empty stomach and low blood sugar associated with morning sickness.

> **TEST-TAKING TIP**—When looking for the false or erroneous option, label each option as true or false and then reread the question. The correct response is usually obvious.
> **EV, APP, 5, Maternity, PhI, and Basic Care and Comfort**

61. (3) The vital signs and urine values indicate that the symptoms are more than a common discomfort and the client is severely dehydrated. **Answer 1** is incorrect because the assessment findings indicate a significant complication, hyperemesis. **Answer 2** is incorrect because the assessment findings indicate a significant complication, hyperemesis. **Answer 4** is incorrect because the assessment findings indicate a significant complication, hyperemesis. Added oral intake will only aggravate the problem.

> **TEST-TAKING TIP**—Large urine ketones is an abnormal finding indicating a serious complication, usually either hyperemesis or diabetic acidosis.
> **AN, ANL, 6, Maternity, PhI, Physiological Adaptation**

62. (1) Progesterone does decrease tone of smooth muscle, and fiber is an effective intestinal stimulant. **Answer 2** is incorrect because sodium and water retention affects cardiovascular volume and edema, *not* fluid in the GI tract. Fluids *are* encouraged in pregnancy. **Answer 3** is incorrect because, although the statement is true, it does *not relate* to *constipation* in pregnancy. **Answer 4** is incorrect because it is *not* a concept regarding *nutrition.*

> **TEST-TAKING TIP**—Read the question carefully to eliminate options, such as **Answers 3** and **4**, that may be *true but not related* to the topics in the question.
> **IMP, APP, 4, Maternity, PhI, and Basic Care and Comfort**

63. (1) The *normal* discomfort of ankle edema in late pregnancy is attributed to poor venous return from the legs, which is relieved after lying down to sleep, preferably on her side. **Answer 2** is incorrect because sitting or lying flat on the back would decrease venous return and *increase* ankle edema. **Answer 3** is incorrect because the normal discomfort of ankle edema in late pregnancy should be improved after a night's rest, *not* made worse. **Answer 4** is incorrect because edema plus headache in late pregnancy is *not* a normal discomfort and may be an early sign of *preeclampsia.*

> **TEST-TAKING TIP**—Stating that something makes ankle edema worse sounds like the wrong answer, but it is a correct statement of normal physiology. Making the right answer sound wrong is a common question-writing strategy.
> **AN, APP, 6, Maternity, HPM, Health Promotion and Maintenance**

64. (3) Shortness of breath may be caused by the enlarging uterus displacing the diaphragm and lungs. Hot flashes may be relieved by removing excessive clothing. **Answer 1** is incorrect because, although some of these discomforts are caused by hormonal shifts in pregnancy and probably cannot be eliminated, there *are* effective self-help measures to reduce discomfort. **Answer 2** is incorrect because a demanding exercise program may increase heat intolerance, shortness of breath, and palpitations. The symptoms described are probably not caused by being out of shape. **Answer 4** is incorrect because sleeping in the supine position (flat on the back) will *increase* pressure of the uterus on the lungs and trigger shortness of breath.

> **TEST-TAKING TIP**—The stem asks for an accurate statement. Look for and eliminate the *false* statements.
> **AN, ANL, 5, Maternity, HPM, Health Promotion and Maintenance**

65. (4) Foods high in roughage stimulate peristalsis, and dark green vegetables are good natural, nonconstipating sources of iron. **Answer 1** is incorrect because taking iron at bedtime will *increase* discomfort from heartburn and have *no* effect on constipation. **Answer 2** is incorrect because avoiding foods high in roughage will make constipation *worse*. **Answer 3** is incorrect because taking a laxative regularly will decrease natural bowel motility and create a dependency habit.

> **TEST-TAKING TIP**—The problem is constipation. Look at the two contradictory options: "avoid roughage" versus "eat roughage."
> **IMP, APP, 4, Maternity, HPM, Health Promotion and Maintenance**

66. (3) Bending from the waist in pregnancy tends to make backache worse. **Answer 1** is incorrect because walking *is* an excellent toning exercise, and good posture prevents lower backache. **Answer 2** is incorrect because pelvic rock *does ease* the spasm in lower back muscles, and squatting strengthens thighs and legs. **Answer 4** is incorrect because swimming and leg kicking *are good* toning exercises, and being in water reduces the pull of gravity on the back and eases sore muscles.

TEST-TAKING TIP—Read the stem carefully to spot the key word: "avoided." The option may sound correct but not for the problem described in the stem.
PL, APP, 3, Maternity, HPM, Health Promotion and Maintenance

67. (2) It validates the woman's feelings and encourages an in-depth response. **Answer 1** is incorrect because it *minimizes* her problems and offers false reassurance. **Answer 3** is incorrect because, although the statement is true, it *fails* to address the *self-image problem* that the woman has described. **Answer 4** is incorrect because these feelings in pregnancy are *not* associated with a depression that must be treated pharmacologically. Mood-altering drugs should be *avoided* in pregnancy if possible.

TEST-TAKING TIP—In communication questions, look for the open-ended, neutral response that validates concerns expressed by the client.
IMP, APP, 7, Maternity, PsI, Psychosocial Integrity

68. (3) The incidence of preterm labor is significantly higher among women with a prior preterm birth. **Answer 1** is incorrect because two prior abortions and a preterm birth do *not* predict possible *fast* labors. **Answer 2** is incorrect because zero prior full-term pregnancies does *not* predict a *slow* labor. **Answer 4** is incorrect because the woman has *no* living children.

TEST-TAKING TIP—When one option is worded in a different way from the other options, it can often (but not always) be discarded as wrong.
AN, ANL, 5, Maternity, PhI, Reduction of Risk Potential

69. (1) The rapid pulse and respirations and dyspnea with common tasks plus periorbital edema may be early signs of a significant complication of pregnancy. **Answer 2** is incorrect because the rapid pulse and respirations and dyspnea with common tasks plus periorbital edema may be early signs of a significant complication of pregnancy. **Answer 3** is incorrect because the rapid pulse and respirations and dyspnea with common tasks plus periorbital edema may be early signs of a significant complication of pregnancy. **Answer 4** is incorrect because the rapid pulse and respirations and dyspnea with common tasks plus periorbital edema may be early signs of a significant complication of pregnancy.

TEST-TAKING TIP—When offered vitals signs and physical assessment data, check carefully for subtle but significant deviations from normal.
AN, ANL, 6, Maternity, PhI, Physiological Adaptation

70. (4) Breathing and relaxation exercises are very important in reducing cardiovascular strain from fear and anxiety, and enhancing the ability to cope with contractions. **Answer 1** is incorrect because regional anesthesia is often used to *avoid* cardiovascular strain from painful contractions and pushing. **Answer 2** is incorrect because excessive pushing is *avoided* in order to reduce cardiovascular strain. **Answer 3** is incorrect because strong emotional support by the family *is* needed in labor to enhance relaxation and to reduce cardiovascular strain from excessive fear and anxiety.

TEST-TAKING TIP—Read the stem carefully for the key words, the specific problem described, to select the right option.
AN, APP, 3, Maternity, HPM, Health Promotion and Maintenance

71. (1) The necessary elements for Rh sensitization are a mother who is Rh-negative, a baby who is Rh-positive, and no

maternal Rh antibodies. **Answer 2** is incorrect because the baby who is Rh-negative does *not* have an antigen to trigger maternal Rh sensitization. **Answer 3** is incorrect because it is the immune system of the *mother* that attacks the red blood cells of the baby. **Answer 4** is incorrect because it is the immune system of the *mother* that attacks the red blood cells of the baby.

TEST-TAKING TIP—Examine conflicting answers and eliminate answers where RhoGam would not be used (**Answers 2** and **4**). Eliminate **Answer 4** because the mother isn't protected by RhoGam.
IMP, APP, 1, Maternity, PhI, Reduction of Risk Potential

72. (3) The anti-insulin effects of pregnancy hormones do not become significant until after the first trimester, and then the woman's insulin requirements increase throughout the remainder of pregnancy. **Answer 1** is incorrect because pregnancy hormones have an *anti*-insulin effect. **Answer 2** is incorrect because many who have diabetes experience a *decrease* in insulin requirements in the first trimester. The anti-insulin effects of pregnancy hormones do not become significant until after the first trimester. **Answer 4** is incorrect because, once the placenta has been delivered, the anti-insulin effects of pregnancy hormones are abruptly terminated and insulin requirements tend to *quickly* return to prepregnancy levels.

TEST-TAKING TIP—Options with absolute words such as "no effect" are usually wrong.
IMP, APP, 4, Maternity, PhI, Reduction of Risk Potential

73. (2) Fetal size is better controlled by keeping glucose levels under 120 mg/dL, and fetal well-being is enhanced by avoiding extremes in serum glucose, hypoglycemia, and ketoacidosis. **Answer 1** is incorrect because merely controlling *weight gain* does *not* avoid hypoglycemia or ketoacidosis. **Answer 3** is incorrect because maintaining good sleep and exercise patterns does *not* avoid hypoglycemia and ketoacidosis. **Answer 4** is incorrect because fetal organ damage can be caused *after* the first trimester by hypoglycemia and ketoacidosis, and fetal macrosomia is influenced by high glucose levels.

TEST-TAKING TIP—Note that the stem asks for the "most important factor." Three of the four options are correct, but the second option is the most important.
IMP, APP, 4, Maternity, PhI, Reduction of Risk Potential

74. (1, 3, 4) **Answer 1** is correct because the fetus with an earlier gestation is more likely to be breech or transverse than a fetus at term. **Answer 3** is correct because the head of a fetus who is premature is extremely fragile, and trauma such as vaginal birth can cause intraventricular hemorrhage. **Answer 4** is correct because antibiotics are recommended to prevent infections in infants who are premature, who have immature immune systems. **Answer 2** is incorrect because cord compression is *common* when amniotic fluid is decreased, as in premature rupture of membranes. **Answer 5** is incorrect because not *all* preterm labor is *caused* by infections.

TEST-TAKING TIP—With multiple-multiples (multiple response questions), think "true-false" for *each* of the options; eliminate any options that are false. Eliminate **Answer 5** because of the "all" in the answer.
AN, APP, 5, Maternity, HPM, Health Promotion and Maintenance

75. (4) The newborn assessment indicates that the baby has several significant signs of dehydration (sunken fontanels, yellow urine, only one or two wet diapers), which can be a

life-threatening problem at this age. **Answer 1** is incorrect because it fails to identify or manage the problem of dehydration. **Answer 2** is incorrect because it fails to recognize or manage the problem of dehydration, and it assumes supplements will be sufficient for the infant's volume needs. **Answer 3** is incorrect because it is outside of the role of the nurse to instruct a new mother to switch to formula when she wants to breastfeed.

> **TEST-TAKING TIP**—Whenever physical assessment data are given, review it carefully, as well as any other words in the stem that might indicate a subtle abnormality (e.g., fontanels).
> **AN, ANL, 4, Newborn, PhI, Reduction of Risk Potential**

76. **(1)** Feelings of fear after a fetal loss are normal, and the response of the nurse encourages the woman to share her feelings in more depth before the nurse makes a specific response that may be inappropriate. **Answer 2** is incorrect because, although it recognizes that the feeling is normal, it *minimizes* the concern of the woman and blocks further communication. **Answer 3** is incorrect because it offers *false reassurance* and blocks further communication. **Answer 4** is incorrect because it implies that the nurse is an inappropriate person with whom to share feelings, and it blocks further communication.

> **TEST-TAKING TIP**—With communication questions, generally the preference is for open-ended neutral responses that encourage communication.
> **IMP, APP, 7, Maternity, PsI, Psychosocial Integrity**

77. **(3)** Preterm labor must be detected early enough to be stopped. Waiting for contractions, show, leaking fluid, or perineal pressure would significantly reduce the chances of successfully stopping the preterm labor process. **Answer 1** is incorrect because these symptoms probably mean that the preterm labor process is too advanced to successfully stop the labor. **Answer 2** is incorrect because these symptoms probably mean that the preterm labor process is too advanced to successfully stop the labor. **Answer 4** is incorrect because these symptoms probably mean that the preterm labor process is too advanced to successfully stop the labor.

> **TEST-TAKING TIP**—Read the stem carefully for key words. Here the key words, "preterm birth," should alert you to look for a response that applies specifically to preterm rather than term labor.
> **AN, APP, 1, Maternity, HPM, Health Promotion and Maintenance**

78. **(3)** It is an accurate statement of the risks of *Chlamydia* in pregnancy and stresses the importance of effective early treatment. **Answer 1** is incorrect because *Chlamydia* is often asymptomatic but has serious consequences for the well-being of the baby (preterm birth and newborn pneumonia). **Answer 2** is incorrect because chlamydia is associated with a higher incidence of preterm labor; it is necessary to treat it early in pregnancy. *Chlamydia* does not reoccur after treatment unless the client is exposed to the infection again by a partner who is infected. **Answer 4** is incorrect because the woman must be treated *regardless* of her partner's test result. It is important to have all partners tested and treated to avoid reinfection.

> **TEST-TAKING TIP**—Read the stem carefully for key words. Here the key word, "chlamydia," should alert you to look for a response that applies uniquely to *Chlamydia*; in this case, it is associated with preterm birth.
> **IMP, APP, 1, Maternity, SECE, Safety/Infection Control**

79. **(2)** The serological test for syphilis (RPR) becomes positive in the presence of reagin, which may be from an old treated infection or other circumstances that cause a false positive. It is necessary to do a second test that is diagnostic for active syphilis infection, such as the fluorescent treponemal antibody absorbed (FTA-ABS) and microhemagglutination assay for antibody to *Treponema pallidum* (MHA-TP). **Answer 1** is incorrect because syphilis does not cross the placenta *until after the 16th–18th week* of gestation when the protective Langhans' layer in the chorion begins to atrophy. **Answer 3** is incorrect because the serological test for syphilis is a screening test and the diagnosis must be confirmed by other tests. **Answer 4** is incorrect because syphilis is transmitted to the fetus by crossing the placenta. Delaying treatment until late in pregnancy places both the mother and fetus at risk for significant complications.

> **TEST-TAKING TIP**—Read the stem carefully for key words. Here the key word, "syphilis," should alert you to look for a response that applies uniquely to syphilis; in this case, it requires *two* tests for a positive diagnosis.
> **IMP, APP, 1, Maternity, SECE, Safety/Infection Control**

80. **(3)** The blood pressure has increased 30/15 from the baseline at the first prenatal visit. This adolescent is at increased risk for pregnancy-induced hypertension because of her age and parity. **Answer 1** is incorrect because there is a significant elevation in blood pressure in a woman who is at risk for preeclampsia. **Answer 2** is incorrect because the changes in pulse and respirations are not significantly higher than the baseline. **Answer 4** is incorrect because the blood pressure in second-trimester pregnancy usually *remains* at the baseline or *decreases* slightly. Pregnancy is a state of decreased peripheral resistance; therefore, increased blood pressure should be evaluated further.

> **TEST-TAKING TIP**—Whenever physical assessment data are given, review the findings carefully and look for words in the stem that might suggest a subtle deviation from normal; in this case, there is an adolescent with a low baseline blood pressure. Note that two options state that this is OK (normal) and one does not. Choose the answer that is different.
> **IMP, ANL, 6, Maternity, PhI, Reduction of Risk Potential**

81. **(2)** Protein loss in the urine in women who are pregnant with hypertension complications can reach significant levels and make it difficult for the body to replace it from nutritional sources. **Answer 1** is incorrect because, although the adolescent is growing and needs more protein, that added protein *has* been provided (according to the stem). **Answer 3** is incorrect because the exact etiology of hypertension complications in pregnancy is *unknown*. **Answer 4** is incorrect because the reduced placental circulation from vasospasm and hypertension will *not be affected* by added protein.

> **TEST-TAKING TIP**—Of the two potentially correct responses (**Answers 1** and **2**), only **Answer 2** relates directly to the problem addressed in the question.
> **AN, APP, 4, Maternity, HPM, Health Promotion and Maintenance**

82. **(3)** All three signs are related directly to vasospasm and tissue perfusion. **Answer 1** is incorrect because ankle edema is *normal* in pregnancy and polyuria is *not* related to decreased renal perfusion, but rather *increased* renal perfusion. **Answer 2** is incorrect because dysuria is *not* related to vasospasm and decreased tissue perfusion. **Answer 4** is incorrect because edema of the *ankles* is considered *normal* in pregnancy and is associated with increased pressure on the veins of the legs.

> **TEST-TAKING TIP**—When lists of signs are given in the answer options, it may be helpful to first eliminate the ones that you know are wrong (**Answers 1** and **4**).
> **AS, APP, 6, Maternity, PhI, Physiological Adaptation**

83. **(2)** Vasospasm and reduced tissue perfusion may cause organ damage and failure. This problem often involves the kidneys. **Answer 1** is incorrect because hypertensive disorders in pregnancy do *not* automatically resolve with delivery of the fetus and placenta and, in fact, may become worse. **Answer 3** is incorrect because, although it is true that magnesium sulfate is cleared by the kidneys, the purpose of fluid restriction is to *prevent fluid overload* if the kidneys have become damaged. **Answer 4** is incorrect because it is an inaccurate reading of the order. The order reads "fluid restriction," which is interpreted to include all fluids.

> **TEST-TAKING TIP**—When an answer includes a "because" statement, read the "because" statement carefully. It may give the wrong rationale. In this case the "because" statement in **Answer 2** is correct; but in **Answer 3**, the statement supports drug administration, *not* fluid restriction.
> **AN, APP, 6, Maternity, PhI, Reduction of Risk Potential**

84. **(4)** The abdominal pain might be the result of uterine contractions and the bright-red bleeding might be show. **Answer 1** is incorrect because placenta previa is generally *painless* vaginal bleeding. **Answer 2** is incorrect because, while it *may* be an abruption, this option states "*must* be." Placental abruption may involve a massive hemorrhage that is completely obscured by the placenta, with *no* vaginal bleeding. **Answer 3** is incorrect because, although pain and bleeding are signs of infection, in pregnancy they do not necessarily occur together.

> **TEST-TAKING TIP**—Answers that contain absolute terms such as "must" (**Answers 1** and **2**) are often wrong.
> **AN, ANL, 6, Maternity, PhI, Physiological Adaptation**

85. **(1)** Backache and cramping are early signs of labor that might trigger a significant hemorrhage. If she is in labor, the physician should be notified. **Answer 2** is incorrect because the possibility of labor and an associated hemorrhage must be avoided with placenta previa. The nurse should check for bleeding and notify the physician. **Answer 3** is incorrect because the nurse fails to recognize the possibility of labor and the need to check for bleeding. Straining should be avoided while having a bowel movement since it can cause vaginal bleeding. **Answer 4** is incorrect because a vaginal exam might perforate the placenta and cause a massive hemorrhage. Vaginal and rectal exams are *prohibited* in placenta previa.

> **TEST-TAKING TIP**—When physical signs and symptoms are given in the stem, check the stem carefully for key words, such as "placenta previa," that might alter the interpretation of the signs and symptoms.
> **AS, ANL, 6, Maternity, PhI, Reduction of Risk Potential**

86. **(2)** The assessment signs of severe pain and rigidity of the abdomen suggest placental abruption, and the labor process with uterine contractions is often obscured. **Answer 1** is incorrect because vaginal bleeding may accompany *placental abruption*, and the physical assessment signs suggest placental abruption *rather than* placenta previa. **Answer 3** is incorrect because the physical assessment signs are *outside* the range of normal for labor. **Answer 4** is incorrect because, although rupture of membranes should be noted, it is not as important as the presence of labor when it is a threat to maternal and fetal well-being.

> **TEST-TAKING TIP**—When given physical assessment signs in the stem, evaluate carefully for deviations from normal and make sure that the deviations noted are consistent with the options included in the responses.
> **AS, ANL, 6, Maternity, PhI, Reduction of Risk Potential**

87. **(3)** A large amount of bright-red vaginal bleeding is abnormal at the beginning of labor and suggests a placenta problem, probably placenta previa. **Answer 1** is incorrect because, although fetal movement is important, it is a priority to determine the position and condition of the placenta with bright-red bleeding in order to determine whether to do a cesarean delivery. **Answer 2** is incorrect because, although the reaction of the fetal heart rate to stress is important, it is a priority to determine the position and condition of the placenta with bright-red bleeding in order to determine whether to do a cesarean delivery. **Answer 4** is incorrect because, although signs of labor are important, it is a priority to determine the position and condition of the placenta with bright-red bleeding in order to determine whether to do a cesarean delivery.

> **TEST-TAKING TIP**—When all of the responses sound reasonable, which one would directly determine the presence of a life-threatening condition?
> **PL, APP, 6, Maternity, PhI, Reduction of Risk Potential**

88. **(3)** The pressure of the enlarged uterus is taken off of the vena cava and diaphragm. Both respiratory and cardiovascular function are improved. **Answer 1** is incorrect because it is the enlargement of the uterus, *not* the position, that increases the risk of preterm labor. **Answer 2** is incorrect because in lateral Sims' position the fetal body will fall toward the mattress and away from the abdominal surface, which may make it harder to monitor. **Answer 4** is incorrect because, although the discomfort from backache may be lessened, the position has more important effects on respiratory and cardiovascular function.

> **TEST-TAKING TIP**—**Answer 3** describes an *immediate* and lifesaving effect, whereas the other options involve ease for the nurse, client comfort, and prevention of future problems.
> **PL, APP, 3, Maternity, PhI, Reduction of Risk Potential**

89. **(3)** The massive rush of fluid out of the vagina may sweep a loop of cord with it past the baby's presenting part and out of the cervix. Then, as the baby rapidly descends, the cord is compressed and the baby can die. **Answer 1** is incorrect because, although it is a possibility, the immediate and actual risk to the fetus is prolapsed cord. **Answer 2** is incorrect because, although it is a possibility, the immediate and actual risk to the fetus is prolapsed cord. **Answer 4** is incorrect because, although it is a possibility, the immediate and actual risk to the fetus is prolapsed cord.

> **TEST-TAKING TIP**—When prioritizing care or anticipating problems, place the immediate and life-threatening ones first as most important. Think about *actual* risk, *not* every *potential* risk.
> **AN, ANL, 1, Maternity, PhI, Physiological Adaptation**

90. **(4)** The nonstress test tests the autonomic control of the heart rate, which should speed up during increased demand for oxygen. **Answer 1** is incorrect because the presence of muscle mass is *not* the basis for the nonstress test. **Answer 2** is incorrect because the nonstress test is testing neural control of the heart rate. **Answer 3** is incorrect because many babies move slowly and are *normal*. The nonstress test is testing *reaction* to movement, *not* number of movements.

TEST-TAKING TIP—The only option that deals directly with fetal movement and fetal heart rate is **Answer 4**.
IMP, ANL, 3, Maternity, PhI, Reduction of Risk Potential

91. **(4)** The nonstress test is used as a screening test and is an indicator of an intact fetal autonomic nervous system. The contraction stress test is used to confirm the reduction of fetal cardiovascular reserves as a result of reduced uteroplacental function. **Answer 1** is incorrect because the contraction stress test confirms the screening test and may well be *normal,* indicating a baby with adequate cardiovascular reserves. **Answer 2** is incorrect because other techniques are used to wake up the fetus who is sleeping before the contraction stress test is indicated. **Answer 3** is incorrect because techniques such as nipple stimulation are used to simulate contractions *without* the presence of labor.

TEST-TAKING TIP—Sometimes the response that is the most precise (and may be the longest response) is the correct one.
EV, APP, 1, Maternity, PhI, Reduction of Risk Potential

92. **(2)** The volume of amniotic fluid is often reduced with a postmature pregnancy. This test measures amniotic fluid volume. **Answer 1** is incorrect because this test measures the relationship between fetal movement and heart rate (the nonstress test). **Answer 3** is incorrect because this test does *not* measure serial fetal growth. **Answer 4** is incorrect because this test does *not* determine the presence of gross fetal anatomical abnormalities.

TEST-TAKING TIP—The only option that directly relates to the length of pregnancy is **Answer 2**.
AS, APP, 1, Maternity, PhI, Reduction of Risk Potential

93. **(4)** Chorionic villus sampling may be done as early as 10 weeks of gestation, but there is insufficient amniotic fluid to do an amniocentesis before 14 weeks of gestation. **Answer 1** is incorrect because *both* tests look directly at fetal cells. **Answer 2** is incorrect because chorionic villus sampling may be done as early as 10 weeks of gestation. **Answer 3** is incorrect because *both* tests involve the potential of hemorrhage, spontaneous abortion, and fetal trauma.

TEST-TAKING TIP—Responses that offer absolute terms such as "must be done" and "no risk" are usually wrong.
IMP, APP, 6, Maternity, PhI, Reduction of Risk Potential

94. **(2)** Lightening occurs in primiparas about 2–3 weeks before labor begins. **Answer 1** is incorrect because second labors are *not always* shorter than first labors. **Answer 3** is incorrect because a small amount of vaginal bleeding might be show, an early sign of the onset of labor. **Answer 4** is incorrect because the membranes may *not* rupture until the birth of the baby or may rupture spontaneously during pregnancy *before* fetal descent.

TEST-TAKING TIP—Be cautious about "always" in **Answer 1**. Absolute words usually indicate that the option is wrong. Eliminate the false options.
IMP, APP, 5, Maternity, HPM, Health Promotion and Maintenance

95. **(1, 3, 5)** **Answer 1** is correct because preeclampsia is more common in women carrying twins. **Answer 3** is correct because in multiple gestation, 38 weeks is considered term, rather than 40 weeks in a singleton gestation; uterine overdistention and other factors usually lead to delivery before the EDD. **Answer 5** is correct because uterine overdistention is a risk factor for postpartum hemorrhage. **Answer 2** is incorrect because PIH is *more* common rather than *less* common in women carrying twins. **Answer 4** is incorrect because nonstress tells nothing about *growth* of the fetus. The best test is an ultrasound.

TEST-TAKING TIP—The question asks for risk factors in twin gestation. With multiple-multiples (multiple-choice questions), think "true-false" for *each* of the options; eliminate any options that are false.
AN, APP, 5, Maternity, HPM, Health Promotion and Maintenance

96. **(1)** Lightening or descent of the fetus puts added pressure on the bladder, causing frequency. **Answer 2** is incorrect because lightening or descent of the fetus actually relieves pressure on the diaphragm, causing *easier* breathing. **Answer 3** is incorrect because lightening or descent of the fetus actually relieves pressure on the upper gastrointestinal tract, *decreasing* heartburn. **Answer 4** is incorrect because, although descent of the fetus may actually press on the lower colon, passage of soft stool is not obstructed. Lightening has *no* effect on absorption of fluid from the lower bowel, which results in constipation.

TEST-TAKING TIP—The only option that is associated with the onset of labor (involving descent of the fetus) is **Answer 1**.
AS, APP, 5, Maternity, HPM, Health Promotion and Maintenance

97. **(4)** Dilation without effacement is normal for a multipara, and regular contractions 5 minutes apart suggest the onset of active phase. **Answer 1** is incorrect because the Friedman curve for multiparas would suggest that she could deliver *before* 8 hours. Multiparous labors are very unpredictable. **Answer 2** is incorrect because a multipara with contractions 5 minutes apart is most likely in active labor and may deliver very quickly. **Answer 3** is incorrect because dilation without effacement is *normal* for multiparas.

TEST-TAKING TIP—The key in this question is knowledge about parity. The assessment signs must be interpreted with parity in mind, noting the unique features of multiparous labor.
AN, ANL, 5, Maternity, HPM, Health Promotion and Maintenance

98. **(1)** Voluntary forces in labor are composed of abdominal pushing, which is most effective after complete cervical dilation and effacement. **Answer 2** is incorrect because pushing *before* second stage may cause excessive pressure on the fetal head and swelling of the cervix. **Answer 3** is incorrect because analgesics may *not* eliminate the urge to push in doses that are safe for the fetus. **Answer 4** is incorrect because relaxing between contractions and proper positioning to assist the force of gravity to aid descent *are* two of many ways to assist involuntary forces.

TEST-TAKING TIP—Absolute statements ("*every* contraction," **Answer 2**; "*no* way," **Answer 4**) are usually wrong.
PL, APP, 3, Maternity, HPM, Health Promotion and Maintenance

99. **(2)** Forceful uncomfortable contractions, irritability, and withdrawal are normal signs of transition that are stressful for the support person. **Answer 1** is incorrect because he may not have been there many hours and it cannot be assumed that he is bored and restless. **Answer 3** is incorrect because it may be several hours before second stage is reached, followed by 1–2 hours more labor before birth. **Answer 4** is incorrect because transition is in first-stage labor, and voluntary pushing should *not* be used in first-stage labor.

TEST-TAKING TIP—Key word: "transition." **Answer 2** is the only option that describes transition.
AS, ANL, 7, Maternity, PsI, Psychosocial Integrity

100. **(3)** Ambulation would *increase* back discomfort by increasing fetal descent. **Answer 1** is incorrect because massage to the back muscles between contractions may *help* loosen and relax them and decrease pain. **Answer 2** is incorrect because external pressure to the sacrum may *relieve* pressure on the

sacral joints from the descending presenting part. **Answer 4** is incorrect because lying on the side supported by pillows *relieves* pressure on the back and may help the fetus rotate to an anterior position.

TEST-TAKING TIP—Note that the question asks for an "ineffective" means of enhancing comfort. Therefore look for the false answer.
IMP, APP, 3, Maternity, PhI, Basic Care and Comfort

Nursing Care of Children and Families

Kathleen Snider

INTRODUCTION

The revised NCLEX-RN® Test Plan includes content that has been covered in this unit, but often raises concern in candidates. This section assists NCLEX® candidates to think about this content in terms of the current test plan, in a concrete and specific manner through the clinical examples given.

Management of Care of Infants, Children, and Adolescents

The role of the pediatric nurse in *management of care* includes the following:

1. Serving as an *advocate* for the child and family, such as informing child and family of all treatments and procedures.
2. Coordinating clinical *case management* to provide access to high-quality clinical resources appropriate to the level of care needed, such as referring child to acute rehabilitation facility following spinal cord injury.
3. Coordinating *continuity of care* across the health-care delivery continuum, such as discussing needs of child and family with home care nurse before child's discharge in a spica cast.
4. *Delegating* care to and *supervising* care among various members of the health-care delivery team, such as assigning a float nurse to care for selected clients on the pediatrics unit.
5. Completing *incident/irregular occurrence/variance reports* as needed, including filing, monitoring, and analyzing reports of drug reactions to a new medication.
6. Working toward *continuous quality improvement*, such as studying incident reports of accidents on the pediatrics unit to determine what changes in practice are needed to increase client safety.
7. Suggesting *organ donation* to selected families when appropriate—for example, asking the family whose 16-year-old has been declared brain dead about the possibility of organ donation.
8. Collaborating with other members of the health-care team *in consultation and referrals,* such as requesting a psychiatric consultation for a child who is depressed.
9. Coordinating *resource management,* such as reminding the UAP to stamp all equipment charge forms used for each child.

Safety and Infection Control for Infants, Children, and Adolescents

The role of the pediatric nurse in *safety and infection control* includes the following:

1. Engaging in *disaster planning* activities—for example, the nurse reads and thoroughly reviews the disaster plan for the health-care facility in which the nurse is practicing.
2. Engaging in activities designed to *prevent errors,* such as identifying pediatric clients only by their name bands or by a reliable adult who knows the child.
3. *Handling hazardous and infectious materials* appropriately—for example, always disposing of contaminated waste in a clearly marked biohazard container.
4. Using *medical and surgical asepsis,* such as using sterile gloves and technique when changing a surgical incision dressing.

Prevention and Early Detection of Disease in Infants, Children, and Adolescents

The role of the pediatric nurse in the *prevention and early detection of disease* includes the following:

1. Engaging in *disease prevention* activities (e.g., washing hands thoroughly before and after providing client care).
2. Participating in *health promotion programs,* such as teach-

ing a class on accident prevention to parents of infants and young children.

3. Conducting *health screening* as needed, such as performing Denver Developmental Screening Test (DDST) on age-appropriate clients (1 mo–6 yr) in the pediatric clinic as part of routine screening.

4. Teaching families about and administering *immunizations* as ordered—signs/symptoms of reactions, providing parents with an immunization record card after administering immunization(s).

5. Discussing *lifestyle choices* with older children and adolescents, as appropriate (e.g., discussing risks associated with body piercing and tattooing).

Coping and Adaptation in Infants, Children, and Adolescents

The role of the pediatric nurse in *coping and adaptation* includes the following:

1. Understanding and respecting *religious and spiritual influences on children's health* (e.g., allowing families to engage in dying and death rituals according to their spiritual beliefs). See **Table 5.1**.

2. Helping clients engage in problem solving related to *situational role changes,* such as discussing transportation and child care issues with the parents of a child who is newly diagnosed with leukemia.

GROWTH AND DEVELOPMENT

I. Infant (28 days–1 year)
   A. Erikson's theory of personality development
      1. *Central task:* basic trust vs. mistrust; central person: primary caregiver/maternal person.
      2. *Behavioral indicators:*
         a. Crying is only means of communicating needs.

TABLE 5.1	Stages of Spiritual Development in Childhood
Infancy (Stage 0: *undifferentiated*)	▪ No concept of right/wrong ▪ No convictions to guide behavior ▪ Beginnings of a faith are established with the development of basic trust through relationships with the primary caregiver
Toddler/Preschooler (Stage 1: *intuitive-projective*)	**Toddlers:** ▪ Imitate the religious gestures and behaviors of others without comprehending the meaning or significance of the activities **Preschoolers:** ▪ Assimilate some of the values and beliefs of their parents ▪ Parents' attitudes toward moral codes and religious beliefs convey to child what they consider good and bad ▪ Follow parental beliefs as part of daily lives rather than through an understanding of their basic concepts
School-age (Stage 2: *mythical-literal*)	▪ Spiritual development parallels cognitive development ▪ Closely related to child's experiences and social interactions ▪ Develop strong interest in religion ▪ Accept existence of a deity ▪ Petitions to an omnipotent being are important and expected to be answered ▪ Good behavior is rewarded/bad behavior is punished ▪ Conscience is bothered when they disobey ▪ Have reverence for many thoughts and matters ▪ Able to articulate own faith ▪ May even question validity of faith
Preadolescent (Stage 3: *synthetic-convention*)	▪ Become increasingly aware of spiritual disappointments ▪ Recognize that prayers are not always answered (at least on their own terms) ▪ Begin to reason, to question some of the established parental religious standards ▪ May drop or modify some religious practices
Adolescent (Stage 4: *individuating-reflexive*)	▪ Become more skeptical ▪ Begin to compare parent's religious standards with the standards of others ▪ Attempt to determine which to adopt and incorporate into their own set of values ▪ Begin to compare religious standards with the scientific viewpoint ▪ Time of "searching" rather than "reaching" ▪ Uncertain about many religious ideas but will not achieve profound insights until late adolescence or early adulthood

b. Quieting usually means needs are met.

c. Fear of strangers at 6–8 mo.

3. **Parental guidance/teaching**

a. Must meet infant's needs consistently—cannot "spoil" infant by holding, comforting.

b. Neonatal *reflexes* fade between 4 and 6 mo, replaced with increase in purposeful behavior, e.g., babbling, reaching.

c. *Fear of strangers* is normal—indicates attachment between infant and primary caregiver.

d. Child may repeat over and over newly learned behaviors, e.g., sitting or standing.

e. *Weaning* can begin around the time child begins walking.

f. Review preventive care timeline and Recommended Health Screenings (**Tables 5.2 and 5.3**) with parents of infants.

4. For additional information about behavioral concerns for each age group, see **Tables 5.4** and **5.5**.

B. **Physical growth** (by 1 yr)

1. *Height* (length): 50% increase by first birthday.

2. *Weight:*

a. Doubles by 4 to 7 mo, triples by 1 yr.

b. Gains 5–7 oz/wk in first 6 mo of life.

c. Gains 3–5 oz/wk in second 6 mo of life.

3. *Vital signs:* see **Table 5.6**.

4. *Cardiac system:*

a. Heart begins to function effectively.

b. Decreased heart rate, increased blood pressure from neonatal values.

5. *Pulmonary system:*

a. Predisposed to upper respiratory infections due to anatomical differences (e.g., eustachian tube is shorter and straighter in infant).

b. Decreased respiratory rate from neonatal values.

6. *Gastrointestinal system:*

a. Swallowing improves.

b. Stomach enlarges to hold greater volume.

c. Digests more complex foods as enzymes increase (by 4–6 mo).

7. *Genitourinary system:*

a. Immature; waste products poorly eliminated.

b. Easily prone to fluid and electrolyte imbalances.

8. *Immune system:*

a. Functional by 2 mo.

b. Produces IgG and IgM antibodies.

9. *Neurological system:*

a. Fontanels:

(1) Anterior—open or patent through first 12 mo.

(2) Posterior—closed by 2 mo.

b. Head circumference increases as brain grows rapidly.

c. Neurological reflexes (e.g., Landau, parachute) appear; neonatal reflexes (e.g., Moro, rooting) disappear.

10. *Sensory:*

a. Hearing improves from "quieting" to a sound, to locating a sound easily and turning toward it.

b. Vision improves from 8 to 18 in, to searching for hidden objects and following moving objects.

11. *Teething:*

a. Generally begins around 6 mo.

b. First two teeth: lower central incisors.

c. By 1 yr: six to eight teeth.

C. **Denver Developmental Screening Test (DDST):** See **Table 5.7**.

1. *Birth to 3 mo*

a. Personal-social: smiles responsively, then spontaneously.

b. Fine motor-adaptive:

(1) Follows 180 degrees, past midline.

(2) Grasps rattle.

(3) Holds hands together.

c. Language: laughs/squeals; vocalizes without crying.

d. Gross motor: while on stomach, lifts head 45 to 90 degrees, able to hold head steady and erect; rolls over, from stomach to back.

2. *4–6 mo*

a. Personal-social: works for toy; feeds self (bottle).

b. Fine motor-adaptive: palmar grasp, reaches for objects.

c. Language: turns toward voice, imitates speech.

d. Gross motor: some weightbearing on legs; no head lag when pulled to sitting; sits with support.

3. *7–9 mo*

a. Personal-social

(1) Indicates wants.

(2) Plays pat-a-cake, waves bye-bye.

b. Fine motor-adaptive: takes two cubes in hands and bangs them together; passes cube hand to hand; crude pincer grasp.

c. Language: "dada," "mama," nonspecific, jabbers.

d. Gross motor: creeps on hands and knees; gets self up to sitting; pulls self to standing; stands holding on.

4. *10–12 mo*

a. Personal-social

(1) Plays ball.

(2) Imitates activities.

(3) Drinks from cup.

b. Fine motor-adaptive: neat pincer grasp.

c. Language: "dada," "mama," specific.

d. Gross motor: stands alone well; walks holding on; stoops and recovers.

◆ D. **Nursing interventions/parental guidance, teaching:**

1. *Play*

a. First year—generally solitary.

b. Visual stimulation

(1) Best color: red.

(2) *Toys:* mirrors, brightly colored pictures.

TABLE 5.2   Child Preventive Care Timeline

Clinical Preventive Services for Normal-Risk Children

IMMUNIZATION

Month/Years of Age	B	1m	2m	3m	4m	5m	6m	12m	15m	18m	Y E A R S	2yr	4yr	6yr	11yr	12yr	14yr	16yr	18yr‡
Hepatitis B	Dose 1	Dose 1	Dose 2				Dose 3												
Polio (IPV)*			Dose 1		Dose 2			Dose 3						Dose 4	Doses 3				
Haemophilus Influenzae type B (HIB)*			Dose 1		Dose 2		Dose 3	Dose 4											
Diphtheria, Tetanus, Pertussis (DTaP, Td)			Dose 1		Dose 2		Dose 3		Dose 4				Dose 5			Td Once			
Measles, Mumps, Rubella (MMR)								Dose 1					Dose 2		or Dose 2			
Chickenpox (VZV)								Once					or Once					
Hepatitis A												Once in selected areas						
Pneumococcal Disease (Prevnar)			Dose 1		Dose 2		Dose 3		Dose 4										

SCREENING

Years of Age	B	1y	2y	3y	4y	5y	6y	7y	8y	9y	10y	11y	12y	13y	14y	15y	16y	17y	18y
Newborn Screening: PKU, Sickle cell, Hemoglobinopathies, Hypothyroidism	■																		
Hearing		Periodically																	
Head Circumference																			
Height and weight		Periodically																	
Lead			■																
Vision Screening					■														
Blood Pressure				Periodically															
Dental Health				Periodically															
Alcohol use														Adolescents					
Chlamydia														Adolescents					

COUNSELING

Years of Age	B	1y	2y	3y	4y	5y	6y	7y	8y	9y	10y	11y	12y	13y	14y	15y	16y	17y	18y
Development, nutrition, physical activity, safety, unintentional injuries and poisonings, Violent behaviors and firearms, STDs and HIV, family planning, Tobacco use, drug use					As appropriate for age														

■ **Recommended by most U.S. authorities**

‡ Also see Table 5.18. To keep current on vaccine recommendations, please go to the website: www.cdc.gov/nip/acip.
*Schedules may vary according to vaccine type.

From *Child health guide: Put prevention into practice*, Department of Health and Human Services. The information on immunizations is based on recommendations issued by the Advisory Committee on Immunization Practices, the American Academy of Pediatrics, and the American Academy of Family Physicians.

TABLE 5.3	🧪	Recommended Health Screenings for Infants, Children, and Adolescents: Specific Conditions

Area of Concern	Screening Method	Recommendations
Neonatal metabolic and genetic screening: Hypothyroidism Sickle cell anemia PKU	Blood tests: Serum T_3/T_4 levels ↓ Sickledex ↓ Phenylalanine levels ↓	All are done in immediate neonatal period, within first few days of life. Testing for PKU must be done after infant has ingested formula or breast milk for 48–72 hours.
Lead poisoning (see **Table 5.2**)	Blood-lead level (BLL)	Centers for Disease Control and Prevention (CDC) recommends universal or targeted screening for all children. At a minimum, all children should have BLL drawn between 1–2 yr, or earlier if needed. BLL should also be done on any child between 3–6 yr who has never been tested. Those children at high risk (e.g., live in older home with lead in paint and plumbing, have sibling or friend with lead poisoning) should be screened earlier and more frequently.
Hyperlipidemia	Serum cholesterol levels	Routinely at 2–4 yr, 6 yr, 10 yr, 11–14 yr, 15–17 yr, and 18–21 yr. May be done earlier or more frequently with risk factors such as diabetes, hypertension, parent with high cholesterol level.
Cystic fibrosis	Genetic studies, sweat test	Screen children who have sibling or other family members with CF. Screen family members of child with CF.
Tuberculosis	Mantoux or PPD	First test done at age 12–15 mo; repeated prn based on risk and exposure.
Latex allergies	Health history	During each routine visit, but especially important preoperatively or before procedures or children with ongoing urinary catheterizations (e.g. in myelomeningocele).

TABLE 5.4	Pediatric Behavioral Concerns: Nursing Implications and Parental Guidance

Behavioral Concern	Nursing Implications/Parental Guidance
Teething	Begins around age 4 mo—infant may seem unusually fussy and irritable but should *not* run a fever. Provide relief with teething rings, acetaminophen, topical preparations.
Thumb sucking	Need to "suck" varies: may be due to hunger, frustration, loneliness. Do *not* stop *infant* from doing this—usually stops by preschool years. If behavior persists, evaluate need for attention, peer play.
Temper tantrums	Normal in the *toddler*—occurs in response to frustration. *Avoid* abrupt end to play or making excessive demands. Offer only allowable choices. Once a decision is verbalized, *avoid* sudden changes of mind. Provide diversion to achieve cooperation. If it occurs, best means to handle is to *ignore* the outburst.
Toilet training	Assess child for readiness: awareness of body functions, form of mutual communication, physical control over sphincters. Use child-size seat. *No* distractions (food, toys, books). Offer praise for success *or* efforts (never shame accidents).
Discipline	*Not* for infant. Can begin with *toddler*, within limits. Be consistent and clear. *Avoid* excessively strict measures.
Sibling rivalry	Fairly common, normal. Allow older child to "help." Give each child "special" time, with individual attention.

(Continued on following page)

TABLE 5.4	Pediatric Behavioral Concerns: Nursing Implications and Parental Guidance *(Continued)*
Behavioral Concern	**Nursing Implications/Parental Guidance**
Masturbation	Normal, common in *preschooler*. Set firm limits. *Avoid* overreacting.
Lying	*In preschooler:* not deliberate; child is often unable to differentiate between "real" and "lie," and by speaking something often feels it makes a thing real. *In older child:* may indicate problems and need for professional attention if persists. Serve as role model—no "white lies."
Cursing	*Avoid* overreacting. Defuse use of "the word" by simply stating "not here, not now." Distract, change subject, substitute activity. Serve as role model by own language.
"Accidents" (enuresis)	*Occasional*—common and normal through preschool. *If frequent*—need complete physical exam to rule out pathology. "Training": after dinner—*avoid* fluids; before bed—toilet (perhaps awaken once during night). *Never* put back into diapers or attempt to shame.
Smoking/drinking	May begin in *older school-age* child or adolescent. Serve as role model with own habits.

TABLE 5.5	Pediatric Sleep and Rest Norms: Nursing Implications and Parental Guidance
Pediatric Sleep and Rest Norms	**Nursing Implications/Parental Guidance**
INFANT: 16–20 hr/day	
3 mo: nocturnal pattern	No set schedule can be predetermined
6 mo: 1–2 naps, with 12 hr at night	If waking at night after age 3 mo, investigate hunger as a probable cause
12 mo: 1 nap, with 12 hr at night	Monitor behavior to determine sleep needs: alert and active? Growing, developing? Routine fairly well established
TODDLER: 12–14 hr/night	
"Dawdles" at bedtime	Set firm, realistic limits
Dependency on security object	Place favorite blanket or toy in crib/bed
May ask to sleep with bottle	**Avoid** "bottle mouth syndrome" (caries)
May rebel against going to sleep	Establish bedtime "ritual"
PRESCHOOL: 10–12 hr/night	
Gives up afternoon nap	May regress in behavior when tired; provide "quiet time" in place of nap
Difficulty falling asleep/nighttime waking	**Avoid** overstimulation in evening
Fear of dark	Leave night-light on, door open
Enuresis	Occasional accidents are normal
May begin to have nightmares	Comfort child but leave in own bed
SCHOOL-AGE: 8–12 hr/night	
Nightmares common	Comfort child but leave in own bed
Awakens early in morning	Important that child play/relax after school
May not be aware he or she is tired	Remind about bedtime
Likes to stay up late	"Privilege" of later bedtime can be "awarded" as child gets older
Slumber parties	Permit, as good opportunity to socialize
ADOLESCENT: 10–14 hr/night	
Need for sleep increases greatly	Needs vary greatly among individuals
May complain of excessive fatigue	Rapid growth rate Related to rapid growth and overall increased activity

TABLE 5.6	Normal Vital Signs: Measurements and Variations with Age		
Age (yr)	Heart (beats/min)	Respiratory Rate(breaths/min)	Blood Pressure(mm Hg)
Newborn	120–160	30–40	70/55
1	100–140	25–35	90/55
2	80–120	20–30	90/56
5	70–100	18–24	95/56
10	60–90	18–22	102/62
14	55–90	16–20	110/65
18	55–90	16–18	116/68

Source: Adapted from Wong, D: Whaley and Wong's Nursing Care of Infants and Children, ed. 7. Mosby, St. Louis.

c. Auditory stimulation
   (1) Talk and sing to infant.
   (2) *Toys:* musical mobiles, rattles, bells.
d. Tactile stimulation
   (1) Hold, pat, touch, cuddle, swaddle/keep warm; rub body with lotion.
   (2) *Toys:* various textures; nesting and stacking; plastic milk bottle with blocks to dump in, out.
e. Kinetic stimulation
   (1) Cradle, stroller, carriage, infant seat, car rides, wind-up infant swing, furniture strategically placed for walking.
   (2) *Toys:* cradle gym, push-pull.
2. *Safety*
   a. Refer to **Tables 5.8, 5.9,** and **5.10** for additional information on safety and infection control.
   b. *Note:* Most common accident during first 12 mo is the aspiration of foreign bodies.
      (1) Keep small objects out of reach.
      (2) Use one-piece pacifier only.
      (3) *No* nuts, raisins, hot dogs, popcorn.
      (4) *No* toys with small, removable parts.
      (5) *No* balloons or plastic bags.

c. *Falls*
   (1) Raise crib rails.
   (2) *Never* place child on high surface unsupervised.
   (3) Use restraining straps in seats, swings, highchairs, etc.
d. *Poisoning*
   (1) Check that paint on toys/furniture is *lead-free.*
   (2) Treat all medications as drugs, never as "candy."
   (3) Store all poisonous substances in locked cabinet, closet.
   (4) Have telephone number of poison control center on hand.
   (5) Instruct in use of syrup of ipecac, if indicated. The use of syrup of ipecac is controversial in infants. (see **p. 316**).
e. *Burns*
   (1) Use microwave oven to heat refrigerated formula only; heat only 4 oz or more for about 30 sec. Test formula on top of your hand, not inside wrist.
   (2) Check temperature of bath water; *never* leave infant alone in bath.

(see **p. 316**).

TABLE 5.7	Facts About the Denver Developmental Screening Test (DDST)
Parents' Questions	**Nurse's Best Response**
"Will this be used as a measure of my child's IQ?"	"No, it is a screening test for your child's development."
"What ages can be tested?"	"Infants through preschoolers, *or* from 1 month to 6 years."
"What will they test?"	"There are four areas: personal-social, fine motor-adaptive, language, gross motor."
"Can I stay with my child?"	"Yes, in fact it is preferred you be there."
"If my child fails, does it mean he is retarded?"	"No, this is not a diagnostic tool but rather a screening test."
"If he fails, what do we do?"	"Repeat the test in a week or two to rule out temporary factors."
"Why didn't my child accomplish everything?"	"He is not expected to."
"Why did my child score so poorly?"	"Perhaps it's a bad day for the child, he isn't feeling up to par, etc."

Pediatrics

TABLE 5.8	Safety Considerations When Caring for Hospitalized Infants, Children, and Adolescents
Area of Concern	**Safety Interventions**
Security	■ Be alert to all visitors; restrict prn ■ Monitor/report suspicious visitors ■ Assess high-risk children (e.g., custody disputes) ■ Identify person to whom child is discharged ■ All staff to wear photo ID, especially when transporting child ■ Transport one child at a time; *never* leave child unattended during transport ■ Do *not* allow visitors to borrow scrubs or lab coat ■ Infants placed near nurses station, in direct line of vision ■ Access to pediatrics unit limited; doors alarmed to indicate when someone enters or leaves the unit
Electrical equipment (e.g., apnea monitor, ECG monitor, respirator)	■ Maintain all equipment in good working order ■ Remove leads when not attached to monitor ■ Unplug power cord when not connected to equipment ■ Keep equipment away from moisture (e.g., puddle of water, tub) ■ Do *not* turn off alarm for any reason ■ Always check the child when an alarm sounds; *never* ignore the alarm ■ Teach other children *not* to touch or play with the equipment **Home care:** ■ CPR guidelines posted near bed ■ Emergency numbers posted near phone ■ Notify electric company, get on priority service list in case of power outage ■ Use intercom or monitoring system
Environment	■ Keep unused electrical outlets covered with child-proof caps ■ Secure screens on all windows ■ Strap infant securely into infant seat, high chair, stroller ■ Discourage use of walkers ■ Crib rails up at all times when infant or young child is alone ■ When a crib rail is down, keep one hand on the infant or young child at all times ■ Keep plants or flowers out of the reach of infants or young children ■ *No* small or sharp objects within reach of infants or young children; no pins on diapers ■ *No* small or removable parts of toys of infants or young children ■ Keep all medications out of the reach of infants or young children ■ *Never* leave an infant or young child alone in a bath or near water

(3) Special care with cigarettes, hot liquids.

(4) Do *not* leave infant in sun.

(5) Cover all electrical sockets.

(6) Keep electrical wires out of sight/reach.

(7) *Avoid* tablecloths with overhang.

(8) Put guards around heating devices.

  f. *Motor vehicles*

(1) Use only federally approved car seat for all car rides; safest position is rear-facing in middle of back seat (from *birth to 20 pounds,* and as close to *1 year* of age as possible).

(2) *Never* leave stroller behind parked car.

(3) Do *not* allow infant to crawl near parked cars or in driveway.

II. Toddler (1–3 yr)

A. Erikson's theory of personality development

1. *Central task:* autonomy vs. shame and doubt; central person(s): parent(s)

2. *Behavioral indicators*

  a. Does not separate easily from parents.

  b. Negativistic.

  c. Prefers rituals and routine activities.

  d. Active physical explorer of environment.

  e. Begins attempts at self-assertion.

  f. Easily frustrated by limits.

  g. Temper tantrums.

  h. May have favorite "security object."

  i. Uses "mine" for everything—does not understand concept of sharing.

3. **Parental guidance/teaching**

  a. *Avoid* periods of prolonged separation if possible.

  b. *Avoid* constantly saying "no" to toddler.

  c. *Avoid* "yes/no" questions.

  d. Stress that child may use "no" even when he or she means "yes."

  e. Establish and maintain rituals, e.g., toilet training, going to sleep.

  f. Offer opportunities for play, *with* supervision.

  g. Allow child to feed self.

  h. Offer only allowable choices.

  i. Best method to handle temper tantrums: ignore them.

TABLE 5.9	Safety and Injury Prevention—Home Safety

These safety measures should be used in homes where children live and in homes they frequently visit, e.g., grandparents or babysitters.

Burns, Electrical, and Fire	**Falls**
■ Guards in front of or around heating appliances, fireplace, furnace (including floor furnace) ■ Electrical wires in good repair and out of reach ■ Electrical outlets "capped" ■ Smoke detectors operational ■ Matches out of reach ■ All heated appliances/objects placed out of child's reach and disconnected when not in use ■ Hot water heater set at 49° C (120° F) or lower ■ Pot handles turned toward back of stove or toward center of table ■ Cool, *not* hot, mist vaporizer used ■ Fire extinguisher(s) available and operational ■ Family escape plan (in case of fire) current ■ "9-1-1" and address of home with nearest cross street posted near phone	■ Exits, halls, stairs free of obstructions and well lighted ■ Nonskid mats and safety strips in tubs and showers and on stairs ■ Decals on glass doors/walls ■ Safety glass in doors/walls/windows ■ Gates at doors/stairwells ■ Guard rails on upstairs windows ■ Safety locks/latches that prevent/limit opening in use on doors/windows ■ Crib rails raised to full height and mattress kept in low position ■ Restraints used in high chairs and other infant/child furniture ■ Pediatrician's phone number posted near phone
Aspiration and Suffocation	**Bodily Injury**
■ Small objects stored out of reach and hanging objects (e.g., mobile) placed out of reach ■ Toys inspected for broken or removable parts ■ Plastic bags and plastic-covered pillow/mattress not accessible or in use ■ Cribs with slats meet federal regulations (slats < $2\frac{3}{8}$ inches (6 cm) apart with snug fitted mattress) ■ Bathroom and kitchen faucets firmly turned off ■ Toilet seats in down position or latched shut ■ Locked gates by fenced-in pools, spas, etc. ■ Proper safety equipment by pools, spas, etc. ■ Wading pools kept empty when not in use ■ Doors to dishwashers, refrigerators, washing machines, and dryers kept closed ■ Food cut into "sticks" rather than "coins" ■ Adult family member trained in CPR and Heimlich maneuver	■ Knives, unloaded firearms, power tools stored in locked cabinet ■ Pets properly restrained and immunized for rabies ■ Outdoor play equipment kept in safe, working condition ■ Yard free of glass, nails, litter, etc. ■ Nearest emergency department's phone number posted near phone
Poisoning	
■ Toxic substances placed on high shelf in locked cabinet ■ "Extra" quantities of toxic substances *not* stored in the house ■ Used containers of poisonous substances *not* accessible by the child ■ Household cleaners/disinfectants kept in original containers, separate from food and out of reach ■ Medications clearly labeled in childproof containers and stored out of reach ■ Poison Control Center phone number and address of home with nearest cross street posted near phone	

Adapted from Hockenberry, M: Wong's Clinical Manual of Pediatric Nursing, ed. 6, Mosby, St. Louis.

j. Keep security object with child, if so desired.
k. Do not force toddler "to share."
l. Review Recommended Health Screenings (see **Tables 5.2** and **5.3**) with parents of toddlers.
4. Additional information about behavioral concerns for each age group may be found in **Tables 5.4** and **5.5**.

B. **Physical growth** (by 3 yr)
1. *Height*
a. Slow, steady growth at 2–4 in/yr, mainly in *legs* rather than trunk.

TABLE 5.10	Infection Control When Caring for Infants, Children, and Adolescents		
Type	**Definition**	**Equipment**	**Clinical Applications**
Standard precautions	Reduce the risk of transmission of infection from all recognized and unrecognized sources of infection (formerly termed *universal precautions*)	▪ Gloves ▪ Protective eyewear ▪ Gown ▪ Mask	▪ Blood ▪ Body fluids ▪ Secretions ▪ Excretions ▪ Any break in skin or mucous membranes
Airborne precautions	Reduce the risk of airborne transmission of infectious agents	▪ Special air handling systems ▪ Ventilation systems: HEPA filter masks, N95 Respirator	▪ Measles ▪ Varicella ▪ Tuberculosis
Droplet precautions	Reduce the risk of airborne transmission of infectious agents transmitted by large particle droplets	▪ Surgical mask	▪ *Haemophilus influenzae* type B ▪ Pertussis ▪ Streptococcal pharyngitis ▪ Scarlet fever
Contact precautions	Reduce the risk of transmission of infectious agents by direct client contact or indirect contact with contaminated items in the client's environment	▪ Gloves ▪ Gown	▪ Enteric infections ▪ Skin/wound infections ▪ Respiratory syncytial virus (RSV) ▪ Herpes simplex ▪ Impetigo ▪ Viral hemorrhagic conjunctivitis

b. Adult height is roughly *twice* child's height at 2 yr of age.

2. *Weight*
   a. Slow, steady growth at 4–6 lb/yr.
   b. Birth weight *quadruples* by 2.5 years of age.

3. *Vital signs:* refer to **Table 5.6**.

4. *Cardiac system*
   a. Heart begins to function more efficiently.
   b. Decreased heart rate, slight increase in blood pressure from infant values.

5. *Pulmonary system*
   a. Mainly abdominal breathing.
   b. Lumina of bronchial vessels ↑ in size → decrease in lower respiratory system infections.
   c. Decreased respiratory rate from infant values.

6. *Gastrointestinal system*
   a. Increased capacity → three meals a day feeding schedule.
   b. Gastric juices increase in acidity → decrease in GI infections.
   c. Possible voluntary control of anal sphincter.

7. *Genitourinary system*
   a. Bladder capacity increases; to determine bladder capacity in ounces, add 2 to the child's age (e.g., 2-year-old has a bladder capacity of 4 oz or 120 mL).
   b. Ability to "hold" urine increases.
   c. Possible voluntary control of urethral sphincter.

8. *Immune system*
   a. Possible immunity from intrauterine life/maternal transfer disappears.
   b. Gradual increase in IgA, IgD, and IgE antibodies.

9. *Neurological system*
   a. Anterior fontanel closed by 18 mo.
   b. Brain increases to 90% of adult size.
   c. Progressive increase in intelligence.
   d. Myelinization of spinal cord is complete.

10. *Sensory system*
    a. Hearing evidences basic auditory skills.
    b. Vision shows evidence of convergence and accommodation; full binocular vision developed; visual acuity: 20/40.

11. *Teething*
    a. Introduce toothbrushing as a "ritual."
    b. By 30 mo: all 20 primary teeth present.
    c. First dental checkup should be between 12 and 18 mo.

12. *Musculoskeletal system*
    a. Lordosis: abdomen protrudes.
    b. Walks like a duck: wide-based gait, side-to-side.

C. **DDST** (see **Table 5.7**)
   1. *12–18 mo*
      a. Personal-social
         (1) Imitates housework.
         (2) Uses spoon, spilling little.
         (3) Removes own clothes.
         (4) Drinks from cup.
         (5) Feeds doll.
      b. Fine motor-adaptive
         (1) Scribbles spontaneously.
         (2) Builds tower with two to four cubes.
      c. Language
         (1) Three to six words other than "mama," "dada."
         (2) Points to at least one named body part.

d. Gross motor
    (1) Kicks ball forward.
    (2) Walks up steps.
2. *19–24 mo*
    a. Personal-social
        (1) Puts on clothing.
        (2) Washes and dries hands.
        (3) Brushes teeth with help.
    b. Fine motor-adaptive
        (1) Builds tower with four to six cubes.
        (2) Imitates vertical line.
    c. Language
        (1) Combines two or three words.
        (2) Speech partially understandable.
        (3) Names picture.
    d. Gross motor
        (1) Throws ball overhand.
        (2) Jumps in place.
3. *2–3 yr*
    a. Personal-social
        (1) Puts on T-shirt.
        (2) Can name a friend.
    b. Fine motor-adaptive
        (1) Thumb wiggles.
        (2) Builds tower of eight cubes.
    c. Language
        (1) Knows two verbs and two adjectives.
        (2) Names one color.
    d. Gross motor
        (1) Balances on one foot briefly.
        (2) Pedals tricycle.
◆ **D. Nursing interventions/parental guidance:**
    1. *Play:* toddler years—generally parallel.
    2. *Toys*—stimulate multiple senses simultaneously:
        a. Push-pull.
        b. Riding toys, e.g., straddle horse or car.
        c. Small, low slide or gym.
        d. Balls, in various sizes.
        e. Blocks—multiple shapes, sizes, colors.
        f. Dolls, trucks, dress-up clothes.
        g. Drums, horns, cymbals, xylophones, toy piano.
        h. Pounding board and hammer, clay.
        i. Finger paints, chalk and board, thick crayons.
        j. Wooden puzzles with large pieces.
        k. Toy record player with kiddie records.
        l. Talking toys: dolls, See 'n Say, phones.
        m. Sand, water, soap bubbles.
        n. Picture books, photo albums.
        o. Nursery rhymes, songs, music.
    3. *Safety*
        a. Refer to **Tables 5.8, 5.9,** and **5.10** for additional information on safety and infection control.
        b. Accidents are the leading cause of death among toddlers.
        c. *Motor vehicles:* most accidental deaths in children under age 3 are related to motor vehicles.

(1) Use only federally approved car seat for all car rides, through age 8 or 60 lb.
(2) Follow manufacturer directions carefully.
(3) Make car seat part of routine for toddler.
d. *Drowning*
    (1) Always supervise child near water: tub, pool, Jacuzzi, lake, ocean.
    (2) Keep bathroom locked to prevent drowning in toilet.
e. *Burns*
    (1) Turn pot handles *in* when cooking.
    (2) Do *not* allow child to play with electrical appliances.
    (3) Decrease water temperature in house to avoid scald burns.
f. *Poisonings:* most common in 2-year-olds.
    (1) Consider every nonfood substance a hazard and place out of child's sight/reach.
    (2) Keep all medications, cleaning materials, etc., in clearly marked containers in locked cabinets.
    (3) Instruct in use of syrup of ipecac, if indicated (see **p. 316**).
g. *Falls*
    (1) Provide barriers on open windows.
    (2) *Avoid* gates on stairs—child can strangle on gate.
    (3) Move from crib to bed.
h. *Choking: avoid* food on which child might choke:
    (1) Fish with bones.
    (2) Fruit with seeds, pits, or "skin."
    (3) Nuts, raisins.
    (4) Hot dogs.
    (5) Chewing gum.
    (6) Hard candy.
    (7) "Coin-cut" foods.
III. **Preschooler (3–5 yr)**
    A. **Erikson's theory of personality development**
        1. *Central task:* initiative vs. guilt; central person(s): basic family unit.
        2. *Behavioral indicators*
            a. Attempts to perform activities of daily living (ADL) independently.
            b. Attempts to make things for self/others.
            c. Tries to "help."
            d. Talks constantly: verbal exploration of the world ("Why?").
            e. Extremely active, highly creative imagination: fantasy and magical thinking.
            f. May demonstrate fears: "monsters," dark rooms, etc.
            g. Able to tolerate short periods of separation.
        3. **Parental guidance/teaching**
            a. Encourage child to dress self by providing simple clothing.
            b. Remind to go to bathroom (tends to "forget").

c. Assign small, simple tasks or errands.

d. Answer questions patiently, simply; do *not* offer child more information than he or she is asking for.

e. Normal to have "imaginary playmates."

f. Offer realistic support and reassurance with regard to fears.

g. Expose to a variety of experiences: zoo, train ride, shopping, sleigh riding, etc.

h. Enroll in preschool/nursery school program; kindergarten at 5 yr.

i. Review *Recommended Health Screenings* (see **Tables 5.2** and **5.3**) with parents of preschoolers.

4. Additional information about behavioral concerns for each age group may be found in **Tables 5.4** and **5.5**.

B. Physical growth (by 5 yr)

1. *Height and weight*

a. Continued slow, steady growth.

b. Generally grows more in *height* than weight.

c. Posture: appears taller and thinner; "lordosis" of toddler gradually *disappears*.

2. *Vital signs:* see **Table 5.6**.

3. *Cardiac system*

a. Increased heart size (4 times larger than at birth); heart function is comparable to a healthy adult (by 5 yr).

b. Heart assumes vertical position in thoracic cavity.

c. May hear "splitting" of heart sounds, as well as innocent murmurs on auscultation.

d. Decreased heart rate, steady blood pressure from toddler values.

4. *Pulmonary system*

a. Increase in amount of lung tissue.

b. Adult-like lung sounds heard on auscultation.

c. Decreased respiratory rate from toddler values.

5. *Gastrointestinal system*

a. Continued increase in size.

b. Position is straighter and more upright than adult stomach → more rapid emptying (defecation, vomiting).

c. Lining still sensitive to roughage and spices.

d. Elimination controlled.

6. *Genitourinary systems*

a. Bladder remains palpable above symphysis pubis.

b. Needs to void frequently, or "accidents" may occur despite sphincter control.

c. Low-grade urinary tract infections common.

7. *Immune system*

a. Growth of lymphoid tissue (especially tonsils).

b. Illnesses (especially respiratory) tend to be more localized.

c. Continued increase in IgA and IgG.

8. *Neurological system*

a. "Handedness" (right or left) is established.

9. *Sensory*

a. Vision—far-sightedness is improving; visual acuity: 20/30.

b. Vision and hearing screening should be conducted before kindergarten, and annually thereafter.

10. *Teeth*

a. All 20 primary or deciduous teeth ("baby teeth") should be present.

b. Annual dental checkups; continue daily brushing.

C. DDST/developmental norms: see **Table 5.7**

1. *3 yr*

a. Personal-social

(1) Dresses without help.

(2) Plays board/card games.

b. Fine motor-adaptive

(1) Picks longer of two lines.

(2) Copies circle, intersecting lines.

(3) Draws person, three parts.

c. Language

(1) Comprehends "cold," "tired," "hungry."

(2) Comprehends prepositions: "over," "under."

(3) Names four colors.

d. Gross motor

(1) Pedals tricycle; hops, skips on alternating feet.

(2) Broad jumps, jumps in place.

(3) Balances on one foot.

2. *4 yr*

a. Personal-social

(1) Brushes own teeth, combs own hair.

(2) Dresses without supervision.

(3) Knows own age and birthday.

(4) Ties own shoes.

b. Fine motor-adaptive

(1) Draws person with six body parts.

(2) Copies square.

c. Language

(1) Knows opposite analogies (two of three).

(2) Defines seven words.

d. Gross motor

(1) Balances on each foot for 5 sec.

(2) Can walk heel-to-toe.

3. *5 yr*

a. Personal-social

(1) Interested in money.

(2) Knows days of week, seasons.

b. Fine motor-adaptive

(1) Prints name.

c. Language

(1) Counts to 10.

(2) Verbalizes number sequences (e.g., telephone number).

d. Gross motor

(1) Attempts to ride bike.

(2) Rollerskates, jumps rope, bounces ball.

(3) Backward heel-toe walk.

◆ **D. Nursing interventions/parental guidance:**

1. *Play:* preschool years—associative and cooperative.

a. Likes to play house, "work," school, firehouse.

b. "Arts and crafts": color, draw, paint dot-to-dot, color by number, cut and paste, simple sewing kits.

c. Ball, rollerskate, jump rope, jacks.

d. Swimming.

e. Puzzles, blocks (e.g., Lego blocks).

f. Tricycle, then bicycle (with/without training wheels).

g. Simple card games and board games.

h. Costumes and dress-up: "make-believe."

2. *Safety:* Emphasis shifts from protective supervision to teaching simple safety rules. Preschoolers are "the great imitators" of parents, who now serve as role models.

a. Refer to **Tables 5.8, 5.9,** and **5.10** for additional information on safety and infection control.

b. Teach child car/*street* safety rules.

c. Convertible safety seats should be used until child weighs at least 40 lb.

d. Teach child not to go with strangers or accept gifts or candy from strangers.

e. Teach child danger of *fire,* matches, flame: "drop and roll."

f. Teach child rules of *water* safety; provide swimming lessons.

g. Provide adult supervision, frequent checks on activity/location. Despite safety teaching, preschooler is still a child and may be unreliable.

IV. School age (6–12 yr)

A. Erikson's theory of personality development

1. *Central task:* industry vs. inferiority; central person(s): school, neighborhood friend(s).

2. *Behavioral indicators*

a. Moving toward complete independence in ADL.

b. May be very competitive—wants to achieve in school, at play.

c. Likes to be alone occasionally, may seem shy.

d. Prefers friends and peers to siblings.

3. **Parental guidance/teaching**

a. Be accepting of the child as he or she *is.*

b. Offer consistent support and guidance.

c. *Avoid* authoritative or excessive demands on child.

d. Respect need for privacy.

e. Assign household tasks, errands, chores.

f. Review *Recommended Health Screenings* (see **Tables 5.2** and **5.3**) with parents of school-age children.

4. Additional information about behavioral concerns for each age group may be found in **Tables 5.4** and **5.5.**

B. Physical growth (by 12 yr)

1. *Height and weight*

a. Almost *double* in weight from 6 to 12 yr.

b. Period of slow, steady growth.

c. 1 to 2 in/yr.

d. 3 to 6 lb/yr.

e. Girls and boys differ in size at end of school-age years.

2. *Vital signs:* refer to **Table 5.6.**

3. *Cardiac system*

a. Increased size of left ventricle (to meet demands for increased blood to growing structures).

b. Decreased heart rate, increased blood pressure from preschool values.

4. *Pulmonary system*

a. Front sinuses develop (by 7 yr).

b. Lymphatic tissue completes growth (by 9 yr).

c. Remains well oxygenated on exertion.

d. Continued decrease in respiratory rate from preschool values; using intercostal muscles more effectively for breathing.

5. *Gastrointestinal system*

a. Higher metabolic rate requires adequate food and fluids to ensure nutrition and hydration.

b. Food retained in stomach for longer periods of time.

6. *Genitourinary system*

a. Bladder capacity increase continues.

b. Kidneys mature.

c. Less likely to have fluid and electrolyte (F/E) imbalance as increased conservation of water occurs.

7. *Immune system*

a. Growth of lymphoid tissue increases, then plateaus, then decreases.

b. Continued improvement noted with body's increased ability to localize infections.

8. *Neurological system*

a. Central nervous system matures.

b. Myelinization continues → increase in both fine motor-adaptive and gross motor skills.

9. *Sensory*

a. Vision: 20/20 vision well established between 9 and 11 yr.

b. Should be screened for vision/hearing annually, usually in school.

10. *Teeth*

a. Begins to lose primary teeth around sixth birthday.

b. Eruption of permanent teeth, including molars; 28 permanent teeth (by 12 yr).

c. Dental screening annually, daily brushing.

11. *Pubescence* (preliminary physical changes of adolescence)

a. Average age of onset: girls at 10, boys at 12.

b. Beginning of growth spurt.

c. Some sexual changes may start to occur.

C. **Developmental norms**
1. *6 to 8 yr*
   a. Dramatic, exuberant, boundless energy.
   b. Alternating periods: quiet, private behavior.
   c. Conscientious, punctual.
   d. Wants to care for own needs but needs reminders, supervision.
   e. Oriented to time and space.
   f. Learns to read, tell time, follow map.
   g. Interested in money—asks for "allowance."
   h. Eagerly anticipates upcoming events, trips.
   i. Can bicycle, swim, play ball.
2. *9 to 11 years*
   a. Worries over tasks; takes things seriously, yet also developing sense of humor—likes to tell jokes.
   b. Keeps room, clothes, toys relatively tidy.
   c. Enjoys physical activity, has great stamina.
   d. Very enthusiastic at work and play; has lots of energy—may fidget, drum fingers, tap foot.
   e. Wants to work to earn money: mow lawn, babysit, deliver papers.
   f. Loves secrets (secret clubs).
   g. Very well behaved outside own home (or with company).
   h. Uses tools, equipment; follows directions, recipes.
   i. By twelfth birthday: paradoxical stormy behavior, onset of adolescent conflicts.

◆ D. **Nursing interventions/parental guidance:**
1. *Play*
   a. Wants to win, likes competitive games.
   b. Prefers to play with same-sex children.
   c. Enjoys group, team play.
   d. Loves to do magic tricks and other "show-off" activities (e.g., puppet shows, plays, singing).
   e. Likes to collect things: cards, compact discs.
   f. Does simple scientific experiments, computer games.
   g. Has hobbies: needlework, woodwork, models.
   h. Enjoys pop music, musical instruments, radio, audiotapes, videos, posters.
2. *Safety*
   a. As passenger: use specially designed car restraints until age 8 or 60 lbs, then safety belts. Teach child not to distract driver.
   b. As pedestrian: teach bike, street safety.
   c. Teach how to swim, rules of water safety.
   d. Sports: teach safety rules.
   e. Adult supervision still necessary; serve as role model for safe activities.
   f. Suggest Red Cross courses on first aid, water safety, babysitting, etc.
   g. Refer to **Tables 5.8, 5.9,** and **5.10** for additional information on safety and infection control.

V. **Adolescent (12–18 yr)**
A. **Erikson's theory of personality development**
1. *Central task:* identity vs. role confusion; central person(s): peer group.

2. **Behavioral indicators**
   a. Changes in body image related to sexual development.
   b. Awkward and uncoordinated in the beginning.
   c. Much interest in opposite sex: girls become romantic.
   d. Wants to be exactly like peers.
   e. Becomes hostile toward parents, adults, family.
   f. Concerned with vocation, life after high school.
3. **Parental guidance/teaching**
   a. Offer firm but realistic limits on behavior.
   b. Continue to offer guidance, support.
   c. Allow child to earn own money, control own finances.
   d. Assist adolescent to develop positive self-image.
   e. Review *Recommended Health Screenings* (see **Tables 5.2** and **5.3**) with parents of adolescents.
4. Additional information about behavioral concerns for each age group may be found in **Tables 5.4** and **5.5.**
B. **Physical growth** (by 18 yr)
1. *Height and weight*
   a. Adolescent growth spurt lasts 24–36 mo.
   b. Growth in height commonly *ceases* at 16–17 yr in girls, 18–20 yr in boys.
   c. Boys gain more weight than girls, are generally taller and heavier.
2. *Vital signs* approximately those of the adult (see **Table 5.6**).
3. *Cardiac system*
   a. Increased heart size and strength to near-adult values.
   b. Decreased heart rate, increased blood pressure from school-age values.
4. *Pulmonary system*
   a. Lungs increase in size to near-adult levels, but not as rapidly as other body systems (may explain lack of energy).
   b. System is "mature" by 12 yr.
   c. Continued decreased respiratory rate from school-age values.
5. *Gastrointestinal system*
   a. Continued need for increased calories.
6. *Genitourinary system*
   a. Fully developed; bladder can hold 700 mL.
7. *Immune system*
   a. Fully developed; infections become increasingly rare in an adolescent who is healthy.
   b. Lymphoid tissue matures and regresses.
8. *Neurological system*
   a. Fully developed.
9. *Sensory*
   a. Fully developed.
10. *Teeth:* 32 permanent teeth by 18–21 yr.
11. *Sexual changes*

a. *Girls*
  (1) Changes in nipple and areola; development of breast buds.
  (2) Growth of pubic hair.
  (3) Change in vaginal secretions.
  (4) Menstruation—12.8 yr (average); range 10.5–15 yr
  (5) Growth of axillary hair.
  (6) Ovulation.
b. *Boys*
  (1) Enlargement of genitalia.
  (2) Growth of pubic, axillary, facial, and body hair.
  (3) Lowering of voice.
  (4) Production of sperm; nocturnal emission ("wet dreams").

C. **Developmental norms**
  1. *Motor development*
    a. *Early (12–15 yr)*—awkward, uncoordinated, poor posture, decrease in energy and stamina.
    b. *Later (15–18 yr)*—increased coordination and better posture; more energy and stamina.
  2. *Cognitive*
    a. Academic ability and interest vary greatly.
    b. "Think about thinking"—period of introspection.
  3. *Emotional*
    a. Same-sex best friend, leading to strong friendship bonds.
    b. Highly romantic period for boys and girls.
    c. May be moody, unpredictable, inconsistent.
  4. *Social*
    a. Periods of highs and lows, sociability and loneliness.
    b. Turmoil with parents—related to changing roles, desire for increased independence.
    c. Peer group is important socializing agent—conformity increases sense of belonging.
    d. Friendships: same-sex best friend advancing to heterosexual "relationships."

◆ D. **Nursing interventions/parental guidance:**
  1. *Play*
    a. School-related group activities and sports.
    b. Develops talents, skills, and abilities.
    c. Television—watches soap operas, romantic movies, sports.
    d. Develops interest in art, writing, poetry, musical instrument.
    e. Girls: increased interest in makeup and clothes.
    f. Boys: increased interest in mechanical and electronic devices.
  2. *Safety*—motor vehicles (cars and motorcycles)—as *passenger* or as *driver*
    a. Encourage driver education; serve as positive role model.
    b. Teach rules of safety for water sports.
    c. Wants to earn money but still needs guidance: advocate safe job, reasonable hours.
    d. Refer to **Tables 5.8, 5.9,** and **5.10** for additional information on safety and infection control.

Developmental Disabilities

I. **Down syndrome**
  A. *Introduction:* Down syndrome (trisomy 21; mongolism) is a chromosomal abnormality involving an extra chromosome #21 and resulting in 47 chromosomes instead of the normal 46 chromosomes. As a consequence, the child usually has varying degrees of mental retardation, characteristic facial and physical features, and other congenital anomalies. Down syndrome is the most common chromosomal disorder, occurring in approximately 1 of 800 to 1000 live births. Perinatal risk factors include advanced maternal age, especially with the first pregnancy; paternal age is thought to be a related factor. Multiple causality is suspected.

◆ B. **Assessment:**
  1. *Physical characteristics*
    a. Brachycephalic (small, round *head*) with oblique palpebral fissures (Oriental *eyes*) and *Brushfield's* spots (speckling of *iris*)—depressed *nasal* bridge ("saddle nose") and small, low-set *ears*.
    b. Mouth
      (1) Small oral cavity with protruding tongue causes difficulty sucking and swallowing.
      (2) Delayed eruption/misalignment of teeth.
    c. Hands
      (1) Clinodactyly—in-curved little finger.
      (2) Simian crease—transverse palmar crease.
    d. Muscles: hypotonic ("floppy baby") with hyperextensible joints.
    e. Skin: dry, cracked.
  2. Genetic studies reveal an extra chromosome #21 ("trisomy 21").
  3. *Intellectual characteristics*
    a. Mental retardation—varies from severely retarded to low-average intelligence.
    b. Most fall within "trainable" range, or IQ of 36–51 ("moderate mental retardation").
  4. *Congenital anomalies/diseases*
    a. 40%–45% have congenital heart defects: mortality highest in clients with Down syndrome and cyanotic heart disease.
    b. GI: tracheoesophageal fistula (TEF), Hirschsprung's disease.
    c. Thyroid dysfunction, especially hypothroidism.
    d. Visual defects: cataracts, strabismus.
    e. Hearing loss.
    f. Increased incidence of leukemia.
  5. *Growth and development*
    a. Slow growth, especially in height.
    b. Delay in developmental milestones.
  6. *Sexual development*
    a. Delayed or incomplete.
    b. Women—small number have had offspring (majority have had abnormality).
    c. Men—infertile.
  7. *Aging*
    a. Premature aging, with shortened life expectancy.

b. Death—generally related to respiratory complications: repeated infections, pneumonia, lung disease.

◆ **C. Analysis/nursing diagnosis:**
1. *Risk for aspiration* related to hypotonia.
2. *Altered nutrition, less than body requirements,* related to hypotonia or congenital anomalies.
3. *Altered growth and development* related to Down syndrome.
4. *Self-care deficit* related to Down syndrome.
5. *Altered family processes* related to birth of an infant with a congenital defect.
6. *Knowledge deficit* related to Down syndrome.

◆ **D. Nursing care plan/implementation:**
1. Goal: *prevent physical complications.*
   a. Respiratory
      (1) Use bulb syringe to clear nose, mouth.
      (2) Vaporizer.
      (3) Frequent position changes.
      (4) *Avoid* contact with people with upper-respiratory infections.
   b. Aspiration
      (1) Small, more frequent feedings.
      (2) Burp well during/after infant feedings.
      (3) Allow sufficient time to eat.
      (4) *Position after meals:* head of bed elevated, right side—or on stomach, with head to side.
   c. Observe for signs and symptoms of heart disease, constipation/GI obstruction, leukemia, thyroid dysfunction.
2. Goal: *meet nutritional needs.*
   ▶ a. Suction (before meals) to clear airway.
   b. Adapt feeding techniques to meet special needs of infant/child; e.g., use long, straight-handled spoon.
   c. Monitor height and weight.
   d. As child grows, monitor caloric intake (tends toward obesity).
   🍽 e. Offer foods *high in bulk* to prevent constipation related to hypotonia.
3. Goal: *promote optimal growth and development.*
   a. Encourage parents to enroll infant/toddler in early stimulation program and to follow through with suggested exercises at home.
   b. Preschool/school-age: special education classes.
   c. Screen frequently, using DDST to monitor development.
   d. Help parents focus on "normal" or positive aspects of infant/child.
   e. Help parents work toward realistic goals with their child.
4. Goal: *health teaching.*
   a. Explain that tongue-thrust behavior is normal and that child should be refed.
   b. Before adolescence—counsel parents and child about delay in sexual development, decreased libido, marriage and family relations.
   c. In severe cases, assist parents to deal with issue of placement/institutionalization.

◆ **E. Evaluation/outcome criteria:**
1. Physical complications are prevented.
2. Adequate nutrition is maintained.
3. Child attains optimal level of growth and development.

II. Attention deficit–hyperactivity disorder (ADHD); behavioral disorder (DSM-IV)
A. *Introduction:* As defined by the American Psychiatric Association (APA), this diagnostic term includes a persistent pattern of inattention or hyperactivity-impulsivity. The exact cause and pathophysiology remain unknown. The major symptoms include a greatly shortened attention span and difficulty in integrating and synthesizing information. This disorder is 3 times more common in boys than girls, with onset before age 7; the diagnosis is based on the child's history rather than on any specific diagnostic test.

◆ **B. Assessment:**
1. The behaviors exhibited by children with ADHD are not unusual behaviors seen in children. The behavior of children with ADHD *differs* from the behavior of non-ADHD children in both *quality* and *appropriateness:*
   a. Motor activity is excessive.
   b. Developmentally "younger" than chronological age.
2. Inattention
   a. Does not pay attention to detail.
   b. Does not listen when spoken to.
   c. Does not do what he or she is told to do.
3. Hyperactivity
   a. Fidgets and squirms excessively.
   b. Cannot sit quietly.
   c. Has difficulty playing quietly.
   d. Seems to be constantly in motion, moving or talking; always "on."
4. Impulsiveness
   a. Blurts out answers before question is completed.
   b. Has difficulty awaiting turn. Interrupts others.

◆ **C. Analysis/nursing diagnosis:**
1. *Altered thought processes* related to inattention and impulsiveness.
2. *Impaired physical mobility* related to hyperactivity.
3. *Risk for injury* related to impulsivity.
4. *Self-esteem disturbance* related to hyperactivity and impulsivity.
5. *Knowledge deficit* related to behavioral modification program, medications, and follow-up care.

◆ **D. Nursing care plan/implementation:**
1. Goal: *teach family and child about ADHD.*
   a. Provide complete explanation about disorder, probable course, treatment, and prognosis.
   b. Answer questions directly, simply.
   c. Encourage family to verbalize; offer support.
2. Goal: *provide therapeutic environment* using principles of behavior modification and/or psychotherapy.
   a. Reduce extraneous or distracting stimuli.
   b. Reduce stress by decreasing environmental expectations (home, school).

c. Provide firm, consistent limits.

d. Special education programs.

e. Special attention to safety needs.

3. *Goal: reduce symptoms by means of prescribed medication.*

   a. Medications: *Ritalin* and *Cylert*—both are CNS stimulants but have a paradoxical calming effect on the child's behavior. *Tofranil* and *Norpramin*—both are tricyclic antidepressants that ↑ action of norepinephrine and serotonin in nerve cells, but also can have paradoxical calming effect on child's behavior. Must monitor for development of tics and arrhythmias.

   b. *Health teaching* (child *and* parents).

     (1) Need to take medication regularly, as ordered. *Avoid* taking medication late in the day because it may cause insomnia; monitor neurological and cardiac status. Assess for ↓ appetite → ↓weight; *avoid* caffeine.

     (2) Need for long-term administration, with probable decreased need as child nears adolescence.

4. *Goal: provide safe outlet for excess energy.*

   a. Alternate planned periods of outdoor play with schoolwork or quiet indoor play.

   b. Channel energies toward safe, large-muscle activities: running track, swimming, bicycling, hiking.

◆ E. **Evaluation/outcome criteria:**

1. Family and child verbalize understanding of "attention deficit disorders."

2. Therapeutic environment enhances socially acceptable behavior.

3. Medication taken regularly, with behavioral improvements noted.

4. Excess energy directed appropriately.

PSYCHOSOCIAL-CULTURAL FUNCTIONS

Refer to **Table 5.11** for information on the nursing care of hospitalized infants and children as it relates to key developmental differences.

DISORDERS AFFECTING FLUID-GAS TRANSPORT

Cardiovascular Disorders

Congenital Heart Disease (CHD)

I. *Introduction:* There are more than 35 documented types of congenital heart defects, which occur in 5 to 8 per 1000 live births. For the purpose of this review, only 5 *major* defects are given. These are presented in **Figures 5.1** through **5.5.** *Note:* The content has been

TABLE 5.11	Nursing Care of Hospitalized Infants and Children: Key Developmental Differences	
Age	◆ **Assessment: Reaction to Hospitalization**	◆ **Nursing Care Plan/Implementation: Key Nursing Behaviors**
INFANT	Difficult to assess needs, pain Wants primary caretaker	Close observation, must look at behavioral cues Rooming-in
TODDLER	Separation anxiety Frustration, loss of autonomy Regression Fears intrusive procedures	Rooming-in Punching bag, pounding board, clay Behavior modification Axillary temperatures
PRESCHOOLER	Fearful Fantasy about illness/hospitalization (may feel punished, abandoned) Peak of body mutilation fear Behavior problems: aggressive, manipulative Regression	Therapeutic play with puppets, dolls Therapeutic play with puppets, dolls Care with dressings, casts, IMs; invasive procedures Clear, consistent limits Behavior modification
SCHOOL AGE	Cooperative Quiet, may withdraw May complain of being bored	Use diagrams, models to teach Indirect interview: tell story, draw picture Involve in competitive game with peer; encourage peers to call, send get well cards, and visit
ADOLESCENT	Fears loss of control Competitive—afraid of "failing" Difficulty with body image Does not want to be separated from peers Rebellious behavior	Provide privacy; allow to make some decisions Provide tutor prn; get books and homework Provide own clothes; give realistic feedback Telephone in room; liberal visiting; teen lounge Set clear rules; form teen support group

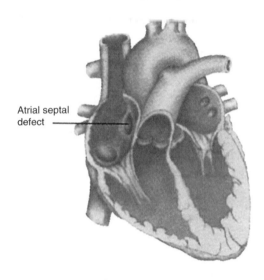

FIGURE 5.1   Atrial septal defect. An opening between the two atria, allowing oxygenated blood and unoxygenated blood to mix. Left-to-right shunting of blood occurs due to the higher pressure on the left side of the heart. (From Ashwill, JW, and Droske, SC: Nursing Care of Children: Principles and Practice. WB Saunders, Philadelphia.)

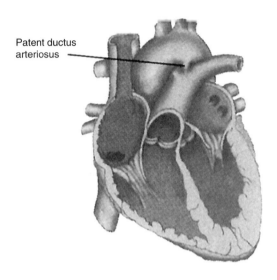

FIGURE 5.3   Patent ductus arteriosus. An artery that connects the aorta and the pulmonary artery during fetal life. It generally closes spontaneously within a few hours to several days after birth. Allows abnormal blood flow from the high-pressure aorta to the low-pressure pulmonary artery, resulting in a left-to-right shunt. (From Ashwill, JW, and Droske, SC: Nursing Care of Children: Principles and Practice. WB Saunders, Philadelphia.)

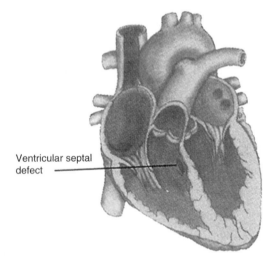

FIGURE 5.2   Ventricular septal defect. An opening between the two ventricles, allowing oxygenated and unoxygenated blood to mix. Shunting of blood occurs due to the higher pressure on the left side of the heart. Ventricular septal defects are classified as membranous or muscular according to location in the septum. (From Ashwill, JW, and Droske, SC: Nursing Care of Children: Principles and Practice. WB Saunders, Philadelphia.)

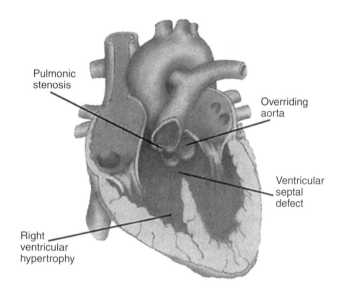

FIGURE 5.4   Tetralogy of Fallot. Four cardiac anomalies make up tetralogy of Fallot: a ventricular septal defect, pulmonary stenosis, an overriding aorta, and right ventricular hypertrophy. There are other associated defects in certain cases. Pulmonary stenosis results in reduction of pulmonary blood flow; the ventricular septal defect allows mixing of oxygenated and unoxygenated blood. (From Ashwill, JW, and Droske, SC: Nursing Care of Children: Principles and Practice. WB Saunders, Philadelphia.)

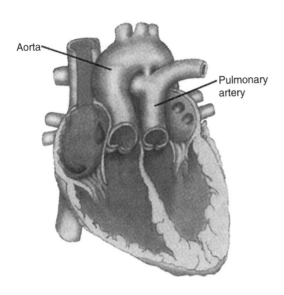

FIGURE 5.5   Transposition of the great arteries. The aorta and the pulmonary artery are reversed; i.e., the aorta rises from the right instead of the left ventricle, and the pulmonary artery arises from the left instead of the right ventricle. Systemic venous blood (unoxygenated blood) returns to the right side of the heart to pass through the aorta back to the body without being oxygenated because of bypassing the lungs. The pulmonary venous blood (oxygenated blood) enters the left side of the heart, returning to the lungs via the pulmonary artery. The systemic (unoxygenated) and pulmonary (oxygenated) circulations are totally separate. There must be some opening (i.e., patent ductus arteriosus or septal defect) to allow blood to mix. (From Ashwill, JW, and Droske, SC: Nursing Care of Children: Principles and Practice. WB Saunders, Philadelphia.)

synthesized for ease in review and recall; for additional study aids, the student may wish to refer to **Tables 5.12** and **5.13**. **Unit 7** also contains information on congestive heart failure, and **Unit 10** covers the most commonly used drugs, including digoxin and furosemide (*Lasix*).

◆ **II. Assessment:**

A. Exact cause unknown, but related factors include:
1. Familial history of CHD, especially in siblings, parents.
2. Presence of other genetic defects in infant, e.g., Down syndrome, trisomy 13 or 18.
3. History of maternal prenatal infection with rubella, cytomegalovirus, etc.
4. High-risk maternal factors:
   a. Age: under 18 yr, over 40 yr.
   b. Weight: under 100 lb, over 200 lb.
   c. Maternal insulin-dependent diabetes.
5. Maternal history of drinking during pregnancy, with resultant "fetal alcohol syndrome."
6. Extracardiac defects including tracheoesophageal fistula, renal agenesis, and diaphragmatic hernia.

B. Most frequent parental complaint: *difficulty feeding.*
1. Infant must be awakened to feed.
2. Has weak suck.
3. May turn blue when eating, especially with cyanotic defects.
4. Infant takes overly long time to feed.
5. Falls asleep during feeding, without finishing.

◆ C. Nursing observations
1. *Most frequent symptom*—tachycardia, as body attempts to compensate for lack of oxygen (hypoxia), i.e., heart rate over 160 beats/min.
2. Tachypnea, corresponding to heart rate, i.e., respirations over 60 breaths/min.
3. Cyanosis due to hypoxia:
   a. *Not* with acyanotic defects (unless CHF is present).
   b. *Always* with cyanotic defects ("blue infants").
4. Failure to grow at a normal rate, i.e., slow weight gain, height and weight below the norm due to difficulty feeding and hypoxia.
5. Developmental delays related to weakened physical condition.
6. Frequent respiratory infections associated with increased pulmonary blood flow or aspiration.
7. Dyspnea on exertion due to hypoxia, shunting of blood.
8. Murmurs may or may not be present, e.g., patent ductus arteriosus (PDA) machinery murmur.
9. Changes in blood pressure, e.g., coarctation—

Pediatrics

TABLE 5.12	Comparison of Acyanotic and Cyanotic Heart Disease	
Feature	**Acyanotic**	**Cyanotic**
Shunting of blood	L → R	R → L
Cyanosis	*Not usual* (unless congestive heart failure)	*Always;* "blue babies"
Surgery	Usually done in one stage—technically simple	Usually done in several stages—technically complex
Prognosis	Very good/excellent	Guarded
Major types	1. Atrial septal defect (ASD) 2. Ventricular septal defect (VSD) 3. Patent ductus arteriosus (PDA) 4. Coarctation of the aorta (COA)	1. Tetralogy of Fallot (TOF) 2. Transposition of the great vessels (TGV)

TABLE 5.13	Overview of the Most Common Types of Congenital Heart Disease		
Type of Defect	**Medical Treatment**	**Surgical Treatment**	**Prognosis**
ACYANOTIC			
Atrial septal defect (ASD)	Clinical trials using device closure during cardiac catheterization	Open chest/open heart surgery with closure through patch (recommended age: preschooler).	Excellent, with survival rate greater than 99%
Ventricular septal defect (VSD)	Clinical trials using device closure during cardiac catheterization	*Palliative treatment:* pulmonary banding; *definitive repair:* same as for **ASD**	Excellent, with 95% or greater survival rate
Patent ductus arteriosus (PDA)	In newborns, attempt pharmacological closure with indomethacin (prostaglandin inhibitor)	Open chest: surgical division or ligation of the patent ductus	Excellent, with survival rate greater than 99%
Coarctation of the aorta (COA)	Infants or children with CHF: digoxin and diuretics	Open chest: resection of coarcted portion of aorta with end-to-end anastomosis within first 2 years of life Nonsurgical: balloon angioplasty	Fair—less than 5% mortality rate
CYANOTIC			
Tetralogy of Fallot (ToF)	None—supportive prn	Often done in *stages* with definitive repair accomplished within first year of life	Fair—less than 5% mortality rate
Transposition of the great vessels (TGV)	None—supportive prn	Arterial switch procedure during first weeks of life	Guarded—5%–10% mortality rate

increased blood pressure in arms; *decreased* blood pressure in legs.

10. Possible congestive heart failure—refer to **Unit 7.** *Note:* Infants may *not* demonstrate distended neck veins.

11. Cyanotic heart defects:
  a. **"Tet. spells"**—choking spells with paroxysmal dyspnea: severe hypoxia, deepening cyanosis; relieved by placing infant in knee-chest position, which alters cardiopulmonary dynamics, thus increasing the flow of blood to the lungs.
  b. Clubbing of fingers and toes—due to chronic hypoxia.
  c. Polycythemia (increased red blood cells [RBCs]) with possible thrombi/emboli formation.

◆ III. **Analysis/nursing diagnosis:**
  A. *Ineffective breathing pattern* related to tachypnea and respiratory infection.
  B. *Activity intolerance* related to tachycardia and hypoxia.
  C. *Altered nutrition, less than body requirements,* related to difficulty in feeding.
  D. *Risk for infection* related to poor nutritional status.
  E. *Knowledge deficit* related to diagnostic procedures, condition, surgical/medical treatments, prognosis.

◆ IV. **Nursing care plan/implementation:**
  A. Goal: *promote adequate oxygenation.*
  ▶ 1. Administer oxygen per physician's order/prn.
    2. Use loose-fitting clothing; tape diapers loosely to *avoid* pressure on abdominal organs, which could impinge on diaphragm and impede respiration.
    3. *Position:* neck slightly hyperextended to keep airway patent; place in knee-chest position to relieve "Tet. spell" (choking spell).
  ▶ 4. Suction prn to clear the airway.
    5. Administer *digoxin,* per physician's order, to slow and strengthen heart's pumping action (refer to **Unit 10** and to **Table 5.6** for pediatric pulse rate norms).
    6. Monitor pulse oximetry, as ordered.
  B. Goal: *reduce workload of heart to conserve energy.*
    1. *Position:* infant seat, semi-Fowler's to promote maximum expansion of the lungs.
    2. Provide pacifier to promote psychological rest.
    3. Organize nursing care to provide periods of uninterrupted rest.
    4. Adjust physical activity according to child's condition, capabilities to conserve energy.
    5. Provide diversion, as tolerated, to meet developmental needs yet conserve energy.

6. *Avoid* extremes of temperature to avoid the stress of hypothermia/hyperthermia, which will increase the body's demand for oxygen.

7. Administer diuretics (*Lasix*), per physician's order, to eliminate excess fluids, which increase the heart's workload. *Note:* Refer to **Unit 10.**

C. Goal: *provide for adequate nutrition.*

1. May need standard infant formula with ↑ caloric density to minimize fluid retention and meet nutritional needs.

2. Discourage foods with high or added sodium to minimize fluid retention.

3. I&O, daily/weekly weights, and monitor for rate of growth.

4. Limit PO feedings to 20 min to *avoid* overtiring infant. Supplement PO feeding with gavage feeding (prn with physician's order) to meet fluid and caloric needs.

5. Encourage foods *high in potassium* (prevent hypokalemia) and *high in iron* (prevent anemia). *Note:* Refer to **Unit 9.**

D. Goal: *prevent infection.*

1. Standard precautions to prevent infection.
2. Use good handwashing technique.
3. Limit contact with staff/visitors (especially children) with infections.
4. Monitor for early symptoms and signs of infection; report STAT.

E. Goal: *meet teaching needs of client, family.*

1. Explain diagnostic procedures: blood tests, x-rays, urine, ECG, echocardiogram, cardiac catheterization.
2. Explain condition/treatment/prognosis (see **Table 5.13**).
3. Review nutrition and medications.
4. Discuss how to adjust realistically to life with congenital heart disease, activity restrictions, etc.

V. Evaluation/outcome criteria:

A. Child's level of oxygenation is maintained, as evidenced by pink color in nailbeds and mucous membranes (for both light- and dark-skinned children) and ease in respiratory effort.

B. Energy is conserved, thus reducing the heart's workload as evidenced by vital signs within normal limits.

C. The child's fluid and caloric requirements are met, allowing for physical growth to occur at normal or near-normal rate.

D. The family (and child, when old enough) verbalize their understanding of the type of CHD, its treatment, and prognosis.

E. The family and child demonstrate adequate coping mechanisms to deal with CHD.

Disorders of the Blood

I. Leukemia

A. *Introduction:* Known as "cancer of the blood," leukemia is the most common form of childhood cancer, with an incidence of 4/100,000. Acute leukemia is basically a malignant proliferation of white blood cell (WBC) precursors triggered by an unknown cause and affecting all blood-forming organs and systems throughout the body. The onset is typically insidious, and the disease is most common in preschoolers (age 2–6 yr).

B. **Assessment:**

1. Major problem—leukopenia: *decreased* WBC/*increased* blasts (overproduction of immature, poorly functioning white blood cells).

2. Bone marrow dysfunction results in:

   a. *Neutropenia:* multiple prolonged infections.
   b. *Anemia:* pallor, weakness, irritability, shortness of breath.
   c. *Thrombocytopenia:* bleeding tendencies (petechiae, epistaxis, bruising).

3. Infiltration of reticuloendothelial system (RES): hepatosplenomegaly, abdominal pain, lymphadenopathy.

4. Leukemic invasion of CNS: increased intracranial pressure/leukemic meningitis.

5. Leukemic invasion of bone: pain, pathological fractures, hemarthrosis.

C. **Analysis/nursing diagnosis:**

1. *Risk for infection* related to neutropenia.
2. *Risk for injury* related to thrombocytopenia.
3. *Altered nutrition, less than body requirements,* related to loss of appetite, vomiting, mouth ulcers.
4. *Pain* related to disease process and treatments (e.g., hemarthrosis, bone pain, bone marrow aspiration).
5. *Activity intolerance* related to infection and anemia.
6. *Self-esteem disturbance* related to disease process and treatments (e.g., loss of hair with chemotherapy, moon face with prednisone).
7. *Anticipatory grieving* related to life-threatening illness.
8. *Knowledge deficit* related to diagnosis, treatment, prognosis.

D. **Nursing care plan/implementation:**

1. Goal: *maintain infection-free state.*

   a. Standard precautions to prevent infection.
   b. Use good handwashing technique.
   c. Ongoing evaluation of sites for potential infection, e.g., gums.
   d. Provide meticulous oral hygiene.
   e. Keep record of vital signs, especially temperature.
   f. Provide good skin care.
   g. Screen staff and visitors (especially children)—restrict anyone with infection.
   h. *Protective isolation/reverse isolation* to minimize exposure to potentially life-threatening infection.
   i. Discharge planning: return to school, but isolate from chickenpox or known communicable diseases.

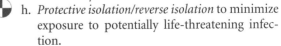

2. Goal: *prevent injury.*

a. *Avoid* IMs/IVs if possible, due to bruising and bleeding tendencies.

b. Do *not* give aspirin or medications containing aspirin, which will interfere with platelet formation, thus increasing the risk of bleeding.

c. Use soft toothbrush to *avoid* trauma to gums, which may cause bleeding and infection.

d. *Avoid* "per rectum" suppositories, due to probable rectal ulcers.

e. Supervise play/activity carefully to promote safety and prevent excessive bruising or bleeding.

3. Goal: *promote adequate nutrition.*

a. *Diet:* high *calorie*, high *protein*, high *iron*.

b. Encourage *extra fluids* to prevent constipation or dehydration.

c. I&O, daily weights, to monitor fluid and nutritional status.

d. Allow child to be involved with food selection/preparation; allow child almost any food he or she tolerates, to encourage better dietary intake.

e. Thoroughly wash/peel fresh fruits and vegetables if child is neutropenic (or *avoid* eating these foods).

f. Serve frequent, small snacks to increase fluid and caloric consumption.

g. Offer dietary supplements to increase caloric intake.

h. Encourage local anesthetics such as dextromethorphan throat lozenges (*Chloraseptic*) before meals to allow child to eat without pain from oral mucous membrane ulcers.

4. Goal: *relieve pain.*

a. Offer supportive alternatives: extra company, back rub. Offer complementary therapies: meditation, visualization (if age appropriate).

b. Administer medications regularly, before pain becomes excessive.

c. Use bean bag chair for positional changes.

d. *Avoid* excessive stimulation (noise, light), which may heighten perception of pain.

5. Goal: *promote self-esteem.*

a. Stress what child can still do to keep the child as independent as possible.

b. Encourage performance of ADL as much as possible to foster a sense of independence.

c. Provide diversion/activity as tolerated.

d. Give lots of positive reinforcement to enhance a sense of accomplishment.

e. Provide realistic feedback on child's appearance; offer suggestions, such as a wig or cap to cover alopecia secondary to chemotherapy.

f. Encourage early return to peers/school to avoid social isolation.

6. Goal: *prevent complications related to leukemia/prolonged immobility/treatments.*

a. Inspect skin for breakdown, especially over bony prominences, due to poor nutritional intake and limited mobility due to bone pain.

b. Anticipate need for and administer (per physi-

cian's order) multiple transfusions of platelets, packed RBCs, etc.

c. Check for hemorrhagic cystitis; *push fluids* (especially with *cytoxan*).

d. Check for constipation or peripheral neuropathy (especially with vincristine). Refer to **Unit 10** for specific information on chemotherapy.

7. Goal: *assist child and parents to cope with life-threatening illness.*

a. Teach rationale for repeated hospitalizations, multiple invasive tests/treatments, long-term follow-up care.

b. Encourage compliance with all aspects of therapy, to increase chances of survival.

c. Support family members and their coping mechanisms.

d. Offer factual information regarding ultimate prognosis ("80% cure" for acute lymphocytic leukemia [ALL]).

e. If death appears imminent, assist family to cope with dying and death.

◆ **E. Evaluation/outcome criteria:**

1. Child is maintained in infection-free state.

2. Injuries are prevented or kept to a minimum.

3. Adequate nutrition is maintained.

4. Child is free from pain or can live with minimum level of pain.

5. Child's self-esteem is maintained; child is treated as living (not dying).

6. Complications are prevented or kept to a minimum.

7. Child and family use positive coping mechanisms to deal with illness.

II. Sickle cell anemia

A. *Introduction:* Sickle cell anemia is a congenital hemolytic anemia resulting from a defective hemoglobin (Hgb) molecule (hemoglobin S). It is most common in African Americans (8% have sickle cell trait) and in people of Mediterranean, Hispanic, and Middle Eastern descent. The diagnosis is usually made during the toddler or preschool years, during the first crisis episode following an infection. There is also the need to differentiate between *sickle cell trait* (Sickledex test) and *sickle cell anemia* (hemoglobin electrophoresis). Sickle cell anemia has no known cure.

◆ **B. Assessment:**

1. Increased susceptibility to infection (cause: unknown; most common cause of death in children under 5 yr).

2. Inherited as autosomal recessive disorder (**Figure 5.6**).

3. Precipitated by conditions of low oxygen tension, dehydration, vascular obstruction, increased blood viscosity, infection.

4. Signs of anemia:

a. Pallor (in dark-skinned children, do not rely on pallor alone—check hemoglobin [Hgb] and hematocrit [Hct]).

b. Jaundice, due to excessive hemolysis.

c. Irritability, lethargy, anorexia, malaise.

(A) Normal parent and parent who carries trait

	A	A
A	AA	AA
S	AS	AS

1:2 (or 2:4) chance offspring will carry trait.

(B) Two parents who carry trait

	A	S
A	AA	AS
S	AS	SS

1:4 chance offspring will be normal.
1:4 chance offspring will have sickle cell anemia.
1:2 (or 2:4) chance offspring will carry trait.

(C) Normal parent and parent with sickle cell anemia

	A	A
S	AS	AS
S	AS	AS

4:4 (100%) chance offspring will carry trait.

(D) Parent with sickle cell anemia and parent who carries trait

	A	S
S	AS	SS
S	AS	SS

1:2 chance offspring will carry trait.
1:2 chance offspring will have sickle cell anemia.

(E) Two parents with sickle cell anemia

	S	S
S	SS	SS
S	SS	SS

4:4 (100%) chance offspring will have sickle cell anemia.

Key   AA   = normal hemoglobin
AS   = sickle cell trait
SS   = sickle cell disease (anemia)

Note: The odds cited here are for *each* pregnancy.

FIGURE 5.6   Genetic transmission of sickle cell anemia.

5. **Vaso-occlusive crisis:** severe pain (variable sites, e.g., chest, back, abdomen), fever, swelling of hands and feet, joint pain and swelling, all related to hypoxia, ischemia, and necrosis at the cellular level. Most common; usually non–life threatening.
6. **Splenic sequestration crisis:** blood is sequestered (pooled) in spleen; precipitous drop in hemoglobin levels and blood pressure, increased pulse rate, shock, and ultimately death from profound anemia and cardiovascular collapse.

◆ **C. Analysis/nursing diagnosis:**
   1. *Altered tissue perfusion* related to anemia and occlusion of vessels.
   2. *Pain* related to vaso-occlusion.
   3. *Impaired physical mobility* related to pain, immobility.
   4. *Knowledge deficit* related to disease process and treatment (e.g., prevention of sickling or infection; genetic counseling).

◆ **D. Nursing care plan/implementation:**
   1. Goal: *prevent sickling.*
      a. *Avoid* conditions of low oxygen tension (hypoxia), which causes RBCs to assume a sickled shape.
      b. Provide continuous *extra fluids* to prevent dehydration, which causes sluggish circulation. State

specific amounts to be consumed rather than "encourage fluids." *Avoid* temperature extremes.
      c. *Avoid* activities that may result in overheating, to prevent dehydration; suggest appropriate clothes; limit time in sun.
      d. If dehydrated due to acute illness, supplement with IV fluids and additional oral fluids to reestablish fluid balance.
   2. Goal: *maintain infection-free state.*
      a. *Standard precautions* to prevent infection.
      b. Use good handwashing technique.
      c. Evaluate carefully, check continually for potential infection sites, which may either lead to death due to sepsis or precipitate sickle cell crisis.
      d. Teach importance of prevention of sickle cell crisis: adequate fluids and nutrition; frequent medical checkups; keep away from known sources of infection.
      e. Stress need to report early signs of infection (Acute Chest Syndrome) promptly to physician.
      f. Need to balance prevention of infection with child's need for a "normal" life.
       g. Administer yearly influenza vaccine.
   3. Goal: *provide supportive therapy during crisis.*
      a. Provide bedrest/hospitalization during crisis to decrease the body's demand for oxygen.
      b. Relieve pain due to infarction of tissues by

administering pain medications as ordered; handle gently and use proper positioning techniques.

   ▶ c. Apply heat *(never cold)* to affected painful areas to increase blood flow (vasodilation) and oxygen supply.

   ▶ d. Administer oxygen, as ordered, to relieve hypoxia and prevent further sickling.

   ⬤▢ e. Administer blood transfusions, as ordered, to correct severe anemia. *Complication:* If hypertransfusion programs are implemented, child

   ⬤▢ may develop "iron overload." *Desferal* chelates the iron so that it can be excreted through the urine or bile to help reduce this complication.

   ⬤▢ f. Standard meds: hydroxyurea, folic acid.

   🧪 g. Monitor fluid and electrolyte balance: I&O, weight, electrolytes.

   h. Perform ADL for child if unable to care for own needs; encourage self-care as soon as possible to promote independence. *Avoid* stress and fatigue.

4. Goal: *teach child and family about sickle cell anemia.*

   a. Provide factual information based on child's developmental level.

   b. When asked, offer information regarding prognosis (no known cure).

   c. Encourage child to live as normally as possible.

   d. Genetic screening and counseling (see **Figure 5.6**).

◆ **E. Evaluation/outcome criteria:**

1. Sickling is prevented or kept to a minimum.
2. Child is maintained in infection-free state.
3. Child/family verbalize that they can cope adequately with crisis.
4. Child/family verbalize their understanding about disease, its management, and its prognosis.

III. Hemophilia

   A. *Introduction:* Hemophilia is a bleeding disorder inherited as a sex-linked (X-linked) recessive trait; i.e., it occurs only in men but is transmitted by women carriers who are symptom free (**Figure 5.7**). Hemophilia results in a deficiency of one or more clotting factors; it is necessary to determine which clotting factor is deficient and to what extent. Classic hemophilia (hemophilia A), a lack of clotting factor VIII, accounts for 75% of all cases of hemophilia.

◆ **B. Assessment:**

1. Major problem is bleeding.

   a. In *newborn* boy: abnormal bleeding from umbilical cord, prolonged bleeding from circumcision site.

   b. In *toddler* boy: excessive bruising, possible intracranial bleeding, prolonged bleeding from cuts or lacerations.

   c. *General:* hemarthrosis, petechiae, epistaxis, frank hemorrhage anywhere in body, anemia.

2. Need to determine which clotting factor is deficient/missing and extent of deficiency:

   a. *Mild:* child has 5%–50% of normal amount of clotting factor.

   b. *Moderate:* child has 1%–5% of normal amount of clotting factor.

   c. *Severe:* child has less than 1% of normal amount of clotting factor.

   🧪 3. Definitive test: PTT

◆ **C. Analysis/nursing diagnosis:**

1. *Risk for injury* related to bleeding tendencies.
2. *Pain* related to hemarthrosis.
3. *Impaired physical mobility* related to bleeding and pain.
4. *Knowledge deficit* related to home care and follow-up.

(A) "Normal" male and female with trait

	X	Y
X*	X*X	X*Y
X	XX	XY

1:4 chance will be female with trait.
1:4 chance will be male with hemophilia.
1:2 (or 2:4) chance will be "normal" female/male.

(B) Male with hemophilia and "normal" female

	X*	Y
X	XX*	XY
X	XX*	XY

1:2 (or 2:4) chance will be female with trait.
1:2 (or 2:4) chance will be "normal" male.

(C) Male with hemophilia and female with trait

	X*	Y
X*	X*X*	X*Y
X	X*X	XY

1:2 (or 2:4) chance will be female with trait.
1:4 chance will be "normal" male.
1:4 chance will be male with hemophilia.

Key

XY	= normal male
X*Y	= male with hemophilia
XX	= normal female
X*X	= female carrying hemophilia trait
X*X*	= female with possible relative lack of clotting factor—*not* a true hemophiliac (von Willebrand's disease).

Note: The odds cited here are for *each* pregnancy.

FIGURE 5.7 **Genetic transmission of hemophilia.**

◆ **D. Nursing care plan/implementation:**

1. Goal: *prevent injury and possible bleeding.*

   a. Provide an environment that is as safe as possible, e.g., toys with no sharp edges, child's safety scissors.

   b. Use soft toothbrush to prevent trauma to gums. Wear safety equipment in PE; no contact sports.

   c. When old enough to shave, use only electric razor (no straight-edge razors).

   d. *Avoid* IMs/IVs—but when absolutely necessary, treat as arterial puncture; that is, apply direct pressure to the site for at least 5 min after withdrawing needle.

   e. Do **not** use aspirin or medication containing aspirin (prolongs bleeding/clotting time). Caution with NSAIDs (inhibit platelet function).

2. Goal: *control bleeding episodes when they occur.*

   a. Local measures: *RICE* (**R**est, **I**ce, **C**ompression, **E**levation); keep immobilized during acute bleeding episodes only. For epistaxis: child should sit up and lean slightly forward.

   b. Systemic measures: administer clotting *antihemophilic factor* (Factor VIII or DDVAP) via IV infusion. *Note:* These are blood products, so a transfusion reaction is possible.

   c. *Note:* cryoprecipitate (a blood product) is no longer used due to risk of transmission of hepatitis and HIV.

3. Goal: *prevent long-term disability related to joint degeneration.*

   a. Keep *immobilized* during period of acute bleeding and for 24 to 48 hr afterward to allow blood to clot and to prevent dislodging the clot.

   b. Administer prescribed pain medications *before* physical therapy sessions.

   c. Begin prescribed exercise program, starting with passive range of motion (ROM) and gradually advancing to active ROM, then full exercise program, as tolerated, to maintain maximum joint function. Monitor weight to prevent ↑ strain on joints (especially knees).

   d. **Avoid:** prolonged immobility, braces, splints—which can lead to permanent deformities and loss of mobility.

4. Goal: *promote independence in management of own care.*

   a. Encourage child to assume responsibility for choosing safe activities.

   b. Encourage child to attend regular school as much as possible; provide support through school nurse.

   c. Advise child to wear MedicAlert bracelet.

   d. Caution parents to *avoid* overprotecting child.

   e. Offer child chance to self-limit activities within appropriate limits (parents can offer guidance).

   f. Assist child to cope with life-threatening disorder with no known cure.

5. Goal: *health teaching.*

   a. Between 9 and 12 years of age: child can be taught to self-administer clotting factor IV (before this, family can perform).

   b. As child enters adolescence: begin to discuss issues such as realistic vocations, insurance coverage, genetic transmission (see **Figure 5.7**).

◆ **E. Evaluation/outcome criteria:**

1. Serious injuries are prevented; bleeding is kept to a minimum.

2. Episodes of bleeding controlled by prompt, effective intervention.

3. There are no long-term disabilities.

4. Child is able to manage own care independently, with minimum supervision.

Pulmonary Disorders

I. Cystic fibrosis

A. *Introduction:* Cystic fibrosis is a generalized dysfunction of the exocrine glands that produces multisystem involvement. The disorder is inherited as an autosomal recessive defect. The mutated gene responsible for CF is located on the long arm of chromosome 7 (CFTR). The basic problem is one of *thick, sticky, tenacious mucous secretions that obstruct* the ducts of the exocrine glands, thus affecting their ability to function. Cystic fibrosis is found in all races and socioeconomic groups, although there is a significantly lower incidence in Asians and African Americans. It is a chronic disease with no known cure and guarded prognosis; median age at death in the United States is 31 years. Those born in the late 1990s can be expected to survive into their forties with new therapies.

◆ **B. Assessment:**

1. Newborn: *meconium ileus.*

2. Frequent, recurrent *pulmonary infections:* bronchitis, bronchopneumonia, pneumonia, and ultimately chronic obstructive pulmonary disease (COPD) due to mechanical obstruction of respiratory tract caused by thick, tenacious mucous gland secretions.

3. *Malabsorption syndrome:* failure to gain weight, distended abdomen, thin arms and legs, lack of subcutaneous fat due to disturbed absorption of nutrients that results from the inability of pancreatic enzymes to reach intestinal tract.

4. *Steatorrhea:* bulky, foul-smelling, frothy, fatty stools in increased amounts and frequency (predisposed to rectal prolapse).

5. Parents may note that child *"tastes salty"* when kissed, due to excessive loss of sodium and chloride in sweat.

6. *Sweat test* reveals high sodium and chloride levels in child's sweat, unique to children with cystic fibrosis.

7. Sexual development:

a. *Boys/Men:* sterile (due to aspermia).

b. *Girls/Women:* difficulty conceiving and bearing children (due to increased viscosity of cervical mucus, which acts as a plug in the cervical os and mechanically blocks the entry of sperm).

◆ **C. Analysis/nursing diagnosis:**

1. *Ineffective breathing patterns* related to thick, viscid secretions.

2. *Altered nutrition, less than body requirements,* related to diarrhea and poor intestinal absorption of nutrients.

3. *Decreased cardiac output* related to COPD and decreased compliance of lungs.

4. *Activity intolerance* related to respiratory compromise.

5. *Self-esteem disturbance* related to body image changes.

6. *Knowledge deficit* related to disease process, treatments, medications, genetics.

7. *Risk for noncompliance* related to complicated and prolonged treatment regimen.

◆ **D. Nursing care plan/implementation:**

1. Goal: *assist child to expectorate sputum.*

   ▶ a. Perform postural drainage and percussion as prescribed: first thing in morning, between meals, before bedtime, *not* after meals to prevent aspiration.

   b. Administer nebulizer treatments, expectorants, mucolytics, bronchodilators. *Avoid* or limit use of medications that suppress cough mechanism.

   c. Provide for exercises that promote position changes and keep sputum moving up and out.

   d. Encourage *high fluid intake* to keep secretions liquefied.

   ▶ e. Suction, administer oxygen prn.

2. Goal: *prevent infection.*

   a. Standard precautions to prevent infection.

   b. Evaluate carefully, check continually for potential infection (especially respiratory); report to physician promptly.

   c. Limit contact with staff or visitors (especially children) with infection.

   d. Administer antibiotics as ordered, to *treat* respiratory infections and *prevent* overwhelming sepsis.

   e. May be placed on *prophylactic* antibiotic therapy *between* episodes of infection.

   f. Teach importance of prevention of infection at home: adequate nutrition, frequent medical checkups, stay away from known sources of infection.

3. Goal: *maintain adequate nutrition.*

   a. *Diet:* well balanced, *high calorie* and *protein* to prevent malnutrition. Fat content in diet is controversial and must be individualized.

   b. Administer *pancreatic enzyme* (Viokase, Pancreatin) immediately before *every* meal and *every* snack to enhance the absorption of vital nutrients, especially fats.

   c. If child is unable to swallow capsules, take capsule apart and sprinkle on food at beginning of meal or mix with chilled applesauce.

   d. Administer water-miscible preparations of *fat-soluble vitamins* (A, D, E, K), multivitamins, and iron.

   e. Encourage *extra salt* intake to compensate for excessive sodium losses in sweat (unless CHF is present); especially important in hot weather, after physical exertion, febrile periods.

   f. Encourage *extra fluid* intake (e.g., *Gatorade*) to *prevent* dehydration/electrolyte imbalance, ↑ thickening of mucous secretions.

   g. Daily I&O and weights to monitor nutritional and hydration status.

   h. Encourage child to assume gradually increasing responsibility for choosing own foods within dietary restrictions.

4. Goal: *teach child and family about cystic fibrosis.*

   a. Discuss diagnostic procedures: sweat test, stool specimens.

   b. Review multiple medications: use, effects, side/toxic effects.

   c. Stress need to care for pulmonary system (major cause of mortality/morbidity).

   ▶ d. Teach various treatments: postural drainage, nebulizers, oxygen therapy, breathing exercise.

   e. Encourage child to assume as much responsibility for own care as possible: medications, treatments, diet.

   f. Promote development of healthy attitude toward disease/prognosis (no known cure). Heart/lung transplant may be considered as an option.

   g. Refer to appropriate community agencies for assistance with home care.

   h. Assist with genetic counseling.

   i. Discuss sexual concerns with adolescent.

5. Goal: *promote compliance with treatment regimen.*

   a. Encourage child to verbalize anger or frustration at being "different"/body image alterations.

   b. Suggest alternatives to chest physical therapy (CPT), e.g., yoga/standing on head.

   c. Offer "rewards" for compliance: going swimming with friends or other types of peer activities.

◆ **E. Evaluation/outcome criteria:**

1. Child can clear own airway, expectorate sputum.

2. Child is maintained in infection-free state.

3. Adequate nutrition is maintained.

4. Child and family verbalize understanding of the disease.

5. Child complies with rigors of treatment.

II. Pediatric respiratory infections

◆ **A. Assessment:** general assessment of infant/child with respiratory distress. *Note:* Additional information about specific respiratory infections may be found in **Table 5.14.**

TABLE 5.14	Pediatric Respiratory Infections

Name	Definition	Age Group	Etiology	◆ Assessment: Definitive Clinical Signs and Symptoms	◆ Plan: Specifics Treatment	Prognosis
Bronchiolitis/ respiratory syncytial virus (RSV)	Acute viral infection of lower respiratory tract (small, low bronchioles), with resultant trapping of air	Infants 2–12 mo (peak at 2–5 mo)	Respiratory syncytial virus 80% of cases	Hyperinflation of alveoli Scattered areas of atelectasis Acute, severe respiratory distress for first 48–72 hr, followed by rapid recovery	Supportive care during acute phase: ■ Hospitalization ■ High humidity ■ Clear liquids ■ Ribavirin, RespiGam if causative agent is RSV	Excellent (less than 1% mortality rate)
Croup (acute spasmodic laryngitis)	Paroxysmal attacks (spasms of larynx)	3 mo–3 yr	Viral (possible allergy or psychogenic)	Most common onset at night Inspiratory stridor "Croupy" barking cough Dyspnea Anxiety	Teach parents— turn on hot water in bathroom and close door (steam); warm temperature will not relieve the congestion Common to treat at home	Excellent (but likely to recur)
Laryngo-tracheo-bronchitis (LTB)	Acute infection of lower respiratory tract: larynx, trachea, and bronchi	3 mo–8 yr	Viral (possible secondary bacterial infection)	Inspiratory stridor High fever Signs and symptoms of severe respiratory distress Hoarseness, progressing to aphonia and respiratory arrest without treatment	Hospitalization: ■ Tracheostomy set at bedside ■ Racemic epinephrine/steroids ■ Antibiotics if cultures are positive	Good
Epiglottitis	Extremely acute, severe, and rapid, progressive swelling (due to infection) of epiglottis and surrounding tissue	1–8 yr	Bacterial (*H. influenzae* type b)	Abrupt onset— rapid progression; **medical emergency** Dyspnea, Dysphagia Sit up/chin thrust/mouth open Thick muffled voice Cherry red, swollen epiglottis	Do *not* visualize epiglottis unless airway support is immediately available Will need endotracheal tube or tracheostomy for 24–48 hr to maintain patent airway IV ampicillin for 10–14 days to treat bacterial infection IV corticosteroids (e.g., Solu-Cortef) to reduce inflammation	Very good if detected and treated early Prevent via Hib immunization

1. Restlessness—*earliest* sign of hypoxia.
2. Difficulty sucking/eating—parents may state the infant or child has "poor appetite."
3. Expiratory grunt, flaring of nasal alae, retractions.
4. Changes in vital signs: fever, tachycardia, tachypnea.
5. Cough: productive/nonproductive.
6. Wheeze; expiratory/inspiratory.
7. Hoarseness or aphonic crying.
8. Dyspnea or prostration.
9. Dehydration—related to increase in sensible fluid loss and poor PO intake.
10. Color change (pallor, cyanosis)—*later* sign of respiratory distress.

◆ **B. Analysis/nursing diagnosis:**
1. *Ineffective airway clearance* related to infection or obstruction.
2. *Fluid volume deficit* related to excessive losses through normal routes, discomfort and inability to swallow.
3. *Anxiety* related to hypoxia.
4. *Risk for injury* related to spread of infection.
5. *Knowledge deficit* related to disease process, infection control, home care, and follow-up.

◆ **C. Nursing care plan/implementation:**
1. Goal: *relieve respiratory distress by reducing swelling and edema and liquefying secretions.*
   ▶ a. Environment: age- and disease-appropriate oxygen delivery system (see **Table 5.15**).
   b. Administer oxygen as ordered.

   c. Position: semi-Fowler's or in infant seat to promote maximum expansion of the lungs; small blanket or diaper roll under neck to keep airway patent; change position at least q2h to prevent pooling of secretions.
   ▶ d. Suction/postural drainage and percussion prn.
   e. Tape diapers loosely and use only loose-fitting clothing to *avoid* pressure on abdominal organs, which could impinge on diaphragm and impede respirations.
   f. Administer medications: antibiotics, bronchodilators, steroids.
   ▶ g. Monitor temperature q4h/prn; reduce fever with acetaminophen, cool sponges, hypothermia blanket.
2. Goal: *observe for potential respiratory failure related to exhaustion or complete airway obstruction.*
   a. Place in room near nurses' station for maximum observation.
   b. Monitor vital signs: q1h during acute phase, then q4h.
   ▶ c. Place emergency equipment near bedside prn: endotracheal tube, tracheostomy set.
   d. Monitor closely for signs of impending respiratory failure: increased rapid, shallow respirations, progressive hoarseness/aphonia, deepening cyanosis.
   e. Report adverse changes in condition STAT to physician.

TABLE 5.15	Comparison of Common Oxygen Delivery Systems

System	Advantages	Disadvantages
Cannula	▪ Provides low-moderate oxygen concentration (22%–40%) ▪ Child can talk/eat without altering FIO_2 ▪ Possibility of more complete observation of child because nose/mouth remain unobstructed ▪ Relatively comfortable and inexpensive	▪ Difficulty in controlling O_2 concentrations if child breathes through mouth ▪ Must have patent nasal passages ▪ Possibility of causing abdominal distention/discomfort/vomiting ▪ Can cause drying/bleeding of nasal mucosa
Hood	▪ Achievement of high O_2 concentrations; FIO_2 up to 1.00 ▪ Quick recovery time of FIO_2 ▪ Free access to infant's chest for assessment	▪ Moist environment may lead to skin irritation and prevent quick assessment of color or respiratory effort ▪ Need to remove infant for feeding and weighing
Mask	▪ Various sizes available ▪ Delivers higher, more precise FIO_2 concentrations than cannula ▪ Comfortable for older children who are quiet and do not struggle	▪ Accumulation of moisture on face leading to skin irritation ▪ Possibility of aspiration of vomitus ▪ Eating disrupts O_2 delivery ▪ Not well tolerated by most children due to fear of suffocation
Tent	▪ Achievement of lower O_2 concentrations (FIO_2 of 0.3–0.5) ▪ Child receives increased inspired O_2 concentrations even while eating ▪ Child can move around in bed and play while receiving O_2 and humidity	▪ Necessity for tight fit around bed to prevent leakage of O_2 and maintain specific O_2 concentrations ▪ Child is difficult to see/assess ▪ Cool/wet tent environment will decrease body temperature, increasing O_2 requirements ▪ Inspired O_2 levels will fall whenever tent is entered for caregiving purposes

Pediatrics

3. Goal: *maintain normal fluid balance.*
   a. May be NPO initially to prevent aspiration.
   b. IVs until severe distress subsides and child is able to suck and swallow.
   c. Monitor hydration status: I&O, urine specific gravity, weight.
   d. When resuming PO fluids—start with sips of clear liquids, advance slowly as tolerated: Pedialyte, clear broth, gelatin, popsicles, fruit juices, ginger ale.
   e. **Avoid** milk/milk products, which may cause increased mucous production.
4. Goal: *provide calm, secure environment.*
   a. During acute distress: remain with child/family (do **not** leave unattended).
   b. Keep crying to a minimum to prevent severe hypoxia and to reduce the body's demand for oxygen.
   c. *Avoid* painful/intrusive procedures if possible.
   d. Organize nursing care to provide planned periods of uninterrupted rest.
   e. Allow parents to room-in, and encourage their participation in care of their child to keep the child relatively calm and reduce anxiety.
   f. Allow child to keep favorite toy or security object.
5. Goal: *provide parents with teaching, as necessary.*
   a. *Short term:* discuss equipment, treatments, procedures; offer frequent progress reports, answer parents' questions.
   b. *Long term:* how to handle recurrences, how to check temperature at home, medications for fever, when to call physician about respiratory problem.

◆ D. **Evaluation/outcome criteria:**
1. No further evidence of respiratory distress.
2. Resumption of normal respiratory pattern.
3. Normal fluid balance maintained/restored.
4. Parents verbalize their concerns and express confidence in their ability to care for their child after discharge.

III. Apnea-related disorders
A. **Apnea of infancy**
1. *Introduction:* Apnea of infancy is the unexplained cessation of breathing for 20 sec or longer in an apparently healthy, full-term infant who is more than 37 weeks of gestation. It is usually diagnosed by the second month of life and is generally thought to resolve during the first 12–15 mo of life. The exact cause is unknown. The association between apnea of infancy and sudden infant death syndrome (SIDS) is still controversial. However, infants experiencing significant apnea without a known cause are thought to be at increased risk for SIDS and must be treated accordingly. The diagnosis of apnea of infancy (AOI) is made when no identifiable cause for

the apparent life-threatening event (ALTE) is found.

◆ 2. **Assessment:**
   a. Unexplained cessation of breathing (apnea) for 20 sec or longer.
   b. Bradycardia.
   c. Color change: cyanosis or pallor.
   d. Limp, hypotonic.
   e. Diagnostic tests including cardiopneumogram, pneumocardiogram, and polysomnography.

◆ 3. **Analysis/nursing diagnosis:**
   a. *Ineffective breathing patterns* related to apnea.
   b. *Anxiety, fear* related to apnea and threat of infant's death.
   c. *Knowledge deficit* regarding home care of infant on an apnea monitor and infant cardiopulmonary resuscitation (CPR).

◆ 4. **Nursing care plan/intervention:**
   a. Goal: *maintain effective breathing pattern.*
   ▶ (1) Apnea monitor on infant at all times, including at home.
   (2) Place in room near nurses' station for maximum observation with a nurse or parent present at all times.
   (3) Suction, oxygen, and resuscitation equipment readily available if needed.
   (4) Observe for apnea or bradycardia; note duration and associated symptoms—color change, change in muscle tone.
   ▶ (5) If apnea occurs, use gentle stimulation to start infant breathing again. If ineffective, begin CPR (**Figures 5.8** through **5.11**).
   ▶ (6) If suctioning is needed, do it gently for the shortest time and least number of times possible to maintain patent airway. *Note:* Repeated, vigorous suctioning is associated with prolonged periods of apnea.
   (7) Medications: respiratory stimulant drugs (such as theophylline or caffeine) may be given until 2–3 months have passed without an episode of apnea.
   (8) *Positions:* side-lying or supine; *never* prone, to prevent SIDS.
   (9) Feedings: smaller and more frequent; *avoid* overfeeding, which can lead to reflux and apnea.
   b. Goal: *teach parents how to care for their infant at home* (**Table 5.16**).
   (1) Thoroughly explain discharge plans to parents; encourage questions and discussion.
   (2) Begin teaching use of apnea monitor and infant CPR techniques several days before discharge; allow parents to handle the monitor and become thoroughly familiar with its use.

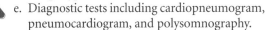

	Objectives	ACTIONS		
		Adult (over 8 yr)	**Child (1 to 8 yr)**	**Infant (under 1 yr)**
A. AIRWAY	1. Assessment: Determine unresponsiveness.	Tap or gently shake shoulder.		
		Say, "Are you okay?"		Speak loudly.
	2. Get help.	Activate EMS.	Shout for help. If second rescuer available, have person activate EMS.	
	3. Position the victim.	Turn on back as a unit, supporting head and neck if necessary (4-10 sec).		
	4. Open the airway.	Head tilt/chin lift.		
B. BREATHING	5. Assessment: Determine breathlessness.	Maintain open airway. Place ear over mouth, observing chest. Look, listen, feel for normal breathing (no more than 10 sec).*		
	6. Give 2 rescue breaths.	Maintain open airway.		
		Pinch nose, seal mouth to mouth.		Mouth to nose and mouth.
		Give 2 slow effective breaths. Observe chest rise. Allow lung deflation between breaths.		
		2 sec each	1 to $1\frac{1}{2}$ sec each	
	7. Option for obstructed airway.	a. Reposition victim's head. Try again to give rescue breaths.		
			b. Activate EMS.	
		c. Give 5 subdiaphragmatic abdominal thrusts (the Heimlich maneuver).		c. Give 5 back blows.
				c. Give 5 chest thrusts.
		d. Tongue-jaw lift and finger sweep.	d. Tongue-jaw lift, but finger sweep only if you see a foreign object.	
		If unsuccessful, repeat a, c, and d until successful.		
C. CIRCULATION	8. Assessment: Determine pulselessness.	Feel for carotid pulse with one hand; maintain head-tilt with other hand (no more than 10 sec).		Feel for brachial pulse: keep head tilt.
CPR	Pulse absent: Begin chest compressions: 9. Landmark check.	Use 2–3 fingers to locate lower margin of rib cage. Follow rib margin to base of sternum (xiphoid process).		Imagine a line drawn between the nipples.
	10. Hand position.	Place one hand above fingers of first hand on lower half of sternum.		Place 2 fingers on sternum 1 finger's width below line. Depress $\frac{1}{2}$ - 1 in.†
		Place other hand on top of hand on sternum. Depress $1\frac{1}{2}$-2 in.	Use heel of one hand. Depress 1-$1\frac{1}{2}$ in.	
	11. Compression rate.	80–100 per min	100 per min	At least 100 per min
	12. Compressions to breaths.	2 breaths to every 15 compressions	1 breath to every 5 compressions	
	13. Number of cycles.	4	20 (approximately 1 min)	
	14. Reassessment.	Feel for carotid pulse.		Feel for brachial pulse.
		If no pulse, resume CPR, starting with compressions.	If alone, activate EMS. If no pulse, resume CPR, starting with compressions.	
	Pulse present: not breathing: Begin rescue breathing.	1 breath every 5 sec (12 per min)	1 breath every 3 sec (20 per min)	

FIGURE 5.8   One-rescuer CPR. *If victim is breathing or resumes effective breathing, place in recovery position: (1) move head, shoulders, and torso simultaneously; (2) turn onto side; (3) leg not in contact with ground may be bent and knee moved forward to stabilize victim; (4) victim should not be moved in any way if trauma is suspected and should not be placed in recovery position if rescue breathing or CPR is required. †Use the 2 thumb–encircling hands technique if two rescuers are available for infant CPR. (Modified from Stapleton, ER, and others: Textbook of Basic Life Support for Healthcare Providers, American Heart Association, Dallas, 2001. Published in Wong, D: Whaley and Wong's Nursing Care of Infants and Children, ed 7. Mosby, St Louis, 2003.)

Step	Objective	Actions
1. AIRWAY	**One rescuer (ventilation):** Assessment: Determine unresponsiveness.	Tap or gently shake shoulder.
		Shout, "Are you okay?"
	Call for help.	Activate EMS.
	Position the victim.	Turn on back if necessary (4–10 sec).
	Open the airway.	Use a proper technique to open airway.
2. BREATHING	Assessment: Determine breathlessness.	Look, listen, and feel (3–5 sec).
	Ventilate twice (2 slow breaths).	Observe chest rise: 2 sec/inspiration.
3. CIRCULATION	Assessment: Determine pulselessness.	Feel for carotid pulse (5–10 sec).
	State assessment results.	Say "No pulse."
	Other rescuer (compressor): Get into position for compressions.	Hand, shoulders in correct position.
	Locate position on sternum.	Check hand position.
4. COMPRESSION/ VENTILATION CYCLES	**Compressor:** Begin chest compressions.	Correct ratio compressions/ventilations: 15:2
		Compression rate: 100/min (2 compressions per sec).
		Say any helpful mnemonic (such as "1 and 2 and 3").
		Stop compressing for each ventilation.
	Ventilator: Ventilate twice after 15 compressions and check compression effectiveness. (Minimum of 10 cycles.)	Ventilate 1 time (2 sec/inspiration).
		Check pulse occasionally to assess compressions.
5. CALL FOR SWITCH	**Compressor:** Call for switch when fatigued.	Give clear signal to change.
		Compressor completes 15th compression.
		Ventilator completes ventilation after 15th compression.
6. SWITCH	Simultaneously switch:	
	Ventilator: Move to chest.	Become compressor.
		Get into position for compressions.
		Locate position on sternum and hand position.
	Compressor: Move to head.	Become ventilator.
		Check carotid pulse (5 sec).
		Say "No pulse."
		Ventilate once (2 sec/inspiration).
7. CONTINUE CPR	Resume compression/ventilation cycles.	Resume Step 4.

FIGURE 5.9   Two-rescuer CPR. NOTE: Two-rescuer CPR for children ages 1 to 8 yr can be performed similarly to that for adults with appropriate changes in chest compressions and ventilations. (Modified from Stapleton, ER, and others: *Textbook of Basic Life Support for Healthcare Providers*, American Heart Association, Dallas, 2001. Published in Wong, D: *Whaley and Wong's Nursing Care of Infants and Children*, ed 7. Mosby, St Louis, 2003.)

Pediatrics

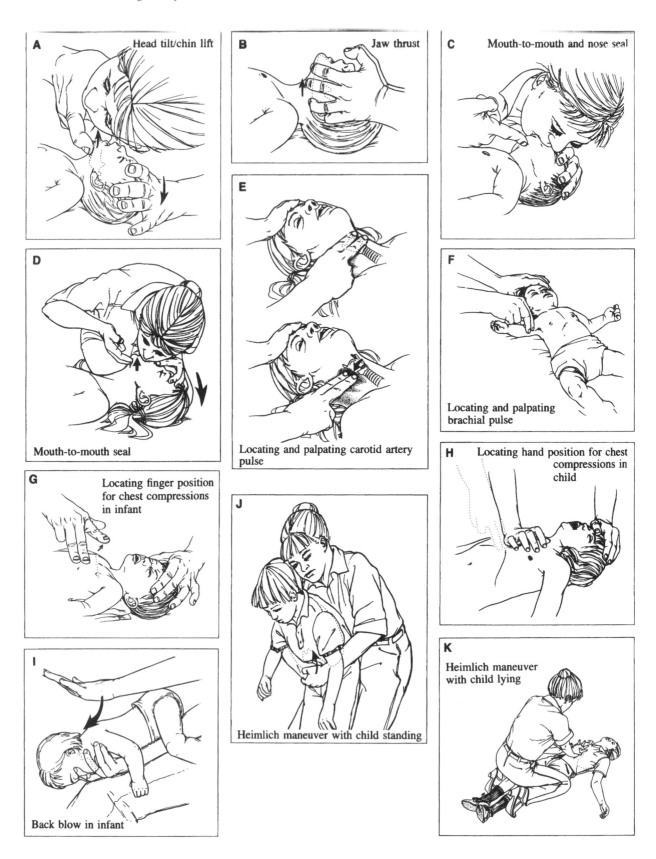

FIGURE 5.10 **CPR and airway. Procedures for cardiopulmonary resuscitation (*A* through *H*) and clearing airway obstruction (*I* through *K*).** (Modified from Chandra, NC, and Hazinski, MF [eds]: Textbook of Basic Life Support for Healthcare Providers, American Heart Association, Dallas, 1997. Published in Wong, D: Whaley and Wong's Nursing Care of Infants and Children, ed. 7. Mosby, St. Louis, 2003.)

Signs of life-threatening obstruction: truly choking child *cannot speak*, *becomes cyanotic*, and *collapses*.

	Objectives	Actions		
		Adult (over 8 yr)	**Child (1 to 8 yr)**	**Infant (under 1 yr)**
CONSCIOUS VICTIM	1. Assessment: Determine airway obstruction.	Ask, "Are you choking?" Determine if victim can cough or speak.		Observe breathing difficulty, ineffective cough, no strong cry.
	2. Act to relieve obstruction.	Perform up to 5 subdiaphragmatic abdominal thrusts (Heimlich maneuver).		Give 5 back blows.
				Give 5 chest thrusts.
	Be persistent.	Repeat Step 2 until obstruction is relieved or victim becomes unconscious.		
VICTIM WHO BECOMES UNCONSCIOUS	3. Position the victim: call for help.	Turn on back as a unit, supporting head and neck, face up, arms by sides. Call out, "Help!" Activate EMS. If second rescuer available, have person activate EMS.		
	4. Check for foreign body.	Perform tongue-jaw lift and finger sweep.	Perform tongue-jaw lift. Remove foreign object only if you actually see it.	
	5. Give rescue breaths.	Open the airway with head-tilt/chin-lift. Try to give rescue breaths. If airway is obstructed, reposition head and try to ventilate again.		
	6. Act to relieve obstruction.	Perform up to 5 subdiaphragmatic abdominal thrusts (Heimlich maneuver).		Give 5 back blows.
				Give 5 chest thrusts.
	Be persistent.	Repeat steps 4-6 until obstruction is relieved.		
UNCONSCIOUS VICTIM	1. Assessment: Determine unresponsiveness.	Tap or gently shake shoulder. Shout, "Are you okay?"	Tap or gently shake shoulder.	
		If unresponsive, activate EMS.		
	2. Call for help: position the victim.	Turn on back as a unit, supporting head and neck, face up, arms by sides.		
			Call out for help.	
	3. Open the airway.	Head-tilt/chin-lift.		Head-tilt/chin-lift, but do not tilt too far.
	4. Assessment: Determine breathlessness.	Maintain an open airway. Ear over mouth; observe chest. Look, listen, feel for breathing (no more than 10 sec).		
	5. Give rescue breaths.	Make mouth-to-mouth seal.		Make mouth-to-mouth-and-nose seal.
		Try to give rescue breaths.		
	6. If chest not rising, try again to give rescue breaths.	Reposition head. Try rescue breaths again.		
	7. Activate the EMS system.		If airway obstruction not relieved after about 1 min, activate EMS as rapidly as possible.	
	8. Act to relieve obstruction.	Perform up to 5 subdiaphragmatic abdominal thrusts (Heimlich maneuver).		Give 5 back blows.
				Give 5 chest thrusts.
	9. Check for foreign body.	Perform tongue-jaw lift and finger sweep.	Perform tongue-jaw lift. Remove foreign object only if you actually see it.	
	10. Rescue breaths.	Open the airway with head-tilt/chin-lift. Try again to give rescue breaths. If airway is obstructed, reposition head and try to ventilate again.		
	Be persistent.	Repeat steps 8-10 until obstruction is relieved.		

Pediatrics

FIGURE 5.11   Foreign body airway obstruction management. (Modified from Stapleton, ER, and others: Textbook of Basic Life Support for Healthcare Providers, American Heart Association, Dallas, 2001. Published in Wong, D: Whaley and Wong's Nursing Care of Infants and Children, ed. 7. Mosby, St. Louis, 2003.)

TABLE 5.16	Guidelines for Home Care of Infant on Apnea Monitor

1. Show the parents how to connect the monitor leads.

2. Remind parents to remove the leads unless they are connected to the infant.

3. Stress that the infant must be on the monitor whenever respirations are not being directly observed and that a trained person must be present in the home at all times in case the alarm sounds.

4. Teach parents **not** to adjust the monitor to eliminate false alarms.

5. Explain that the infant will need direct observation whenever loud noises could obscure the monitor alarm, e.g., dishwasher, vacuum.

6. Teach parents what to look for when alarm sounds, i.e., loose monitor leads vs. apnea.

7. Teach parents how to assess the infant for an episode of apnea, i.e., lack of respirations, duration, color, muscle tone.

8. Teach the parents to first use gentle physical stimulation if the infant experiences an apnea spell, e.g., touching the face or stroking the soles of the feet.

9. Demonstrate infant CPR to be used if tactile stimulation is not effective in reestablishing respirations.

10. Encourage parents to keep emergency numbers posted near the telephone.

11. Explain that monitor will not interfere with normal growth and development. Encourage the parents to promote normal growth and development as much as possible.

Also refer to **Table 5–8**: Safety Considerations, p. 272.

(3) Provide parents with emergency response numbers and community health nurse referral.

(4) Stress need for at least *1 year of ongoing care* with constant use of monitor, or 2–3 months without an episode requiring intervention.

(5) Discuss need for support and refer to local self-help/support group.

(6) Encourage parents to take time for themselves if a reliable caregiver is available who is trained in use of monitor and infant CPR.

◆ 5. **Evaluation/outcome criteria:**
   a. Effective breathing pattern is established.
   b. Parents verbalize their concerns and express confidence in their ability to care for their infant at home.

B. **Sudden infant death syndrome**
   1. *Introduction:* SIDS is the *sudden, unexpected* death of an apparently healthy infant under 1 year of age, which remains *unexplained* after a complete postmortem examination. Various theories have been suggested, none proved; research is ongoing. It is the third leading cause of death between 1 mo and 1 yr, affecting almost 2500 infants annually.

◆ 2. **Assessment:**
   a. Sudden, unexplained death in otherwise "normal" infant; occurs exclusively during sleep.

   b. Note overall appearance of infant (differentiate from child abuse).
   c. Obtain history from parents—note affect or how parents are dealing with grief.

◆ 3. **Analysis/nursing diagnosis:**
   a. *Dysfunctional grieving* related to loss of infant.
   b. *Knowledge deficit* related to SIDS.

◆ 4. **Nursing care plan/implementation:**
   a. *Immediate goal:* support parents who are grieving.
     (1) Stress that nothing could have been done to prevent the death.
     (2) Allow parents to express grief emotions; provide privacy.
     (3) Offer parents opportunity to see, hold infant.
     (4) Explain purpose of autopsy (physician to obtain consent).
     (5) Contact spiritual advisor: priest, rabbi, minister.
     (6) Assist parents to plan what to tell siblings.
   b. *Ongoing goal:* provide factual information regarding SIDS.
     (1) Offer information that is known about SIDS in simple, direct terms (**Table 5.17**).
     (2) Answer questions honestly.
     (3) Give parents printed literature on SIDS.
     (4) Refer to local/national SIDS foundation group.
   c. *Long-term goal:* assist family to resolve grief.

TABLE 5.17	SIDS: What to Tell Families

Concern	Facts
Cause	Unknown (possibly related to delayed maturation of cardiorespiratory system)
Incidence	Almost 2500 cases annually; leading cause of death between ages 1 mo and 1 yr
When	Occurs during *sleep* (nap, night)
Age	Peak at 2–4 mo; 95% of cases occur by age *6 mo*
Sex	More common in boys
Race	More common in African Americans, Native Americans and Hispanics
Season	More common in *winter*, peaks in January
Siblings	May have greater incidence
Perinatal	More common in preterm infants, in *multiple* births, in infants with *low Apgar scores*, and with maternal smoking
Socioeconomic	More common in lower socioeconomic classes
Feeding habits	More common in infants who are bottle-fed, less common in infants who are breastfed.
Means of Prevention	*Supine* (on back) sleeping position (mnemonic: "back to sleep"); *avoid* soft bedding and overheating during sleep

(1) Track progress of other siblings.
(2) Refer to local perinatal bereavement group.
(3) Consider subsequent pregnancy to be at risk for:
   (a) Attachment/bonding.
   (b) SIDS recurrence.

5. **Evaluation/outcome criteria:**
   a. Parents are able to express their grief and receive adequate support.
   b. Parents raise questions about SIDS and can understand answers.
   c. Family's grief is resolved; in time, normal family dynamics resume.

DISORDERS AFFECTING PROTECTIVE FUNCTIONS

Immunity and Communicable Diseases

I. **Recommended schedule for active immunization of healthy infants and children (Table 5.18).**

II. **Assessment:** common side effects of immunizations (occur 24–48 hr after immunization except as noted):
   A. Soreness, redness, tenderness, or lump at injection site.
   B. Fever: brief, mild to moderate.
   C. Crankiness and fussiness; anorexia; drowsiness.
   D. Measles—coryza and rash 7–10 days after immunization.
   E. Rubella—arthralgia and arthritis-like symptoms 2 wk after immunization.

III. **Nursing interventions/home care** for infant or child who has been immunized:
   A. Explain to parents the reason for each immunization and common side effects.
   B. Suggest acetaminophen for fever or discomfort.
   C. Extra affection and closeness—cuddling, soothing, rocking.
   D. Teach parents to notify MD of untoward, serious, or prolonged side effects.

IV. **Contraindications/precautions to immunizations:**
   A. Child who has a severe febrile illness (e.g., upper respiratory infection [URI], gastroenteritis, or any fever).
   B. Child with alteration in skin integrity: rash, eczema.
   C. Child with alteration in immune system; steroids; chemotherapy, radiation therapy; human immunodeficiency virus (HIV)/acquired immunodeficiency syndrome (AIDS) (no live virus vaccine).
   D. Child with a known allergic reaction to previous immunization or substance in the immunization.
   E. Recent recipient of blood/blood products.

V. **Childhood communicable diseases (Table 5.19).** Basic principles of care:
   A. Standard precautions to prevent communicability/infection.
   B. Fever control with acetaminophen.
   C. Extra fluids for hydration.
   D. General home care procedures: comfort measures/supportive care.

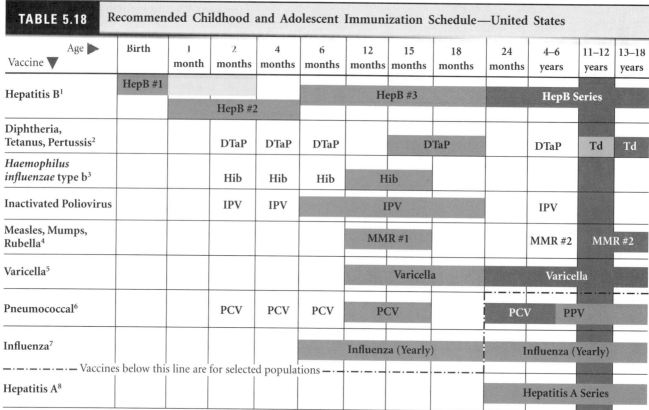

Vaccine ▼ / Age ▶	Birth	1 month	2 months	4 months	6 months	12 months	15 months	18 months	24 months	4–6 years	11–12 years	13–18 years
Hepatitis B¹	HepB #1	HepB #2			HepB #3						HepB Series	
Diphtheria, Tetanus, Pertussis²			DTaP	DTaP	DTaP		DTaP			DTaP	Td	Td
Haemophilus influenzae type b³			Hib	Hib	Hib	Hib						
Inactivated Poliovirus			IPV	IPV		IPV				IPV		
Measles, Mumps, Rubella⁴						MMR #1				MMR #2		MMR #2
Varicella⁵						Varicella					Varicella	
Pneumococcal⁶			PCV	PCV	PCV	PCV			PCV	PPV		
Influenza⁷					Influenza (Yearly)					Influenza (Yearly)		
⎯·⎯·⎯·⎯ Vaccines below this line are for selected populations ⎯·⎯·⎯·												
Hepatitis A⁸									Hepatitis A Series			

This is an example of a typical schedule that indicates the recommended ages for routine administration of currently licensed childhood vaccines for children through age 18 years. Any dose not administered at the recommended age should be administered at any subsequent visit when indicated and feasible. **Keep current on vaccine recommendations by going to websites listed** ▨ Indicates age groups that warrant special effort to administer those vaccines not previously administered. Additional vaccines may be licensed and recommended during the year. Licensed combination vaccines may be used whenever any components of the combination are indicated and other components of the vaccine are not contraindicated. Providers should consult the manufacturers' package inserts for detailed recommendations. Clinically significant adverse events that follow immunization should be reported to the Vaccine Adverse Event Reporting System (VAERS). Guidance about how to obtain and complete a VAERS form are available at www.vaers.org or by telephone, **800-822-7967.**

▨ Range of recommended ages   ▨ Only if mother HBsAg(–)

▨ Preadolescent assessment   ▨ Catch-up immunization

The Childhood and Adolescent Immunization Schedule is approved by:
Advisory Committee on Immunization Practices www.cdc.gov/nip/acip
American Academy of Pediatrics www.aap.org
American Academy of Family Physicians www.aafp.org

1. **Hepatitis B (HepB) vaccine.** All infants should receive the first dose of HepB vaccine soon after birth and before hospital discharge; the first dose may also be administered by age 2 months if the mother is hepatitis B surface antigen (HBsAg) negative. Only monovalent HepB may be used for the birth dose. Monovalent or combination vaccine containing HepB may be used to complete the series. Four doses of vaccine may be administered when a birth dose is given. The second dose should be administered at least 4 weeks after the first dose, except for combination vaccines which cannot be administered before age 6 weeks. The third dose should be given at least 16 weeks after the first dose and at least 8 weeks after the second dose. The last dose in the vaccination series (third or fourth dose) should not be administered before age 24 weeks.
    Infants born to HBsAg-positive mothers should receive HepB and 0.5 mL of hepatitis B immune globulin (HBIG) at separate sites within 12 hours of birth. The second dose is recommended at age 1–2 months. The final dose in the immunization series should not be administered before age 24 weeks. These infants should be tested for HBsAg and antibody to HBsAg (anti-HBs) at age 9–15 months.
    Infants born to mothers whose HBsAg status is unknown should receive the first dose of the HepB series within 12 hours of birth. Maternal blood should be drawn as soon as possible to determine the mother's HBsAg status; if the HBsAg test is positive, the infant should receive HBIG as soon as possible (no later than age 1 week). The second dose is recommended at age 1–2 months. The last dose in the immunization series should not be administered before age 24 weeks.
2. **Diphtheria and tetanus toxoids and acellular pertussis (DTaP) vaccine.** The fourth dose of DTaP may be administered as early as age 12 months, provided 6 months have elapsed since the third dose and the child is unlikely to return at age 15–18 months. The final dose in the series should be given at age ≥ 4 years. **Tetanus and diphtheria toxoid (Td)** is recommended at age 11–12 years if at least 5 years have elapsed since the last dose of tetanus and diphtheria toxoid-containing vaccine. Subsequent routine Td boosters are recommended every 10 years.
3. *Haemophilus influenzae* type b (Hib) conjugate vaccine. Three Hib conjugate vaccines are licensed for infant use. If PRP-OMP (PedvaxHIB® or ComVax® [Merck]) is administered at ages 2 and 4 months, a dose at age 6 months is not required. DTaP/Hib combination products should not be used for primary immunization in infants at ages 2, 4 or 6 months but can be used as boosters after any Hib vaccine. The final dose in the series should be administered at age ≥ 12 months.
4. **Measles, mumps, and rubella vaccine (MMR).** The second dose of MMR is recommended routinely at age 4–6 years but may be administered during any visit, provided at least 4 weeks have elapsed since the first dose and both doses are administered beginning at or after age 12 months. Those who have not previously received the second dose should complete the schedule by age 11–12 years.
5. **Varicella vaccine.** Varicella vaccine is recommended at any visit at or after age 12 months for susceptible children (i.e., those who lack a reliable history of chickenpox). Susceptible persons aged ≥ 13 years should receive 2 doses administered at least 4 weeks apart.
6. **Pneumococcal vaccine.** The heptavalent **pneumococcal conjugate vaccine (PCV)** is recommended for all children aged 2–23 months and for certain children aged 24–59 months. The final dose in the series should be given at age ≥ 12 months. **Pneumococcal polysaccharide vaccine (PPV)** is recommended in addition to PCV for certain high-risk groups.
7. **Influenza vaccine.** Influenza vaccine is recommended annually for children aged ≥ 6 months with certain risk factors (including, but not limited to, asthma, cardiac disease, sickle cell disease, human immunodeficiency virus [HIV], and diabetes), healthcare workers, and other persons (including household members) in close contact with persons in groups at high risk. In addition, healthy children aged 6–23 months and close contacts of healthy children aged 0–23 months are recommended to receive influenza vaccine because children in this age group are at substantially increased risk for influenza-related hospitalizations. For healthy persons aged 5–49 years, the intranasally administered, live, attenuated influenza vaccine (LAIV) is an acceptable alternative to the intramuscular trivalent inactivated influenza vaccine (TIV). Children receiving TIV should be administered a dosage appropriate for their age (0.25 mL if aged 6–35 months or 0.5 mL if aged ≥ 3 years). Children aged ≤ 8 years who are receiving influenza vaccine for the first time should receive 2 doses (separated by at least 4 weeks for TIV and at least 6 weeks for LAIV).
8. **Hepatitis A vaccine.** Hepatitis A vaccine is recommended for children and adolescents in selected states and regions and for certain high-risk groups; consult your local public health authority. Children and adolescents in these states, regions, and high-risk groups who have not been immunized against hepatitis A can begin the hepatitis A immunization series during any visit. The 2 doses in the series should be administered at least 6 months apart.

Reye Syndrome

I. *Introduction:* Reye syndrome, first described as a disease entity in the mid-1960s, is a multisystem disorder primarily affecting children between 6 and 12 years of age. Although **not** truly a "communicable disease," studies have confirmed a relationship between aspirin administration during a viral illness (e.g., chickenpox, flu) and the onset of Reye syndrome. The exact cause remains unknown. Reye syndrome is characterized by acute metabolic encephalopathy and fatty degeneration of the visceral organs, particularly the liver. Earlier diagnosis, more sophisticated monitoring equipment, and more aggressive treatment have greatly improved the survival rate of children with Reye syndrome. Recovery is generally rapid in those children who do survive, though they may suffer certain deficits.

II. **Assessment:**
   A. Onset typically follows a viral illness, just as child appears to be recovering.
   B. *Early signs and symptoms:*
      1. Rapidly progressing behavioral changes: irritability, agitation, combativeness, hostility, confusion, apathy, lethargy.
      2. Vomiting, which becomes progressively worse.
   C. Rapidly progressive neurological deterioration:
      1. Cerebral edema and increased intracranial pressure.
      2. Alteration in level of consciousness from lethargy through coma, decerebrate posturing, and respiratory arrest.
   D. Liver biopsy reveals liver dysfunction, necrosis, and failure:

      1. *Elevated* serum alanine aminotransferase (ALT), (serum glutamic-oxaloacetic transaminase [SGOT]), aspartate aminotransferase (AST), (serum glutamate pyruvate transaminase [SGPT]), lactate dehydrogenase (LDH), serum-ammonia levels.
      2. Severe hypoglycemia.
      3. *Increased* prothrombin time, coagulation defects, and bleeding.

III. **Analysis/nursing diagnosis:**
   A. *Altered cerebral tissue perfusion* related to cerebral edema and increased intracranial pressure.
   B. *Altered hepatic tissue perfusion* related to fatty degeneration of the liver.
   C. *Risk for injury* related to coagulation defects and bleeding.
   D. *Knowledge deficit* related to diagnosis, course of disease, treatment, and prognosis.

IV. **Nursing care plan/implementation:**
   A. Goal: *reduce intracranial pressure.*
      1. Child is admitted to pediatric intensive care unit (PICU) for intensive nursing care, continuous observation, and monitoring.
      2. Monitor neurological status and vital signs continuously.
      3. Assist with/prepare for numerous invasive procedures, including endotracheal (ET) tube/mechanical ventilation and intracranial pressure monitor.
      4. Monitor closely for the development of seizures; institute seizure precautions.
      5. *Position:* elevate head of bed (HOB) 30 to 45 degrees.
      6. Administer medications as ordered:
         a. Osmotic diuretics (e.g., mannitol) to decrease ICP.
         b. Diuretics (e.g., *Lasix*) to decrease cerebrospinal fluid (CSF) production.
         c. Anticonvulsants (e.g., *Dilantin,* phenobarbital).
         d. Vitamin K, fresh frozen plasma, or platelet transfusions for overt or covert bleeding.
   B. Goal: *restore and maintain fluid and electrolyte balance, including perfusion of liver.*
      1. Administer IV fluids per physician's order—usually 10% glucose (or higher).
      2. Strict I&O.
      3. Prepare for/assist with Foley catheter placement, CVP, ICP monitor, NG tube, etc.
      4. Monitor serum electrolyte lab values.
   C. Goal: *prevent injury and possible bleeding.*
      1. Observe child for petechiae, unusual bruising, oozing from body orifices or tubes, frank hemorrhage.
      2. Check all urine and stool for occult blood.
      3. Monitor lab values, including prothrombin time (PT), partial thromboplastin time (PTT), platelets.
      4. Administer blood products per physician's order.
   D. Goal: *provide parents with thorough understanding of Reye syndrome.*
      1. Primary nurse assigned to provide care and follow through with teaching.
      2. Encourage parents' presence, even in PICU—explain all equipment and procedures in simple, direct terms.
      3. Provide factual, honest, and complete information regarding disease, diagnosis, and prognosis.

V. **Evaluation/outcome criteria:**
   A. Intracranial pressure is reduced and normal neurological functioning is restored.
   B. Fluid and electrolyte balance is restored.
   C. No clinical evidence of bleeding is found.
   D. Parents express understanding of Reye syndrome.

Autoimmune Disorders

Streptococcus Infections/Sequelae

Introduction: Group A beta-hemolytic streptococcus is a common infectious organism that causes illness in children and is highly contagious. In themselves, the diseases caused by streptococcus do not seem very serious: e.g., strep throat, otitis media, impetigo, or scarlet fever. The most common treatment for strep is a full course of antibiotic therapy: 10 days of penicillin (or, if allergic, erythromycin). With adequate therapy, generally no sequelae are seen. If the strep is *not* treated, or is only partially treated, the sequelae include serious systemic diseases, with potentially long-term

(Continued on page 308)

Pediatrics

TABLE 5.19	Communicable Diseases of Childhood

Disease

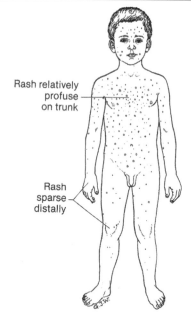

Rash relatively profuse on trunk

Rash sparse distally

Chickenpox (Varicella)
Agent: Varicella zoster virus (VZV)
Source: Primary secretions of respiratory tract of person who is infected and to a lesser degree skin lesions (scabs not infectious)
Transmission: Direct contact, droplet (airborne) spread, and contaminated objects
Incubation period: 2–3 wk, usually 13–17 days
Period of communicability: Probably 1 day before eruption of lesions (prodromal period) to 6 days after first crop of vesicles when crusts have formed

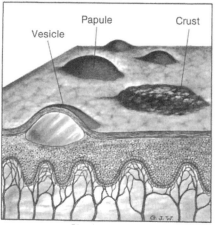

Simultaneous stages of lesions in chickenpox

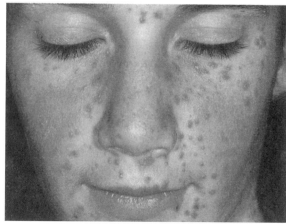

Chickenpox (varicella). (From Habif TP: Clinical dermatology: A color guide to diagnosis and therapy, ed. 3, St. Louis, Mosby.)

Pediatrics

TABLE 5.19	Communicable Diseases of Childhood *(Continued)*

Clinical Manifestations	Therapeutic Management/ Complications	◆ Nursing Considerations
Prodromal stage: Slight fever, malaise, and anorexia for first 24 hours; rash highly pruritic; begins as macule, rapidly progresses to papule and then vesicle (surrounded by erythematous base, becomes umbilicated and cloudy, breaks easily and forms crusts); all three stages (papule, vesicle, crust) present in varying degrees at one time. *Distribution:* Centripetal, spreading to face and proximal extremities but sparse on distal limbs and less on areas not exposed to heat (i.e., from clothing or sun) *Constitutional signs and symptoms:* Elevated temperature from lymphadenopathy, irritability from pruritus	*Specific:* Antiviral agent acyclovir (Zovirax), varicella-zoster immune globulin (VZIG) after exposure in children who are high-risk. *Supportive:* Diphenhydramine hydrochloride or antihistamines to relieve itching; skin care to prevent secondary bacterial infection *Complications:* Secondary bacterial infections (abscesses, cellulitis, pneumonia, sepsis) Encephalitis Varicella pneumonia Hemorrhagic varicella (tiny hemorrhages in vesicles and numerous petechiae in skin) Chronic or transient thrombocytopenia	Maintain strict isolation in hospital Isolate child in home until vesicles have dried (usually 1 wk after onset of disease), and isolate children who are high-risk from children who are infected Administer skin care: give bath and change clothes and linens daily; administer topical calamine lotion; keep child's fingernails short and clean; apply mittens if child scratches Keep child cool (may decrease number of lesions) Lessen pruritus; keep child occupied Remove loose crusts that rub and irritate skin Teach child to apply pressure to pruritic area rather than scratch it If older child, reason with child regarding danger of scar formation from scratching *Avoid* use of aspirin; use of acetaminophen controversial

(Continued on following page)

Pediatrics

TABLE 5.19	Communicable Diseases of Childhood *(Continued)*

Disease

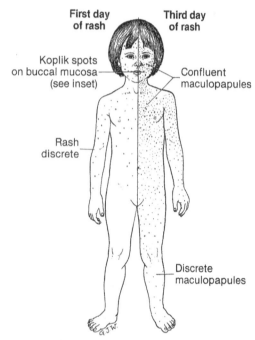

First day of rash / **Third day of rash**

Koplik spots on buccal mucosa (see inset)

Confluent maculopapules

Rash discrete

Discrete maculopapules

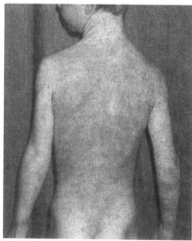

Measles (Rubeola)

Agent: Virus

Source: Respiratory tract secretions, blood, and urine of person who is infected

Transmission: Usually by direct contact with droplets of person who is infected

Incubation period: 10 to 20 days

Period of communicability: From 4 days before to 5 days after rash appears but mainly during prodromal (catarrhal) stage

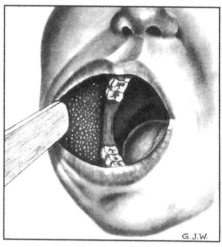

Koplik spots

Mumps

Agent: Paramyxovirus

Source: Saliva of people who are infected

Transmission: Direct contact with or droplet spread from a person who is infected

Incubation period: 14–21 days

Period of communicability: Most communicable immediately *before* and *after* swelling begins

Measles (rubeola). (From Seidel HM and others: Mosby's guide to physical examination, ed. 3, St. Louis.).

TABLE 5.19	Communicable Diseases of Childhood *(Continued)*

Clinical Manifestations	Therapeutic Management/ Complications	◆ Nursing Considerations

Prodromal (catarrhal) stage: Fever and malaise, followed in 24 hours by coryza, cough, conjunctivitis, *Koplik spots* (small, irregular red spots with a minute, bluish white center first seen on buccal mucosa opposite molars 2 days before rash); symptoms gradually increase in severity until second day after rash appears, when they begin to subside
 	
Rash: Appears 3–4 days after onset of prodromal stage; begins as erythematous maculopapular eruption on face and gradually spreads downward; more severe in earlier sites (appears confluent) and less intense in later sites (appears discrete); after 3–4 days assumes brownish appearance, and fine desquamation occurs over areas of extensive involvement
 	
Constitutional signs and symptoms: Anorexia, malaise, generalized lymphadenopathy
	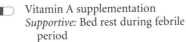 Vitamin A supplementation
	Supportive: Bed rest during febrile period
	Antipyretics
	Antibiotics to prevent secondary bacterial infection in high-risk children
	Complications:
	  Otitis media
	  Pneumonia
	  Bronchiolitis
	  Obstructive laryngitis and laryngotracheitis
	  Encephalitis
		Isolation until fifth day of rash; if hospitalized, institute respiratory precautions
		Maintain bedrest during prodromal stage; provide quiet activity
		Fever: Instruct parents to administer antipyretics; *avoid* chilling; if child is prone to seizures, institute appropriate precautions (fever spikes to 104°F [40°C] between fourth and fifth days)
		Eye care: Dim lights if photophobia present; clean eyelids with warm saline solution to remove secretions or crusts; keep child from rubbing eyes; examine cornea for signs of ulceration
		Coryza/cough: Use cool mist vaporizer; protect skin around nares with layer of petrolatum; encourage fluids and soft, bland foods
		Skin care: Keep skin clean; use tepid baths as necessary

Prodromal stage: Fever, headache, malaise, and anorexia for 24 hours, followed by "earache" that is aggravated by chewing
 	
Parotitis: By third day, parotid gland(s) (either unilateral or bilateral) enlarge(s) and reach(es) maximum size in 1–3 days; accompanied by pain and tenderness
 	
Other manifestations: Submaxillary and sublingual infection, orchitis, and meningoencephalitis
	Symptomatic and supportive:
	Analgesics for pain and antipyretics for fever
	Intravenous fluid may be necessary for child who refuses to drink or vomits because of meningoencephalitis
	Complications:
	  Sensorineural deafness
	  Postinfectious encephalitis
	  Myocarditis
	  Arthritis
	  Hepatitis
	  Epididymo-orchitis
	  Sterility (extremely rare in adult men)
		Isolation during period of communicability; institute respiratory precautions during hospitalization
		Maintain bed rest during prodromal phase until swelling subsides
		Give analgesics for pain; if child is unwilling to chew medication, use elixir form
		Encourage fluids and soft, bland foods; *avoid* foods that require chewing
		Apply hot or cold compresses to neck, whichever is more comforting
		To relieve orchitis, provide warmth and local support with tight-fitting underpants (stretch bathing suit works well)

(Continued on following page)

Pediatrics

TABLE 5.19	**Communicable Diseases of Childhood** *(Continued)*

Disease

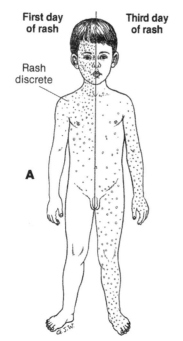

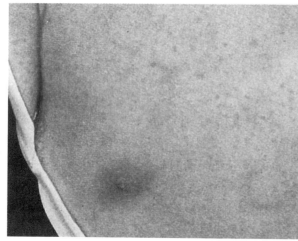

Rubella (German Measles). **A,** Progression of rash. **B,** Appearance of rash. (Source: Habif TP: *Clinical dermatology: A color guide to diagnosis and therapy,* ed. 3, St. Louis, Mosby.)

Rubella (German Measles)
Agent: Rubella virus
Source: Primarily nasopharyngeal secretions of persons with apparent or inapparent infection; virus also present in blood, stool, and urine
Transmission: Direct contact and spread via person who is infected; indirectly via articles freshly contaminated with nasopharyngeal secretions, feces, or urine
Incubation period: 14–21 days
Period of communicability: 7 days *before* to approximately 5 days *after* appearance of rash

Scarlet Fever
Agent: Group A β-hemolytic streptococci
Source: Usually from nasopharyngeal secretions of person who is infected and carriers
Transmission: Direct contact with person who is infected, or droplet spread indirectly by contact with contaminated articles, ingestion of contaminated milk or other food
Incubation period: 2–4 days, with range of 1–7 days
Period of communicability: During incubation period and clinical illness approximately 10 days; during first 2 weeks of carrier phase although may persist for months

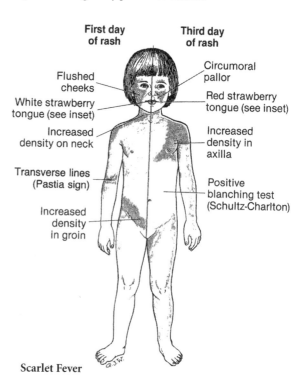

Scarlet Fever

TABLE 5.19	Communicable Diseases of Childhood *(Continued)*

Clinical Manifestations	Therapeutic Management/ Complications	◆ Nursing Considerations
Prodromal stage: Absent in children, present in adults and adolescents; consists of: low-grade fever, headache, malaise, anorexia, mild conjunctivitis, coryza, sore throat, cough, and lymphadenopathy; lasts for 1–5 days, subsides 1 day after appearance of rash *Rash:* First appears on face and rapidly spreads downward to neck, arms, trunk, and legs; by end of first day, body is covered with a discrete, pinkish red maculopapular exanthema; disappears in same order as it began and is usually gone by third day *Constitutional signs and symptoms:* Occasionally low-grade fever, headache, malaise, and lymphadenopathy	No treatment necessary other than antipyretics for low-grade fever and analgesics for discomfort *Complications:* Rare (arthritis, encephalitis, or purpura); most benign of all childhood communicable diseases; greatest danger is teratogenic effect on fetus	Reassure parents of benign nature of illness in child who is affected Use comfort measures as necessary Isolate child from women who are pregnant
Prodromal stage: Abrupt high fever, pulse increased out of proportion to fever, vomiting, headache, chills, malaise, abdominal pain *Enanthema:* Tonsils enlarged, edematous, reddened, and covered with patches of exudate; in severe cases appearance resembles membrane seen in diphtheria; pharynx is edematous and beefy red; during first 1–2 days tongue is coated and papillae become red and swollen (white strawberry tongue); by fourth or fifth day white coat sloughs off, leaving prominent papillae (red strawberry tongue); palate is covered with erythematous punctate lesions *Exanthema:* Rash appears within 12 hours after prodromal stage; red pinhead-sized punctate lesions rapidly become generalized but are absent on face, which becomes flushed with striking circumoral pallor; rash is more intense in folds of joints; by end of first week desquamation begins (fine, sandpaper-like on torso; sheetlike sloughing on palms and soles), which may be complete by 3 weeks or longer	Treatment of choice is a full course of penicillin (or erythromycin for children who are penicillin-sensitive); fever should subside 24 hr after beginning therapy Antibiotic therapy for newly diagnosed carriers (nose or throat cultures positive for streptococci) *Supportive measures:* Bedrest during febrile phase, analgesics for sore throat *Complications:* Otitis media Peritonsillar abscess Sinusitis Glomerulonephritis Carditis, polyarthritis (uncommon)	Institute respiratory precautions until 24 hr after initiation of treatment Ensure compliance with oral antibiotic therapy (intramuscular benzathine penicillin G [Bicillin] may be given if parents' reliability in giving oral drugs is questionable) Maintain bedrest during febrile phase; provide quiet activity during convalescent period Relieve discomfort of sore throat with analgesics, gargles, lozenges, antiseptic throat sprays (*Chloraseptic*), and inhalation of cool mist Encourage fluids during febrile phase; *avoid* irritating liquids (citrus juices) or rough foods; when child is able to eat, begin with soft diet Advise parents to consult practitioner if fever persists after beginning therapy Discuss procedures for preventing spread of infection

First day

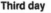

Third day

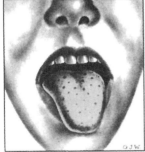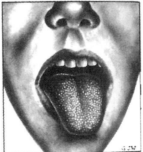

White strawberry tongue   Red strawberry tongue

Source: Wong, D: Whaley and Wong's Nursing Care of Infants and Children, ed. 7. Mosby, St. Louis.

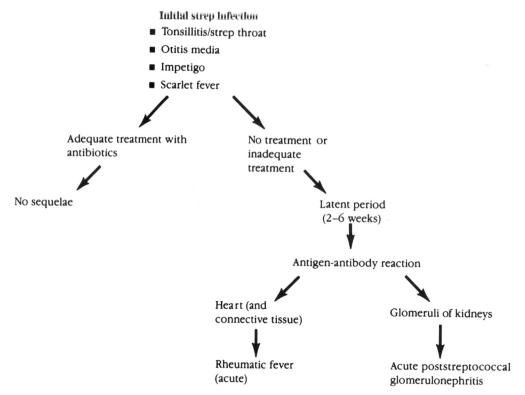

Initial strep Infection

- Tonsillitis/strep throat
- Otitis media
- Impetigo
- Scarlet fever

Adequate treatment with antibiotics

No treatment or inadequate treatment

No sequelae

Latent period (2–6 weeks)

Antigen-antibody reaction

Heart (and connective tissue)

Glomeruli of kidneys

Rheumatic fever (acute)

Acute poststreptococcal glomerulonephritis

FIGURE 5.12   Sequelae of strep infections.

effects. If the effect is manifested primarily in the *heart (carditis),* it is *acute rheumatic fever.* If the effect is manifested primarily in the *kidneys,* it is *acute glomerulonephritis* (**Figure 5.12**).

I. Rheumatic fever

  A. *Introduction:* Rheumatic fever is an acute, systemic, inflammatory disease affecting multiple organs and systems: heart, joints, CNS, collagenous tissue, etc. Thought to be autoimmune in nature, it most commonly follows a streptococcus infection (see **Figure 5.12**) and occurs primarily in school-age children. In addition, it tends to recur, and the risk of permanent heart damage increases with each subsequent attack of rheumatic fever.

  ◆ **B. Assessment:**

    1. *Major manifestations* (modified Jones criteria)

      a. *Carditis:* tachycardia, cardiomegaly, murmur, congestive heart failure (CHF).

      b. *Migratory polyarthritis:* swollen, hot, red, and excruciatingly painful large joints; migratory and reversible.

      c. *Sydenham chorea* (St. Vitus Dance): sudden, aimless, irregular movements of the extremities; involuntary facial grimaces, speech disturbances, emotional lability, muscle weakness; completely reversible.

      d. *Erythema marginatum:* reddish pink rash most commonly found on the trunk; nonpruritic, macular, clear center, wavy but clearly marked border; transient.

      e. *Subcutaneous nodules:* small, round, freely

movable, and painless swellings usually found over the extensor surfaces of the hands/feet or bony prominences; resolve without any permanent damage.

    2. *Minor manifestations*

      a. Clinical

        (1) Previous history of rheumatic fever.

        (2) Arthralgia.

        (3) Fever—normal in morning, rises in mid-afternoon, normal at night.

      b. Laboratory

        (1) *Increased* erythrocyte sedimentation rate (ESR).

        (2) *Positive* C-reactive protein.

        (3) Leukocytosis.

        (4) Anemia.

        (5) *Prolonged* P-R/Q-T intervals on ECG.

    3. Supportive evidence

      a. Recent history of streptococcus infection:

        (1) Strep throat/tonsillitis.

        (2) Otitis media.

        (3) Impetigo.

        (4) Scarlet fever.

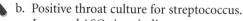   b. Positive throat culture for streptococcus.

      c. *Increased* ASO titer: indicates presence of streptococcus antibodies; begins to rise in 7 days, reaches maximum level in 4–6 wk.

  ◆ **C. Analysis/nursing diagnosis:**

    1. *Decreased cardiac output* related to carditis.

    2. *Pain* related to migratory polyarthritis.

3. *Risk for injury* related to chorea.
4. *Diversional activity deficit* related to lengthy hospitalization and recuperation.
5. *Knowledge deficit* related to preventing cardiac damage, relieving discomfort, and preventing injury.
6. *Ineffective management of therapeutic regimen* with long-term antibiotic therapy and follow-up care.

◆ **D. Nursing care plan/implementation:**
1. Goal: *prevent cardiac damage.*
   a. Hospitalization, with strict bedrest.
   b. Monitor apical pulse for changes in rate, rhythm, murmurs.
   c. Evaluate tolerance of increased activity by apical rate: if heart rate increases by more than 20 beats/min over resting rate, child should return to bed.
   d. Offer *low sodium diet* to prevent fluid retention.
   e. Administer oxygen, digoxin/*Lasix* as ordered (if CHF develops). *Note:* Refer to **Unit 7** for additional information on CHF.
2. Goal: *relieve discomfort.*
   a. Use bed cradle to keep linens from resting on painful joints.
   b. Administer aspirin as ordered to relieve pain.
   c. Move child carefully, minimally—support joints.
   d. Do *not* massage; do *not* perform ROM exercises; do *not* apply splints; do *not* apply heat/cold. All these treatments will cause increased pain and are *not needed,* because *no* permanent deformities will result from this type of arthritis.
3. Goal: *promote safety and prevent injury related to chorea.*
   a. Use side rails: elevated, padded.
   b. Restrain in bed if necessary.
   c. *No* oral temperatures—child may bite thermometer.
   d. Spoon-feed—no forks or knives, to prevent injury to oral cavity.
   e. Assist with all aspects of ADL until child can care for own needs.
4. Goal: *provide diversion as tolerated.*
   a. Encourage quiet diversional activities: hobbies, reading, puzzles.
   b. Get homework, books; provide tutor as condition permits.
   c. Encourage contact with peers: telephone calls, letters, cards.
5. Goal: *encourage child and family to comply with long-term antibiotic therapy.*
   a. Begin antibiotics immediately, to eradicate any lingering streptococcus infection.
   b. Duration of prophylaxis varies (5 yr→ lifelong) and depends on cardiac involvement.
   c. Stress need to adhere to prescribed prophylaxis schedule.
   d. Enlist child's cooperation with therapy, e.g., "hero" badge.

6. Goal: *health teaching.*
   a. To encourage compliance with prolonged bed rest—stress that ultimate prognosis depends on amount of cardiac damage.
   b. Teach necessity for long-term prophylactic therapy, e.g., during dental work, childbirth, surgery (to prevent subacute bacterial endocarditis [SBE]). Instruct adolescents to *avoid* body piercing and tattooing for same rationale.
   c. Teach rationale: permanent cardiac damage (mitral valve) is more likely to occur with subsequent attacks of rheumatic fever.

◆ **E. Evaluation/outcome criteria:**
1. No permanent cardiac damage occurs.
2. Child is free from discomfort or is able to tolerate discomfort.
3. Injuries are avoided.
4. Child's need for diversional activity is met.
5. Child/family comply with long-term antibiotic therapy/prophylactic therapy.

II. Acute poststreptococcal glomerulonephritis

A. *Introduction:* Acute poststreptococcal glomerulonephritis (APSGN) is a bilateral inflammation of the glomeruli of the kidneys and is the most common noninfectious renal disease of childhood. It occurs most frequently in early school-age children, with a peak age of onset of 6–7 yr; it is twice as common in boys as in girls. Like rheumatic fever, acute glomerulonephritis is thought to be the result of an antigen-antibody reaction to a streptococcus infection (see **Figure 5.12**); however, unlike rheumatic fever, it does *not* tend to recur, because specific immunity is conferred following the first episode of APSGN. (Further information about APSGN is found in **Table 5.20.**)

◆ **B. Assessment:**
1. Typical concerns from family about urine: change in color/appearance of urine (thick, reddish brown; decreased amounts).
2. *Acute edematous phase*—usually lasts 4–10 days.

 a. Lab examination of urine:

> (1) Severe **hematuria.**
> (2) Mild proteinuria.
> (3) *Increased* specific gravity.

   b. **Hypertension**
      (1) Headache.
      (2) Potential hypertensive encephalopathy leading to seizures, increased intracranial pressure.
   c. Mild-moderate edema: chiefly periorbital; increased weight due to fluid retention.
   d. General:
      (1) Abdominal pain.
      (2) Malaise.
      (3) Anorexia.
      (4) Vomiting.
      (5) Pallor.
      (6) Irritability.

TABLE 5.20	Comparison of Nephrosis and Acute Poststreptococcal Glomerulonephritis	

Factor	Nephrosis (Nephrotic Syndrome)	Acute Poststreptococcal Glomerulonephritis (APSGN)
Illness type	Chronic	Acute
Illness course	Characterized by periods of exacerbations and remissions during many years	Predictable, self-limiting, typically lasting 4–10 days (acute edematous phase)
Cause	Unknown	Group A β-hemolytic streptococci
Age at onset	2–4 yr	Early school-age children; peaks at 6–7 yr
Sex	More common among boys	More common among boys
Major signs and symptoms:		
General	Syndrome with variable pathology: massive proteinuria, hypoalbuminemia, severe edema, hyperlipidemia	Hematuria, hypertension
Blood pressure	Normal or decreased	Elevated
Edema	Generalized and severe	Periorbital and peripheral
Proteinuria	Massive	Moderate
Serum protein level	*Decreased (6.1–7.9 g/dL)*	Slightly decreased
Serum lipid level	*Elevated*	Normal
Potassium level	Normal (3.5–5 mEq/L)	*Increased*
Treatment	Symptomatic—no known cure; prednisone, cyclophosphamide, furosemide	Penicillin (EES), hydralazine, furosemide (sources are divided regarding use of prophylactic antimicrobials)
Diet	*Decrease* sodium, *increase* protein (unless azotemia develops)	*Decrease* sodium, *decrease* potassium, *decrease* protein (if azotemia develops)
Fluid restrictions	Seldom necessary	Necessary if output is significantly reduced
Specific nursing care	Treat at home if possible; good skin care; prevent infection	Treat in hospital during acute phase; monitor vital signs, especially blood pressure; on discharge, stress need to restrict strenuous activity until microscopic hematuria is gone
Prognosis	Fair; subject to long-term steroid treatment and social isolation related to frequent hospitalizations/confinement during relapses; 20% suffer chronic renal failure	Good; stress that recurrence is *rare* because specific immunity is conferred

(7) Lethargy.

(8) Fever.

3. *Diuresis phase:*

  a. Copious diuresis.

  b. Decreased body weight.

  c. Marked clinical improvement.

  d. Decrease in gross hematuria, but microscopic hematuria may persist for weeks/ months.

◆ C. **Analysis/nursing diagnosis:**

1. *Fluid volume excess* related to decreased urine output.

2. *Pain* related to fluid retention.

3. *Altered nutrition, less than body requirements,* related to anorexia and vomiting.

4. *Impaired skin integrity* related to immobility.

5. *Activity intolerance* related to fatigue.

6. *Knowledge deficit* related to disease process, treatment, and follow-up care.

◆ D. **Nursing care plan/implementation:**

1. Goal: *monitor fluid balance, observing carefully for complications.*

  a. Check and record blood pressure at least every 4 hr to monitor hypertension.

  b. Monitor daily weights.

  c. Urine: strict I&O; specific gravity and dipstick for blood every void.

  d. Note edema: extent, location, progression.

  e. Adhere to fluid restrictions if ordered.

  f. Monitor for possible development of hypertensive encephalopathy (seizures, increased intracranial pressure); report any changes STAT to physician.

  g. Administer medications as ordered:

    (1) *Antibiotics*—eradicate any lingering streptococcus infection; controversial.

    (2) *Antihypertensives,* e.g., Apresoline.

Pediatrics

(3) Rarely use diuretics—limited value.

(4) If CHF develops—may use digoxin.

(5) Refer to **Unit 10** for additional information on medications.

2. Goal: *provide adequate nutrition.*

  a. *Diet: low sodium, low potassium*—to prevent fluid retention and hyperkalemia; *decrease protein* (if azotemia develops). Refer to **Unit 9** for additional information on diets.

  b. Stimulate appetite: offer small portions, attractively prepared; meals with family or other children; offer preferred foods, if possible; encourage parents to bring in special foods, e.g., culturally related preferences.

3. Goal: *provide reasonable measure of comfort.*

  a. Encourage parental visiting.

  b. Provide for positional changes, give good skin care.

  c. Provide appropriate diversion, as tolerated.

4. Goal: *prevent further infection.*

  a. Use good handwashing technique.

  b. Screen staff, other clients, visitors (especially children) to limit contact with people who are infectious.

  c. Administer antibiotics if ordered (usually only for children with positive cultures).

  d. Keep warm and dry, stress good hygiene.

  e. Note possible sites of infection: increased skin breakdown secondary to edema.

5. Goal: *teach child and family about APSGN/ discharge planning.*

  a. Teach how to check urine at home: dipstick for protein and blood. (*Note:* occult hematuria may persist for months.)

  b. Teach activity restriction: **no** strenuous activity until hematuria is completely resolved.

  c. Teach family how to prepare low sodium, low potassium diet.

  d. Arrange for follow-up care: physician, home health nurse.

  e. *Stress:* subsequent recurrences are *rare* because specific immunity is conferred.

◆ **E. Evaluation/outcome criteria:**

1. No permanent renal damage occurs.

2. Normal fluid balance is maintained/restored.

3. Adequate nutrition is maintained.

4. No secondary infections occur.

5. Child/family verbalize their understanding of the disease, its treatment, and its prognosis.

Kawasaki Disease (Mucocutaneous Lymph Node Syndrome)

I. *Introduction:* Kawasaki disease (mucocutaneous lymph node syndrome) is an acute, febrile, multisystem disorder believed to be autoimmune in nature. Affecting primarily the *skin* and *mucous membranes of the respiratory tract, lymph nodes,* and *heart,* Kawasaki disease has a low fatality rate (<2%), although vasculitis and cardiac involvement (coronary artery changes) may result in major complications in as many as 20 to 25% of children with this disease. The disease is not believed to be communicable, and the exact cause remains unknown; *geographic* (living near fresh water) and *seasonal* (late winter, early spring) outbreaks do occur. Kawasaki disease occurs in *both* boys and girls between 1 and 14 years of age; 80% of cases occur in children *under age 5 years.* It may be preceded by URI or exposure to a freshly cleaned carpet. A complete and apparently *spontaneous* recovery occurs within 3 to 4 wk in the majority of cases. Treatment, which is primarily symptomatic, does not appear to either enhance recovery or prevent complications, although recent research indicates that life-threatening complications and long-term disability may be avoided or minimized with early treatment (i.e., gamma globulin) to reduce cardiovascular damage.

◆ **II. Assessment:**

A. Abrupt onset with high fever (102° to 106°F) lasting more than 5 days that does *not* remit with the administration of antibiotics and antipyretics.

B. Conjunctivitis—bilateral, nonpurulent.

C. Oropharyngeal manifestations:

1. Dry, red, cracked lips.

2. Oropharyngeal reddening and a "strawberry" tongue.

D. Peeling (desquamation) of the palms of the hands and the soles of the feet; begins at the fingertips and the tips of the toes; as peeling progresses, hands and feet become very red, sore, and swollen.

E. Cerivcal lymphadenopathy.

F. Generalized erythematous rash on trunk and extremities, without vesicles or crusts.

G. Irritability, anorexia.

H. Arthralgia and arthritis.

I. Panvasculitis of coronary arteries: formation of aneurysms and thrombi; CHF, myocarditis, pericardial effusion, arrhythmias, mitral insufficiency, myocardial infarction (MI).

J. Three phases: *acute* (onset of fever) → *subacute* (resolution of fever and all outward clinical signs) → *convalescent* (without clinical signs but laboratory values remain abnormal).

K. Laboratory tests:

1. *Elevated*: ESR.

2. *Elevated*: WBC count.

3. *Elevated*: platelet count.

◆ **III. Analysis/nursing diagnosis:**

A. *Hyperthermia* related to high, unremitting fever.

B. *Altered oral mucous membrane and impaired swallowing* related to oropharyngeal manifestations.

C. *Impaired skin integrity* related to desquamation.

D. *Fluid volume deficit* related to high fever and poor oral intake.

E. *Altered tissue perfusion* (cardiovascular, potential/ actual) related to vasculitis or thrombi.

F. *Knowledge deficit* related to disease course, treatment, prognosis.

IV. Nursing care plan/implementation:
A. Goal: *reduce fever.*
 1. Monitor temperature every 2 hr or prn.
 2. Administer **aspirin** (*not* acetaminophen [Tylenol]) per physician's order. (*Note:* aspirin is the drug of choice to reduce fever; also has anti-inflammatory effect and antiplatelet effect. Dose is 100 mg/kg/day in divided doses q6h. Monitor for signs of salicylate toxicity.)
 3. Tepid sponge baths or hypothermia blanket per physician's order.
 4. Offer frequent cool fluids.
 5. Apply cool, loose-fitting clothes; use cotton bed linens only (no heavy blankets).
 6. Seizure precautions.

B. Goal: *provide comfort measures to oral cavity to ease the discomfort of swallowing.*
 1. Good oral hygiene with soft sponge and diluted hydrogen peroxide.
 2. Apply petroleum jelly to lips.
 3. *Bland* foods in small amounts at frequent intervals.
 4. *Avoid* hot, spicy foods.
 5. Offer favorite foods from home or preferred foods from hospital selection.

C. Goal: *prevent infections and promote healing of skin.*
 1. Monitor skin for desquamation, edema, rash.
 2. Keep skin clean, dry, well lubricated.
 3. *Avoid* soap to prevent drying.
 4. Gentle handling of skin to minimize discomfort.
 5. Provide sheepskin to lie on.
 6. Prevent scratching and itching—apply cotton mittens if necessary.
 7. Bedrest; *elevate* edematous extremities.

D. Goal: *prevent dehydration and restore normal fluid balance.*
 1. Strict I&O.
 2. Monitor urine specific gravity q8h for increase (dehydration) or decrease (hydration).
 3. Monitor vital signs for fevers, tachycardia, arrhythmia.
 4. Monitor skin turgor, mucous membranes, anterior fontanel for dehydration.
 5. Force fluids.
 6. IV fluids per physician's order.

E. Goal: *prevent cardiovascular complications.*
 1. EKG monitor—report arrhythmias or tachycardia.
 2. Administer aspirin (see **Goal A**) and high-dose IV gamma globulin.
 3. Monitor for signs and symptoms of CHF: tachycardia, tachypnea, dyspnea, crackles, orthopnea, distended neck veins, dependent edema.
 4. Monitor circulatory status of extremities—check for possible development of thrombi.
 5. Stress need for long-term follow-up, including ECGs and echocardiograms, possible cardiac catheterization (if coronary artery abnormalities exist at 1 year post disease).

V. Evaluation/outcome criteria:
A. Fever returns to normal.
B. Oral cavity heals, and child is able to swallow.
C. Skin heals, and no infection occurs.
D. Normal fluid balance is restored.
E. Normal cardiovascular functioning is reestablished, and no complications occur.
F. Parents/child verbalize their understanding of Kawasaki disease.

Bacterial Infections

Introduction: Acute bacterial ear infection (*acute otitis media*) is common in young children, primarily because their eustachian tube is shorter and straighter than the adult's; this allows for ready drainage of infected mucus from URIs directly into the middle ear. In *some* cases, acute otitis media precedes the onset of *bacterial meningitis,* an extremely serious and potentially fatal disease. Bacterial meningitis is a *medical emergency,* requiring early detection and prompt, aggressive therapy to prevent permanent neurological damage or death. (Refer to section on hydrocephalus, p. 332). Serous otitis (chronic) may result in hearing impairment or loss but is not likely to result in meningitis (Refer to Myringotomy, **Table 5.21**).

I. Acute otitis media
A. Assessment:
 1. Fever.
 2. Pain in affected ear. An infant who is prelingual may not complain of pain but may tug at ear, cry, shake head, refuse to lie down.
 3. Malaise, irritability, anorexia (possibly vomiting).
 4. May have symptoms and signs of URI: rhinorrhea, coryza, cough.
 5. Diminished response to sound.

B. Analysis/nursing diagnosis:
 1. *Pain* related to pressure of pus/purulent material on eardrum.
 2. *Risk for injury/infection* related to complication of meningitis.

C. Nursing care plan/implementation:
 1. Goal: *eradicate infection and prevent further complications (meningitis).* Administer antibiotics as ordered.
 2. Goal: *relieve pain and promote comfort.*
  a. Administer decongestants as ordered.
  b. Offer analgesics/antipyretics to provide symptomatic relief and to decrease fever.
 3. Goal: *health teaching.*
  a. Teach parents that the child needs to finish all medication, even though child will seem clinically better within 24–48 hr.
  b. Review appropriate measures to control fever: antipyretics, cool sponges.

D. Evaluation/outcome criteria:
 1. Infection is eradicated, no complications.
 2. Child appears to be comfortable.

TABLE 5.21	Pediatric Surgery: Nursing Considerations

Surgical Procedure	◆ Specific Nursing Care
TONSILLECTOMY	*Preoperative:* check bleeding and clotting times *Postoperative:* ▪ *Position*—place on abdomen or semiprone with head turned to side to prevent aspiration ▪ *Observe for most frequent complication—hemorrhage* (frequent swallowing, emesis of bright red blood, shock) *Prevent bleeding:* ▪ Do *not* suction—may cause bleeding ▪ Do *not* encourage coughing, clearing throat, or blowing nose—may aggravate operative site and cause bleeding ▪ Minimize crying *Decrease pain:* ▪ Offer ice collar to decrease pain and for vasoconstriction, but do *not* force 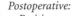 ▪ Acetaminophen for pain (*no* aspirin) *Nutrition:* ▪ NPO initially, then cool, clear fluids such as cool water, crushed ice, flavored icepops, dilute (noncitrus) fruit juice ▪ **No** red or brown fluids (punch, Jell-O, icepops, colas), citrus juices, warm fluids (tea, broth), toast, milk/ice cream/pudding, carbonated sodas; progress to soft, bland foods; milk products can increase production of mucus *Teach parents/discharge planning:* ▪ Signs and symptoms of infection; call physician promptly ▪ 5–10 days postoperatively, expect slight bleeding ▪ Continue soft, bland diet as tolerated
MYRINGOTOMY ("tubes")	*Postoperative:* ▪ *Position*—place with operated ear down, to allow for drainage. Expect moderate amount of purulent drainage initially ▪ Keep external ear canal clean and dry *Teach parents/discharge planning:* ▪ Need to keep water out of ear—use special earplugs when bathing or swimming ▪ "Tubes" will remain in place 3–7 mo and then fall out spontaneously (with healing of eardrum)
APPENDECTOMY (See **Clinical Pathway** for Appendectomy-Perforated)	(Observe same principles of preoperative and postoperative care as for adult GI surgery) NPO until bowel sounds return (24–48 hr) If appendix ruptured preoperatively or intraoperatively, *position* in semi-Fowler's and implement wound precautions; administer antibiotics as ordered Monitor for signs and symptoms of peritonitis Typical course: speedy recovery, with discharge in about 2–3 days and excellent prognosis
HERNIORRHAPHY (umbilical/inguinal)	*Umbilical:* increased incidence in infants who are of African descent. *Inguinal:* increased incidence in boys *Preoperative:* monitor for possible complications of strangulation Routine postoperative GI surgery care Prognosis—excellent, with discharge 24–48 hr postoperatively

Pediatrics

II. Bacterial meningitis

◆ **A. Assessment:**

1. Abrupt onset: initial sign may be a seizure, following an episode of URI/acute otitis media.
2. Chills and fever.
3. Vomiting; may complain of headache, neck pain (older children).
4. Photophobia.
5. Alterations in level of consciousness: delirium, stupor, increased intracranial pressure.
6. Nuchal rigidity (older children).
7. Opisthotonos position: head is drawn backward into overextension; bulging fontanel (most significant finding in infants).
8. Hyperactive reflexes related to CNS irritability.

◆ **B. Analysis/nursing diagnosis:**

1. *Risk for infection* related to communicability of meningitis.
2. *Risk for injury* related to CNS irritability and seizures.
3. *Pain* related to nuchal rigidity, opisthotonos position, increased muscle tension.
4. *Sensory/perceptual alterations* related to seizures and changes in level of consciousness.
5. *Altered nutrition, less than body requirements,* related to fever and poor oral intake.
6. *Knowledge deficit* regarding diagnostic procedures, condition, treatment, prognosis.

◆ **C. Nursing care plan/implementation:**

1. Goal: *prevent spread of infection.*

CLINICAL PATHWAY 5.1: Appendectomy-Perforated

Aspect of Care	Admission Day	Day 2	Day 3	Day 4	Day 5	Day 6	Day 7
Daily Outcome			Ambulating	NG tube out	Afebrile	Eating	Discharge
Tests	■ CBC ■ Electrolytes (+/−) ■ Sonogram (if ind.)	■ Electrolytes (+/-) ■ Gent level (if ind.)		CBC (+/−)	CBC (+/−)	CBC (+/−)	
Consults	Surgeon	Child life therapist/play therapist	Consider home health				
Fluid/Electrolyte Management	I&O	I&O	I&O	I&O	I&O	I&O	I&O
Treatments/Procedures	Appendectomy: ■ NG irrigation ■ Wound care	■ NG irrigation ■ Wound care	■ NG irrigation ■ Wound care	■ Wound care	■ Wound care	■ Wound care	
Medications	IV (pump, site check) ■ *Gentamicin w/clindamycin* **q 8 h** ■ *Ampicillin* **q 6 h** ■ *Methadone or morphine for pain*	IV (pump, site check) ■ *Gentamicin w/clindamycin* **q 8 h** ■ *Ampicillin* **q 6 h** ■ *Methadone or morphine for pain*	IV (pump, site check) ■ *Gentamicin w/clindamycin* **q 8 h** ■ *Ampicillin* **q 6 h** ■ *Methadone or morphine for pain*	IV (pump, site check) ■ *Gentamicin w/clindamycin* **q 8 h** ■ *Ampicillin* **q 6 h** ■ *Methadone or morphine for pain*	Hep lock ■ *Gentamicin w/clindamycin* **q 8 h** ■ *Ampicillin* **q 6 h** ■ *Methadone or morphine for pain*	Hep lock ■ *Gentamicin w/clindamycin* **q 8 h** ■ *Ampicillin* **q 6 h** ■ *Analgesics PO*	Hep lock ■ *Gentamicin w/clindamycin* **q 8 h** ■ *Ampicillin* **q 6 h** ■ *Analgesics PO*
Clinical Support	■ NPO ■ Pain management ■ Parent support ■ Bed/chair Extra client checks Reposition **q 4 h**	■ NPO ■ Pain management ■ Parent support ■ Chair Routine safety Reposition PRN Notify school re: child's absence	■ NPO ■ Pain management ■ Parent support ■ Ambulate Routine safety ■ Begin quiet, in-room play activities	■ NPO/Clear liquids (+/−) ■ Pain management ■ Parent support ■ Ambulate Routine safety ■ Playroom activities	■ Clear liquids/full liquids ■ Pain management ■ Parent support ■ Ambulate Routine safety ■ Playroom activities	■ Regular ■ Pain management ■ Ambulate Routine safety ■ Playroom activities	■ Regular ■ Pain management ■ Ambulate Routine safety ■ Activity ad lib ▶ Wound care Follow-up visit Notify school re: child's return with modified P.E. (no contact sports)

Adapted from Cook Children's Medical Center "Sample Pediatric Clinical Pathways." Published in Ashwill, JW, and Droske, SC: Nursing Care of Children: Principles and Practice. WB Saunders, Philadelphia.

a. Institute standard precautions.

b. Enforce strict handwashing.

 c. Institute and maintain *respiratory isolation* for minimum of 24 hr after starting IV antibiotics, at which time child is no longer considered to be communicable and can be removed from isolation.

d. Supervise all visitors in isolation techniques.

e. Identify family members and others at high risk: do cultures (*Haemophilus influenzae, Escherichia coli,* etc.); possibly begin prophylactic antibiotics, e.g., rifampin. Lumbar puncture (LP) is the definitive diagnostic test.

f. Treat with IV antibiotics (as ordered) as soon as possible after admission (after cultures are obtained); continue 10–14 days (until CSF culture is negative and child appears clinically improved).

g. Anticipate large-dose IV medications only—administer *slowly* in *dilute* form to prevent phlebitis.

h. Restrain as needed to maintain IV.

2. Goal: *promote safety and prevent injury/seizures.*

a. Maintain seizure precautions. Give anticonvulsants, as ordered (e.g., phenytoin).

b. Place child near nurses' station for maximum observation; provide private room for isolation.

c. Minimize stimuli: quiet, calm environment.

d. Restrict visitors to immediate family.

e. *Position:* HOB slightly elevated to decrease intracranial pressure. (If opisthotonos: side-lying, for comfort and safety.)

3. Goal: *maintain adequate nutrition.*

a. NPO or *clear liquids* initially; supplement with IVs, because child may be unable to coordinate sucking and swallowing.

b. Offer diet for age, as tolerated—child may experience anorexia (due to disease) or vomiting (due to increased intracranial pressure).

c. Monitor I&O, daily weights.

◆ **D. Evaluation/outcome criteria:**

1. No spread of infection noted; immunize all children against *H. influenzae* type B

2. Safety maintained.

3. Adequate nutrition and fluid intake maintained.

4. Child recovers without permanent neurological damage (e.g., seizure disorders, hydrocephalus).

III. Infestations

A. Lice (pediculosis)

1. *Introduction:* In children, the most common form of lice is *pediculosis capitis,* or head lice. This parasite feeds on the scalp, and its saliva causes severe itching. Head lice are frequently associated with the sharing of combs and brushes, hats, and clothing; thus, they are more common in girls, especially those with long hair. Lice are also associated with overcrowded conditions and poor hair hygiene.

◆ 2. **Assessment:**

a. Severe itching of scalp.

b. Visible eggs/nits on shafts of hair.

◆ 3. **Analysis/nursing diagnosis:**

a. *Impaired skin integrity* related to infestation of scalp with lice.

b. *Risk for impaired skin integrity* related to severe pruritus of scalp.

c. *Knowledge deficit* related to transmission and prevention of disease and treatment regimen.

◆ 4. **Nursing care plan/implementation:**

a. Goal: *eradicate lice infestation.* Apply permethrin (*Nix*) as drug of choice for infants and children—rub shampoo in for 4 to 5 min, then comb with fine-tooth comb to remove dead lice and nits (eggs).

 b. Goal: *prevent spread of lice.*

(1) Wear gloves and cap to protect self.

(2) Inspect other family members; treat prn with pediculocide.

(3) Wash all clothes and linens to kill any lice that may have fallen off the child's hair.

(4) Encourage short hair, if acceptable.

(5) Teach preventive measures: do *not* share comb, brushes, hats.

◆ 5. **Evaluation/outcome criteria:** lice are eradicated and do not spread.

B. Pinworms (enterobiasis)

1. *Introduction:* In children, the most common helminthic infestation is pinworms. Infestation usually occurs when the child places fingers (and the pinworm eggs) into the mouth. Breaking the *anus-to-mouth* contamination cycle can best be accomplished by good hygiene, especially handwashing before eating and after toileting. If one family member has pinworms, it is highly likely that other family members are also infested; therefore, treat the entire family to eradicate the parasite. Pinworms are easily eradicated with antiparasitic medications.

◆ 2. **Assessment:**

a. Intense perianal itching.

b. Visible pinworms in the stool.

c. Vague abdominal discomfort.

d. Anorexia and weight loss.

◆ 3. **Analysis/nursing diagnosis:**

a. *Risk for infection/injury* related to the anus-to-mouth contamination cycle of pinworm infestation, severe rectal itching.

b. *Knowledge deficit* related to transmission and prevention of disease and treatment regimen.

◆ 4. **Nursing care plan/implementation:**

a. Goal: *eradicate pinworm infestation.* Treat all family members simultaneously with an antiparasitic agent, e.g., *Vermox, Povan.*

b. Goal: *prevent spread of pinworms.*

(1) Launder all underwear, bed linens, and towels in hot soapy water to kill eggs.

(2) Teach family members the importance of good hygiene, especially handwashing before eating (or preparing food) and after toileting. Stress to children to keep their fingers out of their mouths.

◆ 5. **Evaluation/outcome criteria:** Pinworms are eradicated and do not spread; reinfestation does not occur.

Accidents: Ingestions and Poisonings

I. **General principles of treatment for ingestions and poisonings:**

A. *Prevention:* refer to section on toddler safety, **p. 275.**

B. How to induce vomiting:

 1. Drug of choice—*syrup of ipecac* (available over the counter; does not require a physician's order). Families with young children should keep this medication on hand in case of accidental poisoning. Note: safety of ipecac has been questioned due to esophageal tears (when misused) and anorexia nervosa/bulimia (when abused).

2. Dose:

a. 30 mL for adolescents over 12 yr; repeat dosage once if vomiting has not occurred within 20 min.

b. 15 mL for children 1–12 yr; repeat dosage once if vomiting has not occurred within 20 min. *Note:* Do *not* administer to infants *less than 1 yr of age* without physician's order.

c. 10 mL for infants 6–12 mo; do *not* repeat dosage.

3. Follow dose of ipecac with 4 to 8 oz of tap water or as much water as child will drink. In young children, give water first because child may refuse to drink anything else after tasting the ipecac.

4. The child *must* vomit the syrup of ipecac to avoid its being absorbed and causing potentially fatal cardiotoxicity (cardiac arrhythmias, atrial fibrillation, severe heart block). If child does not vomit within 20 min of second dose, summon paramedics; gastric lavage may be indicated upon arrival in Emergency Department. Do **not** manually stimulate gagging because gagging may ↑ vagal response → significant bradycardia.

C. When **not** to induce vomiting:

1. Child is stuporous or comatose.

2. Poison ingested is a corrosive substance or petroleum distillate.

3. Child is having seizures.

4. Child is in severe shock.

5. Child has lost the gag reflex.

II. **Salicylate poisoning**

◆ A. **Assessment:**

1. Determine how much aspirin was ingested, when, which type.

2. Evaluate salicylate levels: normal, 0; therapeutic range = 15–30 mg/dL; *toxic,* >30 mg/dL.

3. *Early* identification of *mild toxicity:*

a. Tinnitus (ringing in the ears).

b. Changes in vision, dizziness.

c. Sweating.

d. Nausea, vomiting, abdominal pain.

4. *Immediate* recognition of salicylate *poisoning:*

a. Hyperventilation (*earliest* sign).

b. Fever—may be extremely high (105° to 106°F).

c. Respiratory alkalosis or metabolic acidosis.

d. *Late* signs: bleeding tendencies, severe electrolyte disturbances, liver or kidney failure.

◆ B. **Analysis/nursing diagnosis:**

1. *Ineffective breathing patterns* related to hyperventilation/respiratory alkalosis.

2. *Fluid volume deficit* (dehydration) related to increased insensible loss of fluids through hyperventilation, increased loss of fluids through vomiting, and increased need for fluids due to hyperpyrexia (fever).

3. *Risk for injury* related to bleeding.

4. *Anxiety* related to parental/child feelings of guilt, uncertainty as to outcome, invasive nature of treatments.

5. *Knowledge deficit* regarding accident prevention.

◆ C. **Nursing care plan/implementation:**

1. Goal: *promote excretion of salicylates.*

 a. If possible, induce vomiting using syrup of ipecac (save, bring to emergency room).

▶ b. Assist with gastric lavage, if appropriate.

c. Administer activated charcoal as early as possible.

d. Administer IV fluids, as ordered.

e. Assist with hemodialysis, as ordered, to promote excretion of salicylates and fluids.

2. Goal: *restore fluid and electrolyte balance.*

a. Monitor I&O, urinalysis, specific gravity.

b. Prepare sodium bicarbonate, administer as ordered to correct metabolic acidosis.

c. Monitor IV fluids and electrolytes.

d. NPO initially (nasogastric [NG] tube).

3. Goal: *reduce temperature.*

a. **No** aspirin or acetaminophen, which might further complicate bleeding tendencies or lead to liver or kidney damage.

▶ b. Supportive measures: cool soaks, ice packs to armpits/groin, hypothermia blanket.

4. Goal: *prevent bleeding and possible hemorrhage.*

a. Monitor urine and stools for occult blood.

▶ b. Insert NG tube to detect gastric bleeding.

c. Observe for petechiae, bruising; monitor laboratory values for Hct and Hgb.

d. Administer vitamin K as ordered to correct bleeding tendencies.

5. Goal: *health education to prevent another accidental poisoning:*

a. Teach principles of poison prevention.

b. Stress need to avoid accidental overdose with over-the-counter medications or dosage mix-ups.

c. Allow child/parents to verbalize guilt, but *avoid* blaming or scapegoating.

◆ **D. Evaluation/outcome criteria:**
1. Aspirin is successfully removed from child's body without permanent damage.
2. Fluid and electrolyte balance is restored and maintained.
3. Child is afebrile.
4. Bleeding is controlled, no hemorrhage occurs.
5. No further episodes of poisoning occur.

III. Acetaminophen poisoning

◆ **A. Assessment:**
1. Determine how much acetaminophen was ingested, when, and which type.

2. Evaluate acetaminophen levels: normal = 0; therapeutic range = 15–30 μg/mL; toxic = 150 μg/mL 4 hr after ingestion.

3. *Initial period* (2–4 hr after ingestion): malaise, nausea, vomiting, anorexia, diaphoresis, pallor.
4. *Latent period* (1–3 days after ingestion): clinical improvement with asymptomatic rise in liver enzymes.
5. *Hepatic involvement* (may last 7 days or may be permanent): pain in right upper quadrant (RUQ), jaundice, confusion, hepatic encephalopathy, clotting abnormalities.
6. Gradual recuperation.

◆ **B. Analysis/nursing diagnosis:**
1. *Altered tissue perfusion* (liver) related to hepatic necrosis.
2. *Fluid volume deficit* related to increased loss of fluids secondary to vomiting and diaphoresis.
3. *Risk for injury* related to bleeding and clotting disorders.
4. *Anxiety* related to parental/child feelings of guilt, uncertainty as to outcome, and invasive nature of treatments.
5. *Knowledge deficit* regarding accident prevention.

◆ **C. Nursing care plan/implementation:**
1. Goal: *promote excretion of acetaminophen.*
   a. If possible, induce vomiting; save, bring to emergency department.
   ▶ b. Assist with gastric lavage, if appropriate.
   c. Administer activated charcoal.
   d. Assist with obtaining acetaminophen level 4 hr after ingestion.
2. Goal: *prevent permanent liver damage.*
   a. Treatment must begin as soon as possible; therapy begun later than 10 hr after ingestion has no value.
   b. Administer the antidote (acetylcysteine [*Mucomyst*]) per physician's order. Usually administered in cola or through NG tube because of offensive odor. Given as one loading dose and 17 maintenance doses.
   c. Monitor hepatic functioning—assist with obtaining specimens and check results frequently; be aware that liver enzymes will

rise and peak within 3 days and then should rapidly return to normal.

3. Goal: *restore fluid and electrolyte balance.*
   a. Monitor vital signs and perform neurological checks every 2–4 hr and prn.
   b. Monitor I&O; urine analysis, including specific gravity; and weight.
   c. Monitor IV fluids as ordered.
4. Goal: *prevent bleeding.*
   a. Assist in monitoring child's PT; notify physician of significant changes.
   b. Monitor urine and stool for occult blood.
   c. Observe for and report any petechiae or unusual bruising.
5. Goal: *health education to prevent another accidental poisoning.* (See **Goal 5, Nursing care plan/ implementation,** Salicylate poisoning.)

◆ **D. Evaluation/outcome criteria:**
1. Acetaminophen is successfully removed from child's body.
2. Normal liver function is reestablished.
3. Fluid and electrolyte balance is restored and maintained.
4. No further episodes of poisoning occur.

IV. Lead poisoning (plumbism)

A. *Introduction:* Lead poisoning is a heavy-metal poisoning that occurs from ingestion or inhalation of lead. In children, this is most common in the *toddler* age group (1–3 yr) and is usually a *chronic* type of poisoning that occurs as the result of repeated ingestions of lead. Older plumbing is one source of lead. Children who engage in the practice of *pica*, the ingestion of nonnutritive substances, often ingest lead in flecks of lead-based paint from plumbing, walls, furniture, or toys. In addition, research demonstrates that the parent–child relationship is a significant variable in lead poisoning; typically, there is a lack of adequate parental supervision that enables the child to engage in pica repeatedly over a fairly long time, until symptoms of lead poisoning become evident. (**Figure 5.13** shows the pathophysiological effects of lead poisoning.)

◆ **B. Assessment:**
1. Investigate history of pica.
2. Evaluate parent-child relationship.
3. *Chronic lead poisoning:* vague, crampy abdominal pain; constipation; anorexia and vomiting; listlessness.
4. Neurological, renal, hematological effects: see **Figure 5.13.**
5. "Blood-lead line"—bluish black line seen in gums.
6. X-rays: lead lines in long bones and flecks of lead in GI tract.
7. *Elevated* serum-blood-lead levels: ≥ 20 μg/dL requires clinical management; ≥ 45 μg/dL requires parenteral chelating therapy.

▶ **C. Analysis/nursing diagnosis:**
1. *Altered thought processes* related to neurotoxicity.

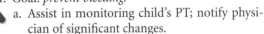
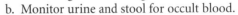
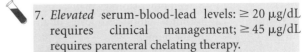

Pediatrics

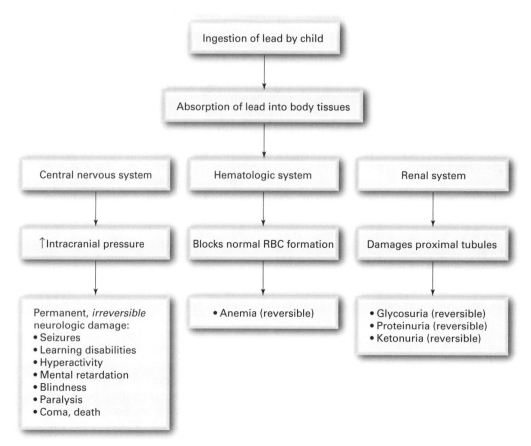

FIGURE 5.13   Pathophysiological effects of lead poisoning.

2. *Activity intolerance* (and *risk for infection*) related to anemia.
3. *Altered urinary elimination* related to excretion of lead by kidneys.
4. *Pain* related to lead poisoning and its treatment.
5. *Knowledge deficit* related to etiology of lead poisoning.

◆ **D. Nursing care plan/implementation:**
  1. Goal: *promote excretion of lead.*
     a. Administer chelating agents (EDTA [IM or IV], BAL [IM only]) as ordered. Chelation therapy typically continues over several days, with multiple treatments daily.
     b. Monitor kidney function carefully: the treatment itself is potentially nephrotoxic. Maintain adequate oral intake of fluids.
  ▶ c. Institute seizure precautions.
  2. Goal: *prevent reingestion of lead.*
     a. Determine primary source of poisoning.
     b. Eliminate source from child's environment before discharge.
     c. Follow up with home care referral.
       (1) Screen other siblings prn.
       (2) Monitor "blood-lead level" of all children in the home.
  3. Goal: *assist child to cope with multiple painful injections when treated with IM chelation therapy.*
     a. Prepare child for treatment regimen.

  b. Stress that this is *not* a punishment.
  c. Rotate sites as much as possible.
  d. May use a local anesthetic, e.g., procaine, injected simultaneously with chelating agent to decrease pain of injections.
  ▶ e. Apply warm soaks to injection sites: may help lessen pain.
  f. Encourage child to self-limit gross muscle activity (which increases pain).
  g. Offer child safe outlets for anger, fear, frustration—punching bag, pounding board, clay.
  h. Offer opportunity for medical play with empty syringes, etc.
  4. Goal: *health teaching.*
     a. Stress (to child and parents) that removing the lead is the only way to prevent permanent, irreversible neurological damage (irreversible damage may have *already* occurred).
     b. Teach that the chelating agent binds with the lead and promotes its excretion through the kidneys.

◆ **E. Evaluation/outcome criteria:**
  1. Lead is successfully removed from child's body without permanent damage.
  2. No further episodes of lead poisoning.
  3. Child copes successfully with the disease and its treatment.

Allergic Response: Threats to Health Status

I. Infantile eczema (atopic dermatitis)

A. *Introduction:* Eczema is an allergic skin reaction, most commonly to foods (e.g., cow's milk, eggs). It is most common in *infants* and young children (under 2 yr). Infantile eczema generally undergoes permanent, spontaneous remission by age 3 yr; however, approximately 50% of children who have had infantile eczema develop asthma during the preschool or school-age years.

◆ **B. Assessment:**

1. Erythematous lesions, beginning on cheeks and spreading to rest of face and scalp.
2. May spread to rest of body, especially in flexor surfaces, e.g., antecubital space.
3. Lesions may ooze or crust over.
4. Severe pruritus, which may lead to secondary infection.
5. Lymphadenopathy near site of rash.
6. Unaffected skin tends to be dry and rough.
7. Systemic manifestations are rare—but child may be irritable, cranky.

◆ **C. Analysis/nursing diagnosis:**

1. *Impaired tissue integrity* related to lesions.
2. *Pain* related to pruritus.
3. *Risk for (secondary) infection* related to breaks in the skin (first line of defense) and itching.
4. *Knowledge deficit* related to care of child with eczema, prognosis, how to prevent exacerbations.

◆ **D. Nursing care plan/implementation:**

1. Goal: *promote healing of lesions.*
   a. *Wet method:* frequent tepid baths (up to 4 times a day) followed by immediate application of a lubricant while the skin is still moist; **no soap** or use very mild, nonperfumed soap (e.g., Dove, Neutrogena); most useful method if child lives in a *dry* climate.
   b. *Dry method:* infrequent baths; cleanse skin with nonlipid, hydrophilic agent (e.g., Cetaphil); most useful method if child lives in a *humid* climate.
   c. Can add cornstarch to bath water to relieve itching and promote healing; keep skin well hydrated by applying emollients containing petrolatum or lanolin, which are occlusive and prevent evaporation of moisture.
   d. Apply wet soaks with Burow's solution (aluminum acetate solution; topical astringent and antiseptic); wet soaks should not be used for more than 3 days at a time.
   e. Protect child from possible sources of infection; standard precautions to prevent infection.
   f. **Absolutely no** immunizations during acute exacerbations of eczema because of the possibility of an overwhelming dermatitis, allergic reaction, shock, or even death.
   g. Apply topical creams/ointments as prescribed: A

and D emollient ointment, hydrocortisone cream to promote healing.

2. Goal: *provide relief from itching/keep child from scratching.*
   a. Administer systemic oral antihistamines as ordered (e.g., *Benadryl* or *Atarax*) to break itch-scratch cycle. Most useful at bedtime when itching tends to increase.
   b. Keep nails trimmed short—may need mittens (preferable not to use elbow restraints, because the antecubital space is a common site for eczema).
   c. Use clothes and bed linens that are nonirritating, i.e., pure cotton (**no** wool or blends).
   d. Institute *elimination/hypoallergenic diet:*
      (1) *No* milk or milk products.
      (2) Change to lactose-free formula, e.g., Isomil.
      (3) *Avoid* eggs, wheat, nuts, beans, chocolate.
   e. *No* stuffed animals or hairy dolls.

3. Goal: *provide discharge planning/teaching for parents and child.*
   a. Include all above information.
   b. Include information on course of disease: characterized by exacerbations and remissions throughout early years.
   c. Include information on prognosis: 50%–60% will go into spontaneous (and permanent) remission during preschool years; 40%–50% will develop asthma/hayfever during school-age years.

◆ **E. Evaluation/outcome criteria:**

1. Lesions heal well, without secondary infection.
2. Adequate relief from itching is achieved.
3. Parents verbalize understanding of eczema, prognosis, and how to prevent exacerbations.

II. Asthma

A. *Introduction:* Asthma is generally considered a chronic, lower airway disorder characterized by heightened airway reactivity with bronchospasm and obstruction. The exact cause of asthma is unknown; however, it is believed to include an allergic reaction to one or more allergens, or "triggers," that either precipitate or aggravate asthmatic exacerbation. The child usually exhibits other symptoms of allergy, such as infantile eczema or hayfever; in addition, 75% of children with asthma have a positive family history for asthma. The onset is usually before age 5 and remains with the child throughout life, although some children experience dramatic improvement in their asthma with the onset of puberty. Most children do *not* require continuous medication. Early relief of symptoms with a combination of drugs can reverse bronchospasm.

◆ **B. Assessment:**

1. Expiratory wheeze.
2. General signs and symptoms of respiratory distress, including: anxiety, cough, shortness of breath, crackles, cyanosis due to obstruction within the respiratory tract, use of accessory muscles of respirations.

3. *Cough:* hacking, paroxysmal, nonproductive; especially at night.
4. *Position* of comfort for breathing: sitting straight up, leaning forward, which is the position for optimal lung expansion.
5. Peak expiratory flow rate (PEFR) is in the *yellow* zone (50%–80% of personal best) or in the *red* zone (<50% of personal best).

◆ **C. Analysis/nursing diagnosis:**
1. *Ineffective airway clearance* related to bronchospasm.
2. *Anxiety* related to breathlessness.
3. *Knowledge deficit,* actual or risk for potential, related to disease process, treatment, and prevention of future asthmatic attacks.
4. *Activity intolerance* related to dyspnea and bronchospasm.

◆ **D. Nursing care plan/implementation:**
Treatment is aimed toward *improvement of ventilation, correction of dehydration and acidosis,* and *management of concurrent infection.*
1. Goal: *provide patent airway and effective breathing patterns.*
   ▶ a. Initiate oxygen therapy (by tent, face mask, or cannula), as ordered, to relieve hypoxia, with high humidity (to liquefy secretions).
   b. Administer bronchodilators, as ordered, to relieve the obstruction: epinephrine (1:1000), nebulized albuterol, *Brethine.* Inhalers may be used with metered dose inhalers (MDIs) to ensure proper delivery of the medication.
   c. Administer corticosteroids as ordered (PO or IV) to reduce inflammation, relieve edema (prednisone, *Decadron*) and decrease bronchial hyperreactivity.
   d. Administer antibiotics as ordered; infection is commonly either a trigger or complication of asthma.
   e. *Note:* methylxanthines (theophylline, aminophylline) are third-line agents that are rarely used to treat asthma.
2. Goal: *relieve anxiety.*
   a. Provide relief from hypoxia (refer to Goal 1), which is the chief source of anxiety.
   b. Remain with child, offer support.
   c. Administer sedation as ordered.
   d. Encourage parents to remain with child.
3. Goal: *teach principles of prophylaxis.*
   a. Review home medications, including cromolyn sodium. See **Unit 10.**
   b. Review breathing exercises.
   c. Discuss precipitating factors ("triggers") and offer suggestions on how to avoid them.
   ▶ d. Teach how to use peak expiratory flowmeter to monitor respiratory status and determine need for treatment.
   e. Introduce need for child to assume control over own care.

◆ **E. Evaluation/outcome criteria:**
1. Adequate oxygenation provided, as evidenced by

pink color of nailbeds and mucous membranes and ease in respiratory effort.
2. Anxiety is relieved.
3. Child verbalizes confidence in, and demonstrates mastery of, skills needed to care for own asthma.

Pediatric Surgery: Nursing Considerations

I. In general, basic care principles for children are the same as for adults having surgery.
II. *Exceptions:*
  A. Children should be prepared according to their developmental level and learning ability.
  B. Children cannot sign own surgical consent form; to be done by parent or legal guardian.
  C. Parents should be actively involved in the child's care.
III. See **Table 5.21,** which reviews specific nursing care for the most common pediatric surgical procedures.

DISORDERS AFFECTING NUTRITIONAL FUNCTIONING

Insulin-Dependent Diabetes Mellitus

Insulin-dependent diabetes mellitus (IDDM) was formerly called juvenile-onset diabetes. Diabetes mellitus is fully covered in **Unit 7.** Only the differences between adults and children are covered in **Table 5.22.**

Upper Gastrointestinal Anomalies

I. Cleft lip and cleft palate
  A. *Introduction:* Cleft lip and cleft palate are congenital facial malformations resulting from faulty embryonic development; there appear to be multiple factors involved in the exact etiology: mutant genes, chromosomal abnormalities, teratogenic agents, etc. The infant may be born with cleft lip alone, cleft palate alone, or with both cleft lip and cleft palate. **Table 5.23** compares these conditions.
◆ **B.** Assessment:
  1. *Cleft lip*—obvious facial defect, readily detectable at time of birth.
  2. *Cleft palate*—must feel inside infant's mouth to check for presence of palatal defect and to note extent of defect: soft palate only or soft palate *and* hard palate.
  3. *Both*—major problems with feeding: difficult to feed, noisy sucking, swallows excessive amounts of air, prone to aspiration.
  4. Parent-infant attachment (bonding) may be adversely affected due to "loss of perfect infant," multiple hospitalizations; note amount and quality of parent-infant interaction.

TABLE 5.22	Differences Between Type 1 (formerly called insulin-dependent) and Type 2 (formerly called non–insulin-dependent) Diabetes Mellitus	
Variable	Type 1 (Insulin-dependent) Diabetes Mellitus	Type 2 (Non–Insulin-dependent) Diabetes Mellitus
Endogenous (naturally occurring) insulin	*Absolute* deficiency of insulin; pancreas produces no insulin	*Relative* insufficiency of insulin
Dependence on exogenous insulin	Total dependence on insulin injections for remainder of life	Varies; disease may be controlled by combination of: diet, exercise, oral hypoglycemics, and insulin injections
Typical onset	Abrupt	Insidious
Age at onset	Anytime during childhood years; usually before age 20	Most common between age 40 and 60 years, but ↑ incidence in children with obesity, lack of exercise, diet high in "junk" food
Weight at onset	Normal or sudden, unexplained loss of weight	Overweight or obese
Gender	Slightly more common in boys than girls	More common in women than men
Ethnicity	More common in Caucasians	More common in Hispanics and Native Americans
Ketoacidosis	Relatively common	Relatively rare
Ease of control/stability	Unstable, difficult to achieve steady blood sugar level	Stable, easier to achieve steady blood sugar level
Presenting symptoms	Polyuria, polyphagia, polydipsia (**"three P's"**)	More commonly related to long-term complications (e.g., changes in vision or kidney function)
Complications	Occur more frequently and at relatively younger age because of younger age at onset of disease; rate 80% or greater	Occur less frequently, and often not seen until later adult years; rate is variable

TABLE 5.23	Comparison of Cleft Lip and Cleft Palate		
Dimension	Cleft Lip Only	Cleft Palate Only	Both Cleft Lip and Cleft Palate
Incidence	1/7800 More common among boys	1/2000 More common among girls	Most common facial malformation More common among boys More common among Caucasians than African Americans
Surgical repair	"Cheiloplasty" (Logan bow) Often done in a single stage Timing: age 6–12 wk	Palatoplasty Often done in staged repairs Timing: age 12–18 mo; (controversial; usually done prior to development of faulty speech habits)	Lip always repaired before palate to enhance parent-infant attachment, bonding
Position postoperatively	*Never* on abdomen	*Always* on abdomen	
Feeding postoperatively	*No* sucking Use Breck feeder or Asepto syringe	*No* sucking Use wide-bowl spoon or plastic cup	
Nursing care postoperatively	Elbow restraints Lessen crying	Elbow restraints Lessen crying	OK to show parents pictures of "before" and "after" repair
Long-term concerns	Bonding, attachment Social adjustment—potential threat to self-image	Defective speech—refer to speech therapist Abnormal dentition—refer to orthodontist Hearing loss—refer to pediatric eye, ear, nose, throat specialist/physician	

Pediatrics

◆ **C. Analysis/nursing diagnosis:**

1. *Altered nutrition, less than body requirements*, related to physical defect.
2. *Impaired physical mobility* (postoperative) related to postoperative care requirements.
3. *Altered parenting* related to birth of child with obvious facial defect.
4. *Knowledge deficit*, actual or risk for, potential, related to treatment and follow-up.

◆ **D. Nursing care plan/implementation:**

1. Goal: *maintain adequate nutrition.*
   a. *Preoperative:* first encourage parents to watch nurse feed infant, then teach parents proper feeding techniques:

   > (1) Use *Breck* feeder or Asepto syringe.
   > (2) Deposit formula on back of tongue to facilitate swallowing and to prevent aspiration.
   > (3) Rinse mouth with sterile water after feedings, to prevent infection.
   > (4) Feed slowly, with child in sitting position, to prevent aspiration.
   > (5) Burp frequently, because infant will swallow air along with formula due to the defect.
   > (6) Monitor weight.

   b. *Postoperative*

   (1) Begin with *clear liquids* when child has fully recovered from anesthesia (see **Table 5.23**).
   (2) Monitor weight gain carefully, to ensure adequate rate of growth.
   (3) **No** sucking for either cleft lip or palate repair until incision is healed.

2. Goal: *promote parent-infant attachment.*
   a. Show no discomfort handling infant; convey acceptance.
   b. Stay with parents the first time they see/hold infant.
   c. Offer positive comments about infant.
   d. Give positive reinforcement to parents' initial attempts at parenting.
   e. Encourage parents to assume increasing independence in care of their infant.
   f. Allow rooming-in on subsequent hospitalizations.

3. Goal: *teach parents particulars of feeding and need for long-term follow-up care.*
   a. Teach parents regarding long-term concerns (see **Table 5.23**).
   b. Make necessary *referrals* before discharge:
      (1) Specialists: speech, dentition, hearing.
      (2) Home health nurse.
      (3) Social service.
      (4) Disabled children's services for financial assistance.
      (5) Local facial-malformations support group.
   c. Refer parents to genetic counseling services because of mixed genetic/environmental etiology.
   d. Encourage parents to promote self-esteem in infant/child as child grows and develops.

◆ **E. Evaluation/outcome criteria:**

1. Adequate nutrition is provided, and infant grows at "normal" rate for age.
2. Parent-infant attachment is formed.
3. Parents verbalize confidence in their ability to care for infant.

II. Tracheoesophageal fistula

A. *Introduction:* Tracheoesophageal fistula (TEF) is a congenital anomaly resulting from faulty embryonic development; although there are numerous "types" of TEF, the major problem is an anatomical defect that results in an abnormal connection between the trachea (respiratory tract) and the esophagus (GI system) (**Figure 5.14**). No exact cause has been identified; however, infants born with TEF are often premature, with a maternal history of polyhydramnios. Diagnosis should be made immediately, within hours after birth, and preferably before feeding (to avoid aspiration pneumonia). Associated anomalies include: CHD, anorectal malformations, and genitourinary anomalies.

◆ **B. Assessment:**

1. Perinatal history: maternal polyhydramnios, premature birth.
2. *Most important system* affected is *respiratory:*
   a. Shortly after birth, infant has excessive amounts of mucus.
   b. Mucus bubbles or froths out of nose and mouth as infant literally "exhales" mucus.
   c. **"Three C's": coughing, choking, cyanosis**—because mucus accumulates in respiratory tract.
   d. "Pinks up" with suctioning, only to experience repeated respiratory distress within a short time as mucus builds up again.
   e. Aspiration pneumonia occurs early.
   f. Respiratory arrest may occur.
3. *Second* system affected is GI:
   a. Abdominal distention because excessive air enters stomach with each breath infant takes.
   b. Inability to aspirate stomach contents when attempting to pass NG tube.
   c. If all these signs are not correctly interpreted and feeding is attempted, infant takes two to three mouthfuls, coughs and gags, and forcefully "exhales" formula through nostrils.

◆ **C. Analysis/nursing diagnosis:**

1. *Ineffective breathing pattern/ineffective airway clearance* related to excess mucus.
2. *Altered nutrition, less than body requirements*, related to inability to take fluids by mouth.
3. *Anxiety* related to surgery, condition, preterm delivery, and uncertain prognosis.
4. *Knowledge deficit* regarding discharge care of infant related to gastrostomy tube, feeding.

◆ **D. Nursing care plan/implementation:**

1. Goal: *prepare neonate for surgery.*
   a. Stress to parents that surgery is *only* possible treatment.
   b. Allow parents to see neonate before surgery to promote bonding and attachment.

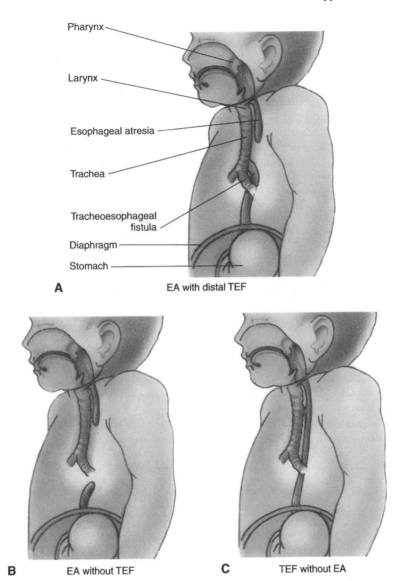

FIGURE 5.14 Esophageal malformations. *(A)* The esophagus ends in a blind pouch with a fistula between the distal esophagus and trachea. *(B)* Esophageal atresia without fistula. *(C)* Tracheoesophageal fistula without esophageal atresia. (From Bowden, VR, Dickey, SB, and Greenberg, CS: Children and Their Families: The Continuum of Care. WB Saunders, Philadelphia, 1999, p 105.)

c. Maintain NPO—provide IV fluids, monitor I&O, gastrostomy tube.

d. *Position:* elevate HOB 20°–30° to prevent aspiration.

e. Administer warmed, humidified oxygen, as ordered, to relieve hypoxia and to prevent cold stress.

2. Goal: *postoperative—maintain patent airway.*

a. *Position:* elevate HOB 20°–30°.

b. Care of chest tubes (open-chest procedure).

c. Care of endotracheal tube/ventilator (neonate frequently requires ventilatory assistance for 24–48 hr postoperatively).

d. Monitor for symptoms and signs of pneumonia (most common postoperative complication):
   (1) Aspiration.
   (2) Hypostatic, secondary to anesthesia.

e. Monitor for symptoms and signs of respiratory distress syndrome (preterm infant).

f. Use special precautions when suctioning: "suction with marked catheter" to avoid exerting undue pressure on newly sutured trachea.

g. Administer prophylactic/therapeutic antibiotics, as ordered.

h. Administer warmed, humidified oxygen, as ordered; monitor arterial blood gases (ABGs).

3. Goal: *maintain adequate nutrition.*

a. Maintain NPO for 10–14 days, until esophagus is fully healed (offer pacifier).

b. 48–72 hr postoperatively: IV fluids only.

c. When condition is stable: begin gastrotomy tube (G-tube) feedings, as ordered.
   (1) Start with small amounts of clear liquids.
   (2) Gradually increase to full-strength formula.

Pediatrics

(3) *Postoperative:* leave G tube open and elevated slightly above level of stomach to prevent aspiration if infant vomits.

(4) Offer pacifier ad lib.

d. Monitor weight, I&O.

e. Between *10th and 14th postoperative day:* begin oral feedings.

(1) Start with clear liquids again.

(2) Note ability to suck and swallow.

(3) Offer small amounts at frequent inter-vals.

(4) May need to supplement postop feeding with G-tube feeding prn.

4. Goal: *prepare parents to successfully care for the infant after discharge.*

a. Teach parents that infant will probably be discharged with G-tube in place; teach care of G-tube at home.

b. Teach parents symptoms and signs of most common long-term problem, i.e., *stricture formation.*

(1) Refusal to eat solids or swallow liquids.

(2) Dysphagia.

(3) Increased coughing or choking.

c. Stress need for long-term follow-up care.

d. Offer realistic encouragement, because prognosis is generally good.

◆ **E. Evaluation/outcome criteria:**

1. Neonate survives immediate surgical repair without untoward difficulties.

2. Patent airway is maintained; adequate oxygenation is provided.

3. Adequate nutrition is maintained; infant begins to gain weight and grow.

4. Parents verbalize confidence in ability to care for infant on discharge.

III. Hypertrophic pyloric stenosis

A. *Introduction:* Hypertrophic pyloric stenosis (HPS) causes obstruction of the upper GI tract, but the infant frequently does not have symptoms until 2–4 wk of age. HPS results in thickening, or hypertrophy, of the pyloric sphincter located at the distal end of the stomach; this causes a mechanical intestinal obstruction that becomes increasingly evident as the infant begins to consume larger amounts of formula during the early weeks of life. Pyloric stenosis is five times more common in *boys* than girls and is most often found in full-term Caucasian infants. The exact etiology remains unknown; however, there does seem to be a genetic predisposition.

◆ **B. Assessment:**

1. Classic symptom is *vomiting:*

a. Begins as nonprojectile at age 2–4 wk.

b. Advances to projectile at age 4–6 wk.

c. Vomitus is non–bile stained (stomach contents only).

d. Most often occurs shortly after a feeding.

e. Major problem is the mechanical obstruction of the flow of stomach contents to the small intestine due to the anatomical defect of stenosis of the pyloric sphincter.

f. No apparent nausea or pain, as evidenced by the fact that infant eagerly accepts a second feeding after episode of vomiting.

g. Metabolic alkalosis develops due to loss of hydrochloric acid.

2. Inspection of abdomen reveals:

a. Palpable olive-shaped *mass* in right upper quadrant.

b. Visible peristaltic *waves,* moving from left to right across upper abdomen.

3. *Weight:* fails to gain or loses.

4. *Stools:* constipated, diminished in number and size—due to loss of fluids with vomiting.

5. Signs of *dehydration* may become evident (**Table 5.24**).

 6. Upper GI series and ultrasonography reveal:

a. Delayed gastric emptying.

b. Elongated and narrowed pyloric canal.

◆ **C. Analysis/nursing diagnosis:**

1. *Fluid volume deficit* related to vomiting.

2. *Altered nutrition, less than body requirements,* related to vomiting.

3. *Risk for injury/infection* related to altered nutritional state.

4. *Impaired skin integrity* related to dehydration and altered nutritional state.

5. *Knowledge deficit* related to cause of disease, treatment and surgery, prognosis, and follow-up care.

◆ **D. Nursing care plan/implementation:**

1. Goal (**preoperative**): *restore fluid and electrolyte balance.*

a. Generally NPO, with IVs preoperatively to provide fluids and electrolytes.

b. Observe and record I&O, including vomiting and stool.

c. Weight: check every 8 hr or daily.

d. Monitor laboratory data.

2. Goal: *provide adequate nutrition.*

a. Maintain NPO with IVs for 4–6 hr postoperatively, as ordered (*can* offer pacifier).

TABLE 5.24	◆ Signs and Symptoms of Dehydration in Infants and Young Children

■ *Weight loss* (most important variable to assess): *mild dehydration* (less than 5% weight loss); *moderate dehydration* (5%–9% weight loss); *severe dehydration* (10%–15% weight loss)

■ *Skin:* gray, cold to touch, poor skin turgor (check skin across abdomen)

■ *Mucous membranes:* dry oral buccal mucosa; salivation absent

■ *Eyes:* sunken eyeballs; absence of tears when crying

■ *Anterior fontanel* (in infant): sunken

■ *Shock: increased* pulse, *increased* respirations, *decreased* blood pressure

■ *Urine:* oliguria, *increased* specific gravity, ammonia odor

■ *Alterations in level of consciousness:* irritability, lethargy, stupor, coma, possible seizures

■ *Metabolic acidosis* (with diarrhea)

■ *Metabolic alkalosis* (with vomiting)

b. Follow specific feeding regimen ordered by doctor—generally start with clear fluids in small amounts hourly, increasing slowly as tolerated. Full feeding schedule reinstated within 48 hr. Offer pacifier between feedings.

c. **Fed only by RN for 24–48 hr,** because vomiting tends to continue in immediate postoperative period.

d. Burp well—before, during, and after feeding.

e. *Position* after feeding: high Fowler's turned to right side; minimal handling after feeding to prevent vomiting.

3. Goal (**preoperative and postoperative**): *institute preventive measures to avoid infection or skin breakdown.*

a. Use good handwashing technique.

▶ b. Administer good skin care, especially in diaper area (urine is highly concentrated); give special care to any reddened areas.

c. Give mouth care when NPO or after vomiting.

d. Tuck diaper down below suture line to prevent contamination with urine (postoperatively).

e. Note condition of suture line—report any redness or discharge immediately.

f. Screen staff and visitors for any sign of infection.

4. Goal: *do discharge teaching to prepare parents to care for infant at home.*

a. Teach parents that defect is anatomical and unrelated to their parenting behavior/skill.

b. Demonstrate feeding techniques, and remind parents that vomiting may still occur.

c. Stress that repair is complete; this condition will *never* recur.

d. Instruct parents in care of the suture line: no baths for 10 days, tuck diaper down, report any signs of infection promptly.

e. Offer follow-up referrals as indicated.

◆ E. **Evaluation/outcome criteria:**

1. Infant survives surgical repair without untoward difficulties (including infection/skin breakdown).

2. Adequate nutrition is maintained, and infant begins to grow and gain weight.

3. Parents verbalize confidence in their ability to care for their infant on discharge.

DISORDERS AFFECTING ELIMINATION

Gastrointestinal Disorders

I. **Lower gastrointestinal anomalies/obstruction**

A. **Hirschsprung's disease** (congenital aganglionic megacolon)

1. *Introduction:* Hirschsprung's disease is a congenital anomaly of the lower GI tract, but the diagnosis often is not established until the infant is 6–12 months old. The major problem is a functional obstruction of the colon caused by the congenital anatomical defect of lack of nerve cells in the walls of the colon, resulting in the *absence* of peristalsis. Hirschsprung's disease is four times more common in *boys* than girls and is frequently noted in children with *Down* syndrome.

◆ 2. **Assessment:**

a. In the newborn, failure to pass meconium (in addition to other signs and symptoms of intestinal obstruction).

b. *Obstinate constipation*—history of inability to pass stool without stool softeners, laxatives, or enemas; persists despite all attempts to treat medically.

c. *Stools* are infrequent and tend to be thin and ribbonlike.

d. *Vomiting:* bile stained, flecked with bits of stool (breath has fecal odor), due to GI obstruction and eventual backing up of stools.

e. Abdominal distention can be severe enough to impinge on respirations, due to GI obstruction and retention of stools.

f. Anorexia, nausea, irritability due to severe constipation.

 g. Malabsorption results in *anemia, hypoproteinemia,* and loss of subcutaneous fat.

h. Visible peristalsis and palpable fecal masses may also be detected.

◆ 3. **Analysis/nursing diagnosis:**

a. *Constipation* related to impaired bowel functioning.

b. *Altered nutrition, less than body requirements,* related to poor absorption of nutrients.

c. *Risk for injury/infection* related to malnutrition.

d. *Pain* related to surgery and treatments.

e. *Knowledge deficit* regarding care of the child with a colostomy and follow-up care.

◆ 4. **Nursing care plan/implementation:**

a. Goal (**preoperative**): *promote optimum nutritional status, fluid and electrolyte balance.*

(1) Monitor for signs and symptoms of progressive intestinal obstruction: measure abdominal girth daily.

(2) Administer IV fluids, as ordered—may include hyperalimentation or intralipids.

(3) Daily weights, I&O, urine specific gravity.

(4) Monitor for possible dehydration.

(5) *Diet:* low residue.

b. Goal (**preoperative**): *assist in preparing bowel for surgery.*

(1) Teach parents what will be done and why—enlist their cooperation as much as possible.

▶ (2) Insert NG tube, connect to low suction to achieve and maintain gastric decompression.

(3) *Position:* semi-Fowler's.

▶ (4) Bowel is cleansed with a series of isotonic saline (0.9%) enemas.

(5) Administer oral antibiotics and colonic irrigations to decrease bacteria.

(6) Take axillary temperatures *only.*

(7) If child can understand, prepare for probable colostomy using pictures, dolls (usual age at surgery is 10–16 mo).

c. Postoperative goals: same as for adult having major abdominal surgery or a colostomy (see **Unit 7**).

d. Goal (**postoperative**): *discharge teaching to prepare parents to care at home for infant with a colostomy.*

　(1) Home care of colostomy of infant is essentially same as for adult (see **Unit 7**).

　(2) Teach parents to keep written records of stools: number, frequency, consistency.

　(3) Teach parents to tape diaper below colostomy to prevent irritation.

　(4) Because colostomy is usually temporary, discuss:

　　(a) Second-stage repair (closure and pull-through) done when the child weighs approximately 20 lb.

　　(b) Possible difficulties in toilet training.

　(5) Stress need for long-term follow-up care.

　(6) Make referral to home care if indicated.

◆ 5. **Evaluation/outcome criteria:**

a. Infant is prepared for surgery and tolerates procedure well.

b. Postoperative recovery is uneventful.

c. Parents verbalize confidence in ability to care at home for infant with a colostomy and verbalize their understanding that second surgery will be needed to close the colostomy.

B. Intussusception

1. *Introduction:* Intussusception is the apparently spontaneous telescoping of one portion of the intestine into another, resulting in a mechanical obstruction of the lower GI tract. There is no known cause, and intussusception is three times more common in *boys* than girls; the child with intussusception is usually between 3 and 36 months of age.

◆ 2. **Assessment:**

a. Typically presents with sudden onset in child who is healthy, thriving.

b. *Pain:* paroxysmal, colicky, abdominal, with intervals when the child appears normal and comfortable.

c. *Stools:* "currant-jelly," bloody, mixed with mucus.

d. *Vomiting* due to intestinal obstruction.

e. *Abdomen:* distended, tender, with palpable, sausage-shaped mass in RUQ.

f. *Late signs:* fever, shock, signs of peritonitis as the compressed bowel wall becomes necrotic and perforates.

◆ 3. **Analysis/nursing diagnosis:**

a. *Fluid volume deficit* related to diarrhea and vomiting.

b. *Pain* related to bowel-wall ischemia, necrosis, and death.

c. *Risk for injury/infection* related to bowel-wall perforation and peritonitis.

d. *Knowledge deficit* regarding the disease, medical or surgical treatment, and prognosis.

◆ 4. **Nursing care plan/implementation:**

a. Goal: *assist with attempts at medical treatment.*

　(1) Explain to parents that a barium enema will be given to the child in an attempt to reduce the telescoping through hydrostatic pressure (succeeds in 75% of cases).

　(2) Stress that if this treatment is not successful, or if perforation of the bowel wall has already occurred, surgery will be necessary.

　(3) If medical treatment is apparently successful, monitor child for 24–36 hr for recurrence before discharge.

b. *Preoperative and postoperative goals:* same as for adult with major abdominal surgery (see **Unit 7**).

c. Goal: *discharge teaching to prepare parents for care of the child at home.*

　(1) Stress that recurrence is rare (10%) and most often occurs within the first 24–36 hr after reduction.

　(2) Other teaching: same as for adult going home after bowel surgery (see **Unit 7**).

◆ 5. **Evaluation/outcome criteria:**

a. Infant tolerates medical-surgical treatment and completely recovers.

b. Parents verbalize confidence in ability to care for infant after discharge.

II. Acute gastroenteritis (AGE)

A. *Introduction:* In infants and young children, gastroenteritis is a common acute illness that can rapidly progress to dehydration, hypovolemic shock, and severe electrolyte disturbances.

◆ **B. Assessment:**

1. Diarrhea: often watery, green, explosive, contains mucus and blood.

2. Abdominal cramping and pain, often accompanied by bouts of diarrhea.

3. Dehydration: see **Table 5.24.**

4. Irritability, restlessness, alterations in level of consciousness.

5. Electrolyte disturbances: see **Unit 7.**

◆ **C. Analysis/nursing diagnosis:**

1. *Fluid volume deficit* related to vomiting and diarrhea.

2. *Altered nutrition, less than body requirements,* related to AGE and its treatment, i.e., dietary restrictions.

3. *Pain* related to abdominal cramping, diarrhea.

4. *Impaired skin integrity* related to diarrhea.

5. *Altered tissue perfusion* related to dehydration and hypovolemia.

6. *Knowledge deficit* regarding diagnosis, dietary restrictions, treatment.

◆ **D. Nursing care plan/implementation:**

1. Goal: *prevent spread of infection.*

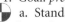 a. Standard precautions to prevent infection.

b. Enforce strict handwashing.

 c. Institute and maintain *enteric precautions—*

follow policies regarding linens, excretions, specimens ("double bag, special tag").

    d. Tape diapers snugly; keep hands out of mouth.

    e. Obtain stool culture to identify causative organism; then administer antibiotics as ordered.

    f. Identify family members and others at high risk, obtain cultures.

2. Goal: *restore fluid and electrolyte balance.*

    a. Administer IV fluids and electrolytes as ordered.

    b. Monitor for appropriate response to therapy: decreased specific gravity, good skin turgor, normal vital signs.

    c. Monitor weight, I&O, specific gravity.

    d. Oral feedings—oral rehydration therapy (ORT) with Pedialyte or comparable solution; resume normal diet as quickly as possible.

    e. Ongoing assessment of stools: note **A**mount, **C**olor, **C**onsistency, **T**iming (**ACCT**).

3. Goal: *maintain or restore skin integrity.*

    a. Frequent diaper changes.

    b. Keep perineal area clean and dry.

    c. Apply protective ointments, e.g., petroleum jelly, A and D emollient ointment.

    d. If feasible, expose reddened buttocks to air (but *not* with explosive diarrhea).

4. Goal: *provide discharge teaching to parents.*

    a. Careful review of diet to be followed at home.

    b. Review principles of food preparation and storage to prevent infection.

    c. Instruct in disposal of stools at home.

    d. Emphasize importance of good hygiene.

◆ **E. Evaluation/outcome criteria:**

1. No spread of infection noted.
2. Fluid and electrolyte balance normal.
3. No skin breakdown noted.
4. Parents verbalize understanding of home care.

Genitourinary Disorders

I. Hypospadias

  A. *Introduction:* Hypospadias is a congenital anatomical defect of the male genitourinary tract, readily detected at birth through simple visual examination. In hypospadias, the urethral opening is located on the ventral surface of the penile shaft; this makes voiding in the standing position virtually impossible, which creates potential for serious psychological problems. Ideally, staged surgical repair should be completed *by 6–18 months of age,* before body image is developed or castration fears are evident.

◆ **B. Assessment:**

1. Urethral opening is located on ventral surface of penis.
2. May be accompanied by "chordee"—ventral curvature of the penis due to a fibrous band of tissue.
3. Rare: ambiguous genitalia, resulting in need for chromosomal studies to determine sex of neonate.

◆ **C. Analysis/nursing diagnosis:**

1. *Altered urinary elimination* related to congenital anatomical defect of penis.
2. *Pain* related to surgery and treatments.
3. *Self-esteem disturbance* related to anatomical defect in penis and resulting disturbance in ability to void standing up.
4. *Knowledge deficit* related to condition, surgeries, outcome.

◆ **D. Nursing care plan/implementation:**

1. Goal: *promote normal urinary function.*

    a. Teach family that surgery is done in several stages, beginning in the early months of life and finishing by age 18 mo.

    b. Provide age-appropriate information to child regarding condition, surgery.

    c. *Preoperative* teaching with child: simulate anticipated postoperative urinary drainage apparatus and dressings on dolls; allow child to handle and play with them *now,* but stress need *not* to touch postoperatively.

    d. *Postoperatively:* Monitor urinary drainage apparatus; note hourly urine output, color, appearance (should be clear yellow, no blood).

2. Goal: *promote self-esteem.*

    a. Do *not* scold child if he exposes penis, dressings, catheters, etc.

    b. Reassure parents that preoccupation with penis is normal and will pass.

    c. Encourage calm, matter-of-fact acceptance of, and *avoid* strict discipline for this behavior, which could affect the child negatively.

◆ **E. Evaluation/outcome criteria:**

1. Child is able to void in normal male pattern.
2. Child does not experience disturbances in self-concept and has normal self-esteem.

II. Wilms' tumor (nephroblastoma)

  A. *Introduction:* Wilms' tumor, a malignant tumor of the kidney, is the most common form of renal cancer in children. Peak incidence occurs at 3 years of age, with a slightly higher incidence in *boys* than girls. Ninety percent of the cases occur unilaterally; the treatment of choice is nephrectomy (and adrenalectomy) followed by chemotherapy and radiation.

◆ **B. Assessment:**

1. Most common sign: abdominal mass (firm, nontender).
2. Most often first found by parent changing diaper; felt as a mass over the kidney area.
3. Intravenous pyelogram (IVP), abdominal ultrasound, and CT confirm the diagnosis.
4. Metastasis occurs most frequently to the lungs: pain in chest, cough, dyspnea.

◆ **C. Analysis/nursing diagnosis:** *altered urinary elimination* (other diagnoses depend on stage of tumor and presence of metastasis—similar to adult with cancer).

◆ **D. Nursing care plan/implementation:**

1. Goal: *promote normal urinary function.*

    a. Inform family that surgery is scheduled as soon as possible after confirmed diagnosis (within 24–48 hr).

b. Explain to family that the preferred surgical approach is nephrectomy (and adrenalectomy).

c. *Preoperative:* do **not palpate abdomen** because the tumor is highly friable, and palpation increases the risk of metastasis.

d. *Postoperative nursing care:* similar to care of adult with nephrectomy (see **Unit 7**).

e. *Postoperative care also includes long-term radiation therapy and chemotherapy* (actinomycin D, vincristine, adriamycin; see **Units 7** and **10**).

2. Goal: *discharge teaching to prepare parents to care for child at home.*

a. Teach parents need for long-term follow-up care with specialists: oncologist, urologist.

b. Answer questions regarding prognosis, offering realistic hope.

(1) Children with localized tumor: 90% survival rate.

(2) Children with metastasis: 50% survival rate.

◆ E. **Evaluation/outcome criteria:**

1. Child is able to maintain normal urinary elimination.

2. Parents verbalize their understanding of home care for the child.

III. Nephrosis. Nephrosis (idiopathic nephrotic syndrome) is a chronic renal disease having no known cause, variable pathology, and no known cure. It is thought that several different pathophysiological processes adversely affect the glomerular membranes of the kidneys, resulting in increased permeability to protein. This "leakage" of protein into the urine results in massive *proteinuria*, severe *hypoproteinemia*, and total body edema. A chronic disease, nephrosis often has its onset during the preschool years but is characterized by periods of exacerbation and remission throughout the childhood years.

The nursing care plan for the child with nephrosis is very similar to that for the adult with compromised renal functioning. Refer to **Units 9** and **10** for additional information about dietary restrictions and medications; refer to **Table 5.20** for a chart comparing nephrosis and nephritis.

DISORDERS AFFECTING COMFORT, REST, ACTIVITY, AND MOBILITY

Musculoskeletal Disorders

Orthopedic conditions in infants and children are many and varied, but treatment is based on basic principles of nursing care. **Table 5.25** and **Figures 5.15** and **5.16** offer a quick review of the major pediatric orthopedic conditions.

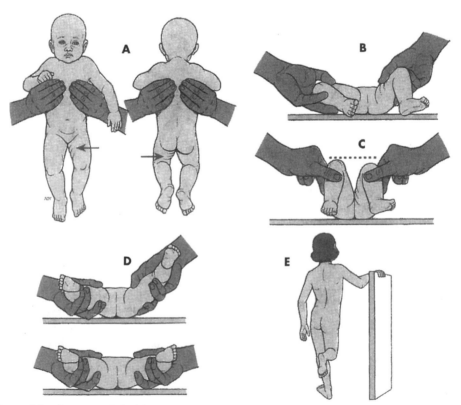

FIGURE 5.15 **Signs of developmental *dysplasia of the hip.*** *(A)* Asymmetry of gluteal and thigh folds. *(B)* Limited hip abduction as seen in flexion. *(C)* Apparent shortening of the femur, as indicated by the level of the knees in flexion. *(D)* Ortolani click (if infant is under 4 weeks of age). *(E)* Positive Trendelenburg sign or gait (if child is weight bearing). (From Wong, D: Whaley and Wong's Nursing Care of Infants and Children, ed. 7. Mosby, St. Louis.)

THORACIC

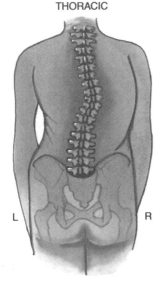

L   R

90% occur on the right side above T-11

LUMBAR

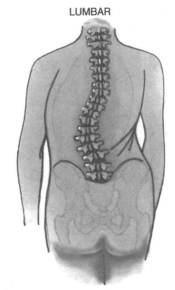

70% occur on the left side at L-1 or lower

THORACOLUMBAR

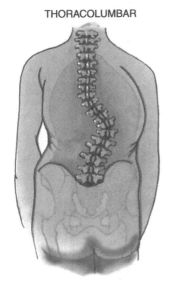

80% occur on the right side at T-11 – T-12

DOUBLE MAJOR

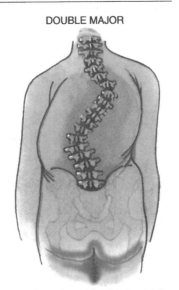

Usually involves right-sided and left-sided lumbar curves

Curve location is determined by the level of the apical vertebra

FIGURE 5.16   The four major curve patterns in idiopathic scoliosis. (From Bowden, VR, Dickey, SB, and Greenberg, CS: Children and Their Families: The Continuum of Care. WB Saunders, Philadelphia.)

Neuromuscular Disorders

I. Cerebral palsy

A. *Introduction: Cerebral palsy (CP) is the most common permanent physical disability of childhood. It is a neuromuscular disorder of the pyramidal motor system resulting in debilitating impaired voluntary muscle control. The damage appears to be fixed and nonprogressive, and the cause is unknown. However, although a variety of factors have been implicated in the etiology of CP, it is now known that CP results more commonly from prenatal brain abnormalities.*

◆ **B. Assessment:**
1. Most common type of cerebral palsy—*spastic.*
   a. Delayed developmental milestones.
   b. Tongue thrust with difficulty swallowing and sucking. Poor weight gain. Aspiration may occur.
   c. Increased muscle tone: "scissoring" (legs crossed, toes pointed).
   d. Persistent neonatal reflexes.
   e. Associated problems:
      (1) Mental retardation in 30% of children with cerebral palsy (70% are normal).
      (2) Sensory impairment: vision, hearing.

TABLE 5.25	Common Pediatric Orthopedic Conditions

Condition	Definition	Age at Onset/ Sex Difference	Treatment	◆ Nursing Considerations
Clubfoot	Downward, inward rotation of one or both feet: talipes equinovarus (95%)	Newborn (congenital); twice as common in *boys*	Series of casts changed weekly followed by *Denis Browne splint* and then corrective shoes (severe cases—surgery)	Care of child in cast/brace Stress need for follow-up Encourage compliance
Developmental hip dysplasia (see Figure 5.15)	Abnormal development of hip joint (most frequently unilateral)	Newborn (congenital); more common in *girls*	*Newborn—Pavlik harness;* older infant or toddler—possible surgery, spica cast	Early identification Care of child in traction/cast: check circulation; turn q2h while cast is wet Encourage compliance Check for other anomalies (e.g., spina bifida)
Osteomyelitis	Most frequently occurring bone infection among children	5–14 yr; twice as common in *boys*	Blood cultures to diagnose causative organisms—select appropriate antibiotic; bedrest, immobilization with splint or cast	Care of child in splint/cast Provide diversion Pain medications/antibiotics per MD order
Legg-Calvé-Perthes	Aseptic necrosis of the head of the femur (cause unknown)	*Peak:* 4–8 yr; *range:* 3–12 yr; 5 times more common in *boys;* 10 times more common in Caucasians than non-Caucasians	Conservative therapy lasts 2–4 yr, usually begins with bed rest and traction, followed by non–weight-bearing devices such as brace, cast	Early identification Care of child in traction/cast: check for frayed pulley ropes Provide diversion Assist child and family to cope with child's prolonged immobility
Juvenile rheumatoid arthritis, a.k.a. juvenile idiopathic arthritis (JIA)	Chronic systemic inflammatory disease (cause unknown)	*Peak:* 1–3 yr and 8–10 yr; more common in *girls*	Prevent joint deformity by exercise, splints, medications (NSAIDs, SAARDs, corticosteroids, biological agents [Etanercept], cytotoxic agents); relieve symptoms (as per adult with arthritis)	Care of child in brace/splint Provide diversion Encourage compliance
Scoliosis (see **Figure 5.16**)	Lateral curvature of the spine (cause unknown)	Adolescence; more common in *girls*	Braces specific to type of curvature; halo-pelvic traction; *Harrington rod;* Luque, Cotrel-Dubousset, or Dwyer/Zielke instrumentation	Care of child in traction/cast/brace Teach that brace is worn 16–23 hr/day, 7 days/wk for 6 mo–2 yr Encourage compliance Promote positive self-image
Osteosarcoma	Most frequently occurring bone cancer among children	Adolescence (10–25 yr); more common in *boys* and men	Limb salvage procedure; amputation→prosthesis; chemotherapy	Prepare child for loss of limb Help cope with prosthesis, life-threatening illness Assist with grieving process

Pediatrics

(3) Orthopedic conditions: congenital dysplasia of hip, clubfoot.

(4) Dental problems: malocclusion.

(5) Seizures.

◆ **C. Analysis/nursing diagnosis:**

1. *Ineffective airway clearance* related to hyperactive gag reflex and possible aspiration.

2. *Altered nutrition, less than body requirements,* related to difficulty sucking and swallowing.

3. *Fluid volume deficit* related to difficulty sucking and swallowing.

4. *Impaired verbal communication* related to difficulty with speech.

5. *Sensory/perceptual alterations* related to potential vision and hearing defects.

6. *Risk for injury* related to difficulty controlling voluntary muscles.

7. *Self-esteem disturbance* related to disability.

8. *Note:* Because the level of disabilities with CP can vary, the nurse must select those diagnoses that apply, and clearly specify the individual child's limitations in any diagnostic statements.

◆ **D. Nursing care plan/implementation:**

1. Goal: *maintain patent airway.*

a. Have suction and oxygen readily available.

▶ b. Use feeding and positioning techniques to maintain patent airway.

c. Institute prompt, aggressive therapy for URIs, to prevent the possible development of pneumonia.

2. Goal: *promote adequate nutrition.*

a. *Diet: high* in *calories* (to meet extra energy demands).

b. Ensure balanced diet of basic foods that can be easily chewed. Refer to dentist for early dental care.

c. Provide feeding utensils that promote independence.

d. Feed in upright position.

e. Relaxed mealtimes, decreased emphasis on manners, cleanliness.

f. Monitor I&O, weight gain.

3. Goal: *facilitate verbal communication.*

a. Refer to speech therapist.

b. Speak slowly, clearly to child.

c. Use pictures or actual objects to reinforce speech.

4. Goal: *prevent injury.* Refer to information on safety throughout growth and development sections, **pp. 271–273, 275, 277–279.**

a. Use individually designed chairs with restraints for positioning and safety.

b. Provide protective helmet to prevent head trauma.

c. Implement seizure precautions.

5. Goal: *provide early detection of and correction for vision and hearing defects.*

a. Arrange for screening tests.

b. Assist family with obtaining corrective devices: eyeglasses, hearing aids.

6. Goal: *promote locomotion.*

a. Encourage "infant stimulation" program to assist infant in reaching developmental milestones.

b. *Refer to physical therapy* for exercise program.

c. Incorporate play into exercise routine.

d. Use devices that promote locomotion: parallel bars, crutches, and braces.

e. Surgical approach may be needed to relieve contractures.

f. Medications: focus on ↓ excessive motion and tension; antianxiety agents, skeletal muscle relaxants, Botox injections, Baclofen pump (IT).

7. Goal: *encourage independence in ADL.*

a. Adapt clothing, feeding utensils, etc., to facilitate self-help.

b. Encourage child to perform ADL as much as possible; offer positive reinforcement.

c. Assist parents to have realistic expectations for their child; *avoid* excessively high expectations that might increase frustration.

8. Goal: *promote self-esteem.*

a. Praise child for each accomplishment or for sincere effort.

b. Help child dress and groom self daily in an attractive "normal" manner for developmental level and age.

c. Encourage child to form friendships with children with similar problems.

d. Enroll child in "special ed" classes to meet his or her needs.

e. Encourage parents to expose child to wide variety of experiences.

◆ **E. Evaluation/outcome criteria:**

1. Patent airway and adequate oxygenation maintained.

2. Adequate nutrition maintained, and child begins to grow and gain weight.

3. Child has an acceptable means of verbal communication.

4. Safety is maintained.

5. Vision and hearing within normal limits using corrective devices prn.

6. Child is as mobile as possible, given disabilities.

7. Child is performing ADL, within capabilities.

8. Child has positive self-image/self-esteem.

II. Spina bifida (myelodysplasia)

A. *Introduction:* Three different types of spina bifida:

1. *Spina bifida occulta*—a "hidden" bony defect without herniation of the meninges or cord; not visible externally, no symptoms are present, and no treatment is needed.

2. Spina bifida cystica—visible defect of the spine with external saclike protrusion.

a. *Meningocele* **Table 5.26.**

b. *Myelomeningocele*—see **Table 5.26.** Most serious type of spina bifida cystica and also most common.

The remainder of this section deals with *myelomeningocele* exclusively.

◆ **B. Assessment:**

1. Congenital defect.

2. Readily detected by visual inspection in delivery room: round, bulging sac filled with fluid, usually in lumbosacral area.

TABLE 5.26	Comparison of Two Major Types of Spina Bifida	
Dimension	**Meningocele**	**Myelomeningocele**
Contents of sac	Meninges and cerebrospinal fluid	Meninges, cerebrospinal fluid, spinal cord
Transillumination	Present	Absent
Percentage of total cases	25%	75%
Motor function	Present	Absent
Sensory function	Present	Absent
Urinary/fecal incontinence	Absent	Present
Associated orthopedic anomalies	Rare	Developmental dysplasia of the hip, *clubfoot*
Other anomalies	Rare	*Hydrocephalus* (90–95%)
Treatment	Surgery	Surgery
Major *short-term* complication	Infection (meningitis)	Infection (meningitis)
Major *long-term* complication	None	Chronic urinary tract infection leading to renal disease/failure
Prognosis	Excellent	Guarded

3. *Sensation and movement:* complete lack below the level of the lesion.

4. *Urinary:* retention, with overflow incontinence.

5. *Fecal:* constipation, fecal impaction, oozing of liquid stool around impaction.

6. 80%–85% develop signs and symptoms of hydrocephalus (see **below**).

7. May have associated orthopedic anomalies: clubfoot, developmental hip dysplasia.

◆ **C. Analysis/nursing diagnosis:**

1. *Risk for injury/infection* related to rupture of the sac.

2. *Altered urinary elimination* related to urinary retention and overflow incontinence.

3. *Impaired skin integrity* related to immobility.

4. *Constipation* related to fecal incontinence and impaired innervation.

◆ **D. Nursing care plan/implementation:**

1. Goal: *prevent rupture of the sac and possible infection (preoperative).*

a. *Position:* no pressure on sac; *prone,* to prevent contamination with urine or stool.

b. *No* clothing or diapers to *avoid* pressure on sac.

▶ c. Place in heated isolette to maintain body temperature. *Avoid* radiant heat, which can dry and crack the sac.

d. Keep sac covered with sterile, moist, nonadherent dressing (sterile normal saline) to prevent drying, cracking, and leakage of CSF; change every 2–4 hr; document appearance of sac with each dressing change to note signs and symptoms of infection, leaks, abrasions, or irritation.

e. Enforce strict aseptic technique to prevent infection (leading cause of morbidity/mortality in neonatal period).

f. *Avoid* repeated latex exposure (e.g., gloves, catheters) to decrease risk of latex allergy.

2. Goal: *prevent infection in postoperative period.*

a. *Position:* prone, side-lying, or partial side-lying.

▶ b. Use myelomeningocele apron (specific type of dressing) to prevent urine or stool from contaminating suture line.

◖ c. Administer antibiotics as ordered.

 d. Use strict aseptic techniques in dressing changes; standard precautions to prevent infection.

3. Goal: *prevent urinary retention and UTI.*

a. Monitor I&O, offer extra fluids to flush kidneys.

b. Keep urethral meatus clean of stool to prevent ascending bacterial infection.

c. Monitor urinary output for retention.

◖ d. Administer antibiotics/urinary tract antiseptics as ordered.

4. Goal: *prevent complications of prolonged immobility or associated orthopedic anomalies.*

a. *Position:* hips abducted.

▶ b. Use positional devices, rotating pressure mattress/flotation mattress.

c. *Refer to physical therapy* for ROM exercises.

d. Make necessary referrals for care of possible clubfoot/developmental hip dysplasia.

5. Goal: *monitor for possible development of hydrocephalus.* Occurs in 90%–95% of infants born with myelomeningocele.

◆ **E. Evaluation/outcome criteria:**

1. Integrity of sac is maintained until surgery is done.

2. No infection occurs.

3. Adequate patterns of urinary and bowel elimination with necessary support.

4. Complications of immobility, orthopedic anomalies are prevented or treated promptly.

DISORDERS AFFECTING SENSORY-PERCEPTUAL FUNCTIONING

I. Hydrocephalus

A. *Introduction:* Hydrocephalus, known to the layperson as "water on the brain," is actually a syndrome resulting from disturbances in the dynamics of CSF. The accumulation of this fluid causes enlargement and dilation of the ventricles of the brain and increased ICP. If untreated, severe brain damage will result; treatment is a surgical shunting procedure that allows

CSF to drain from the ventricles of the brain to another, less harmful area within the body: jugular vein, right atrium of the heart, or peritoneal cavity. Hydrocephalus can develop as the result of a *congenital malformation* (e.g., Arnold-Chiari malformation); can be *associated with other congenital defects* (e.g., spina bifida); or can be acquired secondary to infection (e.g., meningitis), trauma, or neoplasm.

◆ **B. Assessment:**

1. *Head:* increased circumference—earliest sign of hydrocephalus in the infant (more than 1 in/mo).
2. *Fontanels:* tense and bulging without head enlargement.
3. *Veins:* dilated scalp veins.
4. **"Setting-sun" sign:** sclera visible above pupil; pupils are sluggish, with unequal response to light.
5. *Cry:* shrill, high pitched.
6. Developmental milestones: delayed.
7. *Reflexes:* persistence of neonatal reflexes; hyperactive reflexes.
8. Feeds poorly.

9. *Signs of increased ICP:*
   a. Vomiting.
   b. Irritability.
   c. Seizures.
   d. *Decreased* pulse.
   e. *Decreased* respirations.
   f. *Increased* blood pressure.
   g. Widened pulse pressure.

10. History may reveal other CNS defects (e.g., spina bifida), infection (e.g., meningitis), trauma, or neoplasm.

◆ **C. Analysis/nursing diagnosis:**

1. *Altered cerebral tissue perfusion* related to increased intracranial pressure.
2. *Impaired skin integrity* related to enlarged head size and lack of motor coordination.
3. *Altered nutrition, less than body requirements,* related to anorexia and vomiting.
4. *Anxiety* related to diagnosis and uncertain outcome.
5. *Knowledge deficit* regarding care of the child with a shunt and follow-up care.

◆ **D. Nursing care plan/implementation:**

1. Goal: *monitor neurological status.*
   a. Measure head circumference daily, and note any abnormal increase.
   ▶ b. Perform neurological checks at least every 4 hr to monitor for signs of increased ICP.
   c. Report signs of increased ICP **STAT** to physician.
   d. Assist with diagnostic procedures/treatments: *ventricular tap, computed tomography* (CT) scan, etc.
2. Goal: *health teaching to reduce parental anxiety.*
   a. Do preoperative teaching regarding the shunt procedure: stress need to remove excessive CSF to relieve pressure on brain; done as soon as possible after diagnosis is established.

   b. Stress early diagnosis and prompt shunting procedure to minimize the risk of long-term neurological complications.
   c. Offer realistic information regarding prognosis:
      (1) Surgically treated, with continued follow-up care: 80% survival rate.
      (2) Of these survivors, 50% are completely normal and 50% have some degree of neurological disability (such as inattentiveness or hyperactivity).
3. Goal: *provide postoperative shunt care.*
    a. *Position:*
      (1) Flat in bed for 24 hr to prevent subdural hematoma.
      (2) Gradually increase the angle of elevation of HOB, as ordered by surgeon.
      (3) On the *nonoperative side,* to prevent mechanical pressure and obstruction to shunt.
   b. Monitor head circumference daily to note any abnormal increase that might indicate malfunctioning shunt.
   c. Monitor vital signs; monitor for signs of increased ICP.
   d. Monitor for possible complications:
      (1) Infection.
      (2) Malfunction of shunt: increased ICP.
4. Goal: *provide discharge teaching to parents regarding home care of the child with a shunt.*
   a. Stress need for long-term follow-up care.
   b. Discuss feeding techniques, care of skin (especially scalp), need for stimulation.
   c. Prepare parents for shunt revisions to be done periodically as child grows.
   d. Teach parents signs and symptoms of shunt malfunctioning (i.e., of increased ICP or infection) and to report these promptly to physician.
   e. Encourage parents to enroll infant in "early infant stimulation" program to maximize developmental potential.
   f. Stress need to monitor development at frequent intervals, make referrals prn.

◆ **E. Evaluation/outcome criteria:**

1. Neurological functioning is maintained or improved.
2. Adequate nutrition is maintained.
3. No impairment of skin integrity occurs.
4. Parents' anxiety is relieved; they verbalize understanding of how to care for child after discharge.

II. Febrile seizures

A. *Introduction:* Febrile seizures are *transient* neurological disorders of childhood, affecting perhaps as many as 3% of all children. Although the exact cause of febrile seizures remains uncertain, they seem to be a relatively transient problem that occurs exclusively in the presence of high, spiked fevers. Children in the infant and toddler stages (6 mo–3 yr) appear to be most susceptible to febrile seizures, and they are twice as common in boys as in girls. There also

Pediatrics

appears to be an increased susceptibility within families, suggesting a possible genetic predisposition. *Note:* Epilepsy is discussed in **Unit 7.**

◆ **B. Assessment:**
1. History usually reveals presence of URI or gastroenteritis.
2. Occurs with a sudden rise in fever: often spiked and quite high (102°F or higher) vs. prolonged temperature elevation.

◆ **C. Analysis/nursing diagnosis:**
1. *Risk for injury* related to seizures.
2. *Knowledge deficit* related to prevention of future seizures, care of child having a seizure, and possible long-term effects.

◆ **D. Nursing care plan/implementation:**
1. Goal: *reduce fever/prevent further elevation of fever.*
   a. Administer antipyretics, as ordered: acetaminophen only (*not* aspirin).
   b. Use cool, loose, cotton clothes to decrease heat retention.
   c. *Avoid* shivering, which increases metabolic rate and temperature.
   d. Encourage child to drink *cool fluids.*
   e. Monitor temperature hourly.
   f. Minimize stimulation, frustration for child.
2. Goal: *teach parents about care of child who experiences febrile seizure.*
   a. Discuss how to prevent seizures from recurring: best method is to prevent temperature from rising over 102°F (see **Goal 1**).
   b. Discuss how to handle seizures if they do recur: prevent injury, maintain airway, etc.
   c. Answer questions simply and honestly:
      (1) 25% of children with one febrile seizure will experience a recurrence.
      (2) 75% of recurrences occur within 1 year.
      (3) Reassure parents of the benign nature of febrile seizures; 95%–98% of children with febrile seizures do not develop epilepsy or neurological damage.

◆ **E. Evaluation/outcome criteria:**
1. Fever is kept below 102°F; additional seizures are prevented.
2. Parents verbalize their understanding of how to care for child at home.

SELECTED PEDIATRIC EMERGENCIES

For a quick review; use this index to locate content on 19 pediatric emergencies that are covered in this book.

Questions

Select the one best answer for each question, unless otherwise directed.

1. A school-age child with rheumatic fever complains of severe joint pains in the knees and ankles. The best method to provide relief would be for the nurse to:
   1. Give a warm bath or shower.
   2. Apply splints to the affected joints.
   3. Refer the child to physical therapy.
   4. Place a bed cradle over the child's legs.

2. School-age child who is hospitalized is very quiet and seldom talks to the staff. The nurse can best communicate with this child by saying:
   1. "I've noticed you seem very quiet. Is anything troubling you?"
   2. "Let's tell each other a secret; you start by telling me what you are thinking."
   3. "It must be awfully hard to be away from home. Let's call your mom!"
   4. "Draw me some pictures of the things you've seen and done while you've been in the hospital."

3. The nurse reviews a toddler's immunizations with the parents and finds that the child has had all immunizations recommended during the toddler years. The nurse should advise the parents that, at 4–6 years of age, the child should update/receive immunizations for:
   1. MMR (measles, mumps, rubella) and hepatitis B.
   2. Hepatitis B and varicella.
   3. *Haemophilus influenzae* type b and DTaP.
   4. MMR (measles, mumps, rubella), polio, and DTaP.

4. A nurse is working with a group of parents who have infants with various forms of congenital heart disease. The nurse anticipates that the parents will have concerns regarding:
   Select all that apply.
   1. Frequent, severe respiratory infections.
   2. "Slower" development.
   3. Delayed growth.
   4. Feeding difficulties.

5. When performing an infant's admission examination, the nurse notes all the following abnormal findings. Which one is the *most common sign* of heart disease the nurse should assess?
   1. Circumoral cyanosis.
   2. Hypertension.
   3. Diastolic murmur.
   4. Tachycardia.

6. A 7-year-old who has had leukemia for 2 years was in primary remission for 18 months but recently experienced infections, epistaxis, and abdominal petechiae. The doctor suspects the child is no longer in remission and must be admitted to the hospital. In reviewing admitting blood work, the nurse notes

all the following. Which finding should the nurse interpret as the probable cause of the infections?

1. Anemia.
2. Leukopenia.
3. Neutropenia.
4. Thrombocytopenia.

7. A school-age child with rheumatic fever develops heart failure and is placed on digoxin, Lasix, and potassium. The chief purpose for giving potassium is to:
1. Enhance the cardiogenic effect of digoxin.
2. Potentiate the diuretic action of Lasix.
3. Prevent hypokalemia.
4. Pharmacologically induce hyperkalemia.

8. A 12-year-old is admitted to the hospital in status asthmaticus, for the second time. In planning care for this child, the nurse must first assess:
1. What the child knows about asthma.
2. How the child usually does self-care.
3. What the child knows about hospitalization.
4. How the child feels about becoming a teenager.

9. When the nurse begins teaching a teenager with diabetes about insulin, which one fact should be stressed to this teen and the family?
1. Properly controlled dietary management, along with hypoglycemic agents, may eventually be used.
2. Exogenous insulin will be necessary for the rest of the teen's life.
3. Activity level, nutritional intake, and state of health will necessitate daily modifications in the insulin dose.
4. Due to the need for insulin, the teenager should no longer participate in active sports.

10. The nurse performs a Denver Developmental Screening Test (DDST) on a 3-year-old. Which behavior should the nurse expect this child to be capable of doing?
1. Going up stairs on alternate feet.
2. Pedaling a bicycle.
3. Dressing without supervision.
4. Tying shoelaces.

11. The best way for a nurse to perform a DDST on a 9-month-old is to:
1. Take the infant from the mother and ask her to wait in the child's room.
2. Take the infant from the mother and ask her to come with them to the testing area.
3. Briefly talk first with the mother, then take the infant to the testing area alone.
4. Ask the infant's mother to carry the child to the testing area.

12. The parents of a preschool child with leukemia tell the nurse that their daughter frequently has nightmares, and they wonder how to handle this. The nurse would be most correct in advising them to:
1. Comfort her, but leave her in her own bed.
2. Comfort her by bringing her into their bed.
3. Consult a child psychologist to determine why she has recurring sleep disturbances.
4. Encourage the child to draw a picture of her dreams and discuss them with her primary nurse during hospitalization.

13. A lumbar puncture is performed on a child by the doctor. After the procedure, the nurse should position the child:
1. Flat in bed, with no pillow.
2. Flat in bed, with a small pillow.
3. In semi-Fowler's position.
4. Semiprone, with head to the side.

14. When the parents of a newborn with myelomeningocele visit the nursery for the first time, they make no comments about the infant's spinal sac. Instead, they offer many positive observations about size, color, hair, and appearance. The nurse would be most correct in interpreting the parents' behavior as:

1. Attachment.
2. Denial.
3. Immaturity.
4. Love.

15. The mother of a toddler who will have his third, and final, surgical procedure to correct congenital hypospadias questions the need for another surgical procedure while he is still so young. The nurse should stress that:
1. It is the mother's right to refuse surgery at any time.
2. It is in her son's best interest to follow the doctor's recommendations.
3. He can have this third, and final, surgery any time before the onset of puberty.
4. This type of surgery is usually timed to take place between 6 and 18 months of age.

16. The nurse should withhold a 6-year-old's digoxin and notify the physician if the child's pulse was *below*:
1. 80 beats/min.
2. 90 beats/min.
3. 100 beats/min.
4. 110 beats/min.

17. The mother of a hospitalized 3-year-old tells the nurse that he is a very poor eater at home. The best recommendation the nurse can make to increase his nutritional intake would be to:
1. Provide him with a child-size table.
2. Use plastic cups and plates with cartoon characters he likes.
3. Offer him small portions of his favorite foods.
4. Allow him to feed himself.

18. A 3-year-old with hemophilia is to be discharged, and the nurse has completed home care instructions with the child's parents. Which statement by the parents indicates they may have misunderstood the nurse's teaching regarding the care?
1. "If our child gets a fever, we will only give acetaminophen, not aspirin."
2. "We will be sure to supervise our child carefully so that our child doesn't experience another bleeding episode."
3. "I'll order a MedicAlert bracelet for our child as soon as we get home."
4. "It's a relief to know that our younger daughter will not get this disease too."

19. An infant with CHF takes 1.25 oz of formula in 20 minutes. The doctor ordered 2 oz of formula q3h. The *best* action for the nurse to take at this time would be to:
1. Ask the mother to feed the infant when she arrives.
2. Burp the infant and try to stimulate sucking.
3. Continue feeding slowly, allowing as much time as the infant needs to finish.
4. Stop the feeding, and request an order for gavage feedings prn.

20. Between feedings, the nurse should place an infant with CHF in which position?
1. In an infant seat with head elevated.
2. Prone with head turned to side.
3. Supine with head slightly hyperextended.
4. Side-lying with the head of the bed elevated 30 degrees.

21. The doctor attempts to shine a light through a myelomeningocele sac and notes "no transillumination." The nurse should interpret this finding to mean that the sac:
1. Can be easily repaired.
2. Cannot be evaluated by this technique.
3. Contains meninges and CSF.
4. Contains meninges, CSF, and the spinal cord.

22. After administering syrup of ipecac to a toddler, the nurse should also give:
1. Four ounces of warm milk.
2. Activated charcoal powder.
3. As much water as the child will drink.
4. A slice of dry toast.

23. In what position should the nurse place a child in status asthmaticus?
    1. Knee-chest.
    2. High-Fowler's.
    3. Lateral Sims'.
    4. Supine, with neck hyperextended.

24. A teenager hospitalized with diabetes goes to the teen lounge and becomes very boisterous and aggressive, starting a fight with another teen. The *first* question the nurse should consider is:
    1. "Should he be sent to his room?"
    2. "Did he eat breakfast today?"
    3. "What did the other teen do to him?"
    4. "Does he miss his own friends?"

25. The nurse has completed discharge teaching with the parents of an infant with ventricular septal defect (VSD) and CHF. Which one statement by the mother would indicate the need for additional teaching by the nurse?
    1. "I'll be sure to dress our baby in loose-fitting clothes."
    2. "I'll try to keep my house as warm as I can for our baby."
    3. "I'll be at the clinic in 3 days for the appointment."
    4. "I'll put the baby in the playpen at least once a day."

26. A 7-month-old infant is admitted to the pediatrics unit with moderate dehydration secondary to acute gastroenteritis (AGE). The physician writes all the following orders for this infant. Which one should the nurse implement *first*?
    1. Contact precautions.
    2. IV of 5% dextrose in $^1/_3$ normal saline solution at 25 mL/hr.
    3. Urine specific gravity STAT and q4h.
    4. Stool culture every shift × 3.

27. The *best* advice the nurse can give to parents to handle a toddler's temper tantrums would be to:
    1. Allow the toddler to make own choices.
    2. Ignore this behavior.
    3. Change the setting in which they occur.
    4. Give in to the toddler's demands, to nurture autonomy.

28. The parents of a child with epiglottitis tell the nurse that they do not understand what epiglottitis is except that it is "very serious." The nurse's best response would be:
    Select all that apply.
    1. "It is a potentially life-threatening infection."
    2. "It is a form of croup."
    3. "It requires a prolonged stay in the pediatric intensive care unit."
    4. "It can be prevented via immunization."

29. A toddler is admitted to the hospital with classic hemophilia (factor VIII deficiency). Which admission procedure by the nurse would not be the one to do and probably be the most frightening for this child?
    1. Blood pressure.
    2. Rectal temperature.
    3. Urine specimen.
    4. Weight.

30. In writing a nursing care plan for a child with leukemia, the nurse should include all of the following goals. Which goal is *most* important?
    1. Maintain infection-free state.
    2. Prevent injury.
    3. Promote adequate nutrition.
    4. Meet developmental needs.

31. The physician orders sterile moist soaks to a myelomeningocele sac. The major reason for this treatment is to:
    1. Promote comfort.
    2. Prevent infection.
    3. Relieve pressure.
    4. Stimulate neural development.

32. The night before surgery, as he is getting ready for bed, a preschooler asks his father to "check under the bed for monsters." The nurse would be most correct in advising his father to:

1. Ask the child to talk more about these monsters.
2. Leave a light on and let the child check for himself.
3. Make a game of checking under his bed.
4. Tell him that monsters are only make-believe.

33. Following surgery to correct hypospadias, a toddler returns to the unit with a Foley catheter in place. The nurse should expect the drainage to have:
    1. A clear yellow appearance.
    2. Small clots of blood or mucus.
    3. Gross hematuria in moderate amounts.
    4. A brownish tinge.

34. A child with cystic fibrosis is to receive replacement pancreatic enzymes several times daily. The best time for the nurse to plan to administer this medication is:
    1. After every meal or snack.
    2. Between meals and after every snack.
    3. Immediately before meals or snacks.
    4. With meals and before snacks.

35. In addition to administering oxygen, the nurse can also relieve the pain experienced by a teenager in sickle cell crisis by:
    1. Applying warm compresses.
    2. Applying cold compresses.
    3. Performing passive ROM exercises.
    4. Performing ADL as needed.

36. The nurse observes a nursing student fastening an infant's diaper snugly around the abdomen; the infant has CHF. The nurse should:
    1. Ask the student to loosen the diaper.
    2. Do or say nothing, as this is expected behavior for a student.
    3. Loosen the diaper after the student leaves the room.
    4. Praise the student for outstanding attention to detail.

37. Which statement by the parents of a preschooler with nephrosis indicates that they have fully understood the nurse's teaching?
    1. "We will keep him away from other children so he doesn't get a relapse."
    2. "We're so glad this is all over and we don't have to worry any more."
    3. "When we get home, we're going to find it hard to keep him in bed."
    4. "We will watch him for any signs of this starting up again."

38. A child with leukemia is receiving vincristine. The nurse should observe this child closely for the side effect of:
    1. Diarrhea.
    2. Diplopia.
    3. Hemorrhagic cystitis.
    4. Peripheral neuropathy.

39. A 6-year-old with cystic fibrosis refuses to swallow the replacement pancreatic enzyme tablets. The best course of action for the nurse would be to:
    1. Check with the doctor about discontinuing this medication.
    2. Crush the tablets and mix with 1 teaspoon of cold applesauce.
    3. Dissolve the tablets in 4 oz of warm milk.
    4. Offer the child a "special treat" for swallowing the tablets "like a big kid."

40. A school-age child experiences the following signs or symptoms of rheumatic fever. The nurse should plan any interventions based on the knowledge that the only one that may result in *permanent* damage is:
    1. Sydenham's chorea.
    2. Migratory polyarthritis.
    3. Carditis.
    4. Erythema marginatum.

41. The best roommate for a 9-year-old girl with rheumatic fever would be:
    1. An 8-year-old girl with impetigo.
    2. A 9-year-old girl with a tonsillectomy.

3. A 10-year-old girl with a concussion.

4. An 11-year-old girl with a fractured elbow in skeletal traction.

42. The nurse should be aware that the most important nursing diagnosis in caring for a child with diabetes is:
1. *Risk for injury* related to insulin deficiency.
2. *Altered family processes* related to situational crisis (child with chronic disease).
3. *Knowledge deficit* related to care of a child with diabetes.
4. *Altered body image* related to treatment of diabetes.

43. An infant with myelomeningocele is scheduled to have surgery to close the sac. The mother asks the nurse if the infant will be able to move the legs following this operation. The best response for the nurse to make would be:
1. "Not usually, although we can always hope for a miracle."
2. "There is no way to predict. All we can do is watch the baby closely."
3. "No, the surgery is done mainly to prevent infection."
4. "Yes, the surgery will restore the ability to move the legs."

44. The best method to prevent the spread of infection from an infant with AGE to other staff members or visitors would be:
1. Double-bagging all linens.
2. Obtaining stool cultures.
3. Strict handwashing.
4. Wearing disposable gloves.

45. At 7 months of age, an infant exhibits the following skills. The nurse should know that the most recently acquired skill is the ability to:
1. Roll over.
2. Sit up.
3. Bear some weight on legs.
4. Pick up objects with palmar grasp.

46. The most appropriate person to administer a preoperative series of cleansing enemas to a 9-month-old with Hirschsprung's disease would be the:
1. Primary nurse.
2. Mother.
3. Nursing student.
4. Nursing assistant.

47. On admission, the nurse would expect a toddler to demonstrate which two *early* signs of laryngotracheobronchitis (LTB)?
1. Cyanosis and apnea.
2. Hoarseness and croupy cough.
3. Restlessness and tachypnea.
4. Retractions and inspiratory stridor.

48. A diagnosis of bacterial meningitis is confirmed, and the child assumes an opisthotonos position. In which position should the nurse now place this child?
1. Prone.
2. Supine.
3. Side-lying.
4. Trendelenburg.

49. In planning a roommate for a 12-year-old girl who is hospitalized, the nurse should realize that a child of this developmental level will:
1. Prefer another girl her own age.
2. Most likely seek out opportunities to socialize with teenagers.
3. Enjoy being with either a girl or boy, as long as they are the same age.
4. Feel helpful if given the opportunity to look after a slightly younger child.

50. In teaching a teenager how to prevent further episodes of sickle cell crisis, the nurse should stress the need to *avoid:*
1. Moderate emotional stress.
2. Cool weather.
3. Conditions of low oxygen tension.
4. Extra fluid consumption.

51. A new nurse who is being oriented to the Pediatric Unit admits a child with hemophilia. The nurse manager plans to review the new nurse's admission history for the child. The nurse manager anticipates that the new nurse's assessment will include the child's history of:
Select all that apply
1. Excessive hematoma formation.
2. Hemarthrosis.
3. Prolonged bleeding from lacerations.
4. Intracranial bleeding.

52. If a child who was given syrup of ipecac has not vomited within 20 minutes, the nurse should:
1. Manually stimulate the gag reflex, using fingers or back of a spoon.
2. Wait another 20 minutes before doing anything else.
3. Assume the danger is past and no further treatment is needed at this time.
4. Repeat the dose a second time.

53. The physician orders "increase activity as tolerated" for a school-age child with carditis associated with rheumatic fever. After getting the child up into an armchair, the nurse should monitor how well this increase in activity is tolerated by checking the:
1. Apical pulse rate.
2. Breath sounds.
3. Degree of restlessness.
4. Lips and nailbeds.

54. About a week after discharge, a teenager newly diagnosed with diabetes and his mother return to the clinic for a checkup. His mother states, "I'm worried he will make a mistake, so I've been giving him his insulin." The nurse should:
1. Allow the teenager and his mother to work this out on their own.
2. Assist his mother to understand that he must assume this responsibility.
3. Encourage his mother to continue working closely with him.
4. Realize that this is an appropriate response by the mother.

55. The mother of an infant hospitalized with CHF asks the nurse why the infant is sucking on a pacifier. The nurse would be most correct in telling her:
1. "The baby seems to like it."
2. "Most babies prefer a pacifier to their thumb."
3. "This is to keep the baby from crying."
4. "We give all hospitalized babies a pacifier."

56. During the first night in the hospital, a child with hemophilia suffers an episode of epistaxis. In which position should the nurse place this child?
1. Prone, with head turned to side.
2. Semi-Fowler's with two pillows.
3. Sitting up with head tilted backward.
4. Sitting up and leaning forward slightly.

57. The mother of a child with cystic fibrosis tells the nurse that she is thinking of getting pregnant again but is worried that her next child might also have cystic fibrosis. Because her child does have this disease, the nurse should advise this mother that a second child:
1. Could be even more severely affected than her first child.
2. Might also have the disease.
3. Should be "normal," or disease free.
4. Would only carry the trait.

58. A child has had asthma since age 6. In reviewing this child's history, which one factor should the nurse realize may be related to the development of the asthma?
1. Strep throat/tonsillitis at age 2.
2. Eczema at age $3\frac{1}{2}$.
3. Paternal death at age 5.
4. Pneumonia at age 7.

59. Which one behavior should the nurse expect a 5-month-old with CHF to be capable of demonstrating?

1. Rolling over from stomach to back.
2. Sitting with support.
3. Pincer grasp.
4. Bearing some weight on legs.

60. Following surgery to close the myelomeningocele sac, the nurse should place the infant on the:
    1. Abdomen, with head 10 degrees lower than hips.
    2. Abdomen, with head of bed elevated 30 degrees.
    3. Abdomen, with hips 10 degrees lower than head.
    4. Abdomen, flat in bed.

61. Parents of an infant with Hirschsprung's disease ask the nurse how their baby got the disease. The nurse would be most correct in advising them that:
    1. Their infant was born with this condition.
    2. It is the result of the meconium ileus the infant experienced as a newborn.
    3. Their infant spontaneously developed this condition.
    4. It often occurs following the introduction of solid foods due to a genetically inherited metabolic defect.

62. As a toddler recovers from meningitis, for which *long-term* complication should the nurse watch carefully?
    1. Encephalitis.
    2. Hydrocephalus.
    3. Learning disabilities.
    4. Mental retardation.

63. In reviewing what he would do if he experienced a hypoglycemic episode, a teenager correctly states that he would eat a piece of candy or drink a glass of orange juice. The nurse should then instruct him to follow this concentrated sweet with:
    1. A blood glucose level.
    2. A urine dipstick for glucose.
    3. A glass of milk.
    4. 5 U of regular insulin.

64. The mother of a child hospitalized with asthma asks the nurse what causes asthma. The nurse would be most correct in telling her the cause is:
    1. Unknown.
    2. Allergies.
    3. Stress.
    4. Multiple factors.

65. Long-term follow-up care is being planned for a school-age child with rheumatic fever before discharge from the hospital. This *must* include:
    1. Indefinite antibiotic therapy.
    2. Immunization against future attacks.
    3. Cardiac rehabilitation program.
    4. Home schooling.

66. A preschooler has been admitted with a tentative diagnosis of epiglottitis. A medical student wants to look down this child's throat to visualize the epiglottis. The nurse would be most correct in:
    1. Asking the child's mother if she objects to the medical student checking her child.
    2. Telling the medical student that this absolutely cannot be done.
    3. Promising the child a special treat for "opening real wide for the doctor."
    4. Helping restrain the child so the medical student can get a better look.

67. A preschooler with nephrosis is started on prednisone. If the prednisone is having the expected therapeutic effect, the nurse should expect that this child will:
    1. Experience mood swings.
    2. Have sugar in the urine.
    3. Gain weight.
    4. Feel better.

68. In a 2-week-old infant, the earliest sign of hydrocephalus that the nurse would observe is:

1. Bulging anterior fontanel.
2. Increasing head circumference.
3. Shrill, high-pitched cry.
4. Sunset eyes.

69. A child with leukemia who is receiving chemotherapy develops oral ulcers. Three of the following are appropriate nursing interventions; which one is inappropriate?
    1. Encourage the child to use viscous lidocaine (Xylocaine) before meals.
    2. Offer the child a bland, moist, soft diet.
    3. Use a soft toothbrush.
    4. Provide frequent normal saline mouth rinses.

70. A child with nephrosis has a swollen scrotal sac. Which nursing action would be most effective in relieving discomfort?
    1. Apply zinc oxide to scrotum qid.
    2. Cleanse scrotum with warm water only.
    3. Sprinkle medicated powder on scrotum.
    4. Support scrotum with an athletic support.

71. The surgeon orders a preoperative series of cleansing enemas for an infant with Hirschsprung's disease. The nurse should expect the solution ordered for these enemas to be:
    1. Soapsuds enema (SSE).
    2. Normal saline.
    3. Pediatric Fleets.
    4. Tap water.

72. In doing the admission assessment, the nurse should expect to find which signs of dehydration in an infant?
    1. Fever and bradycardia.
    2. Irritability and sunken eyeballs.
    3. Hypotension and anuria.
    4. Dry mucous membranes and bulging anterior fontanel.

73. Prior to administering digoxin to an infant, which pulse would the nurse be most correct in assessing?
    Select all that apply.
    1. Apical.
    2. Radial.
    3. Popliteal.
    4. Femoral.
    5. Brachial.
    6. Pedal.

74. If a toddler were to develop hydrocephalus, which would be the *earliest* sign(s) the nurse would most likely note?
    1. Irritability and poor feeding.
    2. Increasing head circumference.
    3. Headache and diplopia.
    4. Ruptured retinal vessels.

75. The mother of a child with cystic fibrosis asks the nurse if the child will be allowed to participate in any team sports now that he is starting school. The nurse would be most correct in advising her that the child can participate in:
    1. Softball.
    2. Tennis.
    3. Soccer.
    4. Swimming.

76. Parents of a child with sickle cell anemia both have the sickle cell trait. In counseling these parents about having another child, the nurse would be most correct in telling them that future pregnancies will have a:
    1. 1:4 chance of producing a child with sickle cell anemia.
    2. 1:2 chance of producing a child with sickle cell anemia.
    3. 1:4 chance of producing a child with sickle cell trait.
    4. 4:4 chance of producing a child with sickle cell anemia.

77. A child with hemophilia is to receive factor VIII concentrate. During the infusion of this medication, for which potential complications should the nurse plan to observe this child?
    1. Emboli formation.
    2. Fluid volume overload.
    3. Onset of AIDS.
    4. Transfusion reaction.

78. A preschooler with epiglottitis is admitted to the hospital and is to receive Solu-Cortef 100 mg IV q6h. The main purpose for this medication is to:
    1. Provide mild sedation.
    2. Reduce swelling.
    3. Relieve pain.
    4. Treat infection.

79. A child with leukemia is being discharged, and the doctor suggests an immediate return to school. The nurse should be sure to teach the parents to keep this child home if any classmates develop:
    1. Impetigo.
    2. Strep throat.
    3. Pneumonia.
    4. Chickenpox.

80. In doing discharge teaching with the parents of an infant with VSD and CHF, which one visitor should the nurse discourage from touching or holding this infant?
    1. An aunt, who has lupus.
    2. A grandmother, who has a slight cold.
    3. The father, who is a drug addict.
    4. A 3-year-old sister, who is in nursery school.

81. In monitoring a toddler for response to syrup of ipecac, the nurse should base any actions on the knowledge that ipecac is potentially:
    1. Cardiotoxic.
    2. Hepatotoxic.
    3. Nephrotoxic.
    4. Neurotoxic.

82. A mother who lost her first-born to SIDS tells the nurse that she plans to breastfeed her second infant to prevent this from happening again. The nurse should base any response on the knowledge that:
    1. The risk of SIDS is the same however infants are fed.
    2. Breastfeeding *does* seem to prevent SIDS.
    3. SIDS occurs less frequently in infants who are bottle fed.
    4. Breastfeeding is contraindicated for *siblings* of infants who died from SIDS.

83. Normally, an infant's birth weight doubles by age 6 mo and triples by age 1 yr. By what age should the nurse expect the birth weight to *quadruple*?
    1. 18 mo.
    2. 2 yr.
    3. $2^1/_2$ yr.
    4. 3 yr.

84. A mother asks the nurse how tall her child will be when grown up. What answer should the nurse offer?
    1. "This is virtually impossible to predict."
    2. "It will be double the child's height at 2 years of age."
    3. "It will be triple the child's height at 18 months of age."
    4. "Add 2 feet to the child's height at 4 years of age."

85. In teaching principles of poison control to a group of mothers, the nurse would be most correct in stressing that the age group most likely to suffer from accidental ingestions is:
    1. 6–18 mo.
    2. 12 mo–$2^1/_2$ yr.
    3. 2–4 yr.
    4. 3–5 yr.

86. In deciding which *one* type of accident prevention to discuss *first* with the parents of a toddler, the nurse should base the choice on the knowledge that most deaths in children under age 3 are caused by:
    1. Aspiration/suffocation.
    2. Falls.
    3. Motor vehicles.
    4. Poisonings.

87. The following four children are clients in the pediatric unit. Which one should the nurse anticipate will be *most* affected by separation from parents?
    1. A 6-week-old with pyloric stenosis.
    2. A 19-month-old with salicylate poisoning.
    3. A $3^1/_2$-year-old with hypospadias.
    4. A 5-year-old with hemophilia.

88. In assessing the development of a 5-year-old, the nurse would not expect the child to be able to:
    1. Name primary colors.
    2. Count to 100.
    3. Know the days of the week.
    4. Give telephone number and address.

89. The RN is supervising a nurse's aide/UAP who is caring for a child with a multidrug-resistant respiratory infection. Which action by the aide/UAP would be unsafe and would require the RN's immediate attention?
    1. The aide/UAP wears a gown and gloves when entering the child's room.
    2. The aide/UAP removes the gown and gloves before leaving the child's room.
    3. The aide/UAP leaves the sphygmomanometer, thermometer, and stethoscope in the child's room, out of the child's reach.
    4. The aide/UAP washes her hands after removing her gloves, and then leaves the child's room to care for another child in the next room.

90. An adolescent is admitted to the pediatric unit in sickle cell crisis with severe pain in the legs and abdomen. The adolescent asks the nurse why the pediatrician ordered oxygen when there is no trouble breathing. The nurse would be most correct in stating that the main therapeutic effect of oxygen is to: *Select all that apply.*
    1. Reverse sickling of RBCs.
    2. Prevent further sickling.
    3. Prevent respiratory complications.
    4. Increase the oxygen-carrying capacity of RBCs.

91. The RN assigns an LPN/LVN to care for a child with Hirschsprung's disease; the child's abdomen is grossly distended. The RN directs the LPN/LVN to measure the child's abdominal girth. Which action by the LPN/LVN would require the RN's intervention and further direction? The LPN/LVN:
    1. Uses a cloth tape to measure the child's abdominal girth.
    2. Leaves the tape in place after measuring the child's abdominal girth.
    3. Measures the child's abdominal girth at the umbilicus.
    4. Pulls the tape snug, but not tight, around the abdomen when measuring girth.

92. A child with a diagnosis of "rule out meningitis" is admitted to the pediatric unit. The RN assigns this child to an LPN/LVN. Admitting orders include the following: bedrest with vital signs q2h; CBC with chemistry and electrolytes; gentamicin 80 mg IVPB q8h; liquid diet as tolerated; nasopharyngeal culture; and droplet precautions. In what sequence should the RN instruct the LPN/LVN to implement these orders?
    1. Put the child to bed and check vitals, take culture, draw blood, start antibiotics, initiate droplet precautions, order diet.
    2. Offer fluids, draw blood, take culture, put the child to bed and check vitals, start antibiotics, initiate droplet precautions.
    3. Initiate droplet precautions, put child to bed and check vitals, take a culture, start antibiotics, draw blood, order diet.
    4. Draw blood, start antibiotics, initiate droplet precautions, take culture, offer fluids, put child to bed and check vitals.

93. The nursing student is teaching an adolescent who is newly diagnosed with diabetes about the disease and its treatment. Which statement by the student would require the RN's intervention?
    1. "When you use the vial of insulin marked 'U80,' it means that there are 80 units of insulin in that vial."
    2. "Be sure to check in with your doctor right away if you

develop a fever or have an infection. You could develop a complication called ketoacidosis."

3. "When you are getting ready to give yourself insulin, first draw up the short-acting insulin and then draw up the intermediate-acting insulin."

4. "You should check your blood sugar four times a day, just like the MD ordered. The supplies are easily transportable and can go with you wherever you go."

94. The RN instructs the aide to give a child with eczema a bath. Which action by the aide would require the RN to provide additional supervision? The aide:
   1. Adds bath oil to the water.
   2. Bathes the child for 15–20 minutes.
   3. Provides toys for water play.
   4. Applies Lubriderm to the skin immediately after the bath.

95. The nurse is caring for all of the following children. Which child should the nurse recognize is at the highest risk for fluid and electrolyte imbalance?
   1. Infant with acute gastroenteritis.
   2. Toddler with lead poisoning.
   3. Preschooler with leukemia.
   4. School-age child with multiple trauma.

96. The RN should instruct the LPN/LVN or UAP caring for a child with PKU to be sure *not* to give this child:
   1. Green grapes.
   2. Diet soda.
   3. Cheerios.
   4. Cranberry apple juice.

97. An RN can safely delegate three of the following tasks to an LPN/LVN caring for a child with Down syndrome. Which one task should the RN perform personally and not delegate to an LPN/LVN?
   1. Transporting the child to the cardiac catheterization lab.
   2. Taking the child's vital signs, including blood pressure.
   3. Listening to the child's breath sounds bilaterally.
   4. Assisting the child to eat meals and snacks.

98. A nurse's aide/UAP is working with a group of children in the playroom. Which action by the UAP would require the RN to intervene?
   1. The UAP offers a pacifier to an infant who is NPO.
   2. The UAP opens a can of Play-Doh and gives it to a toddler.
   3. The UAP stops a preschooler with terminal cancer from pulling on the braids of another child who is ready to be discharged.
   4. The UAP tells a school-age child that he is too big to be crying for his parents.

99. A nursing student has been assigned to plan the prehospitalization teaching for a group of preschoolers having elective surgery. The nursing student's preceptor should correct the teaching plan if it included which of the following?
   1. Make a list of the things the children could bring from home.
   2. Show the children a video describing activities that will take place during their hospital stay.
   3. Provide a detailed explanation to the children of what they will experience during preadmission testing.
   4. Give the children a tour of the ambulatory surgery unit, followed by a light snack and a chance to talk with the staff.

100. A child with severe pain asks for pain medication. The team caring for this child includes an RN, an LPN/LVN, and a UAP. After assessing the child, the RN administers the pain medication. Who should subsequently evaluate the effectiveness of the pain medication?
   1. The RN only.
   2. The RN and the LPN/LVN.
   3. The LPN/LVN and the UAP.
   4. All of the members of the team caring for this child.

Answers/Rationales/Tips

1. **(4)** For a child experiencing migratory polyarthritis secondary to rheumatic fever, even the weight of a single sheet can cause excruciating pain; therefore, a bed cradle will help keep the linens off the child's joints and provide symptomatic relief. This child is most likely on bed rest, thus making a bath or shower (**Answer 1**) out of the question. Splints or a referral to physical therapy (**Answers 2, 3**) is unnecessary, because this type of arthritis causes no permanent deformities.

> **TEST-TAKING TIP**—Comfort is the priority of care, because of pain associated with migratory polyarthritis.
> **IMP, ANL, 1, PEDS, PhI, Basic Care and Comfort**

2. **(4)** Projective techniques seem to work best with school-age children in getting them to share their thoughts, feelings, and experiences. Direct questioning (**Answer 1**) often proves too threatening, causing the child to become even quieter. Challenging the child directly to "tell secrets" (**Answer 2**) is also too threatening and will likely cause the child to refuse to speak about anything. Calling the child's mother (**Answer 3**) will not necessarily assist the child to communicate with the nurse.

> **TEST-TAKING TIP**—Select the age-appropriate, nonthreatening approach. When in doubt, note the pattern in responses: three are verbal and one is nonverbal (draw). Choose the method that is different.
> **IMP, APP, 7, PEDS, PsI, Psychosocial Integrity**

3. **(4)** At preschool age (4–6 yr), the child should receive immunizations for DTaP, IPV, and MMR. MMR (**Answer 1**) is correct, but hepatitis B is not. Hepatitis (**Answer 2**) is completed by *18 mo*, as is varicella. *Haemophilus influenzae* (**Answer 3**) is completed by *15 mo*, although DTaP is correct.

> **TEST-TAKING TIP**—The best answer is based on knowing the recommended schedule of immunizations.
> **IMP, COM, 1, PEDS, HPM, Health Promotion and Maintenance**

4. **(1, 2, 3, 4)** **Answer 1** is correct because these infants usually have a weak suck and altered cardiopulmonary dynamics, causing the infants to be at risk for aspiration, pneumonia and various respiratory infections. **Answer 2** is correct because these infants usually have a weak suck, causing the infants to have feeding difficulties and delayed weight gain leading to developmental delays. **Answer 3** is correct because these infants usually have a weak suck, causing the infants to have feeding difficulties and delayed weight gain leading to delayed growth. **Answer 4** is correct because these infants usually have a weak suck, causing the infants to have feeding difficulties.

> **TEST-TAKING TIP**—"Feeding difficulties" is the key to the correct answers; it relates to all of the other responses so that they are all correct.
> **AN, APP, 6, PEDS, PhI, Basic Care and Comfort**

KEY TO CODES FOLLOWING RATIONALES *NURSING PROCESS:*

AS, assessment; **AN,** analysis; **PL,** plan; **IMP,** implementation; **EV,** evaluation. *Cognitive level:* **COM,** comprehension; **APP,** application; **ANL,** analysis. *Category of human function:* **1,** protective; **2,** sensory-perceptual; **3,** comfort, rest, activity, and mobility; **4,** nutrition; **5,** growth and development; **6,** fluid-gas transport; **7,** psychosocial-cultural; **8,** elimination. *Client need:* **SECE,** safe, effective care environment; **HPM,** health promotion/maintenance; **PsI,** psychosocial integrity; **PhI,** physiological integrity. (Client subneed appears after Client Need code.) See appendices for full explanation.

5. **(4)** The majority of infants with CHD have tachycardia, or a heart rate above 160 beats/min; this is often the *first* sign of CHD that the nurse can assess. Circumoral cyanosis (**Answer 1**), hypertension (**Answer 2**), and diastolic murmur (**Answer 3**) all *may or may not* be present, depending on the type and severity of the defect.

> **TEST-TAKING TIP**—Note the use of the words "most common sign" in this question. Eliminate the three others that *may not* be present.
> **AS, COM, 6, PEDS, PhI, Physiological Adaptation**

6. **(3)** Neutropenia is an abnormal decrease in the number of neutrophils, the specific type of WBC responsible for phagocytosis and bacterial destruction; as such, the infection in a child with leukemia is most commonly related to neutropenia. These children may also suffer from anemia (**Answer 1**), leukopenia (**Answer 2**), or thrombocytopenia (**Answer 4**), although these blood dyscrasias will result in other signs or symptoms of leukemia.

> **TEST-TAKING TIP**—Look for the cause that is *directly* related.
> **AN, ANL, 1, PEDS, PhI, Reduction of Risk Potential**

7. **(3)** Children receiving digoxin in addition to Lasix are particularly prone to developing hypokalemia, which can result in digoxin toxicity and potentially fatal cardiac dysrhythmias. Potassium supplements are frequently administered to avoid this problem rather than for any of the other reasons cited here (**Answers 1, 2, 4**).

> **TEST-TAKING TIP**—It logically follows that if K$^+$ is given, the purpose is to *replace* K$^+$ and therefore to avoid *low* K$^+$.
> **AN, APP, 1, PEDS, PhI, Pharmacological and Parenteral Therapies**

8. **(3)** In working with children in hospitals, the most important factor for the nurse to *assess first* is the child's experience with illness and hospitalization. This is of special importance with this child, who has been hospitalized previously. *After this* most important factor, the nurse would continue the admitting assessment by determining what the child knows about asthma (**Answer 1**), how the child usually does self-care (**Answer 2**), and how the child feels about becoming a teenager (**Answer 4**).

> **TEST-TAKING TIP**—A major principle of teaching-learning is to start where the client is.
> **AN, ANL, 7, PEDS, PsI, Psychosocial Integrity**

9. **(2)** Because the beta cells of the islets of Langerhans of the pancreas will never again produce a sufficient quantity of insulin, this teenager will remain dependent on insulin injections (exogenous insulin) for the rest of the teenager's life. Clients with type 1 diabetes can never rely on hypoglycemic agents to control diabetes (**Answer 1**), because these drugs work by stimulating the pancreas, and in this case the stimulation would have absolutely no effect. *Daily* modifications generally would not be necessary (**Answer 3**), although *periodic* adjustments in insulin dosage would be needed as this teenager grows. The teenager can continue to participate in sports (**Answer 4**), but should be taught to take some extra foods on those days when actively participating in sports.

> **TEST-TAKING TIP**—To pick the most theoretically correct answer, pull apart the key points about a *time* element: eventually, *for life*, daily, never.
> **IMP, APP, 4, PEDS, PhI, Physiological Adaptation**

10. **(1)** Three-year-olds should be able to coordinate the brain and gross motor activity necessary to go up stairs using alternate feet. They should also be able to pedal a Big Wheel or a tricycle but *not* a bicycle (**Answer 2**). Three-year-olds should also be able to get dressed *with* supervision but not without it (**Answer 3**). They should not be ready to master tying shoelaces (**Answer 4**) for another year or two.

> 💡 **TEST-TAKING TIP**—Remember, *three years = three wheels;* a 3-year-old should be capable of pedaling a tricycle.
> **AN, COM, 6, PEDS, HPM, Health Promotion and Maintenance**

11. **(4)** The instruction manual of the DDST clearly states that the parent should accompany the infant who is to have the DDST and that the examiner should do everything possible to establish rapport with the parent and the infant. With a 9-month-old, this should include allowing the parent to hold the infant rather than separating them for the purpose of testing (**Answers 1, 2, 3**).

> **TEST-TAKING TIP**—Fear of strangers peaks at 8–9 months of age (i.e., keep the mother and infant together). Therefore, eliminate **Answers 1, 2, and 3**.
> **IMP, APP, 5, PEDS, HPM, Health Promotion and Maintenance**

12. **(1)** Most psychologists would recommend that a child be offered comfort in the form of a hug, kiss, or cuddle; however, the child should be left in his or her own bed to avoid overdependence on the parents. (**Answer 2**). For the preschool child, nightmares are a common occurrence and can be accepted as a *normal* part of growth and development; therefore, no professional intervention is necessary at this time (**Answer 3**). It could be difficult for this preschool child to draw a picture of her dreams (**Answer 4**).

> **TEST-TAKING TIP**—Focus on two options with "comfort," which are better than "consult" or "draw." As a general rule, children should sleep in their own beds, not with parents.
> **IMP, APP, 5, PEDS, PsI, Psychosocial Integrity**

13. **(1)** The best position after a spinal tap is flat in bed, with no pillow at all because of headaches related to the loss of CSF during the spinal tap; until the fluid is naturally replaced by the body, a flat position will minimize cerebral irritation and minimize headache; thus, (**Answer 2**) is incorrect. Elevating the HOB (**Answer 3**) will increase headache and is not recommended. There is no need to place the child in a semiprone position (**Answer 4**) at this time.

> **TEST-TAKING TIP**—Focus on two options that are "flat." "Flat" is "flat," meaning *no* pillow. Following a spinal tap, the position should be *flat* in bed.
> **IMP, APP, 1, PEDS, PhI, Reduction of Risk Potential**

14. **(2)** The usual response to the birth of a "defective" infant is denial, which often manifests in the parents' "refusing" to acknowledge the problem; this is a normal response, at least initially. The parents' comments about their infant, in view of this serious defect, should not be interpreted as attachment (**Answer 1**), immaturity (**Answer 3**), or love (**Answer 4**).

> **TEST-TAKING TIP**—*Denying* (in this case, the obvious physical problem) is one of the most commonly seen defense mechanisms.
> **EV, ANL, 7, PEDS, PsI, Psychosocial Integrity**

15. **(4)** The corrective surgery for hypospadias is usually timed to be completed before the child develops body image and castration anxiety, by 18 months of age. Developmental and

psychological factors thus play a crucial role in the timing of this surgery, and other explanations (**Answers 1, 2, 3**) are either incorrect or inappropriate for this child.

> **TEST-TAKING TIP**—Note the two options with "time" (**3, 4**). Select the option that is age specific, (**4**) not "anytime" (**3**).
> **IMP, APP, 8, PEDS, SECE, Management of Care**

16. (**1**) The lower limit of a normal pulse rate for a 6-year-old is 70 to 100 beats/min; the nurse would be most correct in withholding the child's digoxin and notifying the physician if the pulse were below 80. A pulse rate of 90–110 (**Answers 2, 3, 4**) would be considered within normal limits for a 6-year-old, and the nurse would be correct in administering the medication as ordered.

> **TEST-TAKING TIP**—The nurse should know approximate pulse rate norms for children of varying age groups. Key word is *withhold* with age-relevant norm for bradycardia.
> **EV, COM, 6, PEDS, PhI, Pharmacological Therapy**

17. (**4**) For a child just leaving the toddler period of autonomy and just entering the preschool period of initiative, the best suggestion to improve his nutritional intake would be to allow the child to feed himself. Other suggestions would supplement and enhance this primary consideration (**Answers 1, 2, 3**).

> **TEST-TAKING TIP**—The major developmental task of the toddler is autonomy; the major developmental task of the preschooler is initiative. Look at the verbs: "provide," "use," "offer," and "allow." Choose "allow."
> **IMP, APP, 5, PEDS, HPM, Health Promotion and Maintenance**

18. (**2**) It would be impossible to supervise a child with hemophilia so carefully that any other bleeding episodes would be prevented; furthermore, to attempt to do so would cause the parents to restrict the child totally, resulting in extreme overprotection. An acceptable alternative response would be to prevent "major" episodes of bleeding or to promptly recognize signs of a bleeding episode that would require medical intervention. The other statements (**Answers 1, 3, 4**) *are all correct* responses by the parents, indicating they have probably *understood* the nurse's teaching regarding the child's care.

> **TEST-TAKING TIP**—Note the use of the word "misunderstood" in this question, meaning look for the *incorrect* statement.
> **EV, APP, 6, PEDS, HPM, Health Promotion and Maintenance**

19. (**4**) Infants with CHF should be given about 15–20 min per feeding; if the infant is unable to finish the feeding, or if the infant becomes cyanotic or experiences respiratory distress during the feeding, gavage feeding should be used to avoid exhausting the infant and possibly precipitating an episode of apnea. No attempts should be made to continue the feeding (**Answers 1, 2, 3**).

> **TEST-TAKING TIP**—Three options continue the feeding and one option stops the feeding. In this case, choose the option that is different.
> **IMP, ANL, 4, PEDS, PhI, Basic Care and Comfort**

20. (**1**) As with an adult with CHF, the infant should be positioned in a chair/infant seat, in semi-Fowler's position, to provide for maximum expansion of the lungs and to assist the heart. Placing the infant on the stomach (**Answer 2**) might be an acceptable second choice, providing the infant can tolerate this position. The infant should never be placed on the back (**Answer 3**), even with the head slightly hyperextended,

because of the possibility of aspiration and other respiratory complications. A side-lying position (**Answer 4**) would not allow for maximum expansion of the lungs; an infant seat is more appropriate.

> **TEST-TAKING TIP**—Picture the various positions and eliminate **Answers 2** and **3**. Cardiac rest is best promoted by a semi-Fowler's (i.e., head elevated) position, regardless of the infant's age or condition.
> **IMP, APP, 6, PEDS, PhI, Basic Care and Comfort**

21. (**4**) Transillumination, or the procedure of shining a light through the sac, is the usual means for evaluating the contents of the sac. When there is "no transillumination" (the light cannot shine through the sac), this indicates the presence of solid material, or the spinal cord, within the sac. Thus **Answers 2** and **3** are incorrect. Transillumination has no bearing on determining whether the sac can be easily repaired (**Answer 1**).

> **TEST-TAKING TIP**—Break up the word *transillumination* into its respective parts, *trans* and *illumination*, to derive its meaning. Choose the option that is most inclusive (**Answer 3** is included in **Answer 4**).
> **AN, APP, 2, PEDS, PhI, Reduction of Risk Potential**

22. (**3**) Syrup of ipecac is an emetic used to induce vomiting following ingestion of a harmful substance; the usual dose in children is 15 mL PO followed by at least 200 mL of water. The water is thought to enhance the emetic effect of ipecac and stimulate emptying of the stomach, thus ridding the body of the harmful substance. Activated charcoal (**Answer 2**) will *neutralize* the emetic effect and should *not* be given with ipecac, although in some cases it may be given *after* vomiting has occurred. Milk or toast (**Answers 1, 4**) has *little or no effect* and will neither help nor harm; however, if the child does vomit, they may increase the risk of aspiration.

> **TEST-TAKING TIP**—Ipecac should always be administered with water.
> **IMP, APP, 1, PEDS, PhI, Pharmacological and Parenteral Therapies**

23. (**2**) The preferred position for a child with asthma is high Fowler's, or sitting up straight, which allows for maximum expansion of the lungs. Other positions would *not* allow for the maximum expansion of the lungs (**Answers 1, 3, 4**) and would only contribute to this child's hypoxia.

> **TEST-TAKING TIP**—A full upright position allows for maximum expansion of the lungs.
> **IMP, COM, 6, PEDS, PhI, Basic Care and Comfort**

24. (**2**) Juveniles with diabetes (type 1 diabetes) are extremely brittle, or difficult to control, and prone to episodes of hypoglycemia or ketoacidosis. If this teenager were to experience a hypoglycemic episode, the earliest symptoms would often be behavioral: irritability, personality changes, etc. If this teen becomes disruptive, the nurse should first ask if he has eaten his breakfast, how much he ate, and when; other areas (**Answers 1, 3, 4**) would be appropriate to explore *after* this primary consideration.

> **TEST-TAKING TIP**—An underlying physiological cause of a teenager's behavior should be explored first, before looking at behavioral considerations.
> **AN, ANL, 4, PEDS, PhI, Physiological Adaptation**

25. (**2**) Extremes of temperatures, either too warm or too cold, should be avoided for infants with CHD, because this increases the body's demand for oxygen, thus increasing the workload of the heart. The mother would need no further

teaching if she *correctly* stated that this infant should be dressed in loose-fitting clothing (**Answer 1**), should be brought back to the clinic for regularly scheduled appointments (**Answer 3**), and should be placed in a safe play area to stimulate development (**Answer 4**).

> **TEST-TAKING TIP**—Note the use of the phrase "need for additional teaching" in this question (i.e., look for the incorrect statement).
> **EV, ANL, 6, PEDS, HPM, Health Promotion and Maintenance**

26. (**1**) With an infant with a potentially contagious infection such as AGE, the first priority is protection of the nurse and others by observing appropriate infection control measures, including contact precautions. Other interventions can *then* be safely implemented without risk of cross-contamination (**Answers 2, 3, 4**).

> **TEST-TAKING TIP**—Infection control is always a priority of care.
> **AN, ANL, 1, PEDS, SECE, Safety and Infection Control**

27. (**2**) The general recommendation to make to parents on how to handle temper tantrums is to ignore this behavior. If a parent allows a child to make a choice (**Answer 1**) and then does not follow through with this choice either because of personal preference or because the choice is unsafe, tantrums will increase. Changing settings (**Answer 3**) is often a catalyst for a tantrum as the child is moved from one area to another (e.g., from the park to home). Giving in to a toddler's demands (**Answer 4**) is unrealistic; parents should offer only allowable choices to their toddler and then allow the toddler to follow through with these choices.

> **TEST-TAKING TIP**—Paying attention to a temper tantrum will reinforce this behavior.
> **IMP, APP, 5, PEDS, HPM, Health Promotion and Maintenance**

28. (**1, 2, and 4**) Answer 1 is correct because epiglottitis is a bacterial infection of the epiglottis, resulting in rapid airway swelling and obstruction. Without prompt, aggressive treatment it can progress rapidly and result in respiratory arrest within 6–8 hours of onset. **Answer 2** is correct because epiglottitis is a form of croup. Croup syndromes are usually described according to the primary anatomic area affected (i.e. epiglottitis/supraglottitis, laryngotracheobronchitis, and acute spasmodic laryngitis/spasmodic croup). **Answer 4** is correct because epiglottitis can be prevented via immunization. The responsible organism for epiglottitis is usually *H. influenzae*. Therefore, the American Academy of Pediatrics recommends that all children, beginning at 2 months of age, receive the *H. influenzae* type B conjugate vaccine series. **Answer 3** is incorrect because, although epiglottitis is medical emergency and requires immediate attention, usually in the form of a tracheostomy or intubation, the epiglottal swelling usually decreases after 24 hours of antibiotic therapy, and the epiglottitis is near normal by the third day. A prolonged stay in the pediatric intensive care unit is usually not necessary.

> **TEST-TAKING TIP:** Of all of the respiratory condition of childhood, epiglottitis is the most *rapidly* progressive; *quickly* life threatening and *quick* to recover; hence, a *short* stay in the pediatric intensive care unit (PICU).
> **IMP, APP, 6, PEDS, PhI, Physiological Adaptation**

29. (**2**) Toddlers typically fear those procedures that are "intrusive," that is, where something goes into their bodies. Therefore, a rectal temperature would most likely evoke the most anxiety in a toddler. There is also the danger of bleeding

in a child with hemophilia if rectal temperatures are done. Generally, a toddler would be relatively cooperative with getting weighed (**Answer 4**) and giving a urine specimen (**Answer 3**), although having blood pressure taken might also be somewhat threatening (**Answer 1**).

> **TEST-TAKING TIP**—Note the patterns in the answers: three options are nonintrusive procedures, one option *is* intrusive—and therefore most frightening (and dangerous due to bleeding).
> **AN, ANL, 7, PEDS, HPM, Health Promotion and Maintenance**

30. (**1**) The leading cause of morbidity and mortality in children with leukemia is infection; therefore, preventing infection is the most important nursing care plan goal. Preventing injury (**Answer 2**), promoting adequate nutrition (**Answer 3**), and meeting developmental needs (**Answer 4**) are less important goals for the child with leukemia.

> **TEST-TAKING TIP**—Infection control is a high *priority* of care when the immune system is compromised (e.g., in leukemia).
> **PL, ANL, 1, PEDS, SECE, Safety and Infection Control**

31. (**2**) The chief purpose of the moist soaks is to prevent tears or leaks in the sac, which could lead to infection, the number one cause of death during the neonatal period. Promoting comfort (**Answer 1**) and relieving pressure (**Answer 3**) are not reasons for ordering moist soaks for this infant. It is *not* possible to stimulate neural development (**Answer 4**), which is permanently and irreversibly arrested before birth.

> **TEST-TAKING TIP**—Look at the verbs: "promote," "prevent," "relieve," and "stimulate." Choose "prevent."
> **AN, COM, 1, PEDS, SECE, Safety and Infection Control**

32. (**3**) By making a game of "checking for monsters," a potentially frightening situation is relieved, and the child may even begin to realize that there "really" are no monsters. Asking the child to talk about his monsters (**Answer 1**) may make him believe they are real and that his father also believes in them. It would be too frightening to the child to have to look for these monsters by himself (**Answer 2**). Telling a preschooler that his fantasies are not real (**Answer 4**) would not be enough to convince him and might make him become even more convinced they are real.

> **TEST-TAKING TIP**—Preschoolers are in the age of fantasy or magical thinking; therefore choose **Answer 3**, "make a game."
> **IMP, APP, 5, PEDS, HPM, Health Promotion and Maintenance**

33. (**1**) The surgical repair for hypospadias is done on the urethra primarily and also on the urethral meatus. Postoperatively, a urinary drainage apparatus (Foley or suprapubic) will be in place, and the urine is expected to have a clear yellow appearance. There should normally be no blood or mucus (**Answers 2, 3, 4**), which would indicate hemorrhage or infection is present.

> **TEST-TAKING TIP**—Choose the option that is different: three options indicate a problem, one says it is OK (yellow urine is normal).
> **EV, APP, 8, PEDS, PhI, Reduction of Risk Potential**

34. (**3**) To be most effective, pancreatic enzymes should be administered immediately before every meal and every snack; this will facilitate the absorption of fats and proteins contained within the meal. The enzymes will have little or no therapeutic value if given at other times (**Answers 1, 2, 4**).

TEST-TAKING TIP—Key word is "replacement" of what is missing in CF; therefore, the best *time* to aid fat absorption is *before* eating.
PL, COM, 6, PEDS, PhI, Pharmacological and Parenteral Therapies

35. **(1)** Warmth causes vasodilation, thus relieving the occlusion of small vessels and preventing tissue damage. Cold (**Answer 2**) would never be used, because it causes vasoconstriction. Performing ROM exercises (**Answer 3**) or ADL (**Answer 4**) would not relieve pain.

TEST-TAKING TIP—Focus on two options that are contradictory: warmth → vasodilation; cold → vasoconstriction. Occluded blood vessels need vasodilation measures.
IMP, APP, 6, PEDS, PhI, Reduction of Risk Potential

36. **(1)** An infant with CHF should wear loose-fitting clothes, including diapers, to avoid pressure on the abdominal organs, which could impinge on the diaphragm and impede respiratory effort. The nursing student should loosen the diaper and should know the rationale for this action as well. The nurse should not take care of this after the student leaves (**Answer 3**), because the student will repeat the mistake without the nurse's intervention; in addition, pinning the diaper snugly is inappropriate for an infant with CHF (**Answers 2, 4**), and the nurse has the final responsibility for the care this infant receives.

TEST-TAKING TIP—Any child with CHF should wear *loose*-fitting clothes.
EV, APP, 6, PEDS, PhI, Reduction of Risk Potential

37. **(4)** Nephrosis is characterized by periods of exacerbations and remissions that occur throughout the childhood years. The child's parents should watch him closely for exacerbations, which should be reported promptly to the physician. The child should be encouraged to play with other children, not to stay away from them (**Answer 1**) to avoid feelings of social isolation. It is *not* "over" (**Answer 2**), and the child will need to be watched carefully for periods of exacerbation. Once the child is discharged, he generally will not need to remain in bed (**Answer 3**) but rather can convalesce at home with alternating periods of activity and rest.

TEST-TAKING TIP—Note the use of the words "fully understood" in this question; therefore, use a true-false approach to eliminate the three false statements.
EV, APP, 8, PEDS, HPM, Health Promotion and Maintenance

38. **(4)** Vincristine is an antineoplastic *Vinca* alkaloid, which causes numbness, tingling, footdrop, paresthesia, etc. In addition, vincristine may also cause constipation, *not* diarrhea (**Answer 1**). Hemorrhagic cystitis (**Answer 3**) may be caused by cyclophosphamide (Cytoxan), *not* vincristine. Vincristine does *not* cause visual changes (**Answer 2**).

TEST-TAKING TIP—Know the major side effects of vincristine (peripheral neuropathy).
IMP, COM, 6, PEDS, PhI, Pharmacological and Parenteral Therapies

39. **(2)** Pancreatic enzymes *are* enzymes; as such, they break down whatever food or liquid they are mixed with. However, for maximum therapeutic effect, the enzymatic action should be delayed until the medication reaches the stomach. The best food to mix with pancreatic enzyme tablets is cold applesauce. The applesauce should be cold because cold delays the enzymatic action, which is most effective at 98.6°F. Applesauce is used because of its high fiber content, which also delays the enzymatic action of the medication. Any other foods or liquids

the pancreatic enzymes might be mixed with (**Answer 3**) would be less than ideal. Pancreatic enzyme tablets cannot simply be discontinued (**Answer 1**) because a child has difficulty swallowing them; this medication must be taken for the rest of the child's life. It is not appropriate to bribe a child (**Answer 4**) with a reward for desired behavior; children should never be bribed or threatened into taking medication.

TEST-TAKING TIP—Focus on the two options with contradictory terms: cold vs. warm. Cold has the desired effect of delaying enzymatic action.
IMP, ANL, 4, PEDS, PhI, Pharmacological and Parenteral Therapies

40. **(3)** Carditis can lead to permanent, irreversible cardiac damage, specifically, mitral value stenosis. The other manifestations of rheumatic fever (**Answers 1, 2, 4**) are *transient* and do not leave any permanent effects.

TEST-TAKING TIP—Key word is "permanent." Choose the option pertaining to the *heart*.
PL, APP, 1, PEDS, PhI, Physiological Adaptation

41. **(4)** A child with rheumatic fever will be in the hospital for a relatively longer time and will be confined to bed most of the time. The ideal roommate would be another child of the same sex and same developmental level who will also be in the hospital for some time and confined to bed. The best choice is the young girl with the fractured elbow, who will be in skeletal traction and also on bedrest. The child with a tonsillectomy (**Answer 2**) or the child with a concussion (**Answer 3**) will most likely be in the hospital for a very short time and will be out of bed. The child with impetigo, caused by streptococcus (**Answer 1**), would be a most unsatisfactory roommate for this child, because she might reinfect her with strep.

TEST-TAKING TIP—The ideal roommate for any child is another child of the same sex and developmental level.
IMP, ANL, 1, PEDS, HPM, Health Promotion and Maintenance

42. **(1)** The most important nursing diagnosis relates to physiological integrity (i.e., maintaining a normal blood-sugar level). Other diagnoses (**Answers 2, 3, 4**) would be correct but not necessarily of primary concern.

TEST-TAKING TIP—Physiological integrity is always a priority of care.
EV, APP, 4, PEDS, PhI, Physiological Adaptation

43. **(3)** Parents often hope that the surgery done to close the sac will also help the infant move the legs. Surgery will *not* enable the infant to regain motor or sensory functioning; surgery is done primarily to prevent infection. Parents should not be told the infant will move the legs after surgery (**Answer 4**) or be offered false hope (**Answers 1, 2**).

TEST-TAKING TIP—Myelomeningocele results in permanent, irreversible nerve damage.
IMP, APP, 3, PEDS, PsI, Psychosocial Integrity

44. **(3)** The best means to prevent any type of infection in any type of setting is good handwashing. Other techniques are *secondary* (**Answers 1, 2, 4**).

TEST-TAKING TIP—Hand washing is the first line of defense in infection control.
AN, COM, 8, PEDS, SECE, Safety and Infection Control

45. **(2)** At 7 months of age, an infant may either sit with some support or sit alone; either behavior is commonly acquired at this age. Rolling over (**Answer 1**) is usually observed in infants around 3 to 4 months of age, whereas weightbearing

(**Answer 3**) and the palmar grasp (**Answer 4**) are commonly observed in infant between ages 4 and 6 mo.

> **TEST-TAKING TIP**—Note the use of the phrase "most recently acquired skill" in this question.
> **AN, APP, 5, PEDS, HPM, Health Promotion and Maintenance**

46. (**2**) As a 9-mo-old with a chronic bowel problem, this infant has probably become accustomed to mother's administering suppositories or enemas. In addition, fear of strangers is common in this age group. Considering these factors, this infant's mother should at least be offered the opportunity to administer or assist with the enemas. If this is not feasible, another qualified person could take her place (**Answers 1, 3, 4**).

> **TEST-TAKING TIP**—Look at the pattern of responses: three options are staff, one is the mother. Choose the one that is different, especially considering that fear of strangers peaks at 8 to 9 mo.
> **AN, APP, application 6, PEDS, HPM, Health Promotion and Maintenance**

47. (**2**) LTB progresses through four distinct stages, with *early symptoms in the first* stage including fear, hoarseness, croupy cough, and inspiratory stridor only when disturbed. In the *second* stage, the stridor is constant and is accompanied by retractions (**Answer 4**). In the *third* stage, restlessness and tachypnea (**Answer 3**) are seen in addition to anxiety, pallor, and sweating. In the *fourth and final* stage, intermittent or constant cyanosis is followed by the cessation of breathing, or apnea (**Answer 1**).

> **TEST-TAKING TIP**—Note the use of the words "early signs" in this question.
> **AN, ANL, 6, PEDS, PhI, Physiological Adaptation**

48. (**3**) The opisthotonos position occurs in children with severe meningitis due to the pressure on the spinal cord; the child's head is drawn back and the spine is arched backward in an attempt to minimize pressure on the cord. When the child assumes this position, the nurse should place the child in a side-lying position for safety and comfort. Any other position would not work as well (**Answers 1, 2, 4**).

> **TEST-TAKING TIP**—Visualize the condition, and then visualize the options to identify the position for safety and comfort.
> **IMP, ANL, 1, PEDS, PhI, Basic Care and Comfort**

49. (**1**) Younger teenage girls in particular prefer the company of other young girls; they have a definite preference for same-sex, same-age companions. As such, this child would not necessarily seek out older or younger children (**Answers 2, 4**), nor would she have "no preference" regarding the sex of her companion (**Answer 3**).

> **TEST-TAKING TIP**—Know age-relevant stages of psychosocial development. Young teenage girls generally prefer a same sex "best friend."
> **AN, APP, 5, PEDS, HPM, Health Promotion and Maintenance**

50. (**3**) Crises are precipitated by conditions of low oxygen tension; this may include contact with sources of infection. Other sources of low oxygen tension might include *severe* emotional stress (**Answer 1**), *extremely* cold or windy weather (**Answer 2**), or *dehydration* (**Answer 4**), as well as high altitudes.

> **TEST-TAKING TIP**—Note the use of the word "avoid" in this question, and situations that may lead to infections.
> **IMP, APP, 6, PEDS, HPM, Health Promotion and Maintenance**

51. (**1, 2, 3, 4**) Answer 1 is correct because excessive or unusual hematoma formation is a sign of hemophilia. A hematoma is a swelling composed of a mass of extravasated blood (usually clotted) confined to an organ, tissue, or space and caused by a break in a blood vessel. **Answer 2** is correct because hemarthrosis, or bleeding into a joint either spontaneously or following an injury, is considered the hallmark or most typical sign of hemophilia. If the hemarthosis is not treated properly or adequately, permanent joint deformities may result. **Answer 3** is correct because bleeding from a relatively minor injury is a sign of hemophilia. **Answer 4** is correct because intracranial bleeding, usually following a closed head injury, is a sign of hemophilia.

> **TEST-TAKING TIP**—Hemophilia is an inherited bleeding disorder. All of the answers are correct because they all contain some type of bleeding.
> **EV, APP, 6, PEDS, SECE, Management of Care**

52. (**4**) With children (older than 1 yr) who have received a 15 mL dose of syrup of ipecac, if vomiting has not occurred within 20 min, the dose may be repeated once more, although the first dose is generally effective in the majority of cases. If the child does not vomit *after* a second dose, gastric lavage must be promptly initiated to avoid cardiotoxic effects of ipecac. The nurse should *never attempt* to manually stimulate the gag reflex (**Answer 1**). Ipecac works within 15–30 min, and waiting *another* 20 min will not be helpful (**Answer 2**). If the child does not vomit at all, thus not removing either the ipecac or the ingested substance(s), there *is* danger of ipecac toxicity, as well as poisoning from the ingested substance (**Answer 3**).

> **TEST-TAKING TIP**—Eliminate **Answer 2** (important to *not* wait) and **Answer 3** (there *is* a danger) because ipecac is cardiotoxic and can cause complete heart block.
> **IMP, ANL, 1, PEDS, PhI, Pharmacological and Parenteral Therapies**

53. (**1**) Due to this child's carditis, the best means for the nurse to evaluate how well any increase in activity is tolerated would be by monitoring the apical pulse rate. Any increase in pulse rate over 15 to 20 beats/min would indicate that the increase in activity is not tolerated and would be an indication for returning the child to bed immediately. Any other method of evaluating tolerance of increasing activity would be less effective (**Answers 2, 3, 4**).

> **TEST-TAKING TIP**—Activity tolerance in *heart* conditions (carditis in rheumatic fever) is best measured by *heart* rate.
> **IMP, APP, 6, PEDS, HPM, Health Promotion and Maintenance**

54. (**2**) The teenager who is newly diagnosed with diabetes must assume responsibility for his own care as soon as possible; diabetes is a chronic disease with no known cure, so that this teen will have to live with it for the rest of his life. The nurse should discourage his mother from being overly protective of him or from assuming this responsibility (**Answers 1, 3, 4**).

> **TEST-TAKING TIP**—Self-care management is always a client-centered goal.
> **IMP, ANL, 7, PEDS, PsI, Psychosocial Integrity**

55. (**3**) The use of a pacifier for an infant with CHF will promote true psychological rest, thus reducing the body's demand for oxygen and reducing the workload of the heart. This is the *most* important reason that this infant should be offered the pacifier; although it may also be true that the infant seems to

like the pacifier (**Answer 1**), this is not the main reason one should be given. **Answers 2** and **4** are too generalized and not necessarily true.

> **TEST-TAKING TIP**—According to Freud, because infants are in the stage of oral gratification, a pacifier will reduce crying, which is medically significant in this case.
> **IMP, APP, 6, PEDS, PhI, Reduction of Risk Potential**

56. **(4)** Contrary to popular belief, the best position for the nurse to place a child with a nosebleed in is sitting up and leaning forward slightly, with head remaining above the level of the heart; this position will allow the blood to drain freely from the nose and prevent aspiration. Sitting up with the head tilted backward (**Answer 3**) will predispose the child to swallowing or aspirating blood, as will a semi-Fowler's position (**Answer 2**). The prone position (**Answer 1**) might be an acceptable *second* choice if the child were too weak to sit up without assistance.

> **TEST-TAKING TIP**—Preventing aspiration and maintaining a patent airway is always a priority of care.
> **IMP, APP, 6, PEDS, PhI, Reduction of Risk Potential**

57. **(2)** Cystic fibrosis is inherited as an autosomal recessive disorder. The fact that these parents have a child with CF means that they are carriers of the trait, and each subsequent pregnancy might result in a child who also has CF. It would not be correct to advise the mother that a second child would only carry the trait (**Answer 4**) or would be normal (**Answer 3**), although there is a possibility these might occur; the parents should be fully advised of the odds of this happening. In addition, it would needlessly worry the parents to tell them a second child might be more severely affected (**Answer 1**), although this is also a possibility.

> **TEST-TAKING TIP**—Regardless of the genetics, having had one child with this disease, there is always a risk that subsequent children may also have this disease.
> **IMP, ANL, 1, PEDS, HPM, Health Promotion and Maintenance**

58. **(2)** About half the children who have eczema during the toddler or preschool years develop asthma during the school-age or teenage years. Asthma seems to have little or no relation to strep throat or tonsilitis (**Answer 1**). The father's death undoubtedly would have affected this child, but it occurred 1 year before the onset of the asthma (**Answer 3**). The pneumonia experienced at age 4 might have been related to the asthma, but was not the cause of it (**Answer 4**).

> **TEST-TAKING TIP**—Although the etiology of asthma is multifactorial, there is thought to be an allergic predisposition.
> **AN, ANL, 1, PEDS, HPM, Health Promotion and Maintenance**

59. **(1)** Considering this infant's diagnosis, the nurse should anticipate that the infant will most likely have at least some developmental delays; most infants would begin to roll over by 3 months of age, but at 5 mo the infant should be doing this now. Sitting (**Answer 2**) is normally found around 6 mo; this infant will most likely *not* be capable of this behavior at 5 mo. A pincer grasp (**Answer 3**) is normally found at 9–12 mo, and this infant will most likely *not* be capable of this behavior. Weight bearing (**Answer 4**) is typically noted in healthy infants at 4–6 mo; considering this infant's diagnosis, however, this infant may or may not be capable of this more strenuous behavior.

> **TEST-TAKING TIP**—Infants learn to roll over at 3 mo, sit at 6 mo, and crawl at 9 mo. Consider delayed development in congestive heart failure.
> **AS, ANL, 5, PEDS, HPM, Health Promotion and Maintenance**

60. **(1)** The infant is placed on the abdomen postoperatively to prevent trauma or pressure to the sutured area on the back. In addition, the infant's head should be positioned 10 degrees lower than the hips to prevent the pressure of circulating CSF from affecting the suture line on the lower back. An obvious contraindication to this position is the presence of increased ICP, in which case the infant would be positioned flat in bed (**Answer 4**). In general, the head is never higher than the hips (**Answers 2, 3**) during the immediate postoperative period for this type of surgery.

> **TEST-TAKING TIP**—Visualize the positions; know postoperative objectives regarding preventing pressure to suture area.
> **IMP, APP, 3, PEDS, PhI, Reduction of Risk Potential**

61. **(1)** Hirschsprung's disease is a congenital condition. It does not "develop spontaneously," although the diagnosis may not be made until symptoms have been present for several months and some attempts at conservative medical treatment (enemas, stool softeners, etc.) have been made (**Answer 3**). In the newborn with Hirschsprung's disease, there may be an episode of meconium ileus (**Answer 2**), but this occurs as a *result* of the Hirschsprung's disease *rather than as the cause of it*. There is no known metabolic defect (**Answer 4**).

> **TEST-TAKING TIP**—Narrow your option to the one that is different: congenital vs. acquired after birth.
> **IMP, APP, 8, PEDS, PsI, Psychosocial Integrity**

62. **(2)** As healing of the pathways of the CSF occurs following an episode of meningitis, scar tissue naturally forms; this may lead to noncommunicating hydrocephalus. The hydrocephalus might *then* lead to learning disabilities (**Answer 3**) or mental retardation (**Answer 4**). Encephalitis (**Answer 1**) may occur in *conjunction with* the meningitis, but it is *not* a complication.

> **TEST-TAKING TIP**—Note the use of the term *long-term complication* in this question, and select the option that incorporates (leads to two other conditions) or is in conjunction with the other options.
> **AS, ANL, 2, PEDS, HPM, Health Promotion and Maintenance**

63. **(3)** Because concentrated sweets will cause a rise in blood sugar, followed by a precipitous drop, the nurse should teach this teenager that he should follow up this concentrated sweet with a complex carbohydrate such as a glass of milk. Any other action would be inappropriate at this time (**Answers 1, 2, 4**).

> **TEST-TAKING TIP**—The complex carbohydrate will help maintain a steady blood sugar level. Therefore, choose the only option that is not a diagnostic test or pharmacological agent.
> **IMP, APP, 4, PEDS, PhI, Reduction of Risk Potential**

64. **(4)** There are multiple factors involved in the etiology of asthma, including an allergic predisposition (**Answer 2**), precipitation by severe emotional or physical stress (**Answer 3**), and other factors yet to be determined (**Answer 1**).

> **TEST-TAKING TIP**—When more than one option looks correct, choose the more comprehensive answer (multiple answers = "multiple factors").
> **IMP, APP, 1, PEDS, PsI, Psychosocial Integrity**

65. **(1)** Long-term follow-up care for children with rheumatic fever most frequently includes antibiotic therapy with penicillin or erythromycin on an exact schedule for an indefinite time. There is no way to immunize against future attacks (**Answer 2**). This child will be sent home on restricted activity, and cardiac rehabilitation programs are out of the question at this time (**Answer 3**). Home schooling would be fine, but it is not a priority at this time (**Answer 4**).

> **TEST-TAKING TIP**—Medical prevention is the clue to the best choice.
> **IMP, APP, 6, PEDS, PhI, Reduction of Risk Potential**

66. **(2)** In suspected cases of epiglottitis, the visualization of the epiglottis is strictly contraindicated, because it may precipitate laryngospasm and immediate respiratory arrest. It is a nursing responsibility to inform any less knowledgeable health-care providers of this danger; any other action (**Answers 1, 3, 4**) would be inappropriate at this time.

> **TEST-TAKING TIP**—The nurse must always serve as a client advocate. Also note that three responses allow the procedure, but one does not. Choose the one that is different from the others.
> **IMP, ANL, 6, PEDS, PhI, Reduction of Risk Potential**

67. **(4)** There is no known cure for nephrosis; rather, treatment is aimed at providing symptomatic relief. To that effect, prednisone—an anti-inflammatory corticosteroid—is given to relieve symptoms rather than effect a cure. If prednisone has the expected therapeutic effect, the preschooler should report "feeling better" as symptoms are relieved. *Side* effects of prednisone therapy may also include mood swings (**Answer 1**), glucosuria (**Answer 2**), and fluid retention with weight gain (**Answer 3**).

> **TEST-TAKING TIP**—Note the key words "expected therapeutic effects," *not* side effects.
> **EV, APP, 8, PEDS, PhI, Pharmacological and Parenteral Therapies**

68. **(2)** In infants, the earliest sign of hydrocephalus is increasing head circumference, which occurs as the suture lines separate and the fontanels widen to accommodate the extra fluid within the skull. *Later* signs would indicate that no further accommodation can occur and brain tissue is being destroyed; these signs might include bulging anterior fontanel (**Answer 1**), shrill, high-pitched cry (**Answer 3**), and sunset eyes (**Answer 4**).

> **TEST-TAKING TIP**—Note the use of the term *earliest sign* in this question.
> **AN, ANL, 3, PEDS, HPM, Health Promotion and Maintenance**

69. **(1)** Viscous xylocaine is never recommended for children with mucosal ulcerations secondary to chemotherapy, because of the risk of a depressed gag reflex and aspiration. The other interventions (**Answers 2, 3, 4**) *are,* however, all *appropriate* nursing interventions.

> **TEST-TAKING TIP**—Note that this question is asking about an intervention that is *not* appropriate, meaning eliminate the correct statements.
> **IMP, APP, 6, PEDS, PhI, Pharmacological and Parenteral Therapies**

70. **(4)** As generalized edema progresses, in boys the scrotal sac can become extremely swollen, tender, and painful. The best nursing intervention is to use an athletic support while the child is lying in bed. Zinc oxide (**Answer 1**) is not used because the problem is *mechanical* rather than on the skin itself. Cleansing the scrotum (**Answer 2**) is important to prevent infection, because all edematous tissue needs special care to prevent skin breakdown; however, this will *not relieve* the child's discomfort. **Answer 3** is incorrect because powder is **not** used in a pediatric unit.

> **TEST-TAKING TIP**—Providing comfort is the priority of care.
> **IMP, APP, 8, PEDS, PhI, Basic Care and Comfort**

71. **(2)** The only solution that should be used in doing cleansing enemas for a child with Hirschsprung's disease is normal saline, because the child will retain some of this fluid, which will be absorbed through the bowel wall. As an isotonic solution, normal saline will not alter the fluid balance, as a nonisotonic solution almost certainly would (**Answers 1, 3, 4**).

> **TEST-TAKING TIP**—The choice is between isotonic and nonisotonic solutions. Select the isotonic solution because it will not alter fluid balance.
> **AN, ANL, 8, PEDS, PhI, Basic Care and Comfort**

72. **(2)** Signs of dehydration in infants include irritability and sunken, dry eyeballs due to fluid loss. Fever may be present, and tachycardia, *not* bradycardia (**Answer 1**), is also common. Low blood pressure often results, followed by *oliguria;* anuria (**Answer 3**) is rare and would be an ominous sign of renal failure. The oral buccal mucosa may be quite dry, and the anterior fontanel may be *sunken, not* bulging (**Answer 4**).

> **TEST-TAKING TIP**—If part of an answer is right but part of it is wrong, the answer must be wrong.
> **AS, ANL, 6, PEDS, HPM, Health Promotion and Maintenance**

73. **(1)** In infants, the apical impulse (heard through a stethoscope held to the chest at the apex of the heart) is the most reliable in terms of assessing cardiac activity (heartbeat). Having the most reliable pulse rate possible is critical in the safe administration of digoxin to an infant. **Answer 2** is incorrect because an accurate radial pulse can usually only be obtained in children *over 2 years of age.* It would also not reflect cardiac activity (heartbeat) as accurately as an apical pulse. **Answer 3** is incorrect because the popliteal pulse is usually reserved for use during early childhood to detect the presence of circulatory impairment in the *lower extremities.* **Answer 4** is incorrect because the femoral pulse is usually reserved for use during early childhood to detect the presence of circulatory impairment in the *lower extremities.* **Answers 5** and **6** can be used, but are less accurate in children.

> **TEST-TAKING TIP**—In this case, the key words *most correct* mean *most accurately.* Infant's pulses should always be checked apically prior to the administration of digoxin (an anti-arrhythmic drug).
> **AS, APP, 6, PEDS, PhI, Pharmacological and Parenteral Therapies**

74. **(1)** If a toddler were to develop hydrocephalus, the first sign would most likely be irritability and poor feeding due to increased ICP. The head circumference would *not increase* (**Answer 2**), because the fontanels have closed. Headaches or double vision might occur (**Answer 3**), but a toddler is not likely to complain of them. Ruptured retinal vessels (**Answer 4**) is a *later* sign of increased ICP.

> **TEST-TAKING TIP**—Note the use of the word "toddler," not "infant," in this question.
> **AN, ANL, 2, PEDS, HPM, Health Promotion and Maintenance**

75. (4) The best exercise for a child with cystic fibrosis is swimming, which provides needed exercise at an activity level that is not overly taxing for the child. Softball, tennis, and soccer (**Answers 1, 2, 3**) are all generally thought to be too strenuous for a child with CF.

> **TEST-TAKING TIP** — "Swimming" is the option that is different from the others, which all call for ball playing.
> **IMP, ANL, 3, PEDS, HPM, Health Promotion and Maintenance**

76. (1) Because sickle cell anemia is inherited as an autosomal recessive disorder, if both parents have the trait, any future pregnancies would have a 1:4 (not 4:4 as in **Answer 4**) chance of producing a child *with* sickle cell anemia. **Answer 2** is incorrect because each pregnancy would have a 1:2 chance of producing a child *with the trait*. **Answer 3** is incorrect there is a 1:4 chance of producing a *normal* child. **Answer 4** is totally incorrect.

> **TEST-TAKING TIP**—Autosomal recessive disorders have a 1:4 chance of occurring when both parents are carriers of the trait.
> **IMP, ANL, 6, PEDS, HPM, Health Promotion and Maintenance**

77. (4) Factor VIII concentrate is a blood product; a type and crossmatch may be ordered for the child before the IV administration of this medication. Given the relatively small volume of fluid to be administered, it would *not* usually cause fluid volume overload (**Answer 2**). Although there has been some discussion about administering multiple IV medications to a child with hemophilia and the linkage to AIDS (**Answer 3**), this is *not* a concern *during* the actual administration of the medication but rather a long-term concern. Emboli formation (**Answer 1**) can occur with any IV administration and is *not specific* to cryoprecipitate, although the nurse would need to take the necessary precautions to prevent this possibility.

> **TEST-TAKING TIP**—Any child receiving blood or blood products should be closely monitored for a possible transfusion reaction.
> **PL, APP, 6, PEDS, PhI, Pharmacological and Parenteral Therapies**

78. (2) Solu-Cortef is a corticosteroid/antiinflammatory used in epiglottitis to relieve edema. Solu-Cortef does *not* provide sedation (**Answer 1**) or relieve pain (**Answer 3**), and the bacterial infection is treated with *antibiotics* (**Answer 4**).

> **TEST-TAKING TIP**—Recall that this is a steroid; recall its function and recall that edema is a main concern in this condition. Therefore, reduction of swelling to keep airway patent is a priority.
> **AN, APP, 6, PEDS, PhI, Pharmacological and Parenteral Therapies**

79. (4) Although any infection can be life-threatening to a child with leukemia, chickenpox presents a particular danger, because the child may develop encephalitis or sepsis. Infections such as impetigo (**Answer 1**), streptococcus (**Answer 2**), or pneumonia (**Answer 3**) are *less specific* dangers.

> **TEST-TAKING TIP**—Choose the option that can result in encephalitis, a *specific* danger.
> **IMP, ANL, 1, PEDS, SECE, Safety and Infection Control**

80. (2) Because infants with VSD and CHF have a tendency toward respiratory infections, the infant should have limited contact with visitors with URIs, such as the grandmother with her slight cold. In fact, her slight cold might mean an episode of pneumonia for this infant. Lupus (**Answer 1**) in the aunt is not contagious, nor is the father's drug addiction (**Answer 3**). The sister (**Answer 4**) should be allowed to see and touch the infant, unless she herself is sick.

> **TEST-TAKING TIP**—Respiratory infection control is the priority of care because of the danger of pneumonia and ↑ cardiac problems.
> **IMP, ANL, 6, PEDS, SECE, Safety and Infection Control**

81. (1) The chief danger of ipecac absorption into the body is that it can cause cardiac arrhythmias, atrial fibrillation, or severe heart block. There is minimal effect on the liver (**Answer 2**), kidneys (**Answer 3**), or CNS (**Answer 4**).

> **TEST-TAKING TIP**—Ipecac can cause cardiotoxicity.
> **AN, COM, 1, PEDS, PhI, Pharmacological and Parenteral Therapies**

82. (2) The most recent research indicates that *infants who are breastfed do have a lower incidence of SIDS* than infants who are bottle-fed. It is not true that infants who are bottle-fed have a lower risk of SIDS (**Answer 3**), nor is it true that the risk of SIDS is the same (**Answer 1**) however infants are fed. Breastfeeding is not contraindicated for siblings of infants who died from SIDS (**Answer 4**); in fact, breastfeeding in this instance is recommended.

> **TEST-TAKING TIP**—Breastfeeding is generally recommended for all infants whose mothers express an interest and willingness to do so.
> **IMP, APP, 4, PEDS, HPM, Health Promotion and Maintenance**

83. (3) Generally, infants who weigh 7 lb at birth will weigh 28 lb, or quadruple their birthweight, by $2\frac{1}{2}$ years of age. Consequently, the other listed ages are incorrect (**Answers 1, 2, 4**).

> **TEST-TAKING TIP**—Know growth and development milestones to choose the *only* correct answer.
> **EV, APP, 5, PEDS, HPM, Health Promotion and Maintenance**

84. (2) The general rule of thumb to predict a child's height as an adult is to double the child's height at 2 years of age. The other answers (**Answers 1, 3, 4**) are incorrect.

> **TEST-TAKING TIP**—Know developmental milestones to pick the only correct answer.
> **IMP, APP, 5, PEDS, HPM, Health Promotion and Maintenance**

85. (2) Poisoning is most common in toddlers, who have the motor skills necessary to reach the poisons yet lack the intelligence to know not to ingest the poison. The other answers (**Answers 1, 3, 4**) are, therefore, incorrect.

> **TEST-TAKING TIP**—Know age-relevant safety concerns.
> **AN, ANL, 1, PEDS, SECE, Safety and Infection Control**

86. (3) In children under 3 years, most accidental deaths are related to motor vehicles in which the child is a passenger; other types of accidents are not as common or not as likely to result in death (**Answers 1, 2, 4**).

> **TEST-TAKING TIP**—Know age-typical cause of accidental death.
> **AN, COM, 1, PEDS, SECE, Safety and Infection Control**

87. (2) Toddlers always suffer when separated from their parents, more so than any other age group (**Answers 1, 3, 4**). In fact, between ages 1 and 3 yr, children are most likely to suffer separation anxiety.

TEST-TAKING TIP—It is the age, *not* the condition. Toddlers are at the peak age for separation anxiety.
AN, ANL, 5, PEDS, PsI, Psychosocial Integrity

88. **(2)** Five-year-olds may count up to 20 or 25, but seldom beyond this. They should be able to name colors such as red, green, and blue (**Answer 1**). In addition, they should be able to give their phone number and address (**Answer 4**) and have a better sense of temporal relationships, as evidenced by their ability to name days of the week, months of the year, and seasons (**Answer 3**).

TEST-TAKING TIP—The stem asks for what this child is *not* expected to do. The nurse should be familiar with developmental norms found in the DDST.
AS, COM, 5, PEDS, HPM, Health Promotion and Maintenance

89. **(2)** In addition to removing gown and gloves, the aide/UAP should wash hands before leaving the child's room. **Answers 1, 3,** and **4** are incorrect because these actions *are* appropriate and would not require the nurse's immediate attention.

TEST-TAKING TIP—Key word: "unsafe." Use a true-or-false approach to rule out the three approaches that *are* OK.
EV, ANL, 1, PEDS, SECE, Safety and Infection Control

90. **(2)** Sickling of RBCs occurs under conditions of low oxygen tension. Giving the adolescent oxygen will prevent further sickling of RBCs. **Answer 1** is incorrect because oxygen will not reverse the sickling of cells that has already occurred. **Answer 3** is incorrect because oxygen is given to prevent further sickling of RBCs rather than to prevent any respiratory complications. **Answer 4** is incorrect because oxygen does not have an effect on the oxygen-carrying capacity of RBCs.

TEST-TAKING TIP—Focus on the two options with "prevent." Then note that the word "sickle" is in both the stem and **Answer 2** ("sickling").
IMP, APP, 6, PEDS, PhI, Physiological Adaptation

91. **(1)** Cloth tape can stretch over time, eventually resulting in inaccurate measurements. The RN should intervene and direct the LPN/LVN to use paper tape instead of cloth tape. **Answers 2, 3,** and **4** are incorrect because these actions *are* appropriate and would *not* require intervention and further direction.

TEST-TAKING TIP—Key words: "intervention and further direction," implying that the best answer is the *incorrect* action.
EV, ANL, 8, PEDS, SECE, Management of Care

92. **(3)** The nurse should always initiate infection control measures, such as droplet precautions, before administering any other care in order to protect the nurse, other health-care workers, and other children and their families. **Answers 1, 2,** and **4** are not correct because the nurse is not initiating infection control measures first, but is checking vitals or offering fluids or drawing blood first.

TEST-TAKING TIP—Infection control is always a priority of care.
IMP, ANL, 1, PEDS, SECE, Management of Care

93. **(1)** U80 means that there are 80 units of insulin per milliliter, not 80 units of insulin in the vial. **Answers 2, 3,** and **4** are incorrect because these statements *are true* and do not require the RN's intervention.

TEST-TAKING TIP— "U" (units) followed by a number always refers to the number of units of insulin per milliliter.
EV, ANL, 4, PEDS, PhI, Pharmacological and Parenteral Therapies

94. **(1)** The child with eczema should be bathed in plain water, with no oils or soaps, to avoid further damage to the skin. **Answers 2, 3,** and **4** are incorrect because these actions *are* appropriate and require no additional supervision.

TEST-TAKING TIP—Note the use of the words "require... additional supervision" in this question, meaning *incorrect,* or *not* OK.
EV, ANL, 1, PEDS, SECE, Management of Care

95. **(1)** Infants have the greatest percentage of fluid per pound of body weight than any other age group and are at highest risk for fluid and electrolyte imbalance. **Answers 2, 3,** and **4** are incorrect because none of the other conditions is at the *highest* risk for *fluid and electrolyte imbalance.*

TEST-TAKING TIP—It is not an age variable but the *condition* that is at risk.
AN, ANL, 6, PEDS, PhI, Reduction of Risk Potential

96. **(2)** Diet soda contains aspartame (NutraSweet), which metabolizes into phenylalanine. **Answers 1, 3,** and **4** are incorrect because these food items *are* allowed on a *low* phenylalanine diet that this child is undoubtedly on.

TEST-TAKING TIP—Products containing aspartame (NutraSweet) should not be given to anyone with PKU. The stem calls for an elimination approach to selecting what is OK to offer from what is not OK.
IMP, APP, 4, PEDS, PhI, Basic Care and Comfort

97. **(3)** This activity, auscultation of breath sounds, involves assessment skills. Transport (**Answer 1**), taking vital signs (**Answer 2**), and helping with activities of daily living (ADL) (**Answer 4**) do *not* involve assessment and therefore can be safely delegated to an LPN/LVN.

TEST-TAKING TIP—Key concept in delegation: assessments can be done *only* by the RN.
IMP, ANL, 6, PEDS, SECE, Management of Care

98. **(4)** No child should be told not to express his or her feelings. Crying when upset is normal and healthy for any child, regardless of age. **Answers 1, 2,** and **3** are incorrect because these actions *are* age and condition appropriate, and do not require the nurse to intervene.

TEST-TAKING TIP—Concept: therapeutic interventions/communication calls for encouraging children to express their feelings.
IMP, ANL, 7, PEDS, SECE, Management of Care

99. **(3)** Preschoolers, who are at an age of fears and fantasies, should not be given detailed explanations of treatments. **Answers 1, 2,** and **4** are incorrect because these actions *are* age appropriate and do not require the preceptor to correct the teaching plan.

TEST-TAKING TIP—The concept here is an age-appropriate activity. Preschoolers should be given a simple and brief explanation, shortly before the intervention.
EV, ANL, 5, PEDS, SECE, Management of Care

100. **(1)** Only the RN should evaluate the efficacy of pain medication or other treatments/medications. **Answers 2, 3,** and **4** are incorrect because the LPN/LVN and the UAP are not legally responsible for evaluating the efficacy of pain medication.

TEST-TAKING TIP—Recall that the concept of delegation sets responsibility for assessment/evaluation with the RN, not other assistive personnel.
PL, APP, 1, PEDS, SECE, Management of Care

Unit 6

Nursing Care of Behavioral and Emotional Problems Throughout the Life Span (Client Need: Psychosocial Integrity)

Sally L. Lagerquist
Contributor to Selected Sections: Mary St. Jonn Seed

The chief *objective* of this unit is to highlight the most commonly observed behavioral and emotional problems and disorders in the mental health field. The emphasis is on (a) main points for *assessment,* (b) *analysis* of data based on underlying *basic concepts and general principles* drawn from a psychodynamic and interpersonal theoretical framework, and (c) *nursing interventions* based on the therapeutic use of self as the cornerstone of a helping process. Nursing actions are listed in *priority* whenever possible. Hence the **nursing process framework** is followed throughout. Note that nursing interventions are divided into *planning* and *implementation* (covering long-term and short-term *goals* and stressing *priority* of actions) and *health teaching. Evaluation* of results is listed separately, although this step of the nursing process is circular and relates back to "assessment" and "goals."

The categorization of psychiatric-emotional disorders can be complex and controversial. For purposes of clarity and simplicity, an attempt has been made here to capsulize many theoretical principles and component skills of the helping process that these disorders have *in common.* That the term *client* is often used in place of *patient* reflects the interpersonal rather than medical model of psychiatric nursing. The diagnostic categorization of disorders (based on a synthesis of the North American Nursing Diagnosis Association [NANDA], Psychiatric Nursing Diagnosis [PND-I], and American Nurses Association [ANA] classification system for psychiatric nursing diagnoses) is included here to update the reader in current terminology in the mental health field.

The underlying organizational framework for this unit is based on applicable **categories of human functions** (Growth and Development; Protective Functions; Comfort, Rest, Activity, and Mobility; Sensory-Perceptual Functions; and Psychosocial-Cultural Functions; see **Appendices H** and **I**).

These categories have been incorporated into the candidates' performance report (CPR) sent to the NCLEX-RN® examinees as part of a report of their performance on the licensure exam. The categories reflect four **client needs** and **six subneeds** and are based on clusters of nursing activities designed to meet these needs (e.g., protecting clients, assisting clients with mobility needs).

GROWTH AND DEVELOPMENT

Major Theoretical Models

I. Psychodynamic model (Freud)

A. Assumptions and key ideas

1. No human behavior is accidental; each psychic event is determined by preceding ones.
2. Unconscious mental processes occur with great frequency and significance.
3. Psychoanalysis is used to uncover childhood trauma, which may involve conflict and repressed feelings.
4. Psychoanalytic methods are used: therapeutic alliance, transference, regression, dream association, catharsis.

B. *Freud*—shifted from classification of behavior to understanding and explaining in psychological terms and changing behavior under structured conditions.

1. Structure of the mind: id, ego, superego; unconscious, preconscious, conscious.
2. Stages of psychosexual development (**Table 6.1**).
3. Defense mechanisms (see **p. 424**).

TABLE 6.1	Freud's Stages of Psychosexual Development	
Stage	**Age**	**Behaviors**
Oral	Birth–1 yr	Dependency and oral gratification.
Anal	1–3 yr	Creativity, stinginess, cruelty, cleanliness, self-control, punctuality.
Phallic or oedipal	3–6 yr	Sexual, aggressive feelings; guilt.
Latency	6–12 yr	Reactivation of pregenital impulses; intellectual and social growth.
Genital	12–18 yr	Displacement of pregenital impulses; learns responsibility for self; establishes identity.

II. Psychosocial development model (Erikson, Maslow, Piaget, Duvall)

    A. *Erik Erikson—Eight Stages of Man* (1963)

        1. Psychosocial development—interplay of biology with social factors, encompassing total life span, from birth to death, in progressive developmental tasks.

        2. *Stages of life cycle*—life consists of a series of developmental phases (**Table 6.2** and **Table 6.3**).

            a. Universal sequence of biological, social, psychological events.

            b. Each person experiences a series of normative conflicts and crises and thus needs to accomplish specific psychosocial tasks.

TABLE 6.2	Erikson's Stages of the Life Cycle	
Age and Stage of Development	**Conflict Areas Needing Resolution**	◆ **Evaluation: Result of Resolution/Nonresolution**
Infancy (birth–18 mo)	Trust	Shows affection, gratification, recognition; trusts self and others; begins to tolerate frustrations; develops *hope.* Uses primary caregiver as a base for exploration.
	vs.	
	Mistrust	Withdrawn, alienated.
Early childhood (18 mo–3 yr)	Autonomy	Cooperative, self-controlled, self-expressive, can delay gratification; develops *will.*
	vs.	
	Shame and doubt	Exaggerated self-restraint; defiance; compulsive; overly compliant.
Late childhood (3–5 yr)	Initiative	Realistic goals; can evaluate self; explorative; imitates adult, shows imagination; tests reality; anticipates roles; develops *purpose*, self-motivation.
	vs.	
	Guilt	Self-imposed restrictions relative to jealousy, guilt, and denial.
School age (5–12 yr)	Industry	Sense of duty; acquires self-confidence from social and school *competencies;* persevering in real tasks.
	vs.	
	Inferiority	School and social dropout; social loner; incompetent.
Adolescence (12–18 yr)	Identity	Has ideological commitments, self-actualizing; sense of self; experiments with roles; experiences sexual polarizations; develops *fidelity.*
	vs.	
	Role diffusion	Ambivalent, confused, indecisive; may act out (antisocial acts).
Young adulthood (18–25yr)	Intimacy, solidarity	Makes commitments to love, work relationships, a cause or creative effort; able to sustain mutual *love* relationships.
	vs.	
	Isolation	Superficial, impersonal, biased.
Adulthood (25–60 yr)	Generativity	Productive, creative, procreative, concerned for others; develops *care.*
	vs.	
	Self-absorption, stagnation	Self-indulgent.
Late adulthood (60 yr–death)	Ego integrity	Appreciates past, present, and future; self-acceptance of own contribution to others, of own *self-worth*, and of changes in lifestyle and life cycle; can face "not being"; develops *wisdom.*
	vs.	
	Despair	Preoccupied with loss of hope, of purpose; contemptuous, fears death.

Source: ©Lagerquist, S: Nursing Examination Review, ed. 4. Addison-Wesley, Redwood City, Calif.

TABLE 6.3	Summary of Theories of Psychosocial Development Throughout the Life Cycle			
Freud	**Piaget**	**Sullivan**	**Erikson**	
Emphasis on Pathology (intrapsychic)	*Normal* children	Pathology (interpersonal)	Both health and illness	
Anxiety	*No* emphasis on ego, anxiety, identity, libido	Anxiety		
Unconscious, uncontrollable drives	Cognitive development	Unconscious, uncontrollable drives	Problems are manageable and can be solved	
Ego needing defense	Tasks can be accomplished through learning process	Self-system needing defense	Need to integrate individual and society	
Pathological Development Influenced by Early feelings; repressed experiences in unconscious mind	Individual differences and social influences on the mind	Unconscious mind *and* interpersonal relationships (IPR)	Ego, anxiety, identity, libido concepts *combined* with social forces	
Change Possible with Understanding content and meaning of unconscious	Socialization process to facilitate cognitive development	Improved IPR and understanding basic good-bad transformations	Integration of attitudes, libido, and social roles for strong ego identity	
Age Group First 5 yr of life	Middle childhood years	Adolescence	Middle age, old age	
Focus on Emotional development	Cognitive skills	Emotional and interpersonal development; relationships with opposite sex	Emotional, interpersonal, spiritual	
Psychosexual aspects	Cognitive, interactive aspects	Psychosocial aspects; developing sense of identity	Psychosocial aspects	
Cause of Conflicts and Problems Oral, anal, genital stage problems (especially unresolved oedipal/castration conflicts)	Faulty adaptation between individual and environment for intellectual development	Threats to self-system; disturbed communication process; 7 stages not complete	Unresolved conflicts, crises in 8 successive life cycle stages	
Prognosis Few changes possible after age 5	Little change in adult cognitive structure after middle adolescence	Change usually possible with improved IPR	Change not only possible but *expected* throughout life	
Sexual problems part of disturbed behavior	Sex as a variable in learning (age, IQ)	Sexual problems are only one type of faulty IPR affecting behavior	Sexual identity as one of many problems solved by interaction of desire and social process	

c. Two opposing energies (positive and negative forces) coexist and must be synthesized.

d. How each age-specific task is accomplished influences the developmental progress of the next phase and the ability to deal with life.

B. *Abraham Maslow—Hierarchy of Needs* (1962)

1. Beliefs regarding emotional health based on a comprehensive, multidisciplinary approach to human problems, involving all aspects of functioning.

a. *Premise:* mental illness cannot be understood without prior knowledge of mental health.

b. *Focus:* positive aspects of human behavior (e.g., contentment, joy, happiness).

2. *Hierarchy of needs*—physiological, safety, love and belonging, self-esteem and self-recognition, self-actualization, aesthetic. As each stage is mastered, the next stage becomes dominant (**Figure 6.1**).

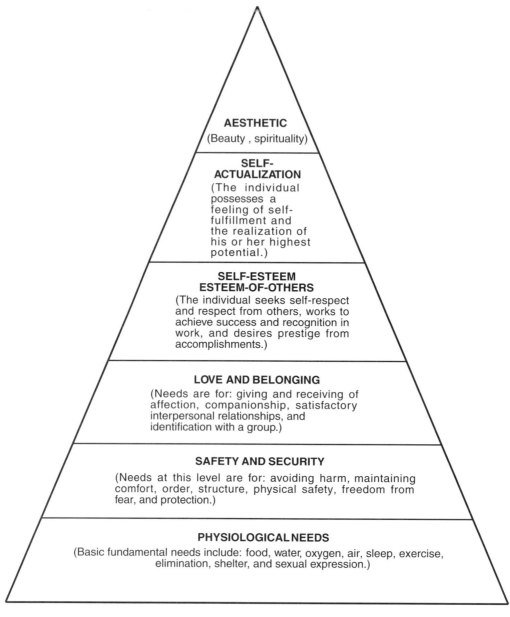

FIGURE 6.1 Maslow's hierarchy of needs. (Modified from Townsend M: Essentials of Psychiatry/Mental Health Nursing. FA Davis, Philadelphia.)

3. *Characteristics of optimal mental health*—keep in mind that *wellness is on a continuum with cultural variations.*
   a. *Self-esteem:* entails self-confidence and self-acceptance.
   b. *Self-knowledge:* involves accurate self-perception of strengths and limitations.
   c. *Satisfying interpersonal relationships:* able to meet reciprocal emotional needs through collaboration rather than by exploitation or power struggles or jealousy; able to make full commitments in close relationships.
   d. *Environmental mastery:* can adapt, change, and solve problems effectively; can make decisions, choose from alternatives, and predict

consequences. Actions are conscious, not impulsive.
   e. *Stress-management:* can delay seeking gratification and relief; does not blame or dwell on past; assumes self-responsibility; either modifies own expectations, seeks substitutes, or withdraws from stressful situation when cannot reduce stress.
C. *Jean Piaget—Cognitive and Intellectual Development* (1963)
   1. **Assumptions**—child development is steered by interaction of environmental and genetic influences; therefore focus is on environmental and social forces. (see **Table 6.3** for comparison with other theories).

2. **Key concepts**
   a. *Assimilation:* process of acquiring new knowledge, skills, and insights by using what they already know and have.
   b. *Accommodation:* adjusts to change by solving previously unsolvable problems because of newly assimilated knowledge.
   c. *Adaptation:* coping process to handle environmental demands.
3. **Age-specific developmental levels**—sensorimotor, preconceptual, intuitive, concrete, formal operational thought (**Table 6.4**).

D. *E. M. Duvall—Family Development* (1971)—developmental tasks are family oriented, presented in eight stages throughout the life cycle (see also **Family Therapy, p. 451**).
   1. *Married couple*
      a. Establishing relationship.
      b. Defining mutual goals.
      c. Developing intimacy: issues of dependence-independence-interdependence.
      d. Establishing mutually satisfying relationship.
      e. Negotiating boundaries of couple with families.
      f. Discussing issue of childbearing.
   2. *Childbearing years*
      a. Working out authority, responsibility, and caregiver roles.
      b. Having children and forming new unit.
      c. Facilitating child's trust.
      d. Need for personal time and space while sharing with each other and child.
   3. *Preschool-age years*
      a. Experiencing changes in energy.
      b. Continuing development as couple, parents, family.
      c. Establishing own family traditions without guilt related to breaks with tradition.
   4. *School-age years*
      a. Establishing new roles in work.
      b. Children's school activities interfering with family activities.
   5. *Teenage years*
      a. Parents continue to develop roles in community other than with children.
      b. Children experience freedom while accepting responsibility for actions.
      c. Struggle with parents in emancipation process.
      d. Family value system is challenged.
      e. Couple relationships may be strong or weak depending on responses to needs.
   6. *Families as launching centers*
      a. Young adults launched with rites of passage.
      b. Changes in couple's relationship due to empty nest and increased leisure time.
      c. Changes in relationship with children away from home.
   7. *Middle-aged parents:* Dealing with issues of aging of own parents.
   8. *Aging family members*
      a. Sense of accomplishment and desire to continue to live fully.
      b. Coping with bereavement and living alone.

III. **Community mental health model (Gerald Kaplan)—levels of prevention**
   A. *Primary prevention*—lower the risk of mental illness and increase capacity to resist contributory influences by providing anticipatory guidance and maximizing strengths.
   B. *Secondary prevention*—decrease disability by shortening its duration and reducing its severity through detection of early-warning signs and effective intervention following case-finding.
   C. *Crisis intervention* (see **p. 393**).
   D. *Tertiary prevention*—avoid permanent disorder through rehabilitation.

IV. **Behavioral model (Pavlov, Watson, Wolpe, Skinner)**
   A. **Assumptions**
      1. Roots in neurophysiology.
      2. Stimulus-response learning can be *conditioned* through *reinforcement.*
      3. Behavior is what one does.
      4. Behavior is observable, describable, predictable, and controllable.
      5. Classification of mental disease is clinically useless, only provides legal labels.

TABLE 6.4	Piaget's Age-Specific Development Levels

Age	Stage	Abilities
Infancy–2 yr	Sensorimotor	Preverbal; uses all senses; coordinates simple motor actions.
2–4 yr	Preconceptual	Can use language; egocentric; imitation in play, parallel play.
4–7 yr	Intuitive	Asks questions; can use symbols and associate subjects with concepts.
7–11 yr	Concrete	Sees relationships, aware of viewpoints; understands cause and effect, can make conclusions; solves concrete problems.
11 yr and older	Formal operational thought	Abstract and conceptual thinking; can check ideas, thoughts, and beliefs; lives in present and nonpresent; can use formal logic and scientific reasoning.

Source: ©Lagerquist, S: Nursing Examination Review, ed. 4. Addison-Wesley, Redwood City, Calif.

   B. **Aim:** change *observable* behavior. There is *no underlying* cause, *no internal* motive.

  V. **Comparison of models** (see **Table 6.3** for comparison of four theories).

Development of Body Image Throughout the Life Cycle

  I. **Definition**—"Mental picture of body's appearance; an interrelated phenomenon which includes the surface, depth, internal and postural picture of the body, as well as the attitudes, emotions, and personality reactions of the individual in relation to his body as an object in space, apart from all others."*

  II. **Operational definition†**

   A. Body image is created by social interaction.
1. Approval given for "normal" and "proper" appearance, gestures, posture, etc.
2. Behavioral and physical deviations from normality not given approval.
3. Body image formed by the person's response to the approval and disapproval of others.
4. Person's values, attitudes, and feelings about self continually evolving and unconsciously integrated.

   B. Self-image, identity, personality, sense of self, and body image are interdependent.

   C. Behavior is determined by body image.

  III. **Concepts related to persons with problems of body image**

   A. Image of self changes with *changing posture* (walking, sitting, gestures).

   B. *Mental picture of self* may not correspond with the actual body; subject to continual but slow revision.

   C. The degree to which people like themselves (good self-concept) is directly related to how well defined they perceive their body image to be.
1. *Vague, indefinite, or distorted body image* correlates with the following personality traits:
   a. Sad, empty, hollow feelings.
   b. Mistrustful of others; poor peer relations.
   c. Low motivation.
   d. Shame, doubt, sense of inferiority, poor self-concept.
   e. Inability to tolerate stress.
2. *Integrated body image* tends to correlate positively with the following personality traits:
   a. Happy, good self-concept.
   b. Good peer relations.
   c. Sense of initiative, industry, autonomy, identity.
   d. Able to complete tasks.
   e. Assertive.

   f. Academically competent; high achievement.
   g. Able to cope with stress.

   D. Child's concept of body image can indicate degree of *ego strength* and personality integration; vague, distorted self-concept may indicate *schizophrenic* processes.

   E. *Successful* completion of various developmental phases determines body concept and degree of *body boundary definiteness* (see **Table 6.6**).

   F. *Physical changes* of height, weight, and body build lead to changes in perception of body appearance and of how body is used.

   G. Success in *using* one's body (motor ability) influences the value one places on self (self-evaluation).

   H. *Secondary sex characteristics* are significant aspects of body image (*too much, too little, too early, too late,* in the *wrong place,* may lead to disturbed body image). Sexual differences in body image are in part related to differences in anatomical structure and body function, as well as to contrasts in lifestyles and cultural roles.

   I. Different *cultures and families* value bodily traits and bodily deviations differently.

   J. Different *body parts* (for example, hair, nose, face, stature, shoulders) have varying personal significance; therefore there is variability in degree of threat, personality integrity, and coping behavior.

   K. *Attitudes* concerning the self will influence and be influenced by person's physical appearance and ability. Society has developed stereotyped ideas regarding outer body structure (body physique) and inner personalities (temperament). Current stereotypes are:
1. *Endomorph*—talkative, sympathetic, good natured, trusting, dependent, lazy, fat.
2. *Mesomorph*—adventuresome, self-reliant, strong, tall.
3. *Ectomorph*—thin, tense and nervous, suspicious, stubborn, pessimistic, quiet.

   L. Person with a *firm ego boundary or body image* is more likely to be independent, striving, goal oriented, influential. Under stress, *may develop skin and muscle disease.*

   M. Person with *poorly integrated body image and weak ego boundary* is more likely to be passive, less goal oriented, less influential, more prone to external pressures. Under stress, *may develop heart and GI diseases.*

   N. Any situation, *illness,* or *injury* that causes a change in body image is a crisis, and the person will go through the *phases of crisis* in an attempt to reintegrate the body image (**Table 6.5**).

 ◆ IV. **Assessment** (Table 6.6)

 ◆ V. **Analysis/nursing diagnosis**—*body image development disturbance may be related to:*

   A. *Obvious loss* of a major body part—amputation of an extremity; hair, teeth, eye, breast.

   B. Surgical procedures in which the relationship of body parts is *visibly* disturbed—colostomy, ileostomy, gastrostomy, ureteroenterostomy.

   C. Surgical procedures in which the loss of body parts is

---

*Adapted from Kolb, L: Disturbances in body image. In Arieti, S (ed): American Handbook of Psychiatry. Basic Books, New York.

†Adapted from Norris, C: Body image. In Carlson, C, and Blackwell, B (eds): Behavioral Concepts and Nursing Intervention, ed. 2. JB Lippincott, Philadelphia.

TABLE 6.5	Four Phases of Body Image Crisis	
Phase	◆ **Assessment**	◆ **Nursing Care Plan/Implementation**
Acute shock	Anxiety, numbness, helplessness.	Provide sustained support, be available to listen, express interest and concern. Allow time for silence and privacy.
Denial	Retreats from reality; fantasy about the wholeness and capability of the body; euphoria; rationalization; refusal to participate in self-care.	Accept denial without reinforcing it. *Avoid* arguing and overloading with reality. Gradually raise questions, reply with doubt to convey unrealistic ideas. Follow client's suggestions for personal-care routine to help increase feelings of adequacy and to decrease helplessness.
Acknowledgment of reality	Grief over loss of valued body part, function, or role; depression, apathy; agitation, bitterness; physical symptoms (insomnia, anorexia, nausea, crying) serve as outlet for feeling; redefinition of body structure and function, with implications for change in lifestyle; acceptance of and cooperation with realistic goals for care and treatment; preoccupation with body functions.	Expect and accept displacement onto nurse of anger, resentment, projection of client's inadequacy. Examine own behavior to see if client's remarks are justified. Simply listen if this is the only way the client can handle feelings at this time. Offer sustained, nonjudgmental listening without being defensive or taking remarks personally. Help dispel anger by encouraging its ventilation. Encourage self-care activities. Support family members as they cope with changes in client's health or body image, role changes, treatment plans.
Resolution and adaptation	Perceives crisis in new light; increased mastery leads to increased self-worth; can look at, feel, and ask questions regarding altered body part; tests others' reactions to changed body; repetitive talk on painful topic of changed self; concentration on *normal* functions in order to increase sense of control.	Teaching and counseling by same nurse in warm, supportive relationship. Assess level of knowledge; begin at that level. Consider motivational state. Provide gradual, nontechnical medical information and specific facts. Repeat instructions frequently, patiently, consistently. Support sense of mastery in self-care; draw on inner resources. Do *not* discourage dependence while gradually encouraging independence. Focus on necessary adaptations of lifestyle due to realistic limitations. Provide follow-up care via referral to community resources after client is discharged.

Source: ©Lagerquist, S: Nursing Examination Review, ed. 4. Addison-Wesley, Redwood City, Calif.

not visible to others—hysterectomy, lung, gallbladder, stomach.

D. Repair procedures (plastic surgery) that do *not* reconstruct body image as assumed—rhinoplasty, plastic surgery to correct large ears, breasts.

E. *Changes in body size and proportion*—obesity, emaciation, acromegaly, gigantism, pregnancy, pubertal changes (*too early, too late, too big, too small, too tall*).

F. Other changes in *external body* surface—hirsutism in women, mammary glands in men.

G. Skin *color* changes—chronic dermatitis, Addison's disease.

H. Skin *texture* changes—scars, thyroid disease, excoriative dermatitis, acne.

I. *Crippling* changes in bones, joints, muscles—arthritis, multiple sclerosis, Parkinson's.

J. Failure of a body part to *function*—quadriplegia, paraplegia, stroke (brain attack).

K. Distorted ideas of structure, function, and significance stemming from *symbolism* of disease seen in terms of *life and death* when heart or lungs are afflicted—heart attacks, asthmatic attacks, pneumonia.

L. *Side effects* of drug therapy—moon face, hirsutism, striated skin, changes in body contours.

M. *Violent attacks* against the body—incest, rape, shooting, knifing, battering.

N. *Mental, emotional disorders*—schizophrenia with depersonalization, somatic delusions, and hallucinations about the body; anorexia nervosa, hypochondriasis; hysteria, malingering.

O. *Diseases requiring isolation* may convey attitude that

TABLE 6.6	Body Image Development and Disturbance Throughout the Life Cycle: ◆ Assessment	
Age Group	**Development of Body Image**	**Developmental Disturbances in Body Image**
Infant and toddler	Becomes aware of body boundaries and separateness of own external body from others through sensory stimulation. Explores external body parts; handles and controls the environment and body through play, bathing, and eating. Experiences pain, shame, fear, and pleasure. Feels doubt or power in mastery of motor skills and strives for autonomy. Learns who one is in relation to the world.	***Infant*** Inadequate somatosensory stimulation → impaired ego development, increased anxiety level, poor foundation for reality testing. Continues to see external objects as extension of self → unrealistic, *distorted* perceptions of significant persons, inability to form normal attachments to others (possessive, engulfing, autistic, withdrawn). ***Toddler*** If body fails to meet parental expectations → shameful, self-deprecating feelings. Failure to master environment and control own body → helplessness, inadequacy, and doubt.
Preschool and school age	Experiences praise, blame, derogation, or criticism for body, its part, or use (pleasure, pain, doubt, or guilt). Explores genitals—discovers anatomical differences between sexes with joy, pride, or shame. Begins awareness of *sexual identity*. Differentiates self as a body and self as a mind. Beginning of *self-concept;* of self as man or woman. Learns mastery of the body (to *do*, to protect *self*, to protect *others*) and environment (run, skip, skate, swim); feels pleasure, competence, worth, or inadequacy.	***Preschool*** Distortion of body image of genital area due to conflict over pleasure versus punishment. If body build does not conform to sex-typed expectations and sex role identification → body image confusion. ***School age*** Physical impairments (speech, poor vision, poor hearing) → feelings of inadequacy and inferiority. Overly self-conscious about, and excessive focus on, body changes in puberty.
Adolescent	Physical self is of more concern than at any other time except old age. Forced body awareness due to physical changes (new senses, proportions, features); feelings of pleasure, power, confidence, or helplessness, pain, inadequacy, doubt, and guilt. Adult body proportions emerge. Anxiety over *ideal self versus emerging/emerged physical self;* body is compared competitively with same-sex peers. Use of body (adolescents' values and attitudes) to relate with opposite sex. Body image crucial for self-concept formation, status achievement, and adequate social relations. Physical changes need to be integrated into evolving body image (strong, competent, powerful, or weak and helpless).	Growth and changes may produce distorted view of self → overemphasis on defects with compensations; inflated ideas of body ability, beauty, perfection; preoccupation with body appearance or body processes, women more likely than men to see body fatter than it is; egocentrism.
Early adulthood	Learns to accept own body without undue preoccupation with its functions or control of these functions. Stability of body image.	Less dependable, less likable body → regression to adolescent behavior and dress due to denial of aging, defeat, depression, self-pity, egocentrism due to fear of loss of sexual identity, withdrawal to early old age.

(Continued on following page)

Age Group	Development of Body Image	Developmental Disturbances in Body Image
Middle age	New challenges due to differential rates of aging in various body parts.	Women more likely to judge themselves uglier than do men or younger and older women.
	Body not functioning as well; unresolved fears, misconceptions, and experiences in relation to body image persist and become recognized.	
Old age	Accelerated physical decline with influence on self-concept and lifestyle.	Ill health → fear of invalidism, hypochondriasis.
	Can accept self and personality as a whole; continued emphasis on physical self, with increased emphasis on inner, emotional self.	Denial related to feelings of threatened incapacity and fear of declining functions.
		Despair over loss of beauty, strength, and youthfulness, with self-disgust about body → projection of criticism onto others.
		Regression.
		Isolation (separation of affect and thought) leads to less intense response to death, disease, aging.
		Compartmentalization (focus on one thing at a time) causes narrowing of consciousness, resistance, rigidity, repetitiveness.
		Resurgence of egocentrism.

Source: ©Lagerquist, S: Nursing Examination Review, ed. 4. Addison-Wesley, Redwood City, Calif.

body is undesirable, unacceptable—tuberculosis, AIDS, malodorous conditions (e.g., gangrene, cancer).

P. *Women's movement and sexual revolution*—use of body for pleasure, not just procreation, sexual freedom, wide range of normality in sex practices, legalized abortion.

Q. *Medical technology*—organ transplants, lifesaving but scar-producing burn treatment, alive but hopeless, alive but debilitated with chronic illnesses.

◆ **VI. General nursing care plan/implementation:**
  A. *Protect from psychological threat* related to impaired *self-attitudes*.
     1. Emphasize person's *normal* aspects.
     2. Encourage self-performance.
  B. *Maintain warm, communicating relationship*.
     1. Encourage awareness of positive responses from others.
     2. Encourage expression of feelings.
  C. *Increase reality perception*.
     1. Provide *reliable* information about health status.
     2. Provide *kinesthetic* feedback to paralyzed part (e.g., "I am raising your leg.").
     3. Provide *perceptual* feedback (e.g., touch, describe, look at scar).
     4. Support a realistic assessment of the situation.
     5. Explore with the client his or her strengths and resources.
  D. *Help achieve positive feelings about self, about adequacy*.
     1. Support strengths *despite* presence of handicaps.
     2. Assist client to look at self in *totality* rather than focus on limitations.

E. *Health teaching*:
   1. Teach client and family about expected changes in functioning.
   2. Explain importance of maintaining a positive self-attitude.
   3. Advise that negative responses from others be regarded with minimum significance.

◆ **VII. Evaluation/outcome criteria:**
  A. Able to resume function in activities of daily living rather than prolonging illness.
  B. Able to accept limits imposed by physical or mental conditions and not attempt unrealistic tasks.
  C. Can shift focus from reminiscence about the healthy past to present and future.
  D. Less verbalized discontent with present body; diminished display of self-displeasure, despair, weeping, and irritability.

Body Image Disturbance— Selected Examples

I. Definition—a body image disturbance arises when a person is unable to accept the body as is and to adapt to it; a conflict develops between the body as it actually is and the body that is pictured mentally, that is, the ideal self.

◆ **II. Analysis/nursing diagnosis:** *body image disturbance* may be related to:
  A. Sensation of *size change* due to obesity, pregnancy, weight loss.
  B. Feelings of being *dirty*—may be imaginary due to hallucinogenic drugs, psychoses.

Mental Health

C. Dual change of body *structure and function* due to trauma, amputation, stroke, etc.
D. Progressive *deformities* due to chronic illness, burns, arthritis.
E. Loss of body boundaries and *depersonalization* due to sensory deprivation, such as blindness, immobility, fatigue, stress, anesthesia. May also be due to psychoses or hallucinogenic drugs.

◆ **III. Assessment** (see **Table 6.6**)

Body Image Disturbance Caused by Amputation

◆ **A. Assessment:**
1. Loss of self-esteem; feelings of helplessness, worthlessness, shame, and guilt.
2. Fear of abandonment may lead to appeals for sympathy by exhibiting helplessness and vulnerability.
3. Feelings of castration (loss of self) and symbolic death; loss of wholeness.
4. Existence of phantom pain (most clients).
5. Passivity, lack of responsibility for use of disabled body parts.

◆ **B. Nursing care plan/implementation:**
1. *Avoid* stereotyping person as being less competent now than previously by *not* referring to client as the "amputee."
2. Foster independence; encourage self-care by assessing what client *can* do for himself or herself.
3. Help person set *realistic* short-term and long-term goals by exploring with the client his or her strengths and resources.
4. *Health teaching:*
   a. Encourage family members to work through their feelings, to accept person as he or she presents self.
   b. Teach how to set realistic goals and limitations.
   c. Explain what phantom pain is; that it is a normal experience.
   d. Explain role and function of prosthetic devices, where and how to obtain them, and how to find assistance in their use.

◆ **C. Evaluation/outcome criteria:**
1. Can acknowledge the loss and move through three stages of mourning (shock and disbelief, developing awareness, and resolution).
2. Can discuss fears and concerns about loss of body part, its meaning, the problem of compensating for the loss, and reaction of persons (repulsion, rejection, and sympathy).

Body Image Disturbance in Brain Attack (Stroke)

◆ **A. Assessment:**
1. Feelings of shame (personal, private, self-judgment of failure) due to loss of bowel and bladder control, speech function.

2. Body image boundaries disrupted; contact with environment is hindered by inability to ambulate or manipulate environment physically; may result in personality deterioration due to diminished number of sensory experiences. Loses orientation to body sphere; feels confused, trapped in own body.

◆ **B. Nursing care plan/implementation:**
1. Reduce frustration and infantilism due to communication problems by:
   a. Rewarding all speech efforts.
   b. Listening and observing for all nonverbal cues.
   c. Restating verbalizations to see if correct meaning is understood.
   d. Speaking slowly, using two- to three-word sentences.
2. Assist *reintegration* of body parts and function; help regain awareness of paralyzed side by:
   a. Tactile stimulation.
   b. Verbal reminders of existence of affected parts.
   c. Direct visual contact via mirrors and grooming.
   d. Use of safety features (e.g., Posey belt).
3. *Health teaching:* control of bowel and bladder function; how to prevent problems of immobility.

◆ **C. Evaluation/outcome criteria:** dignity is maintained while relearning to control elimination.

Body Image Disturbance in Myocardial Infarction

Emotional problems (e.g., anxiety, depression, sleep disturbance, fear of another myocardial infarction [MI]) during convalescence can seriously hamper rehabilitation. The adaptation and convalescence is influenced by the multiple symbolic meanings of the heart, for example:

1. Seat of emotions (love, pride, fear, sadness).
2. Center of the body (one-of-a-kind organ).
3. Life itself (can no longer rely on the heart; failure of the heart means failure of life).

◆ **A. Assessment:**
1. *Attitude*—overly cautious and restrictive; may result in boredom, weakness, insomnia, exaggerated dependency.
2. *Acceptance* of illness—use of denial may result in noncompliance.
3. *Behavior*—self-destructive.
4. *Family conflicts*—related to activity, diet.
5. *Effects of MI on:*
   a. *Changes in lifestyle*—eating, smoking, drinking; activities, employment, sex.
   b. *Family members*—may be anxious, overprotective.
   c. *Role in family*—role reversal may result in loss of incentive for work.
   d. *Dependence-independence*—issues related to family conflicts (especially restrictive attitudes about desirable activity and dietary regimen).

Mental Health

e. *Job*—social pressure to "slow down" may result in loss of job, reassignment, forced early retirement, "has-been" social status.

◆ **B. Nursing care plan/implementation:**
1. Prevent "cardiac cripple" by shaping person's and family's attitude toward damaged organ.
   a. Instill optimism.
   b. Encourage *productive* living rather than inactivity.
2. Set up a physical and mental activity program with client and mate.
3. Provide anticipatory guidance regarding expected weakness, fear, uncertainty.
4. *Health teaching:* nature of coronary disease, interpretation of medical regimen, effect on sexual behavior.

◆ **C. Evaluation/outcome criteria:**
1. Adheres to medical regimen.
2. Modifies lifestyle without becoming overly dependent on others.

Body Image and Obesity (see Unit 7)

A. Definition: body weight exceeding 20% above the norm for person's age, sex, and height constitutes obesity. Body mass index (BMI) is also used. Although a faulty adaptation, obesity may serve as a protection against more severe illness; it represents an effort to function better, be powerful, stay well, or be less sick. The *problem* may *not* be difficulty in losing weight; reducing may *not* be the appropriate *cure.*

◆ **B. Assessment**—characteristics:
1. Age—one out of three persons under 30 years of age is more than 10% overweight.
2. Increase risks for stroke, MI, diabetes.
3. Feelings: self-hate, self-derogation, failure, helplessness; tendency to avoid clothes shopping and mirror reflections.
4. Viewed by others as ugly, repulsive, lacking in will power, weak, unwilling to change, neurotic.
5. Discrepancy between actual body size (real self) and person's concept of it (ideal self).
6. Pattern of successful weight loss followed quickly and repetitively by failure; that is, weight gain.
7. Eating in response to outer environment (e.g., food odor, time of day, food availability, degree of stress, anger); *not inner* environment (hunger, increased gastric motility).
8. Experiences less pleasure in physical activity; less active than others.
9. All people who are obese are *not* the same.
   a. In *newborns and infants,* there is an increased *number* of adipocytes *who are obese* via *hyperplastic* process.
   b. In *adults who are obese,* there may be increased body fat deposits, resulting in increased *size* of adipocytes via *hypertrophic* process.

c. When an *infant who is obese becomes an adult who is obese* the result may be an increased *number* of cells available for fat *storage.*
10. Loss of control of own body or eating behavior.

◆ **C. Analysis/nursing diagnosis:** *defensive coping* related to eating disorder. Contributing factors:
1. Genetic.
2. Thermodynamic.
3. Endocrine.
4. Neuroregulatory.
5. Biochemical factors in metabolism.
6. Ethnic and family practices.
7. *Psychological:*
   a. Compensation for feelings of helplessness and inadequacy.
   b. Maternal overprotection; overfed and force-fed, especially infants who are formula-fed.
   c. Food offered and used to relieve anxiety, frustration, anger, and rage can lead to difficulty in differentiating between hunger and other needs.
   d. As a child, food offered instead of love.
8. *Social:*
   a. Food easily available.
   b. Use of motorized transportation and labor-saving devices.
   c. Refined carbohydrates.
   d. Social aspects of eating.
   e. Restaurant meals high in salt, sugar.

◆ **D. Nursing care plan/implementation:**
1. Encourage *prevention* of lifelong body image problems.
   a. Support *breastfeeding,* where infant determines quantity consumed, *not* mother; work through her feelings against breastfeeding (fear of intimacy, dependence, feelings of repulsion, concern about confinement, and inability to produce enough milk).
   b. Help mothers to *not overfeed* the infant if formula-fed: suggest water between feedings; do *not* start solids until 6 months old or 14 pounds; do *not* enrich the prescribed formula.
   c. Help mothers *differentiate* between hunger and other infant cries; help her to try out different responses to the expressed needs other than offering food.
2. Use *case findings* of infants who are obese, as well as young children, and adolescents.
3. Assess current eating patterns.
4. Identify need to eat, and relate need to preceding events, hopes, fears, or feelings.
5. Employ behavior-modification techniques.
6. Encourage outside interests not related to food or eating.
7. Alleviate guilt, reduce stigma of being obese.
8. *Health teaching:*
   a. Promote awareness of certain *stressful* periods that can produce maladaptive responses such as obesity (e.g., puberty, postnuptial, postpartum, menopause).

b. Assist in drawing up a meal plan for slow, steady weight loss.

c. Advise eating five small meals a day.

◆ **E. Evaluation/outcome criteria:** goal for desired weight is reached; weight-control plan is continued.

Scope of Human Sexuality Throughout the Life Cycle

Human sexuality refers to all the characteristics of an individual (social, personal, and emotional) that are manifest in his or her relationships with others and that reflect gender-genital orientation.

I. Components of sexual system

A. *Biological sexuality*—refers to chromosomes, hormones, primary and secondary sex characteristics, and anatomical structure.

B. *Sexual identity*—based on own feelings and perceptions of how well traits correspond with own feelings and concepts of maleness and femaleness; also includes gender identity.

C. *Gender identity*—a sense of masculinity and femininity shaped by biological, environmental, and intrapsychic forces, as well as cultural traditions and education.

D. *Sex role behavior*—includes components of both sexual identity and gender identity. Aim: sexual fulfillment through masturbation, heterosexual, or homosexual experiences. Selection of behavior is influenced by personal value system and sexual, gender, and biological identity. Gender identity and roles are learned and constantly reinforced by input and feedback regarding social expectations and demands (**Table 6.7**).

II. Concepts and principles of human sexual response

A. Human sexual response involves not only the genitals but the total body.

B. Factors in early postnatal and childhood periods influence gender identity, gender role, sex typing, and sexual responses in later life.

C. Cultural and personally subjective variables influence ways of sexual expression and perception of what is satisfying.

D. Healthy sexual expressions vary widely.

E. Requirements for human sexual response:

1. Intact central and peripheral nervous system to provide *sensory* perception, *motor* reaction.

2. Intact circulatory system to produce *vasocongestive* response.

3. Desirable and interested partner, if sex outlet involves mutuality.

4. *Freedom* from guilt, anxiety, misconceptions, and interfering conditioned responses.

5. Acceptable physical *setting,* usually private.

Sexual-Health Counseling

General Issues

I. Issues in sexual practices with implications for counseling:

A. *Sex education*—need to provide accurate and complete information on all aspects of sexuality to all people.

B. *Sexual-health care*—should be part of total health-care planning for all.

C. *Sexual orientation*—need to avoid discrimination based on sexual orientation (such as homosexuality); the right to satisfying, nonexploitive relationships with others, regardless of gender.

D. *Sex and the law*—sex between consenting adults not a legal concern.

E. *Explicit sexual material* (pornography)—can be useful in fulfilling various needs in life, as in quadriplegia.

TABLE 6.7	Sexual Behavior Throughout the Life Cycle
Age	**Development of Sexual Behavior**
First 18 mo	Major source of pleasure from touch and oral exploration.
18 mo–3 yr	Pleasurable and sexual feelings are associated with genitals (acts of urination and defecation). Masturbation without fantasy or eroticism.
3–6 yr	Beginning resolution of Oedipus and Electra complexes; foundation for heterosexual relationships; masturbation with curiosity about genitals of opposite sex.
6–12 yr	Peer relations with same sex; onset of sex play; morality and sexual attitudes taught and learned; phase of sexual tranquility.
12–18 yr (adolescence)	Onset of puberty with biological development of secondary sex characteristics; menstruation and ejaculation occur.
	Frequent masturbation. Intense anxiety and guilt may occur over heterosexual or homosexual behavior (petting, coitus, masturbation, STD, pregnancy, genital size).
18–23 yr (early adulthood)	Maximum interpersonal and intrapsychic self-consciousness about sexuality. Issues: premarital coitus, sexual freedom.
	Anxiety about: sexual competency, genital size, impotence, fear of pregnancy, rejection.
23–30 yr	Focus on sexual activity in coupling and parenthood; mutual masturbation.

(Continued on following page)

Mental Health

Age	Development of Sexual Behavior
30–45 yr (**middle adulthood**)	For women—peak sexuality without new sexual experiences. Conflict regarding extramarital sex may increase.

Purpose of Intercourse:

Need for body contact (and procreation until age 35+).

Physical expression of trust, love, and affection.

Reaffirmation of self-concept, as sexually desirable and sexually competent due to worry about effects of aging.

Sexual Dysfunctions:

Men: erectile dysfunction, premature ejaculation, decreasing libido.

Women: intermittent lack of orgasmic response, vaginismus, dyspareunia.

For either or both: changes or divergences in degree of sexual interest.

Causes of Sexual Dysfunction (Men):

Overindulgence in food or drink.

Preoccupation with career and economic pursuits.

Mental or physical fatigue.

Boredom with monotony of relationship.

Drug dependency: alcohol, tobacco, certain medications.

Fear of failure.

Chronic illness: diabetes, alcoholism → peripheral neuropathy → impotence (smoking and drinking may result in decreased testosterone production); excessive smoking → vascular constriction → decreased libido; spinal cord injuries; prostatectomy, androgen deprivation therapy (for prostate cancer).

Self-devaluation due to accumulation of role function losses, sexual self-image, and body image.

Past history of lack of sexual enjoyment in younger years.

Causes of Sexual Dysfunction (Women):

Belief in myths regarding "shoulds and should nots" of frequency, variations, and enjoyment.

Widowhood: inhibition and loyalty to deceased.

45–65 yr (**later adulthood**)	Menopause occurs. Little or no fear of pregnancy; evidence of sexual activity differences in men and women: women may have increased pleasure, men take longer to reach orgasm; may prefer less strenuous mutual masturbation.
Over 65 yr (**old age**)	Activity depends on earlier sexual attitude. May suffer guilt and shame when engaging in sex. Can have active and enjoyable sex life with continuing sex needs. Age is not a barrier provided there is opportunity for sexual activity with a partner or for sublimated activities. Women in this age group outnumber men; single women outnumber single men by an even larger margin.

Source: ©Lagerquist, S: Nursing Examination Review, ed. 4. Addison-Wesley, Redwood City, Calif.

Mental Health

F. *Masturbation*—a natural behavior at all ages; can fulfill a variety of needs (see **Masturbation, p. 365**).

G. Availability of *contraception* for minors—the right of access to medical contraceptive care should be available to all ages.

H. *Abortion*—confidentiality for minors.

I. *Treatment for sexually transmitted disease (STD)*—naming of partners as part of STD control.

J. *Sex and the elderly*—need opportunity for sexual expression; need privacy when in communal living setting.

K. *Sex and the disabled*—need to have possible means available for rewarding sexual expressions.

II. Sexual myths*

A. *Myth:* Ignorance is bliss.

Fact: What you don't know *can* hurt you (note the high frequency of STD and abortions); *myths* can perpetuate fears and such misinformation as:

1. *Masturbation causes mental illness.*
2. *Women don't or shouldn't have orgasms.*
3. *Tampons cause STD.*
4. *Plastic wrap works better than condoms.*
5. *Coca-Cola is an effective douche.*

Fact: Lack of knowledge during initial experiences may result in fear and set precedent for future sexual reactions.

*Adapted from Sedgwick, R: Myths in human sexuality: a social-psychological perspective. Nurs Clin North Am 10(3):539–550, Philadelphia, WB Saunders.

B. *Myths:* The planned sex act is not OK and is immoral for "nice" girls. If a woman gets pregnant, it is her own fault. Contraceptives are solely a woman's responsibility.

Fact: Sex and contraception are the prerogative and responsibility of both partners.

C. *Myth:* A good relationship is harmonious, free of conflict and disagreement (which are signs of rejection and incompatibility).

Fact: Conflict can induce growth in self-understanding and in understanding of others.

D. *Myth:* Sexual deviance (such as homosexuality) is a sign of personality disturbance.

Fact: No single sexual behavior is the most desirable, effective, or satisfactory. Personal sexual choice is a fundamental right.

E. *Myth:* A woman's sexual needs and gratification should be secondary to her partner's; a woman's role is to satisfy others.

Fact: A woman has as much right to sexual freedom and experience as a man.

F. *Myth:* Menopause is an affliction signifying the end of sex.

Fact: Many women do not suffer through menopause, and many report renewed sexual interest.

G. *Myth:* Sexual activity past 60 years of age is not essential.

Fact: Sexual activity is therapeutic because it:
1. Affirms identity.
2. Provides communication.
3. Provides companionship.
4. Meets intimacy needs.

H. *Myth:* A woman's sex drive decreases in postmenopausal period.

Fact: The strength of the sex drive becomes greater as androgen overcomes the inhibitory action of estrogen.

I. *Myth:* Men over age 60 cannot achieve an erection.

Fact: According to Masters and Johnson, a major difference between the aging man and the younger man is the duration of each phase of the sexual cycle. The older man is slower in achieving an erection.

J. *Myth:* Regular sexual activity cannot help the aging person's loss of function.

Fact: Research is revealing that "disuse atrophy" may lead to loss of sexual capacity. Regular sexual activity helps preserve sexual function.

III. Basic principles of sexual-health counseling

A. There is *no* universal consensus about acceptable values in human sexuality. Each social group has very definite values regarding sex.

B. Counselors need to examine own feelings, attitudes, values, biases, knowledge base.

C. Help reduce fear, guilt, ignorance.

D. Offer guidance and education rather than indoctrination or pressure to conform.

E. Each person needs to be helped to make personal choices regarding sexual conduct.

IV. Counseling in sexual health

A. **General considerations**
1. Create atmosphere of *trust and acceptance* for objective, nonjudgmental dialogue.
2. Use *language* related to sexual behavior that is mutually comfortable and understood between client and nurse.
   a. Use alternative terms for definitions.
   b. Determine exact meaning of words and phrases because sexual words and expressions have different meanings to people with different backgrounds and experiences.
3. *Desensitize* own stress reaction to the emotional component of taboo topics.
   a. Increase awareness of own sexual values, biases, prejudices, stereotypes, and fears.
   b. *Avoid* overreacting, underreacting.
4. Become sensitively aware of *interrelationships* between sexual needs, fears, and behaviors and other aspects of living.
5. Begin with *commonly* discussed areas (such as menstruation) and progress to discussion of individual sexual experiences (such as masturbation). Move from areas where there is less voluntary control (nocturnal emissions) to more responsibility and voluntary behavior (premature ejaculation).
6. Offer *educational information* to dispel fears, myths; give tacit permission to explore sensitive areas.
7. Bring into awareness possibly *repressed* feelings of guilt, anger, denial, and suppressed sexual feelings.
8. Explore possible *alternatives* of sexual expression.
9. Determine *interrelationships* among mental, social, physical, and sexual well-being.

◆ B. **Assessment parameters:**
1. Self-awareness of body image, values, and attitudes toward human sexuality; comfort with own sexuality.
2. Ability to identify sex problems on basis of own satisfaction or dissatisfaction.
3. Developmental history, sex education, family relationships, cultural and ethnic values, and available support resources.
4. Type and frequency of sexual behavior.
5. Nature and quality of sex relations with others.
6. Attitude toward and satisfaction with sexual activity.
7. Expectations and goals. **Table 6.8** outlines a guideline in conducting an *assessment* interview.

◆ C. **Nursing care plan/implementation:**
1. *Long-term goals*
   a. Increase knowledge of reproductive system and types of sex behavior.
   b. Promote positive view of body and sex needs.
   c. Integrate sex needs into self-identity.
   d. Develop adaptive and satisfying patterns of sexual expression.
   e. Understand effects of physical illness on sexual performance.
2. *Primary sexual health interventions*
   a. Goals: minimize stress factors, strengthen sexual integrity.

TABLE 6.8	Suggested Format for Sexual Assessment Interview

Interview Step	Rationale
1. Open the discussion of sexual matters subtly with an open-ended question: "People with your illness or stresses often experience other difficulties, sometimes with sexual functioning."	This gentle opening lets the client know that other people have difficulties, too. It gives the client permission to talk with the nurse about sexual matters without labeling these matters as problems.
2. Follow up with another open-ended question about the client's current status: "Has your illness or stresses made any difference in what it's like for you to be a wife or husband (lover, boyfriend, girlfriend, sexual partner)?"	The phrasing of this question enables the client to acknowledge a problem without admitting a shortcoming.
3. If the client speaks of having a dysfunction, ask about its effect: "How does this affect you?" or "How do you feel about it?"	This indicates that the nurse is willing to explore sexual matters more completely.
4. Ask about the severity and duration of the dysfunction: "Is it always difficult to control your ejaculation?" "Tell me when you first noticed this."	These questions are directed at identifying the specific problem.
5. Ask about the effects on the client's sexual partner: "Has this affected your relationship with your partner?"	This question is directed toward exploring the interactional aspects of the identified problem.
6. Ask what the client has already done to alleviate the situation: "Have you made any adjustments in your sexual activity?"	This question yields data that will help the nurse to formulate an intervention plan.
7. Ask the client if and how he or she would like the situation changed: "How would you like to change the situation to make it more satisfying?"	This question conveys the negotiated nature of the therapeutic relationship, in which the client's own goals play an important part.

Source: Adapted from the *classic article by* Whitley, MP, and Willingham, W: Adding a sexual assessment to the health interview. Journal of Psychiatric Nursing and Mental Health Services.

b. Provide education to uninformed or misinformed.
c. Identify stress factors (myths, stereotypes, negative parental attitudes).
3. *Secondary sexual health interventions:* identify sexual problems early and refer for treatment.
◆ **D. Evaluation/outcome criteria:**
1. Reduced impairment or dysfunction from acute sex problem or chronic, unresolved sex problem.
2. Evaluate how client's goals were achieved in terms of *positive* thoughts, feelings, and *satisfying* sexual behaviors.

Specific Situations

I. Masturbation
  A. Definition—act of achieving sexual arousal and orgasm through manual or mechanical stimulation of the sex organs.
  B. Characteristics
    1. Can be an interpersonal as well as a solitary activity.
    2. "It is a healthy and appropriate sexual activity, playing an important role in ultimate consolidation of one's sexual identity."*

*Marcus, IM, and Francis, JJ: Masturbation from Infancy to Senescence. International Universities Press, New York.

3. Accompanied by fantasies that are important for:
    a. Physically disabled.
    b. Fatigued.
    c. Compensation for unreachable goals and unfulfilled wishes.
    d. Rehearsal for future sexual relations.
    e. Absence or impersonal action of partner.
4. Can help release tension harmlessly.
  C. Concepts and principles related to masturbation
    1. Staff's feelings and reactions influence their responses to client and affect continuation of masturbation (that is, negative staff actions increase client's frustration, which increases masturbation).
    2. Masturbation is normal and universal, *not* physically or psychologically harmful in itself.
    3. Pleasurable genital sensations are important for increasing *self-pride,* finding *gratification* in *own* body, increasing sense of *personal value* of being lovable, helping to *prepare for adult* sexual role.
    4. Excessive masturbation—some needs not being met through interpersonal relations; may use behavior to *avoid* interpersonal relations.
    5. Activity may be related to:
      a. Curiosity, experimentation.
      b. Tension reduction, pleasure.
      c. Enhanced interest in sexual development.
      d. Fear and avoidance of social relationships.

◆ D. **Nursing care plan:**
   1. *Long-term goals*
      a. Gain insight into *preference* for masturbation.
      b. Relieve accompanying guilt, worry, self-devaluation (**Figure 6.2**).
   2. *Short-term goals*
      a. Clarify myths regarding masturbation.
      b. Help client see masturbation as an acceptable sexual activity for individuals of all ages.
      c. Set limits on masturbation in inappropriate settings.

◆ E. **Nursing implementation:**
   1. Examine, control nurse's own negative feelings; show respect.
   2. *Avoid:* reinforcement of guilt and self-devaluation; scorn; threats, punishment, anger, alarm reaction; use of masturbation for rebellion in power struggle between staff and client.
   3. *Identify* client's unmet needs; consider purpose served by masturbation (may be useful behavior).
   4. *Examine* pattern in which behavior occurs.
   5. Intervene when degree of functioning in other daily life activities is *impaired.*
      a. Remain calm, accepting, but nonsanctioning.
      b. Promptly help clarify client's feelings, thoughts, at stressful time.
      c. Review precipitating events.
      d. Be a neutral "sounding board"; *avoid* evasiveness.
      e. If unable to handle situation, find someone who can.
   6. For clients who masturbate at *inappropriate* times or in inappropriate places:
      a. Give special attention when they are not masturbating.
      b. Encourage new interests and activities, but *not* immediately after observing masturbation.
      c. Keep clients distracted, occupied with interesting activities.
   7. *Health teaching:* explain myths and teach facts regarding cause and effects.

◆ F. **Evaluation/outcome criteria:**
   1. Acknowledges function of own sexual organs.
   2. States sexual experience is satisfying.
   3. Views sexuality as pleasurable and wholesome.
   4. Views sex organs as acceptable, enjoyable, and valued part of body image.

   5. Self-image as fully functioning person is restored and maintained.

II. **Homosexuality**
   A. **Definition**—alternative sexual behavior; applied to sexual relations between persons of the same sex.
   B. **Theories regarding causes**
      1. Hereditary tendencies.
      2. Imbalance of sex hormones.
      3. Environmental influences and conditioning factors, related to learning and psychodynamic theories.
         a. Defense against unsatisfying relationship with father.
         b. Unsatisfactory and threatening early relationships with opposite sex.
         c. Oedipal attachment to parent.
         d. Parent who is seductive (incest).
         e. Castration fear.
         f. Labeling and guilt leading to sexual acting out.
         g. Faulty sex education.
      4. Preferred choice as a lifestyle.
   ◆ C. **Nursing care plan/implementation:**
      1. Nurse needs to be aware of and work through own attitudes that may interfere with providing care.
      2. Accept and respect lifestyle of a client who is gay (man who is homosexual) or lesbian (woman who is homosexual).
      3. Assess and treat for possible sexually transmitted diseases and hepatitis.
      4. *Health teaching:* assess and add to knowledge base about alternatives in sexual behavior.
   ◆ D. **Evaluation/outcome criteria:** expresses self-confidence and positive self-image; able to sustain satisfying sexual behavior with chosen partner and avoid at-risk behaviors for STDs.

III. **Sex and the person who is disabled**
◆ A. **Assessment parameters:**
   1. Previous level of sex functioning and conflict.
   2. Client's view of sex activity (self and mutual pleasure, tension release, procreation, control).
   3. Cultural environment (influence on body image).
   4. Degree of acceptance of illness.

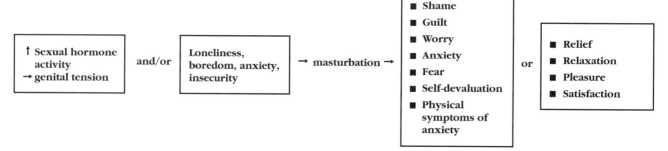

FIGURE 6.2   Operationalization of the behavioral concept of masturbation.

5. Support system (partner, family, support group).
6. Body image and self-esteem.
7. Outlook on future.

◆ **B. Analysis/nursing diagnosis:** *sexual dysfunction* associated with physical illness related to:
 1. Disinterest in sexual activity.
 2. Fear of precipitating or aggravating physical illness through sexual activity.
 3. Use of illness as excuse to avoid feared or undesired sex.
 4. Physical inability or discomfort during sexual activity.

◆ **C. Nursing care plan/implementation:**
 1. Approach with nonjudgmental attitude.
 2. Elicit concerns about current physical state and perceptions of changes in sexuality.
 3. Observe nonverbal clues of concern.
 4. Identify genital assets.
 5. Support client and partner during adjustment to current state.
 6. Explore culturally acceptable sublimation activities.
 7. Promote adjustment to body image change.
 8. *Health teaching:*
  a. Teach self-help skills.
  b. Teach partner to care for client's physical needs.
  c. Teach alternate sex behaviors and acceptable sublimation (touching, for example).

◆ **D. Evaluation/outcome criteria:** attains satisfaction with adaptive alternatives of sexual expressions; has a positive attitude toward self, body, and sexual activity.

IV. Inappropriate sexual behavior

◆ **A. Assessment:** public exhibitions of sexual behaviors that are offensive to others; making sexual advances to other clients or staff.

◆ **B. Analysis/nursing diagnosis:** *conflict with social order* related to:
 1. Acting out angry and hostile feelings.
 2. Lack of awareness of hospital and agency rules regarding acceptable public behavior.
 3. Variation in cultural interpretations of what is acceptable public behavior.
 4. Reaction to unintended seductiveness by person's attire, posture, tone, or choice of terminology.

◆ **C. Nursing care plan/implementation:**
 1. Maintain calm, nonjudgmental attitude.
 2. Set firm limits on unacceptable behavior.
 3. Encourage verbalization of feelings rather than unacceptable physical expression.
 4. Reinforce appropriate behavior.
 5. Provide constructive diversional activity for clients.
 6. *Health teaching:* explain rules regarding public behavior; teach acceptable ways to express anger.

◆ **D. Evaluation/outcome criteria:** verbalizes anger rather than acting out; accepts rules regarding behavior in public.

Concept of Death Throughout the Life Cycle

I. Ages 1–3
 A. No concept per se, but experiences *separation anxiety and abandonment* any time significant other disappears from view over a period of time.
 B. *Coping* means: fear, resentment, anger, aggression, regression, withdrawal.
◆ **C. Nursing care plan/implementation**—help the family:
  1. Facilitate transfer of affectional ties to another nurturing adult.
  2. Decrease separation anxiety of child who is hospitalized by encouraging family visits and by reassuring child that she or he will not be alone.
  3. Provide stable environment through consistent staff assignment.

II. Ages 3–5
 A. Least anxious about death.
 B. Denial of death as inevitable and final process.
 C. Death is separation, being alone.
 D. Death is *sleep* and sleep is death.
 E. "Death" is part of vocabulary; seen as real, gradual, *temporary,* not permanent.
 F. Dead person is seen as alive, but in altered form, that is, lacks movement.
 G. There are *degrees* of death.
 H. Death means not being here anymore.
 I. "Living" and "lifeless" are not yet distinguished.
 J. Illness and death seen as *punishment* for "badness"; fear and guilt about sexual and aggressive impulses.
 K. Death happens, but only to others.
◆ **L. Nursing care plan/implementation** (in addition to previous):
  1. Encourage play for expression of feelings; use clay, dolls, etc.
  2. Encourage verbal expression of feelings using children's books.
  3. Model appropriate grieving behavior.
  4. Protect child from the overstimulation of hysterical adult reactions by limiting contact.
  5. Clearly state what death is—death is final, no breathing, eating, awakening—and that death is *not* sleep.
  6. Check child at night and provide support through holding and staying with child.
  7. Allow a choice of attending the funeral and, if child decides to attend, describe what will take place.
  8. If parents are grieving, have other family or friends attend to child's needs.

III. Ages 5–10
 A. Death is cessation of life; question of what happens after death.
 B. Death seen as definitive, *universal,* inevitable, *irreversible.*
 C. Death occurs to all living things, including self; may express, "It isn't fair."
 D. Death is distant from self (an eventuality).

E. Believe death occurs by accident, happens only to the very *old* or very sick.

F. Death is personified (as a separate person) in fantasies and magical thinking.

G. Death anxiety handled by *nightmares, rituals,* and *superstitions* (related to fear of darkness and sleeping alone because death is an external person, such as a skeleton, who comes and takes people away at night).

H. Dissolution of bodily life seen as a perceptible result.

I. Fear of body mutilation.

◆ J. **Nursing care plan/implementation** (in addition to previous):
1. Allow child to experience the loss of pets, friends, and family members.
2. Help child talk it out and experience the appropriate emotional reactions.
3. Understand need for increase in play, especially competitive play.
4. Involve child in funeral preparation and rituals.
5. Understand and accept regressive or protest behaviors.
6. Rechannel protest behaviors into constructive outlets.

IV. **Adolescence**
A. Death seen as inevitable, *personal,* universal, and *permanent;* corporal life stops; body decomposes.
B. Does not fear death, but concerned with how to *live now,* what death feels like, *body changes.*
C. Experiences *anger, frustration, and despair* over lack of future, lack of fulfillment of adult roles.
D. Openly asks *difficult,* honest, *direct* questions.
E. Anger at healthy peers.
F. Conflict between *developing* body versus *deteriorating* body, *independent* identity versus *dependency.*

◆ G. **Nursing care plan/implementation** (in addition to previous):
1. Facilitate full expression of grief by answering direct questions.
2. Help let out feelings, especially through creative and aesthetic pursuits.
3. Encourage participation in funeral ritual.
4. Encourage full use of peer group support system, by providing opportunities for group talks.

V. **Young adulthood**
A. Death seen as *unwelcome* intrusion, *interruption* of what might have been.
B. Reaction: *rage, frustration, disappointment.*

◆ C. **Nursing care plan/implementation:** all of previous, especially peer group support.

VI. **Middle age**
A. Concerned with *consequences* of own death and that of significant others.
B. Death seen as disruption of involvement, responsibility, and *obligations.*
C. End of plans, projects, experiences.
D. Death is *pain.*

◆ E. **Nursing care plan/implementation** (in addition to previous): assess need for counseling when also in midlife crisis.

VII. **Old age**
A. *Philosophical* rationalizations: death as inevitable, final process of life, when "time runs out."
B. *Religious* view: death represents only the dissolution of life and is a doorway to a new life (a preparatory stage for another life).
C. Time of rest and peace, supreme refuge from turmoil of life.

◆ D. **Nursing care plan/implementation** (in addition to previous):
1. Help person prepare for own death by helping with funeral prearrangements, wills, and sharing of mementos.
2. Facilitate life review and reinforce positive aspects.
3. Provide care and comfort.
4. Be present at death.

Death and Dying

Too often the process of death has had such frightening aspects that people have suffered alone. Today there has been a vast change in attitudes; death and dying are no longer taboo topics. There is a growing realization that we need to accept death as a natural process. Elisabeth Kübler-Ross has written extensively on the process of dying, describing the stages of *denial* ("not me"), *anger* ("why me?"), *bargaining* ("yes me—but"), *depression* ("yes, me"), and *acceptance* ("my time is close now, it's all right"), with implications for the helping person.

I. **Concepts and principles related to death and dying:**
A. Persons may know or *suspect* they are dying and may want to talk about it; often they look for someone to share their fears and the process of dying.
B. Fear of death can be reduced by helping clients feel that they are *not alone.*
C. The dying need the opportunity to live their final experiences to the fullest, in their *own* way.
D. People who are dying remain more or less the *same* as they were during life; their approaches to death are consistent with their approaches to life.
E. Dying persons' need to review their lives may be a purposeful attempt to reconcile themselves to what "was" and what "could have been."
F. *Three ways* of facing death are (a) quiet acceptance with inner strength and peace of mind; (b) restlessness, impatience, anger, and hostility; and (c) depression, withdrawal, and fearfulness.
G. *Four tasks* facing a person who is dying are (a) reviewing life, (b) coping with physical symptoms in the end stage of life, (c) making a transition from known to unknown state, and (d) reaction to separation from loved ones.
H. Crying and tears are an important aspect of the grief process.
I. There are many *blocks* to providing a helping relationship with the dying and bereaved:

1. Nurses' unwillingness to share the process of dying—minimizing their contacts and blocking out their own feelings.
2. Forgetting that a person who is dying may be feeling lonely, abandoned, and afraid of dying.
3. Reacting with irritation and hostility to the person's frequent calls.
4. Nurses' failure to seek help and support from team members when feeling afraid, uneasy, and frustrated in caring for a person who is dying.
5. Not allowing client to talk about death and dying.
6. Nurses' use of technical language or social chit-chat as a defense against their own anxieties.

◆ **II. Assessment of death and dying:**
  A. *Physical*
    1. Observable deterioration of physical and mental capacities—person is unable to fulfill physiological needs, such as eating and elimination.
    2. Circulatory collapse (blood pressure and pulse).
    3. Renal or hepatic failure.
    4. Respiratory decline.
  B. *Psychosocial*
    1. Fear of death is signaled by agitation, restlessness, and sleep disturbances at night.
    2. Anger, agitation, blaming.
    3. Morbid self-pity with feelings of defeat and failure.
    4. Depression and withdrawal.
    5. Introspectiveness and calm acceptance of the inevitable.

◆ **III. Analysis/nursing diagnosis:**
  A. *Terminal illness response.*
  B. *Altered feeling states* related to fear of being alone.
  C. *Altered comfort patterns* related to pain.
  D. *Altered meaningfulness* related to depression, hopelessness, helplessness, powerlessness.
  E. *Altered social interaction* related to withdrawal.

◆ **IV. Nursing care plan/implementation:**
  A. *Long-term goal:* foster environment where person and family can experience dying with dignity.
  B. *Short-term goals:*
    1. Express feelings (person and family).
    2. Support person and family.
    3. Minimize physical discomfort.
  C. Explore your own feelings about death and dying with team members; form support groups.
  D. Be aware of the *normal grief* process.
    1. *Allow* person and family to do the work of grieving and mourning.
    2. Allow crying and mood swings, anger, demands.
    3. Permit yourself to cry.
  E. Allow person to *express* feelings, fears, and concerns.
    1. *Avoid* pat answers to questions about "why."
    2. Pick up symbolic communication.
  F. Provide care and comfort with *relief from pain;* do not isolate person.
  G. Stay *physically close.*
    1. Use touch.
    2. Be available to form a consistent relationship.

  H. *Reduce isolation and abandonment* by assigning person to room in which isolation is less likely to occur and by allowing flexible visiting hours.
  I. Keep activities in room as *near normal* and *constant* as possible.
  J. Speak in *audible* tones, not whispers.
  K. Be alert to cues when person needs to be alone *(disengagement process).*
  L. Leave room for *hope.*
  M. Help person die with peace of mind by lending support and providing opportunities to express anger, pain, and fears to someone who will accept her or him and not censor verbalization.
  N. *Health teaching:* teach grief process to family and friends; teach methods to relieve pain.

◆ **V. Evaluation/outcome criteria:**
  A. Remains comfortable and free of pain as long as possible.
  B. Dies with dignity.

Grief/Bereavement

Grief is a typical reaction to the loss of a source of psychological gratification. It is a syndrome with somatic and psychological symptoms that diminish when grief is resolved. Grief processes have been extensively described by Erich Lindemann and George Engle.*

I. Concepts and principles related to grief:
  A. Cause of grief: reaction to loss (real or imaginary, actual or pending).
  B. Healing process can be interrupted.
  C. Grief is universal.
  D. Uncomplicated grief is a self-limiting process.
  E. Grief responses may vary in degree and kind (e.g., absence of grief, delayed grief, and unresolved grief).
  F. People go through stages similar to stages of death described by Elisabeth Kübler-Ross.
  G. Many factors influence successful outcome of grieving process:
    1. The more *dependent* the person on the lost relationship, the greater the difficulty in resolving the loss.
    2. A *child* has greater difficulty resolving loss.
    3. A person with *few meaningful relationships* also has greater difficulty.
    4. The *more losses* the person has had in the past, the more affected that person will be, because losses tend to be cumulative.
    5. The more *sudden* the loss, the greater the difficulty in resolving it.
    6. The more *ambivalence* (love-hate feelings, with guilt) there was toward the dead, the more difficult the resolution.
    7. *Loss of a child* is harder to resolve than loss of an older person.

---

*Adapted from a *classic* article by George Engel: Grief and grieving. Am J Nurs 9(64):93–98, 1964. American Journal of Nursing.

Mental Health

◆ **II. Assessment—characteristic stages of grief responses:**

    A. *Shock and disbelief* (initial and recurrent stage)

        1. *Denial* of reality. ("No, it can't be.")

        2. Stunned, *numb* feeling.

        3. Feelings of loss, *helplessness,* impotence.

        4. Intellectual acceptance.

    B. *Developing awareness*

        1. Anguish about loss.

          a. *Somatic* distress.

          b. Feelings of emptiness.

        2. *Anger* and hostility toward person or circumstances held responsible.

        3. Guilt feelings—may lead to self-destructive actions.

        4. Tears (inwardly, alone; or inability to cry).

    C. *Restitution*

        1. Funeral *rituals* are an aid to grief resolution by emphasizing the reality of death.

        2. Expression and sharing of feelings by gathered family and friends are a source of acknowledgment of grief and support for the bereaved.

    D. *Resolving the loss*

        1. Increased *dependency* on others as an attempt to deal with painful void.

        2. More aware of own *bodily sensations*—may be identical with symptoms of the deceased.

        3. Complete *preoccupation* with thoughts and memories of the dead person.

    E. *Idealization*

        1. All hostile and negative feelings about the dead are *repressed*.

        2. Mourner may *assume* qualities and attributes of the dead.

        3. Gradual lessening of preoccupation with the dead; *reinvesting* in others.

◆ **III. Analysis (Table 6.9)**

◆ **IV. Nursing care plan/implementation in grief stages:**

    A. *Apply crisis theory and interventions.*

    B. *Demonstrate unconditional respect* for cultural, religious, and social mourning customs.

    C. *Utilize knowledge of the stages of grief* to anticipate reactions and facilitate the grief process.

        1. Anticipate and permit expression of different manifestations of shock, disbelief, and denial.

          a. News of impending death is best communicated to a family group (rather than an individual) in a private setting.

          b. *Let mourners see the dead or dying,* to help them accept reality.

          c. Encourage description of circumstances and nature of loss.

        2. *Accept guilt, anger, and rage* as common responses to coping with guilt and helplessness.

          a. Be aware of potential suicide by the bereaved.

          b. Permit crying; stay with the bereaved.

        3. Mobilize social support system; promote hospital policy that allows gathering of friends and family in a private setting.

        4. Allow dependency on staff for initial decision making while person is attempting to resolve loss.

        5. Respond to somatic complaints.

        6. Permit reminiscence.

        7. Encourage mourner to relate accounts connected with the lost relationship that reflect positive and

TABLE 6.9	◆ Analysis/Nursing Diagnosis: Altered Feeling States Related to Grief	

Problem Classification	Characteristics
1. Somatic distress	Occurs in waves lasting from 20 min–1 hr Deep, sighing respirations most common when discussing grief Lack of strength Loss of appetite and sense of taste Tightness in throat Choking sensation accompanied by shortness of breath
2. Preoccupation with image of deceased	Similar to daydreaming May mistake others for deceased person May be oblivious to surroundings Slight sense of unreality Fear that he or she is becoming "insane"
3. Feelings of guilt	Accuses self of negligence Exaggerates existence and importance of negative thoughts, feelings, and actions toward deceased Views self as having failed deceased—"if I had only…"
4. Feelings of hostility	Irritability, anger, and loss of warmth toward others May attempt to handle feelings of hostility in formalized and stiff manner of social interaction
5. Loss of patterns of conduct	Inability to initiate or maintain organized patterns of activity Restlessness, with aimless movements Loss of zest—tasks and activities are carried on as though with great effort Activities formerly carried on in company of deceased have lost their significance May become strongly dependent on whomever stimulates him or her to activity

negative feelings and remembrances; *place loss in perspective.*

8. Begin to encourage and reinforce new interests and social relations with others by the end of the idealization stage; loosen bonds of attachment.

9. Identify high-risk persons for maladaptive responses (see **I. G.** Many factors influence successful outcome of grieving process **p. 369**).

10. *Health teaching:*
    a. Explain that emotional response is appropriate and common.
    b. Explain and offer hope that emotional pain will diminish with time.
    c. Describe normal grief stages.

◆ **V. Evaluation/outcome criteria:** outcome may take 1 yr or more—can remember comfortably and realistically both pleasurable and disappointing aspects of the lost relationship.

A. Can express feelings of sorrow caused by loss.

B. Can describe ambivalence (love, anger) toward lost person, relationship.

C. Able to review relationship, including pleasures, regrets, etc.

D. Bonds of attachment are loosened and new object relationships are established.

Mental and Emotional Disorders in Children and Adolescents

Children have certain developmental tasks to master in the various stages of development (e.g., learning to trust, control primary instincts, and resolve basic social roles (see **Unit 5**).

I. Concepts and principles related to mental and emotional disorders in children and adolescents

A. Most emotional disorders of children are related to family dynamics and the place the child occupies in the family group.

B. Children must be understood and treated within the context of their *families.*

C. Many disorders are related to the phases of development through which the children are passing. (Erik Erikson's developmental tasks for children are *trust, autonomy, initiative, industry, identity,* and *intimacy.*)

D. Table 6.10 summarizes key age-related disturbances, lists main *symptoms* and *analyses* of causes, and highlights *medical interventions* and *nursing plan/implementation.*

E. Children are not miniature adults; they have special needs.

F. Play and food are important media to make contact with children and help them release emotions in socially acceptable forms, prepare them for traumatic events, and develop skills.

G. Children who are physically or emotionally ill regress, giving up previously useful habits.

H. Adolescents have special problems relating to need for *control* versus need to *rebel, dependency* versus *interdependency,* and search for *identity* and *self-realization.*

I. Adolescents often *act out* their underlying feelings of insecurity, rejection, deprivation, and low self-esteem.

J. Strong feelings may be evoked in nurses working with children; these feelings should be expressed, and each nurse should be supported by team members.

◆ **II. Assessment of** *selected disorders:*

A. *Autistic spectrum disorders* (previously called childhood schizophrenia; most common form of *pervasive developmental disorders* [PDD])—**assessment** (before age 3):

1. Disturbance in how perceptual information is processed (*sensory integrative dysfunction*); normal abilities present.
   a. Behave *as though they cannot* hear, see, etc.
   b. Do *not react to external* stimulus.
   c. Sensory defensiveness:
      (1) Might dislike specific food textures or temperatures.
      (2) Covers ears in response to loud noises.
      (3) Can't concentrate if there are competing noises in environment.
      (4) Might dislike riding or climbing on play equipment.
      (5) Doesn't like people standing too close or being touched.
      (6) Stimuli might be interpreted as threatening or anxiety-provoking.
      (7) Responds in an exaggerated manner (cries, is negative, resistant, or rigid) when a situation makes it difficult for child to process.
   d. Low muscle tone results in inability to maintain stable positions or postures (e.g., standing on one leg); avoids gross and fine motor movement.

2. Lack of self-awareness as a unified whole—may not relate bodily needs or parts as extension of themselves.

3. Severe difficulty in *social interaction* and *communicating* with others—may be mute or echolalic and isolated.

4. Bizarre *restricted* and *repetitive* postures and gestures (banging head, rocking back and forth), and routines.

5. Disturbances in learning: difficulties in understanding and using language.

6. *Etiology* is unknown; but generally accepted that irregularities in brain structure or function may be congenital or acquired.

7. *Prognosis* depends on severity of symptoms and age of onset (can exhibit any combination of symptoms and behaviors).

B. *Other pervasive developmental disorders* include: *Asperger's syndrome* (speak at normal pace and have normal intelligence, but have stunted social skills, limited and obsessive interests), *childhood disintegration disorder (CDD),* and *Rett's disorder.* Characteristics:

1. Hyperactivity.
2. Explosive outbursts.
3. Distractibility.
4. Impulsiveness.

Mental Health

5. Perceptual difficulties (visual distortions, such as figure-ground distortion and mirror reading; body-image problems; difficulty in telling left from right).

6. Receptive or expressive language problems.

C. *Elimination disorders* (functional enuresis)—related to feelings of insecurity due to unmet needs of attention and affection; important to preserve their self-esteem.

D. *Separation anxiety disorders of childhood* (school phobias)—anxiety about school is accompanied by physical distress. Usually observed with fear of leaving home, rejection by mother, fear of loss of mother, or history of separation from mother in early years.

E. *Conduct disorders*—include lying, stealing, running away, truancy, substance abuse, sexual delinquency, vandalism, and fire setting; chief motivating force is either overt or covert hostility; history of disturbed parent-child relations.

III. Analysis/nursing diagnosis:

A. *Altered feeling states:* anxiety, fear, hostility related to personal vulnerability and poorly developed or inappropriate use of defense mechanisms.

B. *Risk for self-mutilation* related to disturbance in self-concept, abnormal response to sensory input, and history of abuse.

C. *Altered interpersonal processes:*
1. *Impaired verbal communication* related to cerebral deficits, withdrawal into self, inability to trust other.
2. *Altered conduct/impulse processes:* aggressive, violent behaviors toward self, others, environment related to feelings of distrust and altered judgment.
3. *Dysfunctional behaviors:* age-inappropriate behaviors, bizarre behaviors; disorganized and unpredictable behaviors related to inability to discharge emotions verbally.
4. *Impaired social interaction:* social isolation/withdrawal related to feelings of suspicion and mistrust, lack of bonding, inadequate sensory stimulation.

D. *Personal identity disturbance* related to lack of development of trust, organic brain dysfunction, maternal deprivation.

E. *Altered parenting* related to ambivalent or dissonant family relationships and failure of child to meet role expectations.

F. *Sensory/perceptual alterations:* altered attention related to disturbed mental activities.

G. *Altered cognition process:* altered decision making, judgment, knowledge, and learning processes; altered thought content and processes related to perceptual or cognitive impairment and emotional dysfunctioning.

IV. Nursing care plan/implementation in mental and emotional disorders in children and adolescents:

A. *General goals:* corrective behavior—*behavior modification.*

B. Help children gain self-awareness.

C. Provide *structured* environment to orient children to reality.

D. Impose *limits* on destructive behavior toward themselves or others without rejecting the children.
1. *Prevent* destructive behavior.
2. *Stop* destructive behavior.
3. *Redirect* nongrowth behavior into constructive channels.

E. Be *consistent.*

F. Meet *developmental and dependency* needs.

G. Recognize and encourage each child's strengths, growth behavior, and reverse regression.

H. Help these children reach the next step in social growth and development scale.

I. Use play and projective media to aid working out feelings and conflicts and in making contact.

J. Offer support to parents and strengthen the parent-child relationship.

K. *Health teaching:* teach parents methods of behavior modification.

V. Evaluation/outcome criteria:

A. Destructive behavior is inhibited.

B. Demonstrates age-appropriate behavior on developmental scale.

TABLE 6.10	**Emotional Disturbances in Children**			
Stage	Disturbance	Assessment: Symptoms or Characteristics	Analysis: Behavior Related To:	Plan/Implementation
Oral (birth–1 yr)	Feeding disturbances	Refusal of food.	1. Rigid feeding schedule. 2. *Psychological* stress. 3. Incompatible formula. 4. *Physiological:* pyloric stenosis.	Pediatric evaluation, especially if infant is not gaining weight or is losing weight. Rule out physiological etiology or incompatible formula. Evaluate *feeding style* of caregiver. Is infant on-demand feeding? Is caregiver sensitive to infant's needs or communications about holding, hunger, or satiation?

(Continued on following page)

Stage	Disturbance	◆ Assessment: Symptoms or Characteristics	◆ Analysis: Behavior Related To:	◆ Plan/Implementation
Oral—Cont'd		*Colic.* Crying is usually confined to one part of day and starts after a feeding. Commonly lasts from first to third month.	Periodic tension in infant's immature nervous system, causing gas and sharp intestinal pains.	Reassure parents and teach about condition and how to relieve it with *hot water bottle, rocking, rubbing back, pacifier,* which may soothe infant.
	Sleeping disturbances	Infant resists being put down for sleep or going to sleep.	1. Need for parental attention. 2. A pattern formed during period of colic or other illness. 3. Emotional disturbance related to *anxiety.*	If it is attention-getting strategy, suggest parental lack of response for a few nights to break pattern. If emotional disturbance is suspected, evaluate *infant-caregiver interaction* and refer for psychotherapeutic intervention.
	Failure to thrive	Infant does not grow or develop over a period of time.	1. *Psychological:* inadequate caretaking. 2. *Physiological:* heart, kidneys, central nervous system (CNS) malfunction.	*Hospitalization* is essential. Assist in evaluation of physiological functioning, especially heart, kidneys, and CNS. *Nurturing plan* for infant, using specifically assigned personnel and the caregiver parent. If the infant grows and develops with nurturing, thus confirming problems of parenting as causative factor, psychotherapeutic and child protective interventions are necessary.
	Severe disturbances	**Pervasive developmental disorders:** Very early onset; lack of response to others; bizarre, repetitive behavior; normal to above normal intelligence; failure to develop language or use communicative speech. Autism is one of the most severe and debilitating psychiatric disturbances.	1. Uncertain etiology; *regression* or *fixation* at earlier developmental stage, before child differentiates "me" from "not me." 2. A "*nature versus nurture*" controversy over the causative factors. These are variously thought to be: a. *Environment only:* Infant is tabula rasa and all disturbance is directly attributable to the environment (primarily the parenting). b. *Heredity only:* For genetic, biochemical, or other predetermined reasons, some infants will be psychotic regardless of the environment.	The child who is severely disturbed requires intensive psychotherapy and often milieu therapy available in residential or daycare programs. Therapy is usually indicated for parents also. Nurses can work on a *primary level* of prevention by assessing parenting skills of prospective parents and *teaching* them these skills. On a *secondary level of prevention,* nurses can be knowledgeable about and *teach* others the early signs of childhood psychosis, making appropriate referrals. The earlier the intervention, the better the prognosis. On a *tertiary level of prevention,* nurses work with children who are severely disturbed and their families in child guidance clinics and residential and daycare settings. *Occupational therapy:* provide tactile, oral-tactile, visual, auditory, gravitational sensory input to normalize response.

(Continued on following page)

Mental Health

TABLE 6.10		Emotional Disturbances in Children *(Continued)*		
Stage	**Disturbance**	◆ **Assessment: Symptoms or Characteristics**	◆ **Analysis: Behavior Related To:**	◆ **Plan/Implementation**
			c. *Combination of environment and heredity* plus *the interaction between them:* An infant who is *susceptible, less* than optimal parenting, and *negative* interaction between parent and infant will combine to produce disturbance.	*Health teaching* would include play activities that foster support, acceptance, and a nonthreatening mode of communication and interaction with a significant other. *Simplify* language by avoiding abstracts and metaphors. Keep gestures clear and simple. Give one instruction at a time, not a sequence. Give time to respond.
		Symbiotic psychosis: Identified later than autistic type, usually between 2 and 5 years of age. These children seem to be unable to function independently of the caregiving parent. A situational stress, such as hospitalization of parent or child or entry into school, may precipitate a psychotic break in the child.	The same "*nature versus nurture*" controversy with respect to the origin of symbiotic psychosis. The child progresses beyond the self-absorbed autistic stage to form an object relationship with another (usually the mother). Having progressed to this stage, the child then *fails to differentiate his or her own identity* from that of the mother.	
Anal (1–3 yr)	Elimination disorders (disturbances related to toilet training)	*Constipation.*	1. *Diet.* 2. Child withholding due to history of one or two painful, *hard bowel movements.* 3. *Psychological* causation: child withholds from parents to *express anger, opposition*, or passage through a very *independent* developmental stage.	Evaluate *diet* and consistency of stools. Fecal softener may be prescribed if necessary. In all cases, *help parent avoid making* an issue of constipation with the child. Enemas are *contraindicated.* If child is withholding, *work with parents* around not forcing rigid toilet training on child. Most children are more cooperative about *toilet training* at 18–24 months.
		Encopresis (soiling).	Child's expression of anger or hostility. It is usually directed toward the parent with whom the child is experiencing conflict and is rarely physiological.	Medical evaluation, then assessment and intervention in the child-parent relationship. Therapy for child and parent may be indicated.
		Enuresis Ordinarily refers to wetting while asleep (nocturnal enuresis), though some children who are enuretic wet themselves during the day also. Enuresis is a *symptom*, not a diagnosis or disease entity.	1. *Faulty toilet training* (especially if child wets during the day also) or 2. *Psychological stress.*	Many approaches have been tried with varying degrees of success. These include *fluid restriction, behavioral intervention* (in which a buzzer wakes the child when the child starts to wet), and psychotherapy.

(Continued on following page)

Stage	Disturbance	Assessment: Symptoms or Characteristics	Analysis: Behavior Related To:	Plan/Implementation
Anal—Cont'd			3. *Physiological* etiology, such as genitourinary (GU) tract infections or CNS disease, is rare. The child *under 4 years* old is usually *not* considered enuretic but is included in this section because bladder training is part of toilet training. Etiology is uncertain.	*Educating parents in bladder training* techniques and attitudes can help solve the problem on a *primary* level. It is important when working with children who are enuretic or their parents to *suggest* ways to help the child *overcome feelings of shame and guilt.* These feelings are often exacerbated by parents who are well-meaning but misguided.
	Excessive rebelliousness	Frequent temper tantrums, fighting, destruction of toys and other objects, consistent oppositional behavior.	1. Fear caused by inconsistency in handling the child, the setting of rigid limits, or the parents' refusal or inability to set limits, which can all create insecurity and fear in the child. 2. Excessive rebelliousness, usually indicating a child who is *frightened;* should not be confused with expression of negativism normal at around age 2, which is a necessary (though trying) developmental stage.	The nurse should offer parent counseling if necessary. When working with the child, the nurse needs to be receptive and sympathetic while establishing and maintaining firm limits.
	Excessive conformity	Lack of spontaneity, anxious desire always to please all adult authority figures, timidity, refusal to assert own needs, passivity.	1. Very rigid control established in an attempt to handle fears. 2. Harsh *toilet training,* resulting in a child who is overcompliant. These children need help as much as children who are overrebellious, but they get it less frequently because their behavior is not a "problem"—that is, it is not difficult for parents to tolerate.	Excessive conformity can lead to *compulsive, ritualistic, or obsessive behavior later.* The nurse needs to be able to identify such a child, then work with the child and parents to encourage *self-expression* in the child. Referral for psychotherapy may be necessary to help the child deal with repressed anger
Oedipal (3–6 yr)	Excessive fears	Child will be frightened even in nonthreatening situations. *Nightmares and other sleep disturbances* occur. Usually, child will be very "clingy" with parents in an attempt to gain reassurance.	*Anxiety* as the causative factor. Anxiety can be induced by many things, such as: 1. Parental *failure to set appropriate limits.* 2. *Physical or psychological abuse.* 3. *Illness.* 4. Fear of *mutilation.*	If possible, identify and deal with the factors that are producing the anxiety. Offer child calm reassurance. *Night-light and open doors* can help allay night fears, but *counsel parents* that it is unwise to allow the child to sleep with the parents, because it may make the child feel that the oedipal retaliation has succeeded.

(Continued on following page)

Mental Health

TABLE 6.10	Emotional Disturbances in Children *(Continued)*		

Stage	Disturbance	◆ Assessment: Symptoms or Characteristics	◆ Analysis: Behavior Related To:	◆ Plan/Implementation
Oedipal —Cont'd			5. *Imaginary* worries that are common at this age (e.g., a 4-year-old who is suddenly afraid of the dark, or dogs, or fire engines is not necessarily suffering from excessive fears).	With the child who is hospitalized, the nurse needs to be aware of and work with the mutilation fears common at this age. Fears around certain procedures (e.g., injections) can often be resolved by helping the child *play out fears.*
	Excessive masturbation	Touching and fondling of genitals excessively, sometimes in a preoccupied or absentminded manner.	1. *Insecurity.* 2. Exploration and stimulation of the genital area, which is *normal* and common in this age group. However, if it is compulsive, the behavior is a signal that the child is *insecure.* 3. Occasionally, a *specific fear.* For example, a boy viewing an infant sister's genitals may have castration fears. These can be dealt with directly.	*Assess* the child's masturbating activity. When does it occur and why? Then help the child develop other *strategies* for defense with anxiety. *Answer questions about sexuality* in an open manner. *Counsel parents* that *threats and shaming are contraindicated,* and help parents deal with *their* feelings about masturbation.
	Regression	Resumption of activities (such as *thumb sucking, soiling and wetting, baby talk*) characteristic of earlier developmental levels.	1. Child's attempt to regain a more comfortable, previous level of development in response to a *threatening* situation (such as a new infant), or 2. A response to difficulty resolving oedipal *conflicts.*	*Counsel parents* not to make an issue of behavior. Offer child emotional support and acceptance, though not approval of regressive behavior.
	Stuttering	Articulation difficulty characterized by many stops and repetitions in speech pattern.	1. Anxiety 2. Frustration. 3. Insecurity. 4. Excitement. Stuttering usually occurs when the affected child feels *anxious, frustrated, insecure,* or *excited.* Parental concerns and attention to stuttering focuses attention on it and increases anxiety. The origins of stuttering are not understood. It is *common around 2-3 years of age* and is *not* a cause for concern at that time.	Speech therapy is usually indicated. Psychotherapy may also be indicated, if stuttering is an expression of anxiety and conflict, persisting *beyond age 6.*

(Continued on following page)

Stage	Disturbance	◆ Assessment: Symptoms or Characteristics	◆ Analysis: Behavior Related To:	◆ Plan/Implementation
Latency (6–12 yr)	**Attention-deficit hyperactivity disorder** (age of onset can occur in preschool children)	Both hyperactivity and hyperkinesis are occasionally observed in school-age children; characterized by a *short attention span*, restlessness, distractibility, and *impulsivity*.	1. An *organic disturbance* of the *CNS*, of uncertain origin, as the basis of *hyperkinesis*. Because the primary symptom—difficulty with attention span—is the same as that presented by the child who is hyperactive, the child who is hyperactive is frequently and incorrectly labeled hyperkinetic. 2. Attempts by child who is *hyperactive* to *control* anxiety through *reducement* (and can attend when interested or relaxed). Does not fit smoothly into environment, but problem may be with the environment *rather* than the child. In other words, the school situation requires a high degree of conformity. The child who does not fit the mold is *not* necessarily emotionally disturbed.	For the child who is *hyperkinetic*, psychopharmaceutical intervention— *Ritalin, Concerta* (long-acting), *Dexedrine*, or *Adderall* (long-acting). Psychotherapy and special education classes may also be indicated. *Ritalin* is also frequently prescribed for the child who is *hyperactive*—which raises the issue of whether an individual should be medicated to fit more smoothly into the environment. Drastic improvement in school performance can be seen with behavioral therapy and medication. Therapy can help the child who is hyperactive *decrease anxiety* and *increase self-esteem*, thus reducing the symptoms.
	Attention-deficit disorder (age of onset can occur throughout adolescence)	Characterized by: a short attention span, distractibility, and subjective feelings of restlessness without hyperactivity.	*Difficulty* with *schoolwork*. Child frequently considered unmotivated or not intelligent.	Psycho-pharmaceutical intervention—*Ritalin, Concerta* (long-acting), *Dexedrine*, or *Adderall* (long-acting)—can drastically increase the attention span. Therapy and behavior modification: work on task for short periods; increase physical energy outlets; tutoring; structure; homework; organizational skills.
	Withdrawal	Reduced body movement and verbalization, lack of close relationships, *detachment*, timidity and seclusiveness.	Need to withdraw as a defensive behavior, through which the child controls anxiety by *reducing contact* with the outer world. Like the child who is overcompliant, the child who is withdrawn frequently not identified as needing help because this behavior is not a "problem."	Offer *positive reinforcement* when child is more active. Help child *assert* self and *experience success* at certain tasks. The nurse needs to work with parents who are overprotective. Therapy may be useful to work through anxiety and provide child with a chance to form a *trusting* relationship with another.
	Psychophysiological symptoms	The child experiences physical symptoms (such as *vomiting, headaches, eczema, asthma, colitis*) with no apparent physiological cause.	*Conversion* of anxiety into physical symptoms.	After medical evaluation has established lack of physiological etiology, psychotherapy is usually indicated. Family therapy may be treatment of choice because *dysfunctional interpersonal family dynamics* are common in these cases.

(Continued on following page)

Mental Health

| TABLE 6.10 | **Emotional Disturbances in Children** *(Continued)* | | | |

Stage	Disturbance	◆ Assessment: Symptoms or Characteristics	◆ Analysis: Behavior Related To:	◆ Plan/Implementation
Latency— Cont'd				The nurse can also provide the child with a healthy interpersonal relationship. Nurses are frequently in a position to talk to parents and teachers about the importance of mental health counseling for children with physical symptoms.
	Separation anxiety disorders (school "phobia")	Sudden and seemingly inexplicable fear of going to school. These children often do not know what it is they fear at school. Frequently occurs *after an illness* and absence from school or birth of sibling.	An *acute anxiety reaction related to separation* from home (not actually a phobia).	If the child is allowed to stay home, the dread of returning to school usually increases. The child and parent should have psychiatric intervention quickly (before the problem becomes worse) to help the child separate from the parent.
	Learning disabilities	Failure or difficulty in learning at school	1. Emotional disorders, which cause school failure. 2. Feelings of *inferiority, discouragement*, and loss of confidence from school failure. Learning disabilities may be caused by many factors or combinations of factors, including *anxiety, poor sensory or sensorimotor integration, dyslexia, receptive aphasia.*	A comprehensive evaluation is essential. Ideally, this would include assessments by a pediatric neurologist, a mental health worker such as a psychiatric nurse or psychiatrist, a learning disabilities teacher specialist, and possibly an occupational therapist trained to work with sensory integration. Treatment is then based on the specific problem or problems.
	Conduct disorders	Behavior that is nonproductive; that is repeated in spite of threats, punishments, or rational argument; and that usually leads to punishment. Persistent *stealing and truancy* are examples.	*Conflicts* that are expressed and communicated through behavior rather than verbally. Child knows what he or she is doing but is unaware of the underlying motivations for the problem behavior.	Counseling or therapy for the child by a child psychiatric nurse or other mental health worker can allow the child to resolve the basic conflict, thus making the problem behavior unnecessary.

Source: Adapted from Wilson, HS, and Kneisl, CR: Psychiatric Nursing, ed. 3. Addison-Wesley, Redwood City, Calif. (out of print).

Midlife Crisis: Phase of Life Problems

Midlife crisis is a time period that marks the passage between early maturity and middle age.

◆ **I. Assessment:**
  A. Commonly occurs between ages 35 and 45.
  B. Preoccupied with *visible* signs of aging, own mortality.
  C. *Feelings: urgency* that time is running out ("last chance") for career achievement and unmet goals; *boredom* with present, *ambivalence, frustration, uncertainty* about the future.
  D. Time of *reevaluation:*
    1. Reassess: meaning of time and parental role (omnipotence as a parent is challenged).

    2. Reexamine and contemplate change in career, marriage, family life.
  E. *Personality changes* may occur. *Women:* traditional definitions of femininity may be challenged as become more assertive. *Men:* may be more introspective, sensitive to emotions, make external changes (younger mate, improve looks, new sports activity), mood swings.
  F. Presence of *helpful elements* necessary to turn life's obstacles into opportunities.
    1. Willingness to take risks.
    2. Strong support system.
    3. Sense of purpose.
    4. Accumulated wisdom.

◆ **II. Analysis/nursing diagnosis:**

A. *Self-esteem disturbance (low self-esteem)* related to loss of youth, faltering physical powers, and facing discrepancy between youthful ambitions and actual achievement (no longer a promising person with potential).

B. *Altered role performance (role reversal)* related to parents who previously provided security and comfort but now need care.

C. *Altered feeling processes (depression)* related to disappointments and diminished optimism as life is reconsidered in light of the reality of aging and death.

◆ **III. Nursing care plan/implementation**—*long-term goal:* help individual to rebuild life structure.

A. Help client reappraise meaning of own life in terms of past, present, and future, and integrate aspects of time. Encourage introspection and reflection with questions:

1. What have I done with my life?
2. What do I really get from and give to my spouse, children, friends, work, community, and self?
3. What are my strengths and liabilities?
4. What have I done with my early dream, and do I want it now?

B. Assist client to complete *four major tasks:*

1. Terminate era of early adulthood by *reappraising* life goals identified and achieved during this era.
2. Initiate movement into middle adulthood by beginning to make *necessary changes* in *unsuccessful* aspects of the current life while trying out new choices.
3. Cope with *polarities* that divide life.
4. Directly confront *death of own parents.*

C. *Health teaching:* stress-management techniques; how to do self-assessment of aptitudes, interests; how to plan for retirement, aloneness, and use of increased leisure time; dietary modification and exercise program.

◆ **IV. Evaluation/outcome criteria:**

A. Gives up *idealized* self of early 20s for more *realistically* attainable self.

1. Talks *less* of early *hopes of eminence* and *more* on modest goal of *competence.*
2. Shifts values from sexuality to platonic relationships: replaces romantic dreams with *satisfying* friendships and companionships.
3. Modifies early illusions about own capacities.
4. Shifts values away from physical attractiveness and strength to *intellectual* abilities.

B. Comes to accept that life is finite and reconciles what *is* with what *might have been;* appreciates everyday human experience rather than glamor or power.

C. Through self-confrontation, self-discovery, and change, experiences time of restabilization; is reinvigorated, adventuresome.

D. Develops *alternative* abilities that release new energies.

E. Tries *less* to please everyone; others' opinions less important.

F. Makes more efficient and well-seasoned decisions from well-developed sense of judgment.

Mental Health Problems of the Aged

In general, problems affecting the elderly are *similar* to those affecting persons of *any* age. This section highlights the *differences* from the viewpoint of etiology, frequency, and prognosis.

I. Concepts and principles related to mental health problems of the aged:

A. The elderly *do* have capacity for growth and change.

B. Human beings, regardless of age, need sense of future and *hope* for things to come.

C. An inalienable right of all individuals should be to make or participate in all decisions concerning themselves and their possessions as long as they can.

D. Physical disability due to the aging process may enforce dependency, which may be unacceptable to elderly clients and may evoke feelings of anger and ambivalence.

E. In an attempt to *reduce feelings of loss,* elderly clients may *cling to concrete things* that most represent, in a *symbolic* sense, all that has been significant to them.

F. As memory diminishes, *familiar objects* in environment and *familiar routines* are important in helping *to keep clients oriented* and in contact with reality.

G. *Familiarity of environment brings security;* routines bring a sense of security about what is to happen.

H. If individuals feel unwanted, they may tell *stories* about their *earlier* achievements.

I. Many of the traits in the elderly result from *cumulative* effect of *past* experiences of frustrations and *present* awareness of limitations rather than from any primary consequences of physiological deficit.

◆ **II. Assessment:**

A. *Psychological characteristics of the aged:*

1. Increasingly *dependent* on others, not only for physical needs but also for emotional security.
2. Concerns focus more and more *inward,* with narrowed outside interests.
   a. Decreased emotional energy for concern with social problems unless these issues affect them.
   b. Tendency to *reminisce.*
   c. May appear selfish and unsympathetic.
3. Sources of pleasure and gratification are more childlike: *food, warmth, and affection,* for example.
   a. Tangible and frequent evidence of affection is important (e.g., letters, cards, and visits).
   b. May hoard articles.
4. *Attention span and memory are short;* may be forgetful and *accuse others of stealing.*
5. Deprivation of any kind is *not* tolerated:
   a. Easily frustrated.
   b. Change is poorly tolerated; need to have favorite chairs and established daily routine, for example.
6. Main *fears* in the aged include fear of *dependency,* chronic *illness, loneliness, boredom,* fear of being

unloved, forgotten, *deserted* by those close to them, fear of *death;* fear of *loss of control* of one's own life; a failing *cognition;* loss of *purpose* and productivity.

7. *Nocturnal delirium* may be due to problems with night vision and inability to perceive *spatial* location.

B. *Psychiatric problems in aging*

1. *Loneliness*—related to *loss* of mate, diminishing circle of friends and family through death and geographic separation, *decline* in physical energy, loss of work (*retirement*), sharp loss of income, and loss of a lifelong lifestyle.

2. *Insomnia*—pattern of sleep changes in significant ways: disappearance of *deep* sleep, frequent *awakening, daytime* sleeping.

3. *Hypochondriasis*—anxiety may shift from concern with finances, job, or social prestige to concern about own bodily function.

4. *Depression*—common problem in the aging, with a *high suicide rate;* partly because of bodily changes that influence the *self-concept,* the older person may direct *hostility toward self* and therefore may be subject to feelings of depression and loneliness.

5. *Senility—four early symptoms:*
   a. Change in attention span.
   b. Memory loss for *recent* events and *names.*
   c. Altered intellectual capacity.
   d. Diminished ability to respond to others.

C. *Successful aging*

1. Being able to *perceive* signs of aging and limitations resulting from the aging process.

2. *Redefining* life in terms of effects on social and physical aspects of living.

3. Seeking *alternatives* for meeting needs and finding sources of pleasure.

4. Adopting a *different outlook* about self-worth.

5. *Reintegrating* values with goals of life.

D. *Causative factors* of mental disorder in the aged related to:

1. *Nutritional* problems and *physical ill health* related to *acute and chronic illness:*
   a. Cardiovascular diseases (heart failure, stroke, hypertension).
   b. Respiratory infection.
   c. Cancer.
   d. Alcohol dependence and abuse.
   e. Dentition problems.

2. Faulty adaptation related to *physical* changes of aging (e.g., depression, hypochondriases).

3. Problems related to *loss, grief, and bereavement.*

4. *Retirement* shock related to loss of status and financial security.

5. Social isolation and loneliness related to *inadequate sensory stimulation.*

6. *Environmental change* (relocation within a community or from home to institution): loss of family, privacy.

7. *Hopelessness, helplessness* related to condition and circumstances.

8. *Altered body image* (negative) related to aging process.

9. Depression related to *helplessness, inability to express anger.*

◆ **III Analysis/nursing diagnosis:**

A. *Self-esteem disturbance* related to body-image disturbance and altered family role.

B. *Impaired social interaction* related to social isolation and environmental changes.

C. *Dysfunctional grieving* related to loss and bereavement.

D. *Altered feeling states and spiritual distress* related to hopelessness, anxiety, fear, powerlessness.

E. *Altered physical regulation processes* related to physical ill health.

F. *Sleep pattern disturbance* related to insomnia and altered sleep/arousal patterns.

◆ **IV. Nursing care plan/implementation:**

A. *Long-term goal:* to help reduce hopelessness and helplessness.

B. *Short-term goal:* to focus on ego assets.

C. Help elderly *preserve* what facet of life they can and *regain* that which has already been lost.
   1. Help *minimize regression* as much as possible.
   2. Help retain their *adult* status.
   3. Help preserve their *self-image* as useful individuals.
   4. Identify and *preserve their abilities* to perform, emphasizing what they *can* do.

D. Attempt to *prevent* loss of dignity and loss of worth—address them by titles, not "Gramps."

E. *Reduce* feelings of *alienation* and loneliness. Provide *sensory* experiences for those with visual problems:
   1. Let them *touch* objects of various textures and consistencies.
   2. Encourage heightened *use of remaining senses* to make up for those that are diminished or lost.

F. *Reduce* depression and feelings of isolation.
   1. Allow time to *reminisce.*
   2. *Avoid changes* in surrounding or routine.

G. *Protect* from rush and excitement.
   1. Use simple, unhurried conversation.
   2. Allow *extra* time to organize thoughts.

H. Be sensitive to *concrete* things they may want to *keep.*

I. *Health teaching:*
   1. How to keep track of time (e.g., by marking off days on a calendar), to promote orientation.
   2. How to keep track of medications.
   3. Exercises to promote blood flow.
   4. *Retirement counseling:*
      a. Obtaining satisfaction from leisure time.
      b. Nurturing relationships with younger generations.
      c. Adjusting to changes: physical health, retirement, loss of loved ones.
      d. Developing connections with own age group.
      e. Taking on new social roles.
      f. Maintaining a satisfactory and appropriate living situation.
      g. Coping with dependence on others, especially one's children.

Mental Health

◆ **V. Evaluation/outcome criteria:**
  A. Less confusion and fewer mood swings.
  B. Increased interest in activities of daily living and interaction with others.
  C. Lessened preoccupation with death, dying, physical symptoms, feelings of sadness.
  D. Reduced insomnia and anorexia.
  E. Expresses feelings of belonging and being needed.

PROTECTIVE FUNCTIONS

Common Behavioral Problems

I. Anger
  A. Definition: feelings of resentment in response to anxiety when threat is perceived; need to discharge tension of anger.
◆ **B. Assessment:**
  1. *Degree of anger and frequency:* scope of anger ranges on a continuum from *everyday mild annoyance* → *frustration* from interference with goal accomplishment → *assertiveness* (behavior used to deal with anger effectively) → *anger* related to helplessness and powerlessness that may interfere with functioning → *rage and fury,* when coping means are depleted or not developed.
  2. *Mode of expression of anger*
    a. *Covert, passive* expression of anger: being overly nice; body language with little or no eye contact, arms close to body, soft voice, little gesturing; sarcasm through humor; *sublimation* through art and music; projection onto others; *denying* and pushing anger out of awareness; *psychosomatic* illness in response to internalized anger (e.g., headache).
    b. *Overt,* active expression of anger: physical activity to work off excess physical energy associated with biological response (e.g., hitting a punching bag, taking a walk); *aggression,* assertiveness.
  3. *Physiological behaviors*—result of secretion of epinephrine and sympathetic nervous system stimulation preparing for fight-flight.
    a. *Cardiovascular* response: increased blood pressure and pulse, increased free fatty acid in blood.
    b. *Gastrointestinal* response: increased nausea, salivation, decreased peristalsis.
    c. *Genitourinary* response: urinary frequency.
    d. *Neuromuscular* response: increased alertness, increased muscle tension and deep-tendon reflexes, ECG changes.
  4. *Positive functions of anger*
    a. Energizes behavior.
    b. Protects positive image.
    c. Provides ego defense during high anxiety.
    d. Gives greater control over situation.
    e. Alerts to need for coping.
    f. A sign of a healthy relationship.

◆ **C. Analysis/nursing diagnosis:** *defensive coping* related to source of stress (stressors):
  1. *Biological stressors*—instinctual drives (Lorenz, on aggressive instincts, and Freud), *endocrine imbalances,* seizures, tumors, *hunger, fatigue.*
  2. *Psychological stressors*—inability to resolve frustration that leads to aggression; real or imagined threatened loss of self-esteem; conflict, lack of control; anger as a learned expression and a reinforced response. Prolonged stress; an attempt to protect self; a desire for retaliation; a normal part of grief process.
  3. *Sociocultural stressors*—lack of early training in self-discipline and social skills; crowding, personal space intrusion; *role modeling of abusive behavior* by significant others and by media personalities.
◆ **D. Nursing care plan/implementation**—*long-term goals:* constructive use of angry energy to accomplish tasks and motivate growth.
  1. *Prevent* and *control* violence.
    a. Approach unhurriedly.
    b. Provide atmosphere of acceptance; listen attentively, refrain from arguing and criticizing.
    c. Encourage expression of feelings.
    d. Offer feedback of client's expressed feelings.
    e. Encourage mutual problem solving.
    f. Encourage realistic perception of others and situation and respect for the rights of others.
  2. *Limit setting:*
    a. Clearly state *expectations* and *consequences* of acts.
    b. Enforce consequences.
    c. Encourage client to assume responsibility for behavior.
    d. Explore reasons and meaning of negative behavior.
  3. Promote *self-awareness* and *problem-solving* abilities. Encourage and assist client to:
    a. Accept self as a person with a right to experience angry feelings.
    b. Explore reasons for anger.
    c. Describe situations where anger was experienced.
    d. Discuss appropriate alternatives for expressing anger (including assertiveness training).
    e. Decide on one feasible solution.
    f. Act on solution.
    g. Evaluate effectiveness.
  4. *Health teaching:*
    a. Explore other ways to express feelings, and provide activities that allow appropriate expression of anger.
    b. Recommend that behavioral limits be set (by the family).
    c. Explain how to set behavioral limits.
    d. Advise against causing defensive patterns in others.
◆ **E. Evaluation/outcome criteria:**
  1. Demonstrates insight (awareness of factors that precipitate anger; identifies disturbing topics,

events, and inappropriate use of coping mechanisms).

2. Uses appropriate coping mechanisms.
3. Reaches out for emotional support before stress level becomes excessive.
4. Evidence of increased reality perception and problem-solving ability.

II. Combative-aggressive behavior
   A. Definition: *acting out* feelings of frustration, anger, anxiety, etc., through *physical or verbal* behavior.
 ◆ **B. Assessment:** recognize *precombative* behavior:
   1. Demanding, fist clenching.
   2. Boisterous, loud.
   3. Vulgar, profane.
   4. Limited attention span.
   5. Sarcastic, taunting, verbal threats.
   6. Restless, agitated, elated.
   7. Frowning.
 ◆ **C. Analysis/nursing diagnosis:** *risk for self-injury* and *violence directed at others* related to:
   1. Frustration as response to *breakdown of self-control* coping mechanisms.
   2. Acting out as customary response to anger (*defensive coping*).
   3. Confusion (*sensory/perceptual alterations*).
   4. Physical restraints, such as when clients are postoperative and discover wrist restraints.
   5. Fear of intimacy, intrusion on emotional and physical space (*altered thought processes*).
   6. Feelings of helplessness, inadequacy (*situational or chronic low self-esteem*).
 ◆ **D. Nursing care plan/implementation:**
   1. *Long-term goal:* channel aggression—help person express feelings rather than act them out.
   2. *Immediate goal: prevent injury to self and others.*
      a. Calmly call for assistance; do *not* try to handle *alone.*
      b. Approach cautiously. Keep client within *eye contact,* observing client's personal space.
      c. *Protect* against self-injury and injury to others; be aware of your position in relation to the weapon, door, escape route.
      d. *Minimize* stimuli, to control the environment—clear the area, close doors, turn off TV so person can hear you.
      e. *Divert* attention from the act; engage in talk and lead away from others.
      f. Assess *triggering* cause.
      g. Identify immediate problem.
      h. Focus on *remedy for immediate* problem.
      i. Choose one individual who has a calm, quiet presence to interact with person; nonauthoritarian, nonthreatening.
      j. Maintain *verbal contact* to keep communication open; offer empathetic ear, but be firm and consistent in setting *limits* on dangerous behavior.
      k. Negotiate, but do not make false promises or argue.

l. *Restraints may be necessary as a last resort.*
      m. Place person in quiet room so he or she can calm down.
   3. *Health teaching:*
      a. Explain how to obtain relief from stress and how to rechannel emotional energy into acceptable activity.
      b. Advise against causing defensive responses in others.
      c. Explain what is justifiable aggression.
      d. Emphasize importance of how to recognize tension in self.
      e. Explain why self-control is important.
      f. Explain to family, staff, how to set behavioral limits.
      g. Explain causes of maladaptive coping related to anger.
      h. Teach how to use problem-solving method.
 ◆ **E. Evaluation/outcome criteria:**
   1. Is aware of causes of anger; can recognize the feeling of anger and use alternative methods of expressing anger.
   2. Expression of anger is appropriate, congruent with the situation.
   3. Replaces aggression and acting out with assertiveness.

III. Confusion/disorientation
   A. Definition: loss of reality orientation as to person, time, place, events, ideas.
 ◆ **B. Assessment:** note unusual behavior:
   1. Picking, stroking movements in the air or on clothing and linens.
   2. Frequent crying or laughing.
   3. Alternating periods of confusion and lucidity (e.g., confused at night, when alone in the dark).
   4. Fluctuating mood, actions, rationality (argumentative, combative, withdrawn).
   5. Increasingly restless, fearful, leading to insomnia, nightmares.
   6. Acts bewildered; has trouble identifying familiar people.
   7. Preoccupied; irritable when interrupted.
   8. Unresponsive to questions; problem with concentration and setting realistic priorities.
   9. Sensitive to noise and light.
   10. Has unrealistic perception of time, place, and situation.
   11. Nurse no longer seen as supportive but as threatening.
 ◆ **C. Analysis/nursing diagnosis:** *altered thought processes and sensory/perceptual alterations* related to:
   1. *Physical and physiological disturbances*—metabolic (uremia, diabetes, hepatic dysfunction), fluid and electrolyte imbalances, cardiac arrhythmias, heart failure; anemia, massive blood loss with low hemoglobin; brain lesions; nutritional deficiency; pain; sleep disturbance; drugs (antidepressants, tranquilizers, sedatives, antihypertensives, diuretics, alcohol, PCP, street drugs).

2. *Unfamiliar environment*—unfamiliar routine and people; procedures that threaten body image; *noisy* equipment.

3. *Loss of sensory acuity* from partial or incomplete reception of orienting stimuli or information.

4. *Disability in screening out* irrelevant and excessive sensory input.

5. *Memory impairment.*

◆ **D. Nursing care plan/implementation:**

1. Check *physical signs* (e.g., vital signs, neurological status, fluid and electrolyte balance, and blood urea nitrogen).

2. Be calm; make contact to *reorient to reality:*
   a. *Avoid* startling if person is alone, in the dark, sedated.
   b. Make sure person can *see, hear, and talk* to you—turn off TV; turn on light, put on client's glasses, hearing aids, dentures.
   c. Call by name, clearly and distinctly.
   d. Approach cautiously, close to *eye* level.
   e. Keep your *hands visible;* for example, on bed.

3. *Take care of immediate problem,* e.g., disconnected IV tube or catheter.
   a. Give instructions slowly and distinctly; *avoid* threatening tone and comments.
   b. *Stay* with person until reoriented.
   c. Put *side rails* up.

4. Use conversation to *reduce* confusion:
   a. Use *simple, concrete phrases;* language the person can understand; *repeat* as needed.
   b. *Avoid:* shouting, arguing, false promises, use of medical abbreviations (e.g., NPO).
   c. Give *more time to concentrate* on what you said.
   d. Focus on *reality-oriented* topics or objects in the environment.

5. *Prevent confusion by establishing a reality-oriented relationship.*
   a. Introduce self by name.
   b. Jointly establish routines to prevent confusion from unpredictable changes and variations. Determine client's usual routine; attempt to incorporate this to lessen disruption in lifestyle.
   c. Explain what to expect in understandable words—where client is and why, what will happen, noises and activities client will hear and see, people client will meet, tests and procedures client will have.
   d. Find out what meaning hospitalization has to client; reduce anxiety related to feelings of apprehension and helplessness.
   e. Spend as much time as possible with client.

6. *Maintain orientation by providing nonthreatening environment.*
   a. Assign to room *near nurse's station.*
   b. Surround with *familiar* objects from home (e.g., photos).
   c. Provide *clock, calendar, and radio.*
   d. Have flexible visiting hours.
   e. Open curtain for *natural light.*
   f. Keep glasses, dentures, hearing aids nearby.

g. Check client often, especially at night.
h. *Avoid* using intercom to answer calls.
i. *Avoid* low-pitched conversation.

7. *Take care of other needs.*
   a. Promote sleep according to usual habits and patterns to *prevent sleep deprivation.*
   b. *Avoid sedatives,* which may lead to or increase confusion.
   c. Promote independent functions, self-help activities, to *maintain dignity.*
   d. Encourage *nutritional* adequacy; incorporate familiar foods, ethnic preferences.
   e. Maintain *routine; avoid* being late with meals, medication, or procedures.
   f. Have *realistic expectations.*
   g. *Discover hidden fears.*
      (1) Do *not* assume confused behavior is unrelated to reality.
      (2) Look for clues to meaning from client's background, occupation.
   h. *Provide support to family.*
      (1) Encourage expression of feelings; *avoid* being judgmental.
      (2) Check what worked in previous situations.

8. *Health teaching:* explain possible causes of confusion. Reassure that it is common. Teach family, friends how to react to confused behavior.

◆ **E. Evaluation/outcome criteria:**

1. Less restlessness, fearfulness, mood lability.

2. More frequent periods of lucidity; oriented to time, place, and person; responds to questions.

IV. Demanding behavior

A. Definition: a strong and persistent struggle to obtain satisfaction of self-oriented needs (e.g., control, self-esteem) or relief from anxiety.

◆ **B. Assessment:**

1. Attention-seeking behavior.

2. Multiple requests.

3. Frequency of questions.

4. Lack of reasonableness; irrationality of request.

◆ **C. Analysis/nursing diagnosis:** *defensive coping and impaired social interaction* related to:

1. Feelings of *helplessness* and *hopelessness.*

2. Feelings of *powerlessness* and *fear.*

3. A way of coping with anxiety.

◆ **D. Nursing care plan/implementation:**

1. *Control* own irritation; assess reasons for own annoyance.

2. *Anticipate* and meet client's needs; set time to discuss requests.

3. *Confront* with behavior; discuss reasons for behavior.

4. *Ignore* negative attention seeking and *reinforce appropriate* requests for attention.

5. Make plans with *entire staff* to set *limits.*

6. Set up *contractual* arrangement for brief, frequent, regular, uninterrupted attention.

7. *Health teaching:* teach appropriate methods for gaining attention.

◆ E. **Evaluation/outcome criteria:** fewer requests for attention; assumes more responsibility for self-care.

V. Denial of illness

A. **Definition:** an attempt or refusal to acknowledge some anxiety-provoking aspect of oneself or external reality. Denial may be an acceptable first phase of coping as an attempt to allow time for adaptation.

◆ B. **Assessment:**
1. Observe for *defense and coping mechanisms* such as dissociation, repression, selective inattention, suppression, displacement of concern to another person.
2. Note behaviors that may indicate *denial* of diagnosis:
   a. Failure to follow treatment plan.
   b. Missed appointment.
   c. Refusal of medication.
   d. Inappropriate cheerfulness.
   e. Ignoring symptoms.
   f. Use of flippant humor.
   g. Use of second or third person in reference to illness.
   h. Flight into wellness, overactivity.
3. Use of earliest and most primitive defense by closing eyes, turning head away to separate from what is unpleasant and anxiety provoking.
4. Note *range* of denial: *explicit* verbal denial of obvious facts, disowning or *ignoring* aspects or *minimizing* by understatement.
5. Be aware of situations such as long-term physical disability that make people more prone to denial of anger. *Denial of illness protects the ego from overwhelming anxiety.*

◆ C. **Analysis/nursing diagnosis:** *ineffective denial* related to:
1. Untenable wishes, needs, ideas, deeds, or reality factors.
2. Inability to adapt to full realization of painful experience or to accept changes in body image or role perception.
3. Intense stress and anxiety.

◆ D. **Nursing care plan/implementation:**
1. *Long-term goal:* understand needs met by denial.
2. *Short-term goals: avoid* reinforcing denial patterns.
   a. Recognize behavioral cues of denial of some reality aspect; be aware of level of awareness and degree to which reality is excluded.
   b. Determine if denial interferes with treatment.
   c. Support moves toward greater reality orientation.
   d. Determine person's stress tolerance.
   e. Supportively help person discuss events leading to, and feelings about, hospitalization.
3. *Health teaching:*
   a. Explain that emotional response is appropriate and common.
   b. Explain to family and staff that emotional adjustment to painful reality is done at own pace.

◆ E. **Evaluation/outcome criteria:** indicates desire to discuss painful experience.

VI. Dependence

A. **Definition:** reliance on other people to meet basic needs, usually for love and affection, security and protection, and support and guidance; *acceptable in early phases* of coping.

◆ B. **Assessment:**
1. Excessive need for advice and answers to problems.
2. Lack of confidence in own decision-making ability and lack of confidence in self-sufficiency.
3. Clinging, too-trusting behavior.
4. Gestures, facial expressions, body posture, recurrent themes conveying "I'm helpless."

◆ C. **Analysis/nursing diagnosis:**
1. *Chronic low self-esteem* related to inability to meet basic needs or role expectations.
2. *Helplessness* and *hopelessness* related to inadvertent reinforcement by staff's expectations.
3. *Powerlessness* related to holding a belief that one's own actions cannot affect life situations.

◆ D. **Nursing care plan/implementation:**
1. *Long-term goal:* increase self-esteem, confidence in own abilities.
2. *Short-term goal:* provide activities that promote independence.
   a. *Limit setting*—clear, firm, consistent; acknowledge when demands are made; accept client but refuse to respond to demands.
   b. *Break cycle* of nurse avoids client when he or she is clinging and demanding → a client's anxiety increases → demands for attention increase → frustration and avoidance on nurse's part increase.
   c. *Give attention before* demand exists.
   d. Use *behavior-modification* approaches:
      (1) *Reward* appropriate behavior (such as making decisions, helping others, caring for own needs) with attention and praise.
      (2) Give *no response* to attention-seeking, dependent, infantile behavior; goal is to increase incidence of mature behavior as client realizes little gratification from dependent behavior.
   e. *Avoid secondary gains* of being cared for, which impede progress toward aforementioned goals.
   f. Assist in developing *ability to control* panic by responding less to client's high anxiety level.
   g. Help client develop ways to seek gratification other than excessive turning to others.
   h. *Resist* urge to act like a parent when client becomes helpless, demanding, and attention seeking.
   i. *Promote decision making* by not giving advice.
   j. *Encourage accountability* for own feelings, thoughts, and behaviors.
      (1) Help identify feelings through nonverbal cues, thoughts, recurrent themes.

(2) Convey expectations that client does have opinions and feelings to share.

(3) Role model how to express feelings.

k. *Reinforce self-esteem* and ability to work out problems independently. (Consistently ask: "How do you feel about …"; "What do you think?")

3. *Health teaching:*

a. Teach family ways of interacting to enforce less dependency.

b. Teach problem-solving skills, assertiveness.

◆ E. Evaluation/outcome criteria:

1. Performs self-care.

2. Asks less for approval and praise.

3. Seeks less attention, proximity, physical contact.

VII. Hostility

A. Definition: a feeling of *intense* anger or an attitude of antagonism or animosity, with the *destructive* component of intent to inflict harm and pain to another or to self; may involve *hate, anger, rage, aggression, regression.*

B. Operational definition:

1. Past experience of frustration, loss of self-esteem, unmet needs for status, prestige, or love.

2. Present expectations of self and others not met.

3. Feelings of humiliation, inadequacy, emotional pain, and conflict.

4. Anxiety experienced and converted into hostility, which can be:

a. Repressed, with result of becoming withdrawn.

b. Disowned to the point of overreaction and extreme compliance.

c. Overtly exhibited: verbal, nonverbal.

C. Concepts and principles:

1. Aggression and violence are two *outward* expressions of hostility.

2. Hostility is often unconscious, automatic response.

3. Hostile wishes and impulses may be underlying motives for many actions.

4. Perceptions may be *distorted* by hostile outlook.

5. Continuum: from extreme politeness to *externalization* as murderous rage or homicide or *internalization* as depression or suicide.

6. Hostility seen as a defense *against* depression, as well as a *cause* of it.

7. Hostility may be repressed, dissociated, or expressed covertly or overtly.

8. *Normal* hostility may come from justifiable fear of *real* danger; *irrational* hostility stems from *anxiety.*

9. Developmental roots of hostility:

a. *Infants* look away, push away, physically move away from threat; give defiant look. Role modeling by parents.

b. *Three-year-olds* replace overt hostility with protective shyness, retreat, and withdrawal. Feel weak, inadequate in face of powerful

person against whom cannot openly ventilate hostility.

c. Frustrated or unmet needs for status, prestige, or power serve as a basis for *adult* hostility.

◆ D. Assessment:

1. Fault-finding, scapegoating, sarcasm, derision.

2. Arguing, swearing, abusiveness, verbal threatening.

3. Deceptive sweetness, joking at other's expense, gossiping.

4. Physical abusiveness, violence, murder, vindictiveness.

◆ E. Analysis/nursing diagnosis:

1. *Causes*

a. *Anxiety* related to a learned means of dealing with an interpersonal threat.

b. *Risk for violence* related to a reaction to *loss of self-esteem* and *powerlessness.*

c. *Defensive coping* related to intense frustration, insecurity, or apprehension.

d. *Impaired social interaction* related to low anxiety tolerance.

2. *Situations with high potential for hostility:*

a. *Enforced illness and hospitalization* cause anxiety, which may be expressed as hostility.

b. Dependency feelings related to acceptance of illness may result in hostility as a coping mechanism.

c. Certain illnesses or physical disabilities may be conducive to hostility:

(1) Client who has *preoperative cancer* and is displacing hostility onto staff and family.

(2) Postoperatively, if diagnosis is *terminal,* the family may displace hostility onto nurse.

(3) Anger, hostility is a *stage of dying* the person may experience.

(4) Client who had *amputation* may focus frustration on others due to dependency and jealousy.

(5) Clients on *hemodialysis* are prone to helplessness, which may be displaced as hostility.

◆ F. Nursing care plan/implementation:

1. *Long-term goal:* help alter response to fear, inadequacy, frustration, threat.

2. *Short-term goal:* express and explore feelings of hostility without injury to self or others.

a. Remain calm, nonthreatening; endure verbal abuse in impartial manner, within limits; speak quietly.

b. *Protect from self-harm,* acting out.

c. Discourage hostile behavior while showing acceptance of client.

d. Offer support to *express* feelings of frustration, anger, and fear *constructively, safely,* and *appropriately.*

e. Explore hostile feelings *without* fear of retaliation, disapproval.

f. *Avoid:* arguing, giving advice, reacting with hostility, punitiveness, finding fault.

g. *Avoid* joking, teasing, which can be misinterpreted.

h. *Avoid* words such as *anger, hostility;* use client's words *(upset, irritated).*

i. Do *not* minimize problem or give client reassurance or hasty, general conclusions.

j. *Do not stop verbal* expression of anger unless detrimental.

k. Respond *matter-of-factly* to attention-seeking behavior, not defensively.

l. *Avoid* physical contact; allow client to set pace in "closeness."

m. Look for clues to antecedent events and focus *directly* on those areas; *do not evade* or ignore.

n. Constantly focus on *here and now* and affective component of message rather than on content.

o. Reconstruct what happened and why, discuss client's reactions; seek observations, *not* inferences.

p. Learn how client would like to be treated.

q. Look for ways to help client relate better without defensiveness, *when ready.*

r. Plan to channel feelings into *motor* outlets (occupational and recreational therapy, physical activity, games, debates).

s. Explain procedures beforehand; approach frequently.

t. Withdraw attention, *set limits,* when acting out.

3. *Health teaching:* teach acceptable motor outlets for tension.

◆ **G. Evaluation/outcome criteria:** identifies sources of threat and experiences success in dealing with threat.

VIII. Manipulation

A. Definition: process of playing on and using others by unfair, insidious means to serve own purpose without regard for others' needs; may take many forms; occurs consciously, unconsciously to some extent, in all interpersonal relations.

B. Operational definition (Figure 6.3):

1. Conflicting needs, goals exist between client and other person (e.g., nurse).

2. Other person perceives need as unacceptable, unreasonable.

3. Other person refuses to accept client's need.

4. Client's tension increases, and he or she begins to relate to others as objects.

5. Client increases attempts to influence others to fulfill his or her needs.

   a. Appears unaware of others' needs.

   b. Exhibits excessive dependency, helplessness, demands.

   c. Sets others at odds (especially staff).

   d. *Rationalizes,* gives logical reasons.

   e. Uses deception, false promises, insincerity.

   f. Questions and *defies nurse's authority* and competence.

6. Nurse feels powerless and angry at having been used.

◆ **C. Assessment:**

1. Acts out sexually, physically.

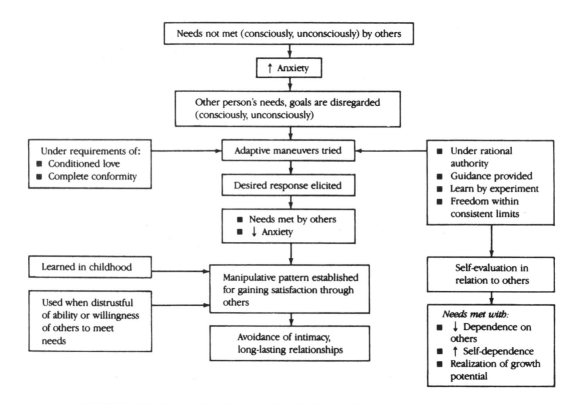

FIGURE 6.3 Operationalization of the behavioral concept of manipulation.

2. Dawdles, always last minute.
3. Uses insincere flattery; expects special favors, privileges.
4. Exploits generosity and fears of others.
5. Feels no guilt.
6. Plays one staff member against another.
7. *Tests limits.*
8. Finds weaknesses in others.
9. Makes excessive, unreasonable, unnecessary *demands* for staff time.
10. *Pretends* to be helpless, lonely, distraught, tearful.
11. Cannot distinguish between truth and falsehood.
12. *Plays on sympathy* or *guilt.*
13. Offers many excuses, lacks insight.
14. Pursues unpleasant issues without genuine regard for or feelings of individuals involved.
15. *Intimidates,* derogates, threatens, bargains, cajoles, violates rules to obtain reactions or privileges.
16. Betrays information.
17. Uses communication as a medium for manipulation, as verbal, nonverbal means to get others to cooperate, to behave in certain way, to get something from another for own use.
18. May be coercive, illogical, or skillfully deceptive.
19. *Unable to learn from experience,* i.e., repeats unacceptable behaviors despite negative consequences.

◆ **D. Analysis/nursing diagnosis:** *ineffective individual coping and impaired adjustment* related to:
  1. Mistrust and contemptuous view of others' motivations.
  2. Life experience of rejection, deception.
  3. Low anxiety tolerance.
  4. Inability to cope with tension.
  5. Unmet dependency needs.
  6. Need to avoid anxiety when cannot obtain gratification.
  7. Need to obtain something that is forbidden, or need for *instant gratification.*
  8. Attempt to put something over on another when no real advantage exists.
  9. *Intolerance of intimacy,* maneuvering effectively to keep others at a safe distance to dilute the relationship by withdrawing and frustrating others or distracting attention away from self.
  10. Attempt to demand attention, approval, disapproval.

◆ **E. Nursing care plan/implementation:**
  1. *Long-term goal:* define relationship as a mutual experience in *learning and trust* rather than a struggle for *power and control.*
  2. *Short-term goals:* increase awareness of self and others; increase self-control; learn to accept limitations.
  3. Promote use of **"three C's"**—*cooperation, compromise, collaboration*—rather than exploitation or deception.

4. *Decrease level and extent of manipulation.*
  a. Set *firm, realistic goals,* with clear, consistent expectations and limits.
  b. *Confront* client regarding exploitation attempts; examine, discuss behavior.
  c. Give *positive reinforcement* with concrete reinforcers for nonmanipulation, to lessen need for exploitive, deceptive, and self-destructive behaviors.
  d. *Ignore* "wooden-leg" behavior (feigning illness to evoke sympathy).
  e. *Allow verbal* anger; do *not* be intimidated; *avoid* giving desired response to obvious attempts to irritate.
  f. Set *consistent, firm, enforceable limits* on *destructive,* aggressive behavior that impinges on others' health, rights, and interests, and on excessive dependency; *give reasons* when you cannot meet requests.
  g. Keep staff informed of rules and reasons; obtain staff *consensus.*
  h. Enforce *direct* communication; encourage openness about *real* needs, feelings.
  i. Do *not* accept gifts, favors, flattery, or other guises of manipulation.
5. Increase responsibility for *self-control* of actions.
  a. Decide who (client, nurse) is responsible for what.
  b. Provide opportunities for *success* to increase self-esteem, experiencing acceptance by others.
  c. Evaluate actions, *not* verbal behavior; point out the difference between talk and action.
  d. Support efforts to be responsible.
  e. Assist client to increase emotional repertoire; explore *alternative* ways of relating interpersonally.
  f. *Avoid submission* to control based on fear of punishment, retaliation, loss of affection.
6. Facilitate awareness of, and *responsibility* for, manipulative behavior and its *effects on others.*
  a. Reflect back client's behavior.
  b. Discourage distortion and misuse of information.
  c. *Increase tolerance* for differences and *delayed gratification* through behavior modification.
  d. Insist on clear, consistent staff communication.
7. *Avoid:*
  a. Labeling client as a "problem."
  b. Hostile, negative attitude.
  c. Making a public issue of client's behavior.
  d. Being excessively rigid or permissive, inconsistent or ambiguous, argumentative or accusatory.
8. *Health teaching:* act as a role model; demonstrate how to deal with mistakes, human imperfections, by admitting mistakes in nonshameful, nonvirtuous ways.

◆ 1. **Evaluation/outcome criteria:** accepts limits; able to compromise, cooperate rather than deceive and exploit; acts responsibly, self-dependent.

IX. Noncompliance and uncooperative behavior

    A. **Definition:** consistently failing to meet the requirements of the prescribed treatment regimen (e.g., refusing to adhere to dietary restrictions or take required medications).

◆ B. **Assessment:**
      1. Refuses to participate in routine or planned activities.
      2. Refuses medication.
      3. Violates rules, ignores limits, and abuses privileges; acts out anger and frustration.

◆ C. **Analysis/nursing diagnosis:** *noncompliance* related to:
      1. *Psychological factors:* lack of knowledge; attitudes, beliefs, and values; denial of illness; rigid, defensive personality type; anxiety level (very high or very low); cannot accept limits or dependency (rebellious counterdependency).
      2. *Environmental factors:* finances, transportation, lack of support system.
      3. *Health care agent-client relationship:* client feels discounted and like an "object"; sees staff as uncaring, authoritative, controlling.
      4. *Health care regimen:* too complicated; not enough benefit from following regimen; results in social stigma or social isolation; unpleasant side effects.

◆ D. **Nursing care plan/implementation:**
      1. *General goal:* reduce need to act out by nonadherence.
        a. Take *preventive* action—be alert to signs of noncompliance, such as intent to leave against medical advice.
        b. *Explore* feelings and reasons for lack of cooperation.
        c. Assess and *allay fears* in client in reassuring manner.
        d. Provide *adequate* information about, and reasons for, rules and procedures.
        e. *Avoid* threats or physical restraints; maintain calm composure.
        f. Demonstrate *tact and firmness* when confronting violations.
        g. Offer *alternatives.*
        h. Firmly insist on cooperation in selected important activities but not all activities.
      2. *Health teaching:* increase knowledge base regarding health-related problem, procedures, or treatments and consequences.

◆ E. **Evaluation/outcome criteria:** follows prescribed regimen.

Psychiatric Emergencies*

  I. **Definition:** sudden onset (days or weeks, not years) of unusual (for that individual), disordered (without pattern or purpose), or socially inappropriate behavior caused by emotional or physiological situation. Examples include: suicidal feelings or attempts, overdose, acute psychotic reaction, acute alcohol withdrawal, acute anxiety.

  II. **General characteristics:**

◆ A. **Assessment:** the presence of great distress without reasonable explanation; *extreme* behavior in comparison with antecedent event.
      1. *Fear*—related to a *particular* person, activity, or place.
      2. *Anxiety*—fearful feeling without any obvious reason, *not* specifically related to a particular person, activity, or place (e.g., adolescent turmoil).
      3. *Depression*—continual pessimism, easily moved to tears, hopelessness, and isolation (e.g., student despondency around exam time, middle-aged crisis, elderly who feel hopelessness).
      4. *Mania*—unrealistic optimism.
      5. *Anger*—many events seen as deliberate insults.
      6. *Confusion*—diminished awareness of who and where one is; memory loss.
      7. *Loss of reality contact*—hallucinations or delusion (as in acute psychosis).
      8. *Withdrawal*—neglect or giving away of belongings and neglect of appearance; loss of interest in activities; apathy.

◆ B. **Analysis/nursing diagnosis:** *ineffective individual coping* related to degree of seriousness:
      1. *Life-threatening emergencies*—violence toward self or others (e.g., suicide, homicide).
      2. *Serious emergencies*—confused and unable to care for or protect self from dangerous situations (as in substance abuse).
      3. *Potentially serious emergencies*—anxious and in pain; disorganized behavior; can become worse or better (as in grief reaction).

◆ C. **General nursing care plan/implementation:**
      1. *Remove* from stressful situation and persons.
      2. Engage in *dialogue* at a nonthreatening distance, to offer help.
      3. Use *calm, slow, deliberate* approach to relieve stress and disorganization.
      4. *Explain* what will be done about the problem and the likely outcome.
      5. *Avoid* using force, threat, or counterthreat.
      6. Use *confident, firm, reasonable* approach.
      7. Encourage client to relate.
      8. Elicit *details.*
      9. Encourage *ventilation* of feelings without interruption.
      10. Accept distortions of reality *without arguing.*
      11. Give form and *structure* to the conversation.
      12. Contact significant others to gain information and to be with client, including previous therapist.
      13. Treat emergency as *temporary* and *readily resolved.*

---

*Adapted from Aguilera, D, and Messick, J: Crisis Intervention, ed. 5. Mosby, St. Louis (out of print).

14. Check every half hour if cannot remain with client.

III. Categories of psychiatric emergencies:

A. *Acute nonpsychotic reactions,* such as acute anxiety attack or panic reaction (for symptoms, see **Anxiety and Anxiety Disorders**).

◆ 1. **Assessment** includes differentiating hyperventilation that is anxiety-connected from asthma, angina, and heart disease.

◆ 2. **Nursing care plan/implementation** in hyperventilation syndrome—*goal:* prevent paresthesia, tetanic contractions, disturbance in awareness; reassure client that vital organs are not impaired.
   a. Increase CO_2 in lungs by rebreathing from paper bag.
   b. Minimize secondary gains; *avoid* reinforcing behavior.
   c. *Health teaching:* demonstrate how to slow down breathing rate.

◆ 3. **Evaluation/outcome criteria:** respirations slowed down; no evidence of effect of hyperventilation.

B. *Delirium*—conditions produced by changes in the cerebral chemistry or tissue by metabolic toxins, direct trauma to the brain, drug effects, or withdrawal.

1. *Acute alcohol intoxication* (see also **Alcohol Abuse and Dependence**).

◆ a. **Assessment:** signs of head or other injury (past and recent), emotional lability, memory defects, loss of judgment, disorientation.

◆ b. **Nursing care plan/implementation:**
   (1) Observe, monitor *vital signs.*
   (2) *Prevent aspiration* of vomitus by positioning.
   (3) *Decrease* environmental stimuli:
      (a) Place in quiet area of emergency department.
      (b) Speak and handle calmly.
   (4) Give medication (benzodiazepines) to control agitation.

◆ c. **Evaluation/outcome criteria:** oriented to time, place, person; appears calmer.

2. *Hallucinogenic drug intoxication*—LSD, mescaline, amphetamines, cocaine, scopolamine, and belladonna.

◆ a. **Assessment:**
   (1) Perceptual and cognitive distortions (e.g., feels heart stopped beating).
   (2) Anxiety (apprehension → panic).
   (3) Subjective feelings (omnipotence → worthlessness).
   (4) Interrelationship of dose, potency, setting, expectations and experiences of user.
   (5) Eyes: *red*—marijuana; *dilated*—LSD, mescaline, belladonna; *constricted*—heroin and derivatives.

◆ b. **Nursing care plan/implementation:**
   (1) "Talk down."
      (a) Establish *verbal* contact, attempt to have client verbally express what is being experienced.

(b) *Environment*—few people, normal lights, calm, supportive.
(c) Allay fears.
(d) Encourage to keep eyes *open.*
(e) Have client focus on *inanimate* objects in room as a bridge to reality contact.
(f) Use simple, *concrete, repetitive* statements.
(g) *Repetitively* orient to time, place, and temporary nature.
(h) Do *not* moralize, challenge beliefs, or probe into lifestyle.
(i) Emphasize confidentiality.

(2) *Medication (minor tranquilizer or benzodiazepines):*
(a) Allay anxiety.
(b) Reduce aggressive behavior.
(c) Reduce suicidal potential; check client every 5–15 min.
(d) *Avoid* anticholinergic crisis (precipitated by use of phenothiazines, belladonna, and scopolamine ingestion) with 2–4 mg IM or PO of physostigmine salicylate.

(3) *Hospitalization:* if hallucinations, delusions last more than 12–18 hr; if client has been injecting amphetamines for extended time; if client is paranoid and depressed.

◆ c. **Evaluation/outcome criteria:** less frightened; oriented to time, place, person.

3. *Acute delirium*—seen in postoperative electrolyte imbalance, systemic infections, renal and hepatic failure, oversedation, metastatic cancer.

◆ a. **Assessment:**
   (1) Disorientation regarding time, at night.
   (2) Hallucinations, delusions, illusions.
   (3) Alterations in mood.
   (4) Increased emotional lability.
   (5) Agitation.
   (6) Lack of cooperation.
   (7) Withdrawal.
   (8) Sleep pattern reversal.
   (9) Alterations in food intake.

◆ b. **Nursing care plan/implementation:**
   (1) Identify and remove *toxic* substance.
   (2) Reality orientation—well-lit room; constant attendance to *repetitively* inform of place and time and to *protect* from injury to self and others.
   (3) Simplify environment.
   (4) *Avoid* excessive medication and restraints; use low-dose phenothiazines; do *not* give barbiturates or sedatives (these increase agitation, confusion, disorientation).

◆ c. **Evaluation/outcome criteria:** oriented to time, place, person; cooperative; less agitated.

C. *Acute psychotic reactions*—disorders of mood or thinking characterized by hallucinations, delusions, excessive euphoria (mania), or depression.

1. *Acute schizophrenic reaction* (see also **Schizophrenic and Other Psychotic Disorders**).

  ◆ a. **Assessment:**
    (1) History of previous hospitalization, illicit drug ingestion; use of major tranquilizers and recent withdrawal from them or alcohol.
    (2) Auditory hallucinations and delusions.
    (3) Violent, assaultive, suicidal behavior directed by auditory hallucinations.
    (4) Assault, withdrawal, and panic related to paranoid delusions of persecution; fear of harm.
    (5) Disturbance in mental status (associative thought disorder).

  ◆ b. **Nursing care plan/implementation** (see also **II. C. Hallucinations**).
    (1) Hospitalization.
    (2) Medication: phenothiazines or atypical antipsychotics.
    (3) *Avoid* physical restraints or touch when fears and delusions of sexual attack exist.
    (4) Allow client to *diffuse* anger and intensity of panic through talk.
    (5) Use simple, *concrete* terms, *avoid* figures of speech or content subject to multiple interpretations.
    (6) Do *not* agree with reality distortions; point out that client's thoughts are difficult to understand but you are willing to listen.

  ◆ c. **Evaluation/outcome criteria:** does not hear frightening voices; less fearful and combative behavior.

2. *Manic reaction* (see also **Bipolar Disorders,** pp.).

  ◆ a. **Assessment:**
    (1) History of depression requiring antidepressants.
    (2) *Thought disorder* (flight of ideas, delusions of grandeur).
    (3) *Affect* (elated, irritable, irrational anger).
    (4) *Speech* (loud, pressured).
    (5) *Behavior* (rapid, erratic, chaotic).

  ◆ b. **Nursing care plan/implementation:**
    (1) Hospitalization to protect from injury to self and others.
    (2) Medication: *lithium carbonate.*
    (3) Same as for acute schizophrenic reaction, *except do not encourage talk,* because of need to decrease stimulation.
    (4) Provide food and fluids that can be consumed while "on the go."

  ◆ c. **Evaluation/outcome criteria:** speech and activity slowed down; thoughts less disordered.

D. *Homicidal or assaultive reaction*—seen in acutely drug-intoxicated, delirious, paranoid, acutely excited manic, or acute anxiety-panic conditions.

  ◆ 1. **Assessment:** history of obvious antisocial behavior, paranoid psychosis, previous violence, sexual conflict, rivalry, substance abuse, recent moodiness, and withdrawal.

  ◆ 2. **Nursing care plan/implementation:**
    a. Physically restrain if client has a weapon; use group of trained people to help.
    b. Allow person to "save face" in giving up weapon.
    c. *Separate* from intended victims.
    d. Approach: calm, unhurried; *one person* to offer support and reassurance; use clear, unambiguous statements.
    e. Immediate and rapid admission procedures.
    f. Observe for *suicidal* behavior that may follow homicidal attempt.

  ◆ 3. **Evaluation/outcome criteria:** client regains impulse control.

◆ **E.** *Suicidal ideation*—seen in anxiety attacks, substance intoxication, toxic delirium, schizophrenic auditory hallucinations, and depressive reactions.

  1. **Concepts and principles related to suicide:**
    a. *Based on social theory:* suicidal tendency is a result of collective social forces rather than isolated individual motives (Durkheim's *Le Suicide*).
      (1) Common factor: increased *alienation* between person and social group; psychological isolation, called "anomie," when links between groups are weakened.
      (2) "Egoistic" suicide: results from lack of integration of individual with others.
      (3) "Altruistic" suicide: results from insufficient individualization.
      (4) *Implication:* increase group cohesiveness and mutual interdependence, making group more coherent and consistent in fulfilling needs of each member.
    b. *Based on symbolic interaction theory:*
      (1) Person evaluates self according to *others' assessment.*
      (2) Thus, suicide stems from *social rejection* and disrupted social relations.
      (3) Perceived failure in relationships with others may be inaccurate but seen as real by the individual.
      (4) *Implication:* need to recognize difference in perception of alienation between own viewpoint and others'.
    c. *Based on psychoanalytic theory:*
      (1) Suicide stems mainly from the individual, with external events only as precipitants.
      (2) There is a strong life urge in people.
      (3) *Universal death instinct* is always present (Freud).
      (4) Person may be balancing life wishes and death wishes. When self-preservation instincts are diminished, death instincts may find direct outlet via suicide.

(5) When *love instinct* is frustrated, *hate* impulse takes over (Menninger).
  (a) Desire to kill → desire to be killed → desire to kill oneself.
  (b) Suicide may be an act of extreme hostility, manipulation, and revenge to elicit guilt and remorse in significant others.
  (c) Suicide may also be act of self-punishment to handle own guilt or to control fate.

d. *Based on synthesis of social and psychoanalytic theories:*
  (1) Suicide is seen as *running away* from an intolerable situation to interrupt it, rather than *running to* something more desirable.
  (2) Process *defined in operational terms* involves:
    (a) Despair over inability to cope.
    (b) Inability to feel hope or adequacy.
    (c) Frustration with others when others cannot fill needs.
    (d) Rage and aggression experienced toward significant other is turned inward.
    (e) Psychic blow acts as precipitant.
    (f) Life seen as harder to cope with, with no chance of improvement in life situation.
    (g) *Implication:* persons who experience suicidal impulses can gain a certain amount of control over these impulses through the support they gain from meaningful relationships with others.

e. *Based on crisis theory (Dublin):* concept of emotional disequilibrium:
  (1) Everyone at some point in life is in a crisis, with temporary inability to solve problems or to master the crisis.
  (2) Usual coping mechanisms do not function.
  (3) Person unable to relate to others.
  (4) Person searches consciously and unconsciously for useful coping techniques, with suicide as one of various solutions.
  (5) With inadequate communication of needs and isolation, suicide is possible.

f. *Based on the view that suicide is an individual's personal reaction and decision, a final response to own situation:*
  (1) *Process* of anger turned inward → self-inflicted, destructive action.
  (2) *Definition* of concept in operational steps:
    (a) Frustration of individual needs → anger.
    (b) Anger turned inward → feelings of guilt, despair, depression, incompetence, hopelessness, and exhaustion.
    (c) Stress felt and perceived as unbearable and overwhelming.

(d) Attempt to communicate hopelessness and defeat to others.
(e) Others do not provide hope.
(f) Sudden change in behavior, as noted when depression appears to lift, may indicate *danger,* as person has more energy to act on suicidal thoughts and feelings.
(g) Decision to end life → plan of action → self-induced, self-destructive behavior.

(3) May be *pseudosuicide* attempts, where there is no actual or realistic desire to achieve finality of death. Intentions or causes may be:
  (a) "Cry for help," where nonlethal attempt notifies others of deeper intentions.
  (b) Desire to *manipulate* others.
  (c) Need for *attention and pity.*
  (d) Self-punishment.
  (e) Symbol of *utter frustration.*
  (f) Wish to *punish* others.
  (g) *Misuse* of alcohol and other drugs.

(4) Other reasons for self-destruction, where the individual *gives his or her life* rather than takes it, include:
  (a) Strong parental love that can overcome fear and instinct of self-preservation to save child's life.
  (b) "Sacrificial death" during war, such as kamikaze pilots in World War II.
  (c) Submission to death for religious beliefs (martyrdom).

◆ 2. **Assessment of suicide:**
  a. *Assessment of risk regarding statistical probability of suicide—composite picture:* male, older than 45 years, unemployed, divorced, living alone, depressed (weight loss, somatic delusions, sleep disturbance, preoccupied with suicide), history of substance abuse and suicide within family.
  b. *Ten factors* to predict potential suicide and assess risk:
    (1) *Age, sex, and race*—teenage and young adult (ages 15 to 24), older age; more women make attempts; more men complete suicide act. *Highest risk:* older women rather than young boys; older men rather than young girls. Suicide occurs in all races and socioeconomic groups.
    (2) *Recent stress* related to *loss*—family problems: death, divorce, separation, alienation; financial pressures; loss of job; loss of status; failing grades.
    (3) *Clues to suicide:* suicidal thoughts are usually time limited and do not last forever. Early assessment of behavioral and verbal clues is important.*

(a) *Verbal clues—direct:* "I am going to shoot myself." *Indirect:* "It's more than I can bear." *Coded:* "This is the last time you'll ever see me." "I want you to have my coin collection."

(b) *Behavioral clues—direct:* trial run with pills or razor, for example. *Indirect:* sudden lifting of depression, buying a casket, giving away cherished belongings, putting affairs in order, writing a will.

(c) *Syndromes—dependent-dissatisfied:* emotionally dependent but dislikes dependent state, irritable, helpless. *Depressed:* detachment from life; feels life is a burden; hopelessness, futility. *Disoriented:* delusions or hallucinations, confusion, delirium tremens, organic brain syndromes. *Willful-defiant:* active need to direct and control environment and life situation, with low frustration tolerance and rigid mind-set, rage, shame.

(4) *Suicidal plan*—the *more details* about method, timing, and place, and preoccupation with thoughts of suicide plan, the *higher* the risk.

(5) *Previous suicidal behavior*—history of prior attempt increases risk. Eight out of ten suicide attempts give verbal and behavioral warnings as listed previously.

(6) *Medical and psychiatric status*—chronic ailments, terminal illness, and pain increase suicidal risk; people with bipolar disorder, and when emerging from depression.

(7) *Communication*—the more disorganized thinking, anxious, hostile, and withdrawn and apathetic, the greater the potential for suicide, unless extreme psychomotor retardation is present.

(8) *Style of life*—high risks include *substance abusers*, those with sexual-identity conflicts, unstable relationships (personal and job related). Suicidal tendencies are not inherited but learned from family and other interpersonal relationships.

(9) *Alcohol*—can reinforce helpless and hopeless feelings; may be *lethal* if *used with barbiturates*; can decrease inhibitions, result in impulsive behavior.

(10) *Resources*—the *fewer* the resources, the *higher* the suicide potential. Examples of resources: family, friends, colleagues, religion, pets, meaningful recreational outlets, satisfying employment.

c. Assess *needs* commonly communicated by individuals who are suicidal:

(1) To trust.

(2) To be accepted

(3) To bolster self-esteem.

(4) To "fit in" with groups.

(5) To experience success and interrupt the failure syndrome.

(6) To expand capacity for pleasure.

(7) To increase autonomy and sense of self-mastery.

(8) To work out an acceptable sexual identity.

◆ 3. **Analysis/nursing diagnosis:** *risk for self-directed violence* related to:

a. Feelings of *alienation.*

b. Feelings of *rejection.*

c. Feelings of *hopelessness, despair.*

d. Feelings of *frustration and rage.*

◆ 4. **Nursing care plan/implementation:**

a. *Long-term goals*

(1) Increase client's self-reliance.

(2) Help client achieve more realistic and positive feelings of self-esteem, self-respect, acceptance by others, and sense of belonging.

(3) Help client experience success, interrupt failure pattern, and expand views about pleasure.

b. *Short-term goals*

▶ (1) Medical: assist as necessary with gastric lavage; provide respiratory and vascular support; assist in repair of inflicted wounds.

(2) Provide a safe environment for protection from self-destruction until client is able to assume this responsibility.

(3) *Allow outward* and *constructive* expression of hostile and aggressive feelings.

(4) Provide for physical needs.

c. *Suicide precautions* to institute under emergency conditions:

(1) One-to-one supervision at *all* times for maximum precautions; check whereabouts every 15 min, if on basic suicide precautions.

(2) Before instituting these measures, explain to client what you will be doing and why; MD must also explain; document this explanation.

(3) Do *not* allow client to leave the unit for tests, procedures.

(4) Look through client's *belongings with* the client and remove any potentially harmful objects (e.g., pills, knife, gun, matches, belts, razors, glass, tweezers).

(5) Allow visitors and phone calls, but maintain one-to-one supervision during visits.

(6) Check that visitors do not leave potentially harmful objects in the client's room.

(7) Serve meals in an isolation meal tray that contains no glass or metal silverware.

(8) Do *not* discontinue these measures without an order.

d. *General approaches*
   (1) *Observe* closely at all times to assess suicide potential.
   (2) *Be available.*
       (a) Demonstrate concern, acceptance, and respect for client as a person.
       (b) Be sensitive, warm, and consistent.
       (c) Listen with empathy.
       (d) *Avoid* imposing your own feelings of reality on client.
       (e) *Avoid* extremes in your own mood when with client (especially exaggerated cheerfulness).
   (3) *Focus directly* on client's self-destructive ideas.
       (a) Reduce alienation and immobilization by discussing this "taboo" topic.
       (b) Acknowledge suicidal threats with calmness and without reproach—do *not* ignore or minimize threat.
       (c) *Find out details* about suicide plan and reduce environmental hazards.
       (d) Help client verbalize aggressive, hostile, and hopeless *feelings.*
       (e) *Explore death fantasies*—try to take "romance" out of death.
   (4) Acknowledge that suicide is one of several options and that there are alternatives.
   (5) *Make a contract* with the client, and structure a plan of alternatives for coping when next confronted with the need to commit suicide (e.g., the client could call someone, express feeling of anger outwardly, or ask for help).
   (6) Point out client's *self-responsibility* for suicidal act.
       (a) *Avoid* manipulation by client who says, "You are responsible for stopping me from killing myself."
       (b) Emphasize protection against self-destruction *rather than* punishment.
   (7) *Support* the part of the client that wants to live.
       (a) Focus on *ambivalence.*
       (b) Emphasize meaningful past relationships and events.
       (c) Look for reasons left for wanting to live. Elicit what is meaningful to the client at the moment.
       (d) Point out effect of client's death on others.
   (8) *Remove sources of stress.*
       (a) Decrease uncomfortable feelings of *alienation* by initiating one-to-one interactions.
       (b) Make all *decisions* when client is in severe depression.
       (c) Progressively let client make simple decisions: what to eat, what to watch on TV, etc.
   (9) *Provide hope.*
       (a) Let client know that problems can be solved with help.
       (b) Bring in new resources for help.
       (c) Talk about likely changes in client's life.
       (d) Review past effective coping behaviors.
   (10) *Provide with opportunity to be useful.* Reduce self-centeredness and brooding by planning diversional activities within the client's capabilities.
   (11) *Involve as many people as possible.*
        (a) Gradually bring in others, for instance, other therapists, friends, staff, clergy, family, co-workers.
        (b) Prevent staff "burnout," found when only one nurse is working with client who is suicidal.
   (12) *Health teaching:* teach client and staff principles of crisis intervention and resolution. Teach new coping skills.
◆ 5. **Evaluation/outcome criteria:** physical condition is stabilized; client able to verbalize feelings rather than acting them out.

Crisis Intervention

Crisis intervention is a type of brief psychiatric treatment in which individuals or their families are helped in their efforts to forestall the process of mental decompensation in reaction to severe emotional stress by direct and immediate supportive approaches.

I. **Definition of crisis:** sudden event in one's life that disturbs homeostasis, during which usual coping mechanisms cannot resolve the problem. Types of crisis:
   A. *Maturational* (internal): see Erik Erikson's eight stages of developmental crises anticipated in the development of the infant, child, adolescent, and adult (see **Unit 5**).
   B. *Situational* (external): occurs at any time (e.g., loss of job, loss of income, death of significant person, illness, hospitalization).

II. **Concepts and principles related to crisis intervention:**
   A. Crises are turning points where changes in behavior patterns and lifestyles can occur; individuals in crisis are most amenable to altering old and unsuccessful coping mechanisms and are most likely to learn new and more functional behaviors.
   B. Social milieu and its structure are contributing factors in both the development of psychiatric symptoms and eventual recovery from them.
   C. If crisis is handled effectively, the person's mental stability will be maintained; individual may return to a precrisis state or better.
   D. If crisis is not handled effectively, individual may progress to a worse state with exacerbations of earlier conflicts; future crises may not be handled well.

E. There are a number of universal developmental crisis periods (maturational crises) in every individual's life.

F. Each person tries to maintain equilibrium through use of adaptive behaviors.

G. When individuals face a problem they cannot solve, tension, anxiety, narrowed perception, and disorganized functioning occur.

H. *Immediate relief* of symptoms produced by crisis is more urgent than *exploring* their cause.

III. Characteristics of crisis intervention:

A. Acute, sudden onset related to a stressful precipitating event of which individual is aware but which immobilizes previous coping abilities.

B. Responsive to brief therapy with focus on immediate problem.

C. Focus shifted from the psyche in the individual to the *individual in the environment;* deemphasis on intrapsychic aspects.

D. Crisis period is *time limited* (usually up to 6 wk).

◆ IV. Nursing care plan/implementation in crises:

A. General goals:
1. *Avoid* hospitalization if possible.
2. Return to precrisis level and preserve ability to function.
3. Assist in problem solving, with *here-and-now* focus.

B. *Assess* the crisis:
1. Identify stressful *precipitating* events: duration, problems created, and degree of significance.
2. Assess *suicidal and homicidal risk.*
3. Assess amount of *disruption* in individual's life and effect on significant others.
4. Assess *current coping skills,* strengths, and general level of functioning.

C. *Plan* the intervention:
1. Consider *past coping* mechanisms.
2. Propose *alternatives* and untried coping methods.

D. *Implementation:*
1. Help client relate the crisis event to current feelings.
2. Encourage expression of all feelings related to disruption.
3. Explore past coping skills and *reinforce adaptive* ones.
4. Use all means available in *social network* to take care of client's *immediate needs* (e.g., significant others, law enforcement agencies, housing, welfare, employment, medical, and school).
5. Set limits.
6. *Health teaching:* teach additional problem-solving approaches.

◆ V. Evaluation/outcome criteria:

A. Client returns to precrisis level of functioning.
B. Client learns new, more effective coping skills.
C. Client can describe realistic plans for future in terms of own perception of progress, support system, and coping mechanisms.

Selected Specific Crisis Situations: Problems Related to Abuse

I. Domestic violence[*]

A. **Characteristics**
1. *Victims:* feel helpless, powerless to prevent assault; blame themselves; ambivalent about leaving the relationship.
2. *Abusers:* often blame the victims; have poor impulse control; use power (physical strength or weapon) to threaten and subject victims to their assault.
3. *Cycle* of stages, with increase in severity of the battering:
   a. *Buildup of tension* (through verbal abuse): abuser is often drinking or taking other drugs; victim blames self.
   b. *Battering:* abuser does not remember brutal beating; victim is in shock and detached.
   c. *Calm:* abuser "makes up," apologizes, and promises "never again"; victim believes and forgives the abuser, and feels loved.

B. **Risk factors**
1. *Learned responses:* abuser and victim have had past experience with violence in family; victim has "learned helplessness."
2. Women who are *pregnant* and those with one or more *preschool children,* who see no alternative to staying in the battering relationship.
3. Women who *fear* punishment from the abuser.

◆ C. Assessment:
1. Injury to parts of body, especially face, head, genitals (e.g., welts, bruises, fracture of nose).
2. Presents in the emergency department with report of "accidental injury."
3. Severe anxiety.
4. Depression.

◆ D. Analysis/nursing diagnosis:
1. *Risk for injury* related to physical harm.
2. *Posttraumatic response* related to assault.
3. *Fear* related to threat of death or change in health status.
4. *Pain* related to physical and psychological harm.
5. *Powerlessness* related to interpersonal interaction.
6. *Ineffective individual coping* related to situational crisis.
7. *Spiritual distress* related to intense suffering and challenged value system.

◆ E. Nursing care plan/implementation:
1. Provide safe environment; refer to community resources for shelter.
2. Treat physical injuries.
3. Document injuries.
4. Supportive, nonjudgmental approach: identify woman's strengths; help her to accept that she cannot control the abuser; encourage description of home situation; help her to see choices.

---

[*]Source: ©Lagerquist, S: In NurseNotes Psychiatric-Mental Health, A.T.I.

5. Encourage individual and family therapy for victim and abuser.

◆ **F. Evaluation/outcome criteria:**
1. Physical symptoms have been treated.
2. Discusses plans for safety (for self and any children) to protect against further injury.

II. Rape-trauma syndrome
A. Definition: forcible perpetration of an act of sexual intercourse on the body of an unwilling person.

◆ **B. Assessment:**
1. *Signs of physical trauma*—physical findings of entry.
2. *Symptoms of physical trauma*—verbatim statements regarding type of sexual attack.
3. *Signs of emotional trauma*—tears, hyperventilation, extreme anxiety, withdrawal, self-blame, anger, embarrassment, fears, sleeping and eating disturbances, desire for revenge.
4. *Symptoms of emotional trauma*—statements regarding method of force used and threats made.

◆ **C. Analysis/nursing diagnosis:** *rape-trauma syndrome* related to phases of response to rape:
1. *Acute response:* volatility, disorganization, disbelief, shock, incoherence, agitated motor activity, nightmares, guilt (feels that should have been able to protect self), phobias (crowds, being alone, sex).
2. *Outward coping:* denial and suppression of anxiety and fear (silent rape syndrome), feelings appear controlled.

3. *Integration and resolution:* confronts anger with attacker; realistic perspective.

◆ **D. Nursing care plan/implementation** in counseling victims of rape. **Figure 6.4** is a summary of self-care decisions a victim faces the first night following a sexual assault.
1. Overall goals:
   a. Protect legal (forensic) evidence.
   b. Acknowledge feelings.
   c. Face feelings.
   d. Resolve feelings.
   e. Maintain and restore *self-respect, dignity, integrity,* and *self-determination.*
2. Work through issues:
   a. Handle *legal* matters and police contacts.
   b. Clarify facts.
   c. Assist medical examiner in collecting DNA evidence.
   d. Get *medical* attention if needed.
   e. Notify *family and friends.*
   f. Understand emotional reaction.
   g. Attend to *practical* concerns.
   h. Evaluate need for psychiatric consultations.
3. *Acute phase:*
   a. Decrease victim's stress, anxiety, fear.
   b. Seek medical care.
   c. Increase self-confidence and self-esteem.
   d. Identify and accept feelings and needs (to be in control, cared about, to achieve).

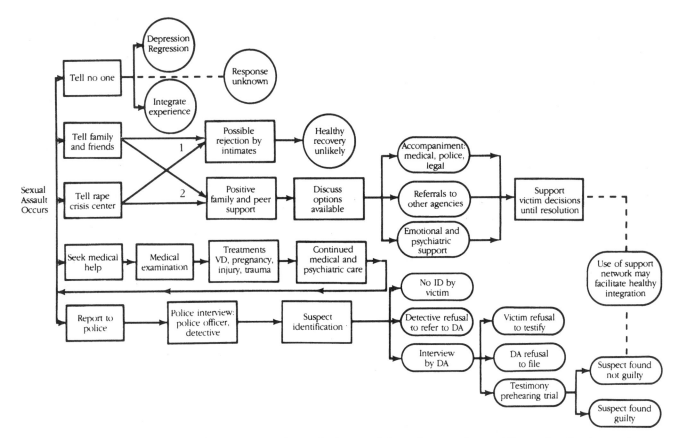

FIGURE 6.4 Victim decisions following a sexual assault. (From Violence Intervention and Prevention Services at the YWCA of Greater Harrisburg, Pa.)

c. Reorient perceptions, feelings, and statements about self.

f. Help resume normal lifestyle.

4. *Outward coping phase:*

a. Remain available and supportive.

b. Reflect words, feelings, and thoughts.

c. Explore real problems.

d. Explore alternatives regarding contraception, legal issues.

e. Evaluate response of family and friends to victim and rape.

5. *Integration and resolution phase:*

a. Assist exploration of feelings (anger) regarding attacker.

b. Explore feelings (guilt and shame) regarding self.

c. Assist in making own decisions regarding health care.

6. Maintain confidentiality and neutrality—facilitate person's own decision.

7. Search for alternatives to giving advice.

8. *Health teaching:*

a. Explain procedures and services to victim.

b. Counsel to avoid isolated areas and being helpful to strangers.

c. Counsel where and how to resist attack (scream, run unless assailant has weapon).

d. Teach what to do if pregnancy or STD is outcome.

◆ E. **Evaluation/outcome criteria:** little or no evidence of possible long-term effects of rape (guilt, shame, phobias, denial).

III. Child who is victim of violence

◆ A. **Assessment**—clues to the identification of a child who is a victim of violence[*]

1. Clues in the *history*

a. Significant *delay* in seeking medical care.

b. Major *discrepancies* in the history:

(1) Discrepancy between different people's versions of the story.

(2) Discrepancy between the history and the observed injuries.

(3) Discrepancy between the history and the child's developmental capabilities.

c. History of multiple emergency department visits for various injuries.

d. A story that is *vague* and *contradictory*.

2. Clues in the *physical examination*

a. Child who seems withdrawn, apathetic, and *does not cry* despite the injuries.

b. Child who *does not turn to parents for comfort;* or unusual desire to please parent; unusual fear of parent(s).

c. *Child who is poorly nourished* and *poorly cared for.*

d. The presence of *bruises: multiple bruises*, welts, and abrasions, especially around the trunk and

TABLE 6.11	Estimation of Time at Which Soft Tissue Injury Occurred
Injury Occurred	**Color**
0–2 hr	No discoloration (may have edema and pain)
1–5 days	Red/blue
5–7 days	Green
7–10 days	Yellow
10–14 days	Brown

buttocks; lesions resembling bites or fingernail marks; *old bruises in addition to fresh ones* (**Table 6.11**).

e. The presence of *suspicious burns:*

(1) Cigarette burns.

(2) Scalds without splash marks or involving the buttocks, hands, or feet but sparing skinfolds.

(3) Rope marks.

f. Clues in parent behavior—exaggerate care and concern.

g. X-rays: old fractures, especially in child under 3 yr.

◆ B. **Analysis/nursing diagnosis:**

1. Same as for *domestic violence* p. xxx.

2. *Altered parenting* related to poor role model/identity, unrealistic expectations, presence of stressors and lack of support.

3. *Low self-esteem* related to deprivation and negative feedback.

◆ C. **Nursing care plan/implementation:**

1. Same as for *domestic violence.*

2. Report suspected child abuse to appropriate source.

3. Conduct assessment interview in private, with child and parent separated.

4. Be supportive and nonjudgmental.

◆ D. **Evaluation/outcome criteria:**

1. Same as *domestic violence.*

2. Child safety has been ensured.

3. Parent(s) or caregivers have agreed to seek help.

IV. Sexual abuse of children

◆ A. **Assessment**—characteristic behaviors:

1. *Relationship* of offender to victim: many filling paternal role (uncle, grandfather, cousin) with repeated, unquestioned access to the child.

2. Methods of *pressuring* victim into sexual activity: offering material goods, misrepresenting moral standards ("it's OK"), exploiting need for human contact and warmth.

3. Method of pressuring victim to *secrecy* (to conceal the act) is inducing fear of punishment, not being believed, rejection, being blamed for the activity, abandonment.

4. Disclosure of sexual activity via:

a. Direct visual or verbal confrontation and *observation* by others.

b. *Verbalization* of act by victim.

---

[*]Adapted from Caroline, N: *Emergency Care in the Streets*, ed. 5. Little, Brown, Boston, out of print).

c. *Visible clues:* excess money and candy, new clothes, pictures, notes; enlarged vaginal or rectal orifice; stains and/or blood on underwear.

d. *Signs and symptoms:* bed-wetting, excessive bathing, tears, avoiding school, somatic distress (*GI and urinary* tract pains). Genital irritation (itching, bruised, bleeding, pain); unusual sexual behavior.

e. Overly solicitous parental attitude toward child.

◆ **B. Analysis/nursing diagnosis:**

1. *Altered protection* related to inflicted pain.
2. *Risk for injury* related to neglect, abuse.
3. *Personal identity disturbance* related to abuse as child and feeling guilty and responsible for being a victim.
4. *Ineffective individual coping* related to high stress level.
5. *Sleep pattern disturbance* related to traumatic sexual experiences.
6. *Ineffective family coping.*
7. *Altered family processes* related to use of violence.
8. *Altered parenting* related to violence.
9. *Powerlessness* related to feelings of being dependent on abuser.
10. *Social isolation/withdrawal* related to shame about family violence.
11. *Risk for altered abuse response patterns.*

◆ **C. Nursing care plan/implementation:**

1. Establish safe environment and the termination of trauma.
2. Encourage child to verbalize feelings about incident to dispel tension built up by secrecy.
3. Ask child to draw a picture or use dolls and toys to show what happened.
4. Observe for symptoms over a period of time.
   a. *Phobic* reactions when seeing or hearing offender's name.
   b. *Sleep pattern* changes, recurrent dreams, nightmares.
5. Look for *silent reaction* to being an accessory to sex (i.e., child keeping burden of the secret activity within self); help deal with unresolved issues.
6. Establish therapeutic alliance with parent who is abusive.
7. *Health teaching:*
   a. Teach child that his (her) body is private and to inform a responsible adult when someone violates privacy without consent.
   b. Teach adults in family to respond to victim with sensitivity, support, and concern.

◆ **D. Evaluation/outcome criteria:**

1. Child's needs for affection, attention, personal recognition, or love met without sexual exploitation.
2. Perpetrator accepts therapy.
3. Conspiracy of silence is broken.

E. Summary: signs that are common to both *physical* and *sexual abuse:*

1. Parental behaviors
   a. Blaming child or sibling for injury.
   b. Anger (rather than providing comfort) toward child for injury.
   c. Hostility toward health-care providers.
   d. Exaggeration or absence of response from parent regarding child's injury.
2. Child (toddler or preschooler)
   a. No protest when parent leaves.
   b. Shows preference for health-care provider over parent.
   c. Signs of "failure to thrive" syndrome.
3. Other signs
   a. History: inconsistent with stages of growth and development.
   b. Inconsistent details of injury between one person and another.

V. Elder abuse/neglect

A. Definition: battering, psychological abuse, sexual assault, or any act or omission by personal caregiver, family, or legal guardian that results in harm or threatened harm.

B. Concepts, principles, and characteristics:

1. Elders who are currently being abused often abused their abusers—their offspring. Violence is a learned behavior.
2. *Victim characteristics:* diminished self-esteem, feeling responsibility for the abuse, isolated.
3. *Abuser characteristics:* usually has physical or psychosocial stressors related to marital or fiscal difficulties; substance abuse.
4. *Legal:* most states have mandatory laws to report elder abuse, although many cases are not reported because of shame, fear of more abuse, cultural/religious beliefs, optimism, loyalty, financial dependency.
5. Types of abuse:
   a. *Financial* abuse (e.g., fraudulent monetary schemes, theft [money, property, or both]).
   b. *Neglect* (e.g., lack of food, clean clothing, medications; no provision for assistive devices [dentures, hearing aids, glasses, canes]).
   c. *Psychological* abuse (e.g., verbal abuse).
   d. *Physical* abuse (e.g., beating, physical restraints, rape).

◆ **C. Assessment:**

1. *Risk factors:*

Victim:	Abuser:
▪ Poor health	▪ Substance abuse
▪ Isolated	▪ Stressful life events
▪ Impaired memory, thinking	▪ Interpersonal problems
◀—— Hx: Mental illness ——▶	
◀—— Hx: Family violence ——▶	
◀—— Financial difficulties ——▶	
◀—— Dependency ——▶	
◀—— Share living space ——▶	

Mental Health

2. *Behavioral clues:* agitation, anger, denial, fear, confusion, depression, withdrawal, unbelievable stories about causes of injuries.
3. *Physical indicators:* weight loss; unexplained cuts, bruises, puncture wounds; untreated injuries; unkempt; noncompliance with medical plan of care.
4. *Financial matters* (e.g., recent changes in will; unusual banking activity; missing checks, personal belongings; forged signatures; unwillingness to spend money on the elder).

◆ D. **Analysis/nursing diagnosis:**
1. *Risk for injury* related to neglect, abuse.
2. *Fear.*
3. *Powerlessness* related to dependency on abuser.
4. *Unilateral neglect.*
5. *Spiritual distress.*
6. *Altered family processes* related to use of violence.

◆ E. **Nursing care plan/implementation:**
1. *Primary prevention:*
   a. Early case finding; early treatment.
   b. Referral to community services for caregiver (e.g., respite care) before serious abuse occurs.
2. *Secondary prevention:*
   a. Report case to law enforcement agencies.
   b. Provide elder with phone number for confidential hotline.
   c. Plan for safety of elder (e.g., shelter).
3. *Tertiary prevention:*
   a. Counseling, support, and self-help groups for victim.
   b. Legal action against abuser.

◆ F. **Evaluation/outcome criteria:**
1. Elder develops trust in caregivers, without fear of further abuse.
2. Spiritual well-being is enhanced, with diminished feelings of guilt, hopelessness, and powerlessness.

COMFORT, REST, ACTIVITY, AND MOBILITY FUNCTIONS

Sleep Disturbance

I. **Types of sleep:**
A. *Rapid eye movement (REM) sleep:* colorful, dramatic, emotional, implausible dreams.
B. *Non-REM sleep—stages:*
1. Stage 1: lasts 30 sec–7 min—falls asleep, drowsy; easily awakened; fleeting thoughts.
2. Stage 2: more relaxed; no eye movements, clearly asleep but readily awakens; 45% of total sleep time spent in this stage.
3. Stage 3 (delta sleep): deep muscle relaxation; decreased temperature, pulse, respiration (TPR).
4. Stage 4 (delta sleep): very relaxed; rarely moves.
C. *Sleep cycle*—common progression of sleep stages:
1. Stages 1, 2, 3, 4, 3, 2, REM, 2, 3, 4, etc.
2. *Delta* sleep most common during first third of night, with *REM* sleep periods increasing in dura-

tion during night from 1–2 min at start to 20–30 min by early morning.
3. REM sleep varies.
   a. Adolescents spend 30% of total sleep time in REM sleep.
   b. Adults spend 15% of total sleep time in REM sleep.

II. **Sleep deprivation (dyssomnias):**
◆ A. **Assessment:**
1. *Non-REM sleep loss:* physical fatigue due to less time spent in normal deep sleep.
2. *REM sleep loss:* psychological effects—irritability, confusion, anxiety, short-term memory loss, paranoia, hallucinations.
3. *Desynchronized sleep:* occurs when sleep shifts more than 2 hr from normal sleep period. Irritability, anoxia, decreased stress tolerance.

◆ B. **Analysis/nursing diagnosis:** *sleep pattern disturbance* may be related to:
1. Interrupted sleep cycles before 90 min sleep cycle is completed.
2. Unfamiliar sleeping environment.
3. Alterations in normal sleep/activity cycles (e.g., jet lag).
4. Preexisting sleep deficits before hospital admission.
5. Medications (e.g., alcohol withdrawal or abruptly discontinuing the use of hypnotic or antidepressant medications).
6. Pain.

◆ C. **Nursing care plan/implementation:**
1. Obtain sleep history as part of nursing assessment. Determine normal sleep hours, bedtime rituals, factors that promote or interrupt sleep.
2. Duplicate normal bedtime rituals when possible.
3. Make *environment* conducive to sleep: lighting, noise, temperature.
   a. Close door, dim lights, turn off unneeded machinery.
   b. Encourage staff to muffle conversation at night.
4. Encourage *daytime* exercise periods.
5. Allow *uninterrupted periods of 90 min of sleep.* Group nighttime treatments and observations that require touching the client.
6. *Minimize* use of hypnotic medications.
   a. Substitute back rubs, warm milk, relaxation exercises.
   b. Encourage physician to consider prescribing hypnotics that minimize sleep disruption (e.g., chloral hydrate and flurazepam HCl [Dalmane]).
   c. *Taper* off hypnotics rather than abruptly discontinuing.
7. Observe client while asleep.
   a. Evaluate quality of sleep.
   b. It may be sleep apnea if client is extremely restless and snoring heavily.
8. *Health teaching: avoid* caffeine and hyperstimulation at bedtime; teach how to promote sleep-inducing environment, relaxation techniques.

◆ **D. Evaluation/outcome criteria:** verbalizes satisfaction with amount, quality of sleep.

EATING DISORDERS

Anorexia Nervosa/Bulimia Nervosa

Anorexia nervosa is an illness of starvation related to a severe disturbance of body image and a morbid fear of obesity; it is an eating disorder, usually seen in adolescence, when a person is underweight and emaciated and refuses to eat. It can result in death due to irreversible metabolic processes.

Bulimia nervosa is another type of eating disorder (binge-purge syndrome) also encountered primarily in late adolescence or early adulthood. It is characterized by at least two binge-eating episodes of large quantities of high calorie food over a couple of hours followed by disparaging self-criticism and depression. Self-induced vomiting, abuse of laxatives, and abuse of diuretics are commonly associated because they decrease physical pain of abdominal distention, may reduce postbinge anguish, and may provide a method of self-control. Bulimic episodes may occur as part of anorexia nervosa, but these clients rarely become emaciated, and not all have a body-image disturbance.

I. **Concepts and principles related to anorexia nervosa:**
  A. *Not* due to lack of appetite or problem with appetite center in hypothalamus.
  B. Normal stomach hunger is *repressed, denied, depersonalized;* no conscious awareness of hunger sensation.

◆ II. **Assessment of anorexia nervosa:**
  A. *Body-image disturbance*—delusional, obsessive (e.g., does not see self as thin and is bewildered by others' concern).
  B. Usually *preoccupied* with food, yet dreads gaining too much weight. *Ambivalence:* avoids food, hoards food.
  C. Feels ineffectual, with low sex drive. *Repudiation of sexuality.*
  D. *Pregnancy* fears, including misconceptions of oral impregnation through food.
  E. *Self-punitive* behavior leading to starvation; suppression of anger.
  F. *Physical signs and symptoms*
    1. Weight loss (20% of previous "normal" body weight).
    2. Amenorrhea and secondary sex organ atrophy.
    3. *Hyperactivity;* compulsiveness; excessive gum chewing.
    4. Constipation.
    5. *Hypotension, bradycardia,* hypothermia.
    6. Skin: hyperkeratosis, poor turgor, dry.
    7. Blood: leukopenia, anemia, hypoglycemia, hypoproteinemia, hypocholesterolemia, hypokalemia, hyponatremia, *decreased* magnesium, *decreased* chloride, *increased* BUN; EKG: T-wave inversion.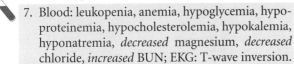

◆ III. **Analysis/nursing diagnosis:**
  A. *Altered nutrition, less than body requirements,* and *fluid volume deficit* related to attempts to vomit food after eating, overuse of laxatives/diuretics, and refusal to eat, related to need to demonstrate control.

  B. *Risk for altered physical regulation processes/risk for or actual fluid volume deficit:* amenorrhea related to starvation; hypotension, bradycardia; metabolic alkalosis.
  C. *Risk for self-inflicted injury* related to starvation from refusal to eat or ambivalence about food.
  D. *Altered eating* related to altered thought processes: binge-purge syndrome.
  E. *Body-image disturbance/chronic low self-esteem* related to anxiety over assuming an adult role and concern with sexual identity; unmet dependency needs, personal vulnerability; perceived loss of control in some aspect of life; dysfunctional family system.
  F. *Compulsive behaviors* related to need to maintain control of self, represented by losing weight.

◆ IV. **Nursing care plan/implementation:**
  A. Help reestablish connections between body sensations (hunger) and responses (eating). Use *stimulus-response conditioning* methods to set up eating regimen.
    1. *Weigh* regularly, at same time and with same amount of clothing, with back to scale.
    2. Make sure water drinking is *avoided* before weighing.
    3. Give one-to-one supervision during and 30 min after mealtimes to *prevent* attempts to vomit food.
    4. Monitor exercise program and set limits on physical activity.
  B. *Monitor* physiological signs and symptoms (amenorrhea, constipation, hypoproteinemia, hypoglycemia, anemia, eroded tooth enamel, inflamed buccal cavity, brittle nails, dull hair, secondary sexual organ atrophy, hypothermia, hypotension, leg cramps and other signs of hypokalemia).
  C. *Health teaching:*
    1. Explain normal sexual growth and development to improve knowledge deficit and confront sexual fears.
    2. Use behavior modification to reestablish awareness of hunger sensation and to relate it to the clock and regular meal times.
    3. Teach parents skills in communication related to dependence/independence needs of adolescent; allow client to assume control in areas other than dieting, weight loss (e.g., management of daily activities, work, leisure choices).

◆ V. **Evaluation/outcome criteria:**
  A. Attains and maintains minimal normal weight for age and height.
  B. Eats regular meal (standard nutritional diet).
  C. No incidence of self-induced vomiting, bulimia, or compulsive physical activity.
  D. Acts on increased internal emotional awareness and recognition of body sensation of hunger (i.e., talks about being hungry and feeling hunger pangs).
  E. Relates increased sense of effectiveness with less need to control food intake.

◆ VI. See sample **Clinical Pathway 6.1: Eating Disorders**

Mental Health

CLINICAL PATHWAY 6.1: Eating Disorders

Nursing Diagnosis and Categories of Care	Time Dimension	Goals/Actions	Time Dimension	Goals/Actions	Time Dimension	Goals/Actions
Altered nutrition: less than body requirements R/T inadequate intake, self-induced vomiting, laxative use	Ongoing	Gain 3 lb/wk as indicated (or 0.5 lb/day)	Day 2–28	Consume at least 75% of food provided at each meal	Day 15–28	Demonstrate ability to select foods to meet at least 80% of nutritional needs
Risk for fluid volume deficit	Ongoing	Be free of signs/symptoms of dehydration	Day 2–28	Ingest at least 1000 mL fluid/day	Day 22–28	Refrain from self-induced vomiting
		Display balanced I&O	Day 3	Vital signs WNL	Day 28	Be free of signs/ symptoms of malnutrition with all labora-tory results WNL
Referral	Day 1 and prn	Dietitian				
Diagnostic studies	Day 1	Electrolytes, CBC, BUN/creatinine Thyroid function UA ECG as indicated	Day 14	Repeat selected studies		
Additional assessments	Day 1–2	Vital signs/I&O every shift	Day 3–7 q A.M.		Day 8–28	As indicated
	Day 1	Weight	Day 7, 14	7:30 A.M., same clothes		
	Day 1–28	Types and amount of food/fluid in-take Behavior/purging following meals Level of activity				
Medications and Allergies:	Day 1–28	Periactin Antidepressant medications Vitamin supple-ment				
Client education	Day 1 and prn	Orient to unit and schedule Behavior modifica-tion program Minimum weight goal and initial nutritional needs	Day 7–14	Principles of nutri-tion; foods for maintenance of wellness	Day 21–28	Incorporate nutri-tional plan into lifestyle and home setting
Additional nursing actions	Day 1–3	Assist client with formulation of behavioral contract and monitoring of cooperation	Day 7–28	Involve mother/signifi-cant other as appropriate in nutritional coun-seling and plan-ning for future		
	Day 1–7 ▶	Administer tube feeding/blend-erized food as indicated				

(Continued on following page)

Nursing Diagnosis and Categories of Care	Time Dimension	Goals/Actions	Time Dimension	Goals/Actions	Time Dimension	Goals/Actions
Additional nursing actions—cont'd	Day 1–21	Bathroom locked for 1 hr after meals				
	Day 1–28	Provide social setting for meals				
Ineffective denial R/T presence of overwhelming anxiety-producing feelings, learned response pattern, personal/family value system	Ongoing	Participate in behavior modification program and adhere to unit policies	Day 8–28	Attend and contribute to group sessions	Day 18–28	Verbalize acceptance of reality that eating behaviors are maladaptive Demonstrate ability to cope more adaptively
			Day 14	Develop trusting relationship with at least one staff member on each shift		
	Day 2–28	Cooperate with therapy to restore nutritional well-being			Day 28	Identify ways to gain control in life situation Refrain from use of manipulation of others to achieve control Plan in place to meet postdischarge needs
Referrals	Day 5 (or when physical condition stable)	Psychologist Social worker Psychodramatist	Day 8–28	Group psychotherapy daily sessions	Day 25	Community resource contact person(s)
					Day 28	Verbalizes ways to gain control in life situation
◆ Additional assessments	Day 1/ ongoing	Degree and stage of denial Perception of situation	Day 5–7	Readiness to participate in group sessions		
	Day 1–17	Assess ability to trust; use of manipulation to achieve control	Day 7–28	Congruence between verbalizations and behaviors (insight)		
			Day 8–28	Degree/quality of nonmanipulative involvement in group sessions; trusting relationship with at least one staff member per shift		
Client education	Day 1 and prn	Privileges and responsibilities of behavior modification Consequences of behaviors	Day 3/ ongoing	Eating disorder and consequences of eating behavior	Day 21	Role of support groups/community resources

(Continued on following page)

Mental Health

CLINICAL PATHWAY 6.1: Eating Disorders (Continued)

Nursing Diagnosis and Categories of Care	Time Dimension	Goals/Actions	Time Dimension	Goals/Actions	Time Dimension	Goals/Actions
					Day 28	Client and family verbalize intention to attend support group
◆ Additional nursing actions—cont'd	Day 1/ ongoing	Encourage expression of feelings *Avoid* agreeing with inaccurate statements/perceptions Provide positive feedback for desired insight/behaviors Set limits on maladaptive behavior	Day 5–28 Day 8–28	Promote involvement in unit activities Support interactions with family members Encourage interactions in group sessions	Day 21–28	Involve family (as appropriate) in long-range planning for meeting individual needs
Body-image disturbance/chronic low self-esteem R/T perceived loss of control, unmet dependency needs, personal vulnerability, negative evaluation of self	Day 7	Acknowledge that attention will not be given to discussion of body image and food	Day 21	Acknowledge misperception of body image as fat Verbalize positive self-attributes	Day 28	Demonstrate realistic body image and self-awareness Verbalize acceptance of self, including "imperfections" Acknowledge self as sexual assault Not obsessed with food
Referrals	Day 1 (or when physical condition stable)	Therapists: occupational, recreational, music, art	Day 14	Image consultant	Day 28	Therapist to address issues of sexuality after discharge, as indicated
◆ Additional assessments	Day 1–7 Day 3 Day 3–28	Suicidal ideation/behaviors Sexual history, including abuse Perceptions of body image Family patterns of interaction	Day 8 Day 8–28	Individual strengths/weaknesses Congruency of feelings/perceptions with actions		
Client education	Day 1–28 Day 7–28	Responsibility for self in family setting Clarify misconceptions of body image	Day 8–10 Day 8–28	General wellness needs Human behavior and interactions with family/others—transactional analysis (TA)	Day 21–28	Sex education reflecting individual sexuality and needs

(Continued on following page)

Mental Health

Nursing Diagnosis and Categories of Care	Time Dimension	Goals/Actions	Time Dimension	Goals/Actions	Time Dimension	Goals/Actions
Client education—cont'd			Day 14	Personal appearance and grooming		
			Day 14–28	Alternative coping strategies for dealing with feelings		
Additional nursing actions	Day 1	Develop therapeutic relationship	Day 7	Compare actual measurements of client's body with client's perceptions; clarify discrepancies	Day 14–28	Have client keep diary of feelings, especially when thinking of food Role-play new behaviors for dealing with feelings and conflicts
	Day 1–28	Provide positive feedback for participation and independent decision making				
	Day 3–5	Confront sabotage behavior by family members Encourage control in areas other than diet	Day 7–9	Assist with planning to meet individual goals	Day 28	Demonstrates adaptive coping strategies not related to eating and for dealing with feelings
	Day 4–6	Support development of goals and adaptive behaviors not related to eating	Day 8–28	Involve in physical activity/exercise program		

Source: Adapted from Doenges. M: Nursing Care Plans. ed. 4. FA Davis, Philadelphia.

SENSORY-PERCEPTUAL FUNCTIONS

Sensory Disturbance

I. **Types of sensory disturbance:**
   A. *Sensory deprivation*—amount of stimuli *less* than required, such as isolation in bed or room, deafness, victim of stroke.
   B. *Sensory overload*—receives *more* stimuli than can be tolerated, e.g., bright lights, noise, strange machinery, barrage of visitors.
   C. *Sensory deficit*—impairment in functioning of sensory or perceptual processes (e.g., blindness, changes in tactile perceptions).

II. **Assessment**—based on awareness of behavioral changes:
   A. *Sensory deprivation*—boredom, daydreaming, increasing sleep, thought slowness, inactivity, thought disorganization, hallucinations.
   B. *Sensory overload*—same as sensory deprivation, plus restlessness and agitation, confusion.
   C. *Sensory deficit*—may not be able to distinguish sounds, odors, and tastes or differentiate tactile sensations.

III. **Analysis/nursing diagnosis:** problems related to sensory disturbance:
   A. *Altered thought processes.*
   B. *Confusion.*

   C. *Anger, aggression.*
   D. *Body-image disturbance.*
   E. *Sleep pattern disturbance.*

IV. **Nursing care plan/implementation:**
   A. *Management of existing* sensory disturbances in:
      1. *Acute sensory deprivation*
         a. Increase interaction with staff.
         b. Use TV.
         c. Provide touch.
         d. Help clients choose menus that have aromas, varied tastes, temperatures, colors, textures.
         e. Use light cologne or after-shave lotion, bath powder.
      2. *Sensory overload*
         a. Restrict number of visitors and length of stay.
         b. Reduce noise and lights.
         c. Reduce newness by establishing and following routine.
         d. Organize care to provide for extended rest periods with minimal input.
      3. *Sensory deficits*
         a. Report observations about hearing, vision.
         b. May imply need for new glasses, medical diagnosis, or therapy.
   B. *Health teaching: prevention* of sensory disturbance involves *education* of parents during child's growth and development regarding tactile, auditory, and visual stimulation.
      1. Hold, talk, and play with infant when awake.
      2. Provide bright toys with different designs for children to hold.

Mental Health

3. Change environment.
4. Provide music and auditory stimuli.
5. Give foods with variety of textures, tastes, colors.

◆ **V. Evaluation/outcome criteria:**
   A. Client is oriented to time, place, person.
   B. Little or no evidence of mood or sleep disturbance.

Delirium, Dementia, and Amnestic and Other Cognitive Disorders

These disorders include etiology associated with (1) the *aging process* (dementias arising in the senium or presenium, including primary degenerative dementia of the Alzheimer type and multi-infarct dementia), (2) *substance-related disorders* (e.g., alcohol, barbiturates, opioids, cocaine, amphetamines, PCP, hallucinogens, *cannabis,* nicotine, and caffeine), and (3) general medical conditions.

I. Concepts, principles, and subtypes:
   A. Course may be progressive, with steady deterioration.
   B. Alternative pathways and compensatory mechanisms may develop to show a clinical picture of remissions and exacerbations.
   C. *Delirium* is characterized by a *disturbance of consciousness* with reduced ability to focus, sustain, or shift attention; and a *change in cognition* (e.g., memory deficit, disorientation [time and place], language disturbance); or *development of perceptual disturbance* (e.g., illusions, hallucinations) that develop over a *short* time (hours or days) and *fluctuate* during the course of the day. *Etiology:* a direct physiological consequence of a general medical condition, substance intoxication or withdrawal, use of a medication, or toxin exposure. *Diagnostic feature:* cannot repeat sequential string of information (e.g., digit span).
   D. *Dementia* is characterized by persistent *multiple cognitive deficits* (e.g., aphasia, apraxia, agnosia, disturbance in executive functioning) accompanied by memory impairment and mood and sleep disturbances. *Possible etiology:* vascular dementia, HIV infection, head trauma, Parkinson's disease, Pick's disease, Alzheimer's disease, Huntington's disease, substance induced, toxin exposure, medication, infections, nutritional deficiencies (hypoglycemia), endocrine conditions (hypothyroidism) brain tumors, seizure disorders, hepatic and renal failure; cardiopulmonary insufficiencies; fluid and electrolyte imbalances. *Diagnostic features:* cannot learn (register) new information (e.g., a list of words), or retain, recall, or recognize information.
     1. **Alzheimer's disease:** progressive; irreversible loss of cerebral function due to cortical atrophy; exists in 2%–4% of people over age 65 yr; may have a genetic component; may begin at ages 40–65; may lead to death within 2 yr. Average duration from onset of symptoms to death: 8–10 yr.
       a. Progressive decline in intellectual capacity (recent and remote memory, judgment), affect and motor coordination (apraxia); loss of social sense; apathy or restlessness.
       b. *Problems with* speech (aphasia), recognition of familiar objects (agnosia), disorientation to self (even parts of *own* body).
     2. **Pick's disease:** unknown cause; may have genetic component. Onset: middle age; women affected more than men. *Pathology:* atrophy in frontal and temporal lobes of brain. Clinical picture similar to Alzheimer's.
     3. **Creutzfeldt-Jakob disease:** uncommon, extremely rapid neurodegeneration caused by transmissible "slow" virus (prion); genetic component in 5%–15%. Clinical picture: typical dementia, with muscle rigidity, ataxia, involuntary movements. Occurrence: ages 40–60 yr. Death within 1 yr.
   E. *Amnestic disorder* is characterized by *severe* memory impairment *without* other significant impairments of cognitive functioning (i.e., without aphasia, apraxia, or agnosia). *Diagnostic features:* memory impairment is always manifested by impairment in the ability to learn *new* information and sometimes problems remembering previously learned information or past events. May result in *disorientation* to place and time, but *rarely* to self. Appears bewildered or befuddled.
     1. *Etiology:* due to direct physiological effects of a general medical condition (e.g., physical trauma or vitamin deficiency) or due to persisting effects of a substance (e.g., drug of abuse, a medication, or toxin exposure).
     2. Memory disturbance: sufficiently severe to cause marked impairment in social or occupational functioning and represents a significant decline from a previous level of functioning. May require supervised living situation to ensure appropriate feeding and care.
     3. Lacks insight into own memory deficit and may explicitly deny the presence of severe memory impairment despite evidence to the contrary.
     4. Altered personality function: apathy, lack of initiative, emotional blandness, shallow range of expression.

◆ **II. Assessment:**
   A. *Most common areas of difficulty* can be grouped under the mnemonic term *JOCAM: J*—judgment, *O*—orientation, *C*—confabulation, *A*—affect, and *M*—memory.
     1. *Judgment:* impaired, resulting in socially inappropriate behavior (such as hypersexuality toward inappropriate objects) and inability to carry out activities of daily living.
     2. *Orientation:* confused, disoriented; perceptual disturbances (e.g., illusions, misidentification of other persons and objects; misperception to make unfamiliar more familiar; *visual, tactile, and audi-*

tory hallucinations may appear as images and voices or disorganized light and sound patterns). *Paranoid delusions* of persecution.

3. *Confabulation:* common use of this defense mechanism to fill in memory gaps with invented stories.

4. *Affect:* mood changes and unstable emotions; quarrelsome, with outbursts of morbid anger (as in cerebral arteriosclerosis); tearful; withdrawn from social contact; *depression* is a frequent reaction to loss of physical and social function.

5. *Memory:* impaired, especially for names and *recent* events; may compensate by confabulating and by using *circumstantiality and tangential* speaking patterns.

B. *Other areas of difficulty:*

1. *Seizures* (e.g., in Alzheimer's disease and cerebral arteriosclerosis).

2. *Intellectual capacities diminished.*

   a. Difficulty with *abstract* thought.

   b. Compensatory mechanism is to stay with familiar topics; repetition.

   c. Short concentration periods.

3. *Personality changes.*

   a. Loss of ego flexibility; adoption of more rigid attitudes.

   b. *Ritualism* in daily activities.

   c. Hoarding.

   d. Somatic preoccupations (hypochondriases).

   e. *Restlessness,* wandering away.

   f. Impaired impulse control.

   g. *Aphasia* (in severe dementia).

   h. *Apraxia* (inability to carry out motor activities).

C. *Diagnostic tests:*

1. *Neurological* exam: perform maneuvers or answer questions that are aimed at eliciting information about condition of specific parts of brain or peripheral nerves.

   a. Assessment of mental status and alertness.

   b. Muscle strength and reflexes.

   c. Sensory-perception.

   d. Language skills.

   e. Coordination.

2. *Laboratory* tests:

   a. *Blood, urine* to test for: infections, hepatic and renal dysfunction, diabetes, electrolyte imbalances, metabolic/endocrine disorders, nutritional deficiencies, and presence of toxic substances (e.g., drugs).

   b. Electroencephalography (EEG) to check brain's electrical activity.

   c. Computed tomography (CT) scan—image of brain size and shape.

   d. Positron emission tomography (PET)—reveals metabolic activity of brain (important for diagnosis of Alzheimer's).

   e. Magnetic resonance imaging (MRI)—computerized image of soft tissue, with sharply detailed picture of brain tissues.

◆ III. **Analysis/nursing diagnosis:**

A. *Risk for trauma* related to cognitive deficits (inability to recognize/identify danger in the environment; confusion; impaired judgment) and altered motor behavior (restlessness, hyperactivity, muscular incoordination).

B. *Altered thought processes/confusion (altered abstract thinking and altered knowledge processes [agnosia])* related to destruction of cerebral tissue, inability to use information to make judgments and transmit messages, and memory deficits.

C. *Sensory/perceptual alterations:* visual, auditory, kinesthetic, gustatory, tactile, olfactory related to neurological deficit.

D. *Sleep pattern disturbance* resulting in disorientation at night, related to confusion; increased aimless wandering (day/night reversal).

E. *Self-care deficit* (feeding, bathing/hygiene, dressing, toileting) related to physical impairments (poor vision, uncoordination, forgetfulness), disorientation, and confusion.

F. *Altered nutrition, more or less than body requirements,* related to confusion.

G. *Total incontinence* related to sensory/perceptual alterations.

H. *Altered attention and memory* related to progressive neurological losses.

I. *Altered conduct/impulse processes* (irritability and aggressiveness) related to neurological impairment.

J. *Impaired communication* related to poverty of speech and withdrawal behavior, progressive neurological losses, and cerebral impairment.

K. *Caregiver role strain* related to long-term illness and complexity of home care needs.

L. *Relocation stress syndrome* related to separation from support systems, physical deterioration, and changes in daily routine.

◆ IV. **Nursing care plan/implementation** (see also interventions in **III. Confusion/disorientation p. 382**).

A. *Long-term goal:* minimize regression related to memory impairment.

B. *Short-term goal:* provide structure and consistency to increase security.

C. Make *brief, frequent* contacts, because attention span is short.

D. Allow clients *time* to talk and to complete projects.

E. Stimulate *associative* patterns to improve recall (by repeating, summarizing, and focusing).

F. Allow clients to *review* their lives and focus on the past.

G. Use *concrete* questions in interviewing.

H. *Reinforce* reality-oriented comments.

I. Keep environment structured the *same* as much as possible (e.g., same room and placement of furniture); *routine* is important to diminish stress.

J. Recognize the importance of *compensatory* mechanisms (e.g., confabulation) to increase self-esteem; build psychological reserve.

K. Give recognition for each accomplishment.

Mental Health

L. Use *recreational* and physical therapy.

M. *Health teaching:* give *specific* instructions for diet, medication (e.g., tacrine [Cognex], donepezil [Aricept] for improving cognition), and treatment; how to use many sensory approaches to learn new information; how to use existing knowledge, old learning, and habitual approaches to deal with new situations.

◆ V. **Evaluation/outcome criteria:**

A. Symptoms occur *less* frequently and are less severe in areas of: emotional lability and appropriateness; false perceptions; self-care ability; disorientation, memory, and judgment; and decision making.

B. Client is able to preserve optimum level of functioning and independence while allowing basic needs to be met.

C. Stays relatively calm and noncombative when upset or fearful.

D. Accepts own irritability and frustrations as part of illness.

E. Asks for assistance with self-care activities.

F. Knows and adheres to daily routine; knows own nurse, location of room, bathroom, clocks, calendars.

G. Uses supportive community services.

Substance-Related Disorders

I. **Definition:** ingesting in any manner a chemical that has an effect on the body.

◆ II. **General assessment:**

A. *Behavioral* changes exist while under the influence of substance.

B. Engages in regular *use* of substance.

1. *Substance abuse:*

a. Pattern of *pathological* use (i.e., day-long intoxication; inability to stop use, even when contraindicated by serious physical disorder; overpowering need or desire to take the drug despite legal, social, or medical problems); daily need of substance for functioning; repeated medical complications from use.

b. *Interference* with social, occupational functioning.

c. Willingness to obtain substance by any means, including illegal.

d. Pathological use for more than 1 mo.

2. *Substance dependence:*

a. More severe than substance abuse; body *requires* substance to continue functioning.

b. Physiological dependence (i.e., either develops a *tolerance*—must increase dose to obtain desired effect—or has *physical withdrawal symptoms* when substance intake is reduced or stopped).

c. Person feels it is impossible to get along without drug.

C. Effects of substance on *central nervous system (CNS).*

◆ III. **General analysis:** only in recent years has substance abuse been viewed as an illness rather than moral delinquency or criminal behavior. The disorders are very complex and little understood. There are physiological, psychological, and social aspects to their causality, dynamics, symptoms, and treatment, where personality disorder has a major part.

A. *Physiological aspects*—current unproven theories include "allergic" reaction to alcohol, disturbance in metabolism, genetic susceptibility to dependency, and hypofunction of adrenal cortex. There are *organic effects* of chronic excessive use.

B. *Psychological aspects*—disrupted parent-child relationship and family dynamics; deleterious effect on ego function.

C. *Social and cultural aspects*—local customs and attitudes vary about what is excessive.

D. *Maladaptive behavior related to:*

1. Low self-esteem.

2. Anger.

3. Denial.

4. Rationalization.

5. Social isolation.

6. A rigid pattern of coping.

7. Poorly defined philosophy of life, values, mores.

◆ E. *Nursing diagnosis* in **acute phase of abuse, intoxication:**

1. *Risk for ineffective breathing patterns* related to pneumonia caused by aspiration, malnutrition; depressed immune system.

2. *Risk for decreased cardiac output* related to effect of substances on cardiac muscle; electrolyte imbalance.

3. *Risk for injury* related to impaired coordination, disorientation, and altered judgment (worse at night).

4. *Risk for violence:* self-directed or directed at others, related to misinterpretation of stimuli and feelings of suspicion or distrust of others.

5. *Sensory/perceptual alterations:* visual, kinesthetic, tactile, related to intake of mind-altering substances.

6. *Altered nutrition,* less than body requirements.

7. *Altered thought processes* (delusions, incoherence) related to misinterpretation of stimuli due to severe panic and fear.

8. *Sleep pattern disturbance* related to mind-altering substance.

9. *Ineffective individual coping* related to inability to tolerate frustration and to meet basic needs or role expectations, resulting in unpredictable behaviors.

10. *Noncompliance* with abstinence and supportive therapy, related to inability to stop using substance because of dependence and refusal to alter lifestyle.

11. *Impaired communication* related to mental confusion or CNS depression due to substance use.

12. *Impaired health maintenance management* related to failure to recognize that a problem exists and inability to take responsibility for health needs.

Alcohol Use Disorders: Alcohol Abuse and Dependence

I. Definitions:

A. *Alcohol dependence* is a primary and chronic disorder that is progressive and often fatal, in which the individual is unable, for physical or psychological reasons or both, to refrain from frequent consumption of alcohol in quantities that produce intoxication and disrupt health and ability to perform daily functions.

B. *Alcohol abuse* is a separate diagnosis, and is defined as a maladaptive pattern of use with one or more of the following over a one-year period:

1. Repeated alcohol consumption that results in an inability to fulfill obligations at home, school, or work.
2. Repeated alcohol consumption when it could be physically dangerous (e.g., driving a car).
3. Repeated alcohol-related legal problems (e.g., arrests).
4. Continued drinking despite interpersonal or social problems caused or made worse by drinking.

II. Concepts and principles related to alcohol abuse and dependence:

A. Alcohol affects cerebral cortical functions:
1. Memory.
2. Judgment.
3. Reasoning.

B. Alcohol is a *depressant:*
1. Relaxes the individual.
2. Lessens use of repression of unconscious conflict.
3. Releases inhibitions, hostility, and primitive drives.

C. Drinking represents a tension-reducing device and a relief from feelings of insecurity. Strength of drinking habit equals degree of anxiety and frustration intolerance.

D. Alcohol dependence is not a *symptom* but rather a disease in itself.

E. Underlying fear and anxiety, associated with inner conflict, motivate the person who is alcoholic to drink.

F. People with alcohol use disorder can *never* be cured to drink normally; cure is to be a "sober alcoholic," with total abstinence.

G. The spouse of the person with alcohol use disorder often unconsciously contributes to the drinking behavior because of own emotional needs (*co-alcoholic* or *co-dependent*).

H. Intoxication occurs with a blood-alcohol level of 0.08% or above. *Signs of intoxication* are:

1. Incoordination.
2. Slurred speech.
3. Dulled perception.

I. Tolerance occurs with alcohol dependence. Increasing amounts of alcohol must be consumed to obtain the desired effect.

◆ III. Assessment:

A. *Vicious cycle*—(a) low tolerance for coping with frustration; tension, *guilt* and shame, resentment; (b) uses alcohol for relief; (c) new problems created by drinking; (d) new anxieties; and (e) more drinking.

B. Coping mechanisms used: *denial, rationalization, projection.*

C. *Complications of abuse and dependence.*

1. ***Alcohol withdrawal delirium (delirium tremens [DTs])* (Figure 6.5)**—result of nutritional deficiencies and toxins; requires sedation and constant watchfulness against unintentional suicide and convulsions.

   a. *Impending* signs relate to *CNS*—marked nervousness and restlessness, increased irritability; gross tremors of hands, face, lips; weakness; also *cardiovascular*—increased blood pressure, tachycardia, diaphoresis, dysrhythmias; *depression; gastrointestinal*—nausea, vomiting, anorexia.

   b. *Actual*—*serious* symptoms of mental confusion, convulsions, hallucinations (visual, olfactory, auditory, tactile). Without treatment, *15%–25%* may die due to cardiac dysrhythmias, respiratory arrest, severe dehydration, massive infection.

2. ***Wernicke's syndrome***—a neurological disturbance manifested by confusion, ataxia, eye movement abnormalities, and memory impairment. Other problems include:

   a. Disturbed vision (diplopia).
   b. Wandering mind.
   c. Stupor and coma.

3. ***Alcohol amnestic syndrome (Korsakoff's syndrome)***—degenerative neuritis due to *thiamine* deficiency.

   a. Impaired thoughts.
   b. Confusion, loss of sense of time and place.
   c. Use of confabulation to fill in severe recent memory loss.
   d. Follows episode of *Wernicke's encephalopathy.*

4. *Polyneuropathy*—weak, irregular, rapid peripheral pulses; sensory and motor nerve endings are involved, causing pain, itching, and loss of limb control.

5. Related concerns—chronic heart failure (generalized tissue edema), *gastritis, esophageal varices, cirrhosis, pancreatitis, diabetes,* pneumonia, REM sleep deprivation, *malnutrition,* cancer of mouth, pharynx, and larynx.

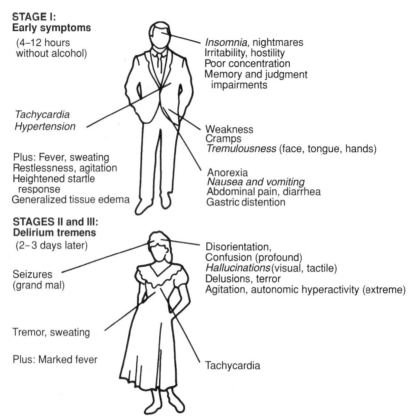

STAGE I:
Early symptoms

(4–12 hours
without alcohol)

Insomnia, nightmares
Irritability, hostility
Poor concentration
Memory and judgment
  impairments

Tachycardia
Hypertension

Weakness
Cramps
Tremulousness (face, tongue, hands)

Plus: Fever, sweating
Restlessness, agitation
Heightened startle
  response
Generalized tissue edema

Anorexia
Nausea and vomiting
Abdominal pain, diarrhea
Gastric distention

STAGES II and III:
Delirium tremens

(2–3 days later)

Disorientation,
Confusion (profound)
Hallucinations (visual, tactile)
Delusions, terror
Agitation, autonomic hyperactivity (extreme)

Seizures
(grand mal)

Tremor, sweating

Plus: Marked fever

Tachycardia

FIGURE 6.5 **Symptoms associated with alcohol withdrawal.** (Adapted from Wilson, HS, and Kneisl, CR: Psychiatric Nursing, ed. 2. Addison-Wesley, Menlo Park, Calif., out of print.)

D. Diagnostic tests
  1. *Blood tests:*
     a. *CBC: decreased* Hgb/Hct to detect iron-deficiency anemia or acute/chronic GI bleeding; *increased* WBC (infection); *decreased* WBC (if immunosuppressed).
     b. *Glucose:* hyperglycemia/hypoglycemia may be present (pancreatitis, malnutrition, or depletion of liver glycogen stores).
     c. *Electrolytes: decreased* potassium and magnesium.
     d. *Liver function tests* are classic toxic markers that alcohol use leaves on body: *increased* CPK, LDH, AST, ALT, and amylase (liver or pancreatic problem).
     e. *Nutritional tests: decreased* albumin and total protein; *decreased* vitamins A, C, D, E, K, and B (malnutrition/malabsorption).
  2. *Urinalysis:* infection; ketones due to breakdown of fatty acids in malnutrition (pseudodiabetic condition).
  3. *Chest x-ray:* rule out right lower lobe pneumonia (related to malnutrition, depressed immune system, aspiration).
  4. *EKG:* dysrhythmias, cardiomyopathies, or ischemia due to direct effect of alcohol on the cardiac muscle or conduction system, as well as effects of electrolyte imbalance.
  5. *Other screening studies* (e.g., hepatitis, HIV, TB): dependent on general condition, individual risk factors, and care setting.

◆ IV. **Analysis/nursing diagnosis:**
  A. *Risk for injury (self-directed violence):* tendency for *self-destructive* acts related to intake of mind-altering substances and chronic low self-esteem.
  B. *Altered nutrition, less than body requirements,* related to a lack of interest in food, interference with absorption/metabolism of nutrients and amino acids.
  C. *Ineffective individual coping: denial/defensive coping* related to tendency to be domineering and critical, with difficulties in *interpersonal* relationships.
  D. *Conflict with social order* related to extreme dependence coupled with resentment of *authority.*
  E. *Spiritual distress* or general dissatisfaction with life related to feelings of powerlessness, *low frustration* tolerance, and demand for immediate need satisfaction.

F. *Dysfunctional behaviors/sexual dysfunction* related to tendency for *excess* in work, sex, recreation, marked *narcissistic* behavior.

G. *Social isolation* related to use of coping mechanisms that are primarily *escapist.*

H. *Knowledge deficit* (learning need) regarding condition, prognosis, treatment, self-care, discharge needs.

◆ **V. Nursing care plan/implementation:**

A. *Detoxification phase*—maintain physiological stability.

1. *Administer adequate sedation* to control anxiety, insomnia, agitation, tremors.

2. *Administer anticonvulsants* to prevent *withdrawal seizures* (Valium, Librium, phenobarbital, magnesium sulfate).

3. *Control nausea and vomiting* to avoid massive GI bleeding or rupture of esophageal varices (antiemetics, antacids).

4. *Assess for* hypertension, tachycardia, increased temperature, Kussmaul's respirations.

5. *Assess fluid and electrolyte balance* for dehydration (may need IV fluids) or overhydration (may need a diuretic).

6. *Reestablish proper nutrition: high protein* (as long as no severe liver damage), carbohydrate, *thiamine, vitamins B complex and C.*

7. *Promote client safety—provide quiet, calm, safe environment:* bedrest *with rails,* and head of bed *elevated;* well-lit room to reduce illusions; constant supervision and reassurance about fears and hallucinations; assess depression for suicide potential.

B. *Recovery-rehabilitation phase:* encourage participation in *group* activities; *avoid sympathy* when client tends to rationalize behavior and seeks special privileges—use acceptance and a *nonjudgmental,* consistent, firm, but kind approach; *avoid:* scorn, contempt, and moralizing or punitive and rejecting behaviors; do *not* reinforce feelings of worthlessness, self-contempt, hopelessness, or low self-esteem.

C. *Problem behaviors:*

1. *Manipulative*—be firm and consistent; *avoid* "bid for sympathy."

2. *Demanding*—set limits.

3. *Acting out*—set limits, enforce rules and regulations, strengthen impulse control and ability to delay gratification.

4. *Dependency*—place responsibility on client; *avoid* giving advice.

5. *Superficiality*—help client make realistic self-appraisals and expectations in lieu of grandiose promises and trite verbalizations; encourage formation of lasting interpersonal relationships.

D. *Common reactions among staff:*

1. *Disappointment*—instead, set realistic goals, take one step at a time.

2. Moral judgment—instead, support each other.

3. Hostility—instead, offer support to each other when feeling frustrated from lack of results.

E. Refer client from hospital to *community resources* for follow-up treatment with social, economic, and psychological problems, as well as to self-help groups, to reduce "revolving door" situation in which client comes in, is treated, goes out, and comes in again the next night.

1. *Alcoholics Anonymous (AA)*—a self-help group of addicted drinkers who confront, instruct, and support fellow drinkers in their efforts to stay sober 1 day at a time through fellowship and acceptance.

2. *Alanon*—support group for *families* of clients with alcoholic use disorder. *Alateen*—support group for *teenagers* when parent is alcoholic.

3. *Aversion therapy*—client is subjected to revulsion-producing or pain-inducing stimuli at the same time he or she takes a drink, to establish alcohol rejection behavior. Most common is disulfiram *(Antabuse),* a drug that works by blocking an enzyme that helps metabolize alcohol. It produces: intense headache, severe flushing, extreme nausea, vomiting, palpitations, hypotension, dyspnea, and blurred vision when alcohol is consumed while person is taking this drug.

4. *Other drug therapy*—naltrexone (ReVia) is a drug that works by blocking endorphin receptors and interfering in alcohol-induced brain reward circuitry that is involved in good feelings people get from drinking.

a. *Benefit:* reduces alcohol relapse and decreases total amount of drinking per day.

b. Dose: 50 mg PO/day.

c. Common side effects: transitory dizziness, diarrhea, nausea. Does not have extreme side effects of Antabuse.

5. *Group psychotherapy*—the goals of group psychotherapy are for the client to give up alcohol as a tension reliever, identify cause of stress, build different means for coping with stress, and accept drinking as a serious symptom.

F. *Health teaching:* teach improved coping patterns to tolerate increased stress; teach substitute tension-reducing strategies; prepare in advance for difficult, painful events; teach how to reduce irritating or frustrating environmental stress.

◆ **VI. Evaluation/outcome criteria:** complications prevented, resolved; everyday living patterns are restructured for a satisfactory life without alcohol; demonstrates feelings of increased self-worth, confidence, and reliance.

VII. See sample **Clinical Pathway 6.2: Alcohol Withdrawal Program**

CLINICAL PATHWAY 6.2:   Alcohol Withdrawal Program

Nursing Diagnosis and Categories of Care	Time Dimension	Goals/Actions	Time Dimension	Goals/Actions	Time Dimension	Goals/Actions
Risk for injury (varied autonomic and sensory responses)	Day 1	Verbalize understanding of unit policies, procedures, and safety concerns relative to individual needs Cooperate with therapeutic regimen	Day 3 Day 4	Vital signs stable I&O balanced Display marked decrease in objective symptoms	Day 7	Discharge: Be free of injury resulting from alcohol withdrawal Display no objective symptoms of withdrawal

Referrals	Day 1	RN-NP or MD
		If indicated:
		  Internist
		  Cardiologist
		  Neurologist				

Diagnostic studies	Day 1	Blood alcohol level
		Drug screen (urine and blood)
		If indicated:
		  Chest x-ray
		  Pulse oximetry
		  ECG
			Day 2	SMA 20: serum Mg, amylase
				Urinalysis
					Day 4	Repeat of selected studies as indicated

Additional assessments	Day 1	VS, temperature, respiratory status/breath sounds q4h	Day 2–3	VS q8h if stable	Day 4–7	VS qd
	Day 1–4	I&O q8h Motor activity, body language, verbalizations, need for/type of restraint			Day 6	Discontinue I&O
	Ongoing	**Withdrawal symptoms:**		Marked decrease in objective symptoms		
	Stage I	Tremors, N/V, hypertension, tachycardia, diaphoresis, sleeplessness				
	Stage II	Increased hyperactivity, hallucinations, seizure activity				
	Stage III	Extreme autonomic hyperactivity, profound confusion, anxiety, fever				

(Continued on following page)

Mental Health

Nursing Diagnosis and Categories of Care	Time Dimension	Goals/Actions	Time Dimension	Goals/Actions	Time Dimension	Goals/Actions
Medications, Allergies:	Day 1	Librium 200 mg PO	Day 3	Librium 120 mg PO	Day 5	Librium 40 mg PO
	Day 1–4	Thiamine 100 mg IM	Day 4	Librium 80 mg PO		
	Day 2	Librium 160 mg PO				
Client education	Day 1	Orient to room/unit, schedule, procedures	Day 5	Need for ongoing therapy Goals/availability of AA program	Day 7	Schedule of follow-up visits if indicated
Additional nursing actions	Day 1	Bedrest 12 hr if in withdrawal *Position* change, HOB elevated Cough, deep breathe Exercise if on bedrest	Day 3–7	Activity as tolerated		
	Day 1–2	Assist with ambulation, self-care as needed Encourage fluids if free of N/V				
	Ongoing	Provide environmental safety measures Seizure precautions as indicated Reorient as needed				
Ineffective individual coping R/T personal vulnerability, situational crisis, inadequate coping methods	Day 1–7	Participate in development/ evaluation of treatment plan	Day 3	Verbalize understanding of relationship of alcohol abuse to current situation	Day 7	Plan in place to meet postdischarge needs
	Day 2–7	Interact in group sessions	Day 6	Identify/make contact with potential resources, support groups		
Referrals	Day 1	Psychiatrist	Day 5	Community classes: assertiveness training Stress management		
	Day 2–7	Group sessions				
Additional assessments	Day 1	Understanding of current situation Drinking pattern, previous withdrawal, other drug use, attitudes toward substance use	Day 2–3	Previous coping strategies/ consequences Perception of drug use on life, employment, legal issues		

Mental Health

(Continued on following page)

CLINICAL PATHWAY 6.2: Alcohol Withdrawal Program *(Continued)*

Nursing Diagnosis and Categories of Care	Time Dimension	Goals/Actions	Time Dimension	Goals/Actions	Time Dimension	Goals/Actions
	Day 1–2	History of violence Relationships with others: personal, work/school Readiness for group activities	Day 3–7	Congruency of actions based on insight		
Medications			Day 5–7	Naltrexone 50 mg/day if indicated		
Client education	Day 1	Physical effects of alcohol abuse	Day 3–7	Human behavior and interactions with others/ transactional analysis (TA)	Day 7	Medication dose, frequency, side effects Written instructions for therapeutic program
	Day 1–2	Types/use of relaxation techniques				
	Day 2	Consequences of alcohol abuse	Day 5–6	Community resources for self/family		
Additional nursing actions	Day 1–7	Support client's taking responsibility for own recovery Provide consistent approach/expectations for behavior Set limits/confront inappropriate behaviors	Day 2–5	Identify goals for change Discuss alternative solutions Provide positive feedback for efforts		
			Day 2–7	Support during confrontation by peer group Encourage verbalization of feelings, personal reflection		
Altered nutrition: less than body requirements R/T poor intake, effects of alcohol on digestive system, and hypermetabolic response to withdrawal	Day 2–7	Select foods appropriately to meet individual dietary needs	Day 4	Verbalize understandings of effects of alcohol abuse and reduced dietary intake on nutritional status	Day 7	Display stable weight or initial weight gain as appropriate, and laboratory results WNL
Referrals	Day 1 and prn	Dietitian				
Diagnostic studies	Day 1	CBC, liver function studies Serum albumin, transferrin	Day 2–7	Fingerstick glucose prn		

(Continued on following page)

Mental Health

◆ Nursing Diagnosis and Categories of Care	Time Dimension	Goals/Actions	Time Dimension	Goals/Actions	Time Dimension	Goals/Actions
◆ Additional assessments	Day 1	Weight, skin turgor, condition of mucous membranes, muscle tone			Day 7	Weight
	Day 1–2	Bowel sounds, characteristics of stools				
	Day 1–7	Appetite, dietary intake				
Medications	Day 1–7	Antacid ac and hs (e.g., Maalox) Imodium 2 mg prn	Day 2–7	Multivitamin tablet qd		
Client education	Day 1–2	Individual nutritional needs	Day 4	Principles of nutrition, foods for maintenance of wellness		
Additional nursing actions	Day 1	Liquid/bland diet as tolerated	Day 2–7	Advance diet as tolerated		
	Day 1–7	Encourage small, frequent, nutritious meals/snacks Encourage good oral hygiene pc and hs				

Source: Adapted from Doenges, M: Nursing Care Plans, ed. 4. FA Davis, Philadelphia.

Other Substance-Related Disorders

I. Concepts and principles:

A. *Three* interacting key factors give rise to dependence—*psychopathology* of the individual; frustrating *environment*; and *availability* of powerful, addicting, and temporarily satisfying drug.

B. According to conditioning principles, substance abuse and dependence proceed in *several phases:*

1. *Use* of sedatives-hypnotics, CNS stimulants, hallucinogens and narcotics, for relief from daily tensions and discomforts or anticipated withdrawal symptoms.
2. Habit is *reinforced* with each relief by drug use.
3. Development of *dependency*—drug has less and less efficiency in reducing tensions.
4. Dependency is further reinforced as addict *fails* to maintain adequate drug intake—increase in frequency and duration of periods of tension and discomfort.

◆ II. Assessment:

A. Abuse

1. *Hallucinogens* (LSD, marijuana, ecstasy, STP, PCP, peyote): euphoria and rapid mood swings, flight of ideas; perceptual impairment, feelings of omnipotence, "bad trip" (panic, loss of control, paranoia), flashbacks, suicide.

2. *CNS stimulants* (*amphetamines* and *cocaine* abuse): euphoria, hyperactivity, hyperalertness, irritability, persecutory delusions; insomnia, anorexia → weight loss; tachycardia; tremulousness; hypertension; hyperthermia → convulsions.

3. *Narcotics* (*opium* and its derivatives [morphine, heroin, codeine, meperidine HCl [Demerol]): used by "snorting," "skin popping," and "mainlining." May lead to abscesses and hepatitis. Decreased pain response, respiratory depression; apathy, detachment from reality; impaired judgment; loss of sexual activity; pinpoint pupils.

4. *Sedatives-hypnotics (barbiturate abuse):* similar to alcohol-induced behavior (e.g., euphoria) followed by depression, hostility; decreased inhibitions; impaired judgment; staggering gait; slurred speech; drowsiness; poor concentration; progressive respiratory depression.

B. *Withdrawal symptoms*

1. *Narcotics* (e.g., heroin): begins within 12 hr of last dose, peaks in 24–36 hr, subsides in 72 hr, and disappears in 5–6 days.
   a. Pupil *dilation.*
   b. Muscle: twitches, tremors, aches, pains.
   c. Goose flesh (piloerection).
   d. *Lacrimation, rhinorrhea, sneezing, yawning.*
   e. *Diaphoresis*, chills.
   f. Potential for fever.

Mental Health

g. Vomiting, abdominal distress.
h. Dehydration.
i. Rapid weight loss.
j. Sleep disturbance.
2. *Barbiturates:* may be gradual or abrupt ("cold turkey"); latter is dangerous or *life-threatening;* should be hospitalized.
   a. *Gradual* withdrawal reaction from barbiturates:
      (1) Postural hypotension.
      (2) Tachycardia.
      (3) Elevated temperature.
      (4) Insomnia.
      (5) Tremors.
      (6) Agitation, restlessness.
   b. *Abrupt* withdrawal from barbiturates:
      (1) Apprehension.
      (2) Muscular weakness.
      (3) Tremors.
      (4) Postural hypotension.
      (5) Twitching.
      (6) Anorexia.
      (7) *Grand mal seizures.*
      (8) *Psychosis-delirium.*
3. *Amphetamines:* depression, lack of energy, somnolence.
4. *Marijuana:* psychological dependency includes craving the "high," and irritability without the drug. Physical withdrawal occurs with heavy daily use; symptoms include: insomnia, anxiety, and loss of appetite.

C. *Difference* between alcohol and other abused substances (e.g., opioid).
1. Other abused substances may need to be obtained by illegal means, making it a legal and criminal problem as well as a medical and social problem; *not* so with alcohol abuse and dependency.
2. Opium and its derivatives *inhibit* aggression; whereas alcohol *releases* aggression.
3. As long as she or he is on large enough doses to avoid withdrawal symptoms, abuser of narcotics, sedatives, or hypnotics is comfortable and functions well; whereas chronically intoxicated abuser of alcohol *cannot* function normally.
4. Direct physiological effects of long-term opioid abuse and dependence on other abused substances are much *less critical* than those with chronic alcohol dependence.

◆ III. **Analysis/nursing diagnosis:**
A. *Risk for altered physical regulation processes* (cardiac, circulatory, gastrointestinal, sleep pattern disturbance) related to use of mind-altering drugs.
B. *Risk for injury* due to *altered judgment* related to misinterpretation of sensory stimuli and low frustration tolerance.
C. *Altered conduct/impulse processes* related to rebellious attitudes toward authority.
D. *Altered social interaction* (manipulation, dependency) related to hostility and personal insecurity.

E. *Altered feeling states* (denial) related to underlying self-doubt and personal insecurity.

◆ IV. **Nursing care plan/implementation:** generally the same as in treating antisocial personality and alcohol abuse and dependence.
A. Maintain *safety* and optimum level of *physical* comfort. Supportive physical care: vital signs, nutrition, hydration, seizure precautions.
B. *Assist with medical treatment* and offer support and *reality orientation* to reduce feelings of panic.
1. *Detoxification (or dechemicalization)*—give medications according to detoxification schedule.
2. *Withdrawal*—may be gradual (barbiturates, hypnotics, tranquilizers) or abrupt ("cold turkey" for heroin). Observe for symptoms and report immediately.
3. *Methadone (Dolophine)*—person must have been dependent on narcotics at least 2 yr and have failed at other methods of withdrawal before admission to program of readdiction by methadone.
   a. *Characteristics:*
      (1) Synthetic.
      (2) Appeases desire for narcotics without producing euphoria of narcotics.
      (3) Given by mouth.
      (4) Distributed under federal control (**N**arcotic **A**ddict **R**ehabilitation **A**ct).
      (5) Given with urinary surveillance.
   b. *Advantages:*
      (1) Prevents narcotic withdrawal reaction.
      (2) Tolerance not built up.
      (3) Person remains out of prison.
      (4) Lessens perceived need for heroin or morphine.
C. *Participation in group therapy—goals:* peer pressure, support, and identification.
D. *Rehabilitation phase:*
1. Refer to halfway house and group living.
2. Support *employment* as therapy (work training).
3. Expand client's *range of interests* to relieve characteristic boredom and stimulus hunger.
   a. Provide *structured* environment and planned routine.
   b. Provide educational therapy (academic and vocational).
   c. Arrange activities to include current events discussion groups, lectures, drama, music, and art appreciation.
E. Achieve role of *stabilizer and supportive* authoritative figure; this can be achieved through frequent, regular contacts with the same client.
F. *Health teaching:* how to cope with pain, fatigue, and anxiety without drugs.

◆ V. **Evaluation/outcome criteria:** replaces addictive lifestyle with self-reliant behavior and a plan formulated to maintain a substance-free life.

Mental Health

PSYCHOSOCIAL-CULTURAL FUNCTIONS

Mental Status Assessment

I. Components of mental status exam
A. *Appearance*—appropriate dress, grooming, facial expression, stereotyped movements, tremors, tics, gestures, gait, mannerisms, rigidity.
B. *Behavior*—anxiety level, congruence with situation, impulse control (aggression, sexual), co-operativeness, openness, hostility, reaction to interview (guarded, defensive, apathetic), consistency.
C. *Speech characteristics*—relevance, coherence, meaning, repetitiveness, qualitative (*what* is said), quantitative (*how much* is said), abnormalities, inflections, affectations, congruence with level of education, impediments (e.g., stutter), tone quality.
D. *Mood*—appropriateness, intensity, hostility turned inwards or toward others, swings, guilty, despairing, irritable, sad, depressed, anxious, fearful.
E. *Thought content*—delusions, hallucinations, obsessive ideas, suicidal, homicidal, paranoid, religiosity, magical, phobic ideas, themes, areas of concern, self-concept.
F. *Thought processes*—organization and association of ideas, coherence, ability to abstract and understand symbols.
G. *Sensorium:*
1. *Orientation* to person, time and place, situation.
2. *Memory*—immediate, rote, remote, and recent.
3. *Attention and concentration*—susceptibility to distraction.
4. *Information and intelligence*—account of general knowledge, history, and reasoning powers.
5. *Comprehension*—concrete and *abstract*.
6. *Stage of consciousness*—alert/awake, somnolent, lethargic, delirious, stuporous, comatose.
H. *Insight and judgment*
1. Extent to which client sees self as having problems, needing treatment.
2. Client awareness of intrapsychic nature of own difficulties.
3. Soundness of judgment, problem solving, decision making.

◆ **II. Individual assessment—consider the following (Table 6.12):**
A. Physical and intellectual factors.
B. Socioeconomic factors.
C. Personal values and goals.
D. Adaptive functioning and response to present involvement.
E. Developmental factors.

◆ **III. Cultural assessment (see Unit 3):**
A. Knowledge of ethnic beliefs and cultural practices can assist the nurse in the planning and implementation of holistic care.

B. Consider the following:
1. *Demographic data:* is this an "ethnic neighborhood"?
2. *Socioeconomic status:* occupation, education (formal and informal), income level; who is employed?
3. *Ethnic/racial orientation:* ethnic identity, value orientation.

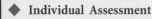

TABLE 6.12	◆ Individual Assessment

Physical and Intellectual
1. Presence of physical illness or disability.
2. Appearance and energy level.
3. Current and potential levels of intellectual functioning.
4. How client sees personal world, translates events around self; client's perceptual abilities.
5. Cause-and-effect reasoning, ability to focus.

Socioeconomic Factors
1. Economic factors—level of income, adequacy of subsistence; how this affects lifestyle, sense of adequacy, self-worth.
2. Employment and attitudes about it.
3. Racial, cultural, and ethnic identification; sense of identity and belonging.
4. Religious identification and link to significant value systems, norms, and practices.

Personal Values and Goals
1. Presence or absence of congruence between values and their expression in action; meaning of values to individual.
2. Congruence between individual's values and goals and the immediate systems with which client interacts.
3. Congruence between individual's values and assessor's values; meaning of this for intervention process.

Adaptive Functioning and Response to Present Involvement
1. Manner in which individual presents self to others—grooming, appearance, posture.
2. Emotional tone and change or constancy of levels.
3. Style of communication—verbal and nonverbal; ability to express appropriate emotion, follow train of thought; factors of dissonance, confusion, uncertainty.
4. Symptoms or symptomatic behavior.
5. Quality of relationship individual seeks to establish—direction, purposes, and uses of such relationships for individual.
6. Perception of self.
7. Social roles that are assumed or ascribed; competence in fulfilling these roles.
8. Relational behavior:
   a. Capacity for intimacy.
   b. Dependence-independence balance.
   c. Power and control conflicts.
   d. Exploitiveness.
   e. Openness.

Developmental Factors
1. Role performance equated with life stage.
2. How developmental experiences have been interpreted and used.
3. How individual has dealt with past conflicts, tasks, and problems.
4. Uniqueness of present problem in life experience.

Adapted from Wilson, HS, and Kneisl, CR: Psychiatric Nursing, ed. 2. Addison-Wesley, Menlo Park, Calif. (out of print).

Mental Health

4. *Country of immigration:* date of immigration; where were the family members born? Where has the family lived?
5. *Languages spoken:* does family speak English? Language and dialect preferences.
6. *Family relationships:* what are the formal roles? Who makes the decisions within the family? What is the family lifestyle and living arrangements?
7. *Degree of acculturation* of family members: how are the family customs and beliefs similar to or different from the dominant culture?
8. *Communication patterns:* social customs, nonverbal behaviors.
9. *Religious preferences:* what role do beliefs, rituals, and taboos play in health and illness? Is there a significant religious person? Are there any dietary symbolisms or preferences or restrictions due to religious beliefs?
10. *Cultural practices related to health and illness:* does the family use folk medicine practices or a folk healer? Are there specific dietary practices related to health and illness?
11. *Support systems:* do extended family members provide support?
12. *Health beliefs:* response to pain and hospitalization; disease predisposition and resistance.
13. Other significant factors related to ethnic identity: what health-care facilities does the family use?
14. Communication barriers:
    a. Differences in language.
    b. Technical languages.
    c. Inappropriate place for discussion.
    d. Personality or gender of the nurse.
    e. Distrust of the nurse.
    f. Time-orientation differences.
    g. Differences in pain perception and expression.
    h. Variable attitudes toward death and dying.

Interviewing

I. **Definition:** a goal-directed method of communicating facts, feelings, and meanings. For interviewing to be successful, interaction between two persons involved must be effective.

II. **Nine principles of verbal interaction**
   A. *Client's initiative* begins the discussion.
   B. *Indirect approach,* moving from the periphery to the core.
   C. *Open-ended* statements, using incomplete forms of statements such as "You were saying ..." to prompt rather than close off an exchange.
   D. *Minimal verbal activity* in order not to obstruct thought process and client's responses.
   E. *Spontaneity,* rather than fixed interview topics, may bring out much more relevant data.
   F. *Facilitate expression of feelings* to help assess events and reactions by asking, for example, "What was that like for you?"

G. *Focus on emotional areas* about which client may be in conflict, as noted by repetitive themes.
H. *Pick up cues, clues, and signals from client,* such as facial expressions and gestures, behavior, emphatic tones, and flushed face.
I. *Introduce material related to content* already brought up by client; do *not* bring in a tangential focus from "left field."

III. **Purpose and goals of interviewing**
   A. *Initiate and maintain a positive nurse-client relationship,* which can decrease symptoms, lessen demands, and move client toward optimum health when nurse demonstrates understanding and sharing of client's concerns.
   B. *Determine client's view of nurse's role* in order to utilize it or change it.
   C. *Collect information on emotional crisis* to plan goals and approaches in order to increase effectiveness of nursing interventions.
   D. *Identify and resolve crisis;* the act of eliciting cause or antecedent event may in itself be therapeutic.
   E. *Channel feelings directly* by exploring interrelated events, feelings, and behaviors in order to discourage displacement of feelings onto somatic and behavioral symptoms.
   F. *Channel communication* and transfer significant information to the physician and other team members.
   G. *Prepare for health teaching* in order to help the client function as effectively as possible.

General Principles of Health Teaching

One key nursing function is to promote and restore health. This involves teaching clients new psychomotor skills, general knowledge, coping attitudes, and social skills related to health and illness (e.g., proper diet, exercises, colostomy care, wound care, insulin injections, urine testing). The teaching function of the nurse is vital in assisting normal development and helping clients meet health-related needs.

I. **Purpose of health teaching**
   A. *General goal:* motivate health-oriented behavior.
   B. *Nursing interventions*
      1. Fill in *gaps* in information.
      2. *Clarify* misinformation.
      3. Teach necessary *skills.*
      4. *Modify* attitudes.

II. **Educational theories** on which effective health teaching is based:
   A. *Motivation theory*
      1. Health-oriented behavior is determined by the degree to which person sees health problem as *threatening,* with *serious consequences, high probability of occurrence,* and *belief in availability of effective course of action.*
      2. Nonhealth-related motives may *supersede* health-related motives.
      3. Health-related motives may not always give rise to health-related behavior, and vice versa.

4. Motivation may be influenced by:
   a. *Phases of adaptation* to crisis (poor motivation in early phase).
   b. *Anxiety and awareness of need* to learn. (Mild anxiety is highly motivating.)
   c. *Mutual* versus externally imposed goal setting.
   d. Perceived *meaningfulness* of information and material. (If within client's frame of reference, both meaningfulness and motivation increase.)
B. *Theory of planned change*
   1. *Unfreeze* present level of behavior—develop awareness of problem.
   2. Establish *need* for change and relationship of trust and respect.
   3. *Move* toward change—examine alternatives, develop intentions into real efforts.
   4. *Freeze* on a new level—generalize behavior, stabilize change.
C. Elements of *learning theory*
   1. *Drive* must be present based on experiencing uncertainty, frustration, concern, or curiosity; hierarchy of needs exists.
   2. *Response* is a learned behavior that is elicited when associated stimulus is present.
   3. *Reward and reinforcement* are necessary for response (behavior) to occur and remain.
   4. *Extinction of response,* that is, elimination of undesirable behavior, can be attained through conditioning.
   5. Memorization is the easiest level of learning, but least effective in changing behavior.
   6. Understanding involves the incorporation of generalizations and specific facts.
   7. After introduction of new material, there is a period of floundering when assimilation and insight occur.
   8. Learning is a two-way process between learner and teacher; defensive behavior in either makes both activities difficult, if not impossible.
   9. Learning flourishes when client feels respected, accepted by nurse who is enthusiastic; learning occurs best when differing value systems are accepted.
   10. Feedback increases learning.
   11. Successful learning leads to more successes in learning.
   12. Teaching and learning should take place in the area where *targeted activity* normally occurs.
   13. Priorities for learning are dependent on client's *physical and psychological status.*
   14. Decreased visual and auditory perception leads to decreased readiness to learn.
   15. Content, terminology, pacing, and spacing of learning must correspond to client's *capabilities, maturity level, feelings, attitudes, and experiences.*

◆ III. **Assessment of the client-learner:**
   A. *Characteristics:* age, sex, race, medical diagnosis, prognosis.

B. *Sociocultural-economic:* ethnic, religious group beliefs and practices; family situation (roles, support); job (type, history, options, stress); financial situation, living situation (facilities).
C. *Psychological:* own and family's response to illness; premorbid personality; current self-image.
D. *Educational:*
   1. Client's *perception* of current situation: what is wrong? Cause? How will lifestyle be affected?
   2. *Past experience:* previous hospitalization and treatment; past compliance.
   3. *Level of knowledge:* what has client been told? From what source? How accurate? Known others with the same illness?
   4. *Goals:* what client *wants* to know.
   5. *Needs:* what nurse thinks client *should* know for self-care.
   6. Readiness for learning.
   7. *Educational* background; ability to read and learn.

◆ IV. **Analysis of factors influencing learning:**
   A. *Internal*
      1. Physical condition.
      2. Senses (sight, hearing, touch).
      3. Age.
      4. Anxiety.
      5. Motivation.
      6. Experience.
      7. Values (cultural, religious, personal).
      8. Comprehension.
      9. Education and language deficiency.
   B. *External*
      1. Physical environment (heat, light, noise, comfort).
      2. Timing, duration, interval.
      3. Teaching methods and aids.
      4. Content, vocabulary.

◆ V. **Teaching plan** must be:
   A. Compatible with the *three* domains of learning:
      1. *Cognitive* (knowledge, concepts): use written and audiovisual materials, discussion.
      2. *Psychomotor* (skills): use demonstrations, illustrations, role models.
      3. *Affective* (attitudes): use discussions, maintain atmosphere conducive to change; use role models.
   B. Appropriate to educational material.
   C. Related to client's abilities and perceptions.
   D. Related to objectives of teaching.

◆ VI. **Implementation**—*teaching guidelines* to use with clients:
   A. Select conducive *environment* and best *timing* for activity.
   B. Assess the client's *needs,* interests, *perceptions,* motivations, and *readiness* for learning.
   C. State purpose and *realistic goals* of planned teaching/learning activity.
   D. Actually involve the client by giving him or her the opportunity to *do, react, experience,* and *ask questions.*
   E. Make sure that the client views the activity as useful and worthwhile and that it is within the client's grasp.

Mental Health

F. Use comprehensible terminology.

G. Proceed from the *known to the unknown*, from *specific to general* information.

H. Provide opportunity for client to *see results* and progress.

I. Give *feedback* and *positive reinforcement*.

J. Provide opportunities to achieve *success*.

K. Offer repeated practice in *real-life* situations.

L. *Space and distribute* learning sessions over a period of time.

◆ **VII. Evaluation/outcome criteria**

A. Client's deficit of knowledge is lessened.

B. Increased compliance to treatment.

C. Length of hospital stay is reduced.

D. Rate of readmission to hospital is reduced.

The Therapeutic Nursing Process*

A *therapeutic nursing process* involves an interaction between the nurse and client in which the nurse offers a series of planned, goal-directed activities that are useful to a particular client in relieving discomfort, promoting growth, and satisfying interpersonal relationships.

I. **Characteristics** of therapeutic nursing:

A. Movement from first contact through final outcome:

1. *Eight general phases* occur in a typical unfolding of a natural process of problem solving.

2. Stages are not always in the same sequence.

3. Not all stages are present in a relationship.

B. **Phases†**

1. *Beginning* the relationship. *Goal:* build trust.

2. *Formulating* and clarifying a problem and concern. *Goal:* clarify client's statements.

3. *Setting a contract* or working agreement. *Goal:* decide on terms of the relationship.

4. *Building* the relationship. *Goal:* increase depth of relationship and degree of commitment.

5. *Exploring goals* and solutions, gathering data, expressing feelings. *Goals:* (a) maintain and enhance relationship (trust and safety), (b) explore blocks to goal, (c) expand self-awareness, and (d) learn skills necessary to reach goal.

6. *Developing action plan. Goals:* (a) clarify feelings, (b) focus on and choose between alternative courses of action, and (c) practice new skills.

7. *Working through* conflicts or disturbing feelings. *Goals:* (a) channel earlier discussions into specific course of action and (b) work through unresolved feelings.

8. *Ending* the relationship. *Goals:* (a) evaluation of goal attainment; (b) pointing out assets and gains; and (c) leave-taking reactions (repression, regression, anger, withdrawal, acting out).

II. **Therapeutic nurse-client interactions**

◆ A. **Plans/goals:**

1. Demonstrate unconditional *acceptance*, interest, concern, and respect.

2. Develop trust—be *consistent and congruent.*

3. Make *frequent* contacts with the client.

4. Be *honest* and *direct, authentic* and spontaneous.

5. Offer support, security, and empathy, *not* sympathy.

6. Focus comments on concerns of client (*client centered*), not self (social responses). *Refocus* when client changes subject.

7. Encourage expression of *feelings;* focus on feelings and *here-and-now* behavior.

8. Give attention to a client who complains.

9. Give information at client's level of understanding, at appropriate time and place.

10. Use open-ended questions; ask *how, what, where, who,* and *when* questions; avoid *why* questions; *avoid* questions that can be answered by *yes* or *no.*

11. Use feedback or reflective listening.

12. Maintain hope, but *avoid* false reassurances, clichés, and pat responses.

13. *Avoid* verbalizing value judgments, giving personal opinions, or moralizing.

14. Do *not* change the subject *unless* the client is redundant or focusing on physical illness.

15. Point out *reality;* help the client leave "inner world."

16. Set *limits* on behavior when client is acting out unacceptable behavior that is self-destructive or harmful to others.

17. Assist clients in arriving at their own decisions by demonstrating problem solving or involving them in the process.

18. Do *not* talk if it is not indicated.

19. Approach, sit, or walk with clients who are agitated; stay with the person who is upset, if he or she can tolerate it.

20. Focus on nonverbal communication.

21. Remember the *psyche has a soma!* Do *not* neglect appropriate physical symptoms.

B. Examples of **therapeutic** responses as interventions:

1. Being *silent*—being able to sit in silence with a person can connote acceptance and acknowledgment that the person has the right to silence. (*Dangers:* The nurse may wrongly give the client the impression that there is a lack of interest, or the nurse may discourage verbalization if acceptance of this behavior is prolonged; it is not necessarily helpful with acutely psychotic behavior.)

2. Using *nonverbal communication*—for example, nodding head, moving closer to the client, and leaning forward; use as a way to encourage client to speak.

3. Give encouragement to continue with *openended leads*—nurse's responses: "Then what?" "Go on," "For instance," "Tell me more," "Talk about that."

---

*Source: ©Lagerquist, S: Addison-Wesley's Nursing Examination Review, ed. 4. Addison-Wesley, Redwood City, Calif.

†Adapted from Brammer, LM: The Helping Relationship; Process and Skills. Prentice Hall, Englewood Cliffs, NJ (out of print).

4. *Accepting, acknowledging*—nurse's responses: "I hear your anger," or "I see that you are sitting in the corner."

5. *Commenting on nonverbal behavior* of client—nurse's responses: "I notice that you are swinging your leg," "I see that you are tapping your foot," or "I notice that you are wetting your lips." Client may respond with, "So what?" If she or he does, the nurse needs to reply why the comment was made—for example, "It is distracting," "I am giving the nonverbal behavior meaning," "Swinging your leg makes it difficult for me to concentrate on what you are saying," or "I think when people tap their feet it means they are impatient. Are you impatient?"

6. Encouraging clients to *notice with their senses* what is going on—nurse's response: "What did you see (or hear)?" or "What did you notice?"

7. Encouraging *recall and description* of details of a particular experience—nurse's response: "Give me an example," "Please describe the experience further," "Tell me more," or "What did you say then?"

8. *Giving feedback by reflecting, restating, and paraphrasing* feelings and content:
Client: I cried when he didn't come to see me.
Nurse: You cried. You were expecting him to come and he didn't?

9. *Picking up on latent content* (what is implied)—nurse's response: "You were disappointed. I think it may have hurt when he didn't come."

10. *Focusing, pinpointing,* asking "what" questions:
Client: They didn't come.
Nurse: Who are "they"?
Client: [Rambling.]
Nurse: Tell it to me in a sentence or two. What is your main point? What would you say is your main concern?"

11. *Clarifying*—nurse's response: "What do you mean by 'they'?" "What caused this?" or "I didn't understand. Please say it again."

12. *Focusing on reality* by expressing doubt on "unreal" perceptions:
Client: Run! There are giant ants flying around after us.
Nurse: That is unusual. I don't see giant ants flying.

13. *Focusing on feelings,* encouraging client to be aware of and describe personal feelings:
Client: Worms are in my head.
Nurse: That must be a frightening feeling. What did you feel at that time? Tell me about that feeling.

14. Helping client to *sort and classify impressions, make speculations, abstract* and *generalize* by making connections, seeing common elements and similarities, making comparisons, and placing events in logical sequence—nurse's responses: "What are the common elements in what you just told me?" "How is this similar to …?" "What

happened just before?" or "What is the connection between this and …?"

15. *Pointing out discrepancies* between thoughts, feelings, and actions—nurse's response: "You say you were feeling sad when she yelled at you, yet you laughed. Your feelings and actions do not seem to fit together."

16. *Checking perceptions* and *seeking agreement* on how the issue is seen, *checking* with the client to see if the message sent is the same one that was received—nurse's response: "Let me restate what I heard you say," "Are you saying that …?" "Did I hear you correctly?" "Is this what you mean?" or "It seems that you were saying …?"

17. *Encouraging client to consider alternatives*—nurse's response: "What else could you say?" or "Instead of hitting him, what else might you do?"

18. *Planning a course of action*—nurse's response: "Now that we have talked about your on-the-job activities and you have thought of several choices, which are you going to try out?" or "What would you do next time?"

19. *Imparting information*—give additional data as new input to help client (e.g., state facts and reality-based data that client may lack).

20. *Summing up*—nurse's response: "Today we have talked about your feelings toward your boss, how you express your anger, and about your fear of being rejected by your family."

21. *Encouraging client to appraise and evaluate* the experience or outcome—nurse's response: "How did it turn out?" "What was it like?" "What was your part in it?" "What difference did it make?" or "How will this help you later"?

C. Examples of **nontherapeutic** responses:

1. *Changing the subject, tangential response,* moving away from problem or focusing on incidental, superficial content:
Client: I hate you.
Nurse: Would you like to take your shower now?
Suggested responses: use reflection: "You hate me; tell me about this," or "You hate me; what does hate mean to you?"
Client: I want to kill myself today.
Nurse: Isn't today the day your mother is supposed to come?
Suggested responses: (a) give open-ended lead, (b) give feedback: "I hear you saying today that you want to kill yourself," or (c) clarifying: "Tell me more about this feeling of wanting to kill yourself."

2. *Moralizing:* saying with approval or disapproval that the person's behavior is good or bad, right or wrong; *arguing* with stated belief of person; directly opposing the person:
Nurse: That's good. It's wrong to shoot yourself.
Client: I have nothing to live for.

Nurse: You certainly do have a lot!
Suggested responses: similar to those in **C.1.** previous.

3. *Agreeing with client's autistic inventions:*
   Client: The eggs are flying saucers.
   Nurse: Yes, I see. Go on.
   Suggested response: use clarifying response first: "I don't understand," and then, depending on client's response, use either *accepting and acknowledging, focusing on reality,* or *focusing on feelings.*

4. *Agreeing with client's negative view of self:*
   Client: I have made a mess of my life.
   Nurse: Yes, you have.
   Suggested response: use clarifying response about "mess of my life"—"Give me an example of one time where you feel you messed up in your life."

5. *Complimenting, flattering:*
   Client: I have made a mess of my life.
   Nurse: How could you? You are such an attractive, intelligent, generous person.
   Suggested response: same as in **C.4.**

6. *Giving opinions and advice* concerning client's life situation—examples of poor responses include: "In my opinion …" "I think you should …" or "Why not?"
   Suggested responses: (a) encourage the client to consider alternatives ("What else do you think you could try?"); (b) encourage the client to appraise and evaluate for himself or herself ("What is it like for you?").

7. *Seeking agreement* from client with nurse's personal opinion—examples of poor responses include: "I think …don't you?" and "Isn't that right?"
   Suggested responses: (a) it is best to keep personal opinion to oneself and only give information that would aid the client's orientation to reality; (b) if you give an opinion as a *model* of orienting to reality, ask client to *state his or her* opinion ("My opinion is …what is your opinion?").

8. *Probing* or *offering premature solutions and interpretations;* jumping to conclusions:
   Client: I can't find a job.
   Nurse: You could go to an employment agency.
   Client: I'd rather not talk about it.
   Nurse: What are you unconsciously doing when you say that? What you really mean is…
   Client: I don't want to live alone.
   Nurse: Are you afraid of starting to drink again?
   Suggested responses: use responses that seek clarification and elicit more data.

9. *Changing client's words* without prior validation:
   Client: I am *not feeling well* today.
   Nurse: What makes you feel so *depressed?*
   Suggested response: "In what way are you not feeling well?" Use the same language as the client.

10. *Following vague content* as if understood or using vague global pronouns, adverbs, and adjectives:
    Client: People are so *unfair.*
    Nurse: I know what you mean.
    Suggested response: clarify vague referents such as "people" and "unfair."
    Client: I feel sad.
    Nurse: Everyone feels that way at one time or another.
    Suggested response: "What are you sad about?"

11. *Questioning on different topics without waiting for a reply:*
    Client: [Remains silent.]
    Nurse: What makes you so silent? Are you angry? Would you like to be alone?
    Suggested response: choose one of the above and wait for a response before asking the next question.

12. *Ignoring client's questions or comments:*
    Client: Am I crazy, nurse?
    Nurse: [Walking away as if he or she did not hear the client.]
    Suggested responses: "I can't understand what makes you bring this up at this time," or "Tell me what makes you bring this up at this time." Ignoring questions or comments usually implies that the nurse is feeling uncomfortable. It is important not to "run away" from the client.

13. *Closing off exploration* with questions that can be answered by *yes* or *no:*
    Client: I'll never get better.
    Nurse: Is something making you feel that way?
    Suggested response: "What makes you feel that way?" Use open-ended questions that start with *what, who, when, where,* etc.

14. *Using clichés* or stereotyped expressions:
    Client: The doctor took away my weekend pass.
    Nurse: The doctor is only doing what's best for you. Doctor knows best. [Comment: also an example of moralizing.]
    Suggested response: "Tell me what happened when the doctor took away your weekend pass."

15. *Overloading:* giving too much information at one time:
    Nurse: Hello, I'm Mr. Brown. I'm a nurse here. I'll be here today, but I'm off tomorrow. Ms. Anderson will assign you another nurse tomorrow. This unit has five RNs, three LVNs, and students from three nursing schools who will all be taking care of you at some time.
    Suggested response: "Hello, I'm Mr. Brown, your nurse today." Keep your initial orienting information simple and brief.

16. *Underloading:* not giving enough information, so that meaning is not clear; withholding information:
    Client: What are visiting hours like here?

Nurse: They are flexible and liberal.

Suggested response: "They are flexible and liberal, from 10 A.M. to 12 noon and from 6 to 8 P.M." Use specific terms and give specific information.

17. *Saying no without saying no:*

    Client: Can we go for a walk soon?

    Nurse: We'll see. Perhaps. Maybe. Later.

    Suggested response: "I will check the schedule in the nursing office and let you know within an hour." Vague, ambiguous responses can be seen as "putting the client off." It is best to be clear, specific, and direct.

18. *Using double-bind communication:* sending conflicting messages that do not have "mutual fit," or are incongruent:

    Nurse: [Continuing to stay and talk with the client.] It's time for you to rest.

    Suggested response: "It's time for you to rest and for me to leave [proceeding to leave]."

19. *Protecting:* defending someone else while talking with client; implying client has no right to personal opinions and feelings:

    Client: This hospital is no good. No one cares here.

    Nurse: This is an excellent hospital. All the staff were chosen for their warmth and concern for people.

    Suggested response: focus on feeling tone or on clarifying information.

20. *Asking "why" questions* implies that the person has immediate conscious awareness of the reasons for his or her feelings and behaviors. Examples of this include: "Why don't you?" "Why did you do that?" or "Why do you feel this way?"

    Suggested response: ask clarifying questions using *how, what,* etc.

21. *Coercion:* using the interaction between people to force someone to do *your* will, with the implication that if he or she does not "do it for your sake," you will not love or stay with him or her:

    Client: I refuse to talk with him.

    Nurse: *Do it for my sake,* before it's too late.

    Suggested response: "Something keeps you from wanting to talk with him?"

22. Focusing on *negative* feelings, thoughts, actions:

    Client: I can't sleep; I can't eat; I can't think; I can't do anything.

    Nurse: How long have you not been sleeping, eating, or thinking well?

    Suggested response: "What *do* you do?"

23. *Rejecting* client's behavior or ideas:

    Client: Let's talk about incest.

    Nurse: Incest is a bad thing to talk about; I don't want to.

    Suggested response: "What do you want to say about incest?"

24. *Accusing, belittling:*

    Client: I've had to wait five minutes for you to change my dressing.

    Nurse: Don't be so demanding. Don't you see that I have several people who need me?

    Suggested response: "It must have been hard to wait for me to come when you wanted it to be right away."

25. *Evading a response* by asking a question in return:

    Client: I want to know your opinion, nurse. Am I crazy?

    Nurse: Do you think you are crazy?

    Suggested response: "I don't know. What do you mean by 'crazy'?"

26. *Circumstantiality:* communicating in such a way that the main point is reached only after many side comments, details, and additions:

    Client: Will you go out on a date with me?

    Nurse: I work every evening. On my day off I usually go out of town. I have a steady boyfriend. Besides that, I am a nurse and you are a client. Thank you for asking me, but no, I will not date you.

    Suggested response: abbreviate your response to: "Thank you for asking me, but no, I will not date you."

27. *Making assumptions* without checking them:

    Client: [Standing in the kitchen by the sink, peeling onions, with tears in the eyes.]

    Nurse: What's making you so sad?

    Client: I'm not sad. Peeling onions always makes my eyes water.

    Suggested response: use simple acknowledgment and acceptance initially, such as "I notice you have tears in your eyes."

28. *Giving false, premature reassurance:*

    Client: I'm scared.

    Nurse: Don't worry; everything will be all right. There's nothing to be afraid of.

    Suggested response: "I'd like to hear about what you're afraid of, so that together we can see what could be done to help you." Open the way for clarification and exploration, and offer yourself as a helping person—not someone with magic answers.

Alterations in Self-Concept

I. **Assessment:**

A. Self-derisive; self-diminution; and self-critical.

B. Denies own pleasure due to need to punish self; doomed to failure.

C. Disturbed interpersonal relationships (cruel, demeaning, exploitive of others; passive-dependent).

D. Exaggerated self-worth or rejects personal capabilities.

E. Feels guilty, worries (nightmares, *phobias, obsessions*).

F. Sets unrealistic goals.

G. Withdraws from reality with intense self-rejection (*delusional, suspicious,* jealous).

H. Views life as either-or, worst-or-best, wrong-or-right.

I. Postpones decisions due to ambivalence (procrastination).

J. Physical complaints *(psychosomatic)*.

K. Self-destructive *(substance abuse* or other destructiveness).

◆ **II. Analysis/nursing diagnosis:** *Altered self-concept may be related to:*

A. *Low self-esteem* that is related to parental rejection, unrealistic parental expectations, repeated failures.

B. *Altered personal identity (negative):* self-rejection and self-hate related to unrealistic self-ideals.

C. *Identity confusion* related to role conflict, role overload, and role ambiguity.

D. *Feelings of helplessness, hopelessness,* worthlessness, fear, vulnerability, inadequacy related to extreme *dependency* on others and *lack of personal responsibility*.

E. *Disturbed body image*.

F. Depersonalization.

G. Physiological factors that produce self-concept distortions (e.g., fatigue, oxygen and sensory deprivation, toxic drugs, isolation, biochemical imbalance).

◆ **III. Nursing care plan/implementation:**

A. *Long-term goal:* Facilitate client's self-actualization by helping him or her to grow, develop, and realize potential while compensating for impairments.

B. *Short-term goals:*

1. Expand client's *self-awareness:*

   a. Establish open, trusting relationship to *reduce fear* of interpersonal relationships.
      (1) Offer unconditional acceptance.
      (2) Nonjudgmental response.
      (3) Listen and encourage discussion of thoughts, feelings.
      (4) Convey that client is valued as a person, is responsible for self *and* able to help self.

   b. Strengthen client's capacity for *reality-testing, self-control,* and *ego integration*.
      (1) Identify ego strengths.
      (2) Confirm identity.
      (3) Reduce panic level of anxiety.
      (4) Use undemanding approach.
      (5) Accept and clarify communication.
      (6) Prevent isolation.
      (7) Establish simple routine.
      (8) Set limits on inappropriate behavior.
      (9) Orient to reality.
      (10) Activities: gradual increase; provide positive experiences.
      (11) Encourage self-care; assist in grooming.

   c. Maximize *participation in decision making* related to self.
      (1) Gradually increase participation in own care.
      (2) Convey expectation of ultimate self-responsibility.

2. Encourage client's *self-exploration*.

   a. Accept client's feelings and assist *self-acceptance* of emotions, beliefs, behaviors, and thoughts.

   b. Help *clarify* self-concept and relationship to others.
      (1) Elicit client's perception of own strengths and weaknesses.
      (2) Ask client to describe: ideal self, how client believes he or she relates to other people and events.

   c. Nurse needs to be aware of *own* feelings as a model of behavior and to limit countertransference.
      (1) Accept own positive and negative feelings.
      (2) Share own perception of client's feelings.

   d. Respond with *empathy,* not sympathy, with the belief that client is subject to own control.
      (1) Monitor sympathy and self-pity by client.
      (2) Reaffirm that client is *not* helpless or powerless but is responsible for own choice of maladaptive or adaptive coping responses.
      (3) Discuss: alternatives, areas of ego *strength,* available coping resources.
      (4) Use family and group-support system for self-exploration of client's conflicts and maladaptive coping responses.

3. Assist client in *self-evaluation*.

   a. Help to clearly *define* problem.
      (1) Identify relevant stressors.
      (2) Mutually identify: faulty beliefs, misperceptions, distortions, unrealistic goals, areas of strength.

   b. Explore use of adaptive *and* maladaptive coping responses and their positive and negative *consequences:*

4. Assist client to formulate a *realistic action plan*.

   a. Identify alternative solutions to client's *inconsistent perceptions* by helping him or her to change:
      (1) Own beliefs, ideals, to bring closer to reality.
      (2) Environment, to make consistent with beliefs.

   b. Identify alternative solutions to client's *self-concept not consistent with his or her behavior* by helping him or her to change:
      (1) Own behavior to conform to self-concept.
      (2) Underlying beliefs.
      (3) Self-ideal.

   c. Help client set and clearly define *goals* with *expected concrete* changes. Use role rehearsal, role modeling, and role playing to see practical, reality-based, emotional consequences of each goal.

5. Assist client to become committed to decision to *take necessary action* to replace maladaptive coping responses and maintain adaptive responses.

   a. Provide opportunity for success and give assistance (vocational, financial, and social support).

b. Provide positive reinforcement; strengths, skills, healthy aspects of client's personality.

c. Allow enough time for change.

6. *Health teaching:* how to focus on strengths rather than limitations; how to apply reality-oriented approach.

◆ **IV. Evaluation/outcome criteria**

A. Client able to discuss perception of self and accept aspects of own personality.

B. Client assumes increased responsibility for own behavior.

C. Client able to transfer new perceptions into possible solutions, alternative behavior.

Anxiety

Anxiety is a subjective warning of danger in which the specific nature of the danger is usually not known. It occurs when a person faces a new, unknown, or untried situation. Anxiety is also felt when a person perceives threat in terms of past experiences. It is a general concept underlying most disease states. In its milder form, anxiety can contribute to learning and is necessary for problem solving. In its severe form, anxiety can impede a client's treatment and recovery. The general feelings elicited on all levels of anxiety are nervousness, tension, and apprehension.

It is essential that nurses recognize their own sources of anxiety and behavior in response to anxiety, as well as help clients recognize the manifestations of anxiety in themselves.

◆ **I. Assessment:**

A. *Physiological* manifestations:

1. Increased heart rate and palpitations.
2. Increased rate and depth of respiration.
3. Increased urinary frequency and diarrhea.
4. Dry mouth.
5. Decreased appetite.
6. Cold sweat and pale appearance.
7. Increased menstrual flow.
8. Increased or decreased body temperature.
9. Increased or decreased blood pressure.
10. Dilated pupils.

B. *Behavioral* manifestations—stages of anxiety:

1. *Mild anxiety:*
   a. Increased perception (visual and auditory).
   b. Increased awareness of meanings and relationships.
   c. Increased alertness (notice more).
   d. Ability to use problem-solving process.

2. *Moderate anxiety:*
   a. Selective inattention (e.g., may not hear someone talking).
   b. Decreased perceptual field.
   c. Concentration on relevant data; "tunnel vision."
   d. Muscular tension, perspiration, GI discomfort.

3. *Severe anxiety:*
   a. Focus on many fragmented details.

b. Physical and emotional discomfort (headache, nausea, dizziness, dread, horror, trembling).

c. Not aware of total environment.

d. Automatic behavior aimed at getting immediate relief instead of problem solving.

e. Poor recall.

f. Inability to see connections between details.

g. Drastically reduced awareness.

4. *Panic state of anxiety:*
   a. Increased speed of scatter; does not notice what goes on.
   b. Increased distortion and exaggeration of details.
   c. Feeling of terror.
   d. Dissociation (hallucinations, loss of reality, and little memory).
   e. Inability to cope with any problems; no self-control.

C. *Reactions in response to anxiety:*

1. *Fight:*
   a. Aggression.
   b. Hostility, derogation, belittling.
   c. Anger.

2. *Flight:*
   a. Withdrawal.
   b. Depression.

3. *Somatization* (psychosomatic disorder).

4. *Impaired cognition:* blocking, forgetfulness, poor concentration, errors in judgment.

5. *Learning* about or searching for causes of anxiety, and identifying behavior.

◆ **II. Analysis/nursing diagnosis:** *Anxiety related to*:

A. *Physical causes:* threats to biological well-being (e.g., sleep disturbances, interference with sexual functioning, food, drink, pain, fever).

B. *Psychological causes: disturbance in self-esteem* related to:

1. Unmet wishes or expectations.
2. Unmet needs for prestige and status.
3. *Impaired adjustment:* inability to cope with environment.
4. *Altered role performance:* not using own full potential.
5. *Altered meaningfulness:* alienation.
6. *Conflict with social order:* value conflicts.
7. Anticipated disapproval from a significant other.
8. *Altered feeling states:* guilt.

◆ **III. Nursing care plan/implementation:**

A. *Moderate to severe anxiety*

1. Provide *motor outlet* for tension energy, such as working at a simple, concrete task, walking, crying, or talking.

2. Help clients *recognize* their anxieties by talking about how they are behaving and by exploring their underlying feelings.

3. Help clients *gain insight* into their anxieties by helping them to understand how their behavior has been an expression of anxiety and to recognize the threat that lies behind this anxiety.

4. Help clients cope with the threat behind their anxieties by reevaluating the threats and learning new ways to deal with them.
5. *Health teaching:*
   a. Explain and offer hope that emotional pain will decrease with time.
   b. Explain that some tension is normal.
   c. Explain how to channel emotional energy into activity.
   d. Explain need to recognize highly stressful situations and to recognize tension within oneself.

B. *Panic state*
1. Give simple, clear, *concise* directions.
2. *Avoid* decision making by client. Do *not* try to reason with client, because he or she is irrational and cannot cooperate.
3. *Stay* with client.
   a. Do *not* isolate.
   b. *Avoid* touching.
4. Allow client to seek *motor* outlets (walking, pacing).
5. *Health teaching:* advise activity that requires no thought.

◆ **IV. Evaluation/outcome criteria:**
A. Uses more positive thinking and problem-solving activities and is less preoccupied with worrying.
B. Uses values clarification to resolve conflicts and establish realistic goals.
C. Demonstrates regained perspective, self-esteem, and morale; expresses feeling more in control, more hopeful.
D. Fewer or absent physical symptoms of anxiety.

Patterns of Adjustment (Defense Mechanisms)

Defense mechanisms (ego defense mechanisms or mental mechanisms) consist of all the *coping* means used unconsciously by individuals to seek relief from emotional conflict and *to ward off excessive anxiety.*

I. Definitions

blocking a disturbance in the rate of speech when a person's thoughts and speech are proceeding at an average rate but are suddenly and completely interrupted, perhaps even in the middle of a sentence. The gap may last from several seconds up to a minute. Blocking is often a part of the thought disorder found in *schizophrenic* disorders.

compensation making up for real or imagined handicap, limitation, or lack of gratification in one area of personality by overemphasis in another area to counter the effects of failure, frustration, and limitation (e.g., the person who is blind compensates by increased sensitivity in hearing; the student who is unpopular compensates by becoming an outstanding scholar; men who are small compensate for short stature by demanding a great deal of attention and respect; a nurse who does not have manual dexterity chooses to go into psychiatric nursing).

confabulating filling in gaps of memory by inventing what appear to be suitable memories as replacements. This symptom may occur in various *amnestic disorders* but is most often seen in *Korsakoff's syndrome* (deterioration due to alcohol) and in *dementia.*

conversion psychological difficulties are translated into physical symptoms ***without conscious*** will or knowledge (e.g., pain and immobility on moving your writing arm the day of the exam).

denial an intolerable thought, wish, need, or reality factor, is disowned automatically (e.g., a student, when told of a failing grade, acts as if he never heard of such a possibility).

displacement transferring the emotional component from one idea, object, or situation to another, more acceptable one. Displacement occurs because these are painful or dangerous feelings that cannot be expressed toward the original object (e.g., kicking the dog after a bad day at school or work; anger with a clinical instructor gets transferred to a classmate who was late to meet you for lunch).

dissociation splitting off or separation of differing elements of the mind from each other. There can be separation of ideas, concepts, emotions, or experiences from the rest of the mind. Dissociated material is deeply repressed and becomes encapsulated and inaccessible to the rest of the mind. This usually occurs as a result of some very painful experience (e.g., split of affect from idea in *anxiety disorders* and *schizophrenia*).

fixation a state in which personality development is arrested in one or more aspects at a level short of maturity (e.g., "She is anally fixated" [controlling, stingy, holding onto things and memories]).

idealization overestimation of some admired aspect or attribute of another person (e.g., "She was a perfect human being").

ideas of reference fixed, false ideas and interpretations of external events as though they had direct reference to self (e.g., client thinks that TV news announcer is reporting a story about client).

identification the wish to be like another person; situation in which qualities of another are unconsciously transferred to oneself (e.g., boy identifies with his father and learns to become a man; a woman may fear she will die in childbirth because her mother did; a student adopts attitudes and behavior of her favorite teacher).

introjection incorporation into the personality, without assimilation, of emotionally charged impulses or objects; a quality or an attribute of another person is taken into and made part of self (e.g., a girl in love introjects the personality of her lover into herself—his ideas become hers, his tastes and wishes are hers; this is also seen in *severe depression* following death of someone close—client may assume many of deceased's characteristics; similarly, working in a psychiatric unit with a suicidal person brings out depression in the nurse).

isolation temporary or long-term splitting off of certain feelings or ideas from others; separating emotional and intellectual content (e.g., talking emotionlessly about a traumatic accident).

projection attributes and transfers own feelings, attitudes, impulses, wishes, or thoughts to another person or object in the environment, especially when ideas or impulses are too painful to be acknowledged as belonging to oneself (e.g., in *hallucinations* and *delusions* by people who use/abuse alcohol; or, "I flunked the course because the teacher doesn't know how to teach"; "I hate him" reversed into "He hates me"; or a student impatiently accusing an instructor of being intolerant).

rationalization justification of behavior by formulating a logical, socially approved reason for past, present, or proposed behavior. Commonly used, conscious or unconscious, with false or real reason (e.g., after losing a class election, a student states that she really did not want all the extra work and is glad she lost).

reaction formation going to the opposite extreme from what one wishes to do or is afraid one might do (e.g., being overly concerned with cleanliness when one wishes to be messy; being a mother who is overly protective through fear of own hostility to child; or showing great concern for a person whom you dislike by going out of your way to do special favors).

regression when individuals fail to solve a problem with the usual methods at their command, they may resort to modes of behavior that they have outgrown but that proved successful at an earlier stage of development; retracing developmental steps; going back to earlier interests or modes of gratification (e.g., a senior nursing student about to graduate becomes dependent on a clinical instructor for directions).

repression involuntary exclusion of painful and unacceptable thoughts and impulses from awareness. *Forgetting* these things solves the situation by not solving it (e.g., by not remembering what was on the difficult exam after it was over).

sublimation channeling a destructive or instinctual impulse that cannot be realized into a *socially acceptable,* practical, and less dangerous outlet, with some relation to the original impulse for emotional satisfaction to be obtained (e.g., sublimation of sexual energy into other creative activities [art, music, literature], or hostility and aggression into sports or business competition; or a person who is infertile puts all energies into pediatric nursing).

substitution when individuals cannot have what they wish and accept something else in its place for symbolic satisfaction (e.g., pin-up pictures in absence of sexual object; or a person who failed an RN exam signs up for an LVN/LPN exam).

suppression a deliberate process of blocking from the conscious mind thoughts, feelings, acts, or impulses that are undesirable (e.g., "I don't want to talk about it," "Don't mention his name to me," or "I'll think about it some other time"; or willfully refusing to think about or discuss disappointment with exam results).

symbolism sign language that stands for related ideas and feelings, conscious and unconscious. Used extensively by children, people from primitive cultures, and clients who are psychotic. There is meaning attached to this sign language that makes it very important to the individual (e.g., a student wears dark, somber clothing to the exam site).

undoing a mechanism against anxiety, usually unconscious, designed to negate or neutralize a previous act (e.g., Lady Macbeth's attempt to wash her hands [of guilt] after the murder). A repetitive, symbolic acting out, in reverse of an unacceptable act already completed. Responsible for *compulsions* and magical thinking.

II. **Characteristics** of defense mechanisms:
  A. Defense mechanisms are used to some degree by everyone occasionally; they are normal processes by which the ego reestablishes equilibrium—unless they are used to an extreme degree, in which case they interfere with maintenance of self-integrity.
  B. Much overlapping:
    1. Same behavior can be explained by more than one mechanism.
    2. May be used in combination (e.g., isolation and repression, denial and projection).
  C. Common defense mechanisms compatible with mental well-being.
    1. Compensation.
    2. Compromise.
    3. Identification.
    4. Rationalization.
    5. Sublimation.
    6. Substitution.
  D. Typical defense mechanisms in:
    1. *Paranoid disorders*—denial, projection.
    2. *Dissociative disorders*—denial, repression, dissociation.
    3. *Obsessive-compulsive behaviors*—displacement, reaction-formation, isolation, denial, repression, undoing.
    4. *Phobic disorders*—displacement, rationalization, repression.
    5. *Conversion disorders*—symbolization, dissociation, repression, isolation, denial.
    6. *Major depression*—displacement.
    7. *Bipolar disorder, manic episode*—reaction-formation, denial, projection, introjection.
    8. *Schizophrenic disorders*—symbolization, repression, dissociation, denial, fantasy, regression, projection, isolation.
    9. *Dementia*—regression.

III. **Concepts and principles related to defense mechanisms:**
  A. Unconscious process—defense mechanisms are used as a substitute for more effective problem-solving behavior.
  B. *Main functions*—increase *self-esteem; decrease,* inhibit, minimize, alleviate, avoid, or eliminate *anxiety;* maintain feelings of personal worth and adequacy and soften failures; *protect the ego; increase security.*

C. Drawbacks—involve high degree of self-deception and reality distortion; may be maladaptive because they superficially eliminate or disguise conflicts, leaving conflicts unresolved but still influencing behavior.

◆ IV. **Nursing care plan/implementation** with defense mechanisms:

A. Accept defense mechanisms as normal, but not when overused.

B. Look beyond the behavior to the need that is expressed by the use of the defense mechanism.

C. Discuss alternative defense mechanisms that may be more compatible with mental health.

D. Assist the person to translate defensive thinking into nondefensive, direct thinking; a problem-solving approach to conflicts minimizes the need to use defense mechanisms.

Anxiety Disorders (Anxiety and Phobic Neuroses)

I. **Definition:** emotional illnesses characterized by *fear* and *autonomic nervous system symptoms* (palpitations, tachycardia, dizziness, tremor); related to *intrapsychic conflict* and psychogenic origin where instinctual impulse (related to sexuality, aggression, or dependence) may be in conflict with the ego, superego, or sociocultural environment; related to sudden object loss.

An *anxiety disorder* is a mild to moderately severe functional disorder of personality in which *repressed* inner conflicts between drives and fears are manifested in behavior patterns, including *generalized anxiety* and *phobic, obsessive-compulsive disorders.* (Other related disorders are *dissociative, conversion,* and *hypochondriasis.*)

II. **General concepts and principles related to anxiety disorders:**

A. Behavior may be an attempt to "bind" anxiety: to *fix* it in some particular area (hypochondriasis) or to *displace* it from the rest of personality (phobic, conversion, and dissociative disorders—amnesia, fugue, obsessive-compulsive disorders).

B. *Purpose of symptoms:*

1. To intensify *repression* as a defense.

2. To exhibit some repressed content in *symbolic* form.

◆ III. **General assessment of anxiety disorders:**

A. Uses behavior to *avoid* tense situations.

B. Frightened, suggestible.

C. Prone to *minor* physical complaints (e.g., fatigue, headaches, and indigestion) and reluctance to admit recovery from physical illnesses.

D. Attitude of martyrdom.

E. Often feels helpless, insecure, inferior, inadequate.

F. Uses *repression, displacement,* and *symbolism* as key defense mechanisms.

Anxiety Disorders

I. *Generalized anxiety disorder (GAD):*

◆ A. **Assessment:**

1. Persistent, diffuse, free-floating, painful anxiety for at least 1 mo; not supported by imminent threat or danger. More than everyday worry.

2. Motor tension, autonomic hyperactivity.

3. Hyperattentiveness expressed through vigilance and scanning and avoidance, with minimal risk-taking.

◆ B. **Analysis/nursing diagnosis:**

1. *Anxiety/powerlessness: excessive worry* related to real or perceived threat to security, unmet needs.

2. *Altered attention* related to overwhelming anxiety out of proportion to actual situation.

3. *Fear* related to sudden object loss.

4. *Guilt* related to inability to meet role expectations.

5. *Risk for alteration in self-concept* related to feelings of inadequacy and worries about own competence.

6. *Altered role performance* related to inadequate support system.

7. *Impaired social interaction* related to use of avoidance in tense situations.

8. *Distractibility* related to pervasive anxiety.

9. *Hopelessness* related to feelings of inadequacy.

10. *Sleep pattern disturbance.*

◆ C. **Nursing care plan/implementation:**

1. Fulfill needs as promptly as possible.

2. Listen attentively.

3. Stay with client.

4. *Avoid* decision making and competitive situations.

5. Promote rest; decrease environmental stimuli.

6. *Health teaching:* teach steps of anxiety reduction.

◆ D. **Evaluation/outcome criteria:** symptoms are diminished.

II. *Panic disorder:*

◆ A. **Assessment:**

1. Three acute, terrifying panic attacks within 3 wk period, *unrelated* to marked physical exertion, life-threatening situation, presence of organic illness, or exposure to specific phobic stimulus.

2. Discrete periods of apprehension, fearfulness (lasting from few moments to an hour).

3. *Mimics cardiac* disease: dyspnea, chest pain, smothering or choking sensations, palpitations, tachycardia, dizziness, fainting, sweating.

4. Feelings of unreality, paresthesias.

5. Hot, cold flashes and dilated pupils.

6. Trembling, sense of impending doom and death, fear of becoming insane.

◆ B. **Analysis/nursing diagnosis:**

1. *Ineffective individual coping* related to undeveloped interpersonal processes.

2. *Altered comfort pattern:* distress, anxiety, fear related to threat to security.

3. *Decisional conflict* related to apprehension.
4. *Altered thought processes* related to impaired concentration.

◆ **C. Nursing care plan/implementation:**
1. *Reduce immediate anxiety* to more moderate and manageable levels.
   a. Stay *physically close* to reduce feelings of alienation and terror.
   b. *Communication approach:* calm, serene manner; short, simple sentences; firm voice to convey that nurse will provide external controls.
   c. *Physical environment:* remove to smaller room to minimize stimuli.
2. Provide *motor outlet* for diffuse energy generated at high anxiety levels (e.g., moving furniture, scrubbing floors).
3. Administer *antianxiety medications* as ordered.
4. *Health teaching:* recommend more effective methods of coping; let client know that panic is time-limited and highly treatable.

◆ **D. Evaluation/outcome criteria:** can endure anxiety while searching out its causes.

III. *Obsessive-compulsive disorder:*
◆ **A. Assessment**—chief characteristic: fear that client can harm someone or something.
1. *Obsessions*—recurrent, persistent, unwanted, involuntary, senseless *thoughts, images, ideas,* or *impulses* that may be trivial or morbid (e.g., fear of germs, doubts as to performance of an act, thoughts of hurting family member, death, suicide; vague fear that "something bad may happen" if routine activities are not done "correctly").
2. *Compulsions*—uncontrollable, persistent urge to perform repetitive, stereotyped *behaviors* that provide relief from unbearable anxiety (e.g., hand-washing, counting, touching, checking and rechecking doors to see if locked, elaborate dressing and undressing rituals, excessive collecting, always doing things in "sets," avoiding certain numbers).

◆ **B. Analysis/nursing diagnosis:**
1. *Ineffective individual coping* related to:
   a. *Intellectualization and avoidance* of awareness of feelings.
   b. Limited ability to express emotions (may be disguised or delayed).
   c. Exaggerated feelings of *dependence and helplessness.*
   d. High need to *control* self, others, and environment.
   e. Rigidity in thinking and behavior.
   f. Poor ability to tolerate anxiety and depression.
2. *Social isolation* related to:
   a. Resentment.
   b. Self-doubt.
   c. Exclusion of pleasure.

◆ **C. Nursing care plan/implementation:**
1. *Accept* rituals permissively (e.g., excessive hand-washing); stopping ritual will increase anxiety.

2. *Avoid* criticism or "punishment," making demands, or showing impatience with client.
3. *Allow* extra time for slowness and client's need for precision.
4. *Protect* from rejection by *others.*
5. *Protect* from *self-inflicted* harmful acts.
6. Engage in nursing therapy *after* the ritual is over, when client is most comfortable.
7. *Redirect* client's actions into substitute outlets.
8. *Health teaching:* teach how to prevent health problems related to rituals (e.g., use rubber gloves, hand lotion).

◆ **D. Evaluation/outcome criteria:** avoids situations that increase tension and thus reduces need for ritualistic behavior as outlet for tension.

IV. *Phobic disorders*—intense, *irrational, persistent* specific fear in response to *external* object, activity, or situation (e.g., *agoraphobia*—fear of being alone or in public places; *claustrophobia*—fear of closed places; *acrophobia*—fear of heights; *simple phobias* such as *mysophobia*—fear of germs; *social phobias:* fear of situations that may be humiliating or embarrassing). *Dynamics: displacement* of anxiety from original source onto avoidable, *symbolic,* external, and specific object (or activity or situation); that is, phobias help person control intensity of anxiety by providing specific object to attach it to, which he or she can then avoid.

◆ **A. Assessment:** same as for anxiety symptoms; fear that someone or something will harm them.

◆ **B. Analysis/nursing diagnosis:** *social isolation;* avoidance; irrational *fear* out of proportion to actual danger; *defensive coping* with high need to control self, others, environment.

◆ **C. Nursing care plan/implementation:** promote psychological and physical calm:
1. *Use systematic desensitization:* never force contact with feared object or situation.
2. *Health teaching:* progressive relaxation, meditation, biofeedback training, or other behavioral conditioning techniques.

◆ **D. Evaluation/outcome criteria:** phobia is eliminated (i.e., able to come into contact with feared object with lessened degree of anxiety).

V. *Acute stress disorder and posttraumatic stress disorder:*
◆ **A. Assessment:**
1. *Acute stress disorder:* symptoms occur *within 1 mo* of extreme stressor.
2. *Posttraumatic stress disorder (PTSD):* symptoms occur *after* 1 mo.
3. Precipitant: severe, threatening, terrifying traumatic event (natural or man-made disaster) that is not an ordinary occurrence (e.g., rape, fire, flood, earthquake, tornado, bombing, torture, kidnapping).
4. Self-report of reexperiencing incident; intrusive memories (e.g., "flashbacks").
5. Numb, unresponsive, detached, estranged reaction to external world (unable to feel tenderness, intimacy).

Mental Health

6. Change in sleep pattern (insomnia, recurrent dreams, nightmares), memory loss, hyperalertness (startle response).
7. Guilt rumination about survival.
8. Avoids activities reminiscent of trauma; phobic responses.
9. Difficulty with task completion and concentration.
10. Depression.
11. Increased irritability may result in unpredictable, explosive outbursts.
12. Impulsive behavior, sudden lifestyle changes.

◆ **B. Analysis/nursing diagnosis:**
1. *Posttrauma response* related to overwhelming traumatic event.
2. *Anxiety* (severe to panic)/*fear* related to memory of environmental stressor, threat to self-concept, negative self-talk.
3. *Risk for violence directed at self/others* related to a startle reaction, use of drugs to produce a psychic numbing.
4. *Sleep pattern disturbance* related to fear and rumination.

5. *Decisional conflict (impaired decision making)* related to perceived threat to personal values and beliefs.
6. *Guilt* related to lack of social support system.
7. *Altered feeling-states:* emotional lability related to diminished sense of control over self and environment.

◆ **C. Nursing care plan/implementation:**
1. Crisis counseling (listen with concern and empathy).
   a. Ease way for client to *talk out* the experience and express fear.
   b. Help client to become aware and accepting of what happened.
2. *Health teaching:* suggest how to resume concrete activity and reconstruct life with available social, physical, and emotional resources. Help make contact with friends, relatives, and other resources.

◆ **D. Evaluation/outcome criteria:** can cry and express anger, loss, frustration, and despair; begins process of social and physical reconstruction.

E. See **Clinical Pathway 6.3: Client who is Posttrauma.**

CLINICAL PATHWAY 6.3: Client who is Posttrauma

Estimated length of stay: 14 days—variations from designated pathway should be documented in progress notes

Nursing Diagnosis and Categories of Care	Time Dimension	Goals/Actions	Time Dimension	Goals/Actions	Time Dimension	Discharge Outcome
Posttrauma response	Day 1	Reassurance of client safety	Ongoing	Environment is made safe for client.	Day 14	Client is able to carry out activities of daily living. Fewer flashbacks, nightmares.
Referrals	Day 1	Psychiatrist Psychologist Social worker Clinical nurse specialist Music therapist Occupational therapist Recreational therapist Chaplain			Day 14	Discharge with follow-up appointments as required.
Diagnostic studies	Day 1	Drug screen ECG EEG				
	Day 2–5	MMPI Impact of event scale (IES)				
Medications	Day 1	Antidepressant medication as ordered (tricyclics or MAO inhibitors)	Day 1–14	Assess for effectiveness and side effects of medications.	Day 14	Discharged with medications as ordered by MD (e.g., antidepressants, clonidine, propranolol).

(Continued on following page)

Nursing Diagnosis and Categories of Care	Time Dimension	Goals/Actions	Time Dimension	Goals/Actions	Time Dimension	Discharge Outcome
Medications (*Cont'd*)		Antianxiety medication, as ordered (benzodiazepines); may be given prn because of addictive quality Clonidine or propranolol (for intrusive thoughts and hyperarousal) Sedative-hypnotics for sleep disturbances; may be given prn		Administer addictive medications judiciously and taper dosage.		
◆ Additional assessments	Day 1	VS every shift Assess: ■ Mental status ■ Mood swings ■ Anxiety level ■ Social interaction ■ Ability to carry out activities of daily living ■ Suicide ideation ■ Sleep disturbances ■ Flashbacks ■ Presence of guilt feelings	Day 2–14 Day 2–13	VS daily if stable. Ongoing assessments.	Day 14	Anxiety is maintained at manageable level. Mood is appropriate. Interacts with others. Carries out activities of daily living independently. Denies suicide ideation. Sleeps without medication. Is able to interrupt flashbacks with adaptive, coping strategies. Has worked through feelings of guilt.
Diet	Day 1	■ Client's choice or low tyramine if taking MAO inhibitors	Day 2–14	Same.	Day 14	Client eats well-balanced diet.
Client education	Day 1	■ Orient to unit	Day 5–12	Stages of grief. Side effects of medications. Coping strategies. Low tyramine diet. Community resources. Support group. Importance of not mixing drugs and alcohol.	Day 14	Client is discharged. Verbalizes understanding of information presented before discharge.
			Day 12–13	Reinforce teaching.		

Source: Adapted from Townsend, M: Essentials of Psychiatric–Mental Health Nursing. FA Davis, Philadelphia.

Mental Health

Dissociative Disorders (Hysterical Neuroses, Dissociative Type)

◆ **I. Assessment:**

   A. *Dissociative amnesia:* partial or total inability to recall the past; occurs during highly stressful events; client may have conscious desire to escape but be unable to accept escape as a solution; uses *repression.*

   B. *Dissociative fugue:* client not only forgets but also *flees* from stress.

   C. *Dissociative identity disorder:* client exhibits two or more complete personality systems, each very different from the other; alternates from one personality to the other without awareness of change (*one personality may be aware of others*); each personality has well-developed emotions and thought processes that are in conflict; uses *repression.*

   D. *Depersonalization disorder:* loss of sense of self; feeling of self-estrangement (as if in a dream); fear of going insane.

◆ **II. Analysis/nursing diagnosis:**

   A. Sudden *alteration in:*

      1. *Memory* (short- and *long-term memory loss:* cannot recall important personal events) related to repression.

      2. *Personal and social identity* (amnesia: forgets own identity; becomes another identity) related to intense anxiety, childhood trauma/abuse, threat to physical integrity, underdeveloped ego.

   B. *Sensory/perceptual alteration* of external environment related to repression and escapism.

   C. *Confusion* related to use of repression.

   D. *Spiritual despair* related to conversion of conflict into physical or mental flights.

   E. *Altered meaningfulness* (hopelessness, helplessness, powerlessness) related to lack of control over situation.

◆ **III. Nursing care plan/implementation:**

   A. *Remove* client from immediate environment to reduce pressure.

   B. *Alleviate* symptoms using behavior-modification strategies.

   C. *Divert* attention to topics other than symptoms (not remembering names, addresses, and events).

   D. Encourage *socialization* rather than isolation.

   E. *Avoid* sympathy, pity, and oversolicitous approach.

   F. *Health teaching:* teach families to avoid reinforcing dissociative behavior; teach client problem solving, with goal of minimizing stressful aspects of environment.

◆ **IV. Evaluation/outcome criteria:** recall returns to conscious awareness; anxiety kept within manageable limits.

Somatoform Disorders

   I. **Main characteristic:** involuntary, physical symptoms *without* demonstrable organic findings or identifiable physiological bases; involve psychological factors or nonspecific conflicts.

◆ **II. General assessment:**

   A. *Precipitant:* major emotional, interpersonal stress.

   B. Occurrence of secondary gain from illness.

◆ **III. General analysis/nursing diagnosis:**

   A. *Fear* related to loss of dependent relationships.

   B. *Powerlessness* related to chronic resentment over frustration of dependency needs.

   C. *Altered feeling states:* inhibition of anger, which is discharged physiologically and is related to control of anxiety.

   D. *Impaired judgment* related to denial of existence of any conflicts or relationship to physical symptoms.

   E. *Altered role performance:* regression related to not having dependency needs met.

Somatization Disorder

Repeated, multiple, vague or exaggerated physical complaints of several years' duration *without* identifiable physical cause; clients constantly seek medical attention, undergo numerous tests; at risk for unnecessary surgery or drug abuse.

◆ **A. Assessment:**

   1. Onset and occurrence—teen years, more common in women.

   2. Reports illness most of life.

      a. *Neuromuscular* symptoms—fainting, seizures, dysphagia, difficulty walking, back pain, urinary retention.

      b. *Gastrointestinal* symptoms—nausea, vomiting, flatus, food intolerance, constipation or diarrhea.

      c. *Female reproductive* symptoms—dysmenorrhea, hyperemesis gravidarum.

      d. *Psychosexual* symptoms—sexual indifference, dyspareunia.

      e. *Cardiopulmonary* symptoms—palpitations, shortness of breath, chest pain.

      f. *Rule out:* multiple sclerosis, systemic lupus erythematosus, porphyria, hyperparathyroidism.

   3. Appears anxious and depressed.

◆ **B. Analysis/nursing diagnosis:**

   1. *Anxiety* (severe) related to threat to security, unmet dependency needs, and inability to meet role expectations.

   2. *Self-care deficit* related to development of physical symptoms to escape stressful situations.

   3. *Impaired social interaction* related to inability to accept that physical symptoms lack a physiological basis; preoccupation with self and physical symptoms, chronic pain; rejection by others.

   4. *Body-image disturbance and altered role performance* related to passive acceptance of disabling symptoms.

Conversion Disorder (Hysterical Neuroses, Conversion Type)

Sudden symptoms of *symbolic* nature developed under *extreme* psychological stress (e.g., war, loss, natural disaster) that *disappear* through hypnosis.

◆ **A. Assessment:**
1. *Neurological* symptoms—paralysis, aphonia, tunnel vision, seizures, blindness, paresthesias, anesthesias.
2. *Endocrinological* symptoms—pseudocyesis.
3. Hysterical, dependent *personality profile:* exhibitionistic dress and language; self-indulgent; suggestible; impulsive and global impressions and hunches; little capacity to concentrate, integrate, and organize thoughts or plan action or outcomes; little concern for symptoms, despite severe impairment ("La Belle Indifference").

◆ **B. Analysis/nursing diagnosis:**
1. Prolonged *loss or alteration of physiological processes* related to severe psychological stress and conflict that results in disuse, atrophy, contractures. *Primary gain*—internal conflict or need is kept out of awareness; there is a close relationship in time between stressor and occurrence of symbolic symptoms.
2. *Impaired social interaction:* chronic sick role related to attention seeking.
3. *Noncompliance* with expected routines related to *secondary gain*—avoidance of upsetting situation, with support obtained from others.
4. *Impaired adjustment* related to *repression* of feelings through somatic symptoms, *regression, denial* and *isolation,* and *externalization.*
5. *Ineffective individual coping* (e.g., day-dreaming, fantasizing, superficial warmth and seductiveness related to inability to control symptoms voluntarily or to explain them by known physical disorder).

Hypochondriasis (Hypochondriacal Neurosis)

Exaggerated concern for one's physical health; *unrealistic* interpretation of signs or sensations as abnormal; *preoccupation with fear* of having serious disease, *despite* medical reassurance of no diagnosis of physical disorder.

◆ **A. Assessment:**
1. Preoccupation with symptoms: sweating, peristalsis, heartbeat, coughing, muscular soreness, skin eruptions.
2. Occurs in both men and women in adolescence, 30s, or 40s.
3. History of long, complicated shopping for doctors and refusal of mental health care.
4. *Organ neurosis* may occur (e.g., cardiac neurosis).
5. Personality trait: *compulsive.*
6. Prevalence of anxiety and depression.
7. *Controls* relationships through physical complaints.

◆ **B. Analysis/nursing diagnosis:**
1. *Personal identity disturbance* related to perception of self as ill in order to meet needs for dependency, attention, affection.
2. Displaced *anxiety* related to inability to verbalize feelings.
3. *Fear* related to not being believed.
4. *Powerlessness* related to feelings of insecurity.
5. *Altered role performance:* disruption in work and interpersonal relations related to regression and

need gratification through preoccupation with fantasized illness; and related to control over others through physical complaints.

◆ **IV. General nursing care plans/implementation** for somatoform disorders:
A. *Long-term goals:*
1. Develop interests *outside* of self. Introduce to new activities and people.
2. Facilitate experiences of increased feelings of *independence.*
3. Increase *reality perception* and *problem-solving ability.*
4. Emphasize *positive* outlook and promote positive thinking. Reassure that symptoms are anxiety related, not a result of physical disease.
5. Develop mature ways for meeting *affection* needs.
B. *Short-term goals:*
1. *Prevent* anxiety from mounting and becoming uncontrollable by recognizing symptoms, for early intervention.
2. *Environment:* warm, caring, supportive interactions; instill hope that anxiety can be mastered.
3. Encourage client to *express* somatic concerns verbally. Encourage awareness of body processes.
4. Provide *diversional* activities.
5. Develop ability to relax rather than ruminate or worry. Help find palliative relief through anxiety reduction (slower breathing, exercise).
C. *Health teaching:*
1. Relaxation training as self-help measures.
2. Increase knowledge of appropriate and correct information on physiological responses that accompany anxiety.

◆ **V. General evaluation/outcome criteria:**
A. Does not isolate self.
B. Discusses fears, concerns, conflicts that are self-originated and not likely to be serious.
C. Decides which aspects of situation can be overcome and ways to meet conflicting obligations.
D. Looks for things of importance and value.
E. Deliberately engages in new activities other than ruminating or worrying.
F. Talks self out of fears.
G. Decrease in physical symptoms; is able to sleep, feels less restless.
H. Makes fewer statements of feeling helpless.
I. Can freely express angry feelings in *overt* way and not through symptoms.

Other Conditions in Which Psychological Factors Affect Medical Conditions (Psychophysiological Disorders)

This group of disorders occurs in various organs and systems, whereby emotions are expressed by affecting body organs.

I. Concepts and principles related to psychological factors affecting physical conditions:
  A. Majority of organs involved are usually under control of *autonomic* nervous system.
  B. Defense mechanisms
    1. *Repression or suppression* of unpleasant emotional experiences.
    2. *Introjection*—illness seen as punishment.
    3. *Projection*—others blamed for illness.
    4. *Conversion*—physical symptoms rather than underlying emotional stresses are emphasized.
  C. Clients often exhibit the following underlying *needs in excess:*
    1. Dependency.
    2. Attention.
    3. Love.
    4. Success.
    5. Recognition.
    6. Security.
  D. Need to distinguish between:
    1. Factitious disorders—deliberate, *conscious* exhibit of physical or psychological illness to avoid an uncomfortable situation.
    2. *Conversion disorder*—affecting *sensory* and skeletal-muscular systems that are usually under *voluntary* control; generally *non–life-threatening;* symptoms are symbolic solution to anxiety; *no* demonstrable *organic* pathology.
    3. *Psychological factors affecting physical condition* (e.g., psychophysiological disorders); under *autonomic* nervous system control; structural *organic* changes; may be life threatening.
  E. A *decrease in emotional security* tends to produce an *increase in symptoms.*
  F. When treatment is confined to physical symptoms, emotional problems are *not* usually relieved.

II. Assessment of physiological factors:
  A. Persistent psychological factors may produce structural *organic* changes resulting in *chronic diseases,* which may be *life threatening* if untreated.
  B. *All* body systems are affected:
    1. Skin (e.g., pruritus, acne, dermatitis).
    2. Musculoskeletal (e.g., *backache,* muscle cramps, rheumatoid arthritis).
    3. Respiratory (e.g., *asthma,* hiccups, hay fever).
    4. Gastrointestinal (e.g., *ulcers,* ulcerative colitis, irritable bowel syndrome, heartburn, constipation, diarrhea).
    5. Cardiovascular (e.g., cardiospasm, angina, paroxysmal tachycardia, *migraines,* palpitations, hypertension).
    6. Genitourinary (e.g., impotence, enuresis, amenorrhea, dysuria, *dysmenorrhea*).
    7. Endocrine (e.g., hypoglycemia, hyperglycemia, hyperthyroidism).
    8. Nervous system (e.g., general fatigue, anorexia, exhaustion).

III. Analysis/nursing diagnosis: *ineffective individual coping* related to inappropriate need-gratification

through illness (actual illness used as means of meeting needs for attention and affection). Absence of life experiences that gratify needs for attention and affection.

IV. Nursing care plan/implementation in disorders in which psychological factors affect physical conditions:
  A. *Long-term goal: release* of feelings through verbalization.
  B. *Short-term goals:*
    1. Take care of *physical* problems during acute phase.
    2. *Remove* client from anxiety-producing stimuli.
  C. Prompt attention in meeting clients' *basic needs,* to gratify appropriate needs for dependency, attention, and security.
  D. Maintain an attitude of *respect and concern;* clients' pains and worries are very real and upsetting to them; do *not* belittle the symptoms. Do *not* say, "There is nothing wrong with you" because emotions do in fact cause somatic disabilities.
  E. *Treat organic* problems as necessary, but without undue emphasis (i.e., do *not* reinforce preoccupation with bodily complaints).
  F. Help clients *express their feelings,* especially anger, hostility, guilt, resentment, or humiliation, which may be related to such issues as sexual difficulties, family problems, religious conflicts, and job difficulties. Help clients recognize that when stress and anxiety are not released through some channel such as verbal expression, the body will release the tension through *"organ language."*
  G. Provide *outlets* for release of tensions and diversions from preoccupation with physical complaints.
    1. Provide social and recreational activities to decrease time for preoccupation with illness.
    2. Encourage clients to use physical and intellectual capabilities in constructive ways.
  H. *Protect* clients from any disturbing stimuli; help the healing process in the acute phase of illnesses (e.g., myocardial infarct).
  I. Help clients feel *in control* of situations and be as independent as possible.
  J. Be *supportive;* assist clients to bear painful feelings through a helping relationship.
  K. *Health teaching:*
    1. Teach how to express feelings.
    2. Teach more effective ways of responding to stressful life situations.
    3. Teach the family supportive relationships.

V. Evaluation/outcome criteria: can verbalize feelings more fully.

Schizophrenia and Other Psychotic Disorders

Schizophrenia is a group of interrelated symptoms with a number of common features involving disorders of *mood, thought content, feelings, perception,* and *behavior.* The term means "splitting of the mind," alluding to the discrepancy between the content of *thought processes* and their emotional expression; this should *not* be confused with "multiple personality" (dissociative reaction).

Half of the clients in mental hospitals are diagnosed as schizophrenic; many more with schizophrenic disorder live in the community. The onset of symptoms for this disorder generally occurs between 15 and 27 years of age.

Genetics and neurochemical imbalances of dopamine and serotonin play a significant role in the etiology of schizophrenia. Clients with schizophrenia have larger brain ventricles, and the prefrontal cortex and limbic cortex are not fully developed. Whether the brain structure changes cause the disorder or are a result of the chemical changes that occur with schizophrenia remains unclear. Other causal theories include prenatal exposure to the influenza virus.

I. **Common subtypes of schizophrenia** (without clear-cut differentiation):

disorganized type disordered, thinking ("word salad"), *inappropriate affect* (blunted, silly), regressive behavior, incoherent speech, preoccupied and withdrawn.

catatonic type disorder of muscle tension, with rigidity, *waxy flexibility, posturing, mutism, violent rage* outbursts, negativism, and frenzied activity. Marked decrease in involvement with environment and in spontaneous movement.

paranoid type disturbed perceptions leading to disturbance in thought content of *persecutory, grandiose,* or hostile nature; *projection* is key mechanism, with religion a common preoccupation.

residual continued difficulty in thinking, mood, perception, and behavior after schizophrenic episode.

undifferentiated type unclassifiable schizophrenic-like disturbance with mixed symptoms of delusions, hallucinations, incoherence, gross disorganization.

II. **Concepts and principles related to schizophrenic disorders:**

A. *General:*

1. *Symbolic* language used expresses life, pain, and progress toward health; all symbols used have meaning.
2. *Physical care* provides media for relationship; nurturance may be initial focus.
3. *Consistency, reliability,* and *empathic* understanding build trust.
4. *Denial, regression,* and *projection* are key defense mechanisms.
5. Felt anxiety gives rise to distorted thinking.
6. Attempts to engage in verbal communication may result in tension, apprehensiveness, and defensiveness.
7. Person *rejects real world* of painful experiences and *creates fantasy* world through illness.

B. *Withdrawal:*

1. Withdrawal from and resistance to forming relationships are attempts to reduce anxiety related to:
   a. Loss of ability to experience satisfying human relationships.
   b. Fear of rejection.
   c. Lack of self-confidence.
   d. Need for protection and restraint against potential destructiveness of *hostile* impulses (toward self and others).
2. *Ambivalence* results from need to *approach* a relationship and need to *avoid* it.
   a. Cannot tolerate swift emotional or physical closeness.
   b. Needs more time than usual to establish a relationship; time to test sincerity and interest of nurse.
3. Avoidance of client by others, especially staff, will reinforce withdrawal, thereby creating problem of mutual withdrawal and fear.

C. *Hallucinations:*

1. It is possible to replace hallucinations with satisfying interactions.
2. Person can relearn to focus attention on real things and people.
3. Hallucinations originate during *extreme* emotional stress when unable to cope.
4. Hallucinations are very real to client.
5. Client will react as the situation is perceived, *regardless* of reality or consensus.
6. Concrete experiences, *not* argument or confrontation, will correct sensory distortion.
7. Hallucinations are *substitutes* for human relations.
8. Purposes served by or expressed in falsification of reality:
   a. Reflection of problem in inner life.
   b. Statement of criticism, censure, self-punishment.
   c. Promotion of self-esteem.
   d. Satisfaction of instinctual strivings.
   e. Projection of unacceptable unconscious content in disguised form.
9. Perceptions *not* as *totally* disturbed as they seem.
10. Client attempts to restructure reality through hallucinations to *protect remaining ego integrity.*
11. Hallucinations may result from a variety of psychological and biological conditions (e.g., extreme fatigue, drugs, pyrexia, organic brain disease).
12. Person who hallucinates needs to feel free to describe his or her perceptions if he or she is to be understood by the nurse.

III. **Assessment of schizophrenic disorders:**

A. Some clinicians prefer to describe signs and symptoms of schizophrenia as "positive" or "negative."

1. "**Positive**" **symptoms**: reflect an *excess* or distortion of normal functions; are associated with *normal* brain structures on CT scans, with *relatively good* responses to treatment.
   a. *Delusions* (see definitions in **B.** following)
      (1) Persecution.
      (2) Grandeur.
      (3) Ideas of reference.
      (4) Somatic.

b. *Hallucinations* (see descriptions in **B.** following)
   (1) Auditory.
   (2) Visual.
   (3) Olfactory.
   (4) Gustatory.
   (5) Tactile.
c. *Disorganized thinking/speech* (see descriptions in **B.** following)
   (1) Associative looseness.
   (2) Clang associations.
   (3) Word salad.
   (4) Incoherence.
   (5) Neologisms.
   (6) Concrete thinking.
   (7) Echolalia.
   (8) Tangentiality.
   (9) Circumstantiality.
d. *Disorganized behavior*
   (1) Appearance: disheveled.
   (2) Behavior: restless agitated; inappropriate sexual behavior.
   (3) Waxy flexibility.

2. **"Negative" symptoms: four A's** reflect a loss or diminuition of normal functions; CT scans often show structural brain abnormalities, with poor response to treatment.
   a. **A**ffective flattening
      (1) Facial expression: unchanged.
      (2) Eye contact: poor.
      (3) Body language: reduced.
      (4) Emotional expression: diminished.
      (5) Affect: inappropriate.
   b. **A**logia (poverty of speech)
      (1) Responses: brief, empty.
      (2) Speech: decreased content and fluency.
   c. **A**volition/**A**pathy
      (1) Grooming/hygiene: impaired.
      (2) Activities: little or no interest (in work or other activities).
      (3) Inability to initiate goal-oriented actions.
   d. **A**nhedonia
      (1) Absence of pleasure in social activities.
      (2) Diminished interest in intimacy/sexual activities.
   e. *Social withdrawal* (see **C.** following)

B. Eugene Bleuler described four classic and primary symptoms as the **"four A's"**:
   1. *Associative looseness*—impairment of logical thought progression, resulting in confused, bizarre, and abrupt thinking. *Neologisms*—making up new words or condensing words into one.
   2. *Affect*—exaggerated, apathetic, blunt, flat, inappropriate, inconsistent feeling tone that is communicated through face and body posture.
   3. *Ambivalence*—simultaneous, conflicting feelings or attitudes toward person, object, or situation; *need-fear dilemma.*
      a. Stormy outbursts.
      b. Poor, weak interpersonal relations.
      c. Difficulty even with simple decisions.

4. *Autism—withdrawal* from external world; preoccupation with fantasies and idiosyncratic thoughts.
   a. *Delusions*—false, fixed beliefs, not corrected by logic; a defense against intolerable feeling. The two most common delusions are:
      (1) *Delusions of grandeur*—conviction in a belief related to being famous, important, or wealthy.
      (2) *Delusions of persecution*—belief that one's thoughts, moods, or actions are controlled or influenced by strange forces or by others.
   b. *Hallucinations*—false sensory impressions without observable external stimuli.
      (1) *Auditory*—affecting hearing (e.g., hears voices).
      (2) *Visual*—affecting vision (e.g., sees snakes).
      (3) *Tactile*—affecting touch (e.g., feels electric charges in body).
      (4) *Olfactory*—affecting smell (e.g., smells rotting flesh).
      (5) *Gustatory*—affecting taste (e.g., food tastes like poison).
   c. *Ideas of reference*—clients interpret cues in the environment as having reference to them. Ideas *symbolize guilt, insecurity,* and *alienation;* may become delusions, if severe.
   d. *Depersonalization*—feelings of strangeness and unreality about self or environment or both; difficulty in differentiating boundaries between self and environment.

C. *Prodromal or residual symptoms:*
   1. Social isolation, *withdrawal; regression:* **extreme withdrawal** and social isolation.
   2. Marked impairment in *role* functioning (e.g., as student, employee).
   3. Markedly *peculiar* behavior (e.g., collecting garbage).
   4. Marked impairment in personal *hygiene.*
   5. *Affect:* blunt, inappropriate.
   6. *Speech:* vague, overelaborate, circumstantial, metaphorical.
   7. *Thinking:* bizarre ideation or magical thinking (e.g., ideas of reference, "others can feel my feelings").
   8. Unusual *perceptual* experiences (e.g., sensing the presence of a force or person not physically there).

D. Rule out general medical conditions/substances that may cause psychotic symptoms.
   1. *Neurological* conditions: neoplasms, cardiovascular disease, epilepsy, Huntington's disease, deafness, migraine headaches, CNS infections.
   2. *Endocrine* conditions: hypothyroidism or hyperthyroidism, hypoparathyroidism or hyperparathyroidism, hypoadrenocorticism.
   3. *Metabolic* conditions: hypoxia, hypoglycemia, hypercarbia.
   4. *Autoimmune* disorders: SLE.

5. *Other conditions:* hepatic or renal disease.
6. *Substances: drugs of abuse* (alcohol, amphetamines, cannabis, cocaine, hallucinogens, inhalants); anesthetics; chemotherapeutic agents; corticosteroids; *toxins* (nerve gases, carbon monoxide, carbon dioxide, fuel or paint, insecticides).

◆ **IV. Analysis/nursing diagnosis:**

A. *Sensory/perceptual alterations* related to inability to define reality and distinguish the real from the unreal (hallucinations, illusions) and misinterpretation of stimuli, disintegration of ego boundaries.

B. *Altered thought processes* related to intense anxiety and blocking (delusions), ambivalence or conflict.

C. *Risk for violence to self or others* related to fear and distortion of reality.

D. *Altered communication process* with inability to *verbally* express needs and wishes related to difficulty with processing information and unique patterns of speech.

E. *Self-care deficit* with *inappropriate* dress and poor physical hygiene related to perceptual or cognitive impairment or immobility.

F. *Altered feeling states* related to anxiety about others (*inappropriate emotions*).

G. *Altered judgment* related to lack of trust, fear of rejection, and doubts regarding competence of others.

H. *Altered self-concept* related to *feelings of inadequacy* in coping with the real world.

I. *Body-image disturbance* related to inappropriate use of defense mechanisms.

J. *Disorganized behaviors:* impaired relatedness to others, related to withdrawal, distortions of reality, and lack of trust.

K. *Diversional activity deficit* related to personal ambivalence.

◆ **V. Nursing care plan/implementation in schizophrenic disorders:**

A. *General:*
1. Set *short-term* goals, realistic to client's levels of functioning.
2. Use *nonverbal* level of communication to demonstrate concern, caring, and warmth, because client often distrusts words.
3. Set climate for free expression of *feelings* in whatever mode, without fear of retaliation, ridicule, or rejection.
4. Seek client out in his or her own fantasy world.
5. Try to understand meaning of symbolic language; help him or her communicate less symbolically.
6. Provide *distance,* because client needs to feel safe and to observe nurses for sources of threat or promises of security.
7. Help client tolerate nurses' presence and learn to *trust* nurses enough to move out of isolation and share painful and often unacceptable (to client) feelings and thoughts.
8. Anticipate and accept negativism; do *not* personalize.

9. *Avoid* joking, abstract terms, and figures of speech when client's thinking is literal.
10. Give antipsychotic medications.

B. *Withdrawn behavior:*
1. *Long-term goal:* develop satisfying interpersonal relationships.
2. *Short-term goal:* help client feel safe in *one-to-one* relationship.
3. Seek client out at every chance, and establish some bond.
   a. Stay with client, in silence.
   b. Initiate talk when he or she is ready.
   c. Draw out, but do *not* demand, response.
   d. Do *not* avoid the client.
4. Use *simple language, specific words.*
5. Use an *object or activity* as medium for relationship; initiate activity.
6. Focus on *everyday* experiences.
7. *Delay* decision making.
8. *Accept one-sided* conversation, with silence from the client; *avoid* pressuring to respond.
9. Accept the client's outward attempts to respond and inappropriate social behavior, without remarks or disdain; teach social skills.
10. *Avoid* making demands on client or exposing client to failure.
11. *Protect* from persons who are aggressive and from impulsive attacks on self and others.
12. Attend to *nutrition, elimination, exercise,* hygiene, and signs of physical illness.
13. Add structure to the day; tell him or her, "This is your 9 A.M. medication."
14. *Health teaching:* assist family to understand client's needs, to see small sign of progress; teach client to perform simple tasks of self-care to meet own biological needs.

C. *Hallucinatory behavior:*
1. *Long-term goal:* establish satisfying relationships with *real* persons.
2. *Short-term goal:* interrupt *pattern* of hallucinations.
3. Provide a *structured* environment with routine activities. Use *real* objects to keep client's interest or to stimulate new interest (e.g., in painting or crafts).
4. *Protect* against injury to self and others resulting from "voices" client thinks he or she hears.
5. *Short, frequent* contacts initially, increasing social interaction gradually (one person → small groups).
6. Ask person to describe experiences as hallucinations occur.
7. *Respond to anything real* the client says (e.g., with acknowledgment or reflection). Focus more on *feelings,* not on delusional, hallucinatory content.
8. *Distract* client's attention to something real when he or she hallucinates.
9. *Avoid* direct confrontation that voices are coming from client himself or herself; do *not* argue, but listen.

10. *Clarify* who "they" are:
    a. Use personal pronouns, *avoid* universal and global pronouns.
    b. Nurse's own language must be clear and unambiguous.
11. Use one sentence, ask only one question, at a time.
12. Encourage *consensual validation*. Point out that experience is not shared by you; voice doubt.
13. *Health teaching:*
    a. Recommend more effective ways of coping (e.g., consensual validation).
    b. Advise that highly emotional situations be avoided.
    c. Explain the causes of misperceptions.
    d. Recommend methods for reducing sensory stimulation.

D. *Delusions* (see **IV. Nursing care plan/implementation in paranoid disorders**, in following section p. 438).

◆ **VI. Evaluation/outcome criteria:**
  A. Small behavioral changes occur (e.g., eye contact, better grooming).
  B. Evidence of beginning trust in nurse (keeping appointments).
  C. Initiates conversation with others; participates in activities.
  D. Decreases amount of time spent alone.
  E. Demonstrates appropriate behavior in public places.
  F. Articulates relationship between feelings of discomfort and autistic behavior.
  G. Makes positive statements.

VII. See sample **Clinical Pathway 6.4: Client with Schizophrenic Psychosis.**

CLINICAL PATHWAY 6.4: Client with Schizophrenic Psychosis

Estimated length of stay: 14 days—variations from designated pathway should be documented in progress notes

◆ Nursing Diagnosis and Categories of Care	Time Dimension	Goals/Actions	Time Dimension	Goals/Actions	Time Dimension	Discharge Outcome
Alteration in thought processes/ sensory-perceptual alteration			Day 7	Client is able to differentiate between what is real and what is not.	Day 14	Client experiences no delusional thinking or hallucinations.
Referrals	Day 1	Psychiatrist Psychologist Social worker Clinical nurse specialist Music therapist Occupational therapist Recreational therapist			Day 14	Discharge with follow-up appointments as required.
Diagnostic studies	Day 1	Drug screen				
	Day 3–5	CT, MRI, PET, EEG (may be ordered to examine structure and function of the brain)				
◆ Additional assessments	Day 1	VS every shift Assess for:	Day 2–14	Ongoing assessments.	Day 2–14	VS daily if stable.
		■ Delusions ■ Hallucinations ■ Loose associations ■ Inappropriate affect ■ Excitement/stupor ■ Panic anxiety ■ Suspiciousness	Day 2–5	Establish trust with at least one person.	Day 14	No evidence of: delusions, hallucinations, loose associations, inappropriate affect, excitement/stupor, panic anxiety, suspiciousness.

(Continued on following page)

Mental Health

Nursing Diagnosis and Categories of Care	Time Dimension	Goals/Actions	Time Dimension	Goals/Actions	Time Dimension	Discharge Outcome
Medications	Day 1	Antipsychotic medication (scheduled and prn); may need order for concentrate and injectable form Antiparkinsonian medication prn	Day 1–14	Assess for effectiveness and side effects of medications.	Day 14	Client is discharged with medications.
Client education			Day 7	Discuss correlation between increased anxiety and psychotic symptoms. Discuss ways to deescalate anxiety.	Day 12–13	Reinforce teaching.
			Day 10	Discuss importance of taking medications regularly, even when feeling well. Discuss possible side effects of medications and when to see the doctor.	Day 14	Client verbalizes understanding information presented before charge.
Risk for violence: Self-directed or directed at others	Day 1	Environment safe for client and others	Ongoing	Client does not harm self or others.	Day 14	Client is discharged without harm to self or others.
Referrals	Day 1	Alert hostility management team for the admission of a client who is potentially violent For relaxation therapy: Music therapist Clinical nurse specialist Stress management specialist Psychiatrist: May give order for mechanical restraints to be used if needed			Day 14	Discharge with follow-up, appointments as required.
Additional assessments	Day 1	Assess for signs of impending violent behaviors: ▪ Increase in psychomotor activity ▪ Angry affect ▪ Verbalized persecutory delusions or frightening hallucinations.	Day 2–14	Ongoing assessments.		

Mental Health

(Continued on following page)

CLINICAL PATHWAY 6.4: Client with Schizophrenic Psychosis *(Continued)*

Nursing Diagnosis and Categories of Care	Time Dimension	Goals/Actions	Time Dimension	Goals/Actions	Time Dimension	Discharge Outcome
Medications	Day 1	Antipsychotic medications, prn, when signs of agitation begin	Day 1–14	Use of medications, isolation/seclusion, or mechanical restraints. If client refuses medications, administer meds after application of restraints.	Day 14	Client is discharged with medications.
Client education			Day 3–12	Teach relaxation techniques; discuss activities in which client could participate to relieve pent-up tension. Discuss signs and symptoms of escalating anxiety.	Day 12–13 Day 14	Reinforce teaching. Client verbalizes understanding of information presented before discharge.

Source: Townsend, M: Essentials of Psychiatric–Mental Health Nursing. FA Davis, Philadelphia.
CT, computed tomography, *EEG,* electroencephalogram; *MRI,* magnetic resonance imaging; *PET,* positron–emission tomography.

Delusional (Paranoid) Disorders

Paranoid disorders have a concrete and pervasive delusional system, usually *persecutory. Projection* is a chief defense mechanism of this disorder.

I. **Concepts and principles related to paranoid disorders:**
   A. Delusions are attempts to cope with stresses and problems.
   B. May be a means of allegorical or symbolic communication and of testing others for their trustworthiness.
   C. Interactions with others and activities interrupt delusional thinking.
   D. To establish a rational therapeutic relationship, gross distortions, misorientation, misinterpretation, and misidentification need to be overcome.
   E. People with delusions have extreme need to maintain self-esteem.
   F. False beliefs cannot be changed without first changing experiences.
   G. A delusion is held because it *performs a function.*
   H. When people who are experiencing delusions become at ease and comfortable with people, delusions will not be needed.
   I. Delusions are misjudgments of reality based on a series of mental mechanisms: (a) *denial,* followed by (b) *projection* and (c) *rationalization.*
   J. There is a *kernel of truth* in delusions.
   K. Behind the anger and suspicion in a person who is paranoid, there is a person who is *lonely* and *terrified* and who *feels vulnerable* and *inadequate.*

II. **Assessment** of paranoid disorders:
   A. Chronically *suspicious,* distrustful (thinks "people are out to get me").
   B. Distant, but *not* withdrawn.
   C. Poor insight; blames others *(projects).*
   D. Misinterprets and *distorts reality.*
   E. Difficulty in admitting own errors; takes pride in intelligence and in being correct (superiority).
   F. Maintains false persecutory belief despite evidence or proof (may refuse food and medicine, insisting they are poisoned).
   G. Literal thinking *(rigid).*
   H. Dominating and provocative.
   I. Hypercritical and intolerant of others; *hostile,* quarrelsome, and aggressive.
   J. *Very sensitive* in perceiving minor injustices, errors, and contradictions.
   K. Evasive.

III. **Analysis/nursing diagnosis:**
   A. *Altered thought processes* related to lack of insight, conflict, increased fear and anxiety.
   B. *Severe anxiety* related to projection of threatening, aggressive impulses and misinterpretation of stimuli.
   C. *Ineffective individual coping* (misuse of power and force) related to lack of trust, fear of close human contact.
   D. *Impaired cognitive functioning* related to rigidity of thought.
   E. *Chronic low self-esteem* related to feelings of inadequacy, powerlessness.
   F. *Impaired social interaction* related to lack of tender, kind feelings, feelings of grandiosity or persecution.

IV. **Nursing care plan/implementation** in paranoid disorders:
   A. *Long-term goals:* gain clear, correct perceptions and interpretations through corrective experiences.
   B. *Short-term goals:*

1. Help client recognize distortions, misinterpretations.
2. Help client feel safe in exploring reality.

C. Help client learn to *trust self;* help to develop self-confidence and ego assets through positive reinforcement.

D. Help to *trust others.*
   1. Be consistent and honest at all times.
   2. *Do not whisper, act secretive, or laugh with others* in client's presence when he or she cannot hear what is said.
   3. Do *not* mix medicines with food.
   4. Keep promises.
   5. Let client know ahead of time what he or she can expect from others.
   6. Give *reasons* and careful, complete, and *repetitive* explanations.
   7. Ask permission to contact others.
   8. Consult client first about all decisions concerning him or her.

E. Help to *test reality.*
   1. Present and repeat reality of the situation.
   2. Do *not* confirm or approve distortions.
   3. Help accept responsibility for own behavior rather than project.
   4. *Divert* from delusions to reality-centered focus.
   5. Let client know when behavior does not seem appropriate.
   6. Assume nothing and leave no room for assumptions.
   7. *Structure* time and activities to limit delusional thought, behavior.
   8. Set limit for *not* discussing delusional content.
   9. Look for underlying needs expressed in delusional content.

F. Provide *outlets* for anger and aggressive drives.
   1. Listen matter-of-factly to angry outbursts.
   2. *Accept* rebuffs and abusive talk as symptoms.
   3. *Do not* argue, disagree, or debate.
   4. *Allow* expression of negative feelings without fear of punishment.

G. Provide *successful group experience.*
   1. *Avoid competitive* sports involving *close physical* contact.
   2. Give recognition to skills and work well done.
   3. Use *managerial* talents.
   4. Respect client's intellect and engage him or her in activities with others requiring *intellect* (e.g., chess, puzzles, Scrabble).

H. *Limit* physical contact.

I. *Health teaching:* teach a more rational basis for deciding whom to trust by identifying behaviors characteristic of trusting and people who are trustworthy.

◆ **V. Evaluation/outcome criteria:** able to differentiate people who are trustworthy from untrustworthy; growing self-awareness, and able to share this awareness with others; accepting of others without need to criticize or change them; is open to new experiences; able to delay gratification.

Personality Disorders

Subtypes of personality disorders include *borderline, paranoid, schizoid, schizotypal, obsessive-compulsive, antisocial, histrionic, narcissistic, avoidant,* and *dependent personalities.* A *personality disorder* is a syndrome in which the person's inner difficulties are revealed through general behaviors and by a pattern of living that seeks *immediate gratification of impulses* and instinctual needs without regard to society's laws, mores, and customs and *without censorship* of personal conscience. *Borderline* and *antisocial personality* disorders are the most significant in interactions with the nurse.

Borderline personality disorder is a subtype in which the client is unstable in many areas: she or he has unstable but intense interpersonal relationships, *impulsive* and unpredictable behavior, wide *mood swings,* chronic feelings of boredom or emptiness, intolerance of being alone, and uncertainty about identity, and is physically *self-damaging.*

I. **Concepts and principles related to** antisocial personality disorders:
   A. One defense against severe anxiety is "acting out," or dealing with distressful feelings or issues through action.
   B. Faulty or arrested emotional development in preoedipal period has interfered with development of adequate social control or superego.
   C. Because there is a malfunctioning or *weakened superego,* there is little internal demand and therefore no tension between ego and superego to evoke guilt feelings.
   D. The defect is *not* intellectual; person shows *lack of moral responsibility, inability to control emotions* and impulses, and *deficiency in normal feeling* responses.
   E. "Pleasure principle" is dominant.
   F. Initial stage of treatment is most crucial; treatment situation is very threatening because it mobilizes client's anxiety, and client ends treatment abruptly. Key underlying emotion: *fear of closeness,* with threat of *exploitation, control,* and *abandonment.*

◆ II. **Assessment** of antisocial personality disorders:
   A. Onset *before* age 15.
   B. History of behavior that *conflicts with society:* truancy, expulsion, or suspension from school for misconduct; delinquency, thefts, vandalism, running away from home; persistent lying; repeated substance abuse; initiating fights; chronic violation of rules at home or school; school grades below IQ level.
   C. Inability to sustain consistent *work* behavior (e.g., frequent job changes or absenteeism).
   D. Lack of ability to function as parent who is *responsible* (evidence of child's malnutrition or illness due to lack of minimal hygiene standards; failure to obtain medical care for child who is seriously ill; failure to arrange for caregiver when parent is away from home).
   E. Failure to accept *social norms* with respect to *lawful* behavior (e.g., thefts, multiple arrests).
   F. Inability to maintain enduring *intimate* relationship (e.g., multiple relations, desertion, multiple divorces); lack of respect or loyalty.

G. *Irritability* and *aggressiveness* (spouse, child abuse; repeated physical fights).

H. Failure to honor *financial* obligations.

I. Failure to *plan ahead.*

J. *Disregard for truth* (lying, "conning" others for personal gain).

K. *Recklessness* (driving while intoxicated, recurrent speeding).

L. *Violating* rights of others.

M. Does not appear to profit from experience; *repeats* same punishable or antisocial behavior; usually does not feel guilt or depression.

N. Exhibits *poor judgment;* may have intellectual, but not emotional, insight to guide judgments. Inadequate problem solving and reality testing.

O. Uses *manipulative* behavior patterns in treatment setting (see **VIII. Manipulation, p. 386**).
   1. Demands and controls.
   2. Pressures and coerces, threatens.
   3. Violates rules, routines, procedures.
   4. Requests special privileges.
   5. Betrays confidences and lies.
   6. Ingratiates.
   7. Monopolizes conversation.

◆ III. **Analysis/nursing diagnosis** in personality disorders:

A. *Ineffective individual coping* related to:
   1. Inability to tolerate frustration (altered conduct/impulse processes).
   2. Verbal, nonverbal manipulation *(lying).*
   3. Destructive behavior toward self (e.g., in borderline personality disorder) or others.
   4. Cognitive distortions (e.g., overuse of denial, projection, rationalization, intellectualization, persecutory thoughts).
   5. Inability to learn from experience.

B. *Personal identity disturbance* related to:
   1. *Self-esteem disturbance* as evidenced by grandiosity, depression, extreme mood changes.
   2. Lack of: responsibility, accountability, commitment, tolerance of rejection.
   3. Distancing relationships.

C. *Social intrusiveness* related to fear of real or potential loss.

D. *Noncompliance* related to excess need for independence.

◆ IV. **Nursing care plan/implementation** in personality disorders:

A. *Long-term goal:* help person accept responsibility and consequences of own actions.

B. *Short-term goal: minimize manipulation* and acting out.

C. Set *fair, firm, consistent limits and follow through on consequences* of behavior; let client know what she or he can expect from staff and what the unit's regulations are, as well as the consequences of violations. Be explicit.

D. *Avoid* letting staff be played against one another by a particular client; staff should present a unified approach.

E. Nurses should *control* their *own* feelings of anger and defensiveness aroused by any person's manipulative behavior.

F. Change focus when client persists in raising inappropriate subjects (such as personal life of a nurse).

G. Encourage expression of *feelings* as an alternative to acting out.

H. Aid client in realizing and accepting responsibility for own actions and *social responsibility* to others.

I. Use group therapy as a means of *peer control* and multiple feedback about behavior.

J. *Health teaching:* teach family how to use behavior-modification techniques to reward client's acceptable behavior (i.e., when he or she accepts responsibility for own behavior, is responsive to rights of others, adheres to social and legal norms).

◆ V. **Evaluation/outcome criteria:** less use of lying, blaming others for own behavior; more evidence of following rules; less impulsive, explosive behavior.

Mood Disorders

Mood disorders include (1) *depressive disorders* and (2) *bipolar disorders.* Bipolar disorders are further divided into (a) *manic,* (b) *depressed,* (c) *mixed,* or (d) *cyclothymia.* The mood disturbance may occur in a number of patterns of severity and duration, alone or in combination, where client feels extreme sadness and guilt, withdraws socially, expresses self-deprecatory thoughts *(major depression),* or experiences an elevated, expansive mood with hyperactivity, pressured speech, inflated self-esteem, and decreased need for sleep *(manic episode or disorder).*

Another specific mood disorder is *dysthymic* disorder (depressive neuroses), in which there is a chronic mood disturbance involving a depressed mood or loss of interest and pleasure in all usual activities, but not of sufficient severity or duration to be classified as a *major depressive episode.* **Table 6.13** *summarizes* the main points of *difference between the two types of depression.*

These affective disorders should be *distinguished from grief.* Grief is *realistic* and proportionate to what has been *specifically* lost and involves *no loss of self-esteem.* There is a *constant* feeling of sadness over a period of 3–12 mo or longer, with good reality contact (no delusions).

Major Depressive Disorder

I. **Concepts and principles:**

A. Self-limiting factors—most depressions are self-limiting disturbances, making it important to look for a change in functioning and behavior.

B. *Theories of cause of depression:*
   1. Aggression turned inward—*self-anger.*
   2. Response to separation or object *loss.*
   3. *Genetic* or *neurochemical* basis—impaired neurotransmission system, especially serotonin regulation.
   4. *Cognitive*—negative mindset of hopelessness toward self, world, future; overgeneralizes; focuses on single detail rather than whole picture; draws conclusions on inadequate evidence.

TABLE 6.13	Comparison of the Two Different Types of Depressive Disorders	
Dimension	**Major Depressive Disorder—Melancholic Type**	**Dysthymic Disorder**
Cause	Primary disturbance in structure and function of brain and nervous system	Severe, prolonged stress, unresolved conflicts; chronic anxiety, fears, anger
Onset	Rapid and *without* apparent cause	Gradual
Form of depression	Restlessness and agitation, *or* psychomotor retardation; severe; tends to be *worse in morning* and better in evening	Mixed; mild to severe; unpredictable mood; usually optimistic in morning and *depressed in evening*
Sleep	Insomnia after being awakened; early-morning awakening	Easily awakened, but goes back to deep sleep in morning
Appetite	Anorexia leading to weight *loss*	Varied (anorexia leading to compulsive eating)
Activity	Chronically tired; needs structure at all times	Occasional energy bursts (feels embarrassed at lack of energy)
Self-esteem	Very low	Fluctuates from high to low
Fears	Intense fear of being alone	Multiple fears about present and future
Decision making	Totally indecisive	OK on minor decisions; indecisive on important decisions
Memory	Poor	Unreliable
Contact with reality	Poor; paranoid, self-deprecatory delusions, distorted judgment	Varies

5. *Personality*—negative self-concept, low self-esteem affects belief system and appraisal of stressors; ambivalence, guilt, feeling of failure.
6. *Learned helplessness*—dependency; environment cannot be controlled; powerlessness.
7. *Behavioral*—loss of positive reinforcement; lack of support system.
8. *Integrated*—interaction of chemical, experiential, and behavioral variables acting on diencephalon.

◆ **II. General assessment:**
  A. *Physical:* early-morning awakening, *insomnia* at night, increased need for sleep during the day, fatigue, constipation, *anorexia* with weight loss, loss of sexual interest, *psychomotor retardation*, physical complaints, amenorrhea.
  B. *Psychological:* inability to remember, decreased *concentration,* slowing or blocking of thought, all-or-nothing thinking, *less interest in* and involvement with external world and own appearance, feeling worse at certain times of day or after any sleep, difficulty in enjoying activities, monotonous voice, *repetitive* discussions, *inability to make decisions* due to ambivalence, impaired coping with "practical problems."
  C. *Emotional:* loss of self-esteem, feelings of *hopelessness* and *worthlessness,* shame and self-derogation due to *guilt, irritability,* despair and *futility* (leading to *suicidal* thoughts), alienation, *helplessness,* passivity, avoidance, *inertia,* powerlessness, denied anger; uncooperative, tense, crying, demanding, and *dependent* behavior.

◆ **III. Analysis/nursing diagnosis:**
  A. *Risk for violence* toward self (suicide) related to inability to verbalize emotions.
  B. *Sleep pattern disturbance* (insomnia or excessive sleep) related to unresolved fears and anxieties, biochemical alterations (decreased serotonin).
  C. *Impaired social interaction/social isolation/withdrawal* related to decreased energy/inertia, inadequate personal resources, absence of significant purpose in life.
  D. *Altered nutrition* (anorexia) related to lack of interest in food.
  E. *Self-care deficit* related to disinterest in activities of daily living.
  F. *Chronic low self-esteem* with self-reproaches and blame related to feelings of inadequacy.
  G. *Altered feeling states and meaning patterns* (sadness, loneliness, apathy) related to overwhelming feeling of unworthiness, hopelessness, and *dysfunctional grieving.*

◆ **IV. Nursing care plan/implementation:**
  A. Promote sleep and food intake: take nursing measures to ensure the *physical* well-being of the client.
  B. Provide steady company to assess *suicidal* tendencies and to diminish feelings of loneliness and alienation.
    1. Build trust in a one-to-one relationship.
    2. Interact with client on a nonverbal level if that is his or her immediate mode of communication; this will promote feelings of being recognized, accepted, and understood.
    3. Focus on *today,* not the past or far into the future.

4. Reassure that present state is temporary and that he or she will be protected and helped.

C. Make the *environment* nonchallenging and non-threatening.
   1. Use a kind, firm attitude, with warmth.
   2. See that client has favorite foods; respond to other wishes and likes.
   3. Protect from overstimulation and coercion.

D. Postpone client's *decision making* and resumption of duties.
   1. Allow *more time* than usual to complete activity (dressing, eating) or thought process and speech.
   2. Structure the environment for client to help reestablish a set schedule and predictable *routine* during ambivalence and problems with decisions.

E. *Provide nonintellectual activities* (e.g., sanding wood); *avoid* activities such as chess and crossword puzzles, because thinking capacity at this time tends to be circular.

F. Encourage expression of emotions: denial, hopelessness, helplessness, guilt, regret; provide *outlets for anger* that may be underlying the depression; as client becomes more verbal with anger and recognizes the origin and results of anger, help client resolve feelings—allow client to complain and be *demanding* in initial phases of depression.

G. Discourage *redundancy in speech and thought*: redirect focus from a monologue of painful recounts to an appraisal of more neutral or positive attributes and aspects of situations.

H. Encourage client to *assess own* goals, unrealistic expectations, and perfectionist tendencies.
   1. May need to change goals or give up some goals that are incompatible with abilities and external situations.
   2. Assist client to recapture what was lost through substitution of goals, sublimation, or relinquishment of unrealistic goals—reanchor client's self-respect to other aspects of his or her existence; help him or her free self from *dependency* on one person or single event or idea.

I. Indicate that success is possible and not hopeless.
   1. Explore what steps client has taken to achieve goals and suggest new or alternative ones.
   2. Set *small, immediate goals* to help attain mastery.
   3. Recognize client's efforts to mobilize self.
   4. Provide positive reinforcement for client through exposure to activities in which client can experience a sense of *success, achievement, and completion* to build *self-esteem* and self-confidence.
   5. Help client experience *pleasure*; help client start good relationships in social setting.

J. *Long-term goal*: to encourage interest in external surroundings, outside of self, to increase and strengthen social relationships.
   1. Encourage purposeful activities.
   2. Let client advance to activities at own pace (graded task assignments).
   3. Gradually encourage activities with others.

K. *Health teaching*: explain need to recognize highly stressful situation and fatigue as stress factor; advise that negative responses from others be regarded with minimum significance; explain need to maintain positive self-attitude; advise occasional respite from responsibilities; emphasize need for realistic expectation of others.

◆ V. **Evaluation/outcome criteria:** performs self-care; expresses increased self-confidence; engages in activities with others; accepts positive statements from others; identifies positive attributes and skills in self.

VI. See sample **Clinical Pathway 6.5: Client who is Depressed.**

Bipolar Disorders

Bipolar disorders are major emotional illnesses characterized by mood swings, alternating from depression to elation, with periods of relative normality between episodes. Most persons experience a *single* episode of manic or depressed type; some have *recurrent* depression or recurrent mania or *mixed*. There is increasing evidence that a biochemical disturbance may exist and that most individuals with manic episodes eventually develop depressive episodes.

I. **Concepts and principles related to bipolar disorders:**
   A. The psychodynamics of manic and depressive episodes are related to hostility and guilt.
   B. The struggle between unconscious impulses and moral conscience produces feelings of *hostility, guilt,* and *anxiety.*
   C. To relieve the internal discomfort of these reactions, the person *projects* long-retained hostile feelings onto others or onto objects in the environment during *manic* phase; during *depressive* phase, hostility and guilt are *introjected* toward self.
   D. Demands, irritability, sarcasm, profanity, destructiveness, and threats are signs of the *projection of hostility;* guilt is handled through *persecutory delusions and accusations.*
   E. Feelings of inferiority and fear of rejection are handled by being light and amusing.
   F. Both phases, though appearing distinctly different, have the *same objective: to gain attention, approval, and emotional support.* These objectives and behaviors are unconsciously determined by the client; this behavior may be either biochemically determined or *both biochemically* and *unconsciously* determined.

◆ II. **Assessment** of bipolar disorders:
   A. Manic and depressed types are *opposite* sides of the *same* disorder.
      1. Both are disturbances of mood and self-esteem.
      2. Both have underlying aggression and hostility.
      3. Both are intense.
      4. Both are self-limited in duration.
   B. Comparison of behaviors associated with mania and depression (**Table 6.14**).

(*Text continued on page 445*)

CLINICAL PATHWAY 6.5: Client who is Depressed

Estimated length of stay: 14 days—variations from designated pathway should be documented in progress notes

Nursing Diagnosis and Categories of Care	Time Dimension	Goals/Actions	Time Dimension	Goals/Actions	Time Dimension	Discharge Outcome
Risk for self-directed violence	Day 1	Environment safe for client	Ongoing	Client does not harm self.	Day 14	Client is discharged without harm to self.
Referrals	Day 1	Psychiatrist: May give order to isolate if risk is great or may do ECT For relaxation therapy: Music therapist Clinical nurse specialist Stress management specialist			Day 14	Discharge with follow-up appointments required.
◆ Additional assessments	Day 1	Suicidal assessment: ▪ Ideation ▪ Gestures ▪ Threats ▪ Plan ▪ Means ▪ Anxiety level ▪ Thought disorder	Day 2–14	Ongoing assessments.	Day 14	Client discharged. Denies suicidal ideations.
	Day 1	Secure no-suicide contract				
Medications	Day 1	Antidepressant medication, as ordered Antianxiety agents, prn	Day 1–14	Assess for effectiveness and side effects of medications. Be alert for sudden lifts in mood.	Day 14	Discharged with antidepressant medications.
Client education	Day 3–12	Teach relaxation techniques Discuss resources outside the hospital from whom client may seek assistance when feeling suicidal	Day 12–13	Reinforce teaching.	Day 14	Discharge with understanding of instruction given.
Dysfunctional grieving	Day 1	Assess stage of fixation in grief process			Day 14	Discharge with evidence of progression toward resolution of grief.
Referrals	Day 1	Psychiatrist Psychologist Social worker Clinical nurse specialist Music therapist Occupational therapist Recreational therapist Chaplain			Day 14	Discharge with follow-up appointments required.

Mental Health

(Continued on following page)

CLINICAL PATHWAY 6.5:   Client who is Depressed *(Continued)*

Nursing Diagnosis and Categories of Care	Time Dimension	Goals/Actions	Time Dimension	Goals/Actions	Time Dimension	Discharge Outcome
Diagnostic studies	Day 1 Day 2–3	Any of the following tests *may* be ordered: ■ Drug screen ■ Urine test for norepinephrine and serotonin ■ Dexamethasone suppression test ■ A measure of TSH response to administered TRH ■ Serum and urine studies for nutritional deficiencies				
Medications	Day 1	Antidepressant medication, as ordered Antianxiety agent, prn	Day 1–14	Assess for effectiveness and side effects of medications.	Day 14	Client is discharged with medications.
Diet	Day 1	If antidepressant medication is MAO inhibitor: *low tyramine*			Day 14	Client has experienced no symptoms of hypertensive crisis.
Additional assessments	Day 1	VS every shift Assess: ■ Mental status ■ Mood, affect ■ Thought disorder ■ Communication patterns ■ Level of interest in environment ■ Participation in activities ■ Weight	Day 2–14	VS daily if stable. Ongoing assessments.	Day 14	Mood and affect appropriate. No evidence of thought disorder. Participates willingly and appropriately in activities.
Client education	Day 1	Orient to unit	Day 8	Discuss importance of taking medications regularly even when feeling well or if feeling medication is not helping. Discuss possible side effects of medication and when to see the physician. Teach which foods to eliminate from diet if taking MAO inhibitor.	Day 14	Client is discharged. Verbalizes understanding of information presented before discharge.
			Day 12–13	Reinforce teaching.		

Source: Townsend, M: Essentials of Psychiatric-Mental Health Nursing. F A Davis, Philadelphia.

Mental Health

TABLE 6.14	Behaviors Associated with Mania and Depression

Mania (Periods of Predominantly and Persistently Elevated, Expansive, or Irritable Mood)	Depression (Loss of Interest or Pleasure in Usual Activities)
Affect Lack of shame or guilt; inflated self-esteem; euphoria; intolerance of criticism	Anger, anxiety, apathy, denial, delusions of guilt, helplessness, feelings of doom, hopelessness, loneliness, low self-esteem (self-degradation)
Physiology Insomnia; inadequate nutrition, weight loss	Insomnia; anorexia, constipation, indigestion, nausea, vomiting → weight loss
Cognition Denial of realistic danger *Thoughts:* flight of ideas, loose associations; illusions, delusions of grandeur; lack of judgment; distractibility	Ambivalence, confusion, inability to concentrate, self-blame; loss of interest and motivation; self-destructive (preoccupied with suicide)
Behavior Hyperactivity (social, sexual, work) → irrationality, aggressiveness, sarcasm, exhibitionism, and acting out in behavior and dress Hostile, arrogant, argumentative, demanding, and controlling *Speech:* rapid, rhyming, punning, witty, pressured	Altered activity level, social isolation, substance abuse, overdependency, underachievement, inability to care for self, *psychomotor retardation*

◆ **III. Analysis/nursing diagnosis:**

A. *Risk for violence directed at others/self* related to poor judgment, impulsiveness, irritability, manic excitement.

B. *Altered nutrition, less than body requirements,* related to inability to sit down long enough to eat, metabolic expenditures.

C. *Sleep pattern disturbance:* lack of sleep and rest related to restlessness, hyperactivity, emotional dysfunctioning, lack of recognition of fatigue.

D. *Self-care deficits* related to altered motor behavior due to anxiety.

E. *Sensory/perceptual alterations (overload)* related to endogenous chemical alteration, sleep deprivation.

F. *Altered feeling state* (anger), *judgment, thought content* (magical thinking), *thought processes* (altered concentration and problem solving) related to disturbance in self-concept.

G. *Altered feeling processes* (mood swings).

H. *Altered attention:* hyperalertness.

I. *Impaired social interaction* related to internal and external stimuli (overload, underload).

J. *Impaired verbal communication:* flight of ideas and racing thoughts.

◆ **IV. Nursing care plan/implementation:**

A. *Manic:*

1. Prevent *physical* dangers stemming from suicide and exhaustion—promote rest, sleep, and intake of nourishment.

a. Use *suicide* precautions.

b. Reduce outside stimuli or remove to quieter area.

c. *Diet:* provide *high calorie beverages, finger foods* within sight and reach.

2. Attend to client's personal care.

3. Absorb with understanding and without reproach behaviors such as talkativeness,

provocativeness, criticism, sarcasm, dominance, profanity, and dramatic actions.

a. Allow, postpone, or partially fulfill demands and freedom of expression *within limits* of ordinary social rules, comfort, and safety of client and others.

b. Do *not* cut off manic stream of talk, because this increases anxiety and need for release of hostility.

4. Constructively utilize excessive energies with *activities* that do *not* call for concentration or follow-through.

a. Outdoor walks, gardening, putting, and ball tossing are therapeutic.

b. Exciting, disturbing, and highly *competitive* activities should be *avoided.*

c. Creative occupational therapy activities promote release of hostile impulses, as does creative writing.

5. Give benzodiazepines as ordered until lithium affects symptoms *(3 wk);* then give lithium carbonate as ordered.

6. Help client to recognize and express *feelings* (denial, hopelessness, anger, guilt, blame, helplessness).

7. Encourage realistic self-concept.

8. *Health teaching:* how to monitor effects of lithium; instructions regarding salt intake.

B. *Depressed:*

1. Take routine *suicide* precautions.

2. Give attention to *physical* needs for food and sleep and to hygiene needs. Prepare warm baths and hot beverages to aid sleep.

3. Initiate *frequent* contacts:

a. *Do not allow long periods of silence* to develop or client to remain withdrawn.

b. Use a kind, understanding, but emotionally neutral approach.

Mental Health

4. *Allow dependency* in severe depressive phase. Because dependency is one of the underlying concerns with persons who are depressed, if nurse allows dependency to occur as an initial response, he or she must plan for resolution of the dependency toward himself or herself as an example for the client's other dependent relationships.

5. Slowly repeat simple, direct information.

6. *Assist in daily decision making* until client regains self-confidence.

7. Select *mild* exercise and diversionary *activities* instead of stimulating exercise and competitive games, because they may overtax physical and emotional endurance and lead to feelings of inadequacy and frustration.

8. *Give* antidepressive drugs.

9. *Health teaching:* how to make simple decisions related to health care.

◆ **V. Evaluation/outcome criteria:**

A. *Manic:* speech and activity are slowed down; affect is less hostile; able to sleep; able to eat with others at the table.

B. *Depressed:* takes prescribed medications regularly. Does not engage in self-destructive activities. Able to express feelings of anger, helplessness, hopelessness.

VI. See sample **Clinical Pathway 6.6: Client Experiencing a Manic Episode.**

CLINICAL PATHWAY 6.6: Client Experiencing a Manic Episode

Estimated length of stay: 14 days-variations from designated pathway should be documented in progress notes

Nursing Diagnosis and Categories of Care	Time Dimension	Goals/Actions	Time Dimension	Goals/Actions	Time Dimension	Discharge Outcome
Risk for injury/ violence	Day 1	Environment is made safe for client and others.	Ongoing	Client does not harm self or others.	Day 14	Client has not harmed self or others.
Referrals	Day 1	Psychiatrist Clinical nurse specialist Internist (may need to determine if symptoms are caused by other illness or medication side effects) Neurologist (may want to check for brain lesion) Alert hostility management team			Day 14	Discharge with follow-up appointments as required.
Diagnostic studies	Day 1	Drug screen Electrolytes Lithium level	Day 5 Day 10	Lithium level Lithium level	Day 14	Lithium level and discharge with instructions to return monthly to have level drawn.
◆ Additional assessments	Day 1 Ongoing Ongoing	VS q4h Restraints prn Assess for signs of impending violent behavior: ■ Increase in psychomotor activity ■ Angry affect ■ Verbalized persecutory delusions or frightening hallucinations	Day 2–14	Ongoing assessments		

(Continued on following page)

Nursing Diagnosis and Categories of Care	Time Dimension	Goals/Actions	Time Dimension	Goals/Actions	Time Dimension	Discharge Outcome
Medications	Day 1	Antipsychotic medications, scheduled and prn Lithium carbonate, 600 mg tid or qid	Day 2–14	Administer medications as ordered and observe for effectiveness and side effects.	Day 14	Client is discharged on maintenance dose of lithium carbonate.
Client education			Day 9	Teach about lithium: Continue to take medication even when feeling okay. Teach symptoms of toxicity. Emphasize importance of monthly blood levels.	Day 14	Client is discharged with written instructions and verbalizes understanding of material presented.
			Day 12	Reinforce teaching.		
Altered nutrition: less than body requirements					Day 14	Nutritional condition and weight have stabilized.
Referrals	Day 1	Consult dietitian	Day 1–14	Fulfill nutritional needs.		
Diet	Day 1	High *protein*, high *calorie*, nutritious *finger* foods; juice and snacks as tolerated	As mania subsides	Regular diet with foods of client's choice.		
Diagnostic studies	Day 1	Chemistry profile Urinalysis	Day 2–13	Repeat of selected diagnostic studies as required.		
Additional assessments	Day 1–14	Weight I&O Skin turgor Color of mucous membranes				
Medications	Day 1–14	Multiple vitamin/mineral tablet				
Client education			Day 9	Principles of nutrition, foods for maintenance of wellness, adequate sodium, 6–8 glasses of water per day. Contact dietitian if weight gain becomes a problem.	Day 12–14	Client demonstrates ability to select appropriate foods for healthy diet and verbalizes understanding of material presented.
			Day 12	Reinforce teaching.		

Source: Townsend, M: Essentials of Psychiatric-Mental Health Nursing. FA Davis, Philadelphia.

Mental Health

TREATMENT MODES

Milieu Therapy

Milieu therapy consists of treatment by means of controlled modification of the client's environment to promote positive living experiences.

I. **Concepts and principles related to milieu therapy:**
   A. Everything that happens to clients from the time they are admitted to the hospital or treatment setting has a potential that is either therapeutic or antitherapeutic.
      1. Not only the therapists but all who come in contact with the clients in the treatment setting are important to the clients' recovery.
      2. Emphasis is on the social, economic, and cultural dimension, the interpersonal climate, and the physical environment.
   B. Clients have the right, privilege, and responsibility to make decisions about daily living activities in the treatment setting.

II. **Characteristics** of milieu therapy:
   A. Friendly, warm, trusting, secure, supportive, comforting atmosphere throughout the unit.
   B. An optimistic attitude about prognosis of illness.
   C. Attention to comfort, food, and daily living needs; help with resolving difficulties related to tasks of daily living.
   D. Opportunity for clients to take responsibility for themselves and for the welfare of the unit in gradual steps.
      1. Client government.
      2. Client-planned and client-directed social activities.
   E. Maximum individualization in dealing with clients, especially regarding treatment and privileges in accordance with clients' needs.
   F. Opportunity to live through and test out situations in a realistic way by providing a setting that is a microcosm of the larger world outside.
   G. Opportunity to discuss interpersonal relationships in the unit among clients and between clients and staff (decreased social distance between staff and clients).
   H. Program of carefully selected resocialization activities to prevent regression.

◆ III. **Nursing care plan/implementation** in milieu therapy:
   A. *New structured relationships*—allow clients to develop new abilities and use past skills; support them through new experiences as needed; help build liaisons with others; set limits; help clients modify destructive behavior; encourage group solutions to daily living problems.
   B. *Managerial*—inform clients about expectations; preserve orderliness of events.
   C. *Environmental manipulation*—regulate the outside environment to alter daily surroundings.
      1. Geographically move clients to units more conducive to their needs.
      2. Work with families, clergy, employers, etc.
      3. Control visitors for the benefit of the client.
   D. *Team approach* uses the milieu to meet each client's needs.

◆ IV. **Evaluation/outcomes criteria:**
   A. *Physical dimension:* order, organization.
   B. *Social dimension:* clarity of expectations, practical orientation.
   C. *Emotional dimension:* involvement, support, responsibility, openness, valuing, accepting.

Behavior Modification

Behavior modification is a therapeutic approach involving the application of learning principles so as to change maladaptive behavior.

I. **Definitions:**
   conditioned avoidance (also ***aversion therapy***) a technique whereby there is a purposeful and systematic production of strongly unpleasant responses in situations to which the client has been previously attracted but now wishes to avoid.
   desensitization frequent exposure in small but gradually increasing doses of anxiety-evoking stimuli until undesirable behavior disappears or is lessened (as in phobias).
   token economy desired behavior is reinforced by rewards, such as candy, money, and verbal approval, used as tokens.
   operant conditioning a method designed to elicit and reinforce desirable behavior (especially useful in mental retardation).
   positive reinforcement giving rewards to elicit or strengthen selected behavior or behaviors.

II. **Objectives and process of treatment** in behavior modification:
   A. Emphasis is on changing unacceptable, overt, and observable behavior to that which is acceptable; emphasis is on changed way of *acting* first, not of thinking.
   B. Mental health team determines behavior to change and treatment plan to use.
   C. Therapy is based on the knowledge and application of *learning* principles, that is, *stimulus-response;* the unlearning, or *extinction,* of undesirable behavior; and the *reinforcement* of desirable behavior.
   D. Therapist identifies what events are important in the life history of the client and arranges situations in which the client is therapeutically confronted with them.
   E. Two primary aspects of behavior modification:
      1. *Eliminate* unwanted behavior by *negative reinforcement* (removal of an aversive stimulus, which acts to reinforce the behavior) and *ignoring* (withholding positive reinforcement).
      2. *Create* acceptable new responses to an environmental stimulus by *positive* reinforcement.

F. Useful with: children who are disturbed, victims of rape, dependent and manipulative behaviors, eating disorders, obsessive-compulsive disorders, sexual dysfunction.

III. **Assumptions of behavioral therapy:**
   A. Behavior is what an organism does.
   B. Behavior can be observed, described, and recorded.
   C. It is possible to predict the conditions under which the same behavior may recur.
   D. Undesirable social behavior is not a symptom of mental illness but is behavior that can be modified.
   E. Undesirable behaviors are learned disorders that relate to acute anxiety in a given situation.
   F. Maladaptive behavior is learned in the same way as adaptive behavior.
   G. People tend to behave in ways that "pay off."
   H. *Three ways* in which behavior can be reinforced:
      1. *Positive* reinforcer (adding something pleasurable).
      2. *Negative* reinforcer (removing something unpleasant).
      3. *Adverse* stimuli (punishing).
   I. If an undesired behavior is ignored, it will be extinguished.
   J. Learning process is the same for all; therefore, all conditions (except organic) are accepted for treatment.

◆ IV. **Nursing care plan/implementation** in behavior modification:
   A. Find out what is a "reward" for the person.
   B. Break the goal down into small, successive *steps*.
   C. Maintain *close* and continual observation of the selected behavior or behaviors.
   D. Be *consistent* with on-the-spot, immediate intervention and correction of undesirable behavior.
   E. Record focused observations of behavior frequently.
   F. Participate in close teamwork with the *entire* staff.
   G. Evaluate procedures and results continually.
   H. *Health teaching:* teach preceding steps to colleagues and family.

◆ V. **Evaluation/outcome criteria:** acceptable behavior is increased and maintained; undesirable behavior is decreased or eliminated.

Activity Therapy

Activity therapy consists of a variety of recreational and vocational activities (recreational therapy [RT]; occupational therapy [OT]; and music, art, and dance therapy) designed to test and examine social skills and serve as adjunctive therapies.

I. **Concepts and principles related to activity therapy:**
   A. Socialization counters the regressive aspects of illness.
   B. Activities must be selected for specific psychosocial reasons to achieve specific effects.
   C. Nonverbal means of expression as an additional behavioral outlet add a new dimension to treatment.

D. Sublimation of sexual drives is possible through activities.
   E. Indications for activity therapy: clients with *low self-esteem* who are socially *unresponsive.*

II. **Characteristics of activity therapy:**
   A. Usually planned and coordinated by other team members, such as the recreational therapists or music therapists.
   B. Goals:
      1. Encourage socialization in community and social activities.
      2. Provide pleasurable activities.
      3. Help client release tensions and express feelings.
      4. Teach new skills; help client find new hobbies.
      5. Offer graded series of experiences, from passive spectator role and vicarious experiences to more direct and active experiences.
      6. Free or strengthen physical and creative abilities.
      7. Increase self-esteem.

◆ III. **Nursing care plan/implementation** in activity therapy:
   A. Encourage, support, and cooperate in client's participation in activities planned by the adjunct therapists.
   B. Share knowledge of client's illness, talents, interests, and abilities with others on the team.
   C. *Health teaching:* teach client necessary skills for each activity (e.g., sports, games, crafts).

◆ IV. **Evaluation/outcome criteria:** client develops occupational and leisure-time skills that will help provide a smoother transition back to the community.

Group Therapy

Group therapy is a treatment modality in which two or more clients and one or more therapists interact in a helping process to relieve emotional difficulties, increase self-esteem and insight, and improve behavior in relations with others.

I. **Concepts and principles related to group therapy:**
   A. People's problems usually occur in a social setting; thus they can best be evaluated and corrected in a social setting. **Table 6.15** is a summary of curative factors.
   B. *Not* all are amenable to group therapies. For example:
      1. Brain damaged.
      2. Acutely suicidal.
      3. Acutely psychotic.
      4. Persons with very passive-dependent behavior patterns.
      5. Acutely manic.
   C. It is best to match group members for *complementarity in behaviors* (verbal with nonverbal, withdrawn with outgoing) but for *similarity in problems* (obesity, predischarge group, clients with cancer, prenatal group) to facilitate empathy in the sharing of experiences and to heighten group identification and cohesiveness.

Mental Health

TABLE 6.15	Curative Factors of Group Therapy

Factor	Definition
Instilling of hope	Imbuing the client with optimism for the success of the group therapy experience.
Universality	Disconfirming the client's sense of aloneness or uniqueness in misery or hurt.
Imparting of information	Giving didactic instruction, advice, or suggestions.
Altruism	Finding that the client can be of importance to others; having something of value to give.
Corrective recapitulation of the primary family group	Reviewing and correctively reliving early familial conflicts and growth-inhibiting relationships.
Development of socializing techniques	Acquiring sophisticated social skills, such as being attuned to process, resolving conflicts, and being facilitative toward others.
Imitative behavior	Trying out bits and pieces of the behavior of others and experimenting with those that fit well.
Interpersonal learning	Learning that the client is the author of his or her interpersonal world and moving to alter it.
Group cohesiveness	Being attracted to the group and the other members with a sense of "we"-ness rather than "I"-ness.
Catharsis	Being able to express feelings.
Existential factors	Being able to "be" with others; to be a part of a group.

Source: Adapted from Wilson, HS, and Kneisl, CR: Psychiatric Nursing, ed. 3. Addison-Wesley, Redwood City, Calif. (out of print).

D. Feelings of *acceptance,* belonging, respect, and comfort develop in the group and facilitate change and health.

E. In a group, members can *test reality* by giving and receiving *feedback.*

F. Clients have a chance to experience in the group that they are not alone (concept of *universality*).

G. Expression and *ventilation* of strong emotional feelings (anger, anxiety, fear, and guilt) in the safe setting of a group is an important aspect of the group process aimed at health and change.

H. The group setting and the *interactions* of its members may provide *corrective emotional experiences* for its members. A key mechanism operating in groups is *transference* (strong emotional attachment of one member to another member, to the therapist, or to the entire group).

I. To the degree that people modify their behavior through corrective experiences and identification with others rather than through personal-insight analysis, group therapy may be of special advantage over individual therapy, in that the possible number of interactions is greater in the group and the patterns of behavior are more readily observable.

J. There is a higher client-to-staff ratio, and it is thus less expensive.

◆ **II. General group goals:**

A. Provide opportunity for self-expression of ideas and feelings.

B. Provide a setting for a variety of relationships through group interaction.

C. Explore current behavioral patterns with others and observe dynamics.

D. Provide peer and therapist support and source of strength for the individuals to modify present behavior and try out new behaviors; made possible through development of identity and group identification.

E. Provide on-the-spot, multiple feedback (i.e., incorporate others' reactions to behavior), as well as give feedback to others.

F. Resolve dynamics and provide insight.

◆ **III. Nursing care plan/implementation** in group setting:

A. Nurses need to fill different roles and functions in the group, depending on the type of group, its size, its aims, and the stage in the group's life cycle. The multifaceted roles may include:
   1. Catalyst.
   2. Transference object (of client's positive or negative feelings)
   3. Clarifier.
   4. Interpreter of "here and now."
   5. Role model and resource person.
   6. Supporter.

B. During the *first sessions,* explain the purpose of the group, go over the "contract" (structure, format, and goals of sessions), and facilitate introductions of group members.

C. In *subsequent sessions,* promote greater group cohesiveness.
   1. Focus on *group concerns* and group process rather than on intrapsychic dynamics of individuals.
   2. Demonstrate nonjudgmental acceptance of behaviors within the limits of the group contract.
   3. Help group members handle their anxiety, especially during the initial phase.

4. Encourage members who are silent to interact at their level of comfort.
5. Encourage members to interact verbally without dominating the group discussion.
6. Keep the focus of discussion on related themes; *set limits and interpret group rules.*
7. Facilitate sharing and *communication* among members.
8. Provide *support* to members as they attempt to work through anxiety-provoking ideas and feelings.
9. Set the expectation that the members are to take responsibility for carrying the group discussion and exploring issues on their own.

D. *Termination phase:*
   1. Make early preparation for group termination (end point should be announced at the first meeting).
   2. Anticipate common reactions from group members to separation anxiety and help each member to work through these reactions:
      a. Anger.
      b. Acting-out.
      c. Regressive behavior.
      d. Repression.
      e. Feelings of abandonment.
      f. Sadness.

◆ IV. **Evaluation/outcome criteria:**
   A. *Physical:* shows improvement in daily life activities (eating, rest, work, exercise, recreation).
   B. *Emotional:* asks for and accepts feedback; states feels good about self and others.
   C. *Intellectual:* is reality-oriented; greater awareness of self, others, environment.
   D. *Social:* willing to take a risk in trusting others; sharing self; reaching out to others.

Reality Orientation and Resocialization

Table 6.16 lists the differences between these two modes of therapy.

Family Therapy

Family therapy is a process, method, and technique of psychotherapy in which the focus is not on an individual but the total family as an interactional system (see also **Major Theoretical Models p. 352**).

I. **Developmental tasks of North American family** (Duvall, 1971):
   A. *Physical maintenance*—provide food, shelter, clothing, health care.

TABLE 6.16	Differences Between Reality Orientation and Resocialization
Reality Orientation	**Resocialization**
1. Maximum use of assets.	1. Reality living situation in a community.
2. Structured.	2. Unstructured.
3. Refreshments *may* be served.	3. Refreshments served.
4. Constant reminders of who the clients are, where they are, and why and what is expected of them.	4. Reliving happy experiences; encouragement to participate in home activities.
5. *Group size:* 3–5, depending on degree and level of confusion or disorientation.	5. *Group size:* 5–17, depending on mental and physical capabilities.
6. *Meetings:* 30 minutes daily, same time and place.	6. *Meetings:* 3 times per week for 30 minutes to 1 hour.
7. Planned topics: reality-centered objects.	7. *No* planned topic; group-centered feelings.
8. *Role of leader:* eliciting response of participants.	8. *Role of leader:* clarification and interpretation.
9. Periodic reality-orientation test of participants' level of confusion.	9. Periodic progress note of participants' enjoyment and improvements.
10. *Emphasis:* time, place, person orientation.	10. Any topic freely discussed.
11. Use of mind function still intact.	11. Rely on memories and experiences.
12. Participant is greeted *by name*, thanked for coming, extended a handshake or other physical contact.	12. Participant greeted on arrival, thanked, extended a handshake on leaving.
13. Conducted by trained aides and activity assistants.	13. Conducted by RN, LPN/LVN, aides, program assistants.

Source: Adapted from *the classic article* by Barns, E, Sack, A, and Shore, H: *Gerontologist,* 13:513, 1973.

Mental Health

B. *Resource allocation* (physical and emotional)—allocate material goods, space, and facilities; give affection, respect, and authority.

C. *Division of labor*—decide who earns money, manages household, cares for family.

D. *Socialization*—guidelines to control food intake, elimination, sleep, sexual drives, and aggression.

E. *Reproduction, recruitment, release of family member*—give birth to, or adopt, children; rear children; incorporate in-laws, friends, etc.

F. *Maintenance of order*—ensure conformity to norms.

G. *Placement of members in larger society*—interaction in school, community, etc.

H. *Maintenance of motivation and morale*—reward achievements, develop philosophy for living; create rituals and celebrations to develop family loyalty. Show acceptance, encouragement, affection; meet crises of individuals and family.

II. Basic theoretical concepts related to family therapy:

A. The ill family member (called the *identified client*), by symptoms, sends a message about the "illness" of the family as a *unit.*

B. *Family homeostasis* is the means by which families attempt to maintain the status quo.

C. *Scapegoating* is found in families who are disturbed and is usually focused on one family member at a time, with the intent to keep the family in line.

D. Communication and behavior by some family members bring out communication and behavior in other family members.

1. Mental illness in the identified client is almost always accompanied by emotional illness and disturbance in other family members.

2. Changes occurring in one member will produce changes in another; that is, if the identified client improves, another identified client may emerge, or family may try to place original person back into the role of the identified client.

E. Human communication is a key to emotional stability and instability—to normal and abnormal health. *Conjoint* family therapy is a communication-centered approach that looks at interactions between family members.

F. *Double bind* is a "damned if you do, damned if you don't" situation; it results in helplessness, insecurity; anxiety; fear, frustration, and rage.

G. *Symbiotic tie* usually occurs between one parent and a child, hampering individual ego development and fostering strong dependence and identification with the parent (usually the mother).

H. *Three basic premises* of communication:[*]

1. One cannot *not* communicate; that is, silence is a form of communication.

2. Communication is a *multilevel* phenomenon.

3. The message sent is *not* necessarily the *same* message that is received.

I. Indications for family therapy:

1. Marital conflicts.

2. Severe sibling conflicts.

3. Cross-generational conflicts.

4. Difficulties related to a transitional stage of family life cycle (e.g., retirement, new infant, death).

5. *Dysfunctional family patterns:* mother who is overprotective and father who is distant, with child who is timid or destructive, teenager who is acting out; overfunctioning "superwife" or "superhusband" and the spouse who is underfunctioning, passive, dependent, and compliant; child with poor peer relationships or academic difficulties.

◆ **III. Family assessment** should consider the following factors:

A. *Family assessment: cultural profile* (see also **Unit 3**)[†]

1. *Communication style:*

a. Language and dialect preference (understand concept, meaning of pain, fever, nausea).

b. Nonverbal behaviors (meaning of bowing, touching, speaking softly, smiling).

c. Social customs (acting agreeable or pleasant to avoid the unpleasant, embarrassing).

2. *Orientation:*

a. Ethnic identity and adherence to traditional habits and values.

b. Acculturation: extent.

c. Value orientations:

(1) *Human nature:* evil, good, both.

(2) *Relationship between humans and nature:* subjugated, harmony, mastery.

(3) *Time:* past, present, future.

(4) *Purpose of life:* being, becoming, doing.

(5) *Relationship to one another:* lineal, collateral, individualistic.

3. *Nutrition:*

a. Symbolism of food.

b. Preferences, taboos.

4. *Family relationships:*

a. Role and position of women, men, aged, boys, girls.

b. Decision-making styles/areas: finances, child rearing, health care.

c. Family: nuclear, extended, or tribal.

d. Matriarchal or patriarchal.

e. Lifestyle, living arrangements (crowded; urban/rural; ethnic neighborhood or mixed).

5. *Health beliefs*

a. Alternative health care: self-care, folk medicine; cultural healer: herbalist, medicine man, curandero.

b. Health crisis and illness beliefs concerning causation: germ theory, maladaptation, stress, evil spirits, yin/yang imbalance, envy and hate.

---

[*]Adapted from Watzlawick, P: An Anthology of Human Communication. Science and Behavior Books, Palo Alto, CA (out of print).

[†]Adapted from the *classic* work by Fong, C: Ethnicity and Nursing Practice. Topics in Clinical Nursing, 7(3):4, with permission of Aspen Publishers, Inc. ©1985.

Mental Health

c. Response to pain, hospitalization: stoic endurance, loud cries, quiet withdrawal.

d. Disease predisposition:
   (1) *Blacks:* sickle cell anemia; cardiovascular disease, brain attack (stroke), hypertension; high infant mortality rate; diabetes.
   (2) *Asians:* lactose intolerance, myopia.
   (3) *Hispanics:* cardiovascular, diabetes, cancer, obesity, substance abuse, TB, AIDS, suicide, homicide.
   (4) *Native Americans:* high infant and maternal mortality rates, cirrhosis, fetal alcohol abnormalities, pancreatitis, malnutrition, TB, alcoholism.
   (5) *Jews:* Tay-Sachs.

B. *Family as a social system:*
   1. Family as responsive and contributing unit within network of other social units.
      a. Family boundaries—permeability or rigidity.
      b. Nature of input from other social units.
      c. Extent to which family fits into cultural mold and expectations of larger system.
      d. Degree to which family is considered deviant.
   2. Roles of family members:
      a. Formal roles and role performance (father, child, etc.).
      b. Informal roles and role performance (scapegoat, controller, follower, decision maker).
      c. Degree of family agreement on assignment of roles and their performance.
      d. Interrelationship of various roles—degree of "fit" within total family.
   3. Family rules:
      a. Family rules that foster stability and maintenance.
      b. Family rules that foster maladaptation.
      c. Conformity of rules to family's lifestyle.
      d. How rules are modified; respect for difference.
   4. Communication network:
      a. How family communicates and provides information to members.
      b. Channels of communication—who speaks to whom.
      c. Quality of messages—clarity or ambiguity.

C. *Developmental stage of family:*
   1. Chronological stage of family.
   2. Problems and adaptations of transition.
   3. Shifts in role responsibility over time.
   4. Ways and means of solving problems at earlier stages.

D. *Subsystems operating within family:*
   1. Function of family alliances in family stability.
   2. Conflict or support of other family subsystems and family as a whole.

E. *Physical and emotional needs:*
   1. Level at which family meets essential physical needs.
   2. Level at which family meets social and emotional needs.

   3. Resources within family to meet physical and emotional needs.
   4. Disparities between individual needs and family's willingness or ability to meet them.

F. *Goals, values, and aspirations:*
   1. Extent to which family members' goals and values are articulated and understood by all members.
   2. Extent to which family values reflect resignation or compromise.
   3. Extent to which family will permit pursuit of individual goals and values.

G. *Socioeconomic factors* (see list in **Table 6.12, p. 415**).

◆ **IV. Nursing care plan/implementation** in family therapy:
   A. Establish a family *contract* (who attends, when, duration of sessions, length of therapy, fee, and other expectations).
   B. Encourage family members to identify and clarify own *goals.*
   C. *Set ground rules:*
      1. Focus is on the family as a whole unit, *not* on the identified client.
      2. *No* scapegoating or punishment of members who "reveal all" should be allowed.
      3. Therapists should *not* align themselves with issues or individual family members.
   D. *Use self* to empathetically respond to family's problems; share own emotions openly and directly; function as a role model of interaction.
   E. Point out and encourage the family to *clarify* unclear, inefficient, and ambiguous family communication patterns.
   F. Identify family *strengths.*
   G. Listen for repetitive interpersonal *themes, patterns,* and *attitudes.*
   H. *Attempt to reduce guilt and blame* (important to neutralize the scapegoat phenomenon).
   I. Present possibility of *alternative* roles and rules in family interaction styles.
   J. *Health teaching:* teach clear communication to all family members.

◆ **V. Evaluation/outcome criteria:** each person clearly speaks for self; asks for and receives feedback; communication patterns are clarified; family problems are delineated; members more aware of each other's needs.

Electroconvulsive Therapy

Electroconvulsive therapy (ECT) is a physical treatment that induces grand mal convulsions by applying electric current to the head. It is also called electric shock therapy (EST).

I. Characteristics of electroconvulsive therapy:
   A. Usually used in treating: major depression with severe suicide risk, extreme hyperactivity, severe catatonic stupor, or those with bipolar affective disorders not responsive to psychotropic medication.
   B. Consists of a series of treatments (6–25) over a period of time (e.g., three times per week).

C. Person is asleep through the procedure and for 20–30 minutes afterward.

D. Convulsion may be seen as a series of minor, jerking motions in extremities (e.g., toes). Spasms are reduced by use of muscle-paralyzing drugs.

E. Confusion is present for 30 minutes after treatment.

F. Induces loss of memory for *recent* events.

II. **Views concerning success** of electroconvulsive therapy:

A. Posttreatment sleep is the "curative" factor.

B. Shock treatment is seen as punishment, with an accompanying feeling of absolution from guilt.

C. Chemical alteration of thought patterns results in memory loss, with decrease in redundancy and awareness of painful memories.

III. **Nursing care plan/implementation** in electroconvulsive therapy:

A. *Always* tell the client of the treatment.

B. Inform client about temporary memory loss for recent events after the treatment.

C. *Pretreatment care:*
   1. Take vital signs.
   2. See to client's toileting.
   3. Remove: client's dentures, eyeglasses or contact lenses, and jewelry.
   4. NPO for 8 hours beforehand.
   5. *Atropine sulfate* subcutaneously 30 minutes before treatment to decrease bronchial and tracheal secretions.
   6. Anesthetist gives anesthetic and muscle relaxant IV (succinylcholine chloride [*Anectine*]) and oxygen for 2–3 minutes and inserts airway. Often all three are given close together—anesthetic first, followed by another syringe with *Anectine* and atropine sulfate. Electrodes and treatment must be given within 2 minutes of injections, because *Anectine* is very short acting (2 minutes).

D. *During the convulsion* the nurse must make sure the person is in a safe position to avoid dislocation and compression fractures (although *Anectine* is given to prevent this).

E. *Care during recovery stage:*
   1. Put up side rails while client is confused; side position.
   2. Take blood pressure, pulse (check for bradycardia) and respirations.
   3. Stay until person awakens, responds to questions, and can care for self.
   4. Orient client to time and place and inform that treatment is over when awakens.
   5. Offer support to help client feel more secure and relaxed as the confusion and anxiety decrease.
   6. Medication for nausea and headache, prn.

F. *Health teaching:* teach family members what to expect of client after ECT (confusion, headache, nausea); how to reorient the client.

IV. **Evaluation/outcome criteria:** feelings of worthlessness, helplessness, and hopelessness seem diminished.

COMPLEMENTARY AND ALTERNATIVE MEDICINE (CAM)

(Also see Appendix p for specific conditions where CAM can be integrated into the treatment plan.)

I. **Definitions:**

A. *Complementary therapy*—used to *supplement or augment* conventional therapy (e.g., use of guided imagery, music and relaxation techniques for pain control in combination with drug therapy).

B. *Alternative therapy*—generally used *instead* of conventional treatment (e.g., use of acupuncture instead of analgesic).

II. **Basic beliefs and assumptions** about health, health care:

A. Diseases are *complex, multifaceted* states of imbalance and require an approach that uses *several* strategies for facilitating healing.

B. Individuals can facilitate their own healing process by engaging their *inner resources* and becoming active participants in promoting their health.

C. Holistic nursing can be a major provider of CAM, with an underlying philosophy of *caring* and *healing*.
   1. Use of an approach to the care of others that facilitates the integration, harmony and balance of body, mind and spirit.
   2. Focus is on the *whole* person in the process of healing.
   3. Experience of illness is an opportunity for growth that invites reflection on important dimensions of their lives and to make changes that encourage a more balanced and integrated state of being. *Emphasis* on: self-responsibility and self-care.
   4. Client-nurse relationship is *reciprocal* where each benefits from the interaction and grows in self-awareness.

III. **Areas of practice within CAM.**

A. Mind-body interventions.

B. Bioelectromagnetic applications in medicine.

C. Manual healing methods.

D. Pharmacological and biological treatments.

E. Herbal medicine (see **Units 9** and **10** and **Appendix P**).

F. Diet and nutrition in the prevention and treatment of chronic disease.

IV. **Examples of well-known alternative and complementary therapies.**

A. *Natural healing:*
   1. Aquatherapy.
   2. Aromatherapy.
   3. Color therapy.
   4. Homeopathy.

B. *Plant therapy:*
   1. Flower essence therapy.
   2. Herbal medicine.

C. *Nutrition and diet:*
   1. Diet therapies (see **Unit 9**).
   2. Naturopathic medicine.

D. *Mobility and posture:*
1. Dance therapy.
2. Rolfing.
3. Yoga.
E. *The mind:*
1. Meditation.
2. Music therapy.
3. Visualization, guided imagery.
F. *Massage and touch:*
1. Massage therapy.
2. Reflexology.
3. Energy field therapies, including therapeutic touch.
G. *Eastern therapies:*
1. Acupuncture.
2. Acupressure.
3. Shiatsu.
4. Chinese herbal medicine.

◆ **V. Implication for nursing:**
A. Familiarize yourself with one or two basic therapies (e.g., massage, music, or guided imagery).
B. Try to eliminate own preconceived ideas.
C. Get adequate instruction before using any CAM with clients.
D. Ask clients if they use any CAM and their response to them.
E. *Health teaching:* Nurses can discuss and do teaching based on scientific research about effectiveness of each therapy when clients seek information about alternative and complementary therapies (because they are *noninvasive*, *holistic* [encompass mind and spirit], and *less* expensive). See **Appendix P**. For example:
1. *Physical tension and anxiety*—can be decreased with meditation combined with guided imagery.
2. Effect of coronary heart disease—can be reversed with carefully planned nutrition, exercise and meditation (Dr. Dean Ornish's plan).
3. Coordination—can be improved with yoga.
4. Blood pressure and stress—can be lowered and reduced with massage.
5. Apical heart rate—can be reduced; peripheral blood flow—can be increased with music.
6. Pain in arthritic joints and back—can be relieved by localized healing touch techniques.
7. Headache pain and breaking up congestion—can be aided by healing touch.
8. Prepare client for pre- and postoperative energy and recovery—can be aided by relaxation and energy-balancing methods.

GLOSSARY

affect *feeling* or *mood* communicated through the face and body posture. Can be blunted, blocked, flat, inappropriate, or displaced.

ambivalence coexisting *contradictory* (positive and negative) emotions, desires, or attitudes toward an object or person (e.g., love-hate relationship).

anhedonia inability to experience any pleasure.

amnesia loss of memory due to physical or emotion trauma.

anxiety state of uneasiness or response to a *vague*, unspecific danger cued by a threat to some value that the individual holds essential to existence (or by a threat of loss of control); the danger may be *real or imagined*. *Physiological* manifestations are increased pulse, respiration, and perspiration, with feeling of "butterflies."

associative looseness speaks with unconnected topics (e.g., "no one needs a bus; we all have heaven here"); disorganized thoughts and verbalizations.

autism self-preoccupation and absorption in fantasy, as found with schizophrenia, with a complete *exclusion of reality* and loss of interest in and appreciation of others.

catatonia type of schizophrenia characterized by muscular rigidity; alternates with periods of excitability.

circumstantiality doesn't reach a main point because speaks with too many unnecessary details.

clang association speaks in rhymes in nonsensical pattern.

compulsion an insistent, repetitive, intrusive, and unwanted urge to perform an *act* that is contrary to ordinary conscious wishes or standards.

concrete thinking difficulty with abstract concepts (e.g., "It's raining cats and dogs").

conflict emotional struggle resulting from *opposing* demands and drives of the id, ego, and superego.

coping mechanism a conscious action mobilized by a person to deal with stressful events. Coping mechanisms can be effective or ineffective.

cyclothymia alterations in moods of elation and sadness, with mood swings out of proportion to apparent stimuli.

defense mechanism device used to ward off anxiety or uncomfortable thoughts and feelings; an activity of the ego that operates outside of awareness to hold impulses in check that might cause conflict (e.g., repression, regression).

delusion a false fixed *belief*, idea, or group of ideas that are contrary to what is thought of as real and that cannot be changed by logic; arise out of the individual's needs and are maintained in spite of evidence or facts (e.g., grandeur and persecution).

depression morbid sadness or dejection accompanied by feelings of hopelessness, inadequacy, and unworthiness. *Distinguished from grief*, which is realistic and in proportion to loss.

disorientation loss of awareness of the position of self in relation to time, place, or person.

echolalia automatic repetition of heard *phrases or words.*

echopraxia automatic repetition of observed *movements*.

ego the "I," "self," and "person" as distinguished from "others"; that part of the personality, according to Freudian theory, that *mediates* between the primitive, pleasure-seeking, instinctual drives of the id and the self-critical, prohibitive, restraining forces of the superego; that aspect of the psyche that is *conscious* and most in touch with external reality and is directed by the *reality principle*. The part of the personality that has to make the *decision*. Most of the ego is conscious and represents the *thinking-feeling* part of a person. The *compromises* worked out on an unconscious level help to resolve intrapsychic conflict by keeping thoughts, interpretations, judgments, and behavior practical and efficient.

electroshock electroshock treatment (EST) or electroconvulsive treatment (ECT) is the treatment of certain psychiatric disorders (best suited for *depression*) by therapeutic administration of regulated electrical impulses to the brain to produce convulsions.

empathy an objective awareness of another's thoughts, feelings, or behaviors and their meaning and significance; intellectual identification versus emotional identification (sympathy).

euphoria exaggerated feeling of physical and emotional well-being *not* related to external events or stimuli.

flight of ideas a *thought disorder* in which one thought moves rapidly to another without reaching a main idea or point, as in manic behavior. The next sentence may be triggered by a word in the previous sentence or by something in the environment.

fugue dissociative state involving amnesia and actual *physical flight*.

hallucination *false sensory* perception in the absence of an actual external stimulus. May be due to chemicals or inner needs and may are occur in any of the five senses (auditory and visual are most common). Seen in *psychosis* and *acute* and *chronic* brain disorder.

hypochondriasis state of morbid preoccupation about one's health (somatic concerns).

id psychoanalytic term for that division of the psyche that is unconscious, contains instinctual primitive drives that lead to immediate gratification, and is dominated by the *pleasure principle*. The id wants what it wants when it wants it.

illusion misinterpretation of a real, external sensory stimulus (e.g., a person may see a shadow on the floor and think it is a hole).

insanity *legal* term for mental defect or disease that is of sufficient gravity to bring person under special legal restrictions and immunities.

labile unstable and rapidly shifting (referring to emotions).

manipulation process of influencing another to meet one's own needs, *regardless* of the other's needs.

mental retardation term for mental deficiency or deficit in normal development of intelligence that makes intellectual abilities lower than normal for chronological age. May result from a condition present at birth, from injury during or after birth, or from disease after birth.

mutism inability or refusal to speak.

narcissism *exaggerated self-love* with all attention focused on own comfort, pleasure, abilities, appearance, etc.

neologism a newly coined word or condensed combination of several words not readily understood by others but with symbolic meaning for the person with *schizophrenia*.

neurosis *an older* term for mild to moderately severe illness in which there is a disorder of feeling or behavior but no gross mental disorganization, delusions, or hallucinations, as in serious psychoses. Typical reactions include disproportionate *anxiety, phobias,* and *obsessive-compulsive behavior*.

obsession persistent, unwanted, and uncontrollable *urge* or *idea* that *cannot* be banished by logic or will.

organic psychosis mental disease resulting from defect, damage, infection, tumor, or other *physical cause* that can be *observed* in the body tissues.

paranoid adjective indicating feelings of suspicion and persecution; one type of schizophrenia.

perseveration repeats same word or idea in response to different questions.

personality disorder broad category of illnesses in which inner difficulties are revealed not by specific symptoms but by *antisocial* behavior.

phobia *irrational, persistent,* abnormal, *morbid,* and unrealistic dread of external object or situation displaced from unconscious conflict.

premorbid personality state of an individual's personality *before* the onset of an illness.

psyche synonymous with mind or the *mental and emotional* "self."

psychoanalysis theory of human development and behavior, method of research, and form of treatment described by Freud that attributes abnormal behavior to repressions in the unconscious mind. Treatment involves dream interpretation and free association to bring into awareness the origin and effects of unconscious conflicts in order to eliminate or diminish them.

psychodrama a therapeutic approach that involves a structured, dramatized, and directed *acting-out* of emotional problems and troubled interactions by the client in order to gain insight into individual's own difficulties.

psychogenic symptoms or physical disorders caused by emotional or mental factors, as opposed to organic.

psychopath *older,* inexact term for one of a variety of *personality disorders* in which person has poor impulse control, releasing tension through immediate action, without social or moral conscience.

Mental Health

psychosis severe emotional illness characterized by a disorder of *thinking, feeling, and action* with the following symptoms: loss of contact, denial of reality, bizarre thinking and behavior, perceptual distortion, delusions, hallucinations, and regression.

regression primary ego defense mechanism of retreat to earlier level of development, with childlike mannerisms and comfort techniques.

schizoid form of personality disorder characterized by shyness, introspection, introversion, withdrawal, and aloofness.

schizophrenia severe functional mental illness characterized in general by a disorder in perception, thinking, feeling, behavior, and interpersonal relationships.

sociopathic pertaining to a disorder of behavior in which a person's feelings and behavior are asocial, with impaired judgment and inability to profit from experience; the intellect remains intact. This term is often used interchangeably with "antisocial personality."

soma term meaning the body or *physical* aspects.

superego in psychoanalysis, that part of the mind that incorporates the parental or societal values, ethics, and standards. It guides, restrains, criticizes, and punishes. It is unconscious and learned and is sometimes equated with the term *conscience*.

tangentiality speaks on unrelated topics without getting to the point.

transference unconscious projections of feelings, attitudes, and wishes that were originally associated with early significant others onto persons or events in the present; may be positive or negative transference.

waxy flexibility psychomotor underactivity in which the individual maintains the posture in which he or she is placed.

word salad meaningless and random mixture of phrases and words without any logical connection often seen in *schizophrenic* behavior (e.g., "the rid jams frost wool mix").

Questions

Select the one answer that is best for each question, unless otherwise directed.

1. A client is in a withdrawn catatonic state and exhibits waxy flexibility. During the initial phase of hospitalization for this client, the nurse's first *priority* is to:
   1. Watch for edema and cyanosis of the extremities.
   2. Encourage the client to discuss concerns that led to the catatonic state.
   3. Provide a warm, nurturing relationship, with therapeutic use of touch.
   4. Identify the predisposing factors in the illness.
2. A client who is elderly has dementia related to cerebral arteriosclerosis says to the nurse, "I'm going to the university today to be their guest lecturer on aerodynamics." Which response by the nurse would be most therapeutic?
   1. "Do you know that you are in the hospital now?"
   2. "Are you saying that you would like to be asked to give a lecture at the university?"
   3. "How about watching a movie on television instead?"
   4. "It's more important that you don't tire yourself out."
3. When assessing clients who are exhibiting a depressed episode and those who are exhibiting a manic episode of bipolar mood disorders, which characteristic common to both episodes of the disorder is the nurse likely to note?
   1. Suicidal tendency.
   2. Underlying hostility.
   3. Delusions.
   4. Flight of ideas.
4. A client who is overweight is referred by the physician to the nurse for diet counseling. What action would the nurse take?
   1. Develop a weight control plan, together with the client, that will allow gradual weight loss.
   2. Ask the client to describe his or her eating patterns.
   3. Support the client's interests in other activities.
   4. Put the client on a diet with very limited number of calories so he or she will have an immediate weight loss.
5. A client begins having auditory hallucinations. When the nurse approaches, the client whispers, "Did you hear that terrible man? He is scary!" Which would be the best response for the nurse to make *initially*?
   1. "What is he saying?"
   2. "I didn't hear anything. What scary things is he saying?"
   3. "Who is he? Do you know him?"
   4. "I didn't hear a man's voice, but you look scared."
6. After seeing a number of doctors for nonspecific complaints of chest pains, with no conclusive findings of organic disease, a client is referred to a local mental health center. The client has read extensively about coronary disease and talks continuously about the symptoms in great detail. Which approach by the nurse would be best when meeting this client for the first time?
   1. Allow the client to describe the physical problems to become familiar with them.
   2. Comment on a neutral topic instead of using the usual conversation opener of "How are you today?"
   3. Give the client a simple but direct explanation of the physiological basis for the symptoms.
   4. Let the client know that the nurse is familiar with the psychogenic problems and guide the discussion to other areas.
7. The nurse needs to assess a client for depression. What are the most characteristic signs and symptoms of depression? *Select all that apply.*
   1. Diarrhea.
   2. Constipation.
   3. Sleep disturbance.
   4. Poor appetite.
   5. Increased appetite.
   6. Anhedonia.
8. A 35-year-old married clerk had surgery for ulcerative colitis 3 days ago. The physical symptoms have abated, but the client continues to complain angrily and to be demanding of the nursing staff, making numerous requests such as to open or close the windows and to bring fresh water. The nurse needs to understand that this behavior might be saying:
   1. "You aren't doing your job."
   2. "I am alone and helpless and need to depend on you to take care of me when I need you."
   3. "Everyone needs attention."
   4. "I'm going to get even with you for thinking I'm a crank by making you work."
9. The nurse is aware that the main function confabulation serves in clients, especially those with dementia, is to:

1. Impress others
2. Protect their self-esteem.
3. Control others by distance maneuvers.
4. Maintain a sense of humor.

10. A 19-year-old client is brought to the emergency department because the client slashed both wrists. What is the nurse's *first* concern?
    1. Stabilization of physical condition.
    2. Determination of antecedent, causal factors relevant to the wrist slashing.
    3. Reduction of anxiety.
    4. Obtaining a detailed nursing history.

11. A client who is agitated begins to shout insults and threats at others, and starts demolishing the recreation room. What is the best response or action by the nurse?
    1. Firmly set limits on the behavior.
    2. Allow the client to continue, because the client is seeking to express herself or himself.
    3. Tell the client he or she is trying to intimidate other clients.
    4. Let the client know that he or she does not need to express anger at the nurse by demolishing the recreation room.

12. A client looks at a mirror and cries out, "I look like a bird. My face is no longer me." Which would be the best response by the nurse?
    1. "Which bird?"
    2. "That must be a distressing experience; your face doesn't look different to me."
    3. "Maybe it was the light at that particular time. Would you like to use another mirror?"
    4. "What makes you think that your face looks like a bird?"

13. A 10-year-old child diagnosed with acute leukemia, terminal stage, asks the nurse one morning: "I am going to die, aren't I?" What would be the most appropriate response by the nurse?
    1. "No, you're not. You are getting the latest treatment available, and you have a very good doctor. Your white count was better yesterday."
    2. "We are all going to die sometime."
    3. "What did the doctor tell you?"
    4. "I don't know. You have a serious illness. Do you have feelings that you want to talk about now?"

14. For a client with a diagnosis of a somatoform disorder, which would be the appropriate *initial* nursing goal?
    1. Help the client learn how to live with the functional organic disturbance without using the symptoms to control others.
    2. Assist the client in developing new and varied interests outside of himself or herself at which he or she can be successful.
    3. Accept the client as a person who is sick and needs help.
    4. Help the client see how he or she uses the illness to avoid looking at or dealing with problems.

15. A client who is acutely ill and is hospitalized with metastatic lung carcinoma begs for a pass to attend a son's high school graduation in a city 100 miles from the hospital. "If only I could do this one thing, then I'll be ready to die," the client says. The nurse identifies this behavior as an example of:
    1. Being unrealistic and denying the degree of illness.
    2. Using bargaining as a reaction to death and dying.
    3. Being manipulative to get own way.
    4. Being unaware of the diagnosis.

16. A client who is elderly and hard of hearing repeats, over and over again, the same story of the client's family coming "out West" in a covered wagon. Which interpretation by the nurse would not demonstrate understanding of this behavior?
    1. The client has better recall for past events than for recent ones.
    2. The client enjoys reliving the pleasurable aspects of life, because the present and future are bleak.

3. Repeating stories is one way of interacting, to compensate for a two-way conversation that is difficult for the client to sustain.
4. The client wants to impress others.

17. A nursing care plan for a hospitalized client who is hyperactive in a manic episode must include:
    1. Involvement in a group activity and encouragement to talk.
    2. Attention to adequate food and fluid intake.
    3. Protection against suicide.
    4. Permissive acceptance of bizarre behavior.

18. The nurse finds a client who is elderly and has Alzheimer's in the hallway at 4:00 A.M., trying to open the door to the fire escape. Which response by the nurse would probably indicate the most accurate assessment of the situation?
    1. "You look confused. Would you like to sit down and talk with me?"
    2. "That door leads to the fire escape. Why do you want to go outside now?"
    3. "This is the fire escape door. Are you looking for the bathroom?"
    4. "Something seems to be bothering you. Let's go back to your room and talk about it."

19. Since the death of her infant, a woman has lost weight, will not eat, spends most of her time immobile, and speaks only in monosyllabic responses. She pays little attention to her appearance. One afternoon, this client comes to lunch with her hair combed and traces of lipstick.
    What could the nurse say to reinforce this change of behavior?
    1. "What happened? You combed your hair!"
    2. "This is the first time I've seen you look so good."
    3. "You must be feeling better. You look much better."
    4. "I see that your hair is combed and you have lipstick on."

20. While the nurse is interviewing a teenage client, the client says, "I suppose you have to tell my parents everything." What would be the best response by the nurse?
    1. "What are you going to tell me that is so secret that I can't tell your parents?"
    2. "If you tell me you are going to do something to hurt yourself I will have to tell your parents, but I will tell you first before I tell them."
    3. "Everything you tell me is confidential. I will not tell your parents anything."
    4. "Everything you tell me I will need to tell your parents. They have a right to know."

21. In paranoid disorder, the part of the personality that is weak is called the:
    1. Id.
    2. Ego.
    3. Superego.
    4. "Not me."

22. A key consideration in planning the general care of clients with dementia is that:
    1. They be protected from suicide attempts.
    2. Their capacity for physical activity is diminished.
    3. Team effort be aimed at increasing their independence.
    4. The staff be sympathetic when clients mention their failing abilities.

23. A college student was doing exceptionally well and was complimented by her chemistry professor, who arranged for her to become his lab assistant and to do advanced research. Although very thorough in her work, when given constructive criticism this student becomes angry and stalks out of the lab for a few hours. The most plausible theoretical explanation is that the student:
    1. Knows she is right.
    2. Thinks the professor is jealous of her.
    3. Needs to feel and know that she is perfect.

4. Feels anxiety as a result of a threat to her security and self-image.

24. Which nursing intervention is inappropriate with a person who is expressing anger?
   1. Stating observations of the expressed anger.
   2. Assisting the person to describe the feelings.
   3. Helping the person find out what preceded the anger.
   4. Helping the person refrain from expressing anger verbally.

25. A crisis intervention nurse meets with a young client who was admitted after attempting suicide by slashing the wrists. The nurse's initial goal at this time is to:
   1. Determine the precipitating event, determine how many people are involved in the incident, and determine how angry the client is.
   2. Determine if the client has an immediate support system, determine what the people in the support system think of the client cutting the wrists, and determine how angry the client is.
   3. Determine the precipitating event, determine if the client has an immediate support system, and assess the likelihood of immediate recurrence of the suicidal act.
   4. Assess the likelihood of immediate recurrence of the suicidal act.

26. The nurse discovers a client crouched in a corner, looking pale and frightened, and holding a gushing wrist wound. A razor is nearby on the floor. What should the nurse do *first*?
   1. Sit down on the floor, next to the client, and in a quiet, reassuring tone, say, "You seem frightened. Can I help?"
   2. Ask the aide to watch the client and run to get the doctor.
   3. Apply pressure on the wrist, saying to the client, "You are hurt. I will help you."
   4. Go back down the hall to get the emergency cart.

27. Which characteristic should the nurse recognize as common in a person engaged in gradual self-destructive behavior (such as in obesity, drug addiction, and smoking)?
   1. Acceptance of the death wish.
   2. Denial of possibility of death.
   3. Ability to control own behavior.
   4. Ignorance of the consequences of own behavior.

28. What will the nurse most commonly note in the clinical picture of dementia?
   1. Memory loss for events in the distant past.
   2. Quarrelsome behavior directly related to the extent of lack of blood supply to the brain.
   3. Increased resistance to change.
   4. Insight into one's situation, its probable causes, and its logical consequences.

29. The nurse should refer a client with a problem of alcohol dependency to:
   1. AA
   2. Al-Anon
   3. MADD
   4. SAD

30. A man is hospitalized following a car accident in which his wife died, and he is unable to attend the funeral due to his severe chest injuries. What would the nurse consider in forecasting this surviving spouse's potential for difficulty with grief resolution?
   1. Feelings of anger toward the hospital staff for keeping him hospitalized during the funeral.
   2. Feelings of anger toward himself for having been injured but not killed in the accident.
   3. His inability to participate in the cultural rituals of grief, wherein the reality of his wife's death is emphasized.
   4. His preoccupation with his own physical distress at this time.

31. In evaluating a client who has somatoform symptoms, the nurse is aware that the client will probably show the most improvement when he or she:

1. Accepts the fact that the physical symptoms have an emotional component.
2. Finds more satisfying ways of expressing feelings through verbalization.
3. Becomes involved in group activities and focuses less on the symptoms.
4. Understands that the current way of reacting to stress is not healthy.

32. An important part of the nursing care for a client with dementia would be:
   1. Minimizing regression.
   2. Correcting memory loss.
   3. Rehabilitating toward independent functioning.
   4. Preventing further deterioration.

33. In explaining the goal of therapy in crisis intervention to a new colleague, the nurse states that the goal is to:
   1. Restructure the personality.
   2. Remove specific symptoms.
   3. Remove anxiety.
   4. Resolve immediate problems.

34. A teenager with acting-out behaviors says to the nurse, "I want you to go tell the teacher I am sick and I am to be allowed to do what I want." The nurse determines that this statement best represents:
   1. Insight.
   2. Manipulation.
   3. Dependency.
   4. Trust.

35. A 52-year-old client who appears lucid learns that after surgery, he will wake up in the recovery room without his thick glasses and hearing aid. He immediately states that without these he will be confused and upset. The nurse determines that the client is trying to say that he:
   1. Has periods of confusion and may have a psychiatric problem.
   2. Is psychologically dependent on the hearing aid and glasses.
   3. Needs the hearing aid and glasses to correctly perceive what is going on around him, and misperception will cause confusion.
   4. Needs the hearing aid and glasses because he wants to be sure people are taking proper care of him.

36. A client relates angrily to the nurse that his wife says he is selfish. Which would be the most helpful response by the nurse?
   1. "That's just her opinion."
   2. "I don't think you're that selfish."
   3. "Everybody is a little bit selfish."
   4. "You sound angry—tell me more about what went on."

37. When a client has dementia, it is most important that the nurse plan the daily activities to:
   1. Be highly structured.
   2. Be changed each day to meet the client's needs for variety.
   3. Be simplified as much as possible to avoid problems with decision making.
   4. Provide many opportunities for making choices to stimulate the client's involvement and interest.

38. The crisis nurse explains to a colleague that the focus of treatment in crisis intervention is on the:
   1. Present and on restoration to the usual level of functioning.
   2. Past and on freeing the unconscious.
   3. Past in relation to the present.
   4. Present and on the repression of unconscious drives.

39. A client in the postoperative period following surgery for ulcerative colitis suddenly becomes angry with another client who is monopolizing the group therapy meeting. Which interpretation of this noted change in behavior would indicate that the nurse understands the dynamics of this client's somatoform disorder?

1. The client is intolerant of others.
2. The client has strong competitive drives.
3. The client has his or her own ideas of how the group members should act.
4. The client is repressing fewer feelings.

40. A client has a somatoform disorder, paralysis of the arm. It would not be helpful for the nurse to use logic and reason to divert this client's attention from this physical state because:
    1. The client is not in contact with reality and thus is unable to "hear" or understand the nurse.
    2. The client may need the symptoms to handle feelings of guilt or aggression.
    3. The nature of the client's particular illness makes the client suspicious of all medical personnel.
    4. Paralysis of the arm has become a habitual response to stress.

41. Which feeling is the nurse likely to identify as antecedent of self-destructive behavior?
    1. Omnipotence.
    2. Grandiosity.
    3. Low self-esteem.
    4. Self-satisfaction.

42. Resolution of grief related to death is likely to be complicated when:
    1. There are ambivalent feelings for the deceased.
    2. The death was due to a chronic illness.
    3. It is the first loss to be experienced.
    4. There was little emotional dependency on the deceased.

43. Which behavior might the nurse expect from a client with congestive heart failure who is in the grief stage of developing awareness of the loss of a spouse?
    1. Crying, anger, or both.
    2. Appearing dazed and repeatedly saying, "No, it can't be."
    3. Preoccupation with thoughts of how ideal the marriage had been.
    4. Responding with a brief complaint about the client's own physical pain.

44. What feeling tone is the nurse most likely to see the client demonstrate during major depression with psychotic features?
    1. Suspicion.
    2. Agitation.
    3. Loneliness.
    4. Worthlessness.

45. What are the most significant signs and symptoms indicative of delirium tremens (alcohol withdrawal delirium)?
    1. Decreased BP and pulse, restlessness.
    2. Increased BP and pulse, seizures.
    3. Cramps, nausea, vomiting.
    4. Anorexia, diarrhea, dehydration

46. When a client's behavior is considered abnormal, the nurse first needs to:
    1. Ignore the client.
    2. Serve as a role model.
    3. Point out the client's disturbed behavior.
    4. Focus on the feelings communicated by the client's behavior.

47. To relate therapeutically with a client who is dependent on alcohol, it is important that the nurse base care on the understanding that alcohol dependence:
    1. Is hereditary.
    2. Is due to lack of willpower and true remorse.
    3. Results in always breaking promises.
    4. Cannot be cured.

48. A client uses repetitive handwashing. To help the client use less maladaptive means of handling stress, the nurse could:
    1. Provide varied activities on the unit, because change in routine can break this ritualistic pattern.
    2. Give the client unit assignments that do not require perfection.

3. Tell the client of changes in routine at the last minute to avoid buildup of anxiety.
4. Provide an activity in which positive accomplishment can occur so the client can gain recognition.

49. The most common defense mechanisms used in somatoform disorders are:
    1. Repression and symbolism.
    2. Sublimation and regression.
    3. Substitution and displacement.
    4. Reaction formation and rationalization.

50. It is important for the nurse to be aware that the mental health of an 87-year-old client is most directly influenced by:
    1. The attitude of relatives in providing for the client's needs.
    2. Societal factors such as role change, loss of loved ones, and loss of physical energy.
    3. The client's level of education and economic situation.
    4. The attitudes the client has toward life circumstances.

51. Two days after a mastectomy, a woman is crying and saying, "My husband won't love me anymore." The nurse is aware that this statement might stem from:
    1. The woman's deep insecurity about her marriage.
    2. Preexisting marital disharmony.
    3. The woman's concerns about her body and a resultant change in her beliefs about her own self-worth.
    4. A momentary fear about her husband's fidelity.

52. A client is diagnosed as having a paranoid disorder. What implication might this have for the nurse?
    1. Let the client talk about the suspicions without correcting misinformation.
    2. Avoid talking to other nurses when the client can see them but cannot hear what is being said.
    3. Placate the client by agreeing with what he or she says.
    4. Argue with the client about his or her ideas.

53. A teenage client says to the nurse, "I want you to go tell the teacher I am sick and I am to be allowed to do what I want." What is the nurse's best response?
    1. "Certainly. You are sick and need some relaxation of rules in the classroom."
    2. "I am glad you recognize you are sick."
    3. "No, you are expected to follow the rules of the classroom."
    4. "All teachers are too strict. I agree some rules need to be relaxed."

54. A mother talks about her daughter, who is mentally retarded: "She's really an inspiration to me, do you know what I mean?" Which would be the most appropriate initial comment by the nurse?
    1. "What makes her an inspiration?"
    2. "It seems to be important to you to find something positive about her."
    3. "No, explain more about what you mean."
    4. "Tell me more about her."

55. A mother says to the nurse, "When my baby had asthma 5 years ago, I thought he was going to die." What would be most appropriate for the nurse to say?
    1. "What made you think that the baby was going to die?"
    2. "What did you do?"
    3. "You thought the baby was dying?"
    4. "What were some of your feelings at that time?"

56. In preparing the nursing care plan for an 84-year-old man, the *most* common basic need that must be met is:
    1. Sexual outlet and security.
    2. Unconditional acceptance by others of his impairments and deficits.
    3. Preservation of self-esteem.
    4. Socialization.

57. One effective way for a nurse to start an interaction with a client who is silent is to:

1. Tell the client something about himself or herself and hope that the client does the same.
2. Remain silent, waiting for the client to bring up a topic.
3. Bring up a controversial topic to elicit the client's response.
4. Introduce a neutral topic, giving the client a broad opening.

58. What would be the most realistic statement a nurse could make about a client's prognosis after a course of necessary treatment for ulcerative colitis?
    1. The symptoms will recur.
    2. The ulcerative lesions will heal, but under stress the same symptoms will reappear.
    3. It is not possible to prognosticate the future course.
    4. Ongoing psychotherapy is essential for the client to be free of symptoms.

59. What might be the most therapeutic response the nurse could make to a student who begins crying on hearing that he or she failed an exam?
    1. "You'll make it next time."
    2. "Failing an exam is an upsetting thing to happen."
    3. "How close were you to passing?"
    4. "It won't seem so important 5 years from now."

60. Which adaptive behavior by a client with somatoform disorders might indicate to the nurse the greatest improvement in the client's condition?
    1. The client recognizes that the behavior is unreasonable.
    2. The client agrees to go to occupational therapy and recreational therapy every day.
    3. The symptoms are replaced by expressions of hostility.
    4. The client is verbalizing feelings instead of demonstrating them by pathological body languages.

61. Which is an example of *limit setting* as an effective nursing intervention in ritualistic hand-washing behavior?
    1. "I don't want you to wash your hands so often anymore."
    2. "If you continue to wash your hands so frequently, the skin on your hands will break down."
    3. "You may wash your hands before the group therapy meeting if you wish, but not during group therapy."
    4. "The doctor wrote an order that you are to stop washing your hands so often."

62. Which nursing intervention is effective when clients are severely anxious?
    1. Encourage group participation.
    2. Give detailed instructions before treatment procedures.
    3. Impart information succinctly and concretely.
    4. Increase opportunities for decision making.

63. A nursing care plan for a client with a history of alcohol abuse and dependency must incorporate monitoring which physical consequence?
    1. Cardiac arrhythmia.
    2. Convulsive disorder.
    3. Psychomotor hyperactivity.
    4. Cirrhosis of the liver.

64. A new nurse is assigned to take clients for an outing. A client with an antisocial disorder approaches the nurse and says, "I like you. I'm glad you'll be the one to take us out. My doctor told me that I can go too." Which *initial* response by the nurse is best?
    1. "Since I am new here and not familiar with unit routine, I will go check with the staff and be back."
    2. "It's a beautiful day, and I'm glad that you have ground privileges now."
    3. "When did the doctor tell you that?"
    4. "You seem pleased."

65. Which common physiological reaction occurring in response to anxiety is the nurse likely to note?
    1. Clammy hands and increased perspiration.
    2. Palpitations and pupillary constriction.
    3. Diarrhea and vomiting.
    4. Pupillary dilation and retention of feces and urine.

66. Clients with paranoid behavior use projection. The nurse is aware that this mechanism is chiefly a way to:
    1. Provoke anger in others.
    2. Control delusional thought.
    3. Handle their own unacceptable feelings.
    4. Manipulate others.

67. Which most characteristic behavior of a panic response is the nurse likely to note?
    1. Goal-directed behavior aimed at a "flight" from apparent threat.
    2. Automatic behavior with poor judgment.
    3. A severity of reaction that is not related to the severity of the threat to self-esteem.
    4. A delayed reaction in perceiving the danger.

68. At times, a client seems preoccupied with her own thoughts as she grins, giggles, grimaces, and frowns. Although she is 23 years old, her behavior seems childish and regressed. She is unkempt, voids on the floor, disrobes, and openly masturbates. The main nursing care at this time should be directed toward:
    1. Improving the client's social conduct to meet hospital standards.
    2. Controlling the narcissistic impulses.
    3. Finding out why the client is behaving this way.
    4. Showing acceptance of the client.

69. The nurse is aware that the two major types of precipitating factors in anxiety are:
    1. Fear of disapproval and shame.
    2. Conflicts involving avoidance and pain.
    3. Threats to one's biological integrity and threats to one's self-system.
    4. A person's poor health and poor financial condition.

70. The nurse needs to do ongoing assessment when a client is on haloperidol (Haldol) because of which significant side effects?
    Select all that apply.
    1. Diarrhea.
    2. Constipation.
    3. Orthostatic hypotension.
    4. Urinary retention.
    5. Decreased appetite.
    6. Elevated blood pressure.

71. Psychomotor manifestations of anxiety that a nurse may observe include:
    1. Decreased activity.
    2. Increased activity.
    3. Increased lability of emotions.
    4. Decreased lability of emotions.

72. A client whose significant other recently died shows signs of grief resolution when he or she:
    1. Wants to enter into another relationship soon.
    2. Talks of both the positive and negative aspects of their relationship.
    3. Makes up for deficiencies in the relationship, saying, "Things would have been better if we had only had more time."
    4. Expresses anger toward the deceased.

73. The nurse needs to know that anxiety may increase intellectual functioning because anxiety may:
    1. Increase the perceptual field.
    2. Increase ability to concentrate.
    3. Decrease the perceptual field.
    4. Decrease random activity.

74. In planning client care, a nurse needs to know that self-destructive behavior may be interpreted as the:
    1. Directing of hostile feelings toward self.
    2. Directing of hostile feelings toward others.

3. Directing of hostile feelings toward an internalized love object.
4. Internalization of the fear of death.

75. Based on knowledge of Erikson's stages of growth and development, the nurse determines that the task of old age is primarily concerned with:
1. Ego integrity versus despair.
2. Autonomy versus shame and doubt.
3. Trust versus mistrust.
4. Industry versus inferiority.

76. The nurse must assess for high risk of suicide when a client's behavior suggests:
1. Major depression with melancholia features.
2. Schizophrenic disorders.
3. Bipolar mood disorder, manic episode.
4. Psychological factors affecting physical condition.

77. In working with clients who are depressed, the nurse must know that depression may stem from:
1. A sense of loss—actual, imaginary, or impending.
2. Revived memories of a painful childhood.
3. A confused sexual identity.
4. An unresolved oedipal conflict.

78. When working with a person who is anxious, what is the *overall* goal of nursing intervention?
1. Remove anxiety.
2. Develop the person's awareness of anxiety.
3. Protect the person from anxiety.
4. Develop the person's capacity to tolerate mild anxiety and to use it constructively.

79. In discussions between parents and adolescents about their relationship, a desired outcome is that adolescents benefit because they will be able to:
1. See themselves as the victims.
2. View their parents and themselves realistically.
3. Enlist the therapist's aid as an ally against their parents.
4. See their parents as victims.

80. The main nursing goal with clients with schizophrenic disorders is to:
1. Set limits on their bizarre behavior.
2. Establish a trusting, nonthreatening, reality-based relationship.
3. Quickly establish a warm, close relationship to counteract their aloofness.
4. Protect them from self-destructive impulses.

81. Which activity would be best for the nurse to suggest to a client who is depressed?
1. Folding laundry or stapling paper sheets for charts.
2. Playing checkers.
3. Doing a crossword puzzle.
4. Ice skating.

82. Which activity could a nurse suggest that would be best for a client with hyperactive behavior?
1. Solitary activity, such as reading.
2. Hammering on metal in a jewelry-making class.
3. Playing chess.
4. Competitive games.

83. A client says to his mother, "You are controlling me." The mother asks the nurse what he may have meant. What is the best response by the nurse?
1. "He is upset and thinks you are taking charge of him."
2. "He resents always having to meet your expectations."
3. "I can't tell you. You will have to ask him."
4. "I think you can ask your son that. Do you want me to stay with you while you ask him?"

84. A client who attempted suicide recently remarked to the nurse the next morning, "Let's not think about that now. Maybe I'll feel like thinking about it later." The nurse identifies this as:

1. Blocking.
2. Denial.
3. Suppression.
4. Repression.

85. In conducting an assessment interview, the nurse needs to be aware that self-destructive behavior is determined by:
1. A variety of factors, with the same factors present in each individual.
2. Genetic disturbances.
3. Interpersonal disturbances.
4. A variety of factors, different for each individual.

86. It would be important for the nurse to implement definite suicide precautions for a client who is depressed if the client's mood changed suddenly to one of:
1. Cheerfulness.
2. Psychomotor retardation.
3. Agitation.
4. Hostility.

87. The nurse knows that the most characteristic task of puberty and adolescence, according to Erikson's stages of psychosexual development, is:
1. Identity versus role confusion.
2. Initiative versus guilt.
3. Ego integrity versus despair.
4. Intimacy versus isolation.

88. A person is assessed for signs of apraxia when there is impaired ability to:
1. Recognize or understand familiar words, objects, or people despite intact sensory function.
2. Express thoughts in writing due to organic cerebral pathology.
3. Speak, either a loss or deterioration of language, or incorrect use of words, with excessive use of indefinite terms ("thing," "it").
4. Carry out purposeful motor activities despite intact motor abilities, sensory function, and comprehension of the required task (e.g., inability to use utensils).

89. In assessing the behavior of a child with autism, the nurse notes that a symptom that characteristically differentiates this child from one with Down syndrome is:
1. Retardation of activity.
2. Short attention span.
3. Difficulty in responding to a nurturing relationship.
4. Poor academic performance.

90. The nurse observes for signs of heroin withdrawal, which may include:
1. Rhinorrhea, sneezing, and high fever.
2. Pupillary dilation, diaphoresis, and weight loss.
3. Pupillary constriction, vomiting, and pruritus.
4. Choreiform movements and frequent lip wetting.

91. The nurse will look for what likely outcome of methadone treatment for heroin abuse and dependence?
1. Sedation.
2. Euphoria.
3. Neuritis.
4. Blocking of the euphoric effect of heroin and elimination of craving.

92. A client who is acutely agitated becomes increasingly aggressive. The staff's verbal attempts to stop the aggressive behavior are not effective. The client begins to shout threats at the staff and other clients, throws furniture, breaks windows, and hits, kicks, and bites other clients and staff. The client has a prn order for medication when agitated. Which action should the nurse take *initially*?
1. Orient the client to reality and place the client in a well-lit, quiet room.
2. Give the ordered tranquilizer and put the client in bed with the side rails up.

3. Lock the client in his or her room and call the doctor.
4. Have at least two staff members physically restrain the client and take the client to a quiet room.

93. Several staff members voice their frustrations about a client's constant questions, such as "Should I go to the dayroom or should I stay in my room?" and "Should I have a cup of tea or a cup of coffee?" Which interpretation about this behavior will help the nursing staff deal effectively?
    1. The client's inability to make decisions reflects a basic anxiety about making a mistake and being a failure.
    2. The client's indecisiveness is aimed at testing the staff's reaction and acceptance of him or her.
    3. The client's dependence on others (staff) is a symptom that needs to be interrupted by firm limit setting.
    4. The client's need to ask questions is a bid for attention.

94. In providing dietary instructions to a client who is Orthodox Jewish and is depressed, the nurse needs to know that which practice would be prohibited in dietary kosher laws?
    1. Eating dairy products with meat.
    2. Eating meat from animals with cloven hoofs.
    3. Eating fish with scales and fins.
    4. Eating unleavened bread during the 8 days of Passover.

95. A client with antisocial behavior flatters the nurse. What is the client trying to do?
    1. The client wants something in return.
    2. The client wants the nurse to like him.
    3. The client needs attention.
    4. The client is trying to redirect the focus of the nurse-client interaction.

96. The nurse can anticipate that the person most likely to be at risk for depression is:
    1. A person who is elderly with previous depressive episodes.
    2. A man who is middle-aged and who is a moderate alcohol drinker.
    3. A housewife with three school-age children.
    4. A nursing student at exam time.

97. In admitting a client with Alzheimer's to the unit, which placement variable would have the *highest priority*?
    1. Place the client with a roommate.
    2. Place the client without a roommate.
    3. Place the client close to the nurses' station.
    4. Place the client at a distance from the nurses' station.

98. During a home health assessment visit to an 84-year-old client living alone, which aspect of lifestyle noted by the nurse would be of greatest concern?
    1. The family visits only twice a month.
    2. The family maintains only phone contact daily.
    3. The client uses a cordless telephone rather than a standard phone.
    4. The client prefers not to attend a senior citizen center for meals and recreation.

99. A client hospitalized with Alzheimer's disease is often found wandering in the streets. What measure(s) should be taken in the unit to prevent the client from wandering off?
    1. Place the client in daytime restraints.
    2. Place the client in nighttime restraints.
    3. Provide a security guard at the door.
    4. Use electronic surveillance devices.

100. Which nursing action would be best for a client who is hospitalized, and is constantly upset with the staff, easily angers, and frequently shouts at the nurses?
    1. Request that the client be moved to another unit.
    2. Schedule a conference with the MD, nurse manager, and client about this behavior.
    3. Contact social services to meet with the client and family about the problem.
    4. Involve the client and family in the development of the care plan.

Answers/Rationales/Tips

1. **(1)** Circulation may be severely impaired in a client with waxy flexibility who tends to remain motionless for hours unless moved. **Answer 2** is *not the first* priority. "Touch" is *not* used in this stage, as in **Answer 3. Answer 4** is incorrect because the client is *mute* and also because intellectual discussion of predisposing factors *ignores* the *feelings* of the client.

   > **TEST-TAKING TIP**—Note the key words: *"first* priority." **PL, ANL, 6, Psych, PhI, Physiological Adaptation**

2. **(2)** The best of four poor choices here is an attempt to understand what the client means. The other choices are *not* helpful. **Answers 3** and **4** *switch* the focus and *ignore* the client's statement; **Answer 1** is too brusque an attempt to bring the client back to reality.

   > **TEST-TAKING TIP**—Asking for clarification is a therapeutic communication technique. **IMP, ANL, 2, Psych, PsI, Psychosocial Integrity**

3. **(2)** In the depressed episode, anger is turned inward; in the manic, it is noted in sarcasm, demanding behavior, and angry outbursts. **Answers 3** and **4** occur in the manic episode. **Answer 1** is a particular problem in the depressed phase.

   > **TEST-TAKING TIP**—Remember point of theory: depression may be anger turned *inward* as opposed to expressed *outwardly* (as in manic behavior). **AS, ANL, 2, Psych, PsI, Psychosocial Integrity**

4. **(1)** The nurse should formulate a weight control plan, in *cooperation* with the client, that allows for a *gradual* weight loss, *not immediate* loss as in **Answer 4. Answers 2** and **3** *are incorporated* into **Answer 1.**

   > **TEST-TAKING TIP**—When three options are good, choose the one that covers them all. Also look at two contradictory options: "gradual" vs. "immediate" weight loss. Choose the more realistic option ("gradual"). **IMP, APP, 4, Psych, PhI, Basic Care and Comfort**

5. **(4)** This is a reality-based response, as well as one that acknowledges the client's nonverbal reaction. The other choices are *not* the best because **Answers 1** and **3** focus on "voice," which reinforces the hallucination, and no doubt is raised; in **Answer 2** doubt is raised, but the focus is on "voice" and *not* on client's *feelings*.

   > **TEST-TAKING TIP**—Note the key word "initially," which includes reality orientation and client's feelings. **IMP, APP, 2, Psych, PsI, Psychosocial Integrity**

6. **(1)** It shows acceptance by listening to the client's initial account of the physical problems. Neither a superficial focus nor a technical explanation of physical problems (**Answers 2** and **3**) conveys acceptance of the client as a person; **Answer 4** is too abrupt for an initial response.

KEY TO CODES FOLLOWING RATIONALES:

Nursing process: **AS,** assessment; **AN,** analysis; **PL,** plan; **IMP,** implementation; **EV,** evaluation. *Cognitive level:* **COM,** comprehension; **APP,** application; **ANL,** analysis. *Category of human function:* **1,** protective; **2,** sensory-perceptual; **3,** comfort, rest, activity, and mobility; **4,** nutrition; **5,** growth and development; **6,** fluid-gas transport; **7,** psychosocial-cultural; **8,** elimination. *Client need:* **SECE,** safe, effective care environment; **HPM,** health promotion/maintenance; **PsI,** psychosocial integrity; **PhI,** physiological integrity. (Client subneed appears *after* Client need code.) See appendices for full explanation.

Answers/Rationales

TEST-TAKING TIP—Look at the verbs: "allow," "comment," "give," "let (the client know)." Choose the one that most conveys acceptance.
IMP, APP, 7, Psych, PsI, Psychosocial Integrity

7. **(2, 3, 4, 6)** These are symptoms of depression. **Answer 1** is incorrect because this symptom is not commonly seen in clients who are depressed. **Answer 5** is incorrect because this symptom is not commonly seen in clients who are depressed.

   TEST-TAKING TIP—Remember that in depression everything slows down. The client can not have both an increased and decreased appetite. Only choose the one answer that is the opposite.
   AS, ANL, 7, Psych, PsI, Psychosocial Integrity

8. **(2)** Characteristic underlying needs in somatoform disorders are dependency, attention, and the need for security through trust. **Answers 1** and **4** are incorrect because the client's complaints are not aimed at blaming others or at seeking vengeance, but at expressing dependency needs and seeking security. **Answer 3** is inappropriate because the client is expressing his or her *own* need for attention; the client is not speaking for everyone.

   TEST-TAKING TIP—Apply the process of elimination. Eliminate the two hostile options (**Answers 1** and **4**); next eliminate the global "everyone."
   AN, ANL, 7, Psych, PsI, Psychosocial Integrity

9. **(2)** Because confabulation is a defense mechanism, the best choice is the one that defines one of the main functions of defense mechanisms—to protect self-esteem. **Answers 1** and **3** are incorrect because they focus on *others*, not on self. **Answer 4** is completely *irrelevant*.

   TEST-TAKING TIP—Choose the response that focuses on the *clients*, after eliminating two options that focus on *others* (**Answers 1** and **3**). It's a "client focus vs. others" type of test-taking tip.
   AN, APP, 2, Psych, PsI, Psychosocial Integrity

10. **(1)** Deal first with the *lifesaving* situation. **Answers 2** and **3** are incorrect because they are done *following* stabilization of physical condition. **Answer 4** is incorrect because it is *not* a necessary lifesaving concern.

    TEST-TAKING TIP—Note key words "*first* concern," which is a priority on Maslow's hierarchy of human needs (e.g., physiological needs).
    PL, APP, 7, Psych, PhI, Physiological Adaptation

11. **(1)** The nurse needs to set limits to ensure the safety of the client and others. **Answer 2** is incorrect because the client may hurt herself or himself or others. **Answers 3** and **4** are incorrect because they are interpretations that may or may not be correct, and they do *not* control the *unsafe* behavior.

    TEST-TAKING TIP—Look at two options that are contradictory ("allow" and "limits"). Because the main concern is *safety* when a client is agitated, select **Answer 1**. Avoid interpretive statements (**3 Answers 3** and **4**).
    IMP, APP, 1, Psych, SECE, Safety

12. **(2)** This acknowledges the experience and points out reality as the nurse sees it. **Answers 1, 3,** and **4** do not focus on the client or attempt to explore feelings.

    TEST-TAKING TIP—An effective response to hallucinatory behavior is to support the feeling aspect ("distressing") while also pointing out reality.
    IMP, APP, 2, Psych, PsI, Psychosocial Integrity

13. **(4)** An honest, direct answer that focuses on feelings is the best approach. **Answers 1, 2,** and **3** stop any further exploration of the client's feelings.

    TEST-TAKING TIP—Choose the answer that helps *explore feelings*. Eliminate the other three options that close off communication and focus on facts, not feelings.
    IMP, APP, 7, Psych, PsI, Psychosocial Integrity

14. **(3)** Showing *acceptance* and gaining trust and confidence are usually the key initial nursing goals. You need to show acceptance before *helping* (**Answers 1** and **4**) or *assisting* (**Answer 2**).

    TEST-TAKING TIP—Focus on the phrase "initial nursing goal," which is *acceptance*. Note the lead verb: *accept* before *help* or *assist*.
    PL, APP, 7, Psych, PsI, Psychosocial Integrity

15. **(2)** Refer to Elisabeth Kübler-Ross's emotional stages of death and dying. The client is being neither unrealistic (**Answer 1**), manipulative (**Answer 3**), nor unaware of the diagnosis (**Answer 4**).

    TEST-TAKING TIP—Select the response that typifies a common grief reaction ("bargaining"); eliminate the three responses that have a negative tone ("deny," "manipulative," "unaware").
    EV, COM, 7, Psych, PsI, Psychosocial Integrity

16. **(4)** Redundancy is *not* meant to impress others but is aimed at *pleasure* gained through focus on the *past* and need to *control* the conversation when memory or hearing deficit is present. **Answers 1, 2,** and **3** *would* demonstrate understanding of this behavior.

    TEST-TAKING TIP—Focus on the key phrase "*not* demonstrate understanding"; use a true-or-false approach.
    AN, ANL, 5, Psych, HPM, Health Promotion and Maintenance

17. **(2)** During a manic episode, the client may be too busy to eat and sleep. **Answers 1** and **3** are more appropriate for a depressive episode; **Answer 4** is more appropriate for schizophrenia with bizarre behavior. Clients in manic episode exhibit hyperactive behavior.

    TEST-TAKING TIP—Match characteristic behaviors with other main diagnostic categories: depression with **Answers 1** and **3** and schizophrenia with **Answer 4.**
    PL, ANL, 2, Psych, PsI, Psychosocial Integrity

18. **(3)** Nocturnal urination is a most common need, complicated by disorientation related to the client's age, disorder, and unfamiliar environment at night. To sit down (**Answer 1**) or to go back to the client's room and talk (**Answer 4**) does not take care of the possible problem, the need to urinate. Asking a person "why" questions (**Answer 2**) is not helpful and is too literal a response to the behavior.

    TEST-TAKING TIP—Confusion (Alzheimer's) and age-typical physiological need (nocturia) call for a response that is reality orientation and environmental redirection (to the location of the bathroom).
    IMP, ANL, 7, Psych, HPM, Health Promotion and Maintenance

19. **(4)** A simple acknowledgment of what the nurse sees is the best response. **Answer 3** makes an assumption that the client feels better if she looks better. **Answers 1** and **2** can be taken as a put-down.

    TEST-TAKING TIP—Eliminate put-downs and assumptions. Keep it simple (KIS) and simply acknowledge what the nurse observes.
    IMP, APP, 7, Psych, PsI, Psychosocial Integrity

20. **(2)** Confidentiality cannot be guaranteed if there is a danger to the client or to others. **Answer 1** is incorrect because it is a

sarcastic response and *denies* that the client has serious problems. **Answer 3** *contradicts* **Answer 2. Answer 4** is incorrect because parents do *not* have the right to know the content of therapy sessions except in the circumstances described in **Answer 2.**

> **TEST-TAKING TIP**—Eliminate two options with the global "everything" and one option that can be seen as a put-down.
> IMP, ANL, 7, Psych, SECE, Management of Care

21. **(2)** A diagnosis of a paranoid disorder implies weak *ego* development. **Answers 1, 3,** and **4** are incorrect because a client with a paranoid disorder might have *strong* id, superego, and "not me" components.

> **TEST-TAKING TIP**—Focus on the word "weak" in the stem.
> AN, COM, 5, Psych, PsI, Psychosocial Integrity

22. **(2)** An important principle to remember here is that a program of care should not increase physiological losses by overtaxing the client's physical capacities. It is important to remember that suicide is the *main* concern in *depression* and *not* a key concern in dementia, as in **Answer 1.** Empathy *rather than* sympathy (**Answer 4**) is a helpful behavior. **Answer 3**, increasing independence, is *not realistic; maintaining* it *is*.

> **TEST-TAKING TIP**—Apply the process of elimination. Eliminate **Answer 4** because "sympathy" is not therapeutic; eliminate the unrealistic response in **Answer 3**; eliminate **Answer 1** because it applies to depression, not to general care in dementia.
> PL, ANL, 2, Psych, PhI, Reduction of Risk Potential

23. **(4)** This is the all-inclusive answer. **Answers 1, 2,** and **3** may be part of **Answer 4.**

> **TEST-TAKING TIP**—Choose the "umbrella" answer (i.e., most inclusive) when all four options are correct.
> AN, ANL, 7, Psych, PsI, Psychosocial Integrity

24. **(4)** A person needs to be allowed to express anger appropriately. **Answers 1, 2,** and **3** are *incorrect* choices here because they *are* things the nurse assists a person to do when intervening in anger.

> **TEST-TAKING TIP**—Key word: "inappropriate."
> IMP, ANL, 1, Psych, PsI, Psychosocial Integrity

25. **(3)** It incorporates all information a crisis intervention nurse needs immediately. **Answers 1** and **2** are incorrect because the nurse does not need to know about other people's involvement at this time. **Answer 4** is incorrect because it is *not as complete* as **Answer 3.**

> **TEST-TAKING TIP**—Key words: "initial goal."
> PL, ANL, 7, Psych, PsI, Psychosocial Integrity

26. **(3)** Take care of the bleeding (physical aspects of care) first. In **Answers 1** and **2**, the client could suffer extensive blood loss if the nurse focuses on feelings at this point or leaves the client without first attempting to control the bleeding. In **Answer 4**, the client is left alone, bleeding, frightened, and with a razor still at the side.

> **TEST-TAKING TIP**—Be aware that the stem asks for *first* action.
> AN, APP, 7, Psych, PsI, Psychosocial Integrity

27. **(2)** Persons engaged in self-destructive behavior other than active suicide behavior fantasize that *they can control* their behavior and deny the likelihood of death as a result. Thus **Answers 1, 3,** and **4** are incorrect.

> **TEST-TAKING TIP**—Know theory about gradual self-destructive behaviors and eliminate the three that are theoretically incorrect (**Answers 1, 3** and **4**). Look at two options that are opposites (acceptance and denial) and choose a *most common* defense mechanism (denial).
> AN, APP, 7, Psych, PsI, Psychosocial Integrity

28. **(3)** One of the main needs experienced by most clients with dementia is the need for most things to be the same. The other choices are wrong for the following reasons: there has been no demonstrable evidence of relationship between any behavior symptom and the extent or severity of pathophysiological condition (**Answer 2**); intellectual *blunting* usually occurs, which interferes with ability to deal with insight and abstract thoughts (**Answer 4**); and memory loss is for *recent* events and names, *not* those in the distant past, as in **Answer 1.**

> **TEST-TAKING TIP**—Key words: "most commonly."
> AS, COM, 2, Psych, PsI, Psychosocial Integrity

29. **(1)** Alcoholics Anonymous is the only correct choice because **answer 2** Al-Anon is a support group for family and friends of the person who is alcohol-dependent. **Answer 3** is incorrect because it stands for Mothers Against Drunk Driving. **Answer 4** is incorrect because it stands for Seasonal affective disorders.

> **TEST-TAKING TIP**—Alcoholics Anonymous is the most common self-help group available for clients with alcohol dependency.
> IMP, APP, 7, Psych, SECE, Management of Care

30. **(3)** One way to enhance the development of unresolved grief is *not* to participate in activities that demonstrate death. **Answers 1, 2,** and **4** may occur, but they are *not* the best predictors of grief resolution difficulties.

> **TEST-TAKING TIP**—Apply theory about unresolved grief (which may be related to lack of culturally sanctioned rituals for "letting go").
> AN, ANL, 7, Psych, PsI, Psychosocial Integrity

31. **(2)** All the other choices (**Answers 1, 3** and **4**) are correct but can be dove-tailed into **Answer 2.**

> **TEST-TAKING TIP**—Choose the "umbrella" answer that encompasses the other three choices.
> EV, APP, 7, Psych, PsI, Psychosocial Integrity

32. **(1)** Use of regression as a defense response *can* be minimized. Memory loss is usually permanent, not correctable; thus **Answer 2** is wrong. However, disorientation attributed to loss of memory can be minimized. Clients usually become *more* dependent in the course of illness *and* deteriorate progressively. Thus **Answers 3** and **4** are incorrect.

> **TEST-TAKING TIP**—Know what can and cannot be ameliorated. Whereas the nurse cannot stop the pathological course of Alzheimer's disease (i.e., memory loss is *permanent;* deterioration is *progressive* and rehabilitation is *not* possible), use of a defense mechanism (regression) *can* be minimized.
> PL, APP, 2, Psych, PsI, Psychosocial Integrity

33. **(4)** The major goal of crisis intervention is to resolve immediate problems. **Answer 1** is incorrect because restructuring personality is the goal of *psychoanalytic* therapy. **Answers 2** and **3** are incorrect because they are goals of *brief* psychotherapy, and although they may occur in the resolution of immediate problems, they are *not the* goal.

> **TEST-TAKING TIP**—Note the similarity between the word "crisis" in the stem and "immediate" in the correct option.
> IMP, APP, 7, Psych, PsI, Psychosocial Integrity

Answers/Rationales

34. **(2)** Manipulation is the attempt to control the behavior of others to achieve one's own goals. **Answer 1**, *insight*, is understanding and using understanding to correct one's behavior. **Answers 3** and **4** are incorrect because although the client may be trying to con the nurse into believing he or she *needs* the nurse to do something for him or her and the client *trusts* the nurse, the *real* purpose of the request is manipulation.

> **TEST-TAKING TIP**—Review the concept of manipulation. Eliminate three options that have *no* relationship to "acting out" (insight, dependency, trust).
> **AN, ANL, 7, Psych, PsI, Psychosocial Integrity**

35. **(3)** A person with limited hearing and sight becomes confused and disturbed. **Answers 1** and **4** are *unwarranted* assumptions. **Answer 2** is incorrect because the client's situation is *not psychological* dependency but actual *sensory* need.

> **TEST-TAKING TIP**—Choose the most reasonable explanation and avoid making assumptions (**Answers 1** and **4**).
> **AN, ANL, 2, Psych, PhI, Basic Care and Comfort**

36. **(4)** It is important to pick up on a feeling tone and encourage exploration of the feelings and the situation. **Answer 1** *stops* exploration of the client's feeling. **Answers 2** and **3** *shift* the focus away from feelings to content of selfishness.

> **TEST-TAKING TIP**—Focus on *feelings* and encourage elaboration, with an open-ended statement ("tell me more about …").
> **IMP, APP, 7, Psych, PsI, Psychosocial Integrity**

37. **(1)** Clients with dementia feel more secure when they can count on their environment being the same, predictable, and consistent in detail from day to day (hence, structured) to compensate for feelings of loss of the familiar in terms of body functions, social environment, and so on. **Answers 2** and **4** imply change, not routine. **Answer 3**, although correct, is not the *most* important.

> **TEST-TAKING TIP**—Two options are correct (**Answers 1** and **3**). When the activities are *structured* (the best response), they are usually also *simplified* and avoid decision-making problems. This is a "telescope" answer, in which a broader option subsumes a narrower one.
> **PL, ANL, 6, Psych, SECE, Safety**

38. **(1)** To resolve immediate problems, focus on a person's ability to cope and usual level of functioning. **Answer 2** is incorrect because it is a *psychoanalytic* focus. **Answers 3** and **4** are incorrect because they are the focus of *brief* psychotherapy.

> **TEST-TAKING TIP**—Crisis focuses on the *present* and restoration of *here-and-now* defense.
> **IMP, APP, 7, Psych, PsI, Psychosocial Integrity**

39. **(4)** One defense mechanism often seen in somatoform disorders is repression. As the client is better able to handle the anxiety connected with underlying feelings, the *need for repression lessens*. **Answers 1, 2,** and **3** may be the content of the client's feelings, but they do not explain the dynamics, the *reason* the client is expressing more feelings.

> **TEST-TAKING TIP**—Note the key word: "dynamics." Separate content from dynamics to choose the best answer.
> **AN, ANL, 7, Psych, PsI, Psychosocial Integrity**

40. **(2)** This disorder is an attempt to cope with stress and is a better choice than **Answer 4,** which may be true but is a tangential and irrelevant reason. **Answer 1** is not correct because the client *is* aware of reality but may not understand the *cause* for the somatoform disorder. **Answer 3** is more relevant in a *paranoid* reaction.

> **TEST-TAKING TIP**—Look for the statements that correctly explain somatoform disorders (**Answers 2** and **4**); eliminate **Answer 4** because it is incorporated in **Answer 2.**
> **AN, ANL, 7, Psych, PsI, Psychosocial Integrity**

41. **(3)** When feelings of low self-esteem are prevalent, self-destructive behavior reaches its peak. Hence, **Answers 1, 2,** and **4** are incorrect.

> **TEST-TAKING TIP**—*Low* self-esteem is the option that is different from the three other options (omnipotence, grandiosity, self-satisfaction).
> **AN, ANL, 7, Psych, PsI, Psychosocial Integrity**

42. **(1)** Love-hate feelings take longer to resolve. Reactions to loss tend to be cumulative in effect, in that the more loss experienced in the past, the greater the reaction the next time; thus **Answer 3** is wrong. Reactivation of feelings connected with previous losses by the current loss accounts for the increased intensity of the reaction. Sudden, unexpected death, *rather* than death due to a chronic illness, as in **Answer 2**, is harder to resolve, and strong, *not little,* emotional dependency (as in **Answer 4**) also complicates grief resolution.

> **TEST-TAKING TIP**—Apply your knowledge about grief theory to choose the only correct answer.
> **AN, APP, 7, Psych, PsI, Psychosocial Integrity**

43. **(1)** These behaviors are correct according to Lindemann's and Engle's grief stages. Hence, incorrect are **Answer 2** ("shock" stage), **Answer 3** ("idealization" stage), and **Answer 4** ("resolving the loss" stage).

> **TEST-TAKING TIP**—Review stages of grief to choose the correct stage.
> **AS, COM, 7, Psych, PsI, Psychosocial Integrity**

44. **(4)** Feelings of worthlessness or low self-esteem are the underlying problem in depression. **Answers 1, 2,** and **3** may occur but are *not most* apt.

> **TEST-TAKING TIP**—Note key phrase: "*most* likely to see."
> **AN, COM, 7, Psych, PsI, Psychosocial Integrity**

45. **(2)** Alcohol abuse is the problem here. **Answer 1** is incorrect because although the client with delirium tremens *is* often restless, vital signs are *increased* (BP and pulse) *and* the client may go into seizures if not treated medically as soon as possible. **Answer 3** is incorrect because it focuses on *GI* signs and symptoms; think *neurological* and *cardiovascular* systems for the *most significant* symptoms in this case. **Answer 4** is incorrect because it focuses on *GI* signs and symptoms rather than *significant* neurological and cardiovascular systems.

> **TEST-TAKING TIP**—The key word in the stem is "significant"; in this case, the significant symptoms are *cardiovascular* and *neurological.*
> **AN, ANL, 2, Psych, PhI, Physiological Adaptation**

46. **(4)** Focusing on feelings is usually the best choice. Ignoring the client is rarely an acceptable intervention (**Answer 1**). Pointing out disturbed behavior and role modeling by the nurse are valid, but *not* as first interventions (**Answers 2** and **3**).

> **TEST-TAKING TIP**—Key words: *first need.*
> **PL, APP, 7, Psych, PsI, Psychosocial Integrity**

47. **(4)** Arrest of the disease is possible through abstinence, not through change in psychophysiological response to alcohol. **Answers 1, 2,** and **3** are stereotyped statements, not generally or universally accepted.

TEST-TAKING TIP—Choose the *least* controversial belief: that alcohol dependence cannot be cured. Eliminate the option that has "always"; eliminate the option that is a cliché (**Answer 2**); it has not been universally accepted that alcohol dependency is hereditary.
AN, COM, 7, Psych, PsI, Psychosocial Integrity

48. (4) The *opposite* of what is stated in the first three choices is true. The client seems to do best when *routine* activities are set up and anxiety-provoking changes are avoided (**Answer 1**); *perfection-type* activities bring satisfaction (e.g., cleaning and straightening a linen closet) (**Answer 2**); and the client knows *ahead of time* about changes in routine (**Answer 3**).

TEST-TAKING TIP—By knowing, understanding, and applying theory about dynamics of ritualistic behavior, you can eliminate three options that are theoretically inaccurate. You can also make an educated guess and choose as the best option the answer that includes the phrase "*positive accomplishment can occur.*"
IMP, ANL, 7, Psych, PsI, Psychosocial Integrity

49. (1) The original source of conflict, pain, or guilt is repressed (pushed out of awareness), only to surface in a symbolic way. **Answers 2, 3,** and **4** are only partially correct: in somatoform disorders, regression is common, *not sublimation*; displacement is common, *not substitution*; reaction formation is common, *not rationalization*.

TEST-TAKING TIP—To serve as the best answer, *all* parts must be correct, not just partially correct. Review defense mechanisms as they relate to somatoform disorders.
AN, COM, 7, Psych, PsI, Psychosocial Integrity

50. (4) Although all the other choices (**Answers 1, 2** and **3**) *are* valid and important, **Answer 4** encompasses them all and is therefore the most *comprehensive* answer.

TEST-TAKING TIP—When all four options are correct, choose the "umbrella" answer that includes them all.
AN, ANL, 7, Psych, HPM, Health Promotion and Maintenance

51. (3) A change in body image has made the client feel unloved and unworthy of love. **Answers 1, 2,** and **4** are incorrect because there are *no supporting data*.

TEST-TAKING TIP—Eliminate the three options in which there is lack of information in the stem to support data about problems in the marriage. The best option centers on the *client* and *her* self-concept.
AN, ANL, 7, Psych, PsI, Psychosocial Integrity

52. (2) A client with paranoid disorder is suspicious, so a nurse must make every effort not to engage in behavior the client can misinterpret. **Answers 1** and **3** are incorrect because a nurse *should* give correct information about what the client says and *not* placate him or her (the client will sense the falseness). **Answer 4** is incorrect because arguing just solidifies the client's ideas. In a neutral voice, the nurse should give correct information.

TEST-TAKING TIP—Review interventions with paranoid behavior to choose a response that minimizes distortions and avoids reinforcing the pathology.
IMP, ANL, 7, Psych, PsI, Psychosocial Integrity

53. (3) This response *stops* the manipulation and suggests the client is responsible for his or her own behaviors. **Answers 1, 2,** and **4** are incorrect because they indicate that the nurse has been conned and manipulated.

TEST-TAKING TIP—First, recognize manipulative behavior; next, rule out the three options that may play into this.
IMP, ANL, 5, Psych, PsI, Psychosocial Integrity

54. (3) An appropriate direct response to a "you know what I mean" comment is to say you do *not* automatically know what is meant. **Answers 1, 2,** and **4** are not the best response because they *shift the focus* from the client's experience to the characteristics of the *other* person.

TEST-TAKING TIP—First, choose the answer that directly relates to the mother's question; *then*, seek clarification.
IMP, ANL, 7, Psych, PsI, Psychosocial Integrity

55. (4) Attempts to focus on encouraging the client to describe feelings are important. **Answers 1** and **2** ask for facts rather than focusing on feelings, and **Answer 3** is an example of reflecting—a therapeutic response, but in this case it only reflects a *thought*, not a feeling.

TEST-TAKING TIP—Choose the *feelings*-oriented option.
IMP, APP, 7, Psych, PsI, Psychosocial Integrity

56. (3) Self-esteem is *the most basic* psychological need at *any* age, especially so for the elderly. **Answers 1, 2,** and **4**, although also important, are not the most basic needs.

TEST-TAKING TIP—When you see an option that has "self-esteem," go for it!
PL, ANL, 7, Psych, HPM, Health Promotion and Maintenance

57. (4) This is the least threatening. **Answer 2** is incorrect because the nurse *needs* to intervene into a pattern of silence. It is not therapeutic for the focus to be on the *nurse*, as in **Answers 1** and **3**, and bringing up a *controversial* topic (such as religion or politics) usually results in an exchange of opinions and arguments.

TEST-TAKING TIP—The words "neutral" and "broad opening" in **Answer 4** lead you to the best answer.
PL, APP, 7, Psych, PsI, Psychosocial Integrity

58. (3) This answer is the best choice because the other choices (**Answers 1, 2** and **4**) seem *too certain* for a disorder that, although it has a pattern, can be altered *if* and *when* the client adopts different outlets for expressing emotions.

TEST-TAKING TIP—Choose the most *plausible, tentative* response here rather than the three definitive ones ("will," "essential").
EV, ANL, 7, Psych, PhI, Basic Care and Comfort

59. (2) This response picks up a "here-and-now" underlying feeling tone. **Answers 1** and **4** focus on "there-and-then" rather than "here-and-now" feelings and events, and **Answer 3** is *irrelevant* because the focus is on a *fact* rather than a feeling.

TEST-TAKING TIP—Focus on feelings. Eliminate two options with clichés (**Answers 1** and **4**) and the option that avoids feelings by asking a factual question.
IMP, APP, 7, Psych, PsI, Psychosocial Integrity

60. (4) Expressing feelings *in general* through verbalization is a desired outcome. This answer also incorporates a *specific* feeling in **Answer 3**. Agreement to attend activities (**Answer 2**) does not indicate the *greatest* improvement. The client *already* recognizes that the behavior is irrational but cannot understand the cause or banish the behavior by will, as in **Answer 1**.

TEST-TAKING TIP—When two answers could be correct, choose the one that incorporates both.
EV, ANL, 7, Psych, PsI, Psychosocial Integrity

61. (3) This is the best example of setting limits on the behavior. Answers 1 and 4 may be closely linked to nontherapeutic use of power. Answer 2 is more of an example of a punishment approach.

> TEST-TAKING TIP—You can readily eliminate the three negative options (nurse power in Answer 1; threatening sounding in Answer 2; MD power in Answer 4).
> IMP, APP, 7, Psych, PsI, Psychosocial Integrity

62. (3) Brief and specific information *can* be processed during severe anxiety. In severe anxiety, the person cannot respond to the social environment (as in Answer 1); giving detailed information results in overload, because the client cannot retain and recall data (as in Answer 2). Only directive information that is brief and specific is effective when the client cannot focus on what is happening. Decision making needs to be postponed until the person is less anxious; hence, Answer 4 is wrong.

> 💡 TEST-TAKING TIP—The person who is severely anxious needs to have "KISS" communication—Keep It Simple and Succinct.
> PL, APP, 7, Psych, PsI, Psychosocial Integrity

63. (4) The liver is affected by both the direct effect of alcohol and nutritional deficiencies associated with alcohol abuse and dependence. Answers 1, 2, and 3 are areas not usually affected by alcohol abuse and dependence.

> TEST-TAKING TIP—Review physiological consequences of alcohol abuse.
> AN, APP, 7, Psych, PhI, Reduction of Risk Potential

64. (1) This response aims to prevent use of manipulative patterns. In Answers 2, 3, and 4, the nurse needs to seek validation, and these responses indicate acceptance without validation.

> TEST-TAKING TIP—The team approach for consistent reinforcement of rules is needed when interacting with clients who display manipulative behavior.
> IMP, ANL, 7, Psych, SECE, Management of Care

65. (1) These are typical symptoms/responses to anxiety. Other common reactions are pupillary dilation, *not* constriction (Answer 2); diarrhea, *not* constipation (Answer 4). Vomiting is not typical of an anxiety response (Answer 3).

> TEST-TAKING TIP—Review physiological manifestations of anxiety.
> AS, COM, 7, Psych, PhI, Physiological Adaptation

66. (3) This response refers to the definition of *projection* as a defense mechanism (attributing one's own unacceptable thoughts, feelings, and behaviors to another). Answers 1, 2, and 4 are incorrect because they have nothing to do with the defense mechanism of projection. Defense mechanisms in general function in the service of "self"—that is, they protect the ego and preserve self-esteem in an effort to cope with anxiety; the focus is *not* on *others*, as in Answers 1 and 4. Symptoms of projection do in fact *express* delusional thought rather than *control* it, contrary to Answer 2.

> TEST-TAKING TIP—Select the option that has "feelings."
> AN, COM, 7, Psych, PsI, Psychosocial Integrity

67. (2) In panic, a person is highly suggestible and follows "herd instinct" rather than exercising independent judgment and goal-directed problem solving (Answer 1). Answer 3 is incorrect because the severity of the reaction *is* related to the severity of the threat. The more severe the perceived threat (actual or imaginary), the more intense the reaction to the danger, and *not* delayed as in Answer 4.

> TEST-TAKING TIP—Apply knowledge about panic reaction.
> AN, COM, 7, Psych, PsI, Psychosocial Integrity

68. (4) The primary initial focus of the nurse-client relationship is in showing the client, through acceptance, that it is the *client* one is concerned about, *not* the *symptoms*. Answers 1 and 2 are incorrect because the focus of *initial* nursing care is on the client, not on meeting hospital standards or controlling impulses. Answer 3 is incorrect because it is an attempt to analyze the *whys* of behavior, which is not an appropriate *basic* nursing intervention and *not* an initial aspect of care.

> TEST-TAKING TIP—The key word is "acceptance," a basic tenet of the nurse-client relationship.
> PL, APP, 7, Psych, PsI, Psychosocial Integrity

69. (3) This is the most inclusive answer. Answers 1, 2, and 4 are all *incorporated* into Answer 3.

> TEST-TAKING TIP—When all answers are correct, choose the "umbrella" answer that covers them all.
> AN, COM, 7, Psych, PsI, Psychosocial Integrity

70. (2, 3, 4) Answer 2 is correct because Haldol does produce an anticholinergic response, such as dry mouth and constipation, as well as orthostatic hypotension and urinary retention. Answers 3 and 4 are correct because these side effects are seen when on Haldol. Answer 1 is incorrect because Haldol does not typically cause diarrhea. Answer 5 is incorrect because clients taking Haldol experience an *increase* in appetite, *not* a decrease. Answer 6 is incorrect because high BP is not commonly seen in clients taking Haldol.

> TEST-TAKING TIP—The client usually does not have both an increase and a decrease in blood pressure (Answers 3 and 6) nor both diarrhea and constipation (Answers 1 and 2). Remember to only choose one answer that is the opposite.
> EV, COM, 7, Psych, PhI, Phamacological/Parenteral Therapies

71. (2) Research shows that *increased* activity is a psychomotor manifestation of anxiety; therefore, Answer 1 is incorrect. Answers 3 and 4 are incorrect because emotion is *not* a psychomotor manifestation.

> TEST-TAKING TIP—Note the *similarity* between the word "psychomotor" in the stem and the word "activity" in Answers 1 and 2. Next decide on "increased activity" by applying theory about anxiety.
> AS, COM, 3, Psych, PhI, Physiological Adaptation

72. (2) When the mourner can pass through the idealization stage and be more realistic about the positive and negative aspects of the loss, resolution of grief is beginning. Answers 3 and 4 occur in *earlier* stages of grief. Answer 1 could be a sign of denial of grieving, an initial grief reaction.

> TEST-TAKING TIP—Because all of the answers could be acceptable, you need to review the *stages* of grief to identify the best answer in relation to a *time sequence*. The other three options relate to *earlier* stages.
> EV, APP, 7, Psych, PsI, Psychosocial Integrity

73. (3) Research shows that anxiety *decreases* the perceptual field; therefore, Answer 1 is incorrect. Research also shows that anxiety *decreases* the ability to concentrate and *increases* random activity; therefore, Answers 1, 2, and 4 are incorrect.

TEST-TAKING TIP—Note the two *contradictory* options: "increase perceptual field" vs. "decrease perceptual field." Next, apply knowledge about anxiety to select the *theoretically* correct answer. **Answers 2** and **4** are theoretically incorrect.
AN, COM, 7, Psych, PsI, Psychosocial Integrity

74. (3) This is correct by Freudian theory. **Answers 1, 2,** and **4** are incorrect because they are incomplete.

TEST-TAKING TIP—The correct answer directly stems from a particular theoretical viewpoint—Freudian, which you will need to review.
AN, COM, 7, Psych, PsI, Psychosocial Integrity

75. (1) This is correct according to Erickson. **Answer 2** relates to toddler; **Answer 3,** to infancy; **Answer 4,** to latency period in childhood.

TEST-TAKING TIP—Review and apply your knowledge of the *age-related* stages, which will lead to the only correct answer.
AN, COM, 5, Psych, HPM, Health Promotion and Maintenance

76. (1) Suicide risk is highest in clients with major depression. **Answers 2, 3,** and **4** are incorrect because these diagnoses alone do not indicate suicide risk as does the diagnosis of depression.

TEST-TAKING TIP—Depression is the *most common* direct risk factor for suicide.
AN, ANL, 7, Psych, PsI, Psychosocial Integrity

77. (1) "Loss" is *most basic* to the development of depression. **Answers 2, 3,** and **4** are *not essential* to development of depression.

TEST-TAKING TIP—When in doubt, choose the *least controversial,* more *general* answer ("a sense of loss") rather than pinpointing specific causal factors (e.g., "painful childhood," "confused sexual identity," "unresolved oedipal conflict").
AN, COM, 7, Psych, PsI, Psychosocial Integrity

78. (4) Some anxiety is necessary to learn. **Answer 2** is incorrect because it is *incomplete.* **Answers 1** and **3** are incorrect because anxiety *is necessary* for learning and growth.

TEST-TAKING TIP—When two answers seem right, choose the answer that incorporates the other (i.e., capacity to tolerate anxiety would *also mean* developing awareness of anxiety).
PL, APP, 7, Psych, PsI, Psychosocial Integrity

79. (2) Part of maturing is learning to view one's parents *and* oneself realistically. **Answers 1, 3,** and **4** are incorrect because they represent the *misinformation* that creates problems between individuals.

TEST-TAKING TIP—The key word in the correct option is "realistically."
EV, APP, 7, Psych, HPM, Health Promotion and Maintenance

80. (2) A permissive atmosphere is the key, as well as a *slowly* evolving relationship (not quickly evolving, as in **Answer 3**) with room for *distance.* Self-destruction is *not a persistent* problem requiring *major* focus for concern, as in **Answer 4**. **Answer 1** is not the best response because "acceptance" of *bizarre* behavior is more important than setting limits.

TEST-TAKING TIP—Note the key words in the correct answer: "trusting, nonthreatening, reality-based relationship."
PL, APP, 7, Psych, PsI, Psychosocial Integrity

81. (1) An undemanding task that the client could finish would allow a feeling of successful accomplishment. **Answers 2** and **3** require intellectual activity, which is usually slowed down during a depressive phase. **Answer 4** requires a skill that the client may not have and that might frustrate the client to learn; also, the client may not have the psychomotor energy for ice skating.

TEST-TAKING TIP—Apply the process of elimination. Eliminate the two activities that call for intact cognitive functioning (which is slowed down in depression). The best answer does not involve a great deal of physical exertion, either (**Answer 4**).
IMP, ANL, 3, Psych, PsI, Psychosocial Integrity

82. (2) It will provide energy release without the external stimuli and pressure of *competitive games* (**Answers 3** and **4**). Reading (**Answer 1**) usually requires sitting, which a client who is hyperactive cannot readily do.

TEST-TAKING TIP—Apply theory about manic behavior (hyperactivity) and select the only option that helps the client to externalize the energy (**Answer 2**), without additional stimuli (competitive games).
IMP, ANL, 3, Psych, PsI, Psychosocial Integrity

83. (4) The mother needs to ask the client, not the nurse, but the nurse should also support the mother and encourage her to interact with her son. **Answers 1** and **2** are incorrect because they are *interpretations* that state opinions about the client without his participation. **Answer 3** is incorrect because *no support is given* to the mother.

TEST-TAKING TIP—First, eliminate the two options that are interpretive (**Answers 1** and **2**); then choose the option that *redirects* the mother to the client while providing *support* to the mother (**Answer 4**).
IMP, ANL, 7, Psych, PsI, Psychosocial Integrity

84. (3) By definition, this is the conscious, deliberate effort to avoid talking or thinking about painful, anxiety-producing experiences. **Answers 1, 2,** and **4** are incorrect terms for the example given in the stem.

TEST-TAKING TIP—Review definitions of defense mechanisms in order to select the correct answer.
AN, APP, 7, Psych, PsI, Psychosocial Integrity

85. (4) A variety of factors can cause self-destructive behavior, and these differ for each individual. Hence, **Answers 2** and **3** are not the best choices because, although correct, they are *examples* of a *variety* of factors; **Answer 1** is the opposite of the correct answer.

TEST-TAKING TIP—Choose the most inclusive answer when two options are *examples* of a *main* point. Eliminate **Answer 1,** which is partially the same as **Answer 4** but also the opposite ("same" vs. "different" factors).
AS, ANL, 7, Psych, PsI, Psychosocial Integrity

86. (1) A person who has settled on a plan for suicide may become more cheerful. **Answer 2** is incorrect because a person who is severely retarded in the psychomotor area cannot carry out a suicide act. **Answers 3** and **4** are incorrect because the client is more likely to be hostile and agitated if he or she does not have a suicide plan. Agitated behavior can also represent the need to "repent" for sins thought to be committed.

TEST-TAKING TIP—Look at the two sets of contradictory options: "cheerfulness" (**Answer 1**) vs. "hostility" (**Answer 4**); "psychomotor retardation" (i.e., slowing down)

(**Answer 2**) vs. "agitation" (**Answer 3**). Hostility and agitation can be paired and, therefore, ruled out; that leaves "cheerfulness" as the option that is different, and the one to select ("which of the following is not like the others?").
EV, APP, 7, Psych, PsI, Psychosocial Integrity

87. (1) This is the correct match between age period and developmental task. **Answer 2** refers to preschool age, **Answer 3** is characteristic of "maturity" in later years of life, and **Answer 4** refers to young adulthood.

> **TEST-TAKING TIP**—Review *age*-related psychosocial growth and development stages according to Erikson.
> **AN, COM, 7, Psych, HPM, Health Promotion and Maintenance**

88. (4) This is the correct definition. **Answer 1** is incorrect because it defines agnosia. **Answer 2** is incorrect because it defines agraphia. **Answer 3** is incorrect because it defines aphasia.

> **TEST-TAKING TIP**—Knowing the root words will help you to pick the correct definition (praxis-coordinated movement).
> **AS, COM, 7, Psych, PhI, Physiological Integrity**

89. (3) Most children with Down syndrome are affectionate and enjoy being held and cuddled, whereas the *opposite* is usually the case with a child who is autistic. All other responses (**Answers 1, 2,** and **4**) may apply to *both* Down syndrome and autism.

> **TEST-TAKING TIP**—Apply knowledge about characteristics of Down syndrome and autism to select an important difference related to *interpersonal* behavior.
> **AS, APP, 5, Psych, PsI, Psychosocial Integrity**

90. (2) Note the eyes: when a person is *on* heroin, the pupils are constricted; during *withdrawal*, they are dilated. Withdrawal does *not* usually include high fever, pupillary constriction, or choreiform movements, as in **Answers 1, 3,** and **4**.

> **TEST-TAKING TIP**—Note two *contradictory* options about the eyes ("dilation" vs. "constriction"), and know which applies to *withdrawal* vs. being *on* heroin.
> **AS, APP, 7, Psych, PsI, Psychosocial Integrity**

91. (4) Methadone is a synthetic narcotic and has no euphoric effect. Methadone does not produce sedation (**Answer 1**), euphoria (**Answer 2**), or neuritis (**Answer 3**).

> **TEST-TAKING TIP**—Eliminate the three options that are not related to methadone. Review effects of methadone.
> **EV, COM, 7, Psych, PhI, Pharmacological Therapy**

92. (4) With concern for danger to the other clients, staff, and the environment, it is essential for the client to be restrained at this time. The other choices are incorrect because orientation and a quiet environment *alone* do *not* provide for safety when the client's agitation is out of control (**Answer 1**); the initial *delay* in onset of effectiveness of the tranquilizer does not *immediately* provide for the safety needs of other clients, staff, and the environment (**Answer 2**); and locking the client in his or her room eliminates only the danger to others—additional measures would be needed to provide for the safety of this *client* (**Answer 3**).

> **TEST-TAKING TIP**—Note the key word, "initially." Know *when* it is acceptable to use restraints.
> **IMP, ANL, 1, Psych, SECE, Safety**

93. (3) Limit setting is an important intervention with a client who exhibits excessive, constant dependence on others for

simple, seemingly inconsequential decisions in everyday life. The other choices are wrong because the situation presented provides insufficient data on which to base interpretations related to fear of failure (**Answer 1**), a need to test for staff acceptance (**Answer 2**), or a bid for attention (**Answer 4**).

> **TEST-TAKING TIP**—Eliminate the three options for which there are no data in the stem to validate the interpretations (**Answers 1, 2,** and **4**).
> **AN, ANL, 7, Psych, PsI, Psychosocial Integrity**

94. (1) This is the only correct answer regarding dietary prohibitions. **Answers 2, 3,** and **4** *are allowed.*

> **TEST-TAKING TIP**—Knowledge regarding Orthodox Jewish dietary laws is needed to select the correct option. Note the key word: "prohibited" (i.e., not *not* allowed).
> **AN, COM, 4, Psych, PsI, Psychosocial Integrity**

95. (1) Manipulation is a characteristic antisocial behavior. Flattery is a form of manipulation—with hidden agenda, to get what the client wants, whatever that may be. **Answer 2** may or may not be the agenda behind the flattery. **Answers 3** and **4** are also possible examples of what the client wants.

> **TEST-TAKING TIP**—When more than one answer is plausible, choose the one that covers them all—the "umbrella" answer (**Answer 1**).
> **AN, ANL, 7, Psych, PsI, Psychosocial Integrity**

96. (1) is correct because depressive episodes are often *recurrent.* **Answers 2, 3,** and **4** may or may not experience depression. **Answers 2** and **4** are more likely to experience anxiety. There does not appear to be any reason to expect that a housewife with three children in school would be at risk for any particular emotional distress (**Answer 3**).

> **TEST-TAKING TIP**—Match the key word in the *answers,* "depressive," with the key word in the *stem,* "depression."
> **AN, ANL, 7, Psych, PsI, Psychosocial Integrity**

97. (3) Nursing observation is easier if the client with Alzheimer's is *nearby.* Therefore, **Answer 4** is incorrect. A roommate may (**Answer 1**) or may not (**Answer 2**) be all right, but facilitating nursing observations is the highest priority for a client with memory problems and confusion who is a safety risk for wandering off the unit.

> **TEST-TAKING TIP**—Focus in on the best option by first narrowing choices to two that are contradictory (with/without a roommate; near/at distance from the nurses' station). Then ask, Is it roommate or proximity to nurses' station that is the priority? Next, consider what goal is met by being near the *nurses' station* rather than a roommate. Answer: *safety* from wandering.
> **AN, ANL, 1, Psych, SECE, Management of Care**

98. (1) This is the correct answer because it lets the nurse know that contacts with the person who is elderly are infrequent and that ongoing assessment of needs and health concerns is not likely to occur. **Answer 2** is incorrect because it is *not the greatest concern,* as long as there is the opportunity for assessment by phone. A cordless phone is a *good* idea rather than a great concern (**Answer 3**). Although isolation is further increased by not wanting to go to a senior citizen center, it is not of greatest concern (**Answer 4**).

> **TEST-TAKING TIP**—Put logic and reasoning to work here. Look at patterns in the stem: two options focus on family (**Answers 1** and **2**), one option focuses on a phone instrument (**Answer 3**), and another option focuses on a community agency (**Answer 4**).
> **AN, ANL, 1, Psych, SECE, Management of Care**

99. (4) This answer is concerned with accident prevention and is a means of observation of the client. **Answers 1** and **2** are incorrect because the use of restraints is inappropriate and not justified. Having a security guard is not realistic (**Answer 3**).

> **TEST-TAKING TIP**—Use the process of elimination. Eliminate the two options dealing with restraints; eliminate the most unlikely option (**Answer 3**); **Answer 4,** therefore, is the best answer.
> **IMP, ANL, 1, Psych, SECE, Safety and Infection Control**

100. (4) The client is probably experiencing a loss of control over the hospitalization situation. Initially the client and family should be included in planning care, which returns decision making to the client and decreases frustration. **Answers 1** and **3** shift the problem rather than attempt to resolve the issue. **Answer 2** involves the client but brings in an authority figure (the MD), which may be seen as punishment or "parental" by the client.

> **TEST-TAKING TIP**—Look for the choice that gives the client the most control; do not "pass the buck" to someone else (MD, social services, etc.)
> **PL, ANL, 7, Psych, SECE, Management of Care**

Nursing Care of the Acutely Ill and the Chronically Ill Adult

Robyn Nelson and Debra Brady

ASSESSMENT, ANALYSIS, AND NURSING DIAGNOSIS OF THE ADULT

Assessment is the process of gathering a comprehensive database about the client's present, past, and potential health problems, as well as a description of the client as a whole in his or her environment. It includes a comprehensive nursing history, a physical examination, and laboratory/x-ray data, and it concludes with the formulation of nursing diagnoses.

The Health Insurance Portability and Accountability Act of 1996 (HIPAA) strengthened the privacy protections for consumers. Communications are confidential and the client needs to give permission for other family members to remain in room—particularly when asking sensitive questions on pregnancies, abortions, drug use, or multiple sex partners (see **Unit 3, p 129**).

Subjective Data

Nursing History

The nursing history obtains data for planning and implementing nursing actions.

I. **General health information:** reason for admission; duration of present illness; previous hospitalization; history of illnesses; diagnostic procedures before admission; allergies—type and severity of reactions; medications taken at home—over-the-counter, prescription medications, and alternative/complementary therapies.

II. **Information relative to growth and development:** age; menarche—age at onset; heavy menses; dysmenorrhea; vaginal discharge; date of last Pap smear; pregnancies; abortions; miscarriages.

III. **Information relative to psychosocial functions:** feelings (anger, denial, fear, anxiety, guilt, lifestyle changes); language barriers; family support; spiritual needs; history of trauma/rape.

IV. **Information relative to nutrition:** appetite—normal, changes; dietary habits; food preferences or intolerances; difficulty swallowing or chewing; dentures; use of caffeine/alcohol; weight changes; excessive thirst, hunger, sweating.

V. **Information relative to fluid and gas transport:** difficulty breathing; shortness of breath; home O_2 use; history of cough/smoking; colds; sputum; swelling of extremities; chest pain; palpitations; varicosities; excessive bruising; blood transfusions; excessive bleeding.

VI. **Information relative to protective functions:** skin problems—rash, itch; current treatment; unusual hair loss.

VII. **Information relative to comfort, rest, activity, mobility:** usual activity (activities of daily living [ADL]); present ability and restrictions; rest and sleep pattern; weakness; joint or muscle stiffness, pain, or swelling; occupation; interests.

VIII. **Information relative to elimination:** bowel habits; changes—constipation, diarrhea; ostomy; emesis; nausea; voiding—retention, frequency, dysuria, incontinence.

IX. **Information relative to sensory/perceptual functions:** pain—verbal report; acute/chronic, treatment, quality, location; precipitating factors; duration; limitations in vision (glasses), hearing, touch, smell; orientation to person, place, time; confusion; headaches; fainting; dizziness; convulsions.

Objective Data

◆ I. **General**—provides information on the client as a whole.
   A. *Race, sex, apparent age* in relation to stated age.
   B. *Nutritional status*—well hydrated and developed or obesity, cachexia—include weight.
   C. *Apparent health status*—general good health or mild, moderate, severe debilitation.

D. *Posture and motor activity*—erect, symmetrical, balanced gait and muscle development, or ataxic, circumducted, scissor, or spastic gait; slumped or bent-over posture; mild, moderate, or hyperactive motor responses.

E. *Behavior*—alert; oriented to person, time, place; hears and comprehends instructions, or tense, anxious, angry; uses abusive language; slightly or largely unresponsive; delusions, hallucinations.

F. *Odors*—noncontributory, or acetone, alcohol, fetid breath, incontinent of urine or feces.

◆ II. **Physical assessment**—requires knowledge of normal findings, organization, and keen senses (i.e., visual, auditory, touch, smell). For abnormal findings, refer to the *Assessment* section of each health problem discussed under the categories of human functioning.

A. *Components*
1. *Inspection*—uses observations to detect deviations from normal.
2. *Auscultation*—used to perceive and interpret sounds arising from various organs, particularly heart, lungs, and bowel.
3. *Palpation*—used to assess for discomfort, temperature, pulsations, size, consistency, and texture.
4. *Percussion*—technique used to elicit vibrations produced by underlying organ structures; used less frequently in nursing practice.
   a. Flat—normal percussion; note over muscle or bone.
   b. Dull—normal percussion; note over organs such as liver.
   c. Resonance—normal percussion; note over lungs.
   d. Tympany—normal percussion; note over stomach or bowel.

B. *Approach*—head-to-toe
1. *General appearance*—well or poorly developed or nourished. Color (black, white, jaundiced, pale). In distress (acutely or chronically)?
2. *Vital signs*—blood pressure (which arm or both, orthostatic change). Pulse (regular or irregular, orthostatic change). Respirations (labored or unlabored, wheeze). Temperature (axillary, rectal, temporal [forehead], tympanic membrane, or oral). Weight. Height (**Table 7.1**).

3. *Skin, hair, and nails*—pigmentation, scars, lesions, bruises, turgor. Describe or draw rashes.
   a. Skin color:
      (1) Red—fever, allergic reaction, carbon monoxide (CO) poisoning, burn.
      (2) White (pallor)—excessive blood loss, fright.
      (3) Blue (cyanosis)—hypoxemia, peripheral vasoconstriction, shock.
      (4) Mottled—cardiovascular embarrassment, shock.
   b. Skin temperature:
      (1) Hot, dry—excessive body heat (heatstroke).
      (2) Hot, wet—reaction to increased internal or external temperature.
      (3) Cool, dry—exposure to cold.
      (4) Cool, clammy—shock.
4. *Head*—scalp, skull (configuration), scars, tenderness, bruits.
5. *Neck*—suppleness. Trachea, larynx, thyroid, blood vessels (jugular veins, carotid arteries).
6. *Nodes*—any cervical, supraclavicular, axillary, epitrochlear, inguinal lymphadenopathy? If so, size of nodes (in centimeters), consistency (firm, rubbery, tender), mobile or fixed.
7. *Eyes:*
   a. **External eye.** Conjunctivae, sclerae, lids, cornea, pupils (including reflexes), visual fields, extraocular motions.
   b. **Fundus.** Disk, blood vessels, pigmentation.
8. *Ears*—shape of pinnae, external canal, tympanic membrane, acuity, air conduction versus bone conduction (*Rinne test*), lateralization (*Weber's test*).
9. *Nose*—nares (symmetry), septum, mucosa, polyps.
10. *Mouth and throat*—lips, teeth (loose, dental hygiene, odor), tongue (size, papillation), buccal mucosa, palate, tonsils, oropharynx.
11. *Chest*
    a. **Inspection.** Contour, symmetry, expansion.
    b. **Palpation.** Expansion, rib tenderness, tactile fremitus.
    c. **Percussion.** Diaphragmatic excursion, dullness.
    d. **Auscultation.** Crackles, rubs, wheezes, egophony, pectoriloquy.

TABLE 7.1		Factors Affecting Vital Signs									
Factor	Infection (fever)	↓H&H (hypovolemia)	↓BS (insulin shock)	↑BS/DKA (hyperglycemia)	Narcotic (CNS depression)	Anxiety (fear)	Pain (acute)	Acute MI	↑K⁺ (hyperkalemia)	↓K⁺ (hypokalemia)	Exercise
T	↑	↓	↓	↑	↓	Normal	Normal	Normal	Normal	Normal	↑
HR	↑	↑	Normal/↑	↑	↓	↑	↑	↓	↓	↑	↑
RR	↑	↑	Normal	↑	↓	↑	↑	↑	Shallow	Shallow	↑
BP	Normal	↓	Normal/↑	↓	↓	↑	↑	↓	Normal/↑	↓	↑

From Myers, Ehren: RNotes, FA Davis, Philadelphia, 2003, p. 22.

(1) Use diaphragm or bell. Normal sounds over alveoli—*vesicular.* Large airway or abnormal sounds—*bronchial or bronchovesicular.* Adventitious sounds—*crackles or wheezes.*

(2) *Crackles*—discontinuous noises heard on auscultation; caused by popping open of air spaces; usually associated with increased fluid in the lungs; formerly called *rales* and *rhonchi.*

(3) *Wheezes*—high-pitched, whistling sounds made by air flowing through narrowed airways.

(4) *Stridor*—harsh, high-pitched, heard during inspiration and expiration; life threatening.

12. *Breasts*—symmetry, retraction, lesions, nipples (inverted, everted), masses, tenderness, discharge.

13. *Heart:*
   a. **Inspection.** Point of maximal impulse (PMI), chest contour.
   b. **Palpation.** Point of maximal impulse (PMI), thrills, lifts, thrusts.
   c. **Auscultation.** Heart sounds, gallops, murmurs, rubs. Use diaphragm for high-pitched sounds of normal heart sounds (S_1 and S_2) and bell for abnormal sounds (S_3 and S_4).

14. *Abdomen:*
   a. **Inspection.** Scars (draw these), contour, masses, vein pattern.
   b. **Auscultation.** Bowel sounds, rubs, bruits. Use diaphragm. Auscultate *after* inspection and *before* palpation and percussion. Listen to each quadrant for at least 1 min. If bowel sounds are present, they will be heard in lower right quadrant (area of ileocecal valve). *Hypo*—every minute; *normal*—every 15–20 seconds; *hyper*—about every 3 seconds.
   c. **Percussion**—organomegaly, hepatic dullness.
   d. **Palpation**—tenderness, masses, rigidity, liver, spleen, kidneys.
   e. **Hernia**—femoral, inguinal, ventral.

15. *Genitalia:*
   a. **Male.** Penile lesions, discharge, scrotum, testes. Circumcised?
   b. **Female.** Labia, Bartholin's and Skene's glands, vagina, cervix. Bimanual examination of internal genitalia.

16. *Rectum*—perianal lesions, sphincter tone, tenderness, masses, prostate, stool color, occult blood.

17. *Extremities*—pulses (symmetry, bruits, perfusion). Joints (mobility, deformity). Cyanosis, edema. Varicosities. Muscle mass. Grips equal.

18. *Back*—contour spine, tenderness. Sacral edema.

19. *Neurological:*
   a. **Mental status.** Alertness, memory, judgment, mood.
   b. **Cranial nerves** (I–XII) **(Figure 7.1).**
   c. **Cerebellum.** Gait, finger-nose, heel-shin, tremors.
   d. **Motor.** Muscle mass, strength; deep-tendon reflexes. Pathological or primitive reflexes.

e. **Sensory.** Touch, pain, vibration. Heat and cold as indicated.

III. **Routine laboratory studies**—see **Appendix A** for normal ranges.
   A. *Hematology:*
      1. Complete blood count—detects presence of anemia, infection, allergy, and leukemia.
      2. Prothrombin time—increase may indicate liver disease or cancer.
      3. Serology (VDRL)—determines presence of syphilis; false-positive result may indicate collagen dysfunction.
   B. **Urinalysis:**
      1. Specific gravity—measures ability of kidney to concentrate urine. Fixed specific gravity indicates renal tubular dysfunction.
      2. Protein—indicates glomerular dysfunction.
      3. Albumin, WBC, and pus—indicate renal infection.
      4. Sugar and acetone—presence indicates metabolic disorder.
   C. *Chest x-ray*—detects tuberculosis or other pulmonary dysfunctions, as well as changes in size or configuration of heart.
   D. *Electrocardiogram (ECG or EKG)*—detects rhythm and conduction disturbances, presence of myocardial ischemia or necrosis, and ventricular hypertrophy.
   E. *Blood chemistries*—detect deviation in electrolyte balance, presence of tissue damage, and adequacy of glomerular filtration.

IV. **Preventive Care**
   A. Checkup visits recommended every 1–3 years until age 65 and then yearly thereafter. **Table 7.2** lists suggested timelines.
   B. Individuals with *special risk factors* may need more frequent and additional types of preventive care.
      1. *Diabetes*—eye, foot exams; urine, blood sugar tests.
      2. *Drug abuse*—AIDS, TB tests; hepatitis immunization.
      3. *Alcoholism*—influenza, pneumococcal immunizations; TB test.
      4. *Overweight*—blood sugar test, triglycerides, blood pressure.
      5. *Homeless, recent refugees or immigrant*—TB test.
      6. *High-risk sexual behavior*—AIDS, syphilis, gonorrhea, chlamydia (every year for women who are sexually active), hepatitis tests.
      7. *Pregnancy*—Rubella blood test (prior to first pregnancy).
   C. *Adult immunizations*—prevention of disease and reduction in the severity of disease (**Table 7.3**).

Assessment is followed by *analysis* of data and formulation of a *nursing diagnosis.* Possible nursing diagnoses for each category of human functioning are given in the following sections.

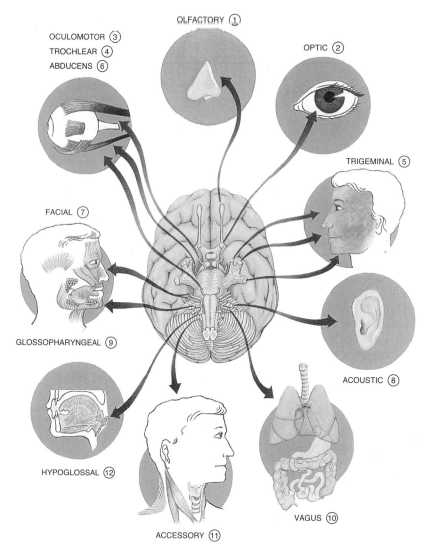

FIGURE 7.1 Cranial nerves and their distributions. (From Venes, D [ed]: Taber's Cyclopedic Medical Dictionary, ed. 20. FA Davis, Philadelphia, 2005.)

TABLE 7.2 — Preventive Care Timelines

Years of Age: 18 · 25 · 30 · 35 · 40 · 45 · 50 · 55 · 60 · 65 · 70 · 75 · <

TESTS

BLOOD PRESSURE	EVERY 2 YEARS
HEIGHT & WEIGHT	PERIODICALLY
CHOLESTEROL	MEN ··· EVERY 2–3 YEARS (MEN & WOMEN)
HEARING	BASELINE ··· PERIODICALLY
MAMMOGRAPHY	YEARLY (WOMEN)
PAP SMEAR (Cervical cancer)	EVERY 1–3 YEARS (WOMEN)
SIGMOIDOSCOPY/COLONOSCOPY	EVERY 3–5 YEARS AND/OR
STOOL OCCULT BLOOD (FOBT)	YEARLY
BLOOD SUGAR	AT LEAST EVERY 3–4 YEARS

EXAMS

Exam	Recommendation
DENTAL, ORAL HEALTH	YEARLY
VISION/GLAUCOMA	EVERY 2–4 YEARS ··· EVERY 1–2 YEARS
BREAST (by doctor)	EVERY 1–3 YEARS (WOMEN) ··· EVERY YEAR (WOMEN)
EXAM FOR CANCER: Thyroid, Mouth, Skin, Ovaries, Testicles (monthly between ages 19–40), Lymph Nodes, Rectum (40+), Prostate (men 50+)	EVERY 3 YEARS ··· YEARLY
BONE DENSITY (Osteoporosis)	EVERY 2 YEARS ··· YEARLY

HEALTH GUIDANCE

PERIODICALLY:
- Smoking, Alcohol & Drugs,
- Sexual Behavior, AIDS,
- Eating Disorders, Nutrition, Physical Activity,
- Weight Management,
- Violence & Guns, Injuries,
- Family Planning,
- Occupational Health,
- Folate (Women 12–45), Aspirin (Men 40+)

Upper age limits should be individualized for each person
- Recommended by most major authorities
- Recommended by some major authorities

Source: Office of Disease Prevention and Health Promotion, in cooperation with the agencies of the Public Health Service, U.S. Department of Health and Human Services.

Adult

477

| TABLE 7.3 | ■ Summary of Recommendations for Adult Immunization |

Vaccine Name and Route	For Whom It Is Recommended	Schedule	Contraindications and Precautions (Mild Illness Is Not a Contraindication)
Influenza ("flu shot")—give IM	■ Adults who are 50 years of age or older. ■ People 6 mo to 65 yr of age with medical problems such as *heart disease, lung disease, diabetes, renal* dysfunction, hemoglobinopathies, *immunosuppression,* or those *living in chronic care facilities.* ■ People (≥6 mo of age) working or living with people who are at risk. ■ All health-care workers and those who provide key community services. ■ Healthy women who are pregnant who will be in their *2nd or 3rd* trimesters during the influenza season. ■ Women who are pregnant who have underlying medical conditions should be vaccinated before the flu season, regardless of the stage of pregnancy. ■ Anyone who wishes to reduce the likelihood of becoming ill with influenza. ■ Travelers to areas where influenza activity exists or when traveling among people from areas of the world where there is current influenza activity.	■ Given *every year.* ■ October through November is the optimal time to receive an annual flu shot to maximize protection, but the vaccine may be given at any time during the influenza season (typically December through March) or at other times when the risk of influenza exits. ■ May be given anytime during the influenza season. ■ May be given with all other vaccines but at a separate site.	■ Previous anaphylactic reaction to this vaccine, to any of its components, or to eggs. ■ Moderate or severe acute illness.
Pneumococcal—give IM or SC	■ Adults who are 65 years of age or older. ■ People 2 yr to 65 yr of age who have chronic illness or other risk factors including chronic cardiac or pulmonary diseases, chronic liver disease, alcoholism, diabetes mellitus, CSF leaks, as well as persons living in special environments or social settings (including Alaska natives and certain American Indian populations). Those at highest risk of fatal pneumococcal infection are persons with anatomical or functional asplenia (including sickle cell disease); persons who are immunocompromised, including those with HIV infection, leukemia, lymphoma, Hodgkin's disease, multiple myeloma, generalized malignancy, chronic renal failure, or nephrotic syndrome; those receiving immunosuppressive chemotherapy (including corticosteroids); and those who received an organ or bone marrow transplant.	■ Routinely given as a *one-time* dose; administer if previous vaccination history is unknown. ■ One-time revaccination is recommended 5 years later for people at highest risk of fatal pneumococcal infection or rapid antibody loss (e.g., renal disease) and for people ≥*65 years* if the 1st dose was given *before age 65* and ≥5 years have elapsed since previous dose. ■ May be given with all other vaccines but at a separate site.	■ Previous anaphylactic reaction to this vaccine or to any of its components. ■ Moderate or severe acute illness.

(Continued on following page)

Adult

Vaccine Name and Route	For Whom It Is Recommended	Schedule	Contraindications and Precautions (Mild Illness Is Not a Contraindication)
Hepatitis B (hep-B)— give IM; brands may be used interchangeably	▪ Adults who are high-risk including household contacts and sex partners of persons who are HBsAg-positive; users of *illicit injectable drugs;* heterosexuals with *more than one sex partner* in 6 months; *men who have sex with men;* people with recently diagnosed STDs; people with multiple piercings/tattoos; clients in *hemodialysis* units and clients with renal disease that may result in dialysis; recipients of certain blood products; health-care workers and public safety workers who are exposed to blood; clients and staff of *institutions for the developmentally disabled; inmates* of long-term correctional facilities; and certain international travelers. *Note:* Prior **serological testing** may be recommended depending on the specific level of risk or likelihood of previous exposure.	▪ *Three* doses are needed on a *0, 1, 6 mo* schedule. ▪ Alternative timing options for vaccination include: 0, 2, 4 months 0, 1, 4 months ▪ There must be 4 wk between doses #1 and #2, and 8 wk between doses #2 and #3. Overall there must be at least 4 mo between doses #1 and #3. ▪ Two-dose formulation available for 11 to 15 yr: 4–6 mo between doses #1 and #2.	▪ Previous anaphylactic reaction to this vaccine or to any of its components. ▪ Moderate or severe acute illness.
	▪ *All adolescents.* *Note:* In 1997, the NIH Consensus Development Conference, a panel of national experts, recommended that hepatitis B vaccination be given to all persons infected with hepatitis C virus. Do *serological screening for people who have emigrated from endemic areas. When persons who are HBsAg-positive are identified, offer them appropriate disease management. In addition, screen their household members and intimate contacts and, if found susceptible, vaccinate.*	▪ **Schedule for those who have fallen behind:** If the series is delayed between doses, do *not* start the series over. Continue from where series left off. ▪ May be given with all other vaccines but at a separate site.	
Hepatitis A (hep-A)— give IM; brands may be used interchangeably	▪ People who travel outside of the United States (except for Northern and Western Europe, New Zealand, Australia, Canada, and Japan).	▪ *Two* doses are needed. ▪ The minimum interval between dose #1 and #2 is 6 mo. ▪ If dose #2 is delayed, do *not* repeat dose #1. Just give dose #2. ▪ May be given with all other vaccines but at a separate site.	▪ Previous anaphylactic reaction to this vaccine or to any of its components. ▪ Moderate or severe acute illness. ▪ Safety during pregnancy has not been determined, so benefits must be weighed against potential risk.

(Continued on following page)

TABLE 7.3	Summary of Recommendations for Adult Immunization *(Continued)*		

Vaccine Name and Route	For Whom It Is Recommended	Schedule	Contraindications and Precautions (Mild Illness Is Not a Contraindication)
Hepatitis A (hep-A)—give IM; brands may be used interchangeably *(continued)*	■ People with *chronic liver disease,* including people with hepatitis C virus infection; people with hepatitis B who have chronic liver disease; *illicit drug users; men who have sex with men;* people with *clotting-factor disorders;* people who work with hepatitis A virus in experimental lab settings (this does not refer to routine medical laboratories); and food handlers where health authorities or private employers determine vaccination to be cost-effective. *Note:* Prevaccination testing is likely to be cost-effective for persons > 40 yr of age, as well as for younger persons in certain groups with a high prevalence of hepatitis A virus infection.		
Td (tetanus, diphtheria)—give IM	■ *All* adolescents and adults. ■ After the primary series has been completed, a booster dose is recommended every 10 years. Make sure clients have received a primary series of 3 doses. ■ A booster dose as early as 5 years later may be needed for the purpose of wound management, so consult ACIP recommendations.	■ Booster dose *every 10 years* after completion of the primary series of three doses. ■ **For those who have fallen behind:** The primary series is three doses: ■ Give dose #2 four weeks after #1. ■ #3 is given 6–12 months after #2. ■ May be given with all other vaccines but at a separate site.	■ Previous anaphylactic or neurological reaction to this vaccine or to any of its components. ■ Moderate or severe acute illness.
MMR (measles, mumps, rubella)—give SC	■ Adults born in 1957 or later who are ≥18 yr of age (including those born outside the United States) should receive at least one dose of MMR if there is no serological proof of immunity or documentation of a dose given on or after 1st birthday.	■ *One* or two doses are needed. ■ If dose #2 is recommended, give it no sooner than 4 wk after dose #1. ■ May be given with all other vaccines but at a separate site. ■ If varicella vaccine and MMR are both needed and are not administered on the same day, space them at least 4 wk apart.	■ Previous anaphylactic reaction to this vaccine or to any of its components. (Anaphylactic reaction to eggs is *no longer* a contraindication to MMR.) ■ Pregnancy or possibility of pregnancy within 3 months. ■ HIV positivity is *not* a contraindication to MMR except for those who are severely immunocompromised. ■ Persons who are immunocompromised due to cancer, leukemia, lymphoma, immunosuppressive drug therapy, including high-dose steroids or radiation therapy.

(Continued on following page)

Vaccine Name and Route	For Whom It Is Recommended	Schedule	Contraindications and Precautions (Mild Illness Is Not a Contraindication)
	• Adults in high-risk groups, such as health-care workers, students entering colleges and other post-high school educational institutions, and international travelers should receive a total of two doses. • All women of childbearing age (i.e., adolescent girls and women who are premenopausal) who do not have acceptable evidence of rubella immunity or vaccination. *Note:* Adults born before 1957 are usually considered immune (naturally infected with measles and mumps), but proof of immunity may be desirable for health-care workers.		• If blood products or immune globulin has been administered during the past 11 months, consult the ACIP recommendations regarding time to wait before vaccinating. • Moderate or severe acute illness. *Note:* MMR is *not* contraindicated if a PPD test was done recently. PPD should be delayed for 4–6 weeks *after* an MMR has been given.
Varicella (var), "chickenpox shot"—give SC	• *All* adults and adolescents who are susceptible should be vaccinated. Make special efforts to vaccinate people who are susceptible and have *close contact with persons at high risk for serious complications* (e.g., health-care workers and family contacts of people who are immunocompromised) and persons who are susceptible who are at *high risk of exposure* (e.g., teachers of young children, daycare employees, residents and staff in institutional settings such as colleges and correctional institutions, military personnel, adolescents and adults living with children, *women who are nonpregnant and are of childbearing age,* and international travelers who do not have evidence of immunity).	• One dose for ages 12 mo–12 yr. • *Two* doses for >12 yrs. Dose #2 is given *4–8 wk after* dose #1. • If the second dose is delayed, do *not* repeat dose #1. Just give dose #2. • May be given with all other vaccines but at a separate site. • If varicella vaccine and MMR are both needed and are not administered on the same day, space them at least 4 wk apart.	• Previous anaphylactic reaction to this vaccine or to any of its components. • Pregnancy, or possibility of pregnancy within 1 month. • People who are immunocompromised due to malignancies and primary or acquired cellular immunodeficiency, including HIV/AIDS. Note: For those on high-dose immunosuppressive therapy, consult ACIP recommendations regarding daily time. • If blood products or immune globulin have been administered during the past 5 months, consult the ACIP recommendations regarding time to wait before vaccinating. • Moderate or severe acute illness. *Note:* Manufacturer recommends that *salicylates be avoided for 6 weeks* after receiving varicella vaccine because of a theoretical risk of Reye syndrome.

Adult

(Continued on following page)

TABLE 7.3 Summary of Recommendations for Adult Immunization *(Continued)*

Vaccine Name and Route	For Whom It Is Recommended	Schedule	Contraindications and Precautions (Mild Illness Is Not a Contraindication)
	Note: People with reliable histories of chickenpox (such as self or parental report of disease) can be assumed to be immune. For adults who have no reliable history, **serological testing** *may be cost-effective* because most adults with a negative or uncertain history of varicella are immune.		
Polio (IPV)—give IM or SC	■ *Not* routinely recommended for persons 18 years of age and older. *Note:* Adults living in the United States who never received or completed a primary series of polio vaccine need *not* be vaccinated unless they intend to travel to areas where exposure to wild-type virus is likely. Adults who have been previously vaccinated should receive *one booster dose if traveling* to polio endemic areas.	■ *Four* doses of inactivated polio vaccine (IPV) at 2, 4, and 6–18 mo, and 4–6 yr. ■ May be given with all other vaccines but at a separate site.	
Lyme disease—give IM	■ Consider for persons 15 to 70 years of age who reside, work, or recreate in areas of high or moderate risk and who engage in activities that result in frequent or prolonged exposure to tick-infested habitat. ■ Persons with a history of previous uncomplicated Lyme disease who are at continued high risk for Lyme disease. (See description in the first bullet). ■ See ACIP statement for a definition of high and moderate risk.	■ *Three* doses are needed. Give at intervals of 0, 1, and 12 mo. Schedule dose #1 (given in year 1) and dose #3 (given in year 2) to be given several weeks before tick season. See ACIP statement for details. ■ Safety of administering Lyme disease vaccine with other vaccines has not been established. ■ ACIP says if it must be administered concurrently with other vaccines, give it at a separate site.	■ Previous anaphylactic reaction to this vaccine or to any of its components. ■ Pregnancy. ■ Moderate or severe acute illness. ■ Persons with treatment-resistant Lyme arthritis. ■ There are not enough data to recommend Lyme disease vaccine to persons with these conditions: immunodeficiency, diseases associated with joint swelling (including rheumatoid arthritis) or diffuse muscular pain, chronic health conditions due to Lyme disease.

Adapted from the Advisory Committee on Immunization Practices (ACIP), Centers for Disease Control, by the Immunization Action Coalition, 2004.

GROWTH AND DEVELOPMENT

Young Adulthood (20–30 Years of Age)

I. **Stage of development—psychosocial stage:** intimacy versus isolation.

II. **Physical development** (see also **Unit 8**)
   A. *At the height* of bodily vigor.
   B. *Maximum* level of strength, muscular development, height, and cardiac and respiratory capacity; also, period of peak sexual capacity for men.

III. **Cognitive development**
   A. Close to *peak* of intelligence, memory, and abstract thought.
   B. Maximum ability to solve problems and learn new skills.

IV. **Socialization**
   A. Has a vision of the future and imagines various possibilities for self.
   B. Defines and tests out what can be accomplished.
   C. Seeks out a mentor to emulate as a guiding, though transitional, figure; the mentor is usually a mixture of parent, teacher, and friend who serves as a role model to support and facilitate the developing vision of self.
   D. Grows from a beginning to a fuller understanding of own authority and autonomy.
   E. Transfers an interest into an occupation or profession; crucial work choice may be made after one has knowledge, judgment, and self-understanding, usually at the end of young adulthood; when the choice is deferred beyond these years, valuable time is lost.
   F. Experiments with and chooses a lifestyle.
   G. Forms mature peer relationships with the opposite sex.
   H. Overcomes guilt and anxiety about the opposite sex and learns to understand the masculine and feminine aspects of self, as well as the adult concept of roles.
   I. Learns to take the opposite sex seriously and may choose someone for a long-term relationship.
   J. Accepts the responsibilities and pleasures of parenthood.

Adulthood (31–45 Years of Age)

I. **Stage of development—psychosocial stage:** generativity versus self-absorption.

II. **Physical development**
   A. Gradual decline in biological functioning, although in the late 30s the individual is still near peak.
   B. Period of peak sexual capacity for women occurs during the mid-30s.
   C. Distinct sense of bodily decline occurs around 40 years of age.
   D. *Circulatory* system begins to slow somewhat after 40 years of age.

III. **Cognitive development**
   A. Takes longer to memorize.
   B. Still at peak in abstract thinking and problem solving.
   C. Generates new levels of awareness.
   D. Gives more meaning to complex tasks.

IV. **Socialization**
   A. Achieves a realistic self-identity.
   B. Perceptions are based on reality.
   C. Acts on decisions and assumes responsibility for actions.
   D. Accepts limitations while developing assets.
   E. Delays immediate gratification in favor of future satisfaction.
   F. Evaluates mistakes, determines reasons and causes, and learns new behavior.
   G. Struggles to establish a place in society.
      1. Begins to settle down.
      2. Pursues long-range plans and goals.
      3. Has a stronger need to be responsible.
      4. Invests self as fully as possible in social structure, including work, family, and community.
   H. Seeks advancement by improving and using skills, becoming more creative, and pursuing ambitions.

Middle Life (46–64 Years of Age)

I. **Stage of development—psychosocial stage:** continuation of generativity versus self-absorption.

II. **Physical development**
   A. Failing *eyesight,* especially for close vision, may be one of the first symptoms of aging.
   B. Hearing loss is very gradual, especially for low sounds; hearing for *high-pitched* sounds is impaired more readily.
   C. There is a gradual loss of *taste* buds in the 50s and gradual loss of sense of *smell* in the 60s, causing the individual to have a diminished sense of taste.
   D. *Muscle strength* declines because of decreased levels of estrogen and testosterone; it takes more time to accomplish the same physical task.
   E. *Lung* capacity is impaired, which adds to decreased endurance.
   F. The *skin* begins to wrinkle, and hair begins graying.
   G. *Postural changes* take place because of loss of calcium and reduced activity.

III. **Cognitive development**
   A. *Memory* begins to decline slowly around age 50 years.
   B. It takes longer to *learn* new tasks, and old tasks take longer to perform.
   C. *Practical judgment* is increased due to experiential background.
   D. May tend to withdraw from mental activity or overcompensate by trying the impossible.

IV. **Socialization**
   A. The middle years can be very rewarding if previous stages have been fulfilled.

Adult

B. The years of responsibility for raising children are over.

C. Husbands and wives usually find a closer bond.

D. There is less financial strain for those with steady employment.

E. Individuals are usually at the height of their careers; the majority of leaders in their field are in this age group.

F. Self-realization is achieved.
  1. There is more inner direction.
  2. There is no longer a need to please everyone.
  3. Individual is less likely to compare self with others.
  4. Individual approves of self without being dependent on standards of others.
  5. There is less fear of failure in life because past failures have been met and dealt with.

Early Late Years (65–79 Years of Age)

I. **Stage of development—psychosocial stage:** ego integrity and acceptance versus despair and disgust.

II. **Physical development**
  A. Continues to decrease in vigor and capacity.
  B. Has more frequent aches and pains.
  C. Likely to have at least one major illness.

III. **Cognitive development**
  A. Mental acuity continues to slow down.
  B. Judgment and problem solving remain intact, but the processes may take longer.
  C. May have problems in remembering *names and dates.*

IV. **Socialization**
  A. Individual is faced with the reality of the experience of physical decline.
  B. Physical and mental changes intensify the feelings of aging and mortality.
  C. Increasing frequency of death and serious illness among friends, relatives, and associates further reinforces the concept of mortality.
  D. Constant reception of medical warnings to follow certain precautions or run serious risks adds to general feeling of decline.
  E. Individual is less interested in obtaining the rewards of society and is more interested in using own inner resources.
  F. Individuals feel that they have earned the right to do what is important for self-satisfaction.
  G. Retirement allows time for expression of own creative energies.
  H. Overcomes the splitting of youth and age; gets along well with adolescents.
  I. Learns to deal with the reality that only old age remains.
  J. Provides moral support to grandchildren; more tolerant of grandchildren than was of own children.
  K. Tends to release major authority of family to children while holding self in the role of consultant.

Later Years (80 Years of Age and Older)

I. **Stage of development—psychosocial stage:** continuation of ego integrity and acceptance versus despair and disgust.

II. **Physical development**
  A. Additional sensory problems occur, including diminished sensation to *touch and pain.*
  B. Increase in loss of muscle tone occurs, including *sphincter* (urinary and anal) control.
  C. Individual is insecure and unsure about orientation to *space* and sense of *balance,* which may result in falls and injury.

III. **Cognitive development**
  A. Has better memory for the *past* than the present.
  B. *Repetition* of memories occurs.
  C. Individual may use *confabulation* to fill in memory gaps.
  D. Forgetfulness may lead to serious *safety* problems, and individual may require constant supervision.
  E. Increased arteriosclerosis may lead to mental illness (dementia and other cognitive disorders).

IV. **Socialization**
  A. Few significant relationships are maintained; deaths of friends, family, and associates cause isolation.
  B. Individual may be preoccupied with immediate bodily needs and personal comforts; the *gastrointestinal tract* frequently becomes the major focus.
  C. Individuals see that they can provide others with an example of wisdom and courage.
  D. Individuals come to terms with themselves.
  E. Individuals are concerned with own immortality.
  F. Individuals come to terms with the process of dying and prepare for own death.

FLUID-GAS TRANSPORT

Conditions Affecting Fluid Transport

I. **Hypertension:** sustained, elevated, systemic, arterial blood pressure; diastolic elevation more serious, reflecting pressure on arterial wall during resting phase of cardiac cycle (**Table 7.4**).
  A. **Pathophysiology:** increased peripheral resistance leading to thickened arterial walls and left ventricular hypertrophy.
  B. **Risk factors:**
    1. Black race (2:1).
    2. Use of birth control pills.
    3. Overweight.
    4. Smoking.
    5. Stress.
    6. Excessive sodium intake or saturated fat.
    7. Lack of activity.

TABLE 7.4	Imbalances in Blood Pressure: Comparative Assessment of Hypotension and Hypertension	
	Hypotension	**Hypertension**
Common Causes		
	Angina pectoris	Essential hypertension
	Myocardial infarction	Iron deficiency anemia
	Acute and chronic pericarditis	Pernicious anemia
	Valvular defects	Arteriosclerosis obliterans
	Heart failure	Polycythemia vera
◆ Assessment		
Behavior	Anxiety, apprehension, decreasing mentation, confusion	Nervousness, mood swings, irritability, difficulty with memory, depression, confusion
Neurological	Essentially noncontributory	Decreased vibratory sensations, increased/decreased reflexes, Babinski reflex, changes in coordination
Head/neck	Distended neck veins, worried expression	Bruits over carotids, distended neck veins, epistaxis, diplopia, ringing in ears, dull occipital headaches on arising
Skin	Pale, cool, moist	Dry, pale, glossy, flaky, cold; decreased or absent hair
GI	Anorexia, nausea, vomiting, constipation	Anorexia, flatulence, diarrhea, constipation
Respiratory	Dyspnea, orthopnea, paroxysmal nocturnal dyspnea, tachypnea, moist crackles, cough	Dyspnea, orthopnea, crackles
Cardiovascular	Tires easily	Decreased exercise tolerance, weakness, palpitations
	Blood pressure—decreased systolic, decreased systolic/diastolic	Blood pressure—increased systolic and/or diastolic
	Pulse—increased/decreased/weak, thready, irregular, arrhythmias	Decreased or absent pedal pulses
Renal	Oliguria	Oliguria, nocturia, proteinuria
Extremities	Dependent edema	Tingling, numbness, or cold hands and feet, dependent edema, ulcers of legs or feet

C. Classifications:

1. *Essential* (primary or idiopathic): occurs in 90%–95% of clients; etiology unknown; diastolic pressure is ≥90 mm Hg, and other causes of hypertension are absent. *Benign* hypertension (diastolic pressure ≤120 mm Hg) considered controllable; asymptomatic until complications develop.
2. *Secondary:* occurs in remaining 5%–10%; usually renal, endocrine, neurogenic, or cardiac in origin.
3. *Malignant hypertension* (diastolic >140–150 mm Hg); uncontrollable. May arise from both types.
4. *Labile* (prehypertensive): a fluctuating blood pressure; increases during stress, otherwise normal or near normal.

◆ D. Assessment:

1. *Subjective data:*
   a. Early-morning headache, usually occipital.
   b. Light-headedness, tinnitus.
   c. Palpitations.
   d. Fatigue, insomnia.
   e. Forgetfulness, irritability.
   f. Altered vision: white spots, blurring, or loss.
2. *Objective data:*
   a. Epistaxis (nosebleeds).
   b. Elevated blood pressure: systolic >140 mm Hg, diastolic >90 mm Hg; narrowed pulse pressure. Rise in diastolic from sitting to standing with *essential;* fall in BP from sitting to standing with *secondary.*
   c. Retinal changes; papilledema.
   d. Shortness of breath on slight exertion.
   e. Cardiac, cerebral, and renal changes.
    f. *Lab data:* UA, ECG, chest x-ray to rule out complications of hypertension.

◆ E. Analysis/nursing diagnosis:

1. *Knowledge deficit* (learning need) regarding condition, treatment plan, and self-care and discharge needs.
2. *Risk for decreased cardiac output* related to ventricular hypertrophy, vasoconstriction, or myocardial ischemia.
3. *Risk for injury* related to complications of hypertension.
4. *Impaired adjustment* related to required lifestyle changes.
5. *Activity intolerance* related to weakness, fatigue.

◆ F. Nursing care plan/implementation:

1. Goal: *provide for physical and emotional rest.*
   a. Rest periods before/after eating, visiting hours; *avoid* upsetting situations.
   b. Give *tranquilizers, sedatives,* as ordered.

Adult

2. Goal: *provide for special safety needs.*
   a. Monitor blood pressure: both arms; standing, sitting, lying positions.
   b. Limit/prevent activities that increase pressure (anxiety, anger, frustration, upsetting visitors, fatigue).
   c. Assist with ambulation; change position gradually to prevent dizziness and light-headedness (postural hypotension).
   d. Monitor for electrolyte imbalance when on low sodium diet, diuretic therapy; I&O to prevent fluid depletion and arrhythmias from potassium loss.
   e. Observe for signs of hemorrhage, shock, stroke, which may occur following surgery.
3. Goal: *health teaching* (client and family).
   a. Procedures to decrease anxiety; relaxation techniques, stress management.
   b. Side effects of hypotensive drugs: initial therapy includes *diuretics* and *beta-blockers*; if response inadequate may use *ACE inhibitors, adrenergic blockers, vasodilators, calcium channel blockers* (faintness, nausea, vomiting, hypotension, sexual dysfunction) (see **Unit 10** for specific pharmacological actions).
   c. Weight control to reduce arterial pressure.
   d. Restrictions: stimulants (tea, coffee, tobacco), sodium, calories, fat.

   e. *Lifestyle adjustments:* daily exercise needed; reduce occupational and environmental stress; importance of rest.
   f. Blood pressure measurement: daily, same conditions, position preference of physician; use of self-monitoring cuff; check at least twice per week.
   g. Signs, symptoms, complications of disease (headache, confusion, visual changes, nausea/vomiting, convulsions).
   h. Causes of intermittent hypotension: alcohol, hot weather, exercise, febrile illness, hot bath.
◆ **G. Evaluation/outcome criteria:**
   1. Blood pressure within normal range for age (diastolic <90 mm Hg)—stable.
   2. Minimal or no pathophysiological or therapeutic complications (e.g., visual changes, stroke, drug side effects).
   3. Reduces weight to reasonable level for height, bone structure.
   4. Takes prescribed medications regularly, even after symptoms have resolved.
   5. Complies with restrictions: no smoking, restricted sodium, fat.
   6. Exercises regularly—program compatible with personal and health-care goals.

II. Cardiac arrhythmias (dysrhythmias): any variations in normal rate, rhythm, or configuration of waves on ECG **(Figure 7.2).**

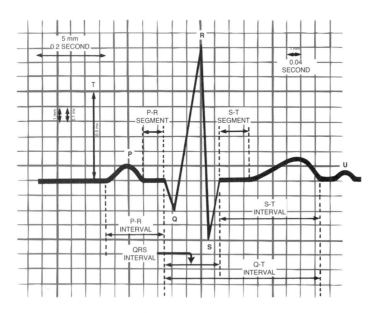

P wave	Depolarization of atrial muscle
QRS complex	Depolarization of ventricular muscle
T wave	Ventricular repolarization
PR interval	Time from start of atrial depolarization to start of ventricular depolarization (12–20 sec)
QRS interval	Total time for ventricular depolarization (6–10 sec)
QT interval	Total time for ventricular depolarization and repolarization
Rate/rhythm	60–100, regular
P-QRS ratio	1:1

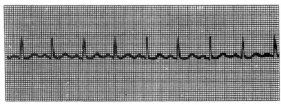

FIGURE 7.2 **Interpretation of normal cardiac cycle.** (From Venes, D [ed]: Taber's Cyclopedic Medical Dictionary, ed. 20. FA Davis, Philadelphia, 2005.)

Adult

A. **Pathophysiology:**
1. Dysfunction of SA node, atria, AV node, or ventricular conduction.
2. Primary heart problem or secondary systemic problem.

B. **Risk factors:**
1. Myocardial infarction.
2. Drug toxicity.
3. Stress.
4. Cardiac surgery.
5. Hypoxia.
6. Congenital.
7. **Table 7.5.**

◆ C. **Assessment:** (see **Table 7.5**) for specific dysrhythmias).

◆ D. **Analysis/nursing diagnosis:**
1. *Decreased cardiac output* related to abnormal ventricular function.

TABLE 7.5	Comparison of Selected Cardiac Dysrhythmias

Dysrhythmia	Description	Etiology	Symptoms/ Consequences	Treatment
Dysrhythmias of Sinus Node				
Sinus dysrhythmia	Phasic shortening then lengthening of P-P and R-R interval	Respiratory variation in impulse initiation by SA node	Usually none	Usually none Atropine if rate below 40 beats/min
Sinus tachycardia	P waves present followed by QRS Rhythm regular Heart rate 100–150 beats/min	Increased metabolic demands Decreased oxygen delivery Heart failure Shock Hemorrhage Anemia	May produce palpitations Prolonged episodes may lead to decreased cardiac output	Treat underlying cause Occasionally sedatives
Sinus bradycardia	P waves present followed by QRS Rhythm regular Heart rate <60 beats/min	Physical fitness Parasympathetic stimulation (sleep) Brain lesions Sinus dysfunction Digitalis excess	Very low rates may cause decreased cardiac output: light-headedness, faintness, chest pain	Atropine if cardiac output is decreased Pacemaker Treat underlying cause if necessary
Atrial Dysrhythmias				
Premature atrial beats	Early P wave QRS may or may not be normal Rhythm irregular	Stress Ischemia Atrial enlargement Caffeine Nicotine	May produce palpitations Frequent episodes may decrease cardiac output Is sign of chamber irritability	Sedation Eliminate nicotine and caffeine May require no other treatment
Atrial tachycardia	P wave present (may merge into previous T wave), QRS usually normal; rapid heart rate usually >150 beats/min	Sympathetic stimulation Chemical stimuli (caffeine, nicotine) Drug toxicity Fluid-electrolyte imbalance Thoracic surgery	Palpitations Possible anxiety Hypotension	Usually none if short burst (<1 min) Prolonged episodes may require carotid artery pressure, vagal stimulation, verapamil, digitalis, beta-blockers, calcium channel blockers
Atrial fibrillation	Rapid, irregular P waves (>350/min) Ventricular rhythm irregularly irregular Ventricular rate varies, may increase to 120–150/min if untreated	Rheumatic heart disease Mitral stenosis Atrial infarction Coronary atherosclerotic heart disease Hypertensive heart disease Thyrotoxicosis	Hypotension Palpitations Pulse deficit Decreased cardiac output if rate is rapid Promotes thrombus formation in atria	Digitalis Cardizem Amiodarone Anticoagulation Cardioversion
Atrial flutter	"Sawtooth" or "picket fence" P waves (220–350 beats/min) Ratio of atrial to ventricular rate constant (3:1, 4: 1, etc.)	Heart failure Mitral valve disease Pulmonary embolus	Occ. palpitations Chest pain	Cardioversion Anticoagulation meds if cardioversion unsuccessful

(Continued on following page)

TABLE 7.5	Comparison of Selected Cardiac Dysrhythmias *(Continued)*			
Dysrhythmia	**Description**	**Etiology**	**Symptoms/ Consequences**	**Treatment**
Ventricular Dysrhythmias				
Premature ventricular beats (PVBs)	Early wide bizarre QRS, not associated with a P wave Rhythm irregular	Stress Acidosis Ventricular enlargement Electrolyte imbalance Myocardial infarction Digitalis toxicity Hypoxemia Hypercapnia	Same as for premature atrial beats	Check Mg^{++}, K$^+$ levels **MEDS:** Procainamide Disopyramide (Norpace) Lidocaine Mexiletine Sodium bicarbonate Potassium Oxygen Treat heart failure
Ventricular tachycardia	No P wave before QRS; QRS wide and bizarre; ventricular rate > 100, usually 140–240	PVB striking during vulnerable period Hypoxemia Drug toxicity Electrolyte imbalance Bradycardia	Decreased cardiac output: hypotension, loss of consciousness, respiratory arrest	**MEDS:** Lidocaine Procainamide Amiodarone Cardioversion Electrolytes
Ventricular fibrillation	Chaotic electrical activity No recognizable QRS complex	Myocardial infarction Electrocution Freshwater drowning Drug toxicity	No cardiac output Absent pulse or respiration Cardiac arrest	Defibrillation **MEDS:** Epinephrine Lidocaine Sodium bicarbonate Bretylium Magnesium sulfate CPR
Pulseless electrical activity (PEA)	Organized ECG rhythm	Electromechanical dissociation Escape rhythms	Pulseless Minimal or no perfusion	CPR Epinephrine Fluid challenge
Ventricular standstill	Can be distinguished from ventricular fibrillation only by ECG P waves *may* be present No QRS "Straight line"	Myocardial infarction Chronic diseases of conducting system	Same as for ventricular fibrillation	CPR Pacemaker Intracardiac epinephrine
Impulse Conduction Deficits				
First-degree atrioventricular [AV] block	PR interval prolonged, >0.20 sec	Rheumatic fever Digitalis toxicity Degenerative changes of coronary atherosclerotic heart disease Infections (e.g., Lyme carditis) Decreased oxygen in AV node	Warns of impaired conduction	Usually none as long as it occurs as an isolated deficit Atropine if PR interval > 0.26 sec or bradycardia
Bundle branch block	Same as normal sinus rhythm (NSR) except QRS duration >0.10 sec	Hypoxia Acute myocardial infarction Heart failure Coronary atherosclerotic heart disease Pulmonary embolus Hypertension	Same as first-degree AV block	Usually none unless severe blockage of left posterior division (see text)

(Continued on following page)

Adult

Dysrhythmia	Description	Etiology	Symptoms/Consequences	Treatment
Second-degree AV blocks	P waves usually occur regularly at rates consistent with SA node initiation (not all P waves followed by QRS; PR interval may lengthen before nonconducted P wave or may be consistent; QRS may be widened)	Acute myocardial infarction Same as first-degree AV block	Serious dysrhythmia that may lead to decreased heart rate and cardiac output, hypotension	May require temporary pacemaker If symptomatic (e.g., hypotension, dizziness), atropine 1 mg
Complete third-degree AV block	Atria and ventricles beat independently P waves have no relation to QRS Ventricular rate may be as low as 20–40 beats/min	Digitalis toxicity Infectious disease Coronary artery disease Myocardial infarction	Very low rates may cause decreased cardiac output: light-headedness, fainting, chest pain	Pacemaker Isoproterenol to increase heart rate Epinephrine if isoproterenol ineffective

Source: Phipps, W, Long, B, Woods, N, and Cassmeyer, V (eds): Medical-Surgical Nursing, ed. 5. Mosby, St. Louis.

2. *Altered tissue perfusion* related to inadequate cardiac functioning.
3. *Knowledge deficit* (learning need) regarding cause/treatment of condition, self-care, and discharge needs.
4. *Anxiety* related to dependence, fear of death.

◆ **E. Nursing care plan/implementation:**
1. Goal: *provide for emotional and safety needs.*
   a. Document ECG tracing for presence of life-threatening arrhythmia.
   b. Encourage discussion of fears, feelings (client and significant other).
   c. *Bedrest:* restricted activities; quiet environment; limit visitors.
   ▶ d. Oxygen, if ordered.
   e. Check vital signs frequently for shock, HF, drug toxicity.
   f. Prepare for cardiac emergency: CPR.
   g. Give cardiac medications; check lab tests for digitalis and potassium levels, to prevent drug toxicity.
2. Goal: *prevent thromboemboli.*
   ▶ a. Apply antiembolic stockings (TED hose); segmental compression device.
   b. Give *anticoagulants* as ordered. (Check for bleeding—gums, urine; monitor *lab tests*—Lee-White clotting time and activated partial thromboplastin time with heparin; prothrombin time with Coumadin.)
   c. Encourage flexion-extension of feet.
3. Goal: *prepare for cardioversion with atrial fibrillation if indicated* (usually if pulse greater than 140 beats/min, symptomatic, or no conversion after 3 days of drug therapy and anticoagulated).
   a. Give Cardizem or amiodarone as ordered at least 24 hr before.
   b. NPO 8 hr before.
   c. Hold digoxin morning of cardioversion per order.
   d. Give *conscious sedation* meds as ordered.

4. Goal: *provide for physical and emotional needs with pacemaker insertion.*
   a. *General concerns:*
      (1) Report excessive bleeding/infection at insertion site—hematoma may contribute to wound infection.
      (2) Encourage verbalization of feelings.
      (3) Report prolonged hiccoughs, which may indicate pacemaker failure.
      (4) Know pacing mode: fixed-rate or demand (most common); type of insertion (temporary or permanent).
   b. *Temporary pacemaker:*
      (1) Limit excessive activity of extremity if antecubital insertion, to prevent displacement; subclavian insertion increases catheter stability.
      (2) Secure wires to chest to prevent tension on catheter.
      (3) Do *not* defibrillate over insertion site, to avoid electrical hazards.
      (4) Electrical safety (grounding; disconnect electric beds/call lights; use battery-operated equipment).
   c. *Permanent pacemaker:*
      (1) Limit activity of shoulder for 48–72 hr post-insertion of transvenous catheter to prevent dislodgement; *avoid* extending arms over head for 8 wk.
      (2) Post-insertion ROM (passive) at least once per shift after 48 hr to prevent frozen shoulder.
      (3) If defibrillation is required, place paddles at least 4 inches from pulse generator.
   d. *Health teaching* following permanent pacemaker:
      (1) Explain procedure: duration, equipment, purpose, type of pacemaker.
      (2) MedicAlert bracelet; pacemaker information card.

Adult

(3) Daily pulse taking on arising (report variation of ±5 beats).

(4) Signs, symptoms of *malfunction* (vertigo, syncope, dyspnea, slowed speech, confusion, fluid retention); *infection* (fever, heat, pain, skin breakdown at insertion site).

(5) **Restrictions:** limit vigorous arm and shoulder motion 6–8 wk; contact sports; electromagnetic interferences (few)—TV/radio transmitters, improperly functioning microwave oven (maintain distance of 3 ft), certain cautery machines; may trigger airport metal-detector alarm.

◆ **F. Evaluation/outcome criteria:**
1. Regular cardiac rhythm, monitors own radial pulse.
2. No complications (e.g., pacemaker malfunction).
3. Returns for regular follow-up of pacemaker function.
4. Tolerates physical or sexual activity.
5. Wears identification bracelet; carries pacemaker identification card.
6. Reports anxiety is reduced to manageable level.

III. Cardiac arrest: sudden unexpected cessation of heartbeat and effective circulation leading to inadequate perfusion and sudden death.

A. Risk factors:
1. Myocardial infarction.
2. Multiple traumas.
3. Respiratory arrest.
4. Drowning.
5. Electrical shock.
6. Drug reactions.

◆ **B. Assessment**—*objective data:*
1. Unresponsive to stimuli (i.e., verbal, painful).
2. Absence of breathing, carotid pulse.
3. Pale or bluish: lips, fingernails, skin.
4. Pupils: dilated.

◆ **C. Analysis/nursing diagnosis:**
1. *Decreased cardiac output* related to heart failure.
2. *Impaired gas exchange* related to breathlessness.
3. *Altered tissue perfusion* related to pulselessness.

◆ **D. Nursing care plan/implementation:**
1. Goal: *prevent irreversible cerebral anoxic damage:*
▶ initiate CPR within 4–6 min; continue until relieved; document assessment factors, effectiveness of actions; presence or absence of pulse at 1 min and every 4–5 min.
2. Goal: *establish effective circulation, respiration* (see **Emergency Nursing Procedures, Table 7.50,** for complete protocols).

◆ **E. Evaluation/outcome criteria:**
1. Carotid pulse present; check after 1 min and every few minutes thereafter.
2. Responds to verbal stimuli.
3. Pupils constrict in response to light.
4. Return of spontaneous respiration; adequate ventilation.

IV. Arteriosclerosis: loss of elasticity, thickening, hardening of arterial walls; symptoms depend on organ system involved; common type—atherosclerosis. Atherosclerosis (coronary heart disease) precedes angina pectoris and myocardial infarction.

A. Pathophysiology:
1. Atherosclerotic plaque, discrete lumpy thickening of arterial wall; cholesterol-lipid-calcium deposits in lining.
2. Narrows lumen, can occlude vessel.

B. Risk factors:
1. Increased serum cholesterol (low-density lipids ≥160 mg/dL).
2. Hypertension.
3. Cigarette smoking.
4. Diabetes mellitus.
5. Family history of premature CHD.
(See **V. Angina pectoris,** and **VI. Myocardial infarction,** following sections, for nursing implications.)

V. Angina pectoris: transient paroxysmal episodes of substernal or precordial pain. Types: *stable* (follows an event, same severity); *unstable* (at rest or minimal exertion, recent onset, increasing severity); *Prinzmetal's variant* (at rest, caused by coronary spasms).

A. Pathophysiology:
1. Insufficient blood flow through coronary arteries. Oxygen demand exceeds supply.
2. Temporary myocardial ischemia.

B. Risk factors:
1. Cardiovascular:
   a. Atherosclerosis.
   b. Thromboangiitis obliterans.
   c. Aortic regurgitation.
   d. Hypertension.
2. Hormonal:
   a. Hypothyroidism.
   b. Diabetes mellitus.
3. Blood disorders:
   a. Anemia.
   b. Polycythemia vera.
4. *Lifestyle choices:*
   a. Smoking.
   b. Obesity.
   c. Cocaine use.
   d. Inactivity.

◆ **C. Assessment:**
1. *Subjective data*
   a. *Pain—typical* (**Table 7.6**).
      (1) *Type:* squeezing, pressing, burning.
      (2) *Location:* retrosternal, substernal, left of sternum, radiates to left arm (**Figure 7.3**).
      (3) *Duration:* short, usually 3–5 min, <30 min.
      (4) *Cause:* emotional stress, overeating, physical exertion, exposure to cold; may occur at rest.
      (5) *Relief:* rest, nitroglycerin.
   b. *Note: Atypical* complaints by women include jaw and upper back pain and persistent gastric upset.
   c. Dyspnea.
   d. Palpitations.

TABLE 7.6	Comparison of Physical Causes of Chest Pain					
Characteristic	Myocardial Infarction	Pericarditis	Gastric Disorders	Angina Pectoris	Dissecting Aneurysm	Pulmonary Embolism
Onset	Gradual or sudden	Sudden	Gradual or sudden	Gradual or sudden	Abrupt, without prodromal symptoms	Gradual or sudden
Precipitating factors	Can occur at rest or after exercise or emotional stress	Breathing deeply, rotating trunk, recumbency, swallowing or yawning	Inflammation of stomach or esophagus; hypersecretion of gastric juices; some medications	Usually after physical exertion, emotional stress, eating, exposure to cold, or defecation; unstable angina occurs at rest	Hypertension	Immobility or prolonged bedrest following surgery, trauma, hip fracture, HF, malignancy, oral contraceptives
Location	Substernal, anterior chest, or midline; rarely back; radiates to jaw or neck	Precordial; radiates to neck or left shoulder and arm	Xiphoid to umbilicus	Substernal, anterior chest; poorly localized	Correlates with site of intimal rupture; anterior chest or back; between shoulder blades	Pleural area, retrosternal area
Quality	Crushing, burning, stabbling, squeezing or vicelike	Pleuritic, sharp	Aching, burning, cramplike, gnawing	Squeezing, feeling of heavy pressure; burning	Sharp, tearing or ripping sensation	Sharp, stabbing
Intensity	Asymptomatic to severe; increases with time	Mild to severe	Mild to severe	Mild to moderate	Severe and unbearable; maximal from onset	Aggravated by breathing
Duration	30 min to 1–2 hr; may wax and wane	Continuous	Periodic	Usually 2–10 min; average 3–5 min	Continuous; does not abate once started	Variable
Relief	Narcotics	Sitting up, leaning forward	Physical and emotional rest, food, antacids, H$_2$-receptor antagonists	Nitroglycerin, rest	Large, repeated doses of narcotics	O$_2$; sitting up morphine
Associated symptoms	Nausea, fatigue, heartburn; peripheral pulses equal	Fever, dyspnea, nausea, anorexia, anxiety	Nausea, vomiting, dysphagia, anorexia, weight loss	Belching, indigestion, dizziness	Syncope, loss of sensations or pulses, oliguria; discrepancy between BP in arms; decrease in femoral or carotid pulse	Dyspnea, tachypnea, diaphoresis, hemoptysis, cough, apprehension

  e. Dizziness; faintness.
  f. Epigastric distress; indigestion; belching.
2. *Objective data*
  a. Tachycardia.
  b. Pallor.
  c. Diaphoresis.
  d. ECG changes during attack.
◆ **D. Analysis/nursing diagnosis:**
1. *Altered cardiopulmonary tissue perfusion* related to insufficient blood flow.

2. *Pain* related to myocardial ischemia.
3. *Activity intolerance* related to onset of pain.
◆ **E. Nursing care plan/implementation:**
1. Goal: *provide relief from pain.*
  a. Rest until pain subsides.
  b. Nitroglycerin or amyl nitrite, beta-adrenergic blockers, as ordered.
  c. Identify precipitating factors: large meals, heavy exercise, stimulants (coffee, smoking), sex when fatigued, cold air.

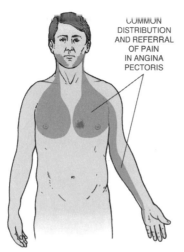

COMMON DISTRIBUTION AND REFERRAL OF PAIN IN ANGINA PECTORIS

FIGURE 7.3 **Angina pectoris.** (From Venes, D [ed]: Taber's Cyclopedic Medical Dictionary, ed. 20. FA Davis, Philadelphia, 2005.)

d. Vital signs: hypotension.

e. Assist with ambulation; dizziness, flushing occurs with nitroglycerin.

2. Goal: *provide emotional support.*

a. Encourage verbalization of feelings, fears.

b. Reassurance; positive self-concept.

c. Acceptance of limitations.

3. Goal: *health teaching.*

a. Pain: alleviation, differentiation of angina from myocardial infarction, precipitating factors (see **Table 7.6**).

b. Medication: frequency, expected effects (headache, flushing); carry fresh nitroglycerin; loses potency after 6 mo ("stings" under tongue when potent); may use nitroglycerin paste—instruct how to apply.

c. *Diet:* restricted calories if weight loss indicated; restricted fat, cholesterol, gas-producing foods; small, frequent meals.

d. *Diagnostic tests* if ordered (e.g., thallium stress test, cardiac catheterization; interventional [stents]; see **p. 497** and **Unit 11**).

e. Exercise: regular, graded, to promote coronary circulation.

f. Prepare for coronary bypass surgery, if necessary.

g. Behavior modification to assist with lifestyle changes (e.g., stress reduction, stop smoking).

◆ **F. Evaluation/outcome criteria:**

1. Relief from pain.

2. Fewer attacks.

3. No myocardial infarction.

4. Alters lifestyle; complies with limitations.

5. No smoking.

VI. Myocardial infarction (MI, heart attack): localized area of necrotic tissue in myocardium from cessation of blood flow; leading cause of death in North America.

A. **Pathophysiology:**

1. Coronary occlusion due to thrombosis, embolism, or hemorrhage adjacent to atherosclerotic plaque.

2. Insufficient blood flow from cardiac hypertrophy, hemorrhage, shock, or severe dehydration.

B. **Risk factors:**

1. Age (35 to 70 yr).

2. Men more than women until menopause.

3. Lifestyle: obesity, smoking, sedentary, amphetamine or cocaine use.

4. Stress or type A personality.

5. High-cholesterol, low-density lipoproteins, and high serum triglyceride levels.

6. Chronic illness (diabetes, hypertension).

◆ C. **Assessment:**

1. *Subjective data*

a. *Pain* (see **Table 7.6**).

(1) *Type:* sudden, severe, crushing, heavy tightness. May be absent in elderly or those who have diabetes.

(2) *Location:* substernal; radiates to one or both arms, jaw, neck. May be confused with indigestion.

(3) *Duration:* >30 min.

(4) *Cause:* unrelated to exercise; frequently occurs when sleeping (REM stage).

(5) *Relief:* oxygen, *narcotics; not* relieved by rest or nitroglycerin.

b. Nausea.

c. Shortness of breath.

d. Apprehension, fear of impending death.

e. History of cardiac disease (family); occupational stress.

2. *Objective data*

a. *Vital signs:* shock; rapid (>100), thready pulse; fall in blood pressure; S₃ gallop; tachypnea, shallow respirations; elevated temperature within 24 hr (100° to 103°F).

b. Skin: ashen or clammy; diaphoretic.

c. Emotional: restless.

 d. Lab data: *increased*—WBC (12,000–15,000/μL), troponin T and I levels, serum enzymes (CK-MB, LDH₁ > LDH₂—"flipped LDH"); *changes*—ECG (*elevated* ST segment, inverted T wave, arrhythmia).

◆ D. **Analysis/nursing diagnosis:**

1. *Decreased cardiac output* related to myocardial damage.

2. *Impaired gas exchange* related to poor perfusion, shock.

3. *Pain* related to myocardial ischemia.

4. *Activity intolerance* related to pain or inadequate oxygenation.

5. *Fear* related to possibility of death.

◆ E. **Nursing care plan/implementation (see also clinical Pathway 7.1: Acute Coronary Syndrome/ Acute MI):**

1. Goal: *reduce pain, discomfort.*
   a. *Narcotics*—morphine; note response. *Avoid* IM.
   b. Humidified oxygen 2 to 4 L/min; mouth care—oxygen is drying.
   c. *Position:* semi-Fowler's to improve ventilation.
2. Goal: *maintain adequate circulation,* stabilize heart rhythm.
   a. Monitor vital signs and urine output; observe for cardiogenic shock.
   b. Monitor ECG for arrhythmias.
   c. Give medications as ordered: *antiarrhythmics*—lidocaine HCl, amiodarone, atropine, beta-blockers, procainamide (Pronestyl), bretylium (Bretylol); propranolol (Inderal); verapamil; *anticoagulants*—heparin sodium, bishydroxycoumarin or dicoumarin; *thrombolytic agents*—streptokinase (tPA), APSAC/anistreplase (Eminase) reteplase followed by IV heparin or a IIB/IIIA inhibitor (Integrilin).
   d. *Diagnostic tests*—prepare for cardiac catheterization, possible interventional cardiology (stents), possible CAB surgery.
   e. Recognize heart failure: edema, cyanosis, dyspnea, cough, crackles.
   f. Check lab data—normal; troponin; serum enzymes (CK 20-220 IU/L depending on gender; CK-MB 0 to 12 IU/L; LDH <115 IU/L; $LDH_1 < LDH_2$); blood gases (pH 7.35 to 7.45; PCO_2 35 to 45 mEq/L; PO_2 80 to 100 mm Hg; HCO_3 22 to 26); electrolytes (K^+ 3.5 to 5.0 mEq/L; Mg^{++} 1.3 to 2.1 mg/dL); clotting time (aPTT 25 to 41 sec; PT 11 to 15 sec).
   g. CVP—zero level at right atrium; fluctuates with respiration; normal range 5 to 15 cm H_2O; note trend; increases with heart failure.
   h. ROM of lower extremities; TED hose/antiembolic stockings.
3. Goal: *decrease oxygen demand/promote oxygenation, reduce cardiac workload.*
   a. O_2 as ordered.
   b. Activity: bedrest (24–48 hr) with bedside commode; planned rest periods; control visitors.
   c. *Position:* semi-Fowler's to facilitate lung expansion and decrease venous return.
   d. Anticipate needs of client: call light, water.
   e. Assist with feeding, turning.
   f. Environment: quiet, comfortable.
   g. Reassurance; stay with client who is anxious.
   h. Give medications as ordered: cardiotonics, calcium channel blockers, vasodilators, vasopressors.
4. Goal: *maintain fluid electrolyte, nutritional status.*
   a. IV (keep vein open); CVP; vital signs
      Urine output—30 mL/hr
   b. Lab data within *normal* limits (Na^+ 135 to 145 mEq/L; K^+ 3.5 to 5.0 mEq/L; Mg^{++} 1.3 to 2.1 mg/dL).

c. Monitor ECG—*hyperkalemia:* peaked T wave; *hypokalemia:* depressed T wave.
   d. *Diet:* progressive *low* calorie, *low* sodium, *low* cholesterol, *low* fat, without caffeine.
5. Goal: *facilitate fecal elimination.*
   a. Medications: *stool softeners* to prevent Valsalva maneuver (straining); mouth breathing during bowel movement; recognize complications of Valsalva maneuver—chest pain, cyanosis, diaphoresis, arrhythmias.
   b. Bedside commode if possible.
6. Goal: *provide emotional support.*
   a. Recognize fear of dying: denial, anger, withdrawal.
   b. Encourage expression of feelings, fears, concerns.
   c. Discuss rehabilitation, lifestyle changes: prevent cardiac-invalid syndrome by promoting self-care activities, independence.
7. Goal: *promote sexual functioning.*
   a. Encourage discussion of concerns regarding activity, inadequacy, limitations, expectations—include partner (usually resume activity 5 to 8 wks after uncomplicated MI or when client can climb two flights of stairs).
   b. Identify need for referral for sexual counseling.
8. Goal: *health teaching.*
   a. Diagnosis and treatment regimen.
   b. *Caution* about when to *avoid* sexual activity: after heavy meal, alcohol ingestion; when fatigued, tense, under stress; with unfamiliar partners; in extreme temperatures.
   c. Information about sexual activity: less fatiguing positions (side to side; noncardiac on top); vasodilators, if ordered, before intercourse; select comfortable, familiar environment.
   d. Referral to available community resources for information, support groups (e.g., American Heart Association, Stop Smoking Clinics).
   e. Medications: administration, importance, untoward effects, pulse taking.
   f. Control risk factors: rest, diet, exercise, no smoking, weight control, stress-reduction techniques.
   g. Need for follow-up care for regulation of medications, evaluating risk factors.
   h. Prepare for angioplasty or coronary bypass if planned.
F. **Evaluation/outcome criteria:**
   1. No complications: stable vital signs; relief of pain.
   2. Adheres to prescribed medication regimen, demonstrates knowledge about medications.
   3. Activity tolerance is increased, participates in program of progressive activity.
   4. Reduction or modification of risk factors. Plans to alter lifestyle (e.g., loses weight, quits smoking).

Adult

Instructions:
Check boxes for items that apply
Draw a line through items that do not apply
Document variances on the opposite side

DATE/	ED	Day 1 ICU/Telemetry	Day 2
	/ /	/ /	/ /
1 Discharge Planning/ Referrals	☐ Initiate Cardiology consult	☐ Evaluation of home situation ☐ Code status_____	☐ SW referral as needed
2 Diagnostic Tests/ Treatments	☐ H & P ☐ BUN ☐ EKG ×2 CXR ☐ CBC ☐ Creatinine ☐ Lipid panel ☐ CK MB #1 ☐ Troponin ☐ PT/PTT ☐ Electrolytes	☐ EKG ☐ CK MB #2 at 8 hr ☐ CK MB #3 at 16 hr ☐ Troponin ☐ PTT per heparin protocol ☐ Platelet count	☐ Transfer to telemetry 24-48 hr after admission Consider cardiac cath or noninvasive test for ischemia prior to discharge
3 Nutrition/Diet	☐ NPO	☐ Cardiac prudent diet	☐ Cardiac prudent diet
4 Treatments and Medications	☐ Medical therapy ☐ MSO$_4$ ☐ Primary PTCA ☐ ASA ☐ Thrombolytic therapy ☐ Beta-blocker ☐ IV fluids/Saline lock ☐ Heparin ☐ O$_2$ OR ☐ Nitrates ☐ Enoxaparin	☐ IV Fluids / Saline lock ☐ ACE Inhibitor ☐ O$_2$ ☐ Heparin ☐ Nitrates or ☐ MSO$_4$ ☐ Enoxaparin ☐ ASA ☐ Stool ☐ Beta-blocker softener	☐ IV to saline lock ☐ Heparin Drip ☐ O$_2$ DC'd if ☐ MSO$_4$ D/C'd indicated ☐ ASA ☐ ACE inhibitor ☐ PO Beta-blockers ☐ Stool softener ☐ IV Beta-blocker DC'd ☐ NTG drip D/C'd
5 Activity Cardiac Rehab	☐ Bedrest with commode	CR step 1: ☐ Bedrest with commode ☐ PT referral	CR step 2: ☐ Begin self care with assistance ☐ PT evaluation

6 Nursing Assessment/ Intervention	VS per ED routine
	I & O
	O$_2$ sat. > 92%
	Cardiac monitor
	Saline lock
		D E N
		☐ EKG monitor/Telemetry ☐ ☐ ☐
		Wt_____
		VS per unit routine ☐ ☐ ☐
		I & O ☐ ☐ ☐
		O$_2$ sat > 92% ☐ ☐ ☐
		Saline lock ☐ ☐ ☐
		A×O ×3, speech clear, memory
		  intact, swallow intact ☐ ☐ ☐
		Abdomen soft nontender,
		  bowel sounds present,
		  tolerates diet ☐ ☐ ☐
		Voiding adequate amounts,
		  urine clear, yellow to amber ☐ ☐ ☐
		Normal ROM and strength
		  appropriate for client ☐ ☐ ☐
		Circulation and sensation intact ☐ ☐ ☐
		Coping appropriately ☐ ☐ ☐
		Communicates needs and concerns,
		  behavior appropriate to age and
		  situation ☐ ☐ ☐
			D E N
			☐ EKG monitor/Telemetry ☐ ☐ ☐
			Wt_____
			VS per unit routine ☐ ☐ ☐
			I & O ☐ ☐ ☐
			O$_2$ sat > 92% ☐ ☐ ☐
			Saline lock ☐ ☐ ☐
			A×O ×3, speech clear, memory
			  intact, swallow intact ☐ ☐ ☐
			Abdomen soft nontender,
			  bowel sounds present,
			  tolerates diet ☐ ☐ ☐
			Voiding adequate amounts,
			  urine clear, yellow to amber ☐ ☐ ☐
			Normal ROM and strength
			  appropriate for client ☐ ☐ ☐
			Circulation and sensation intact ☐ ☐ ☐
			Coping appropriately ☐ ☐ ☐
			Communicates needs and concerns,
			  behavior appropriate to age and
			  situation ☐ ☐ ☐

7 Alteration in Comfort: Pain	☐ Instruct client on pain scale and need to call RN for pain Initial pain level_____	☐ Instruct client on pain scale and need to call RN for pain	☐ Assess for pain
8 Anxiety	Anxiety level identified Low ☐ Med ☐ High ☐ ☐ Appropriate actions taken (see nursing notes for med/high)	☐ Cooperates with care	☐ Receives information about activities ☐ Participates in care ☐ Verbalizes fears and concerns.
9 Knowledge Deficit	☐ Inform client of plan of care ☐ Teach client how to use pain scale	☐ Reinforce use of pain scale ☐ "Recovery After Your Heart Attack" booklet given to client	☐ Knows he/she had an MI and what it means ☐ Cardiovascular disease risk factors reviewed ☐ Medication teaching started
SIGNATURE BOX	A/D: E: P/N:	A/D: E: P/N:	A/D: E: P/N:

(Continued on following page)

Adult

Admitting diagnosis _____

Discharge diagnosis _____

/ /	/ /	/ /	/ /
Day 3	**Day 4**	**Day 5 / Discharge**	**Discharge Outcomes**
☐ Outpatient Cardiac rehab Referral made	☐ Home care referral as needed	☐ Refer family to CPR class	☐ CPR class referral made ☐ Outpt. Cardiac rehab referral made ☐ Home situation adequate/no help ☐ Home care referral completed ☐ Appt. made for f/u MD visit
☐ Nutrition consult			☐ Cardiac evaluation complete
☐ Cardiac prudent diet	☐ Cardiac prudent diet	☐ Cardiac prudent diet	☐ Client/family able to identify elements of cardiac prudent diet ☐ Written materials given
☐ DO O$_2$ ☐ ASA ☐ PO Beta-blockers ☐ ACE inhibitors ☐ Stool softener	☐ Evaluate women for HRT ☐ ASA ☐ PO Beta-blockers ☐ ACE inhibitors ☐ Stool softener	☐ ASA ☐ PO Beta-blockers ☐ ACE inhibitors ☐ Lipid lowering agent	☐ Discharge meds Rx given ☐ Pt. verbalizes understanding how to take d/c medications ☐ Medication teaching sheet completed and signed by client and nurse
CR step 3: Ambulate × 3 without significant change in VS ☐ ☐ ☐ Teach methods to evaluate exertion ☐	CR step 4: Ambulate 5 × day: independent self care ☐ ☐ ☐ ☐ ☐ Stair climbing if appropriate ☐	☐ Verbalizes activity limits	☐ Inpatient Cardiac rehab. complete ☐ ADLs with stable VS
D E N ☐ EKG monitor/Telemetry ☐ ☐ ☐ Wt_____ VS per unit routine ☐ ☐ ☐ I & O ☐ ☐ ☐ O$_2$ sat >92% ☐ ☐ ☐ Saline lock ☐ ☐ ☐ A×O ×3 speech clear, memory intact, swallow intact ☐ ☐ ☐ Abdomen soft nontender, bowel sounds present, tolerates diet ☐ ☐ ☐ Voiding adequate amounts, urine clear, yellow to amber ☐ ☐ ☐ Normal ROM and strength appropriate for client ☐ ☐ ☐ Circulation and sensation intact ☐ ☐ ☐ Coping appropriately ☐ ☐ ☐ Communicates needs and concerns, behavior appropriate to age and situation ☐ ☐ ☐	**D E N** ☐ EKG monitor/Telemetry ☐ ☐ ☐ Wt_____ VS per unit routine ☐ ☐ ☐ I & O ☐ ☐ ☐ O$_2$ sat >92% ☐ ☐ ☐ Saline lock ☐ ☐ ☐ A×O ×3, speech clear, memory intact, swallow intact ☐ ☐ ☐ Abdomen soft nontender, bowel sounds present, tolerates diet ☐ ☐ ☐ Voiding adequate amounts, urine clear, yellow to amber ☐ ☐ ☐ Normal ROM and strength appropriate for client ☐ ☐ ☐ Circulation and sensation intact ☐ ☐ ☐ Coping appropriately ☐ ☐ ☐ Communicates needs and concerns, behavior appropriate to age and situation ☐ ☐ ☐	**D E N** ☐ EKG monitor/Telemetry ☐ ☐ ☐ Wt_____ VS per unit routine ☐ ☐ ☐ I & O ☐ ☐ ☐ O$_2$ sat >92% ☐ ☐ ☐ Saline lock ☐ ☐ ☐ A×O X3, speech clear, memory intact, swallow intact ☐ ☐ ☐ Abdomen soft nontender, bowel sounds present, tolerates diet ☐ ☐ ☐ Voiding adequate amounts, urine clear, yellow to amber ☐ ☐ ☐ Normal ROM and strength appropriate for client ☐ ☐ ☐ Circulation and sensation intact ☐ ☐ ☐ Coping appropriately ☐ ☐ ☐ Communicates needs and concerns, behavior appropriate to age and situation ☐ ☐ ☐	☐ Referral to smoking cessation program made ☐ Referral to stress reduction program made ☐ D/C instructions given to client, verbalizes understanding
☐ Assess for pain	☐ Assess for pain		☐ Client is pain free ☐ Verbalizes appropriate actions to take if chest pain recurs ☐ Verbalizes appropriate use of EMC system
☐ Receives information about activities ☐ Participates in care ☐ Verbalizes fears and concerns	☐ Retains information ☐ Participates in care	☐ Retains information ☐ Participates in care ☐ Verbalizes understanding of appropriate life style changes	☐ Verbalizes ability to manage at home ☐ Continuing care arrangements made if appropriate
☐ "Recovery After Your Heart Attack" booklet reviewed. ☐ Client is able to identify risk factors ☐ Teach pulse taking	☐ Instruct client and family on risk factors reduction ☐ Review "Recovery After Your Heart Attack" booklet ☐ Give D/C instructions	☐ Complete D/C instruction sheet ☐ RN and client sign forms ☐ Client/family member demonstrates pulse taking ☐ Review D/C instructions	☐ MI teaching record complete ☐ DC summary complete
A/D:	A/D:	A/D:	A/D:
E:	E:	E:	E:
P/N:	P/N:	P/N:	P/N:

Source: UCSF Healthcare, San Francisco, Calif. With permission from Jane E. Hirsch, RN, MS, Vice President, Nursing and Patient Care Services.

Adult

VII. Cardiac valvular defects: alteration in the structure of a valve; impede flow of blood or permit regurgitation.

  A. Pathophysiology:

    1. *Stenosis*—narrowing of valvular opening due to adherence, thickening, and rigidity of valve cusp from fibrosis, scarring, and calcification.

    2. *Insufficiency* (incompetence)—incomplete closure of valve due to contraction of chordae tendineae, papillary muscles; or to calcification, scarring of leaflets. Results in regurgitation.

    3. *Mitral stenosis:*

      a. Most common residual cardiac lesion of rheumatic fever.

      b. Affects *women* <45 yr more often than men.

      c. Narrowing of mitral valve.

      d. Interferes with filling of left ventricle.

      e. Produces pulmonary hypertension, right ventricular failure.

    4. *Mitral insufficiency* (incompetence):

      a. Leaking/regurgitation of blood back into left atrium.

      b. Results from rheumatic fever, bacterial endocarditis; less common.

      c. Affects *men* more often.

      d. Produces pulmonary congestion, right ventricular failure.

    5. *Aortic stenosis:*

      a. Fusion of valve flaps between left ventricle and aorta.

      b. Congenital or acquired from atherosclerosis or from rheumatic fever and bacterial endo-

carditis; seen in *men* more often; pulmonary circulation congested, cardiac output decreased.

    6. *Aortic insufficiency:*

      a. Incomplete closure of valve between left ventricle and aorta (regurgitation).

      b. Left ventricular failure leading to right ventricular heart failure.

  B. Risk factors:

    1. Congenital abnormality.

    2. History of rheumatic fever.

    3. Atherosclerosis.

◆ **C. Assessment (Table 7.7).**

◆ **D. Analysis/nursing diagnosis:**

    1. *Decreased cardiac output* related to inadequate ventricular filling.

    2. *Fluid volume excess* related to compensatory response to decreased cardiac output.

    3. *Impaired gas exchange* related to pulmonary congestion.

    4. *Activity intolerance* related to impaired cardiac function.

    5. *Fatigue* related to poor oxygenation.

◆ **E. Nursing care plan/implementation:**

    1. Goal: *reduce cardiac workload.*

    2. Goal: *promote physical comfort and psychological support.*

    3. Goal: *prevent complications.*

    4. Goal: *prepare for surgery* (commissurotomy, valvuloplasty [valvotomy], or valvular replacement, depending on defect and severity of condition).

TABLE 7.7	**Comparison of Symptomatology for Valvular Defects**			
Assessment	**Mitral Stenosis**	**Mitral Insufficiency**	**Aortic Stenosis**	**Aortic Insufficiency**
Subjective Data				
Fatigue	✓	✓	✓	✓
Shortness of breath	✓			
Orthopnea	✓		✓	✓
Paroxysmal nocturnal dyspnea	✓		✓	✓
Cough	✓	✓		
Dyspnea on exertion		✓	✓	✓
Palpitations		✓	✓	
Syncope on exertion			✓	
Angina			✓	✓
Weight loss		✓		
Objective Data				
Vital signs				
Blood pressure:				
Low or normal	✓	✓		
Normal or elevated			✓	✓
Pulse:				
Weak, irregular	✓	✓		
Rapid, "waterhammer"				✓
Respirations:				
Increased, shallow	✓			
Cyanosis	✓			
Jugular vein distention	✓			
Enlarged liver	✓		✓	
Dependent edema	✓		✓	
Murmur	✓	✓	✓	✓

5. See section on cardiac surgery, **pp. 498–500,** for specific nursing actions.

◆ F. **Evaluation/outcome criteria:**
1. Relief of symptoms.
2. Increase in activity level.
3. No complications following surgery.

VIII. Cardiac catheterization: a diagnostic procedure to evaluate cardiac status. Introduces a catheter into the heart, blood vessels; analyzes blood samples for oxygen content, ejection fraction, cardiac output, pulmonary artery blood flow; done before heart surgery; frequently combined with angiography to visualize coronary arteries; also provides access for specialized cardiac techniques (e.g., internal pacing and coronary angioplasty).

A. **Approaches**
1. *Right-heart* catheterization—venous approach (antecubital or femoral)→right atrium→right ventricle→pulmonary artery.
2. *Left-heart* catheterization—retrograde approach: right brachial artery or percutaneous puncture of femoral artery→ascending aorta→ left ventricle.
   a. Transseptal: femoral vein→right atrium→ septum→left atrium→ left ventricle.
   b. Angiography/arteriography: done during left-heart catheterization.

B. **Precatheterization**
◆ 1. **Assessment:**
   a. *Subjective data*
      (1) Allergies: iodine, seafood.
      (2) Anxiety.
   b. *Objective data*
      (1) Vital signs: baseline data.
      (2) Distal pulses: mark for reference after catheterization.
◆ 2. **Analysis/nursing diagnosis:**
   a. *Anxiety* related to fear of unknown.
   b. *Knowledge deficit* (learning need) related to limited exposure to information or sudden need for procedure.
◆ 3. **Nursing care plan/implementation:**
   a. Goal: *provide for safety, comfort.*
      (1) Signed informed consent.
      (2) NPO (except for medications 6 to 8 hr before).
      (3) Have client urinate before going to lab.
      (4) Give *sedatives,* as ordered, 30 min before procedure (e.g., midazolam HCl [Versed] IV, diazepam [Valium] PO).
   b. Goal: *health teaching.*
      (1) Procedure: length (1 to 3 hr).
      (2) Expectations (strapped to table for safety, must lie still, awake but mildly sedated).
      (3) Sensations (hot, flushed feeling in head with dye injection; thudding in chest from premature beats during catheter manipulation; desire to cough, particularly with right-heart angiography and contrast-medium injection).

(4) Alert physician to unusual sensations (coolness, numbness, paresthesia).

C. **Postcatheterization**
◆ 1. **Assessment** (potential complications):
   a. *Subjective data*
      (1) Puncture site: increasing pain, tenderness.
      (2) Palpitations.
      (3) Affected extremity: tingling, numbness, pain from hematoma or nerve damage.
   b. *Objective data*
      (1) Vital signs: shock, respiratory distress (related to pulmonary emboli, allergic reaction).
      (2) Puncture site: bleeding (hematoma).
      (3) ECG: arrhythmias, signs of MI.
      (4) Affected extremity: color, temperature, peripheral pulses.
◆ 2. **Analysis/nursing diagnosis:**
   a. *Decreased cardiac output* related to arrhythmias or MI.
   b. *Altered tissue perfusion* related to bleeding following procedure.
   c. *Pain* related to puncture site tenderness.
◆ 3. **Nursing care plan/implementation:**
   a. Goal: *prevent complications.*
      (1) Bedrest: depends on size of catheter and closure procedure—Perclose dissolvable suture, 30 min; Angioseal (collagen plug), 2 hr; compression pump or 15 min manual compression followed by sandbag, 4 to 5 hr; 12 to 24 hr with sheath or antiplatelet drip (abciximab [ReoPro]).
      (2) Vital signs: record q15min for 1 hr, q30min for 3 hr or until stable; check BP on opposite extremity.
      (3) Puncture site: observe for bleeding, swelling, or tenderness; check pulse distal to insertion site to determine patency of artery; report complaints of coolness, numbness, or paresthesia in extremity.
      (4) ECG: monitor, document rhythm.
      (5) Give medications as ordered: *sedatives; mild narcotics; antiarrhythmics; antiplatelet* (Plavix, aspirin) or *low-molecular-weight heparin* (enoxaparin [Lovenox]) with stent insertion.
   b. Goal: *provide emotional support.*
      (1) Explanations: brief, accurate; client anxious to learn results of test.
      (2) Counseling: refer as indicated.
   c. Goal: *health teaching.*
      (1) Late complications: infection.
      (2) Prepare for surgery if indicated.
      (3) Follow-up medical care.
      (4) Limitations following PTCA (see **IX.**): *no* lifting >10 lb and *no* vigorous exertion for 1 to 2 wk; return to normal work and sexual activity in 2 to 3 days.
◆ 4. **Evaluation/outcome criteria:** no complications (e.g., cardiac arrest, hematoma at insertion site).

Adult

IX. **Percutaneous transluminal coronary angioplasty (PTCA):** a balloon-tipped catheter is threaded to site of coronary occlusion and inflated repeatedly until blood flow increases distal to the obstruction; a nonsurgical alternative to bypass surgery for coronary artery occlusion (**Figure 7.4**); recommended in clients with poorly controlled angina, mild or no symptoms, multiple- or single-vessel disease with a noncalcified, discrete, and proximal lesion that can be reached by the catheter; costs less and requires shorter hospitalization and rehabilitation period; successful in 90% of clients; approximately 30% restenose by 3 months (see **VIII. Cardiac catheterization, p. 497,** for nursing process). **Rotational atherectomy** may also be done; a high-speed drill pulverizes plaque into small particles. An **intravascular stent,** steel mesh or coil spring, may be placed in the coronary artery; the stent acts as a mechanical scaffold to reopen the blocked artery. The client receives low-molecular-weight heparin and/or platelet therapy following the procedure.

X. **Cardiac surgery:** done to alter the structure of the heart or vessels when congenital or acquired disorders interfere with cardiac functioning: septal defects; transposition of great vessels; tetralogy of Fallot; pulmonary/aortic stenosis; coronary artery bypass; valve replacement.

Cardiopulmonary bypass (open-heart surgery): blood from cardiac chambers and great vessels is diverted into a pump oxygenator; allows full visualization of heart during surgery; maintains perfusion and body functioning.

A. **Preoperative**

1. **Assessment:** see specific conditions for preoperative signs and symptoms (i.e., valvular defects, angina, MI); (see also **I. Preoperative preparation, p. 546**). Establish complete baseline: daily weight; vital signs—integrity of all pulses, BP both arms; CVP or pulmonary artery pressures; neurological status; emotional status; nutritional and elimination patterns; *laboratory values* (urine, electrolytes, enzymes, coagulation studies); pulmonary function studies.

2. **Analysis/nursing diagnosis** (see also **VI. Myocardial infarction, p. 492**):
   a. *Decreased cardiac output* related to myocardial damage.
   b. *Activity intolerance* related to poor cardiac function.
   c. *Knowledge deficit* (learning need) related to insufficient time for teaching.
   d. *Anxiety* related to fear of unknown.
   e. *Fear* related to possible death.
   f. *Risk for spiritual distress* related to possible death.

3. **Nursing care plan/implementation:**
   a. Goal: *provide emotional and spiritual support.*
      (1) Arrange for religious consultation if desired.
      (2) Provide opportunity for family visit morning of surgery.
      (3) Encourage verbalization/questions: fear, depression, despair frequently occur.

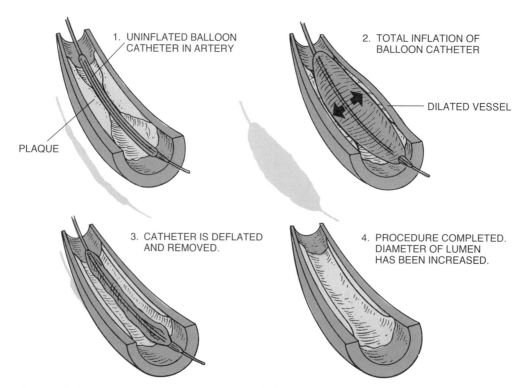

FIGURE 7.4 Arterial balloon angioplasty. (From Venes, D [ed]: Taber's Cyclopedic Medical Dictionary, ed. 20. FA Davis, Philadelphia, 2005.)

b. Goal: *health teaching.*
   (1) Diagnostic procedures, treatments, specifics for surgery (i.e., internal mammarian artery or leg incision with use of saphenous vein in coronary artery bypass surgery) **(Figure 7.5).**
   (2) Postoperative regimen: turn, cough, deep breathe, ROM, equipment used, medication for pain.
   (3) Tour ICU; meet personnel.
   (4) Alternative method of communication while intubated.

◆ **4. Evaluation/outcome criteria:**
   a. Displays moderate anxiety level.
   b. Verbalizes/demonstrates postoperative expectations.
   c. Quits smoking before surgery.

B. Postoperative

◆ **1. Assessment:**
   a. *Subjective data*
      (1) Pain.
      (2) Fatigue—sleep deprivation.
   b. *Objective data*
      (1) *Neurological:* level of consciousness; pupillary reactions; movement of limbs (purposeful, spontaneous).
      (2) *Respiratory:* rate changes (increases occur with obstruction, pain; decreases occur with CO_2 retention); depth (shallow with pain, atelectasis); symmetry; skin *color;* patency/*drainage* from chest tubes, *sputum* (amount, color); endotracheal tube placement (bilateral breath sounds).
      (3) *Cardiovascular:*
         (a) BP—*hypotension* may indicate heart failure, tamponade, hemorrhage, arrhythmias, or thrombosis; *hypertension* may indicate anxiety, hypervolemia.
         (b) Pulse: radial, apical, pedal; rate (>100

may indicate shock, fever, hypoxia, arrhythmias); rhythm, quality.
         (c) CVP or PA catheter (*elevated* in cardiac failure); temperature (normal postop: 98.6° to 101.6°F oral).
      (4) *GI:* nausea, vomiting, distention.
      (5) *Renal:* urine—minimum output (30 mL/hr); color

   > Specific gravity (<1.010 occurs with *over-hydration,* renal tubular damage; >1.020 present with *dehydration,* oliguria, blood in urine).

◆ **2. Analysis/nursing diagnosis:**
   a. *Decreased cardiac output* related to decreased myocardial contractility or postoperative hypothermia.
   b. *Pain* (acute) related to incision.
   c. *Ineffective airway clearance* related to effects of general anesthesia.
   d. *Altered tissue perfusion* related to postoperative bleeding or thromboemboli.
   e. *Fluid volume deficit* related to blood loss.
   f. *Risk for infection* related to wound contamination.
   g. *Altered thought processes* related to anesthesia or stress.
   h. *Altered role performance* related to uncertainty about future.

◆ **3. Nursing care plan/implementation:**
   a. Goal: *provide constant monitoring to prevent complications.*
      (1) *Respiratory:*
         (a) Observe for respiratory distress: restlessness, nasal flaring, *Cheyne-Stokes* respiration, dusky/cyanotic skin; assisted or controlled ventilation via endotracheal tube common 6 to 24 hr; supplemental O_2 after extubation.

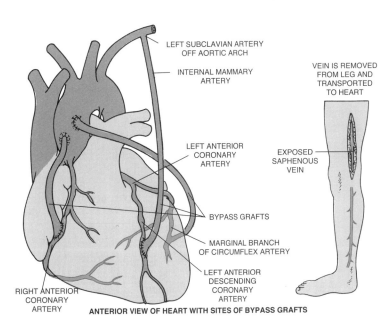

FIGURE 7.5 Bypass. Anterior view of heart with sites of bypass graft. (From Venes, D [ed]: Taber's Cyclopedic Medical Dictionary, ed 20. FA Davis, Philadelphia, 2005.)

LEFT SUBCLAVIAN ARTERY OFF AORTIC ARCH
INTERNAL MAMMARY ARTERY
VEIN IS REMOVED FROM LEG AND TRANSPORTED TO HEART
LEFT ANTERIOR CORONARY ARTERY
EXPOSED SAPHENOUS VEIN
BYPASS GRAFTS
MARGINAL BRANCH OF CIRCUMFLEX ARTERY
LEFT ANTERIOR DESCENDING CORONARY ARTERY
RIGHT ANTERIOR CORONARY ARTERY
ANTERIOR VIEW OF HEART WITH SITES OF BYPASS GRAFTS

Adult

▶ (b) Suctioning; cough, deep breathe.

◤ (c) Elevate *head of bed* at least 30 degrees.

(d) Position chest tube to facilitate drainage; suction maintains patency—do not "milk" chest tube. (see also chest tube care in **Table 11.11**).

(2) *Cardiovascular:*

> (a) Vital signs: BP >80 to 90 mm Hg systolic; *CVP*: range 5 to 15 cm H_2O unless otherwise ordered; pulmonary artery line (PA catheter): mean pressure 4 to 12 mm Hg; I&O: report <30 mL/hr of urine from indwelling urinary catheter.

(b) ECG; PVCs occur most frequently following aortic valve replacement and bypass surgery.

(c) Peripheral pulses if leg veins used for grafting.

(d) Activity: turn q2h; ROM; progressive, early ambulation.

(3) Inspect dressing for bleeding.

(4) Medications according to therapeutic directives—*cardiotonics* (digoxin); *coronary vasodilators* (nitrates); *antibiotics* (penicillin); *analgesics; anticoagulants* (with valve replacements); *antiarrhythmics* (amiodarone, procainamide HCl [Pronestyl]).

b. Goal: *promote comfort, pain relief.*

(1) Medicate: Demerol or morphine sulfate—severe pain lasts 2 to 3 days.

(2) Splint incision when moving or coughing.

(3) Mouth care: frequent, especially if intubated; keep lips moist.

◤ (4) *Position:* use pillows to prevent tension on chest tubes, incision.

c. Goal: *maintain fluid, electrolyte, nutritional balance.*

(1) I&O; urine specific gravity.

(2) Measure chest drainage—should *not* exceed 200 mL/hr for first 4 to 6 hr.

(3) Give fluids as ordered; maintain IV patency.

(4) *Diet:* clear fluids → solid food if no nausea, GI distention; sodium intake *restricted,* low fat.

d. Goal: *promote emotional adjustment.*

(1) Anticipate behavior disturbances (depression, disorientation often occur 3 days postop) related to medications, fear, sleep deprivation.

(2) Calm, oriented, supportive environment, as personalized as possible.

(3) Encourage verbalization of feelings (family and client).

(4) Encourage independence to avoid cardiac-cripple role.

e. Goal: *promote early mobilization.*

(1) Out of bed within first 24 hrs postop.

(2) In chair tid by postop day 2.

f. Goal: *health teaching.*

(1) Alterations in lifestyle; activity, diet, work; resumption of sexual activity usually when client can climb two flights of stairs.

(2) Refer to available community resources for cardiac rehabilitation (e.g., American Heart Association, Mended Hearts).

(3) Drug regimen: purpose, side effects.

(4) Potential complications: dyspnea, pain, palpitations common postoperatively.

◆ 4. **Evaluation/outcome criteria:**

a. No complications; incision heals.

b. Activity level increases—no signs of overexertion (e.g., fatigue, dyspnea, pain).

c. Relief of symptoms.

d. Returns for follow-up medical care.

e. Takes prescribed medications; knows purposes and side effects.

XI. **Minimally invasive direct coronary artery bypass (MIDCAB):** a variation of CABG for clients in whom sternotomy and cardiopulmonary bypass is contraindicated or unnecessary. The left internal mammary is anastomosed to the left anterior descending coronary artery through a thoracic incision without bypass.

XII. **Heart failure (HF):** inability of the heart to meet the peripheral circulatory demands of the body; cardiac decompensation; combined right and left ventricular heart failure.

A. **Pathophysiology:** increased cardiac workload or decreased effective myocardial contractility→ decreased cardiac output (forward effects). Left ventricular failure→pulmonary congestion; right atrial and right ventricular failure→systemic congestion→peripheral edema (backward effects). Compensatory mechanisms in HF include tachycardia, ventricular dilation, and hypertrophy of the myocardium; develops in 50% to 60% of clients with heart disease.

B. **Risk factors:**

1. Decreased myocardial contractility:

a. Myocarditis.

b. MI.

c. Tachyarrhythmias.

d. Bacterial endocarditis.

e. Acute rheumatic fever.

2. Increased cardiac workload:

a. Elevated temperature.

b. Physical/emotional stress.

c. Anemia.

d. Hyperthyroidism (thyrotoxicosis).

e. Valvular defects.

◆ C. **Assessment:**

1. *Subjective data*

a. Shortness of breath.

(1) Orthopnea (sleeps on two or more pillows).

(2) Paroxysmal nocturnal dyspnea (sudden breathlessness during sleep).

(3) Dyspnea on exertion (climbing stairs).

TABLE 7.8	Left Ventricular Compared with Right Ventricular Heart Failure
Left Ventricular Failure	**Right Ventricular Failure**
Pulmonary crackles	Jugular venous distention
Tachypnea	Peripheral edema
S₃ gallop	Perioral and peripheral cyanosis
Cardiac murmurs	Congestive hepatomegaly
Paradoxical splitting of S₂	Ascites
	Hepatojugular reflux

   b. Apprehension; anxiety; irritability.
   c. Fatigue; weakness.
   d. Reported weight gain; feeling of puffiness.
  2. *Objective data* (**Table 7.8**)
   a. *Vital signs:*
    (1) *BP:* decreasing systolic; narrowing pulse pressure.
    (2) *Pulse:* pulsus alternans (alternating strong-weak-strong cardiac contraction), increased.
    (3) *Respirations:* crackles, *Cheyne-Stokes.*
   b. Edema: dependent, pitting (1 + to 4+ mm).
   c. Liver: enlarged, tender.
   d. Neck veins: distended.
   e. Chest x-ray:
    (1) Cardiac enlargement.
    (2) Dilated pulmonary vessels.
    (3) Diffuse interstitial lung edema.
 ◆ **D. Analysis/nursing diagnosis:**
  1. *Decreased cardiac output* related to decreased myocardial contractility.
  2. *Activity intolerance* related to generalized weakness and inadequate oxygenation.
  3. *Fatigue* related to edema and poor oxygenation.
  4. *Altered tissue perfusion* related to peripheral edema and inadequate blood flow.
  5. *Fluid volume excess* related to compensatory mechanisms.
  6. *Impaired gas exchange* related to pulmonary congestion.
  7. *Anxiety* related to shortness of breath.
  8. *Sleep pattern disturbance* related to paroxysmal nocturnal dyspnea.
 ◆ **E. Nursing care plan/implementation (Clinical Pathway 7.2: Congestive Heart Failure):**
  1. Goal: *provide physical rest/reduce emotional stimuli.*
   a. *Position: sitting* or *semi-*Fowler's until tachycardia, dyspnea, edema resolved; change position frequently; pillows for support.
   b. Rest: planned periods; limit visitors, activity, noise. Chair and commode privileges.
   c. Support: stay with client who is anxious; have family member who is supportive present; administer *sedatives/tranquilizers* as ordered.
   d. Warm fluids if appropriate.
  2. Goal: *provide for relief of respiratory distress; reduce cardiac workload.*
   ▶ a. Oxygen: low flow rate; encourage deep breathing (5 to 10 min q2h); auscultate breath sounds for congestion, pulmonary edema.

 b. *Position:* elevating head of bed 20 to 25 cm (8–10 in) alleviates pulmonary congestion.
   c. Medications as ordered:
    (1) *Digitalis* preparations.
    (2) *ACE inhibitors*—captopril, enalapril.
    (3) *Inotropic agent*—dobutamine, dopamine.
    (4) *Diuretics*—thiazides, furosemide, metolazone.
    (5) *Tranquilizers*—phenobarbital, diazepam (Valium), chlordiazepoxide (Librium) HCl.
    (6) *Vasodilators*—hydrolazine, isosorbide.
  3. Goal: *provide for special safety needs.*
   ▶ a. Skin care:
    (1) Inspect, massage, lubricate bony prominences.
    (2) Use foot cradle, heel protectors; sheepskin.
   b. Side rails up if hypoxic (disoriented).
   c. Vital signs: monitor for signs of fatigue, pulmonary emboli.
   d. ROM: active, passive; elastic stockings.
  4. Goal: *maintain fluid and electrolyte balance, nutritional status.*
    a. Urine output: 30 mL/hr minimum; estimate insensible loss in client who is diaphoretic. Monitor BUN, serum creatinine, and electrolytes, b-type natriuretic peptide (BNP).
   b. Daily weight; same time, clothes, scale.
    c. IV: IV infusion pump to avoid circulatory overloading; strict I/O.
   d. Diet:
    (1) *Low* sodium as ordered.
    (2) Small, frequent feedings.
    (3) Discuss food preferences with client.
  5. Goal: *health teaching.*
   a. Diet restrictions; meal preparation.
   b. Activity restrictions, if any; planned rest periods.
   c. Medications: schedule (e.g., diuretic in early morning to limit interruption of sleep) purpose, dosage, side effects (importance of daily pulse taking, daily weights, intake of *potassium*-containing foods).
   d. Refer to available *community resources* for dietary assistance, weight reduction, exercise program.
 ◆ **F. Evaluation/outcome criteria:**
  1. Increase in activity level tolerance—fatigue decreased.
  2. No complications—pulmonary edema, respiratory distress.
  3. Reduction in dependent edema.

XIII. Pulmonary edema: sudden transudation of fluid from pulmonary capillaries into alveoli. **Life-threatening condition.**
  A. Pathophysiology: increased pulmonary capillary permeability; increased hydrostatic pressure (pulmonary hypertension); decreased blood colloidal osmotic pressure; fluid accumulation

Adult

Instructions:
Circle variances and document on opposite side

DATE	/ /	/ /	/ /
	ED	**Day 1**	**Day 2**
1 Discharge Planning/ Referrals	Consider Cardiology consult	☐ Evaluated home situation Identify if client is seen by home care ☐ Yes ☐ No ☐ Code status _____ Advanced directives ☐ Yes ☐ No	☐ SW referral made ☐ Define discharge needs ☐ Notify home care if client was seen by home care before admission
2 Diagnostic Tests/ Treatments	☐ H & P ☐ BUN/Cr ☐ ECG ×2 ☐ Electrolytes ☐ CXR ☐ UA ☐ CBC ☐ PT/INR Consider CK MB and Troponin Consider TSH	☐ Telemetry ☐ BUN/Cr ☐ Electrolytes ☐ ECHO (if not recent or if LV function and valve status are not known) ☐ Fasting lipid panel	☐ Telemetry ☐ BUN/Cr ☐ Electrolytes ☐ Eval. for ischemia completed EF_____ NYHA baseline I II III IV (circle)
3 Nutrition / Diet	☐ NPO	☐ Cardiac prudent diet ☐ Other _____	☐ Cardiac prudent diet ☐ Other _____ ☐ Nutrition consult
4 Treatments and Medications	☐ IV fluids / Saline lock ☐ O_2 ☐ Nitrates ☐ MSO_4 ☐ Furosemide IV/PO	☐ IV fluids / Saline lock ☐ O_2 at _____ L/min. ☐ Nitrates ☐ MSO_4 ☐ ASA ☐ Digoxin ☐ ACE inhibitor/ARBs ☐ Stool softener ☐ Furosemide IV/PO ☐ K supplements IV/PO ☐ Hydralizine ☐ Beta-blocker	☐ IV to saline lock ☐ O_2 at _____ L/min. ☐ ASA ☐ ACE inhibitor/ARBs ☐ Beta-blocker ☐ Nitrates ☐ Furosemide ☐ K supplements ☐ Stool softener ☐ Digoxin
5 Activity/ Cardiac Rehab	☐ Bedrest with commode	☐ Bedrest with commode ☐ PT referral	Begin self care with assistance O_2 pre. ambulation _____ O_2 post. ambulation _____ Client evaluation
6 Nursing Assessment/ Intervention	☐ VS per ED routine ☐ I & O ☐ O_2 sat >92% ☐ Cardiac monitor ☐ Saline lock Wt. _____	A E P Ht _____ Wt _____ Target Wt. (see MD order) _____ VS per unit routine ☐ ☐ ☐ I&O ☐ ☐ ☐ O_2 sat >92% ☐ ☐ ☐ Saline lock ☐ ☐ ☐ A×O × 3, speech clear, memory intact, swallow intact ☐ ☐ ☐ Abdomen soft nontender, bowel sounds present, tolerates diet ☐ ☐ ☐ Voiding adequate amounts, urine clear, yellow to amber ☐ ☐ ☐ Foley cath. draining clear yellow to amber urine ☐ ☐ ☐ Normal ROM and strength appropriate for client ☐ ☐ ☐ Circulation & sensation intact ☐ ☐ ☐	A E P Wt _____ VS per unit routine ☐ ☐ ☐ I&O ☐ ☐ ☐ O_2 sat >92% ☐ ☐ ☐ Saline lock ☐ ☐ ☐ A×O × 3, speech clear, memory intact, swallow intact ☐ ☐ ☐ Abdomen soft nontender, bowel sounds present, tolerates diet ☐ ☐ ☐ Voiding adequate amounts, urine clear, yellow to amber ☐ ☐ ☐ Foley cath. draining clear yellow to amber urine ☐ ☐ ☐ Normal ROM and strength appropriate for client ☐ ☐ ☐ Circulation & sensation intact ☐ ☐ ☐
7 Anxiety	Anxiety level identified Low ☐ Med ☐ High ☐ ☐ Appropriate actions taken (see nursing notes)	☐ Cooperates with care	☐ Receives information about activities ☐ Participates in care ☐ Verbalizes fears and concerns
8 Knowledge Deficit	☐ Inform client of plan of care	☐ CHF client portion of pathway given to client /family ☐ CHF booklet (Krames) given to client ☐ Exacerbation factors identified: _____ _____	☐ Show CHF video ☐ Medication teaching started ☐ Client verbalizes exacerbation factors
Signature	A	A	A
	P	P	P
	N	N	N

(Continued on following page)

Adult

EF NYHA class   I   II   III   IV   (circle)   **Admitting diagnosis** _____

Type of dysfunction _____   **Discharge diagnosis** _____

/ /	/ /	/ /
Day 3	**Day 4/Discharge**	**Day 5 / Discharge**
☐ Home care referral as needed Room air O$_2$ _____ Home O$_2$ at _____		☐ CPR class referral made ☐ Outpt. Cardiac rehab referral made if client has knowledge of CAD ☐ Home situation adequate / no help ☐ Home care referral completed ☐ Appt. made for f/u MD visit
☐ D/c Telemetry		☐ Cardiac evaluation complete EF_____ Type of cardiac dysfunction _____ NYHA class _____ ☐ Lipid status known
☐ Cardiac prudent diet ☐ Other _____	☐ Cardiac prudent diet ☐ Other _____	☐ Client / family able to identify elements of cardiac prudent diet ☐ Written materials given
☐ O$_2$ at _____ L/min. ☐ ASA ☐ Beta-blocker ☐ ACE inhibitor ☐ Nitrates ☐ Furosemide ☐ K supplements ☐ Stool softener ☐ Digoxin	☐ Home O$_2$ at _____ L/min. ☐ ASA ☐ Beta-blocker ☐ ACE inhibitor/ARBs ☐ Nitrates ☐ Furosemide ☐ K supplements ☐ Stool softener ☐ Digoxin	☐ D/C meds R× given ☐ Client verbalized understanding how to take D/C medications ☐ Medication teaching sheet completed and signed by client and nurse ☐ Client identified who will pick up Rx. ☐ Financial considerations addressed ☐ Home O$_2$ arranged if needed
Ambulate × 3 without significant change in VS ☐ ☐ ☐ Client evaluation Teach client methods to evaluate exertion	Ambulate 5 × day ☐ ☐ ☐ ☐ ☐ Independent self care Stair climbing if appropriate ☐ Verbalizes activity limits	☐ Inpatient Cardiac rehab complete ☐ ADLs with stable VS
A E P Wt _____ VS per unit routine ☐ ☐ ☐ I&O ☐ ☐ ☐ O$_2$ sat >92% ☐ ☐ ☐ Saline lock ☐ ☐ ☐ A×O × 3, speech clear, memory intact, swallow intact ☐ ☐ ☐ Abdomen soft nontender, bowel sounds present, tolerates diet ☐ ☐ ☐ Voiding adequate amounts, urine clear, yellow to amber ☐ ☐ ☐ Foley cath. dc'd, voiding without difficulty ☐ ☐ ☐ Normal ROM and strength appropriate for client ☐ ☐ ☐ Circulation & sensation intact ☐ ☐ ☐	A E P Wt _____ VS per unit routine ☐ ☐ ☐ I&O ☐ ☐ ☐ O$_2$ sat >92% ☐ ☐ ☐ Saline lock ☐ ☐ ☐ A×O × 3, speech clear, memory intact, swallow intact ☐ ☐ ☐ Abdomen soft nontender, bowel sounds present, tolerates diet ☐ ☐ ☐ Voiding adequate amounts, urine clear, yellow to amber ☐ ☐ ☐ Foley cath. dc'd, voiding without difficulty ☐ ☐ ☐ Normal ROM and strength appropriate for client ☐ ☐ ☐ Circulation & sensation intact ☐ ☐ ☐	☐ D/C instructions given to client, client verbalizes understanding. ☐ Client at target weight (if known)
☐ Receives information about activities ☐ Participates in care ☐ Verbalizes fears and concerns	☐ Retains information ☐ Participates in care ☐ Verbalizes understanding or proper life style changes	☐ Coping skills adequate ☐ Continuing care arrangements made if appropriate
Symptom management plan: _____ _____ _____ ☐ Medication teaching reviewed ☐ Give D/C instructions	☐ Medication teaching reviewed ☐ Review D/C instructions ☐ Complete D/C instruction sheet ☐ RN and PT sign forms	☐ D/C summary complete ☐ Client verbalizes diagnosis and management plan
A	A	A
P	P	P
N	N	N

Adult

Source: UCSF Healthcare, San Francisco, Calif. With permission from Jane E. Hirsch, RN, MS, Vice President, Nursing and Patient Care Services.

in alveoli → decreased compliance → decreased diffusion of gas → hypoxia, hypercapnea.

B. Risk factors:
1. Left ventricular failure.
2. Pulmonary embolism.
3. Drug overdose.
4. Smoke inhalation.
5. CNS damage.
6. Fluid overload.

◆ **C. Assessment:**
1. *Subjective data*
   a. Anxiety.
   b. Restlessness at onset progressing to agitation.
   c. Stark fear.
   d. Intense dyspnea, orthopnea, fatigue.
2. *Objective data*
   a. *Vital signs:*
      (1) *Pulse:* tachycardia; gallop rhythm.
      (2) *Respiration:* tachypnea, moist, bubbling, wheezing, labored.
      (3) *Temperature:* normal to subnormal.
   b. Skin: pale, cool, diaphoretic, cyanotic.
   c. Auscultation: crackles, wheezes.
   d. Cough: productive of large quantities of pink, frothy sputum.
   e. Right ventricular heart failure: distended (bulging) neck veins, peripheral edema, hepatomegaly, ascites.
   f. Mental status: restless, confused, stuporous.
   g. Arterial blood gases: hypoxia; pulse oximetry: *decreased* O_2 saturation.
   h. Chest x-ray: haziness of lung fields, cardiomegaly.

◆ **D. Analysis/nursing diagnosis:**
1. *Decreased cardiac output* related to decreased myocardial contractility.
2. *Impaired gas exchange* related to pulmonary congestion.
3. *Altered tissue perfusion* related to inadequate blood flow.
4. *Anxiety,* severe, related to difficulty breathing.
5. *Fear* related to life-threatening situation.

◆ **E. Nursing care plan/implementation:**
1. Goal: *promote physical, psychological relaxation measures to relieve anxiety.*
   a. Slow respirations: morphine sulfate 3 to 10 mg IV/SC/IM, as ordered, to reduce respiratory rate, sedate, and produce vasodilation.
   b. Remain with client.
   c. Encourage slow, deep breathing; assist with coughing.
   d. Work calmly, confidently, unhurriedly.
   e. Frequent rest periods.
2. Goal: *improve cardiac function, reduce venous return, relieve hypoxia.*
   a. O_2: slow respiratory rate, provide uniform ventilation via nasal cannula, ventimask, 100% non-rebreather, or intubation, depending on O_2 need. Possibly PEEP.

b. Give aminophylline, as ordered, to lower venous pressure and increase cardiac output.
c. IV: D_5W.
d. *Position: high-Fowler's,* extremities in dependent position, to reduce venous return and facilitate breathing.
e. Medications as ordered: digitalis; *diuretics—* furosemide (Lasix); *inotropic agents —* dobutamine (Dobutrex), dopamine; nitroglycerin, nitroprusside.
f. Vital signs; auscultate breath sounds.
g. *Diet: low* sodium; fluid *restriction* as ordered.
3. Goal: *health teaching* (include family or significant other).
   a. Medications.
      (1) Side effects.
      (2) Potassium supplements if indicated.
      (3) Pulse taking.
   b. Exercise; rest.
   c. *Diet: low* sodium.
   d. *Signs of complications*: edema; weight gain of 2–3 lb (0.9–1.4 kg) in a few days; dyspnea.

◆ **F. Evaluation/outcome criteria:**
1. No complications; vital signs stable; clear breath sounds.
2. No weight gain; weight loss if indicated.
3. Alert, oriented, calm.

XIV. Shock: a critically severe deficiency in nutrients, oxygen, and electrolytes delivered to body tissues, plus deficiency in removal of cellular wastes; results from cardiac failure, insufficient blood volume, or increased vascular bed size.

A. Types, pathophysiology, and risk factors:
1. *Hypovolemic* (hemorrhagic, hematogenic)— markedly decreased **volume** of blood (hemorrhage or plasma loss from intestinal obstruction, burns, physical trauma, or dehydration)→ decreased venous return, cardiac output → decreased → tissue perfusion.
2. *Cardiogenic*—failure of cardiac muscle **pump** (myocardial infarction)→generally decreased cardiac output→pulmonary congestion, hypoxia → inadequate circulation; high mortality rate.
3. *Distributive:*
   a. *Neurogenic*—massive **vasodilation** from reduced vasomotor, vasoconstrictor tone (e.g., spinal shock, head injuries, anesthesia, pain); interruption of sympathetic nervous system; blood volume is normal but inadequate for vessels→decreased venous return→tissue hypoxia.
   b. *Vasogenic* (anaphylactic, septic, endotoxic)— severe reaction to foreign protein (insect bites, drugs, toxic substances, aerobic, gram-negative organisms)→histamine release **vasodilation,** venous stasis→diminished venous return.

TABLE 7.9	Signs of Hypovolemic Shock

Blood Loss (% of Total) ◆	Assessment Data
800–1500 mL (15%–30%)	Restlessness Pulse > 100 Systolic pressure unchanged Diastolic pressure ↑ Urine output ↓
2000 mL (30%–40%)	Mental status ↓ Pulse > 120 Respirations > 30 Systolic pressure ↓
> 2500 mL (>40%)	Cold, clammy skin Pulse > 120 Respirations >30 Narrowed pulse pressure (= systolic minus diastolic)

◆ **B. Assessment:** varies, depending on degree of shock (**Table 7.9**).
1. *Subjective data*
   a. Anxiety; restlessness.
   b. Dizziness; fainting.
   c. Thirst.
   d. Nausea.
2. *Objective data*
   a. *Vital signs:*
      (1) *BP*—hypotension (postural changes in early shock; systolic <70 mm Hg in late shock).
      (2) *Pulse*—tachycardia, thready; irregular *(cardiogenic shock);* could be slow if conduction system of heart damaged.
      (3) *Respirations*—increased depth, rate; wheezing *(anaphylactic shock).*
      (4) *Temperature*—decreased (elevated in *septic shock).*
   b. Skin:
      (1) Pale (or mottled), cool, clammy (warm to touch in *septic shock).*
      (2) Urticaria *(anaphylactic shock).*
   c. Level of consciousness: alert, oriented→unresponsive.
   d. CVP:

   > (1) *Below* 5 cm H₂O with *hypovolemic* shock.
   > (2) *Above* 15 cm H₂O with *cardiogenic*, possibly septic shock.

   e. Urine output: *decreased* (<30 mL/hr).
   f. Capillary refill: slowed; normally nailbed "pinks up" within 2 sec after blanching (nailbed pressure).

◆ **C. Analysis/nursing diagnosis:**
1. *Altered tissue perfusion* related to vasoconstriction or decreased myocardial contractility.
2. *Impaired gas exchange* related to ventilation-perfusion imbalance.

3. *Decreased cardiac output* related to loss of circulating blood volume or diminished cardiac contractility.
4. *Altered urinary elimination* related to decreased renal perfusion.
5. *Fluid volume deficit* related to blood loss.
6. *Anxiety* related to severity of condition.
7. *Risk for injury* related to death.

◆ **D. Nursing care plan/implementation:** Goal: *promote venous return, circulatory perfusion.*
1. *Position:* foot of bed *elevated* 20 degrees (12 to 16 inches), knees straight, trunk horizontal, head slightly elevated; *avoid* Trendelenburg position.
2. Ventilation: monitor respiratory effort, loosen restrictive clothing; O₂ as ordered.
3. Fluids:
   a. Maintain IV infusions—with sepsis, may receive 2–6L to keep CVP >12 mm Hg to prevent end organ hypoxia and organ failure.
   b. Give blood, plasma expanders as ordered (exception—**stop blood immediately** in anaphylactic shock).
4. Vital signs:
   a. CVP (*decreased* with hypovolemia) arterial line, PA catheter (*increased* pulmonary artery wedge pressure indicating cardiac failure).
   b. Urine output (insert catheter for hourly output).
   c. Monitor ECG (increased rate, dysrhythmias).
5. Medications (depending on type of shock) as ordered:
   a. *Vasopressors*—dobutamine, norepinephrine (Levophed), isoproterenol (Isuprel), dopamine (Intropin) (cardiogenic, neurogenic, septic shock).
   b. *Antiarrhythmics* (cardiogenic shock).
   c. *Cardiac glycosides* (cardiogenic shock).
   d. *Adrenocorticoids* (anaphylactic shock).
   e. *Antibiotics* (septic shock).
   f. *Vasodilators*—nitroprusside (cardiogenic shock).
   g. *Antihistamines*—epinephrine (anaphylactic shock).
6. Mechanical support: military (or medical) antishock trousers (MAST) or pneumatic antishock garment (PASG); used to promote internal autotransfusion of blood from legs and abdomen to central circulation; at lower pressures may control bleeding and promote hemostasis; do *not* remove (deflate) suddenly to examine underlying areas or BP will drop precipitously; *compartment syndrome* may result with prolonged use and high pressure; controversial.

◆ **E. Evaluation/outcome criteria:**
1. Vital signs stable, within normal limits.
2. Alert, oriented.
3. Urine output >30 mL/hr.

XV. Disseminated intravascular coagulation (DIC): diffuse or widespread coagulation initially within arterioles and capillaries leading to hemorrhage.

A. Pathophysiology: activation of coagulation system from tissue injury→fibrin microthrombi form throughout the vascular system→microinfarcts, tissue necrosis→red blood cells, platelets, prothrombin, other clotting factors trapped in capillaries, destroyed in process→excessive clotting→release of fibrin split products→inhibition of platelet clotting →profuse bleeding.

B. Risk factors:
1. Obstetric complications (50% of cases).
2. Neoplastic disease.
3. Low perfusion states (e.g., burns, hypothermia); hypovolemia.
4. Infections, sepsis

◆ **C. Assessment**—*objective data:*
1. Skin, mucous membranes: petechiae, ecchymosis.
2. Extremities (fingers, toes): cyanosis.
3. Bleeding: venipuncture sites, wound, oral, rectal, vaginal.
4. Urine output: oliguria→anuria.
5. Level of consciousness: ↓LOC progressing to coma.

6. Lab data: *prolonged*—prothrombin time (PT) >15 sec; *decreased*—platelets, fibrinogen level.

◆ **D. Analysis/nursing diagnosis:**
1. *Altered tissue perfusion* related to peripheral microthrombi.
2. *Risk for injury* (death) related to bleeding.
3. *Risk for impaired skin integrity* related to ischemia.
4. *Altered urinary elimination* related to renal tubular necrosis.

◆ **E. Nursing care plan/implementation:** goal—*prevent and detect further bleeding.*
1. Carry out nursing measures designed to alleviate underlying problem (e.g., shock, birth of fetus, surgery/irradiation for cancer, antibiotics for infection).
2. Medications: heparin sodium IV, 1000 U/hr, if ordered, to reverse abnormal clotting (controversial). Possible human recombient activated protein C.
3. IVs: blood to lessen shock; platelets, cryoprecipitate, fresh plasma to restore clotting factors, fibrinogen.
4. Observe: vital signs, CVP (normal 5 to 15 mm Hg), PAP (normal 20 to 30 systolic and 8 to 12 diastolic), and intake output for signs of shock or fluid overload from frequent infusions; specimens for occult blood (urine, stool).
5. *Precautions: avoid* IM injections if possible; pressure 5 min to venipuncture sites; *no* rectal temperatures.

◆ **F. Evaluation/outcome criteria:**

1. Clotting mechanism restored (increased platelets, normal PT).
2. Renal function restored (urine output >30 mL/hr).
3. Circulation to fingers, toes; no cyanosis.
4. No irreversible damage from renal, cerebral, cardiac, or adrenal hemorrhage.

XVI. Pericarditis: inflammation of parietal or visceral pericardium or both; acute or chronic condition; may occur with or without effusion. Cardiac tamponade may result.

A. Pathophysiology: fibrosis or accumulation of fluid in pericardium→compression of cardiac pumping→decreased cardiac output→increased systemic, pulmonic venous pressure.

B. Risk factors:
1. Bacterial, viral, fungal infections.
2. Tuberculosis.
3. Collagen diseases.
4. Uremia.
5. Transmural MI.
6. Trauma.

◆ **C. Assessment:**
1. *Subjective data*
   a. *Pain:*
      (1) *Type*—sharp, moderate to severe.
      (2) *Location*—wide area of pericardium, may radiate: right arm, jaw/teeth.
      (3) *Precipitating factors*—movement, deep inspiration, swallowing.
   b. Chills; sweating.
   c. Apprehension; anxiety.
   d. Fatigue.
   e. Abdominal pain.
   f. Shortness of breath.
2. *Objective data*
   a. *Vital signs:*
      (1) *BP: decreased* pulse pressure; pulsus paradoxus—abnormal drop in systolic BP of >8 to 10 mm Hg during inspiration.
      (2) *Pulse:* tachycardia.
      (3) *Temperature: elevated*; erratic course; low grade.
   b. Pericardial friction rub.
   c. *Increased* CVP; distended neck veins; dependent pitting edema; liver engorgement.
   d. Restlessness.

   e. Lab data: *elevated* AST (SGOT), WBC; CT or MRI—pericardial thickening
   f. Serial ECGs: *increased* ST segment; echocardiogram: pericardial fluid.

◆ **D. Analysis/nursing diagnosis:**
1. *Decreased cardiac output* related to impaired cardiac muscle contraction.
2. *Pain* related to pericardial inflammation.
3. *Anxiety* related to unknown outcome.
4. *Fatigue* related to inadequate oxygenation.

E. Nursing care plan/implementation:

1. Goal: *promote physical and emotional comfort.*

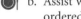 a. *Position:* semi-Fowler's (upright or sitting); bedrest.

b. Vital signs: q2 to 4h and prn; apical and radial pulse; notify physician if heart sounds *decrease* in amplitude or if pulse pressure *narrows,* indicating cardiac tamponade; see **i** below.

c. O₂ as ordered.

d. Medications as ordered:

(1) *Analgesics*—aspirin, morphine sulfate, meperidine or codeine.

(2) *Nonsteroidal antiinflammatory agents*—indomethacin.

(3) *Antimicrobial.*

(4) *Digitalis and diuretics,* if heart failure present.

e. Assist with aspiration of pericardial sac (pericardiocentesis) if needed: medicate as ordered; *elevate* head 60 degrees; monitor ECG; have defibrillator and pacemaker available.

f. Prepare for pericardiectomy (excision of constricting pericardium) as ordered.

g. Continual emotional support.

h. Enhance effects of analgesics: positioning; turning; NPO.

i. Monitor for:

> **Signs of cardiac tamponade:** tachycardia; tachypnea; hypotension; pallor; narrowed pulse pressure; pulsus paradoxus; distended neck veins; ECG changes.

2. Goal: *maintain fluid, electrolyte balance.*

a. Parenteral fluids as ordered; strict I&O.

b. Assist with feedings; *low sodium* diet may be ordered.

F. Evaluation/outcome criteria:

1. Relief of pain, dyspnea.

2. No complications (e.g., cardiac tamponade).

3. Return of normal cardiac functioning.

XVII. Chronic arterial occlusive disease: arteriosclerosis obliterans most common occlusive disorder of the arterial system (aorta, large and medium-size arteries); frequently involves the femoral, iliac, and popliteal arteries (Buerger's disease).

A. Pathophysiology: fatty deposits in intimal, medial layer of arterial walls; plaque formation → narrowed arterial lumens; decreased distensibility → decreased blood flow; ischemic changes in tissues.

B. Risk factors:

1. Age (>50).

2. Sex (men).

3. Diabetes mellitus.

4. Hyperlipidemia—obesity.

5. Cigarette smoking.

6. Hypertension.

7. Family history.

C. Assessment:

1. *Subjective data*

a. *Pain:*

(1) *Type*—cramplike.

(2) *Location*—foot, calf, thigh, buttocks.

(3) *Duration*—variable, may be relieved by rest.

(4) *Precipitating causes*—exercise (intermittent claudication), but occasionally may occur when at rest.

b. Tingling, numbness in toes, feet.

c. Persistent coldness of one or both lower extremities.

2. *Objective data*

a. Lower extremities:

(1) Pedal pulses—absent or diminished.

(2) Skin—shiny, glossy; dry, cold, chalky white, decreased/absent hair, ulcers, gangrene.

 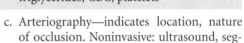 b. Lab data: *increased* serum cholesterol, triglycerides, CBC, platelets

c. Arteriography—indicates location, nature of occlusion. Noninvasive: ultrasound, segmental limb pressure, exercise testing.

D. Analysis/nursing diagnosis:

1. *Altered tissue perfusion* related to peripheral vascular disease.

2. *Risk for activity intolerance* related to pain and sensory changes.

3. *Pain* related to ischemia.

4. *Risk for impaired skin integrity* related to poor circulation.

5. *Risk for injury* related to numbness of extremities.

E. Nursing care plan/implementation:

1. Goal: *promote circulation; decrease discomfort.*

a. *Position:* elevate head of bed on blocks (3 to 6 inches), because gravity aids perfusion to thighs, legs; elevating legs increases pain.

b. Comfort: keep warm: *avoid* chilling or use of heating pads, which may burn skin; apply bed socks.

c. Circulation: check pedal pulses, skin color, temperature qid.

d. Medications:

(1) *Vasodilators.*

(2) *Antiplatelet*—ASA, ticlopidine, dipyridamole.

(3) *Dihydropyridines*—nifedipine, amlodipine.

(4) *Xanthine derivatives*—pentoxifylline.

2. Goal: *prevent infection, injury.*

a. Skin care: use bed cradle, sheepskin, heel pads; mild soap; dry thoroughly; lotion; do *not* massage, to prevent release of thrombus.

b. Foot care: wear properly fitting shoes, slippers when out of bed; inspect for injury or pressure areas; nail care by podiatrist.

3. Goal: *health teaching.*

a. Skin care; inspect daily.

h. Activity; balance exercise, rest to increase collateral circulation; walk only until painful.

c. Exercises: walking, Buerger-Allen exercises (gravity alternately fills and empties blood vessels).

d. *Diet:* low fat, heart-healthy diet to slow disease progression.

e. Lifestyle choices: *avoid* smoking.

f. Recognize and report signs of occlusion (e.g., pain, cramping, numbness in extremities, color changes—white or blue, temperature changes—cool to cold).

◆ **F. Evaluation/outcome criteria:**
1. Decreased pain.
2. Skin integrity preserved; no loss of limb.
3. Quits smoking.
4. Does exercises to increase collateral circulation.

XVIII. Aneurysms (thoracic or abdominal aortic): localized or diffuse dilations/outpouching of a vessel wall, usually an artery; exerts pressure on adjacent structures; affects primarily men over age 60; >6 cm diameter, 50% will rupture; resected surgically, reconstructed with synthetic or vascular graft.

A. Risk factors:
1. Atherosclerosis.
2. Trauma.
3. Syphilis.
4. Congenital weakness.
5. Local infection.
6. Cigarette smoking.

◆ **B. Assessment:**
1. *Subjective data*
   a. *Pain:*
      (1) Constant, boring, neuralgic, intermittent—low back, abdominal.
      (2) Angina—sudden onset may mean rupture or dissection, which are **emergency** conditions.
   b. Dyspnea; orthopnea—pressure on trachea or bronchus.
2. *Objective data*
   a. *Vital signs:*
      (1) Radial pulses differ.
      (2) Tachycardia.
      (3) Hypotension following rupture leading to shock.
   b. Pulsating mass: abdominal, chest wall pulsation; edema of chest wall (thoracic aneurysm); periumbilical (abdominal aneurysm); audible bruit over aorta.
   c. Skin has cyanosis, mottled below level of aneurysm.
   d. Veins: dilated, superficial—neck, chest, arms.
   e. Cough: paroxysmal, brassy.
   f. Diaphoresis, pallor, fainting following rupture.
   g. Peripheral pulses:

(1) Femoral present.
(2) Pedal weak or absent.
h. Stool: bloody from irritation.

◆ **C. Analysis/nursing diagnosis:**
1. *Risk for injury* related to possible aneurysm rupture.
2. *Pain* related to pressure on lumbar nerves.
3. *Anxiety* related to risk of rupture.

D. Nursing care plan/implementation:
1. Goal: *provide emergency care before surgery for dissection or rupture.*
   a. Vital signs: frequent, depending on severity (systolic BP <100 mm Hg and pulse >100 with rupture).
   b. IVs: may have 2 to 4 sites; lactated Ringer's may be ordered.
   c. Urine output: monitored every 15 to 30 min.
   d. O$_2$: usually via nasal prongs.
   e. Medications as ordered: *antihypertensives* to prevent extension of dissection.
   f. Transport to operating room quickly.
   g. See **The Perioperative Experience, p. 546,** for general preoperative care.
2. Goal: *prevent complications postoperatively.*
   a. *Position:* initially flat in bed; *avoid* sharp flexion of hip and knee, which places pressure on femoral and popliteal arteries; turn gently side to side; note erythema on back from pooled blood.
   b. *Vital signs:* CVP; hourly peripheral pulses distal to graft site, including neurovascular check of lower extremities; absent pulses for 6 to 12 hr indicates occlusion; check with Doppler blood flow detector.
   c. *Urine output:* hourly from indwelling catheter.
      (1) Immediately report anuria or oliguria (<30 mL/hr).
      (2) Check color for hematuria.
      (3) Monitor daily blood urea nitrogen (BUN) and creatinine.
   d. Observe *for signs of atheroembolization* (patchy areas of ischemia); report change in color, motor ability, or sensation of lower extremities.
   e. Observe for *signs of bowel ischemia* (decreased/absent bowel sounds, pain, guaiac-positive diarrhea, abdominal distention); may have nasogastric tube.
   f. Measure abdominal girth; increase seen with graft leakage.
3. Goal: *promote comfort.*
   a. *Position:* alignment, comfort; prevent heel ulcers.
   b. Medication: *narcotics.*
4. Goal: *health teaching.*
   a. Minimize recurrence: *avoid* trauma, infection, smoking, high cholesterol diet, obesity.
   b. Regular medical supervision.

◆ **E. Evaluation/outcome criteria:**
1. Surgical intervention before rupture.
2. No loss of renal function.

XIX. Raynaud's phenomenon: a primary vasospastic disease that affects digits of both hands (rarely feet).

 A. **Pathophysiology:** constriction of small arteries and arterioles from vasospasm or obstruction→spasm→hypoxia→hyperthermia as spasm stops.

 B. **Risk factors:**
  1. Cigarette smoking.
  2. Caffeine.
  3. Cold temperature.
  4. Emotional upsets (stress reaction).
  5. Autoimmune conditions:
   a. SLE.
   b. RA.
   c. Scleroderma.
  6. Women between teenage years and age 40.

 ◆ C. **Assessment:**
  1. *Subjective data*
   a. Numbness and sensations of cold.
   b. During "red phase": throbbing, paresthesia, tingling in one or more digits.
  2. *Objective data*
   a. Intermittent *episodes of classic color changes,* occurring in *sequence* in digits: pallor (arterial spasm starts) → bluish (cyanosis from hypoxia) → redness (hyperthermia, as arterial spasm stops).
   b. Skin and subcutaneous tissue: atrophy.
   c. Nails: brittle.

 ◆ D. **Analysis/nursing diagnosis:**
  1. *Pain* (acute/chronic) related to vasospasm/altered perfusion of affected tissues and ischemia of tissues.
  2. *Altered peripheral tissue perfusion* related to vasospastic disease.
  3. *Risk for injury* related to numbness.

 ◆ E. **Nursing care plan/implementation:**
  1. Goal: *maintain warmth in extremities.*
   a. Use wool gloves (when handling cold objects or touching refrigerator/freezer), wool socks and insulated shoes in cold weather.
   b. *Avoid* prolonged exposure to cold material, environment.
  2. Goal: *increase hydrostatic pressure, and therefore circulation.*
   a. Vigorous exercise of arms.
   b. Meds: *vasodilators,* including calcium channel blockers.
  3. Goal: *health teaching:*
   a. *Avoid* smoking.
   b. Biofeedback for stress management.
   c. Identify and *avoid* precipitating factors (e.g., cold, stress).

 ◆ F. **Evaluation/outcome criteria:**
  1. Severity and frequency of attacks are reduced.
  2. Tissue perfusion is maintained.
  3. Verbalization of less numbness and tingling.

XX. Varicose veins: abnormally lengthened, tortuous, dilated superficial veins (saphenous); result of incompetent valves, especially in lower extremities; process is irreversible.

 A. **Pathophysiology:** dilated vein → venous stasis → edema, fibrotic changes, pigmentation of skin, lowered resistance to trauma.

 B. **Risk factors:**
  1. Heredity.
  2. Obesity.
  3. Pregnancy.
  4. Chronic disease (heart, liver).
  5. Occupations requiring long periods of standing.

 ◆ C. **Assessment:**
  1. *Subjective data*
   a. Dull aches; heaviness in legs.
   b. Pain; muscle cramping.
   c. Fatigue in lower extremities, increased with hot weather, high altitude, history of risk factors.
  2. *Objective data*
   a. Nodular protrusions along veins.
   b. Edema.
   c. *Diagnostic tests:* Trendelenburg test; phlebography; Doppler flowmeter.

 ◆ D. **Analysis/nursing diagnosis:**
  1. *Altered tissue perfusion* related to venous valve incompetence.
  2. *Pain* related to edema and muscle cramping.
  3. *Risk for activity intolerance* related to leg discomfort.
  4. *Body image disturbance* related to disfigurement of leg.

 ◆ E. **Nursing care plan/implementation:**
  1. Goal: *promote venous return from lower extremities.*
   a. Activity: walk every hour.
   b. Discourage prolonged sitting, standing, sitting with crossed legs.
   c. *Position:* elevate legs q2 to 3h; elastic stockings or Ace wraps.
  2. Goal: *provide for safety.*
   a. Assist with early ambulation.
   b. *Surgical asepsis* with wounds, leg ulcers.
   c. Observe for hemorrhage—if occurs: *elevate* leg, apply pressure, notify physician.
   d. Observe for allergic reactions if sclerosing drugs used; have *antihistamine* available.
  3. Goal: *health teaching.*
   a. Weight-reducing techniques, dietary approaches if indicated.
   b. Preventive measures: leg elevation; *avoiding* prolonged standing, sitting, high chairs, tight girdles, constrictive clothing; wear support hose.
    c. Expectations for *Trendelenburg test:*
    (1) While client is lying down, *elevate* leg 65 degrees for approximately 1 min to empty veins.
    (2) Apply tourniquet high on upper thigh (do *not* constrict deep veins).
    (3) Client stands with tourniquet in place.
    (4) Filling of veins is observed.
    (5) Normal response is slow filling from

Adult

below in 20 to 30 sec, with no change in
rate when tourniquet is removed.
(6) Incompetent veins distend very quickly
with back flow.

  d. Prepare for sclerotherapy or vein ligation
  and stripping.
◆ **F. Evaluation/outcome criteria:**
  1. Relief or control of symptoms.
  2. Activity without pain.

XXI. **Vein ligation and stripping:** surgical intervention for
advancing varicosities, stasis ulcerations, and
cosmetic needs of client. Procedure involves ligation
of the saphenous vein at the groin, where it joins the
femoral vein; saphenous stripping from the groin to
the ankle; legs are wrapped with a pressure bandage.
Frequently done as outpatient surgery.
◆ **A.** See preceding section on **varicose veins** for *assessment* data and *nursing diagnosis* of the client
requiring surgery.
◆ **B. Nursing care plan/implementation:**
  1. Goal: *prevent complications* after discharge.
  a. *Position: elevate* legs as instructed.
  b. Activity: *No* chair sitting to prevent venous
  pooling, thrombus formation. *Avoid* standing in one place.
  c. Bleeding: report to MD
  2. Goal: *health teaching* to prevent recurrence.
  a. Weight reduction.
  b. *Avoid* constricting garments.
  c. Change positions frequently.
  d. Wear support hose/stockings to enhance
  venous return.
  e. *No* crossing legs at knees.
◆ **C. Evaluation/outcome criteria:**
  1. No complications—hemorrhage, infection,
  nerve damage, deep-vein thrombosis.
  2. No recurrence of varicosities.
  3. Adequate circulation to legs: strong pedal
  pulses.
  4. Resume daily activities; free of pain.

XXII. **Deep vein thrombosis (thrombophlebitis):** formation of a blood clot in an inflamed vein, secondary to
phlebitis or partial obstruction; may lead to venous
insufficiency and pulmonary embolism. Deep vein
thrombosis is most serious form.
  A. Pathophysiology: endothelial inflammation →
  formation of platelet plug (blood clot) → slowing
  of blood flow → increase in procoagulants in local
  area → initiation of clotting mechanisms.
  B. Risk factors:
  1. Immobility/stasis—prolonged sitting, bedrest,
  obesity, pregnancy.
  2. Venous disease.
  3. Age—increased incidence in elderly.
  4. Gender—more often women.
  5. Hypercoagulability of blood.
  6. Intimal damage—IVs, drug abuse.
  7. Fractures.
  8. Oral contraceptives (related to estrogen content).

◆ **C. Assessment:**
  1. *Subjective data*
  a. Calf stiffness, soreness.
  b. Severe pain: walking, dorsiflexion of foot
  (*Homans' sign*—may be unreliable).
  2. *Objective data*
  a. Vein: redness, heat, hardness, threadiness.
  b. Limb: swollen, pale, cold.
  c. *Vital signs:* low-grade fever.
  d. *Diagnostic tests:* venogram, impedance
  plethysmography (electrical resistance to
  blood flow), ultrasonography.
◆ **D. Analysis/nursing diagnosis:**
  1. *Altered peripheral tissue perfusion* related to
  venous stasis.
  2. *Pain* related to inflammation.
  3. *Activity intolerance* related to leg pain.
  4. *Risk for injury* related to potential pulmonary
  emboli.
◆ **E. Nursing care plan/implementation:**
  1. Goal: *provide rest, comfort, and relief from pain.*
  a. Bedrest until therapeutic level of heparin
  reached (5 to 7 days with traditional
  heparin; after 24 hr with low-molecular-
  weight heparin).
  b. *Position:* as ordered; usually extremity
  elevated; watch for pressure points.
  c. Apply warm, moist heat to affected area as
  prescribed (cold may also be ordered).
  d. Assess progress of affected area: swelling,
  pain, soreness, temperature, color.
  e. Administer *analgesics* as ordered.
  2. Goal: *prevent complications.*
  a. Observe for signs of embolism (pain at site
  of embolism); allergic reaction (anaphylactic shock) with streptokinase.
  b. *Precautions: no* rubbing or massage of limb.
  c. Medications: *anticoagulants* (sodium
  heparin, enoxaparin, Coumadin); streptokinase (Varidase), tissue plasminogen acti-
  vator (**Table 7.10**).
  d. Bleeding: hematuria, epistaxis, ecchymosis.
  e. Skin care, to relieve increased redness/
  maceration from hot or cold applications.
  f. ROM: unaffected limb.
  3. Goal: *health teaching.*
  a. *Precautions:* tight garters, girdles; sitting
  with legs crossed; oral contraceptives.
  b. *Preventive* measures: walking daily, swimming several times weekly if possible,
  wading, rest periods with legs *elevated,* elastic stockings (may remove at bedtime).
  c. Medication side effects: *anticoagulants*—
  pink toothbrush, hematuria, easily bruised.
  (1) Carry MedicAlert card/bracelet.
  (2) **Contraindicated** drugs—aspirin, glu-
  tethimide (Doriden), chloramphenicol
  (Chloromycetin), neomycin, phenylbutazone (Butazolidin), barbiturates.
  d. Prepare for surgery (thrombectomy, vein
  ligation).

TABLE 7.10	Nursing Responsibilities with Anticoagulant Therapy		
	Heparin	**Warfarin (Coumadin)**	**Low-Molecular-Weight Heparin (LMWH)**
Monitor	PTT (25–38 sec) (2–3 times baseline)	PT (11–15 sec) ($1^{1}/_{2}$–$2^{1}/_{2}$ times baseline) INR: 2–3.5	Antifactor Xa, CBC, platelets
Inspect	Ecchymosis, bleeding gums, petechiae, hematuria	Bleeding, ecchymosis	Bleeding, hemorrhage, unusual bruising
Administer	With an infusion pump; **never** mix with other drugs; **never** aspirate; **avoid** massaging site	Same time every day; PO	Subcutaneous bid
Avoid	Salicylates and other anticoagulants, e.g., antacids, corticosteroids, penicillin, phenytoin	Same as heparin	Warfarin, platelet aggregation inhibitors (e.g., ASA, NSAIDs, dextran)
Antidote	Protamine sulfate	Vitamin K	Protamine sulfate

◆ **F. Evaluation/outcome criteria:**
1. No complications (e.g., embolism).
2. No recurrence of symptoms.
3. Free of pain—ambulates without discomfort.

XXIII. Peripheral embolism: fragments of thrombi, globules of fat, clumps of tissue, calcified plaques, or air moves in the circulation and lodges in vessel, obstructing blood flow; thrombic emboli most common; may be venous or arterial.

Conditions Affecting Tissue Perfusion

I. Iron deficiency anemia (hypochromic microcytic anemia): inadequate production of red blood cells due to lack of heme (iron); common in infants, women who are pregnant and premenopausal.
  A. Pathophysiology: decreased dietary intake, impaired absorption, or increased utilization of iron decreases the amount of iron bound to plasma transferrin and transported to bone marrow for hemoglobin synthesis; decreased hemoglobin in erythrocytes decreases amount of oxygen delivered to tissues.
  B. Risk factors:
  1. *Excessive menstruation.*
  2. *Gastrointestinal bleeding*—peptic ulcer, hookworm, tumors.
  3. *Inadequate diet*—anorexia, fad diets, cultural practices.
  4. *Poor absorption*—stomach, small intestine disease.
◆ **C. Assessment:**
  1. *Subjective data*
    a. Fatigue: increasing.
    b. Headache.
    c. Change in appetite; difficulty swallowing due to pharyngeal edema/ulceration; heartburn.
    d. Shortness of breath on exercise.
    e. Extremities: numb, tingling.
    f. Flatulence.
    g. Menorrhagia.

  2. *Objective data*
    a. *Vital signs:*
      (1) *BP—increased* systolic, widened pulse pressure.
      (2) *Pulse*—tachycardia.
      (3) *Respirations*—tachypnea.
      (4) *Temperature*—normal or subnormal.
    b. Skin/mucous membranes: pale, dry; tongue—smooth, shiny, bright red; cheilosis (cracked, painful corners of mouth).
    c. Sclera: pearly white.
    d. Nails: brittle, spoon shaped, flattened.
     e. Lab data: *decreased*—hemoglobin (<10 g/dL blood), serum iron (<65 μg/dL blood); *increased* total iron-binding capacity.
◆ **D. Analysis/nursing diagnosis:**
  1. *Altered nutrition, less than body requirements,* related to inadequate iron absorption.
  2. *Altered tissue perfusion* related to reduction in red cells.
  3. *Risk for activity intolerance* related to profound weakness.
  4. *Impaired gas exchange* related to decreased oxygen-carrying capacity.
◆ **E. Nursing care plan/implementation:**
  1. Goal: *promote physical and mental equilibrium.*
    a. *Position:* optimal for respiratory excursion; deep breathing; turn frequently to prevent skin breakdown.
    b. Rest: balance with activity, as tolerated; assist with ambulation.
    c. Medication (*hematinics*):
      (1) Oral iron therapy (ferrous sulfate)—give *with* meals.
      (2) Intramuscular therapy (iron dextran)— use second needle for injection after withdrawal from ampule; use *Z-track method:* inject 0.5 mL of air before withdrawing needle, to prevent tissue necrosis; use 2- to 3-inch needle; rotate sites; do *not* rub site or allow wearing of constricting garments after injection.

Adult

d. Keep warm: no hot water bottles, heating pads, due to decreased sensitivity.

 e. *Diet: high* in protein, iron, vitamins (see **Unit 9**); assistance with feeding, if needed; nonirritating foods with mouth or tongue soreness.

2. Goal: *health teaching.*
   a. Dietary regimen.
   b. Iron therapy: explain purpose, dosage, side effects (black or green stools, constipation, diarrhea); take with meals.
   c. Activity: exercise to tolerance, with planned rest periods.

◆ **F. Evaluation/outcome criteria:**
   1. Hemoglobin and hematocrit level return to normal range.
   2. Tolerates activity without fatigue.
   3. Selects foods appropriate for dietary regimen.

II. Hemolytic anemia (normocytic normochromic anemia): premature destruction (hemolysis) of erythrocytes; occurs extravascularly (autoimmune) or intravascularly (dialysis, heart valves).

A. Risk factors—autoimmune hemolytic anemia:
   1. *Warm reacting* (idiopathic): women, lupus, rheumatoid arthritis, myeloma.
   2. *Cold reacting* (e.g., Raynaud's): older women, Epstein-Barr virus.
   3. *Drug induced:* methyldopa, penicillin, quinine.

◆ **B. Assessment:**
   1. *Subjective data*
      a. Fatigue; physical weakness.
      b. Dizziness.
      c. Shortness of breath.
      d. Diaphoresis on slight exertion.
   2. *Objective data*
      a. Skin: pallor, jaundice.
      b. Posture: drooping.
      c. Lab data:
         (1) *Decreased* hematocrit.
         (2) *Increased* reticulocyte count; bilirubin.
         (3) Direct Coombs' test *positive.*

◆ **C.** See section on **iron deficiency anemia** for analysis, nursing care plan/implementation, and evaluation/outcome criteria.

III. Pernicious anemia (megaloblastic macrocytic anemia) lack of intrinsic factor found in gastric mucosa, which is necessary for vitamin B₁₂ (extrinsic factor) absorption; slow developing, usually after age 50; may be an autoimmune disorder.

A. Pathophysiology: atrophy or surgical removal of glandular mucosa in fundus of stomach → degenerative changes in brain, spinal cord, and peripheral nerves from lack of vitamin B₁₂.

B. Risk factors:
   1. Partial or complete gastric resection.
   2. Prolonged iron deficiency; veganism.
   3. Heredity.

◆ **C. Assessment:**

1. *Subjective data*
   a. Hands, feet: tingling, numbness.
   b. Weakness, fatigue.
   c. Sore tongue, anorexia.
   d. Difficulties with memory, balance.
   e. Irritability, mild depression.
   f. Shortness of breath.
   g. Palpitations.

2. *Objective data*
   a. Skin: pale, flabby, jaundiced.
   b. Sclera: icterus (yellow).
   c. Tongue: smooth, glossy, red, swollen.
   d. *Vital signs:*
      (1) *BP*—normal or elevated.
      (2) *Pulse*—tachycardia.
   e. Nervous system:
      (1) Decreased vibratory sense in lower extremities.
      (2) Loss of coordination.
      (3) *Babinski* present (flaring of toes with stimulation of sole of foot).
      (4) Positive *Romberg* (loses balance when eyes closed).
      (5) Increased or diminished reflexes.
   f. Lab data: *decreased*—hemoglobin, RBCs, platelets, gastric secretions (achlorhydria); *Schilling test* (radioactive vitamin B₁₂ urine test).

◆ **D. Analysis/nursing diagnosis:**
   1. *Altered nutrition, less than body requirements,* related to B₁₂ deficiency.
   2. *Impaired physical mobility* related to numbness of extremities.
   3. *Fatigue* related to decreased oxygen-carrying capacity.
   4. *Altered oral mucous membrane* related to changes in gastric mucosa.
   5. *Altered thought processes* related to progressive neurological degeneration.

◆ **E. Nursing care plan/implementation:**
   1. *Goal: promote physical and emotional comfort.*
      a. Activity: bedrest or activity as tolerated—restrictions depend on neurological or cardiac involvement.
      b. Comfort: keep extremities warm—light blankets, loose-fitting socks.
      c. Medication: vitamin B₁₂ therapy as ordered.
      d. *Diet:*
         (1) Six small feedings.
         (2) *Soft* or *pureed.*
         (3) Organ meats, fish, eggs.
      e. Mouth care: before and after meals, to increase appetite and relieve mouth discomfort.
   2. Goal: *health teaching.*
      a. Medication:
         (1) Lifelong therapy.
         (2) Injection techniques; rotation of sites.
      b. Diet.
      c. Rest; exercise to tolerance.

◆ F. **Evaluation/outcome criteria:**
  1. No irreversible neurological or cardiac complications.
  2. Takes vitamin B$_{12}$ for the rest of life—uses safe injection technique.
  3. Returns for follow-up care.

IV. **Polycythemia vera:** abnormal increase in circulating red blood cells (myeloproliferative disorder); considered to be a form of malignancy; occurs more frequently among middle-aged Jewish men.
  A. **Pathophysiology:** unknown causes→massive increases of erythrocytes, myelocytes (bone marrow leukocytes), and thrombocytes→increased blood viscosity/volume and tissue/organ congestion; increased peripheral vascular resistance; intravascular thrombosis usually develops in middle age, particularly in Jewish men; in contrast, *secondary* polycythemia occurs as a compensatory response to tissue hypoxia associated with prolonged exposure to high altitude, chronic lung disease, and heart disease.
  ◆ B. **Assessment:**
    1. *Subjective data*
      a. Headache; dizziness; ringing in ears.
      b. Weakness; loss of interest.
      c. Feelings of abdominal fullness.
      d. Shortness of breath; orthopnea.
      e. Pruritus, especially after bathing.
      f. Pain: gouty-arthritic.
    2. *Objective data*
      a. Skin: mucosal erythema, ruddy complexion (reddish purple).
      b. Ecchymosis; gingival (gum) bleeding.
      c. Enlarged liver, spleen.
      d. Hypertension.
      e. Lab data:
        (1) *Increased*—hemoglobin, hematocrit, RBCs, leukocytes, platelets, uric acid.
        (2) *Decreased* bone marrow iron.
  ◆ C. **Analysis/nursing diagnosis:**
    1. *Altered tissue perfusion* related to capillary congestion.
    2. *Risk for injury* related to dizziness, weakness.
    3. *Fluid volume excess* related to mass production of red blood cells.
    4. *Risk for impaired skin integrity* related to pruritus.
    5. *Ineffective breathing pattern* related to shortness of breath, orthopnea.
  ◆ D. **Nursing care plan/implementation:**
    1. Goal: *promote comfort and prevent complications.*
      a. Observe for signs of bleeding, thrombosis—stools, urine, gums, skin, ecchymosis.
      b. Reduce occurrence: *avoid* prolonged sitting, knee gatch.
      c. Assist with ambulation.
      d. *Position: elevate* head of bed.
      e. Skin care: cool-water baths to decrease pruritus; may add bicarbonate of soda to water.

      f. Fluids: *force,* to reduce blood viscosity and promote urine excretion;

1500–2500 mL/24 hr

     g. *Diet: avoid* foods high in iron, to reduce RBC production.
      h. Assist with venesection (phlebotomy), as ordered; 350–500 mL blood every other day until Hct low-normal.
    2. Goal: *health teaching.*
    a. *Diet:* foods to *avoid* (e.g., liver, egg yolks); fluids to be increased.
      b. Signs/symptoms of complications: infections, hemorrhage.
      c. *Avoid:* falls, bumps; hot baths/showers (worsens pruritus).
      d. Drugs: *myelosuppressive* agents (busulfan [Myleran], cyclophosphamide [Cytoxan], chlorambucil, radioactive phosphorus); purpose; side effects.
      e. Procedures: venesection (phlebotomy) if ordered.
  ◆ E. **Evaluation/outcome criteria:**
    1. Acceptance of chronic disease.
    2. Reports at prescribed intervals for follow-up.

    3. Remission: reduction of bone marrow activity, blood volume and viscosity (RBC <6,500,000/μL; Hgb <18 g/dL; Hct <45%; WBC <10,000/μL).

    4. No complications (e.g., thrombi, hemorrhage, gout, CHF, leukemia).

V. **Leukemia (acute and chronic):** a neoplastic disease involving the leukopoietic tissue in either the bone marrow or lymphoid areas; acute leukemia occurs in children, young adults; chronic forms occur in later adult life.
  A. **Types:**
    1. *Acute nonlymphocytic (ANLL)*—also known as acute myelogenous leukemia (AML); seen generally in older age (>60 yr).
    2. *Acute lymphoblastic (ALL)*—common in children 2 to 10 yr.
    3. *Chronic lymphocytic (CLL)*—generally affects the elderly.
    4. *Chronic myelogenous (CML)*—also known as chronic granulocytie leukemia (CGL); more likely to occur between 25 and 60 yr.
  B. **Pathophysiology:** displacement of normal marrow cells by proliferating leukemic cells (abnormal, immature leukocytes)→normochromic anemia, thrombocytopenia.
  C. **Risk factors:**
    1. Viruses.
    2. Genetic abnormalities.
    3. Exposure to chemicals.
    4. Radiation.
    5. Treatment for other types of cancer (e.g., alkylating agents).

Adult

◆ **D. Assessment:**
1. *Subjective data*
   a. Fatigue, weakness.
   b. Anorexia, nausea.
   c. *Pain:* joints, bones (acute leukemia).
   d. Night sweats, weight loss, malaise.
2. *Objective data*
   a. Skin: pallor due to anemia; jaundice.
   b. Fever: frequent infections; mouth ulcers.
   c. Bleeding: petechiae, purpura, ecchymosis, epistaxis, gingiva.
   d. Organ enlargement: spleen, liver.
   e. Enlarged lymph nodes; tenderness.
   f. Bone marrow aspiration: increased presence of blasts.
    g. Lab data:
      (1) WBC—abnormally low (<1000/mm³) or extremely high (>200,000/mm³); differential is important.
      (2) RBC—normal to severely *decreased.*
      (3) Hgb—low or normal.
      (4) Platelets—usually low.

◆ **E. Analysis/nursing diagnosis:**
1. *Risk for infection* related to immature or abnormal leukocytes.
2. *Activity intolerance* related to hypoxia and weakness.
3. *Fatigue* related to anemia.
4. *Altered tissue perfusion* related to anemia.
5. *Anxiety* related to diagnosis and treatment.
6. *Altered oral mucous membrane* related to susceptibility to infection.
7. *Fear* related to diagnosis.
8. *Ineffective individual or family coping* related to potentially fatal disease.

◆ **F. Nursing care plan/implementation:**
1. Goal: *prevent, control, and treat infection.*
   a. *Protective isolation* if indicated.
   b. Observe for early signs of infection:
      (1) Inflammation at injection sites.
      (2) Vital sign changes.
      (3) Cough.
      (4) Obtain cultures.
   c. Give *antibiotics* as ordered.
   d. Mouth care: clean q2h, examine for new lesions, *avoid* trauma.
2. Goal: *assess and control bleeding, anemia.*
   a. Activity: *restrict,* to prevent trauma.
   b. Observe for hemorrhage: vital signs; body orifices, stool, urine.
   c. Control localized bleeding: ice, pressure at least 3 to 4 min after needle sticks, positioning.
   d. Use soft-bristle or foam-rubber toothbrush to prevent gingival bleeding.
   e. Give blood/blood components as ordered; observe for transfusion reactions.
3. Goal: *provide rest, comfort, nutrition.*
   a. Activity: 8 hr sleep or rest; daily nap.

b. Comfort measures: flotation mattress, bed cradle, sheepskin.
   c. *Analgesics:* without delay.
      (1) Mild pain (acetaminophen [Tylenol], propoxyphene HCl [Darvon] without aspirin).
      (2) Severe pain (codeine, meperidine HCl [Demerol]).
   d. *Diet:* bland.
      (1) *High* in protein, minerals, vitamins.
      (2) *Low* roughage.
      (3) Small, frequent feedings.
      (4) Favorite foods.
   e. Fluids: 3000–4000 mL/day.
4. Goal: *reduce side effects from therapeutic regimen.*
   a. Nausea: *antiemetics,* usually half-hour *before* chemotherapy.
   b. *Increased* uric acid level: force fluids.
   c. Stomatitis: *antiseptic anesthetic* mouthwashes.
   d. Rectal irritation: meticulous toileting, sitz baths, topical relief (e.g., Tucks).
5. Goal: *provide emotional/spiritual support.*
   a. Contact clergy if client desires.
   b. Allow, encourage client-initiated discussion of death (developmentally appropriate).
   c. Allow family to be involved in care.
   d. If death occurs, provide privacy for family, listening, sharing of grief.
6. Goal: *health teaching.*
   a. Prevent infection.
   b. Limit activity.
   c. Control bleeding.
   d. Reduce nausea.
   e. Mouth care.
   f. Chemotherapy: regimen; side effects.

◆ **G. Evaluation/outcome criteria:**
1. Alleviate symptoms; obtain remission.
2. Prevent complications (e.g., infection).
3. Ventilates emotions—accepts and deals with anger.
4. Experiences peaceful death (e.g., pain free).

VI. Idiopathic thrombocytopenic purpura (ITP): potentially fatal disorder characterized by spontaneous increase in platelet destruction; possible autoimmune response; seen predominantly in 2- to 4-year-olds and girls/women ≥ 10 years old. Remissions occur spontaneously or following splenectomy; in contrast, *secondary thrombocytopenia* (STP) is caused by viral infections, drug hypersensitivity (i.e., *quinidine, sulfonamides*), lupus, or bone marrow failure; treat cause.

◆ **A. Assessment:**
1. *Subjective data*
   a. Spontaneous skin hemorrhages—lower extremities.
   b. Menorrhagia.
   c. Epistaxis.
2. *Objective data*
   a. Bleeding: GI, urinary, nasal; following minor trauma, dental extractions.

b. Petechiae; ecchymosis.

c. *Tourniquet test*—positive, demonstrating increased capillary fragility.

d. Lab data:
   (1) *Decreased* platelets (<100,000/μL).
   (2) *Increased* bleeding time.

◆ **B. Analysis/nursing diagnosis:**
1. *Risk for injury* related to hemorrhage.
2. *Altered tissue perfusion* related to fragile capillaries.
3. *Impaired skin integrity* related to skin hemorrhages.

◆ **C. Nursing care plan/implementation:**
1. Goal: *prevent complications from bleeding tendencies.*
   a. *Precautions:*
   ▶ (1) Injections—use small-bore needles; rotate sites; apply direct pressure.
   (2) *Avoid* bumping, trauma.
   (3) Use swabs for mouth care.
   b. Observe for signs of bleeding, petechiae following blood pressure reading, ecchymosis, purpura.
   c. Administer *steroids* (e.g., prednisone) with ITP to increase platelet count; give platelets for count below 20,000–30,000/μL with STP; high-dose *immunoglobulins.*
2. Goal: *health teaching.*
   a. *Avoid* traumatic activities:
   (1) Contact sports.
   (2) Violent sneezing, coughing, nose blowing.
   (3) Straining at stool.
   (4) Heavy lifting.
   b. *Signs of decreased platelets*—petechiae, ecchymosis, gingival bleeding, hematuria, menorrhagia.
   c. Use MedicAlert tag/card.
   d. *Precautions:* self-medication; particularly *avoid* aspirin-containing drugs.
   e. Prepare for splenectomy if drug therapy unsuccessful (prednisone, cyclophosphamide, azathioprine [Imuran]).

◆ **D. Evaluation/outcome criteria:**
1. Returns for follow-up.
2. No complications (e.g., intracranial hemorrhage).
3. Platelet count >200,000/μL.
4. Skin remains intact.
5. Resumes self-care activities.

VII. Splenectomy: removal of spleen following rupture due to acquired hemolytic anemia, trauma, tumor, or idiopathic thrombocytopenic purpura.

◆ **A. Analysis/nursing diagnosis:**
1. *Risk for fluid volume deficit* related to hemorrhage.
2. *Risk for infection* related to impaired immune response.
3. *Pain* related to abdominal distention.
4. *Ineffective breathing pattern* related to high abdominal incision.

◆ **B. Nursing care plan/implementation:**
1. Goal: *prepare for surgery.*
   a. Give whole blood, as ordered.
   b. Insert nasogastric tube to decrease postoperative abdominal distention, as ordered.
2. Goal: *prevent postoperative complications.*
   a. Observe for:
   (1) *Hemorrhage*—bleeding tendency with thrombocytopenia due to decreased platelet count.
   (2) *Gastrointestinal distention*—removal of enlarged spleen may result in distended stomach and intestines, to fill void.
   b. Recognize 101°F temp as normal for 10 days.
   c. Incision: splint when coughing, to prevent high incidence of atelectasis (common complication), pneumonia with upper-abdominal incision.
3. Goal: *health teaching.*
   a. Increased risk of infection postsplenectomy.
   b. Report signs of infection immediately.

◆ **C. Evaluation/outcome criteria:**
1. No complications (e.g., respiratory, subphrenic abscess or hematoma, thromboemboli, infection).
2. Complete and permanent remission—occurs in 60%–80% of clients.

Fluid and Electrolyte Imbalances

Imbalances in fluid and electrolytes may be due to changes in the total quantity of either substance (deficit or excess), protein deficiencies, or extracellular fluid volume shifts. Clients who are older and very young are particularly susceptible.

I. Fluid volume deficit (dehydration): mechanism that influences fluid balance and sodium levels; decreased quantities of fluid and electrolytes may be caused by *deficient intake* (poor dietary habits, anorexia, and nausea), *excessive output* (vomiting, nasogastric suction, and prolonged diarrhea), or *failure of regulatory mechanism* that influences fluid balance and sodium levels.

A. Pathophysiology: water moves out of the cells to replace a significant water loss; cells eventually become unable to compensate for the lost fluid, and cellular dehydration begins, leading to circulatory collapse.

B. Risk factors:
1. No fluids available.
2. Available fluids not drinkable.
3. Inability to take fluids independently.
4. No response to thirst; does not recognize the need for fluids.
5. Inability to communicate need; does not speak same language.
6. Aphasia.
7. Weakness, comatose.
8. Inability to swallow.
9. Psychological alterations.
10. Overuse of diuretics.

11. Increased vomiting.
12. Fever.
13. Wounds, burns.
14. Blood loss.
15. Endocrine abnormalities

◆ **C. Assessment:**
1. *Subjective data*
   a. Thirst.
   b. Behavioral changes: apprehension, apathy, lethargy, confusion, restlessness.
   c. Dizziness.
   d. Numbness and tingling of hands and feet.
   e. Anorexia and nausea.
   f. Abdominal cramps.
2. *Objective data*
   a. Sudden weight loss of 5%.
   b. *Vital signs:*
      (1) *Decreased* BP; postural changes.
      (2) *Increased* temperature.
      (3) Irregular, weak, rapid pulse.
      (4) *Increased* rate and depth of respirations.
   c. Skin: cool and pale in absence of infection; decreased turgor.
   d. Urine: oliguria to anuria, high specific gravity.
   e. Eyes: soft, sunken.
   f. Tongue: furrows.
   g. Lab data:
      (1) Blood—*increased* hematocrit and BUN.
      (2) Urine—*decreased* 17-ketosteroids.

◆ **D. Analysis/nursing diagnosis:**
1. *Fluid volume deficit* related to inadequate fluid intake.

◆ **E. Nursing care plan/implementation:**
1. Goal: *restore fluid and electrolyte balance—increase* fluid intake to hydrate client.
   a. IVs and blood products as ordered; small, frequent drinks by mouth.
   b. Daily weights (same time of day) to monitor progress of fluid replacement.
   c. I&O, hourly outputs (when in acute state).
   d. *Avoid* hypertonic solutions (may cause fluid shift when compensatory mechanisms begin to function).
2. Goal: *promote comfort.*
   a. Frequent skin care (lack of hydration causes dry skin, which may increase risk for skin breakdown).
   b. *Position:* change every hour to relieve pressure.
   c. Medications as ordered: *antiemetics, antidiarrheal.*
3. Goal: *prevent physical injury.*
   a. Frequent mouth care (mucous membrane dries due to dehydration; therefore, client is at risk for breaks in mucous membrane, halitosis).
   b. Monitor IV flow rate—observe for circulatory overload, pulmonary edema related to potential fluid shift when compensatory mechanisms begin or client is unable to tolerate rate of fluid replacement.

c. Monitor vitals, including level of consciousness (*decreasing* BP and level of consciousness indicate continuation of fluid loss).
d. Prepare for surgery if hemorrhage present (internal bleeding can only be relieved by surgical intervention).

◆ **F. Evaluation/outcome criteria:**
1. Mentally alert.
2. Moist, intact mucous membranes.
3. Urinary output approximately equal to intake.
4. No further weight loss.
5. Gradual weight gain.

II. **Fluid volume excess** (fluid overload): most common cause is an increase in sodium; excessive quantities of fluid and electrolytes may be due to *increased ingestion,* tube feedings, intravenous infusions, multiple tap-water enemas, or a *failure of regulatory systems,* resulting in inability to excrete excesses.

A. Pathophysiology: hypo-osmolar water excess in extracellular compartment leads to intracellular water excess because the concentration of solutes in the intracellular fluid is greater than that in the extracellular fluid. Water moves to equalize concentration, causing swelling of the cells. The most common cause is an increase in sodium.

B. Risk factors:
1. Excessive intake of electrolyte-free fluids.
2. Increased secretion of ADH in response to stress, drugs, anesthetics (**Table 7.11**).
3. Decreased or inadequate output of urine.
4. Psychogenic polydipsia.
5. Certain medical conditions: tuberculosis; encephalitis; meningitis; endocrine disturbances; tumors of lung, pancreas, duodenum, heart failure.
6. Inadequate kidney function or kidney failure.

◆ **C. Assessment:**
1. *Subjective data*
   a. Behavioral changes: irritability, apathy, confusion, disorientation.
   b. Headache.
   c. Anorexia, nausea, cramping.
   d. Fatigue.
   e. Dyspnea.
2. *Objective data*
   a. Vital signs: *elevated* blood pressure.
   b. Skin: warm, moist; edema—eyelids, facial, dependent, pitting.
   c. Sudden weight gain of 5 lb.
   d. Pink, frothy sputum; productive.
   e. Constant, irritating cough.
   f. Crackles in lungs.
   g. Pulse, bounding.
   h. Engorgement of neck veins in sitting position.
   i. Urine: polyuria, nocturia.
   j. Lab data:
      (1) Blood—*decreasing* hematocrit, BUN.
      (2) Urine—*decreasing* specific gravity.

TABLE 7.11	Diabetes Insipidus (DI) Versus Syndrome of Inappropriate Antidiuretic Hormone (SIADH)	
	DI (fluid deficit)	**SIADH (fluid excess)**
Pathophysiology:	▪ Deficiency of ADH → inability to conserve H_2O ▪ Large volumes of hypotonic fluid excreted	▪ Excessive ADH secreted → water retention, hyponatremia, and hypo-osmolality
Risk factors:	▪ Head injury ▪ Brain infection ▪ Posterior pituitary tumors ▪ Drugs that inhibit vasopressin (e.g., glucocorticoids, phenytoin, lithium)	▪ Vasopressin overuse (Rx of DI) or stimulation (chemotherapy) ▪ Small cell carcinoma ▪ Adrenal insufficiency ▪ Myxedema ▪ Anterior pituitary insufficiency
◆ **Assessment:**	▪ Polyuria (up to 18L/day) ▪ Urine specific gravity ↓ ▪ Signs of fluid volume deficit: dry, cool skin; polydipsia; ↓ weight Lab: serum Na^+ ↑ initially, then ↓; serum osmolality ↑ initially, then ↓	▪ Signs of ↓ Na^+—fatigue, headache, ↓ DTR, nausea, anorexia, ↓ mental status ▪ Signs of fluid volume excess: weight gain without edema; tachycardia; tachypnea; crackles
◆ **Nursing care plan/implementation:**	▪ Fluids: IV; I/O ▪ Meds: ADH replacement; Pitressin ▪ Education: prepare for hypophysectomy	▪ Fluids: hypertonic IV (↑ Na^+); I/O ▪ Meds: diuretics; demeclocycline (tetracycline) ▪ Daily weight

◆ **D. Analysis/nursing diagnosis:**
  1. *Fluid volume excess* related to excessive fluid intake or decreased fluid output.
◆ **E. Nursing care plan/implementation:**
  1. Goal: *maintain oxygen to all cells.*
    a. *Position:* semi-Fowler's or Fowler's to facilitate improved gas exchange.
    b. Vital signs: PRN, minimum q4hr.
    c. Fluid restriction.
  2. Goal: *promote excretion of excess fluid.*
    a. Medications as ordered: *diuretics.*
    b. Monitor electrolytes, especially Mg^{++}, K^+
    c. If in kidney failure: may need dialysis; explain procedure.
    d. Assist client during paracentesis, thoracentesis, phlebotomy.
      (1) Monitor vital signs to detect shock.
      (2) Prevent injury by monitoring sterile technique.
      (3) Prevent falling by stabilizing appropriate position during procedure.
      (4) Support client psychologically.
  3. Goal: *obtain/maintain fluid balance.*
    a. Daily weights; 1 kg = 1000 mL fluid.
    b. Measure: all edematous parts, abdominal girth, I&O.
    c. *Limit:* fluids by mouth, IVs, sodium.
    d. Strict monitoring of IV fluids.
  4. Goal: *prevent tissue injury.*
    a. Skin and mouth care as needed.
    b. Evaluate feet for edema and discoloration when client is out of bed.
    c. Observe suture line on surgical clients (potential for evisceration due to excess fluid retention).
    d. IV route preferred for parenteral medications;

Z track if medications are to be given IM (otherwise injected liquid will escape through injection site).
  5. Goal: *health teaching.*
    a. Improve nutritional status with *low sodium* diet.
    b. Identify cause that put client at risk for imbalance, methods to avoid this situation in the future.
    c. Desired and side effects of diuretics and other prescribed medications.
    d. Monitor urinary output, ankle edema; report to health care manager when fluid retention is noticed.
    e. Limit fluid intake when kidney/cardiac function impaired.
◆ **F. Evaluation/outcome criteria:**
  1. Fluid balance obtained.
  2. No respiratory, cardiac complications.
  3. Vital signs within normal limits.
  4. Urinary output improved, no evidence of edema.

III. Common electrolyte imbalances: electrolytes are taken into the body in foods and fluids; normally lost through sweat and urine. May also be lost through hemorrhage, vomiting, and diarrhea. Electrolytes have major influences on: body water regulation and osmolality, acid-base regulation, enzyme reactions, and neuromuscular activity. Clinically important electrolytes are:
A. Sodium (Na^+): normal 135–145 mEq/L. Most prevalent cation in extracellular fluid. Controls osmotic pressure; essential for neuromuscular functioning and intracellular chemical reactions. Aids in maintenance of acid-base balance. Necessary for glucose to be transported into cells.

Adult

1. *Hyponatremia*—sodium deficit, resulting from either a sodium loss or water excess. Serum-sodium level below 135 mEq/L; symptoms usually do not occur until below 120 mEq/L unless rapid drop.
2. *Hypernatremia*—excess sodium in the blood, resulting from either high sodium intake, water loss, or low water intake. Serum-sodium level above 145 mEq/L.

B. **Potassium** (K⁺): normal 3.5–5.0 mEq/L. Direct effect on excitability of nerves and muscles. Contributes to intracellular osmotic pressure and influences acid-base balance. Major cation of the cell. Required for storage of nitrogen as muscle protein.
   1. *Hypokalemia*—potassium deficit related to dehydration, starvation, vomiting, diarrhea, diuretics. Serum-potassium level below 3.5 mEq/L; symptoms may not occur until below 2.5 mEq/L.
   2. *Hyperkalemia*—potassium excess related to severe tissue damage, renal disease, excess administration of oral or IV potassium. Serum-potassium level above 5 mEq/L; symptoms usually occur when above 6.5 mEq/L.

C. **Calcium** (Ca⁺⁺): normal 4.5–5.5 mEq/L. Essential to muscle metabolism, cardiac function, and bone health. Controlled by parathyroid hormone; reciprocal relationship between calcium and phosphorus.
   1. *Hypocalcemia*—loss of calcium related to inadequate intake, vitamin D deficiency, hypoparathyroidism, damage to the parathyroid gland, decreased absorption in the GI tract, excess loss through kidneys. Serum-calcium level below 4.5 mEq/L.
   2. *Hypercalcemia*—calcium excess related to hyperparathyroidism, immobility, bone tumors, renal failure, excess intake of Ca⁺⁺ or vitamin D. Serum-calcium level above 5.5 mEq/L.

D. **Magnesium** (Mg⁺⁺): normal 1.5–2.5 mEq/L. Essential to cellular metabolism of carbohydrates and proteins.
   1. *Hypomagnesemia*—magnesium deficit related to impaired absorption from GI tract, excessive loss through kidneys, and prolonged periods of poor nutritional intake. Hypomagnesemia leads to neuromuscular irritability. Serum-magnesium level below 1.5 mEq/L.
   2. *Hypermagnesemia*—magnesium excess related to renal insufficiency, overdose during replacement therapy, severe dehydration, repeated enemas with Mg⁺⁺ sulfate (epsom salts). Serum-magnesium level above 2.5 mEq/L.

◆ E. **Table 7.12** provides assessment, analysis, nursing diagnosis, nursing care plan/implementation, and evaluation/outcome criteria of the various electrolyte imbalances.

IV. **Acid-base balance:** concentration of hydrogen ions in extracellular fluid is determined by the ratio of bicarbonate to carbonic acid. The normal ratio is 20:1. Even when arterial blood gases are abnormal, if the ratio remains at 20:1, no imbalance will occur. **Table 7.13** shows blood gas variations with acid-base imbalances.

A. **Causes of blood gas abnormalities:** (Table 7.14).
B. **Types of acid-base imbalance:**
   1. *Acidosis:* hydrogen ion concentration *increases* and pH *decreases.*
   2. *Alkalosis:* hydrogen ion concentration *decreases* and pH *increases.*
   3. *Metabolic imbalances:* bicarbonate is the problem. In primary conditions, the level of bicarbonate is directly *proportional* to pH.
      a. *Metabolic acidosis:* excessive acid is produced or added to the body, bicarbonate is lost, or acid is retained due to poorly functioning kidneys. *Deficit* of bicarbonate.
      b. *Metabolic alkalosis:* excessive acid is lost or bicarbonate or alkali is retained. *Excess* of bicarbonate.
      c. As compensatory mechanism, P_{CO_2} will be *low in metabolic acidosis,* as the body attempts to eliminate excess carbonic acid and elevate pH. P_{CO_2} will become *elevated in metabolic alkalosis.*
   4. *Respiratory imbalances:* carbonic acid is the problem. In primary conditions, P_{CO_2} is inversely proportional to the pH.
      a. *Respiratory acidosis:* pulmonary ventilation decreases, causing an elevation in the level of carbon dioxide or carbonic acid. *Excess* of P_{CO_2}.
      b. *Respiratory alkalosis:* pulmonary ventilation increases, causing a decrease in the level of carbon dioxide or carbonic acid. *Deficit* of P_{CO_2}.
      c. As a compensatory mechanism, the level of bicarbonate will *increase in respiratory acidosis* and *decrease in respiratory alkalosis.*

◆ C. **Assessment:** (Table 7.15).
◆ D. **Analysis/nursing diagnosis:**
   1. *Impaired gas exchange* related to hyperventilation.
   2. *Ineffective breathing pattern* related to decreased thoracic movements.
   3. *Ineffective airway clearance* related to retained secretions.
   4. *Risk for injury* related to poorly functioning kidneys.
   5. *Altered renal tissue perfusion* related to dehydration.
   6. *Altered urinary elimination* related to renal failure.
   7. *Fluid volume excess* related to altered kidney function.
   8. *Fluid volume deficit* related to diarrhea or dehydration.
   9. *Knowledge deficit* (learning need) related to self-administration of antacid medications.

◆ E. **Nursing care plan/implementation** (see **Table 7.15**).
◆ F. **Evaluation/outcome criteria** (see **Table 7.15**).

TABLE 7.12	Electrolyte Imbalances			

◆ **Assessment**

Disorder and Related Condition	Subjective Data	Objective Data	◆ Analysis/Nursing Diagnosis	◆ Nursing Care Plan/ Implementation	◆ Evaluation/ Outcome Criteria
Hyponatremia Addison's disease Starvation GI suction Thiazide diuretics Excess water intake,enemas Fever Fluid shifts Ascites Burns Small-bowel obstruction Profuse perspiration	Apathy, apprehension, mental confusion, delirium Fatigue Vertigo, headache Anorexia, nausea Abdominal and muscle cramps	*Pulse:* rapid and weak *BP:* postural hypotension Shock, coma *GI:* weight loss, diarrhea, loss through NG tubes Muscle weakness	*Diarrhea* *Fluid volume excess* *Altered nutrition, less than body requirements* *Sensory-perceptual alteration (kinesthetic)*	*Obtain normal sodium level:* identify cause of deficit, *increase sodium intake* PO (salty foods), IVs–hypertonic solutions *Prevent further sodium loss:* irrigate NG tubes with saline; hourly I&O to monitor kidney output *Prevent injury* related to shock, dizziness, decreased sensorium; dangle before ambulation Skin care	Na⁺ 135–145 mEq/L No complications of shock present Return of muscle strength Alert, oriented Limits intake of plain water
Hypernatremia High sodium intake Low water intake Diarrhea High fever with rapid respirations Impaired renal functions Acute tracheo-bronchitis	Lethargy Restlessness, agitation Confusion	*BP and temperature:* elevated *Neuromuscular:* diminished reflexes *Skin:* flushed; firm turgor *GI:* mucous membrane dry, sticky *GU:* decreased output	*Fluid volume deficit* *Fluid volume excess* *Altered nutrition, less than body requirements* *Sensory-perceptual alteration (kinesthetic)*	*Obtain normal sodium level: decrease sodium intake* I&O to recognize signs and symptoms of complications (e.g., heart failure, pulmonary edema)	Na⁺ 135–145 mEq/L No complaint of thirst Alert, oriented Relaxed in appearance Identifies high sodium foods to avoid
Hypokalemia *Decreased intake:* Poor potassium food intake Excessive dieting Nausea Alcoholism IV fluids without added potassium *Increased loss:* GI suctioning, vomiting, diarrhea Ulcerative colitis Drainage: ostomy; fistulas Medications: potassium-losing diuretics, digoxin, cathartics Increased aldosterone production Renal disorders	Apathy, lethargy, fatigue, weakness Irritability, mental confusion Anorexia, nausea Leg cramps	*Muscles:* weakness, paralysis, paresthesia, hyporeflexia *Respirations:* shallow to respiratory arrest *Cardiac:* decreased BP; elevated, weak, irregular pulse; arrhythmias *ECG:* low, flat T waves; prolonged ST segment; elevated U wave; potential arrest *GI:* vomiting, flatulence, constipation; decreased motility → distention → paralytic ileus *GU:* urine not concentrated; polyuria, nocturia; kidney damage *Speech:* slow	*Decreased cardiac output* *Fatigue* *Altered cardiopulmonary tissue perfusion* *Ineffective breathing patterns* *Constipation* *Bathing/hygiene self-care deficit* *Impaired home maintenance management* *Sensory-perceptual alteration (gustatory)*	*Replace lost potassium:* increase *potassium in diet* (see **Unit 9**); liquid PO potassium medications—dilute in juice to aid taste; give potassium only if kidneys functioning *Prevent injury to tissues:* prevent infiltration, pain, tissue damage *Prevent potassium loss:* Irrigate NG tubes with saline, not water	K⁺ 3.5–5.0 mEq/L Identifies cause of imbalance Lists foods to include in diet Lists signs and symptoms of imbalance Return of muscle strength No cardiac arrhythmias

(Continued on following page)

Adult

TABLE 7.12 Electrolyte Imbalances (Continued)

◆ Assessment

Disorder and Related Condition	Subjective Data	Objective Data	Analysis/Nursing Diagnosis	Nursing Care Plan/ Implementation	Evaluation/ Outcome Criteria
Hyperkalemia Burns Crushing injuries Kidney disease Excessive infusion or ingestion of K+ Adrenal insufficiency Mercurial poisoning	Irritability Weakness, muscle cramps Nausea, intestinal cramps	*Muscles:* paresthesia, flaccid muscle paralysis (later) *Cardiac:* irregular pulse; arrhythmias; bradycardia → asystole *ECG:* high T waves; depressed ST segment; widened QRS complex; diminished or absent P waves; ventricular fibrillation *GI:* explosive diarrhea; hyperactive bowel sounds *Kidney:* scanty to no urine	*Decreased cardiac output* *Altered urinary elimination* *Activity intolerance* *Ineffective breathing patterns* *Diarrhea* *Impaired home maintenance management*	*Decrease amount of potassium in body;* identify and treat cause of imbalance; *give foods low in K+; avoid* drugs or IV fluids containing K+ If kidney failure present, may need to prepare for dialysis	K+ 3.5–5.0 mEq/L No complications (e.g., arrhythmias, acidosis, respiratory failure)
Hypocalcemia Acute pancreatitis Diarrhea Peritonitis Damage to parathyroid during thyroidectomy Hypothyroidism Burns Pregnancy and lactation Low vitamin D intake Multiple blood transfusions Renal disorders Massive infection	Fatigue Tingling/numbness; fingers and circumoral Abdominal cramps Palpitations Dyspnea	*Muscle spasms:* tonic muscles, carpopedal, laryngeal *Neuromuscular:* grimacing, hyperirritable facial nerves Tetany → convulsions *Orthopedic:* osteoporosis → fractures *Cardiac:* arrhythmias → arrest *GI:* diarrhea	*Pain* *Diarrhea* *Altered nutrition, less than body requirements* *Risk for injury* *Sensory-perceptual alteration (gustatory)*	*Prevent tetany* (**medical emergency**): calcium gluconate IV, 2.5–5.0 mL 10% solution; repeated q10min to maximum dose of 30 mL *Prevent tissue injury* due to hypoxia and sloughing; administer slowly; *avoid infiltration* *Prevent injury related to medication administration. Caution:* drug interaction with carbonate, phosphate, digitalis; *avoid hypercalcemia* *In less acute condition:* increase calcium intake—calcium gluconate or lactate	Ca++ 4.5–5.5 mEq/L No signs of tetany Absent *Trousseau's* and *Chvostek's* signs Lists foods high in vitamin D and calcium
Hypercalcemia Parathyroid glands: overactive, tumor Increased immobility Decreased renal function Bone cancer Increased vitamin D and calcium intake *Milk-alkali syndrome*—self-administration of antacids; increased milk in diet to relieve GI symptoms	*Pain:* flank, deep bone, shin splints Muscle weakness, fatigue Anorexia, nausea Headache Thirst → polyuria	*Muscles:* relaxed *GU:* kidney stones *GI:* increased milk intake, constipation, dehydration *Neurological:* stupor → coma	*Decreased cardiac output* *Constipation* *Activity intolerance* *Altered urinary elimination* *Pain*	*Reduce calcium intake:* decrease foods high in calcium; identify cause of imbalance; give steroids, diuretics as ordered; isotonic saline IV *Prevent injury:* prevent pathological fractures (e.g., advanced cancer); prevent renal calculi by *increasing fluid intake*	Ca++ 4.5–5.5 mEq/L No pain reported No fractures/calculi seen on x-ray exam

(Continued on following page)

Hypomagnesemia Impaired GI absorption Prolonged malnutrition or starvation Alcoholism Excess loss of magnesium through kidneys, related to increased aldosterone production Prolonged diarrhea Draining GI fistulas	Agitation Depression Confusion Paresthesia	*Muscles:* irritable, tremors, spasticity, tetany → convulsions *Cardiac:* arrhythmias, tachycardia	*Risk for injury related to seizure activity* *Decreased cardiac output*	Provide safety: prevent injury to client who is disoriented; administer magnesium salts PO or IV *Health teaching:* prevention; diet—high magnesium foods: fruits, green vegetables, whole grain cereals, milk, meats, nuts	Mg^{++} 1.5–2.5 mEq/L
Hypermagnesemia Renal failure Diabetic ketoacidosis Severe dehydration Antacid therapy	Drowsiness, lethargy	*Neuromuscular:* loss of deep tendon reflexes *Respiratory:* depression *Cardiac:* arrest, hypotension	*Ineffective breathing pattern* *Decreased cardiac output* *Fluid volume deficit* *Fluid volume excess* *Altered cardiopulmonary tissue perfusion*	*Obtain normal magnesium level:* IV calcium, fluids; possible dialysis	Mg^{++} 1.5–2.5 mEq/L No complications (e.g., respiratory depression, arrhythmias) Identifies magnesium-based antacids (e.g., Gelusil) Deep-tendon reflexes 2+

TABLE 7.13	Blood Gas Variations with Acid-Base Imbalances

Blood Gas Feature	Normal Value	Value with:			
		Respiratory Acidosis	Respiratory Alkalosis	Metabolic Acidosis	Metabolic Alkalosis
HCO₃ (bicarbonate)	22–26 mm Hg	Normal or ↑	Normal or ↓	↓	↑
Pco₂ (Carbonic acid*)	35–45 mm Hg (1.05–1.35)	↑	↓	Normal or ↓	Normal or ↑
pH (hydrogen-ion concentration)	7.35–7.45	↓	↑	Normal or ↓ ↓	Normal or ↑ ↑

↑ = increased; ↓ = decreased.
*To obtain carbonic acid level, multiply Pco_2 value by 0.03.

TABLE 7.14	Blood Gas Abnormalities: Causes

Decreased Po₂   *Collapsed alveoli* (atelectasis)
  1. Airway obstruction
    a. By the tongue
    b. By a foreign body
  2. Failure to take deep breaths
    a. Pain (rib fracture, pleurisy)
    b. Paralysis of respiratory muscles (spinal cord injury, polio)
    c. Depression of the respiratory center (head injury, drug overdose)
  3. Collapse of the whole lung (pneumothorax)

  Fluid in the alveoli
  1. Pulmonary edema
  2. Pneumonia
  3. Near-drowning
  4. Chest trauma

  Other gases in the alveoli
  1. Smoke inhalation
  2. Inhalation of toxic chemicals
  3. Carbon monoxide poisoning

  Respiratory arrest

Elevated Pco₂   *Decreased CO₂ elimination* (hypoventilation)
  1. Decreased tidal volume
    a. Pain (rib fractures, pleurisy)
    b. Weakness (myasthenia gravis)
    c. Paralysis (spinal cord injury, polio)
  2. Decreased respiratory rate
    a. Head injury
    b. Depressant drugs
    c. Stroke
  Increased CO₂ production
  1. Fever
  2. Muscular exertion
  3. Anaerobic metabolism

TABLE 7.15	Acid-Base Imbalances			
Disorder and Related Conditions	◆ **Assessment**		◆ **Nursing Care Plan/ Implementation**	◆ **Evaluation/ Outcome Criteria**
	Subjective Data	**Objective Data**		
Respiratory Acidosis Acute bronchitis Emphysema Respiratory obstruction Atelectasis Damage to respiratory center Pneumonia Asthmatic attack Drug overdose	Headache Irritability Disorientation Weakness Dyspnea on exertion Nausea	Hypoventilation: ↓rate or rapid and shallow Cyanosis Tachycardia Diaphoresis Dehydration Coma (CO_2 narcosis) Hyperventilation to *compensate* if no pulmonary pathology present HCO_3, normal $Paco_2$, elevated pH <7.35	*Assist with normal breathing:* ▶ encourage coughing; suction airway; postural drainage; pursed-lip breathing; raise HOB *Protect from injury:* oxygen as needed; encourage fluids; *avoid* sedation; medications as ordered—*antibiotics, bronchial dilators* *Health teaching:* identify cause, prevent future episodes; increase awareness regarding risk factors and early signs of impending imbalance; encourage compliance	Normal acid-base balance obtained Respiratory rate: 16–20 No signs of pulmonary infection (e.g., sputum colorless, breath sounds clear) Demonstrates breathing exercises (e.g., diaphragmatic breathing)
Metabolic Acidosis Diabetic ketoacidosis Hyperthyroidism Severe infections Lactic acidosis in shock Renal failure → uremia Prolonged starvation diet; low protein diet Diarrhea, dehydration Hepatitis Burns	Headache Restlessness Apathy, weakness Disorientation Thirst Nausea, abdominal pain	*Kussmaul's* respirations: deep, rapid air hunger; ↑ Temperature Vomiting, diarrhea Dehydration Stupor → convulsions → coma HCO_3, below normal $Paco_2$ normal K^+ > 5 75 pH <7.35	*Restore normal metabolism:* correct underlying problem; sodium bicarbonate PO/IV; sodium lactate; fluid replacement, Ringer's solution; *diet:* high calorie *Prevent complications: regular* insulin for ketoacidosis; hourly outputs; prepare for dialysis if in kidney failure *Health teaching:* identify signs and symptoms of primary illness, prevent complications, cardiac arrest; diet instructions	Normal acid-base balance obtained No rebound respiratory alkalosis following therapy No tetany following return of normal pH Alert, oriented No signs of K^+ excess
Respiratory Alkalosis Hyperventilation—CO_2 loss Hypoxia, high altitudes Fever Metabolic acidosis Increased ICP, encephalitis Salicylate poisoning After intensive exercise	Circumoral paresthesia Weakness Apprehension	Increased respirations Increased neuromuscular irritability; hyperreflexia, muscle twitching, tetany, positive *Chvostek's* sign Convulsions Unconsciousness Hypokalemia HCO_3, normal $Paco_2$, decreased pH >7.45	*Increase carbon dioxide level:* rebreathing into a paper bag; adjusting respirator for CO_2 retention and oxygen inspired; correct hypoxia *Prevent injury:* safety measures for those who are unconscious; hypothermia for elevated temperature *Health teaching:* recognize stressful events; counseling if problem is hysteria	Normal acid-base balance obtained Recognizes psychological and environmental factors causing condition Respiratory rate returns to normal limits No cardiac arrhythmias Alert, oriented
Metabolic Alkalosis Potassium deficiencies Vomiting GI suctioning Intestinal fistulas Inadequate electrolyte replacement Increased use of antacids Diuretic therapy, steroids Increased ingestion/injection of bicarbonates	Lethargy Irritability Disorientation Nausea	*Respirations:* shallow; apnea, decreased thoracic movement; cyanosis *Pulse:* irregular → cardiac arrest *Muscles:* twitching → tetany, convulsions *G. I.:* vomiting, diarrhea, paralytic ileus HCO_3, elevated above 26 $Paco_2$ normal, K^+ <3.5, pH >7.45	*Obtain, maintain acid-base balance:* irrigate NG tubes with saline; monitor I&O; IV saline, potassium added; isotonic solutions PO; monitor vital signs *Prevent physical injury:* monitor for potassium loss, side effects of medications *Health teaching:* increase sodium when loss expected; instructions regarding self-administration of medications (e.g., baking soda)	Normal acid-base balance obtained No signs of potassium deficit Respiratory rate: 16–20 No arrhythmias— pulse regular Lists food sources high in potassium

Adult

Conditions Affecting Gas Transport

I. **Pneumonia:** acute inflammation of lungs with exudate accumulation in alveoli and other respiratory passages that interferes with ventilation process.
  A. **Types:**
    1. *Typical/classic pneumonia: pneumococcal;* related to diminished defense mechanisms, immunocompromised, critically ill, history of smoking, general anesthesia/abdominal surgery, exposure to airborne pathogens, hospitalization, recent respiratory tract infection, viral influenza, increased age, and chronic obstructive pulmonary disease (COPD).
      a. *Lobar pneumonia*—occurs abruptly when an acute bacterial infection affects a large portion of a lobe; causes pleuritic pain, heavy sputum production.
      b. *Bronchopneumonia*—involves patchy infiltration over a general area.
      c. *Alveolar pneumonia*—caused by virus; diffuse bilateral infection without patchy infiltrates.
    2. *Atypical pneumonia:* related to contact with specific organisms.
      a. *Mycoplasma pneumoniae* or *Legionella pneumophila,* if untreated, can lead to serious complications such as adult respiratory distress syndrome (ARDS), disseminated intravascular coagulation (DIC), thrombocytopenic purpura, renal failure, inflammation of the heart, neurological disorders, or possible death.
      b. *Pneumocystis carinii* in conjunction with AIDS.
    3. *Aspiration pneumonia:*
      a. *Noninfectious:* aspiration of fluids (gastric secretions, foods, liquids, tube feedings) into the airways.
      b. *Bacterial aspiration pneumonia:* related to poor cough mechanisms due to anesthesia, coma (mixed flora of upper respiratory tract cause pneumonia).
    4. *Hematogenous pneumonia bacterial infections:* related to spread of bacteria from the bloodstream.
  B. **Pathophysiology:** caused by infectious or noninfectious agents, clotting of an exudate rich in fibrogen, consolidated lung tissue.
  C. **Assessment:**
    1. *Subjective data*
      a. *Pain* location: chest (affected side), referred to abdomen, shoulder, flank.
      b. Irritability, restlessness.
      c. Apprehensiveness.
      d. Nausea, anorexia.
      e. History of exposure.
    2. *Objective data*
      a. Cough
        (1) Productive, rust (blood) or yellowish sputum (greenish with atypical pneumonia).
        (2) Splinting of affected side when coughing.
      b. *Sudden* increased fever, chills.
      c. Nasal flaring, circumoral cyanosis.
      d. Respiratory distress: tachypnea.
      e. Auscultation:
        (1) Decreased breath sounds on *affected* side.
        (2) Exaggerated breath sounds on *unaffected* side.
        (3) Crackles, bronchial breath sounds.
        (4) Dullness on percussion over consolidated area.
        (5) Possible pleural friction rub.
      f. Chest retraction (air hunger in infants).
      g. Vomiting.
      h. Facial herpes simplex.
      i. *Diagnostic studies:*
        (1) Chest x-ray: haziness to consolidation.
        (2) Sputum culture: Gram stain and culture; specific organisms, usually pneumococcus.
        (3) Bronchoscopy if sputum results are inconclusive.
      j. Lab data:
        (1) Blood culture: organism specific except when viral.
        (2) WBC: leukocytosis.
        (3) Sedimentation rate: *elevated.*

    3. Factors contributing to the severity of pneumonia:
      a. *Demographics:*
        (1) Age—severity increased with age
        (2) Gender
        (3) Nursing home resident
      b. *Comorbidities*
        (1) CHF.
        (2) Active cancer.
        (3) Liver disease.
        (4) Renal insufficiency.
        (5) Stroke with residual symptoms.
      c. *Physical exam:*
        (1) Systolic BP <90.
        (2) HR ≥125.
        (3) Respiratory rate ≥30.
        (4) Temperature (PO) ≥104° or <95°.
        (5) Altered LOC.
      d. *Lab results:*
        (1) Hct <30.
        (2) Na <130.
        (3) BUN ≥30.
        (4) Arterial pH <7.35.
        (5) Pleural effusion on chest X-ray.
        (6) Glucose >250 mg/dL.

  D. **Analysis/nursing diagnosis:**
    1. *Ineffective airway clearance* related to retained secretions.
    2. *Activity intolerance* related to inflammatory process.
    3. *Pain* related to continued coughing.
    4. *Knowledge deficit* (learning need) related to proper management of symptoms.
    5. *Risk for fluid volume deficit* related to tachypnea.

◆ **E. Nursing care plan/implementation:**

1. Goal: *promote adequate ventilation.*

   a. Deep breathe, cough.

   ▶ b. Remove respiratory secretions, suction prn.

   c. High humidity with or without oxygen therapy.

   ▶ d. Intermittent positive-pressure breathing (IPPB); incentive spirometry, chest physiotherapy, as ordered and needed to loosen secretions.

   ◖ e. Use of *expectorants* as ordered.

   f. Change position frequently.

   ▶ g. Percussion with postural drainage.

2. Goal: *control infection.*

   a. Monitor vital signs; hypothermia for elevated temperature.

   ◖ b. Administer *antibiotics* as ordered to control infection—broad spectrum, e.g. penicillin, quinolones, aminoglycosides. *Note:* need cultures before starting on antibiotics.

3. Goal: *provide rest and comfort.*

   a. Planned rest periods.

   b. Adequate hydration by mouth, I&O; IVs as needed.

   c. *Diet: high* carbohydrate, *high* protein to meet energy demands and assist in the healing process.

   ◖ d. Mild *analgesics* for pain—*no* opioids.

4. Goal: *prevent potential complications.*

   a. Cross infection: use good handwashing technique.

   b. *Sterile technique* when tracheobronchial suctioning to reduce risk of possible infection.

   c. Hyperthermia: tepid baths, hypothermia blanket.

   d. Respiratory insufficiency and acidosis: clear airway, promote expectoration of secretions.

   e. Assess cardiac and respiratory function.

   f. Remain ambulatory whenever possible.

5. Goal: *health teaching.*

   a. Proper disposal of tissues, cover mouth when coughing.

   b. Expected side effects of prescribed medications.

   c. Need for rest, limited interactions, increased caloric intake.

   d. Need to avoid future respiratory infections. *Immunization:* influenza each year for those at risk. Vaccine for pneumococcal pneumonia every 5 years.

   ◖ e. Correct dosage of antibiotics and the importance of taking entire prescription at prescribed times (times evenly distributed throughout the 24 hr period to maintain blood level of antibiotic) for increased effectiveness.

◆ **F. Evaluation/outcome criteria:**

1. Adheres to medication regimen.

2. Has improved gas exchange as shown by improved pulmonary function tests.

3. No acid-base or fluid imbalance: normal pH.

4. Energy level: increased.

5. Sputum production: decreased, normal color.

6. Vital signs: stable.

7. Breath sounds: clear.

8. Cultures: negative.

9. Reports comfort level increased.

II. Severe Acute Respiratory Syndrome (SARS): viral respiratory illness caused by a coronavirus. Incubation period: 2 to 7 days, maybe as long as 10 to 14 days. Recommend limiting contact after infection until *10 days after fever* has gone.

A. Pathophysiology: little information is known about the SARS-associated coronavirus. May survive in the environment for several days—depends on temperature or humidity, and type of material or body fluid. Spread generally by respiratory droplets—up to 3 ft. May spread through air; other ways not known. Progresses to hypoxia→pneumonia→respiratory distress syndrome.

B. Risk factors:

1. Weakened immune system.

2. Close contact (within 3 ft)—kissing, hugging, sharing utensils.

◆ **C. Assessment:**

1. *Subjective data:*

   a. Headache.

   b. Feeling of discomfort; body aches; chills.

   c. Dyspnea.

2. *Objective data:*

   a. Temp >100.4°F (38.0°C), unless on antipyretics.

   b. Mild respiratory symptoms; dry cough.

   c. Diarrhea in 20%.

   d. Lab: reverse transcription polymerase chain reaction (RT-PCR) of blood, stool, nasal secretions; serologic test for antibodies; viral culture (showing antibodies to virus more than 21 days after onset of illness).

   e. Additional lab findings:

   (1) Leukopenia.

   (2) Lymphopenia.

   (3) Thrombocytopenia.

   (4) ↑ lactose dehydrogenase.

   (5) ↑ aspartate aminotransferase.

   (6) ↑ creatinekinase.

   f. Chest x-ray: focal interstitial infiltrates→ generalized patchy infiltrates → areas of consolidation.

◆ **D. Analysis/nursing diagnosis:**

1. *Ineffective breathing pattern* related to hypoxia and pneumonia.

2. *Risk for spread of infection* related to droplet or airborne transmission.

3. *Impaired gas exchange* related to pneumonia.

◆ **E. Nursing care plan/implementation and evaluation/outcome criteria** (also see **Pneumonia, p. 524**):

 1. Goal: *infection control.*

   a. Standard precautions (e.g., strict hand hygiene).

Adult

b. *Contact* precautions (e.g., gown and gloves) with eye protection.

c. *Airborne* precautions (e.g., isolation room with negative pressure; use of an N-95 filtering disposable respirator for those entering room, or surgical mask).

d. Identify/isolate suspected SARS cases *(quarantine)*.

2. Goal: *supportive care.*

a. Empiric *antibiotic* therapy with broad coverage.

b. *Isolation* (i.e., those without symptoms) for 10 days *after* becoming *afebrile.*

III. Atelectasis: collapsed alveoli in part or all of the lung.

A. Pathophysiology: due to compression (tumor), airway obstruction, decreased surfactant production, or progressive regional hypoventilation.

B. Risk factors:

1. Shallow breathing due to pain, abdominal distention, narcotics, or sedatives.

2. Decreased ciliary action due to anesthesia, smoking.

3. Thickened secretions due to immobility, dehydration.

4. Aspiration of foreign substances.

5. Bronchospasms.

◆ C. Assessment:

1. *Subjective data*

a. Restlessness.

b. Pain.

2. *Objective data*

a. Tachypnea.

b. Tachycardia.

c. Dullness on percussion.

d. Absent bronchial breathing.

e. Crackles at bases as alveoli "pop" open on inspiration.

f. Tactile fremitus in affected area.

g. X-ray:

(1) Patches of consolidation.

(2) Elevated diaphragm.

(3) Mediastinal shift.

◆ D. Analysis/nursing diagnosis:

1. *Impaired gas exchange* related to shallow breathing.

2. *Pain,* acute, related to collapse of lung.

3. *Fear* related to altered respiratory status.

◆ E. Nursing care plan/implementation:

1. Goal: *relieve hypoxia.*

a. Frequent respiratory assessment.

▶ b. Respiratory hygiene measures, cough, deep breathe. Use bedside inspirometer q1h when awake.

▶ c. Oxygen as ordered.

▶ d. Monitor effects of respiratory therapy, ventilators, breathing assistance measures to ensure proper gas exchange.

e. *Position:* on *unaffected* side to allow for lung expansion.

2. Goal: *prevent complications.*

a. *Antibiotics* as ordered.

b. Turn, cough, and deep breathe. Out of bed, ambulation.

c. *Increase fluid* intake to liquefy secretions.

3. Goal: *health teaching.*

a. Need to report signs and symptoms listed in assessment data for early recognition of problem.

b. Importance of coughing and deep breathing to improve present condition and prevent further problems.

◆ F. Evaluation/outcome criteria:

1. Lung expanded on x-ray.

2. Acid-base balance obtained and maintained.

3. No pain on respiration.

4. Activity level increased.

IV. Pulmonary embolism: undissolved mass that travels in bloodstream and occludes a blood vessel; can be thromboemboli, fat, air, or catheter. Constitutes a **critical medical emergency**.

A. Pathophysiology: obstructs blood flow to lung→ increased pressure on pulmonary artery and reflex constriction of pulmonary blood vessels→ poor pulmonary circulation→pulmonary infarction.

B. Risk factors:

1. Thrombophlebitis.

2. Recent surgery.

3. Invasive procedures.

4. Immobility.

5. Obesity

6. Myocardial infarction, heart failure.

7. Smoking.

8. Varicose veins.

9. Hormone replacement therapy.

◆ C. Assessment:

1. *Subjective data*

a. Chest *pain:* substernal, localized; type—crushing, sharp, stabbing with respirations.

b. Sudden onset of profound dyspnea.

c. Restless, irritable, anxious.

d. Sense of impending doom.

2. *Objective data*

a. Respirations: either rapid, shallow or deep, gasping.

b. *Elevated* temperature.

c. Auscultation: friction rub, crackles; diminished breath sounds.

d. Shock:

(1) Tachycardia.

(2) Hypotension.

(3) Skin: cold, clammy.

e. Cough: hemoptysis.

f. X-ray: area of density.

g. ECG changes that reflect right-sided failure.

h. Echocardiogram shows increased pulmonary dynamics.

i. Lung scan. Pulmonary angiography.

> j. Lab data:
>> (1) *Decreased* Paco$_2$.
>> (2) *Elevated* WBC.

◆ **D. Analysis/nursing diagnosis:**
1. *Ineffective breathing pattern* related to shallow respirations.
2. *Impaired gas exchange* related to dyspnea.
3. *Pain* related to decreased tissue perfusion.
4. *Altered peripheral tissue perfusion* related to occlusion of blood vessel.
5. *Fear* related to emergency condition.
6. *Anxiety* related to sense of impending doom.

◆ **E. Nursing care plan/implementation:**
1. Goal: *monitor for signs of respiratory distress.*
   a. Auscultate lungs for areas of decreased/absent breath sounds.
    b. *Elevate head of bed.*
   c. Monitor ABGs.
   d. Monitor pulse oximetry; administer oxygen, supplemental humidification as indicated.
   e. Monitor blood coagulation studies (e.g., aPTT).
   f. Administer *anticoagulation* therapy, *thrombolytic* agents, morphine for *pain, vasopressor* medications.
   g. Fluids: IV/PO as indicated.
   h. Monitor signs: Homans', acidosis.
   i. Ambulate as tolerated/indicated; change position.
   j. Prepare for surgery if peripheral embolectomy is indicated.
2. Goal: *health teaching.*
   a. Prevent further occurrence; importance of antiembolism stockings, intermittent pneumatic compression devices.
   b. Decrease stasis.
   c. If history of thrombophlebitis, *avoid* birth control pills.
   d. Need to continue medication.
   e. Follow-up care.

◆ **F. Evaluation/outcome criteria:**
1. No complications; no further incidence of emboli.
2. Respiratory rate returns to normal.
3. Coagulation studies within normal limits (aPTT 25 to 41 sec, ABGs within normal limits).
4. Reports comfort achieved.

V. Histoplasmosis: infection found mostly in central United States. *Not transmitted from human to human but from dust and contaminated soil.* Progressive histoplasmosis, seen most frequently in middle-aged white men who have COPD, is characterized by cavity formation, fibrosis, and emphysema.

A. Pathophysiology: spores of *Histoplasma capsulatum* (from droppings of infected birds and bats) are inhaled, multiply, and cause fungal infections of respiratory tract. Leads to necrosis and healing by encapsulation.

◆ **B. Assessment:**
1. *Subjective data*
   a. Malaise.
   b. Chest pain, dyspnea.
2. *Objective data*
   a. Weight loss.
   b. Nonproductive cough.
   c. Fever.
   d. Positive skin test for histoplasmosis.
   e. Benign acute pneumonitis.
   f. Chest x-ray: nodular infiltrate.
   g. Sputum culture shows *Histoplasma capsulatum.*
   h. Hepatomegaly, splenomegaly.

◆ **C. Analysis/nursing diagnosis:**
1. *Ineffective airway clearance* related to pneumonitis.
2. *Ineffective breathing pattern* related to dyspnea.
3. *Pain,* acute, related to infectious process.
4. *Risk for infection* related to repeated exposure to fungal spores.
5. *Impaired gas exchange* related to chronic pulmonary disease.
6. *Knowledge deficit* (learning need) related to prevention of disease and potential side effects of medications.

◆ **D. Nursing care plan/implementation:**
1. Goal: *relieve symptoms of the disease:*
   a. Administer medications as ordered.
      (1) Amphotericin B (IV) and ketoconazole.
         (a) Monitor for drug side effects: local phlebitis, renal toxicity, hypokalemia, anemia, anaphylaxis, bone marrow depression.
         (b) *Azotemia* (presence of nitrogen-containing compounds in blood) is monitored by biweekly BUN or creatinine levels.

         > BUN >40 mg/dL or creatinine >3.0 mg/dL Necessitates *stopping* amphotericin B until values return to within normal limits.

      (2) Aspirin, diphenhydramine HCl (Benadryl), promethazine HCl (Phenergan), prochlorperazine (Compazine): used *to decrease systemic toxicity* of chills, fever, aching, nausea, and vomiting.
2. Goal: *health teaching:*
   a. Desired effects and side effects of prescribed medications; importance of taking medications for entire course of therapy (usually from 2 wk to 3 mo).
   b. Importance of follow-up laboratory tests to monitor toxic effects of drug.
   c. Identify source of contamination if possible and *avoid* future contact if possible.
   d. Importance of deep breathing, pursed-lip breathing, coughing (see **VII. Emphysema, p. 529,** for specific care).

Adult

e. Signs and symptoms of chronic histoplasmosis, COPD, drug toxicity, and drug side effects, as in **V. D. I. a.** on **p.527**

◆ **E. Evaluation/outcome criteria:**
1. Complies with treatment plan.
2. Respiratory complications avoided.
3. Symptoms of illness decreased.
4. No further spread of disease.
5. Source of contamination identified and removed.

VI. Tuberculosis: inflammatory, communicable disease that commonly attacks the lungs, although may occur in other body parts.

A. Pathophysiology: exposure to causative organism *(Mycobacterium tuberculosis)* in the alveoli in susceptible individual leads to inflammation. Infection spreads by lymphatics to hilus; antibodies are released, leading to fibrosis, calcification, or inflammation. Exudate formation leads to caseous necrosis, then liquefication of caseous material leads to cavitation.

B. Risk factors:
1. Persons who have inhaled the tubercle bacillus infectious particles called droplet nuclei.
2. Persons who have diseases or therapies known to suppress the immune system.
3. Immigrants from Latin America, Africa, Asia, and Oceania living in the United States for less than 1 year.
4. Americans living in those regions for a prolonged time.
5. Residents of U.S. metropolitan cities such as New York, Miami; those who live in poverty and are in overcrowded, poorly ventilated living conditions.
6. Men >65 yr.
7. Women between ages 26 to 44 yr and >65 yr.
8. Children <5 yr.

◆ **C. Assessment:**
1. *Subjective data*
   a. Loss of appetite, weight loss.
   b. Weakness, loss of energy.
   c. *Pain:* knifelike, chest.
   d. Though client may be symptom free, the disease is found on screening.
2. *Objective data*
   a. Night sweats, chills.
   b. *Fever:* low grade, late afternoon.
   c. *Pulse:* increased.
   d. *Respiratory* assessment:

(1) Productive persistent cough, hemoptsis.
(2) Respirations: normal, increased depth.
(3) Asymmetrical lung expansion.
(4) Increased tactile fremitus.
(5) Dullness to percussion.
(6) Crackles following short cough.

   e. Hoarseness.
   f. Unexplained weight loss.
    g. *Diagnostic tests:*

(1) *Positive tuberculin test (Mantoux)*—reaction to test begins approximately 12 hr after administration with area of redness and a central area of induration. The peak time is 48 hr. Determination of positive or negative is made. A reaction is positive when it measures *10 mm.* Contacts reacting from 5 to 10 mm may need to be treated prophylactically. This test is referred to as purified protein derivative (PPD) or intradermal skin test.
(2) *Sputum:* three specimens tested positive for acid fast (smear and culture). Positive equals greater than 10 AFB per field.
(3) *X-ray:* infiltration cavitation.

h. Lab data: blood—*decreased* RBC, *increased* sedimentation rate.

i. Classification of tuberculosis:
Class Description
0 No TB exposure, not infected.
1 TB exposure, no evidence of infection.
2 TB infection, no disease.
3 TB: current disease (persons with completed diagnostic evidence of TB—both a significant reaction to tuberculin skin test and clinical or x-ray evidence of disease).
4 TB: no current disease (persons with previous history of TB or with abnormal x-ray films but no significant tuberculin skin test reaction or clinical evidence).
5 TB: suspected (diagnosis pending) (used during diagnostic testing period of suspected persons, for no longer than 3 mo).

◆ **D. Analysis/nursing diagnosis:**
1. *Ineffective airway clearance* related to productive cough.
2. *Impaired gas exchange* related to asymmetrical lung expansion.
3. *Pain* related to unresolved disease process.
4. *Body image disturbance* related to feelings about tuberculosis.
5. *Social isolation* related to fear of spreading infection.
6. *Knowledge deficit* (learning need) related to medication regimen.

◆ **E. Nursing care plan/implementation:**
1. Goal: *reduce spread of disease.*
   a. Administer medications: isoniazid (INH), rifampin, pyrazinamide, ethambutol, or streptomycin; or drug combinations such as Rifadin or Rifamate. Client will be treated as an outpatient; may need to go to clinic for directly observed therapy (DOT) to ensure compliance of this long-term medication regimen.

b. The following may need to take 300 mg of INH daily for 1 yr as *prophylactic* measure: positive skin test reactors, including contacts; persons who have diseases or are receiving therapies that affect the immune system; persons who have leukemia, lymphoma, or uncontrolled diabetes or who have had a gastrectomy.

c. *Avoid direct contact with sputum.*

   (1) Use good handwashing technique after contact with client, personal articles.

   (2) Have client cover mouth and nose when coughing and sneezing, and use disposable tissues to collect sputum.

d. *Provide good circulation of fresh air.* (Changes of air dilute the number of organisms. This plus chemotherapy provide protection needed to prevent spread of disease.)

e. Implement *airborne or droplet* precautions (**Table 7.16**).

2. Goal: *promote nutrition.*

a. *Increased protein, calories* to aid in tissue repair and healing.

b. Small, frequent feedings.

c. *Increased fluids,* to liquefy secretions so they can be expectorated.

3. Goal: *promote increased self-esteem.*

a. Encourage client and family to express concerns regarding long-term illness and treatment protocol.

b. Explain methods of disease prevention, and encourage contacts to be tested and treated if necessary.

c. Encourage client to maintain role in family while home treatment is ongoing and to return to work and social contacts as soon as it is determined safe for progress of treatment plan.

4. Goal: *health teaching.*

a. Desired effects and side effects of medications:

   (1) *INH* may affect memory and ability to concentrate. May result in peripheral neuritis, hepatitis, rash, or fever.

   (2) *Streptomycin* may cause eighth cranial nerve damage and vestibular ototoxity, causing hearing loss; may cause labyrinth damage, manifested by vertigo and staggering; also may cause skin rashes, itching, and fever.

   (3) Important for client to know that medication regimen must be adhered to for entire course of treatment.

   (4) Discontinuation of therapy may allow organism to flourish and make the disease more difficult to treat.

b. Need for follow-up, long-term care, and contact identification.

c. Importance of nutritious diet, rest, avoidance of respiratory infections.

d. Identify community agencies for support and follow-up.

e. Inform that this communicable disease must be reported.

F. Evaluation/outcome criteria:

1. Complies with medication regimen.

2. Lists desired effects and side effects of medications prescribed.

3. Gains weight, eats food high in protein and carbohydrates.

4. Sputum culture becomes negative.

5. Retains role in family.

6. No complications (i.e., no hemorrhage, bacillus not spread to others).

VII. Emphysema: chronic disease with excessive inflation of the air spaces distal to the terminal bronchioles, alveolar ducts, and alveoli; characterized by increased airway resistance and decreased diffusing capacity. Emphysema, asthma, and chronic bronchitis together constitute *chronic obstructive pulmonary disease (COPD).*

A. Pathophysiology: imbalance between proteases, which break down lung tissue, and α_1-antitrypsin, which inhibits the breakdown. Increased airway resistance during expiration results in air trapping and hyperinflation→increased residual volumes. Increased dead space→unequal ventilation→perfusion of poorly ventilated alveoli→hypoxia and carbon dioxide retention (hypercapnia). Chronic hypercapnia reduces sensitivity of respiratory center; chemoreception in aortic arch and carotid sinus become principal regulators of respiratory drive (respond to hypoxia).

B. Risk factors:

1. Smoking.

2. Air pollution: long-term exposure to environmental irritants, fumes, dust.

3. Antienzymes and α_1-antitrypsin deficiencies.

4. Destruction of lung parenchyma.

5. Family history and increased age.

TABLE 7.16	**Airborne and Droplet Precautions**

When Used
For infectious diseases that are transmitted through inhalation of airborne particle (e.g., tuberculosis) or infected microorganisms in droplets (e.g., *Haemophilus influenzae*, pertussis)

Precautions
Isolate in private room (clients infected with same disease can be placed in same room)
Client should wear mask if out of room for testing, etc.
Masks to be worn by personnel when working within 3 ft of client
Gowns *not* necessary
Contaminated articles need to be labeled before being sent for decontamination
Provide adequate ventilation in client's room
Careful handwashing

◆ **C. Assessment:**
1. *Subjective data*
   a. Weakness, lethargy.
   b. History of repeated respiratory infections, shortness of breath.
   c. Long-term smoking.
   d. Irritability.
   e. Inability to accept medical diagnosis and treatment plan.
   f. Refusal to stop smoking.
   g. Dyspnea on exertion, dyspnea at rest (**Table 7.17**).
2. *Objective data*
   a. *Increased* BP.
   b. *Increased* pulse
   c. Nostrils: flaring.
   d. Cough: chronic, productive.
   e. Episodes of wheezing, crackles.
   f. Increased anterior-posterior diameter of chest (barrel chest).
   g. Use of accessory respiratory muscles, abdominal and neck.
   h. Asymmetrical thoracic movements, decreased diaphragmatic excursion.
   i. *Position:* sits up, leans forward to compress abdomen and push up diaphragm, increasing intrathoracic pressure, producing more efficient expiration.
   j. Pursed lips for greater expiratory breathing phase (*pink puffer*).
   k. Weight loss due to hypoxia.
   l. Skin: ruddy color, nail clubbing; when combined with bronchitis: cyanosis (*blue bloater*).
   m. Respiratory: *early* disease—alkalosis; *late* disease—acidosis, respiratory failure.
   n. Spontaneous pneumothorax.
   o. Cor pulmonale (**emergency cardiac condition** involving right ventricular failure due to increased pressure within pulmonary artery).
   p. X-ray: hyperinflation of lung, flattened diaphragm; lung scan differentiates between ventilation and perfusion.
   q. Pulmonary function tests:

   > (1) Prolonged rapid, forced exhalation.
   > (2) *Decreased:* vital capacity (<4000 mL); forced expiratory volume.
   > (3) *Increased:* residual volume (may be 200%); total lung capacity.

   r. Lab data:
   (1) $Pao_2 < 80$ mm Hg, pH < 7.35.
   (2) $Paco_2 > 45$ mm Hg.

   Note: In clients whose compensatory mechanisms are functioning, lab values may be out of the normal range, but if a 20:1 ratio of bicarbonate to carbonic acid is maintained, then appropriate acid-base balance also will be maintained. (Carbonic acid value can be obtained by multiplying the Pco_2 value by 0.003.)

◆ **D. Analysis/nursing diagnosis:**
1. *Impaired gas exchange* related to thick pulmonary secretions.
2. *Ineffective breathing pattern* related to hyperinflated alveoli.

TABLE 7.17	Differentiating Between Causes of Dyspnea				
	Asthma	**Chronic Obstructive Pulmonary Disease**	**Pneumothorax**	**Pulmonary Edema**	**Pulmonary Emboli**
Characteristics	Episodic, acute History of allergies Recent cold or flu	History of emphysema, bronchitis Heavy smoker Recent cold or respiratory infection	Chest pain: sudden, sharp *Sudden* onset; associated with coughing, air travel, strenuous exertion	History of myocardial infarction Rapid weight gain Cough Taking diuretics Increasing need for pillows for sleep	*Sudden* dyspnea Sharp chest pain Recent immobilization, surgery, or fracture of lower extremeties History of: thrombophlebitis, use of birth control pills, sickle cell anemia
◆ **Assessment Findings**	Wheezing Hyperresonance Chest may be silent with bronchospasms	Use of pursed-lip breathing Wheezing, crackles "Barrel" chest Uses accessory muscles to breathe	Tracheal deviation Asymmetrical chest motion Diminished breath sounds	Crackles Pink, frothy sputum Gallop (S_3) Air hunger	Tachycardia Hypotension Tachypnea Pleural rub

3. *Ineffective airway clearance* related to pulmonary secretions.
4. *Altered nutrition, less than body requirements,* related to weight loss due to hypoxia.
5. *Infection* related to chronic disease process and decreased ciliary action.
6. *Activity intolerance* related to increased energy demands used for breathing.
7. *Sleep pattern disturbance* related to changes in body positions necessary for breathing.
8. *Anxiety* related to disease progression.
9. *Knowledge deficit* (learning need) related to disease, treatment, and self-care needs.

◆ **E. Nursing care plan/implementation:**
1. Goal: *promote optimal ventilation.*
   a. Institute measures designed to decrease airway resistance and enhance gas exchange.
   ▸ b. *Position:* Fowler's or leaning forward to encourage expiratory phase.
   ▸ c. Oxygen with humidification, as ordered—no more than 2 L/min to prevent depression of hypoxic respiratory drive (see **Oxygen Therapy** in **Unit 11, p. 802**). May need long-term oxygen therapy as disease progresses, to improve quality of life and reduce risk of complications.
   ▸ d. Intermittent positive-pressure breathing (IPPB) with nebulization as ordered.
   e. Assisted ventilation.
   ▸ f. Postural drainage, chest physiotherapy.
   ▸ g. Medications, as ordered:
      (1) *Bronchodilators* to increase airflow through bronchial tree: inhaled: beta$_2$-adrenergic agonists (albuterol, metaproterenol); anticholinergic agent: ipratropium (Atrovent); aminophylline, theophylline, terbutaline, isoproterenol (Isuprel).
      (2) *Antimicrobials* to treat infection (determined by sputum cultures and sensitivity): trimethoprim and sulfamethoxazole (Bactrim, Septra); doxycycline, erythromycin, amoxicillin, cephalosporins, and macrolides (condition deteriorates with respiratory infections).
      (3) *Corticosteroids* to decrease inflammation, mucosal edema, improve pulmonary function during exacerbation; *systemic:* prednisone, methylprednisolone sodium succinate (Solu-Medrol); *inhaled:* trimcinolone acetonide (Azmacort), beclomethasone (Beclovent, Vanceril), flunisolide (AeroBid).
      (4) *Expectorants* (increase water intake to achieve desired effect): glyceryl guaiacolate (Robitussin).
      (5) *Bronchial detergents*/liquefying agents (Mucomyst).
   ▸ h. Immunotherapy: helps ward off life-threatening influenza and pneumonia. Flu vaccination every October or November. Pneumococcal vaccination routinely one dose; revaccinate 5 years later if high risk.

2. Goal: *employ comfort measures and support other body systems.*
   a. Oral hygiene prn; frequently client is mouth breather.
   b. Skin care: waterbed, air mattress, foam pads to prevent skin breakdown.
   ▸ c. Active and passive ROM exercises to prevent thrombus formation; antiembolic stocking or woven elastic (Ace) bandages may be applied.
   d. Increase activities to tolerance.
   e. Adequate rest and sleep periods to prevent mental disturbances due to sleep deprivation and to reduce metabolic rate.

3. Goal: *improve nutritional intake.*
   a. *High protein, high calorie diet* to prevent negative nitrogen balance.
   b. Give small, frequent meals.
   c. Supplement diet with high calorie drinks.
   d. *Push fluids* to 3000 mL/day, unless contraindicated—helps moisten secretions.

4. Goal: *provide emotional support for client and family.*
   a. Identify factors that increase anxiety:
      (1) Fears related to mechanical equipment.
      (2) Loss of body image.
      (3) Fear of dying.
   b. Assist family coping:
      (1) Do *not* reinforce denial or encourage overconcern.
      (2) Give accurate, up-to-date information on client's condition.
      (3) Be open to questioning.
      (4) Encourage client-family communication.
      (5) Provide appropriate diversional activities.

5. Goal: *health teaching.*
   a. Breathing exercises, such as pursed-lip breathing and diaphragmatic breathing.
   b. Stress-management techniques.
   c. Methods to stop smoking.
   d. Importance of avoiding respiratory infections.
   e. Desired effects and side effects of prescribed medications, possible interactions with over-the-counter drugs.
   f. Purposes and techniques for effective bronchial hygiene therapy.
   g. Rest/activity schedule that increases with ability.
   h. Food selection for *high protein, high calorie* diet.
   i. Importance of taking *2500–3000 mL fluid* per day (unless contraindicated by another medical problem).
   j. Importance of medical follow-up.

◆ **F. Evaluation/outcome criteria:**
1. Takes prescribed medication.
2. Participates in rest/activity schedule.
3. Improves nutritional intake, gains appropriate weight for body size.
4. No complications of respiratory failure, cor pulmonale.

Adult

5. No respiratory infections.
6. Acid-base balance maintained through compensatory mechanisms, acidosis prevented.

VIII. **Asthma:** sometimes called reactive airway disease (RAD) or reversible obstructive airway disease (ROAD); a complex inflammatory process that causes increased airway resistance and, over time, airway tissue damage. Characterized by airway inflammation and hyperresponsiveness to a variety of stimuli such as allergens, cold air, dust, smoke, exercise, medications (e.g., aspirin), some food additives, and viral infections. *Immunologic* asthma occurs in childhood and follows other allergic disease. *Nonimmunologic* asthma occurs in adulthood and is associated with a history of recurrent respiratory tract infections.

A. **Pathophysiology:** triggers initiate the release of inflammatory mediators such as histamine, which produce airway obstruction through smooth muscle constriction, microvascular leakage, mucous plugging, and swelling. This process involves *six sequential steps:* (1) triggering—the allergic or antigenic stimuli activate the inflammatory (mast) cells; (2) these mast cells signal the systemic immune system to release proinflammatory substances; (3) migration of circulating inflammatory cells to regions of inflammation in the respiratory tract; (4) migrating cells are activated by the proinflammatory mediators; (5) this results in tissue damage; and (6) resolution. The airways of many clients with asthma are chronically inflamed.

1. *Immunologic,* or allergic asthma in persons who are atopic (hypersensitivity state that is subject to hereditary influences); immunoglobulin E (IgE) usually *elevated.*
2. *Nonimmunologic,* or nonallergic asthma in persons who have a history of repeated respiratory tract infections; age usually >35 yr.
3. *Mixed,* combined immunologic and nonimmunologic; any age, allergen or nonspecific stimuli.

B. **Risk factors:**
1. History of allergies to identified or unidentified irritants; seasonal and environmental inhalants.
2. Recurrent respiratory infection.

◆ C. **Assessment:**
1. *Subjective data*
   a. History: URI, rhinitis, allergies, family history of asthma.
   b. Increasing tightness of the chest→ dyspnea (see **Table 7.17**).
   c. Anxiety, restlessness.
   d. Attack history:
      (1) *Immunologic:* contact with allergen to which person is sensitive; seen most often in children and young adults.
      (2) *Nonimmunologic:* develops in adults >35 yr; aggravated by infections of the sinuses and respiratory tract.

2. *Objective data*
   a. Peak flow meter level drops.
   b. Respiratory assessment: increased rate, audible expiratory wheeze (also inspiratory when severe) on auscultation, hyperresonance on percussion, rib retractions, use of accessory muscles on inspiration.
   c. Tachycardia, tachypnea.
   d. Cough: dry, hacking, persistent.
   e. General appearance: pallor, cyanosis, diaphoresis, chronic barrel chest, elevated shoulders, flattened molar bones, narrow nose, prominent upper teeth, dark circles under eyes, distended neck veins, orthopnea.
   f. Expectoration of tenacious mucoid sputum.
    g. *Diagnostic tests:*
      (1) Forced vital capacity (FVC): *decreased.*
      (2) Forced expiratory volume in 1 second (FEV$_1$): *decreased.*
      (3) Peak expiratory flow rate: *decreased.*
      (4) Residual volume: *increased.*
    h. Lab data: Blood gases—*elevated* P$_{CO_2}$; *decreased* P$_{O_2}$, pH.

   Emergency note: Persons severely affected may develop *status asthmaticus,* a **life-threatening** asthmatic attack in which symptoms of asthma continue and do not respond to usual treatment. Could lead to respiratory failure and hypoxemia.

◆ D. **Analysis/nursing diagnosis:**
1. *Ineffective airway clearance* related to tachypnea.
2. *Impaired gas exchange* related to constricted bronchioles.
3. *Anxiety* related to breathlessness.
4. *Activity intolerance* related to persistent cough.
5. *Knowledge deficit* (learning need) related to causal factors and self-care measures.

◆ E. **Nursing care plan/implementation:**
1. Goal: *promote pulmonary ventilation.*
   a. *Position:* high-Fowler's for comfort.
   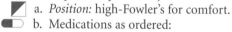 b. Medications as ordered:
      (1) *Rescue* medications: *corticosteroids* (e.g., prednisone, methylprednisolone [Medrol]; beta-adrenergic agonists, such as albuterol [Proventil, Ventolin], metaproterenol [Alupent, Metaprel]).
      (2) *Maintenance* medications: *nonsteroidal* antiinflammatory drugs: cromolyn (Intal), nedocromil (Tilade); *corticosteroids:* beclomethasone (Vanceril), triamcinolone (Azmacort); *leukotriene inhibitors/receptor antagonists:* zafirlukast (Accolate), zileuton (Zyflo); *theophylline* (Theo-Dur, Slo-Bid, Uni-Dur, theophylline ethylenediamino [Aminophylline]); *anticholinergic:* ipratropium (Atrovent); Beta agonists: salmeterol (Serevent); *mast cell stabilizers:* nedocromil sodium (Tilade).
      (3) *Antibiotics* to control infection.

▶ c. Oxygen therapy with increased humidity as ordered.

d. Frequent monitoring for respiratory distress.

e. Rest periods and gradual increase in activity.

2. Goal: *facilitate expectoration.*

a. High humidity.

b. *Increase fluid* intake.

c. Monitor for dehydration.

▶ d. Respiratory therapy: IPPB.

3. Goal: *health teaching to prevent further attacks:*

a. Identify and avoid all asthma triggers.

b. Teach importance of peak flow meter readings.

c. Medications—when to use, how to use, side effects, withdrawals.

▶ d. Using a metered-dose inhaler:

---

(1) Shake vigorously.

(2) Position inhaler about 1 in. in front of mouth. Use 2 fingers to measure the 1-inch distance.

(3) A spacer is recommended: Connect spacer device, shake, press down the canister; place lips on the mouthpiece and take a slow deep breath through mouth. Without spacer, breathe out all the way, open mouth wide and take a slow deep breath through mouth. Press down the canister and continue to breathe in.

(4) Once lungs are full, hold breath for 10 sec if possible.

(5) Exhale normally through pursed lips.

(6) Wait 1 to 2 min between puffs. Depending on the particular medication, may need to rinse mouth with water or mouthwash after each treatment.

---

e. Methods to facilitate expectoration—increase humidity, postural drainage when appropriate, percussion techniques.

f. Breathing techniques to increase expiratory phase.

g. Stress-management techniques.

h. Importance of recognizing early signs of asthma attack and beginning treatment immediately.

i. Steps to take during an attack.

◆ **F. Evaluation/outcome criteria:**

1. No complications.

2. Has fewer attacks.

3. Takes prescribed medications, avoids infections.

4. Adjusts lifestyle.

5. Pulmonary function tests return to normal.

IX. Bronchitis: acute or chronic inflammation of bronchus resulting as a complication from colds and flu. *Acute bronchitis* is caused by an extension of upper-respiratory infection, such as a cold, and can be given to others. It can also result from an irritation from physical or chemical agents. *Chronic bronchitis* is characterized by hypersecretion of mucus and chronic cough for 3 months per year for 2 consecutive years.

A. Pathophysiology: bronchial walls are infiltrated with lymphocytes and macrophages; lumen becomes obstructed due to decreased ciliary action and repeated bronchospasms. Hyperventilation of alveolar sacs occurs. Long-term condition results in respiratory acidosis, recurrent pneumonitis, emphysema, or cor pulmonale.

B. Risk factors:

1. Smoking.

2. Repeated respiratory infections.

3. History of living in area where there is much air pollution.

◆ **C. Assessment:**

1. *Subjective data*

a. History: recurrent, chronic cough, especially when arising in the morning.

b. Anorexia.

2. *Objective data*

a. *Respiratory:*

(1) Shortness of breath.

(2) Use of accessory muscles.

(3) Cyanosis, dusky complexion "blue bloater."

(4) Sputum: excessive, nonpurulent.

(5) Vesicular and bronchovesicular breath sounds; wheezing.

b. Weight loss.

c. Fever.

---

d. Pulmonary function tests:

(1) *Decreased* forced expiratory volume.

(2) $PaO_2 < 90$ mm Hg; $PaCO_2 > 40$ mm Hg.

---

e. Lab data:

(1) RBC: *elevated* to compensate for hypoxia (polycythemia).

(2) WBC: *elevated* to fight infection.

◆ **D. Analysis/nursing diagnosis:**

1. *Ineffective airway clearance* related to excessive sputum.

2. *Ineffective breathing pattern* related to need to use accessory muscles for breathing.

3. *Impaired gas exchange* related to shortness of breath.

4. *Activity intolerance* related to increased energy used for breathing.

◆ **E. Nursing care plan/implementation:**

1. Goal: *assist in optimal respirations.*

a. *Increase* fluid intake.

▶ b. IPPB, chest physiotherapy.

▷ c. Administer medications as ordered:

(1) *Bronchodilators.*

(2) *Antibiotics.*

(3) *Bronchial detergents*, liquefying agents.

2. Goal: *minimize bronchial irritation.*

a. *Avoid* respiratory irritants (e.g., smoke, dust, cold air, allergens).

b. Environment: air-conditioned, increased humidity.

c. Encourage nostril breathing rather than mouth breathing.

3. Goal: *improve nutritional status.*

Adult

a. Diet: soft, *high* calorie.

b. Small, frequent feedings.

4. Goal: *prevent secondary infections.*

a. Administer *antibiotics* as ordered.

b. *Avoid* exposure to infections, crowds.

5. Goal: *health teaching.*

a. *Avoid* respiratory infections.

b. Medications: desired effects and side effects.

c. Methods to stop smoking.

d. Rest and activity balance.

e. Stress management.

◆ **F. Evaluation/outcome criteria:**

1. Stops smoking.

2. Acid-base balance maintained.

3. Respiratory infections less frequent.

X. Acute adult respiratory distress syndrome (ARDS) (formerly called by other names, including *shock lung*): noncardiogenic pulmonary infiltrations resulting in stiff, wet lungs and refractory hypoxemia in an adult who was previously healthy. Acute hypoxemic respiratory failure without hypercapnea.

A. Pathophysiology: damage to alveolar capillary membrane, increased vascular permeability creating noncardiac pulmonary edema, and impaired gas exchange; decreased surfactant production → atelectasis; severe hypoxia; refractory to ↑ Fio_2 → possible death.

B. Risk factors:

1. Primary:

a. Shock, multiple trauma.

b. Infections.

c. Aspiration, inhalation of chemical toxins.

d. Drug overdose.

e. Disseminated intravascular coagulation (DIC).

f. Emboli, especially fat emboli.

2. Secondary:

a. Overaggressive fluid administration.

b. Oxygen toxicity.

◆ **C. Assessment:**

1. *Subjective data*

a. Restlessness, anxiety.

b. History of risk factors.

c. Severe dyspnea (see **Table 7.17**).

2. *Objective data*

a. Cyanosis.

b. Tachycardia.

c. Hypotension.

d. Hypoxemia, acidosis.

e. Crackles.

f. X-ray—bilateral patchy infiltrates.

g. Death if untreated.

◆ **D. Analysis/nursing diagnosis:**

1. *Anxiety* related to serious physical condition.

2. *Ineffective breathing pattern* related to severe dyspnea.

3. *Impaired gas exchange* related to alveolar damage.

4. *Altered tissue perfusion* related to hypoxia.

◆ **E. Nursing care plan/implementation:**

1. Goal: *assist in respirations.*

a. May require mechanical ventilatory support to maintain respirations.

b. May need to be transferred to ICU.

c. May need oxygen to combat hypoxia.

d. Suction prn.

e. Monitor blood gas results to detect early signs of acidosis/alkalosis.

f. If not on ventilator, assess vital signs and respiratory status every 15 min.

g. Cough, deep breathe every hour.

h. May need:

(1) Rotation therapy and/or prone position.

(2) Postural drainage, suction.

(3) *Bronchodilator* medications.

2. Goal: *prevent complications.*

a. Decrease anxiety and provide psychological care:

(1) Maintain a calm atmosphere.

(2) Encourage rest to conserve energy.

(3) Emotional support.

b. Obtain fluid balance:

(1) Slow IV flow rate.

(2) *Diuretics:* rapid acting, low dose.

c. Monitor:

(1) Pulmonary artery and capillary wedge pressure cardiac output.

(2) Central venous pressure (CVP), peripheral perfusion, arterial line BP.

(3) I&O.

(4) Assess for bleeding tendencies, potential for disseminated intravascular coagulation.

d. Protect from infection:

(1) *Strict aseptic* technique.

(2) *Antibiotic* therapy.

(3) Deep vein thrombosis prophylaxis.

e. Provide physiological support:

(1) Maintain nutrition.

(2) Skin care.

3. Goal: *health teaching.*

a. Briefly explain procedures as they are happening (emergency situation can frighten client).

b. Give rationale for follow-up care.

c. Identify risk factors as appropriate for prevention of recurrence.

◆ **F. Evaluation/outcome criteria:**

1. Client survives and is alert.

2. Skin warm to touch.

3. Respiratory rate within normal limits.

4. Lab values and pressures within normal limits.

5. Urinary output >30 mL/hr.

XI. Pneumothorax: presence of air within the pleural cavity; occurs spontaneously or as a result of trauma (**Figure 7.6**).

A. Types:

1. *Closed* (spontaneous): rupture of a subpleural bulla, tuberculous focus, carcinoma, lung abscess, pulmonary infarction, severe coughing attack, or blunt trauma.

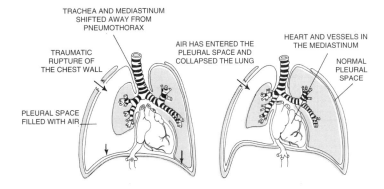

PNEUMOTHORAX
(OPEN —THE CHEST WALL INJURY PERMITS
AIR TO FLOW IN AND OUT OF THE PLEURAL
SPACE ON THE AFFECTED SIDE)

TRACHEA AND MEDIASTINUM
SHIFTED AWAY FROM
PNEUMOTHORAX

TRAUMATIC
RUPTURE OF
THE CHEST WALL

AIR HAS ENTERED THE
PLEURAL SPACE AND
COLLAPSED THE LUNG

HEART AND VESSELS IN
THE MEDIASTINUM

NORMAL
PLEURAL
SPACE

PLEURAL SPACE
FILLED WITH AIR

INHALATION: AIR ENTERS THE INJURED
SIDE, CAUSING COLLAPSE OF THE LUNG
AND SHIFT OF THE MEDIASTINUM AND
HEART TOWARD THE UNAFFECTED SIDE

EXHALATION: THE AIR IS PARTIALLY
FORCED FROM THE AFFECTED SIDE
PLEURAL SPACE AND THE MEDIASTINUM
SHIFT TOWARD THE AFFECTED SIDE

FIGURE 7.6   Pneumothorax. (From Venes, D [ed]: Taber's Cyclopedic Medical Dictionary, ed 20. FA Davis, Philadelphia, 2005.)

2. *Open* (traumatic): communication between atmosphere and pleural space because of opening in chest wall.
3. *Tension:* one-way leak; may occur during mechanical ventilation or CPR, or as a complication of any type of spontaneous or traumatic pneumothorax. Positive pressure within chest cavity resulting from accumulated air that cannot escape during expiration. Leads to collapse of lung, mediastinal shift, and compression of the heart and great vessels.

B. Pathophysiology: pressure builds up in the pleural space, lung on the affected side collapses, and the heart and mediastinum shift toward the unaffected lung.

◆ **C. Assessment:**
   1. *Subjective data*
      a. *Pain*
         (1) Sharp, aggravated by activity.
         (2) Location—chest; may be referred to shoulder, arm on affected side.
      b. Restlessness, anxiety.
      c. Dyspnea (see **Table 7.17**).
   2. *Objective data*
      a. Cough.
      b. Cessation of normal movements on affected side.
      c. Absence of breath sounds on affected side.
      d. Pallor, cyanosis.
      e. Shock.
      f. Tracheal deviation to unaffected side.
      g. X-ray; air in pleural space.

◆ **D. Analysis/nursing diagnosis:**
   1. *Ineffective breathing pattern* related to collapse of lung.
   2. *Impaired gas exchange* related to abnormal thoracic movement.
   3. *Pain* related to trauma to chest area.
   4. *Fear* related to emergency situation.

◆ **E. Nursing care plan/implementation:**
   1. Goal: *prevent damage until medical intervention available.*
      a. Place sterile occlusive gauze dressing over wound.
      b. Tape dressing on three sides to allow air to escape during expiration.
      c. Place client on *affected side* to diminish possibility of tension pneumothorax.
   2. Goal: *protect against injury during thoracentesis.*
      a. Provide sterile equipment.
      b. Explain procedure.
      c. Monitor vital signs for shock.
      d. Monitor for respiratory distress, mediastinal shift.
   3. Goal: *promote respirations.*
      a. *Position:* Fowler's.
      b. Oxygen therapy as ordered.
      c. Encourage slow breathing to improve gas exchange.
      d. Careful administration of narcotics to prevent respiratory depression (*avoid* morphine).
   4. Goal: *prepare client for closed chest drainage, physically and psychologically.*
      a. Explain purpose of the procedure—to provide means for evacuation of air and fluid from pleural cavity; to reestablish negative pressure in pleural space; to promote lung reexpansion.
      b. Explain procedure and apparatus (see chest tubes in **Table 11.11**).
      c. Cleanse skin at tube insertion site; place client in *sitting position,* ensuring safety by having locked over-bed table for client to lean on, or have a nurse stay with client so appropriate position is maintained throughout the procedure.
   5. Goal: *prevent complications with chest tubes.*
      a. Observe for and **immediately report:** crepitations (air under skin, also called *subcutaneous*

Adult

emphysema), labored or shallow breathing, tachypnea, cyanosis, tracheal deviation, or signs of hemorrhage.
b. Monitor for signs of infection.
c. Ensure that tubing stays intact.

▶
d. *Monitor proper tube function.* Attach chest tube to a water-sealed drainage apparatus and use wall suction for negative pressure. Monitor amount and color of tube drainage every 2 hr. Notify MD if bloody drainage exceeds 100 mL/hr. Chest drainage system should be at least 1 ft (30 cm) below the chest tube insertion site. Change dressing at tube insertion site every 48 hr. Air bubbles will continue in the water-seal chamber for 24–48 hr after insertion. Persistent air bubbles indicate an air leak between alveoli and pleural space. Fluctuation of fluid level is expected (when suction is off) because respiration changes the pleural pressure. If a clot forms in the tube, gently squeeze the tube, without occluding it, to move the clot, or follow specific orders as written. Make sure tube is free of kinks. When moving client, do *not* clamp tube; disconnect it from the wall suction. See key points for nursing intervention with chest tubes in Table 11.8.

e. Change position every 1 to 2 hr.
f. Arm and shoulder ROM.
6. Goal: *health teaching.*
a. How to prevent recurrence by avoiding overexertion; *avoid* holding breath.
b. Signs and symptoms of condition.
c. Methods to stop smoking.
d. Encourage follow-up care.

◆ F. **Evaluation/outcome criteria:**
1. No complications noted.
2. Closed system remains intact until chest tubes are removed.
3. Lung reexpands, breath sounds heard, pain diminished, symmetrical thoracic movements.

XII. **Hemothorax:** *presence of blood* in pleural cavity related to trauma or ruptured aortic aneurysm (see

XI. **Pneumothorax** for assessment, analysis/nursing diagnosis, nursing care plan/implementation, and evaluation/outcome criteria). **Table 7.18** compares pneumothorax and hemothorax.

XIII. **Chest trauma**
Flail chest: multiple rib fractures resulting in instability of the chest wall, with subsequent paradoxical breathing (portion of lung under injured chest wall moves in on inspiration while remaining lung expands; on expiration the injured portion of the chest wall expands while unaffected lung tissue contracts).
Sucking chest wound: penetrating wound of chest wall with hemothorax and pneumothorax, resulting in lung collapse and mediastinal shift toward unaffected lung.

◆ A. **Assessment:**
1. *Subjective data*
a. Severe, sudden, sharp pain.
b. Dyspnea.
c. Anxiety, restlessness, fear, weakness.
2. *Objective data*
a. *Vital signs:*
(1) *Pulse:* tachycardia, weak.
(2) *BP:* hypotension.
(3) *Respirations:* shallow, decreased expiratory force, tachypnea, stridor, accessory muscle breathing.
b. Skin color: cyanosis, pallor.
c. *Chest:*
(1) Asymmetrical chest expansion (*paradoxical movement*).
(2) Chest wound, rush of air through trauma site.
(3) Crepitus over trauma site (from air escaping into surrounding tissues).
(4) Lateral deviation of trachea, mediastinal shift.

d. Pneumothorax: documented by absence of breath sounds, x-ray examination.
e. Hemothorax: documented by needle aspiration by physician, x-ray examination.
f. Shock; blood and fluid loss.
g. Hemoptysis.
h. Distended neck veins.

TABLE 7.18	Comparison of Pneumothorax and Hemothorax	
	Pneumothorax (Free Air Between Visceral and Parietal Pleurae)	**Hemothorax (Blood in Pleural Space)**
Cause	*Spontaneous*—air enters without trauma; rupture of bleb (vesicle) on pleura; non–life threatening *Traumatic*—open chest wound: life threatening; closed chest wound—usually non–life threatening unless untreated *Tension*— air cannot escape via route of entry; causes atelectasis	Blunt trauma (assaults, falls) Penetrating trauma (knives, gunshot wounds)
◆ Assessment Findings	Minimal to sudden onset; sharp chest pain; dyspnea; cough; hypotension; tachypnea; tachycardia; mediastinal shift (tracheal deviation)	Asymptomatic or pleuritic pain and dyspnea; decreased or absent breath sounds; often discovered during chest x-ray; in severe cases: shock

◆ B. **Analysis/nursing diagnosis:**
1. *Ineffective airway clearance* related to shallow respirations.
2. *Impaired gas exchange* related to asymmetrical chest expansion.
3. *Pain* related to chest trauma.
4. *Fear* related to emergency situation.
5. *Risk for trauma* related to fractured ribs.
6. *Risk for infection* related to open chest wound.

◆ C. **Nursing care plan/implementation:**
1. Goal: *restore adequate ventilation and prevent further air from entering pleural cavity:* **MEDICAL EMERGENCY.**
   ▶ a. In emergency situation: place air-occlusive dressing or hand over open wound as client exhales forcefully against glottis (*Valsalva maneuver* helps expand collapsed lung by creating positive intrapulmonary pressures); or place client's weight onto *affected* side. Administer oxygen.
   ▶ b. Assist with endotracheal tube insertion; client will be placed on volume-controlled ventilator. (See discussion of ventilators under Oxygen Therapy, **Unit 11.**)
   ▶ c. Assist with thoracentesis and insertion of chest tubes with connection to water-seal drainage as ordered. (See Chest tubes section in **Table 11.11.**)
   d. Monitor vital signs to determine early shock.
   e. Monitor blood gases to determine early acid-base imbalances.
   f. Pain medications given with caution, so as not to depress respiratory center.

◆ D. **Evaluation/outcome criteria:**
1. Respiratory status stabilizes, lung reexpands.
2. Shock and hemorrhage are prevented.
3. No further damage done to surrounding tissues.
4. Pain is controlled.

XIV. **Thoracic surgery:** used for bronchogenic and lung carcinomas, lung abscesses, tuberculosis, bronchiectasis, emphysematous blebs, and benign tumors.
   A. **Types:**
   1. *Thoracotomy*—incision in the chest wall, pleura is entered, lung tissue examined, biopsy secured. *Chest tube is needed postoperatively.*
   2. *Lobectomy*—removal of a lobe of the lung. *Chest tube is needed postoperatively.*
   3. *Pneumonectomy*—removal of an entire lung. *No chest tube is needed postoperatively.*

◆ B. **Analysis/nursing diagnosis:**
1. *Risk for injury* related to chest wound.
2. *Impaired gas exchange* related to pain from surgical procedure.
3. *Ineffective airway clearance* related to decreased willingness to cough due to pain.
4. *Pain* related to surgical incision.
5. *Impaired physical mobility* related to large surgical incision and chest tube drainage apparatus.
6. *Knowledge deficit* (learning need) related to importance of coughing and deep breathing to prevent complications.

◆ C. **Nursing care plan/implementation:**
1. *Preoperative care.*
   a. Goal: *minimize pulmonary secretions.*
      (1) Humidify air to moisten secretions.
      ▶ (2) Use IPPB, as ordered, to improve ventilation.
      (3) Administer *bronchodilators, expectorants,* and *antibiotics* as ordered.
      ▶ (4) Use postural drainage, cupping, and vibration to mobilize secretions.
   b. Goal: *preoperative teaching.*
      (1) Teach client to cough against a closed glottis to increase intrapulmonary pressure for improved expiratory phase.
      ▶ (2) Instruct in diaphragmatic breathing and coughing.
      (3) Encourage to stop smoking.
      ▶ (4) Instruct and supervise practice of postoperative arm exercises—flexion, abduction, and rotation of shoulder—to prevent ankylosis.
      (5) Explain postoperative use of chest tubes, IV, and oxygen therapy.
2. *Postoperative care.*
   a. Goal: *maintain patent airway.*
      ▶ (1) Auscultate chest for breath sounds; report diminished or absent breath sounds on unaffected side (indicates decreased ventilation → respiratory embarrassment).
      (2) Turn, cough, and deep breathe, every 15 min to 1 hr first 24 hr and prn according to pulmonary congestion heard on auscultation.
   b. Goal: *promote gas exchange.*
      (1) Splint chest during coughing—support incision to help *cough up sputum (most important activity postoperatively).*
      (2) *Position:* high-Fowler's.
         (a) Turn client who has had a *pneumonectomy* to *operative* side (*avoid* extreme lateral positioning and mediastinal shift) to allow unaffected lung expansion and drainage of secretions; can also be turned onto back.
         (b) Client who has had a *lobectomy* or *thoracotomy* can be turned on *either* side or back because chest tubes will be in place.
   c. Goal: *reduce incisional stress and discomfort*—pad area around chest tube when turning on operative side to maintain tube patency and promote comfort.
   d. Goal: *prevent complications related to respiratory function.*
      ▶ (1) Maintain chest tubes to water-seal drainage system.

Adult

(2) See Chest tubes section in **Table 11.11.**

(3) Observe for mediastinal shift (trachea should always be midline; movement toward either side indicates shift).

(a) Move client onto back or toward opposite side.

(b) **MEDICAL EMERGENCY:** *Notify physician immediately.*

e. Goal: *maintain fluid and electrolyte balance.*

(1) Administer parenteral infusion *slowly* (risk of pulmonary edema due to decrease in pulmonary vasculature with removal of lung lobe or whole lung).

f. Goal: *postoperative teaching.*

(1) Prevent ankylosis of shoulder—teach passive and active ROM exercises of operative arm.

(2) Importance of early ambulation, as condition permits.

(3) Importance of stopping smoking.

(4) Dietary instructions—nutritious diet to aid in healing process.

(5) Importance of deep breathing, coughing exercises, to prevent stasis of respiratory secretions.

(6) Importance of *increased fluids* in diet to liquefy secretions.

(7) Desired and side effects of prescribed medications.

(8) Importance of rest, *avoidance* of heavy lifting and work during healing process.

(9) Importance of follow-up care; give names of referral agencies where client and family can obtain assistance.

(10) Signs and symptoms of complications.

D. Evaluation/outcome criteria:

1. Client or significant other or both will be able to:

a. Give rationale for activity restriction and demonstrate prescribed exercises.

b. Identify name, dosage, side effects, and schedule of prescribed medications.

c. State plans for necessary modifications in lifestyle, home.

d. Identify support systems.

2. Wound heals without complications.

3. Obtains ROM in affected shoulder.

4. No complications of thoracotomy:

> a. *Respiratory*—pulmonary insufficiency, respiratory acidosis, pneumonitis, atelectasis, pulmonary edema.
> b. *Circulatory*—hemorrhage, hypovolemia, shock, myocardial infarction.
> c. *Mediastinal shift.*
> d. *Renal failure.*
> e. *Gastric distention.*

XV. Tracheostomy: opening into trachea, temporary or permanent. *Rationale:* airway obstruction due to foreign body, edema, tumor, excessive tracheobronchial secretions, respiratory depression, decreased gaseous diffusion at alveolar membrane, increased dead space (e.g., severe emphysema), or failure to wean from mechanical ventilator.

A. Analysis/nursing diagnosis:

1. *Ineffective airway clearance* related to increased secretions and decreased ability to cough effectively.

2. *Ineffective breathing pattern* related to physical condition that necessitated tracheostomy.

3. *Impaired verbal communication* related to inability to speak when tracheostomy tube cuff inflated.

4. *Fear* related to need for specialized equipment to breathe.

B. Nursing care plan/implementation:

1. *Preoperative care:*

a. Goal: *relieve anxiety and fear.*

(1) Explain purpose of procedure and equipment.

(2) Demonstrate suctioning procedure.

(3) Establish means of postoperative communication (e.g., paper and pencil, "magic slate," picture cards, and call bell). Specialized tubes such as a fenestrated tracheostomy tube or a tracheostomy button allow the individual to talk when the external opening is plugged.

(4) Remain with client as much as possible.

2. *Postoperative care:*

a. Goal: *maintain patent airway* (**Table 7.19**).

b. Goal: *alleviate apprehension.*

(1) Remain with client as much as possible.

(2) Encourage client to communicate feelings using preestablished communication system.

c. Goal: *improve nutritional status.*

(1) Provide nutritious foods/liquids the client can swallow.

(2) Give supplemental drinks to maintain necessary calories.

d. Goal: *health teaching.*

(1) Explain all procedures.

(2) Teach alternative methods of communication (best if done before the tracheostomy if it is not an emergency situation).

(3) Teach self-care of tracheostomy as soon as possible.

C. Evaluation/outcome criteria:

1. Airway patent.

2. Acid-base balance maintained.

3. No respiratory infection/obstruction.

PROTECTIVE FUNCTIONS

I. Burns: wounds caused by exposure to excessive heat, chemicals, fire, steam, radiation, or electricity; most often related to carelessness or ignorance; 10,000 to 12,000 deaths annually; survival best at ages 15 to 30 yr and in burns covering less than 20% of total body surface.

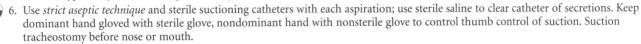

TABLE 7.19 ▶ Tracheostomy Suctioning Procedure

1. Suction as necessary to facilitate respirations. Explain to client what to expect.
2. *Position:* semi-Fowler's to prevent forward flexion of neck, to facilitate respiration, to promote drainage, and to minimize edema.
3. Administer *mist* to tracheostomy because natural humidifying of oropharynx pathways has been eliminated.
4. Auscultate for moist, noisy respirations because nonproductive coughing may indicate need for suctioning.
5. Prevent hypoxia by administering *100% oxygen before suctioning* (unless contraindicated).
6. Use *strict aseptic technique* and sterile suctioning catheters with each aspiration; use sterile saline to clear catheter of secretions. Keep dominant hand gloved with sterile glove, nondominant hand with nonsterile glove to control thumb control of suction. Suction tracheostomy before nose or mouth.
7. *Do not apply suction when inserting* suction catheter to prevent injury to respiratory tract and prevent loss of oxygen. Insert catheter about 5 in (12.5 cm).
8. If client coughs during suctioning, gently remove catheter to permit ejection and suction of mucus.
9. Apply suction intermittently for *no longer* than 5–10 sec because prolonged suction decreases arterial oxygen concentrations. Allow 2–3 min between attempts.
10. Cuff deflation: if high-volume, low-pressure cuffed tube is used, deflation not necessary. If other tracheostomy cuffed tube is used, deflate for 5 min every hour to prevent damage to trachea.
11. Use caution not to dislodge tube when changing dressing or ties that secure tube.

A. **Pathophysiology:**
1. *Emergent phase* (injury to 72 hr): shock due to pain, fright, or terror → fatigue, failure of vasoconstrictor mechanisms → hypotension. Capillary dilation, increased permeability → plasma loss to blisters, edema → hemoconcentration → hypovolemia → hypotension → decreased renal perfusion → potential shutdown.
2. *Acute phase* (3–5 days): interstitial to plasma fluid shift → hemodilution → hypervolemia → diuresis.

◆ B. **Assessment:**
1. *Subjective data:* how the burn occurred.
2. *Objective data:*
   a. Extent of body surface involved: *"rule of nines"*—head and both upper extremities, 9% each; front and back of trunk, 18% each; lower extremities, 18% each; and perineum, 1%. Requires adjustment for variation in size of head and lower extremities according to age.
   b. *Location*—facial, perineal, and hand and foot burns have potentially more complications because of poor vascularization.
   c. *Depth* of burn (**Table 7.20**):
      (1) *First degree (superficial)*—epidermal tissue only; not serious unless large areas involved.
      (2) *Second degree (shallow or deep partial thickness)*—epidermal and dermal tissue, hospitalization required if more than 10% of body surface involved (major burn).
      (3) *Third degree (full thickness)*—destruction of all skin layers; requires immediate hospitalization; involvement of 10% of body surface considered major burn.
      (4) *Fourth degree (deep penetrating)*—muscles (fascia), bone.
   d. Indications of airway burns (e.g., singed nasal hair, progressive hoarseness, sooty expectoration); edema may occur in 1 hr; increased mortality rate.

TABLE 7.20 Burn Characteristics According to Depth of Injury

Classification	Tissue Damage	Appearance	Pain	Clinical Course
Superficial (first degree)	Epidermis	Mild to fiery red erythema; no blisters	Very painful	Ordinarily heals in 3–7 days
Partial thickness; superficial or deep (second degree)	Epidermis and dermis	*Superficial:* mottled, moist, pink or red; may or may not blanch with pressure; usually blisters *Deep:* dry-white or deep red	*Superficial:* extreme pain and hypersensitivity to touch *Deep:* may or may not be painful	Healing takes 10–18 days; if infection develops in deep burn, it converts to full thickness burn *Deep:* often grafted
Full thickness (third degree)	All layers of skin and subcutaneous tissue	Charred, leathery or pale and dry	Usually absent	Heals only with grafting or scarring
*Fourth degree	All layers of skin, subcutaneous tissue, muscle, and bone	Black	Same as full thickness	Same as full thickness

*Used in some classification systems. May require several days after a severe burn to determine fourth degree.

e. Poorer prognosis—*infants*, due to immature immune system and effects of fluid loss; *elderly*, due to degenerative diseases and poor healing.

f. Medical history—presence of hypertension, diabetes, alcohol abuse, or chronic obstructive pulmonary disease increases complication rate.

◆ **C. Analysis/nursing diagnosis:**

1. *Impaired skin integrity* related to thermal injury.
2. *Pain* (depending on type of burn) related to exposure of sensory receptors.
3. *Fluid volume excess or deficit* related to hemodynamic changes.
4. *Risk for infection* related to destruction of protective skin.
5. *Impaired gas exchange* related to airway injury.
6. *Body image disturbance* related to scarring, disfigurement.
7. *Ineffective individual or family* coping related to traumatic experience.

◆ **D. Nursing care plan/implementation:**

1. Goal: *alleviate pain, relieve shock, and maintain fluid and electrolyte balance.*

    a. Medications: give *opioid analgesic* and *anxiolytics* incrementally.

    b. *Fluids:* IV therapy (see **Unit 11**); colloids, crystalloids, or 5% dextrose according to burn formula.

    c. Monitor hydration status:

    ▶ (1) Insert indwelling catheter.
    (2) Note color, odor, and amount of urine hourly.
    (3) *Strict* intake and output; hourly for 36 hr with large burns.
    (4) Check hematocrit. [normal: men > 40%; women > 37%] *Increased* Hct with intravascular fluid depletion.
    (5) Weigh daily.

2. Goal: *prevent physical complications.*

    ▶ a. *Vital signs:* hourly; central venous pressure (CVP) for signs of shock or fluid overload with clients who are at-risk.

    b. Assess respiratory function (particularly with head, neck burns); patent airway; breath sounds.

    c. Give medications as ordered—*tetanus booster; antibiotics* to treat documented infection; *sedatives* and *analgesics; antipyretics*—**avoid** aspirin; H$_2$ blockers.

    d. *Isolation:* protective; contact isolation (handwashing, protective clothing).

    e. *Positioning:* turn q2h; prevent contractures.
    (1) *Head and neck burns*—use pillows under shoulders only for hyperextension of neck.
    (2) *Hand burns*—splints.
    (3) *Arm and hand burns*—keep arms at 90-degree angle from body and slightly above shoulders.
    (4) *Ankle and foot burns*—splints; elevate to prevent edema.

    (5) Splints to maintain functional positions.
    (6) ROM exercises according to therapy guidelines; usually several times per day; active exercises most beneficial.

    f. *Diet:* begin oral fluids at once; food as tolerated—*high* protein, *high* calorie for energy and tissue repair (promote positive nitrogen balance); enteral feedings if protein and calorie goals not met.

    g. Observe for: constriction (circumferential or chest wall burns); check peak inspiratory pressure in client who is intubated—report increased pressure; check pulses in burned extremities every 1 to 2 hr for 24 hr—report loss of pulses.

3. Goal: *promote emotional adjustment and provide supportive therapy.*

    a. Care by same personnel as much as possible, to develop rapport and trust.

    b. Involve client in care plans.

    c. Answer questions clearly, accurately.

    d. Encourage family involvement and participation.

    e. Provide diversional activities and change furnishings or room adornments when possible, to prevent perceptual deprivation related to immobility.

    f. Point out signs of progress (e.g., decreased edema, healing) because client and family tend to become discouraged and cannot see progress.

    g. Encourage self-care to highest level tolerated.

    h. Anticipate psychological changes:
    (1) *Acute period*—severe anxiety: medicate with *anxiolytics* as ordered; maintain eye contact; explain procedures.
    (2) *Intermediate period*—reactions associated with pain, dependency, depression, anger; give medications to decrease pain; explain procedures; have open, nonjudgmental attitude; use consistent approaches to care; contract with client regarding division of responsibilities; encourage self-care.
    (3) *Recuperative period*—grief process reactivated. Anxiety, depression, anger, bargaining, as client tries to cope with altered body image, leaving security of hospital, finances. Encourage verbalization; refer to support group to assist adaptation.

4. Goal: *promote wound healing*—wound care:

    a. *Open method*—exposure of burns to air; useful in burns of face; thin layer (2–4 mm) topical *antimicrobial* ointment applied.

    b. *Closed method*—dressings applied to burned areas, changed 1 to 3 times/day; give PO pain medication 30 min before change; IV pain medication during dressing change; tubbing facilitates removal.

    c. *Multiple dressing change*—common approach; dressings changed bid to q4h depending on wound condition.

TABLE 7.21	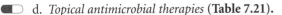 Topical Antimicrobials Used in Burn Care		
Agent	**Advantages**	**Disadvantages**	▶ **Nursing Implications**
Silver sulfadiazine 1% (Silvadene)	Broad-spectrum antimicrobial Antifungal Nonstaining Relatively painless No systemic metabolic abnormalities	Less eschar penetration than mafenide acetate (Sulfamylon) Decreased granulocyte formation; transient leukopenia Macular rash	Check for allergy to sulfa
Mafenide acetate (Sulfamylon) cream or solution	Eschar penetration Effective with *Pseudomonas* Topical of choice for electrical burns Suitable for open or closed method of treatment (cream) Used for gram-negative organisms	Severe pain and burning sensation (lasts 30 min) Metabolic acidosis Carbonic anhydrase inhibitor Ineffective against fungi May cause hypersensitivity rash	Administer pretreatment analgesic Monitor for metabolic acidosis and hyperventilation Check for allergy to sulfa; observe for rash
Silver nitrate	Low cost Broad spectrum Effective with *Candida*	Continuous wet soaks Superficial penetration Black staining of sheets Stinging Electrolyte imbalances (low sodium, low chloride, low calcium, low potassium), alkalosis	Check serum electrolytes daily Rewet dressing to keep moist
Petroleum and mineral oil-based (e.g., Bacitracin, Neosporin, Polysporin)	Bactericidal, gram-positive and gram-negative organisms Painless Prevents drying of wound	Limited ability to penetrate eschar	Apply in thin layer (1mm) Reapply as needed.

d. *Topical antimicrobial therapies* (**Table 7.21**).

e. *Tubbing and debridement.*

(1) Hydrotherapy—body temperature bath water; loosens dressings so some float off; soak 20 to 30 min; encourage limb exercises; do *not* leave unattended; loss of body heat may occur, with chilling and poor perfusion resulting.

(2) Removal of eschar (*débridement*)—done with forceps and curved scissors; medicate for pain before; use *sterile technique;* only loose eschar removed, to prevent bleeding; examine wound for infection, color change, decreased granulation—report changes **immediately.** Chemical debridement also done; agent digests necrotic tissue.

f. Wound coverage, to decrease chances of infection:

(1) Temporary and semipermanent wound coverings (**Table 7.22**).

(2) *Autograft*—client donates skin for wound coverage

(a) Types—free grafts (unattached to donor site) and pedicle grafts (attached to donor site).

(b) Procedure—general anesthesia; donor sites shaved and prepared; graft applied to granulation bed; face, hands, and arms grafted first.

(c) *Post–skin-graft care:*

(i) Sheet grafts: roll cotton-tipped applicator over graft to remove excess exudate; maintain dressings; *aseptic technique;* mesh grafts: irrigate as ordered.

(ii) Third to fifth day—graft takes on pink appearance if it has taken.

(iii) Padding, then splints applied to immobilize grafted extremities.

(iv) Pressure garments worn up to 18 months to decrease hypertrophic scarring.

5. Goal: *health teaching.*

a. Mobility needs: exercise; physical therapy; splints, braces.

b. Community resources: mental health practitioner or psychotherapist if needed for problems with self-image or sexual role; referrals as needed.

c. Techniques to camouflage appearance: slacks, turtlenecks, long sleeves, wigs, makeup.

◆ **E. Evaluation/outcome criteria:**

1. Return of vital signs to preburn levels.

2. Minimal to no hypertrophic scarring.

3. Free of infection; demonstrates wound care.

4. Maintains functional mobility of limbs; no contractures.

5. Adjusts to changes in body image; no depression.

TABLE 7.22	Wound Coverings			
Example	**Advantages**	**Disadvantages**	▶ **Nursing Implication**	
Biological				
Xenograph	Promotes healing of clean wound; relieves pain; readily available; reduces water and heat loss	Easily digested by wound collagenase; allergic reactions	Overlap edges slightly; trim away when skin underneath has healed	
Homograft-cadaver skin	Reduces water and heat loss; relieves pain; used with antimicrobial mesh; may be left in place until rejection occurs	May harbor disease	Observe for signs of infection	
Amnion	Relieves pain; reduces water and heat loss; has bacteriostatic properties	Limited shelf life; requires special preparation for use; may harbor diseases	Change cover dressing q48h; leave on wound until it sloughs	
Biosynthetic (Temporary)				
Biobrane	Protects from microbial penetration; decreases pain; promotes healing in partial-thickness burn	Not effective for preparing a granulation bed	Must be secured to skin with sutures, closure straps, tape, or staples; wrap with gauze; after 48 hr, check for adherence; once adherence has occurred, may be left open to air; check for signs of infection	
Biosynthetic (Semipermanent)				
Integra Artificial Skin	Postexcisional treatment of life-threatening full or deep partial-thickness burns when autograft not available	Infection rate lower than autograft	Maintain integrity of covering; 18–20 days before thin autograft applied. *Avoid* hydrotherapy; observe for infection.	

6. Regains independence; returns to work, social activities.

II. Rheumatoid arthritis:
chronic, systemic, collagen, inflammatory disease; etiology unknown; may be autoimmune, viral, or genetic; affects primarily women age 20 to 40 yr; present in 2% to 3% of total population; follows a course of exacerbations and remissions.

A. Pathophysiology: synovitis with edema → proliferation of various blood material (formation of pannus) → destruction and fibrosis of cartilage (fibrous ankylosis); calcification of fibrous tissue (osseous ankylosis) **(Figure 7.7).**

◆ **B. Assessment:**
1. *Subjective data:*
   a. Joints: pain; morning stiffness; swelling.
   b. Easily fatigues; malaise.
   c. Anorexia; weight loss.
2. *Objective data:*
   a. Subcutaneous nodules over bony prominences.
   b. Bilateral symmetrical involvement of joints: crepitation, creaking, grating.
   c. Deformities: contractures, muscle atrophy.
   d. Lab data: blood: *decreased*—hemoglobin/hematocrit; RBCs;
   increased—WBCs (12,000– 15,000), sedimentation rate (>20 mm/hr), rheumatoid factor.

◆ **C. Analysis/nursing diagnosis:**
1. *Pain* related to joint destruction.
2. *Impaired physical mobility* related to joint contractures.
3. *Risk for injury* related to the inflammatory process.
4. *Body image disturbance* related to joint deformity.
5. *Self-care deficit* related to musculoskeletal impairment.
6. *Risk for activity intolerance* related to fatigue and stiffness.
7. *Altered nutrition, less than body requirements,* related to anorexia and weight loss.
8. *Self-esteem disturbance* related to chronic illness.

◆ **D. Nursing care plan/implementation:**
1. Goal: *prevent or correct deformities.*
   a. Activity:
      (1) Bedrest during exacerbations.
   ▶ (2) Daily ROM—active and passive exercises *even* in acute phase 5 to 10 min periods; *avoid* fatigue and persistent pain.
      (3) Heat or pain medication before exercise.
   b. Medications: *aspirin* (high dosages); *nonsteroidals; steroids; antacids* given for possible GI upset with ASA, steroids; *disease-modifying antirheumatics* (methotrexate, hydroxychloroquine, sulfasalazine).
   c. *Fluids:* at least 1500 mL liquid daily to avoid renal calculi; milk for GI upset.

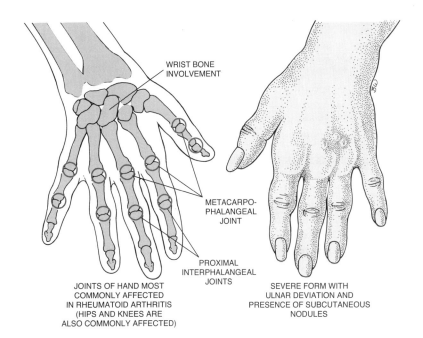

WRIST BONE
INVOLVEMENT

METACARPO-
PHALANGEAL
JOINT

PROXIMAL
INTERPHALANGEAL
JOINTS

JOINTS OF HAND MOST
COMMONLY AFFECTED
IN RHEUMATOID ARTHRITIS
(HIPS AND KNEES ARE
ALSO COMMONLY AFFECTED)

SEVERE FORM WITH
ULNAR DEVIATION AND
PRESENCE OF SUBCUTANEOUS
NODULES

FIGURE 7.7   Rheumatoid arthritis.
(From Venes, D [ed]: Taber's Cyclopedic
Medical Dictionary, ed. 20. FA Davis,
Philadelphia, 2005.)

2. Goal: *health teaching.*
   a. Side effects of medications: tarry stools (GI bleeding); tinnitus (ASA).
   b. Psychosocial aspects: possible need for early retirement; financial hardship; loss of libido; unsatisfactory sexual relations.
   c. Prepare for joint repair or replacement if indicated.

◆ **E. Evaluation/outcome criteria:**
   1. Remains as active as possible; limited loss of mobility; performs self-care activities.
   2. No side effects from drug therapy (e.g., GI bleeding).
   3. Copes with necessary lifestyle changes; complies with treatment regimen.

III. Lupus erythematosus: chronic inflammatory disease of connective tissue; may affect or involve any organ; vague etiology, but genetic factors, viruses, hormones, and drugs are being investigated; occurs primarily in women ages 18 to 35 yr. Two forms: discoid lupus erythematosus (DLE) affects skin only, and systemic lupus erythematosus (SLE) affects multiple organs.

A. Pathophysiology: possible toxic effects from immune complexes deposited in tissue (antibody-antigen trapping in organ capillaries)—fibrinoid necrosis of collagen in connective issue, small arterial walls (kidneys and heart particularly) → cellular death, obstructed blood flow.

◆ **B. Assessment:**
   1. *Subjective data:*
      a. Pain: joints.
      b. Anorexia; weight loss.
      c. Photophobia; sensitivity to sun.
      d. Weakness.
      e. Nausea, vomiting.

2. *Objective data:*
   a. Fever.
   b. Rash: butterfly distribution across nose, cheeks.
   c. Lesions: raised, red, scaling plaques—coinlike (discoid).
   d. Ulceration: oral or nasopharyngeal.

   e. Lab data:
      (1) Blood: *increased* LE cells; *decreased*—RBCs, WBCs, thrombocytes.
      (2) *Urine*—hematuria, proteinuria (nephritis).

◆ **C. Analysis/nursing diagnosis:**
   1. *Risk for injury* related to possible autoimmune disorder.
   2. *Pain* related to joint inflammation.
   3. *Risk for activity intolerance* related to extreme fatigue, anemia.
   4. *Body image disturbance* related to chronic skin eruptions.
   5. *Altered nutrition, less than body requirements,* related to anorexia, nausea, vomiting.
   6. *Altered oral mucous membrane* related to ulcerations.

◆ **D. Nursing care plan/implementation:**
   1. Goal: *minimize or limit immune response and complications.*
      a. Activity: rest; 8 to 10 hr sleep; unhurried environment; assist with stressful activities; ROM to prevent joint immobility and stiffness.
      b. Skin care: hygiene; *topical steroid* cream as ordered for inflammation, pruritus, scaling.
      c. Mouth care: several times daily if stomatitis present; *soft, bland, or liquid diet* to prevent irritation.
      d. *Diet:* low sodium if edematous; *low* protein with renal involvement.

e. Observe for signs of complications:
   (1) *Cardiac/respiratory* (tachycardia, tachypnea, dyspnea, orthopnea).
   (2) *GI* (diarrhea, abdominal pain, distention).
   (3) *Renal* (increased weight, oliguria, *decreased* specific gravity).
   (4) *Neurological* (ptosis, ataxia).
   (5) *Hematological* (malaise, weakness, chills, epistaxis); **report immediately.**

f. Medications, as ordered:
   (1) *Analgesics.*
   (2) *Antiinflammatory* agents (aspirin, prednisone) and *immunosuppressive drugs* (azathioprine [Imuran], cyclophosphamide [Cytoxan]) to control inflammation.
   (3) *Antimalarials* for skin and joint manifestations.

2. Goal: *health teaching.*
   a. Disease process: diagnosis, prognosis, effects of treatment.
   b. *Avoid* precipitating factors:
      (1) Sun (aggravates skin lesions; thus, cover body as much as possible).
      (2) Altering dosage of medications.
      (3) Pregnancy (requires medical clearance).
      (4) Fatigue, stress.
      (5) Infections.
   c. Medications: side effects of immunosuppressives and corticosteroids.
   d. Regular exercise: walking, swimming; but *avoid* fatigue.
   e. Wear MedicAlert bracelet.

◆ **E. Evaluation/outcome criteria:**
   1. Attains a state of remission.
   2. No organ involvement (e.g., no cardiac, renal complications).
   3. Keeps active within limitations.
   4. Continues follow-up medical care—recognizes symptoms requiring immediate attention.

Infectious Diseases

I. **Lyme disease:** a spirochetal illness (syndrome); most common tick-borne infectious disease in United States; prevalent Northeast, upper Midwest, and coastal northern California. Reporting is mandatory. With *early* treatment, recovery is usually quick and complete.
   A. Stages:
   1. *Stage I.* Rash (erythema migrans) at site of tick bite; bull's-eye or target pattern; may appear as hives or cellulitis; common in moist areas (groin, armpit, behind knees). Flulike symptoms may occur (joint pain, chills, fever).
   2. *Stage II.* If untreated, may progress to cardiac problems (10% of clients) or neurological disturbances—Bell's palsy (10% of clients); occasionally meningitis, encephalitis, and eye damage may result.
   3. *Stage III.* From 4 wk to 1 yr after the tick bite, "arthritis," primarily large joint, develops in half

the clients. If untreated, chronic neurological problems may develop.

◆ **B. Assessment** (depends on stage): History is important—where do they live or work? Recent travel? Outdoor activities (gardening, hiking, camping, clearing brush)? Knowledge of tick bite and how removed? Pets?
   1. *Subjective data:*
      a. Malaise (stage I).
      b. Headache (stage I).
      c. Joint, neck, or back pain (stages I and III).
      d. Weakness (stages II and III).
      e. Chest pain (stage II).
      f. Light-headedness (stage II).
      g. Numbness, pain in arms or legs (stage III).
   2. *Objective data:*
      a. Rash—erythema migrans (stage I); at least 5 cm/lesion.
      b. Dysrhythmias; heart block (stage II).
      c. Facial paralysis (stage II).
      d. Conjunctivitis, iritis, optic neuritis (stage II).
      e. Lab data: Lyme titer—*elevated* (stages II and III). Often inconclusive.

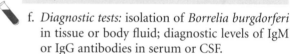

   f. *Diagnostic tests:* isolation of *Borrelia burgdorferi* in tissue or body fluid; diagnostic levels of IgM or IgG antibodies in serum or CSF.

◆ **C. Analysis/nursing diagnosis:**
   1. *Anxiety* related to diagnosis.
   2. *Pain* related to joint inflammation.
   3. *Fatigue* related to viral illness.
   4. *Impaired physical mobility* related to joint pain.
   5. *Altered thought processes* related to neurological deficit.
   6. *Decreased cardiac output* related to dysrhythmias.
   7. *Knowledge deficit* (learning need) related to treatment and course of disease.

◆ **D. Nursing care plan/implementation:**
   1. Goal: *minimize irreversible tissue damage and complications.*
      a. Medications according to presenting symptoms: *stage I—oral antibiotics* for 21 days (doxycycline, amoxicillin, cefotaxime); *stages II and III—oral* (see stage I) or *intravenous antibiotics* for 21 to 28 days (ceftriaxone).
      b. If hospitalized, monitor vital signs q4h for increased temperature, signs of heart failure; check level of consciousness and cranial nerve functioning.
      c. Note treatment response: worsening of symptoms during first 24 hr: redder rash, higher fever, greater pain (*Jarisch-Herxheimer reaction*).
   2. Goal: *alleviate pain, promote comfort.*
      a. Medications: *salicylates, nonsteroidal antiinflammatory agents,* or other *analgesic,* as ordered; observe for side effects (GI irritation).
      b. Rest: give instructions on relaxation techniques; create a quiet environment.
   3. Goal: *maintain physical and psychological well-being.*

a. Activity: ROM at regular intervals; *medicate for pain* before exercise; encourage proper posture to reduce joint stress; rest periods between activities and treatments.

b. Referral: occupational or physical therapy as appropriate.

c. Reassurance: give psychological support; encourage discussion of feelings.

4. Goal: *health teaching.*

a. Information on disease. Transmission from tick not likely if removed before 48 hours of attachment.

b. Instructions for home IV antibiotics with heparin lock, if ordered.

c. Side effects of antibiotics (drug specific); importance of completing therapy.

d. Signs of disease recurrence (later stages of disease: less severe attacks).

e. Preventing subsequent infections: wear proper clothing and tick repellent on clothing (20%–30% DEET); conduct "tick checks" of self, children, and pets; proper tick removal (use tweezers, steady, gentle traction).

f. Start vaccination series (LYMErix); three injections at 0, 1, and 12 months.

◆ E. **Evaluation/outcome criteria:**

1. Achieves reasonable comfort.

2. Regains normal physiological and psychological functioning—no irreversible complications; vital signs within normal limits.

3. Resumes previous activity level; returns to work.

4. Adheres to follow-up care recommendations.

5. Knows ways to minimize risk of reinfection.

II. **Acquired immunodeficiency syndrome (AIDS):** the terminal stage of the disease continuum caused by human immunodeficiency virus (HIV), a retrovirus; typically progresses from asymptomatic seronegative status to asymptomatic seropositive status to subclinical immune deficiency to lymphadenopathy (early AIDS) to AIDS-related complex (middle stage with combination of symptoms) to AIDS; hallmarks of HIV infection include opportunistic infections: *Pneumocystis carinii* pneumonia (PCP); cytomegalovirus (CMV); *Mycobacterium tuberculosis;* hepatitis B; herpes simplex or zoster; candidiasis; may take 7 to 10 yr before signs and symptoms occur.

A. **High-risk populations:**

1. Men, homosexual or bisexual (71%).

2. Injection drug users (IDU)/heterosexual (10%).

3. IDU/homosexual (9%).

4. People who have hemophilia and are recipients of multiple transfusion (1%).

5. Heterosexual (5%).

6. Undetermined/other (4%).

B. **Pathophysiology:** abnormal response to foreign antigen stimulation (acquired immunity) → deficiency in cell-mediated immunity—T lymphocytes, specifically helper cells (T4 cells) and hyperactivity of the humoral system (B cells).

◆ C. **Assessment:**

1. *Subjective data:*

a. Fatigue: prolonged; associated with headache or light-headedness.

b. Unexplained weight loss: >10%.

2. *Objective data:*

a. Fever: prolonged or night sweats >2 wk.

b. Lymphadenopathy.

c. Skin or mucous membrane lesions: purplish-red, nodules *(Kaposi's sarcoma).*

d. Cough: persistent, heavy, dry.

e. Diarrhea: persistent.

f. Tongue/mouth "thrush"; oral hairy leukoplakia.

g. *Diagnostic tests* (with permission of client): enzyme-linked immunosorbent assay (ELISA); Western blot test.

h. Lab data: *decreased*—CD4 (T4) lymphocytes, hematocrit, WBC, platelets. *Seropositive*—syphilis, hepatitis B; ELISA—*positive;* Western blot test—*positive* (mean time for seroconversion is 6 wk after infection).

◆ D. **Analysis/nursing diagnosis:**

1. *Risk for infection* related to immunocompromised state.

2. *Fatigue* related to anemia.

3. *Altered nutrition, less than body requirements,* related to anorexia.

4. *Impaired skin integrity* related to nonhealing viral lesions, Kaposi's sarcoma.

5. *Diarrhea* related to infection or parasites.

6. *Risk for activity* intolerance related to shortness of breath.

7. *Ineffective airway clearance* related to pneumonia.

8. *Visual sensory/perception alteration* related to retinitis.

9. *Risk for altered body temperature* (fever) related to opportunistic infections.

10. *Social isolation* related to stigma attached to AIDS.

11. *Powerlessness* related to inability to control disease progression.

12. *Altered thought processes* related to dementia.

13. *Ineffective individual coping* related to poor prognosis.

14. *Risk for violence, self-directed,* related to anger, panic, or depression.

◆ E. **Nursing care plan/implementation:**

1. Goal: *reduce risk of infection; slow disease progression.*

a. Observe signs of opportunistic infections: weight loss, diarrhea, skin lesions, sore throat.

b. Monitor vital signs (including temperature).

c. Note secretions and excretions: changes in color, consistency, or odor indicating infection.

d. *Diet:* monitor fluid and electrolytes; strict measurement; encourage adequate dietary intake (*high* calorie, *high* protein, *low* bulk); 5 to 10 times RDA for water-soluble vitamins (B complex, C); favorite foods from home; enteral feedings. Six small meals/day.

Adult

e. *Protective isolation,* if indicated, for severe immunocompromise.

f. Antiviral medications, as ordered: nucleoside reverse transcriptase inhibitors (e.g., zidovudine [Retrovir]); nonnucleoside reverse transcriptase inhibitors (e.g., nevirapine [Viramune]); protease inhibitors (e.g., indinavir sulfate [Crixivan]); drug toxicity and numerous side effects likely (rash, GI upset); large number of pills and tight administration schedule; costly; potential for drug resistance.

2. Goal: *prevent the spread of disease.*
   a. Frequent handwashing, even after wearing gloves.
   b. *Avoid* exposure to blood, body fluids of client; wear gloves, gowns; proper disposal of needles, IV catheters (**Table 7.23**).

3. Goal: *provide physical and psychological support.*
   a. Oral care: frequent.
   ▶ b. Cooling bath: 1:10 concentration of isopropyl alcohol with tepid water; *avoid* plastic-backed pads if client has night sweats.
   c. Encourage verbalization of fears, concerns without condemnation; may suffer loss of job, lifestyle, significant other.
   d. Determine status of support network: arrange contact with support group.
   e. Observe for severe emotional symptoms (suicidal tendencies).
   f. Address issues surrounding death to ensure quality of life: advance directive prepared and on file; code blue status; reassurance of comfort and pain control.

4. Goal: *health teaching.*
   a. *Avoidance* of environmental sources of infection (kitty litter, bird cages, tub bathing).
   b. Precautions following discharge: risk-reducing behaviors; condoms (latex), limit number of sexual partners, *avoid* exposure to blood or semen during intercourse.
   c. Family counseling; availability of community resources.
   d. Information on disease progression and life span.
   e. Stress-reduction techniques: visualization, guided imagery, meditation.

f. Expected side effects with drug therapy; importance of compliance.

◆ **F. Evaluation/outcome criteria:**
   1. Relief of symptoms (e.g., afebrile, gains weight).
   2. Resumes self-care activities; returns to work; improved quality of life.
   3. Accepts diagnosis; participates in support group.
   4. Progression of disease slows; improved survival probability.
   5. Retains autonomy, self-worth.
   6. Permitted to die with dignity.

III. Animal-borne diseases (Table 7.24).

IV. Bioterrorism (Table 7.25).

The Perioperative Experience

I. Preoperative preparation
   A. Assessment:
      1. *Subjective data:*
         a. Understanding of proposed surgery—site, type, extent of hospitalization.
         b. Previous experiences with hospitalization.
         c. Age-related factors.
         d. Allergies—iodine, latex, adhesive tape, cleansing solutions, medications.
         e. Medication/substance use—prescribed, OTC, smoking, alcohol, recreational drugs.
         f. Cultural and religious background.
         g. Concerns or feelings about surgery:
            (1) Exaggerated ideas of surgical risk (e.g., fear of colostomy when none is being considered).
            (2) Nature of anesthesia (e.g., fears of going to sleep and not waking up, saying or revealing things of a personal nature).
            (3) Degree of pain (e.g., may be incapacitating).
            (4) Misunderstandings regarding prognosis.
         h. Identification of significant others as a source of client support or care responsibilities postdischarge.
      2. *Objective data:*
         a. Speech patterns indicating anxiety— repetition, changing topics, avoiding talking about feelings.

TABLE 7.23 **Standard Precautions**

- **Wash your hands** and any other skin surfaces immediately and thoroughly if they become contaminated with blood or other body fluids. Use lots of soap and hot water.
- **Wear clean gloves** whenever there is potential exposure to blood or other body fluids except sweat. Wear surgical gloves for performing venipunctures, for touching mucous membranes or nonintact skin, or whenever there is a possibility of exposure to blood or body fluids. **Remove gloves** after contact with each client. **Discard used gloves** immediately after use in an appropriate receptacle (e.g., a plastic bag with a "biohazard" label). **Wash your hands** immediately after removing gloves.
- Use *mask, protective eyewear, face shield, gown* during any procedure that is likely to generate splashes of blood or other body fluids.
- Handle all **needles, intravenous equipment**, and **sharp instruments** with extreme care:
  1. *Never* recap, remove, bend, or break needles after use or manipulate them in any other way by hand.
  2. Dispose of syringes, needles, scalpel blades, and other sharp items in a puncture-resistant container kept within easy reach.

TABLE 7.24	Infectious Diseases: Animal-Borne			

Disease	Caused by	Onset	◆ Symptoms	Treatment
Avian influenza (bird flu) Highly infectious virus affecting millions of birds across Asia (especially Hong Kong, Thailand, Vietnam).	■ Poultry—birds excrete the virus → people inhale fecal dust ■ Human-to-human transmission rare	24–72 hr	■ Eye infection ■ Fever, sore throat, cough ■ In fatal cases: viral pneumonia, severe respiratory problems	▢ ■ Antiviral drug (Tamiflu, Relenza) ■ No vaccine
Lyme disease (see **p. 544**)				
Mad cow disease (bovine spongiform encephalopathy [BSE]) Causes **variant Creutzfeldt-Jakob disease (VCJD)**: a CNS degenerative brain disorder that has killed >100 in past decade, mostly in Britain.	■ Eating meat from cattle (brain, spinal cord, eyes, bone marrow, spleen), or eating contaminated tissue from cattle that ate these parts (have been fed offal)	5 or more years	■ ↓ memory ■ Speech abnormalities ■ Hallucinations ■ Incontinence ■ Difficulty in dressing	■ None ■ Fatal ■ Lasts for several months
Monkey pox Related to smallpox. Fatal in 10% of cases. Found in midwestern U.S. (Illinois, Indiana, Missouri, Wisconsin).	■ Animal bites by or bodily fluids from rats, mice, squirrels, prairie dogs, or imported west African rodent pets ■ *Can* be transmitted human-to-human	7–18 days	■ Lymph adenopathy ■ Fever ■ Headache ■ Fatigue ■ Rash → blisters over entire body	■ None
Rabies Viral disease. 7000 cases/yr in U.S.	■ Bite from infected cat, dog, or wild animal (raccoon, skunk, fox)	Within 24 hours	■ Fever ■ Hypersalivation ■ Dysphagia ■ Partial paralysis ■ Hallucinations ■ Excitation	■ *Postexposure prophylaxis* (PEP): immune globulin for 1 mo.; rabies vaccine ■ No effective therapy after symptoms appear
Salmonella Bacterial disease; kills approx. 1000/yr; 40,000 cases/yr.	■ Drinking contaminated water or eating contaminated chicken or eggs ■ Can be transmitted by reptiles (snakes, turtles, lizards), chicks, ducklings	Hours to 7 days	■ Severe diarrhea ■ Fever ■ Abdominal pain	■ No treatment, as resolved in 5 to 7 days ▢ ■ Antibiotics if infection spreads from intestines
Tularemia (see **IV. Bioterrorism**)				
West Nile virus Fatal in 10% of cases; first found in Uganda.	■ Mosquitoes	3–14 days	■ Flu-like (fever, headache, body aches)	■ IV fluids ■ Prevention of pneumonia as secondary infection

For more information, go to the CDC Web site: www.cdc.gov.

b. Interactions with others—withdrawn or involved.
c. Physical signs of anxiety (i.e., increased pulse, respirations; clammy palms, restlessness).
d. Baseline physiological status: vital signs; breath sounds; peripheral circulation; weight; hydration status (hematocrit, skin turgor, urine output); degree of mobility; muscle strength.

◆ **B. Analysis/nursing diagnosis:**
1. *Anxiety* related to proposed surgery.
2. *Knowledge deficit* (learning need) related to incomplete teaching or lack of understanding.
3. *Fear* related to threat of death or disfigurement.
4. *Risk for injury* related to surgical complications.

5. *Ineffective individual coping* related to anticipatory stress.

◆ **C. Nursing care plan/implementation:**
1. Goal: *reduce preoperative and intraoperative anxiety and prevent postoperative complications.*
    a. *Preoperative teaching:*
       (1) Provide information about hospital nursing routines and preoperative procedures to reduce fear of unknown.
       (2) Explain purpose of diagnostic procedures to enhance ability to cooperate and tolerate procedure.
       (3) Inform about what will occur and what will be expected in the postoperative period:

TABLE 7.25	Recognizing Bioterrorism Agents and Associated Syndromes			
Disease	**Pathophysiology**	**Transmission and Incubation**	◆ **Signs/Symptoms**	**Treatment**
Anthrax—Greek word for "coal" ■ **Cutaneous** ■ **GI** ■ **Inhaled** (most lethal)	■ Caused by *Bacillus anthracis*, a bacterium that is commonly found in grazing animals ■ Forms spores which live in soil for years ■ Man-made form more potent and resistant to treatment	■ Contact with spores through break in skin ■ Eating contaminated meat ■ Inhaling spores ■ *Not* spread from person to person ■ Incubation: 1 to 6 days (inhalation can take up to 42 days)	**Cutaneous:** Skin sores that turn black after a few days **GI:** Nausea, loss of appetite, bloody diarrhea, fever, followed by bad stomach pain **Inhaled:** Cold or flu-like symptoms; cough, fatigue, chest discomfort→ SOB→ severe pneumonia→ severe respiratory distress: diaphoresis, stridor, cyanosis, shock; death in 24 to 36 hours	■ Ciprofloxacin or doxycycline plus one or two additional *antimicrobials* (e.g., rifampin, vancomycin, penicillin, ampicillin, clindamycin [60-day treatment]) ■ Isolation not required ■ Standard precautions
Botulism—a neuroparalytic illness	■ A potent neurotoxin produced from *Clostridium botulinum*, an anaerobic, spore-forming bacterium ■ Characterized by: symmetrical, descending flaccid paralysis of motor and autonomic nerves ■ **Always** begins with cranial nerves	■ Foodborne; ingestion of toxin produced in food (home-canned is most frequent) ■ Fatal in 5% of cases	**Vision:** double, blurred **Eyelids:** drooping **Speech:** slurred **Mouth:** dry **Muscles:** weakness, symmetric flaccid paralysis **Swallowing:** dysphagia If untreated, → descending paralysis of respiratory muscles, arms and legs; death from respiratory failure	■ Botulinum antitoxin from CDC ■ If survive, have SOB and fatigue for years
Plague ■ **Pneumonic** ■ **Bubonic** ■ **Septicemic**	■ Caused by bacterium *Yersinia pestis* (*Y. pestis*); found in rodents and their fleas ■ Easily destroyed by sunlight and drying ■ Will survive up to 1 hr	**Pneumonic:** ■ Infects lungs ■ Airborne transmission ■ Spreads person to person **Bubonic:** ■ Most common form ■ Infected flea bites the skin ■ Does *not* spread person to person **Septicemic:** ■ Often complication of pneumonic or bubonic ■ Does *not* spread from person to person	**Pneumonic:** Fever Headache Weakness Signs of pneumonia for 2 to 4 days (SOB, chest pain, cough, bloody or watery sputum)→ respiratory failure→ shock **Bubonic:** Swollen lymph glands (buboes) Fever Headache Chills Weakness **Septicemic:** Fever Chills Prostration Abdominal pain Shock Bleeding into skin and organs	■ Give *antibiotics within 24 hr* of symptoms—streptomycin, gentamicin, tetracyclines, chloramphenicol ■ Prophylactic antibiotics for 7 days ■ Close-fitting surgical mask to protect against infection

Disease	Description	Transmission	Signs and Symptoms	Treatment
Smallpox—Latin word for "spotted" ■ **Variola major** (severe and most common) ■ **Variola minor**	■ An acute contagious disease caused by variola virus (a member of the orthopoxvirus family)	■ Aerosolized; droplets ■ Direct face-to-face, prolonged contact ■ Incubation: 7 to 21 days—not contagious at this time ■ Lethal in 20%–40% of cases if unvaccinated	*Prodrome* 2 to 4 days (sometimes contagious): flu-like—malaise, fever (101°–104°F), headache, body aches, sometimes vomiting *Early rash* about 4 days (most contagious): small red spots on tongue and mouth; erythema spreads from face/arms to legs, then centrally *Pustular rash:* macules (bellybutton center) → papules → pustular vesicles → scabs	■ No specific treatment ■ Smallpox vaccine effective if given within 3d of exposure ■ Cidofovir possibly effective ■ Ribavirin ■ Victim of attack should be undressed, shower with soap ■ For visible contamination, use 0.5% diluted household bleach
Tuleremia ("rabbit fever")	■ A bacterial zoonosis ■ Caused by *Francisella tularensis*, one of the most infectious pathogenic bacteria ■ Survives for weeks at low temperatures in: *water*, moist soil, hay, straw, and decaying animal carcasses	■ Infects humans through: skin, mucous membranes, GI tract, and lungs ■ Abrupt onset ■ Lower fatality rate than plague or anthrax ■ Aerosol release would be likely in terrorist attack ■ Incubation: 1 to 14 days ■ *Not* transmitted person to person	Skin and oral ulcers Fever (sudden) Headache Chills Rigor Generalized body aches (low back) Coryza Sore throat, dry or slightly productive cough Substernal pain or tightness Atypical *pneumonia* *Pleuritis* Hilar lymphadenopathy	Meds: ■ Streptomycin (drug of choice) ■ Gentamicin (an alternative) ■ Doxycycline and ciprofloxacin in mass casualty ■ Isolation not recommended ■ In hospitals, standard precautions are recommended
Viral hemorrhagic fever (multisystem syndrome) ■ **Ebola** (severe, often fatal) ■ **Lassa** ■ **Hantavirus pulmonary syndrome**	■ Four distinct RNA viruses: arenaviruses, filoviruses, bunyaviruses, and flaviviruses ■ Often animal or insect host, except for *Ebola* (host unknown) ■ Damaged vascular system → bleeding	■ Infected host or vector initially transmits to human; then human to human with **Ebola** or **Lassa**. ***Ebola:*** ■ 2 to 21 days; abrupt onset ***Lassa:*** ■ Spread through contact with body fluids ■ 1 to 3 wks ***Hantavirus:*** ■ Carried by rodents (mice) ■ Aerosolization of virus shed in urine, droppings and saliva ■ *No* person-to-person transmission ■ 1 to 5 wks after exposure	**VHF:** marked fever, fatigue, dizziness, muscle aches, loss of strength, exhaustion. Bleeding: under skin, organs, mouth, eyes, ears (rarely fatal) ***Ebola:*** fever, headache, red eyes, hiccups, joint/muscle aches, sore throat → diarrhea, vomiting, stomach pain ***Lassa:*** 80% may have no symptoms or mild. May be varied; fever, retrosternal pain, sore throat, back pain, cough, abdominal pain, vomiting, diarrhea, conjunctivitis, facial bleeding ***Hantavirus:*** *Early*—fatigue, fever, muscle aches, headache, nausea, vomiting, abdominal pain *Late*—4 to 10 days; cough, SOB, chest tightness, feeling of suffocation	***Ebola:*** ■ Supportive therapy—fluids, electrolytes, O_2 ***Lassa:*** ■ Ribavirin ■ Supportive care ***Hantavirus:*** ■ No specific cure ■ Early admission to ICU—intubation and ventilator support

For more information see www.bioterrorism.uab.edu

Adult

549

      (a) Will return to room, postanesthesia care unit, or intensive care unit.

      (b) Special equipment—monitors, tubes, suction equipment.

      (c) Pain control methods.

  b. *Management of latex allergy if present.* Three forms: *immediate reaction* (most serious, life threatening)—flushing, diaphoresis, pruritus, nausea, vomiting, cramping, hypotension, dyspnea; *delayed response* (most common, discomfort)—localized symptoms 18 to 24 hr after contact; and *contact dermatitis.* Exposure to latex through skin, mucous membranes, inhalation, internal tissue, and intravascular; sources include: gloves, anesthesia masks, tourniquets, ECG electrodes, adhesive tape, warming blankets, elastic bandages, tubes/catheters, irrigation syringes. **Nursing goal:** provide latex-free environment.

2. Goal: *instruct in exercises to reduce complications.*

  ▶ a. *Diaphragmatic breathing*—refers to flattening of diaphragm during inspiration, which results in enlargement of upper abdomen; during expiration the abdominal muscles are contracted, along with the diaphragm.

> (1) The client should be in a *flat, semi-Fowler's,* or *side position,* with knees flexed and hands on the midabdomen.
>
> (2) Have the client take a deep breath through nose and mouth, letting the abdomen rise. Hold breath 3 to 5 seconds.
>
> (3) Have client exhale through nose and mouth, squeezing out all air by contracting the abdominal muscles.
>
> (4) Repeat 10 to 15 times, with a short rest after each five to prevent hyperventilation.
>
> (5) Inform client that this exercise will be repeated 5 to 10 times every hour postoperatively.

  ▶ b. *Coughing*—helps clear chest of secretions and, although uncomfortable, will not harm incision site.

> (1) Have client lean forward slightly from a sitting position, and place client's hands over incisional site; this acts as a splint during coughing.
>
> (2) Have client inhale and exhale slowly several times.
>
> (3) Have client inhale deeply, hold breath 3 seconds, and cough sharply three times while exhaling—client's mouth should be slightly open.
>
> (4) Tell client to inhale again and to cough deeply once or twice. If unable to cough deeply, client should "huff" cough to stimulate cough.

  c. *Turning and leg exercises*—help prevent circulatory stasis, which may lead to thrombus formation, and postoperative flatus or "gas pains," as well as respiratory problems.

> (1) Tell client to turn on one side with uppermost leg flexed; use side rails to facilitate the movement.
>
> (2) In a supine position, have client do five repetitions every hour of: ankle pumps, quad sets, gluteal tightenings, and straight-leg raises.
>
> (3) Apply intermittent pulsatile compression device or sequential compression device to promote venous return.

3. Goal: *reduce the number of bacteria on the skin to eliminate incision contamination.* **Skin preparation:**

> a. Prepare area of skin wider and longer than proposed incision in case a larger incision is necessary.
>
> b. Gently scrub with an *antimicrobial* agent.
>
>   (1) Note possibility of allergy to iodine.
>
>   (2) Hexachlorophene should be left on the skin for 5–10 min.
>
>   (3) If benzalkonium Cl (Zephiran) solution is ordered, do *not* soap skin before use; soap reduces effectiveness of benzalkonium by causing it to precipitate.
>
> c. Hair should remain *unless* it interferes with surgical procedure.
>
>   (1) Note any nicks, cuts, or irritations, potential infection sites.
>
>   (2) Depilatory creams or clipping of hair is preferred to shaving with a razor; nick may result in cancellation of surgery.
>
>   (3) Skin prep may be done in surgery.

4. Goal: *reduce the risk of vomiting and aspiration during anesthesia; prevent contamination of abdominal operative sites by fecal material.* **Gastrointestinal tract preparation:**

  a. *No* food or fluid at least 6 to 8 hr before surgery.

  b. Remove food and water from bedside.

  c. Place NPO signs on bed or door.

  d. Inform kitchen and oncoming nursing staff that client is NPO for surgery.

  e. Give IV infusions up to time of surgery if dehydrated or malnourished.

  ▶ f. Enemas: two or three may be given the evening before surgery with intestinal, colon, or pelvic surgeries; 3 days of cleansing with large-intestine procedures.

  g. Possible *antibiotic* therapy to reduce colonic flora with large-bowel surgery.

  ▶ h. Gastric or intestinal intubation may be inserted the evening before major abdominal surgery.

    (1) Types of tubes:

      (a) *Levin:* single lumen; sufficient to remove fluids and gas from stomach; suction may damage mucosa.

      (b) *Salem-sump:* large lumen; prevents tissue-wall adherence.

(c) *Miller-Abbott:* long single or double lumen; required to remove the contents of jejunum or ileum.

(2) Pressures: *low* setting with Levin and intestinal tubes; *high* setting with Salem-sump; excessive pressures will result in injury to mucosal lining of intestine or stomach.

5. Goal: *promote rest and facilitate reduction of apprehension.*

a. Medications as ordered: on evening before surgery may give *barbiturate*—pentobarbital (Nembutal), secobarbital (Seconal).

b. Quiet environment: eliminate noises, distractions.

c. *Position:* reduce muscle tension.

d. Back rub.

6. Goal: *protect from injury; ensure final preparation for surgery.* Day of surgery:

a. Operative permit signed and on chart; physician responsible for obtaining informed consent. Possible blood products consent.

b. Shower or bathe.

(1) Dress: hospital pajamas.

(2) Remove: hair pins (cover hair); nail polish, to facilitate observation of peripheral circulation; jewelry (or tape wedding bands securely); pierced earrings; contact lenses; dentures (store and give mouth care); give valuable personal items to family; chart disposition of items.

c. Proper identification—check band for secureness and legibility; surgical site (limb) may be marked to prevent error.

d. Vital signs—baseline data.

e. Void, to prevent distention and possible injury to bladder.

f. Give preoperative medication to ensure smooth induction and maintenance of anesthesia—*antianxiety* (e.g., midazolam, diazepam, lorazepam); *narcotics* (e.g., meperidine, morphine, fentanyl); *anticholinergics* (e.g., atropine, glycopyrrolate).

(1) Administered 45 to 75 min before anesthetic induction.

(2) Side rails up (client will begin to feel drowsy and light-headed).

(3) Expect complaint of dry mouth if anticholinergics given.

(4) Observe for side effects—narcotics may cause nausea and vomiting, hypotension, arrhythmias, and/or respiratory depression.

(5) Quiet environment until transported to operating room.

(6) Anticipate antibiotics to start "on call" to OR.

g. Note completeness of chart:

(1) Surgical checklist completed.

(2) Vital signs recorded.

(3) Routine laboratory reports present.

(4) Preoperative medications given.

(5) Significant client observations.

h. Assist client's family in finding proper waiting room.

(1) Inform family members that the surgeon will contact them after the procedure is over.

(2) Explain length of time client is expected to be in recovery room.

(3) Prepare family for any special equipment or devices that may be needed to care for client postoperatively (e.g., oxygen, monitoring equipment, ventilator, blood transfusions).

II. **Intraoperative preparation**—anesthesia: blocks transmission of nerve impulses, suppresses reflexes, promotes muscle relaxation, and in some instances achieves reversible unconsciousness.

A. **Intravenous conscious sedation**—produces sedation and amnesia in ambulatory procedures, short surgical or diagnostic procedures. Allays fear and anxiety, elevates pain threshold, maintains consciousness and protective reflexes, and returns client quickly to normal activities.

Commonly used agents are *benzodiazepines* (midazolam [Versed], diazepam) and *narcotics* (fentanyl [Sublimaze], meperidine, morphine).

B. **Regional anesthesia**—purpose is to block pain reception and transmission in a specified area. Commonly used drugs are lidocaine HCl, tetracaine HCl, cocaine HCl, and procaine HCl. Types of regional anesthetics:

1. *Topical*—applied to mucous membranes or skin; drug anesthetizes the nerves immediately *below* the area. May be used for bronchoscopic or laryngoscopic examinations. *Side effects:* rare anaphylaxis.

2. *Local infiltration*—used for minor procedures; anesthetic drug is injected directly into the area to be incised, manipulated, or sutured. *Side effects:* rare anaphylaxis.

3. *Peripheral nerve block*—regional anesthesia is achieved by injecting drug into or around a nerve after it passes from vertebral column; procedure is named for nerve involved, such as brachial-plexus block. Requires a high degree of anatomical knowledge. *Side effects:* may be absorbed into bloodstream. Observe for: signs of excitability, twitching, changes in vital signs, or respiratory difficulties.

4. *Field block*—a group of nerves is injected with anesthetic as the nerves branch from a major or main nerve trunk. May be used for dental procedures, plastic surgery. *Side effects:* rare.

5. *Epidural anesthesia*—anesthetizing drug is injected into the epidural space of vertebral canal; produces a bandlike anesthesia around body. Frequently used in obstetrics. Rare complications. Slower onset than spinal anesthesia; not dependent on client position for level of anesthesia; no postoperative headaches.

6. *Spinal anesthesia*—anesthetizing drug is injected into the subarachnoid space and mixes with spinal fluid; drug acts on the nerves as they emerge from

the spinal cord, thereby inhibiting conduction in the autonomic, sensory, and motor systems.
  a. *Advantages:* rapid onset; produces excellent muscle relaxation.
  b. Utilization: surgery on lower limbs, inguinal region, perineum, and lower abdomen.
  c. *Disadvantages:*
    (1) Loss of sensation below point of injection for 2 to 8 hr—watch for signs of *bladder distention;* prevent injuries by maintaining alignment, keeping bedclothes straightened.
    (2) Client awake during surgical procedure—*avoid* light or upsetting conversations.
    (3) Leakage of spinal fluid from puncture site—keep flat in bed for 24 to 48 hr to prevent headache. Keep well hydrated to aid in spinal-fluid replacement.
    (4) Depression of vasomotor responses—frequent checks of vital signs.
  7. *Intravenous regional anesthesia*—used in an extremity whose circulation has been interrupted by a tourniquet; the anesthetic is injected into vein, and blockage is presumed to be achieved from extravascular leakage of anesthetic near a major nerve trunk. Precautions as for peripheral nerve block.
C. **General anesthesia**—a reversible state in which the client loses consciousness due to the inhibition of neuronal impulses in the brain by a variety of chemical agents; may be given intravenously, by inhalation, or rectally.
  1. *Side effects:*
    a. Respiratory depression.
    b. Nausea, vomiting.
    c. Excitement.
    d. Restlessness.
    e. Laryngospasm.
    f. Hypotension.
  2. **Nursing care plan/implementation**—Goal: *prevent hazardous drug interactions.*
    a. *Notify anesthesiologist* if client is taking any of the following drugs:
      (1) *Antidepressants,* such as Prozac—long half-life; monitor renal and liver function.
      (2) *Antihypertensives,* such as reserpine, hydralazine, and methyldopa—*potentiate* the hypotensive effects of anesthetic agents.
      (3) *Anticoagulants,* such as heparin, warfarin (Coumadin)—increase bleeding times, which may result in excessive *blood loss* or hemorrhage.
      (4) *Aspirin and NSAIDs*—decrease platelet aggregation and may result in increased *bleeding.*
      (5) *Steroids,* such as cortisone—anti-inflammatory effect may *delay* wound healing.
    b. *Stages of inhalation anesthesia and nursing goals:*

      (1) Stage I—extends from beginning of induction to loss of consciousness. **Nursing goal:** *reduce external stimuli,* because all movement and noises are exaggerated for the client and can be highly distressing.
      (2) Stage II—extends from loss of consciousness to relaxation; stage of delirium and excitement. **Nursing goal:** *prevent injury* by assisting anesthesiologist to restrain client if necessary; maintain a quiet, nonstimulating environment.
      (3) Stage III—extends from loss of lid reflex to cessation of voluntary respirations. **Nursing goal:** *reduce risk of untoward effects* by preparing the operative site, assisting with procedures, and observing for signs of complications.
      (4) Stage IV—indicates overdose and consists of respiratory arrest and vasomotor collapse due to medullary paralysis. **Nursing goal:** *promote restoration of ventilation and vasomotor tone* by assisting with cardiac arrest procedures and by administering *cardiac stimulants* or *narcotic antagonists* as ordered.
D. **Intravenous agents**—rapid and pleasant induction of anesthesia. Three categories: *barbiturates* (thiopental), *narcotics,* and *neuromuscular blocking agents* (succinylcholine, curare, pancuronium). Ketamine also used—may produce *emergence delirium.* IV drugs require liver metabolism and renal excretion.
E. **Hypothermia**—a specialized procedure in which the client's body temperature is lowered to 28°–30°C (82°–86°F).
  1. Reduces tissue metabolism and oxygen requirements.
  2. Used in heart surgery, brain surgery, and surgery on major blood vessels.
  3. **Nursing care plan/implementation:**
    a. Goal: *prevent complications:*
      (1) Monitor vital signs for shock.
      (2) Note level of consciousness.
      (3) Record intake and output accurately.
      (4) Maintain good body alignment; reposition to prevent edema, pressure, or discoloration of skin.
      (5) Maintain patent IV.
    b. Goal: *promote comfort.*
      (1) Apply blankets to rewarm and prevent shivering.
      (2) Mouth care.
    c. Goal: observe for indications of **malignant hyperthermia**—common during induction; may occur 24 to 72 hr postoperatively. Genetic defect of muscle metabolism; early sign is unexplained ventricular dysrhythmia, tachypnea, cyanosis, skin mottling; elevated temperature is not reliable indicator.
      (1) Administer 100% O_2.
      (2) Cool with ice packs or cooling blankets.

(3) Give dantrolene (muscle relaxant) per order.

◆ **F. Evaluation/outcome criteria:** complete reversal of anesthetic effects (e.g., spontaneous respirations, pupils react to light). No indication of intraoperative complications—cardiac arrest, laryngospasm, aspiration, hypotension, malignant hyperthermia.

III. Postoperative experience

◆ **A. Assessment:**
   1. *Subjective data:*
      a. Pain: location, onset, intensity.
      b. Nausea.
   2. *Objective data:*
      a. Operative summary:
         (1) Type of operation performed.
         (2) Pathological findings if known.
         (3) Anesthesia and medications received.
         (4) Problems during surgery that will affect recovery (e.g., arrhythmias, bleeding [estimated blood loss]).
         (5) Fluids received: type, amount.
         (6) Need for drainage or suction apparatus.
      b. Observations:
         (1) Patency of airway.
         (2) Vital signs.
         (3) Skin color and dryness.
         (4) Level of consciousness.
         (5) Status of reflexes.
         (6) Dressings.
         (7) Type and rate of IV infusion and blood transfusion.
         (8) Tubes/drains: urinary, chest, Penrose, Hemovac; note color and amount of drainage.

◆ **B. Analysis/nursing diagnosis:**
   1. *Ineffective breathing pattern* related to general anesthesia.
   2. *Ineffective airway clearance* related to absent or weak cough.
   3. *Risk for aspiration* related to vomiting.
   4. *Pain* related to surgical incision.
   5. *Altered tissue perfusion* related to shock.
   6. *Risk for fluid volume deficit* related to blood loss.
   7. *Risk for injury* related to disorientation.
   8. *Risk for infection* related to disruption of skin integrity.
   9. *Urinary retention* related to anesthetic effects.
   10. *Constipation* related to decreased peristalsis.

◆ **C. Nursing care plan/implementation**—*immediate postanesthesia nursing care:* refers to time following surgery that is usually spent in the recovery room (1 to 2 hr).
   1. Goal: *promote a safe, quiet, nonstressful environment.*
      a. Side rails up at all times.
      b. Nurse in constant attendance.
   2. Goal: *promote lung expansion and gas exchange.*
   3. Goal: *Prevent aspiration and atelectasis.*
      a. *Position:* side or back, HOB 30 degrees, head turned to side to prevent obstruction of airway by tongue; allows for drainage from mouth.
      b. Airway: leave the oropharyngeal or nasopharyngeal airway in place until client awakens and begins to eject; gagging and vomiting may occur if not removed before pharyngeal reflex returns.
      c. After removal of airway: turn on side in a *lateral position;* support upper arm with pillow.
      d. Suction: remove excessive secretions from mouth and pharynx.
      e. Encourage coughing and deep breathing: aids in upward movement of secretions.
      f. Give humidified oxygen as necessary: reduces respiratory irritation and keeps bronchotracheal secretions soft and moist.
      g. Mechanical ventilation: respirators if needed (see Ventilators in **Unit 11, p. 803**).
   4. Goal: *promote and maintain cardiovascular function.*
      a. Vital signs, as ordered: usually q 5 to 15min until stable; continuous pulse oximetry.
         (1) Compare with preoperative vital signs.
         (2) **Immediately report:** systolic blood pressure that *drops 20* mm Hg or more, a pressure *below 80* mm Hg, or a pressure that continually drops 5 to 10 mm Hg over several readings; pulse rates *under 60 or over 110* beats/min, or irregularities; respirations *over 30*/min; becoming shallow, quiet, slow; use of neck and diaphragm muscles (symptoms of *respiratory depression*); stridorous breath sounds.
      b. Observe for other alterations in circulatory function—pallor; thready pulse; cold, moist skin; decreased urine output, restlessness.
         (1) **Immediately** report to physician.
         (2) Initiate oxygen therapy.
         (3) Place client in shock position unless contraindicated—feet elevated, legs straight, head *slightly* elevated to increase venous return.
      c. Intravenous infusions: time, rate, orders for added medications.
      d. Monitor *blood transfusions* if ordered: observe for signs of *reaction* (chills, elevated temperature, urticaria, laryngeal edema, and wheezing). **Table 7.26** illustrates the nursing care plan/implementation.
      e. If reaction occurs, **immediately stop** transfusion and notify physician. Send **STAT** urine to lab.
   5. Goal: *promote psychological equilibrium.*
      a. Reassure on awakening—orient frequently.
      b. Explain procedures even though client does not appear alert.
      c. Answer client's questions briefly and accurately.

Adult

d. Maintain quiet, restful environment.
c. *Comfort measures:*
  (1) Good body alignment.
  (2) Support dependent extremities to *avoid* pressure areas and possible nerve damage.
  (3) Check for constriction: dressings, clothing, bedding.
  (4) Check IV sites frequently for patency and signs of infiltration (swelling, blanching, cool to touch).
6. Goal: *maintain proper function of tubes and apparatus* (see **Table 11.11**).

D. General postoperative nursing care: refers to period of time from admission to the general nursing unit until anticipated recovery and discharge from the hospital (see **Table 7.26** for a review of postoperative complications).

1. Goal: *promote lung expansion, gaseous exchange, and elimination of bronchotracheal secretions.*
  a. Turn, cough, and deep breathe q2h.
  b. Use incentive spirometer as ordered to enable client to observe depth of ventilation.
  c. Administer nebulization as ordered to help mobilize secretions.
  d. Encourage hydration to thin mucous secretions.
  e. Assist in ambulation as soon as allowed.
2. Goal: *provide relief of pain.*
  a. Assess type, location, intensity, and duration; possible causative factors, such as poor body alignment or restrictive bandages.
  b. Observe and evaluate reaction to discomfort. Use scale: 1 to 10 numerical or pictorial.
  c. Use *comfort measures,* such as back rubs and

TABLE 7.26	Postoperative Complications	
Condition and Etiology ◆	**Assessment: Signs and Symptoms** ◆	**Nursing Care Plan/ Implementation**
Respiratory complications —Most common are Atelectasis, Pneumonias (Lobar, Bronchial, and Hypostatic), and Pleuritis; Other Complications are Hemothorax and Pneumothorax		
Atelectasis—undetected preoperative upper respiratory infections, aspiration of vomitus: irritation of the tracheobronchial tree with increased secretions of mucus due to intubation and inhalation anesthesia, a history of heavy smoking, or chronic obstructive pulmonary disease; severe postoperative pain, or high abdominal or thoracic surgery, which inhibits deep breathing; and debilitation or old age, which lowers the client's resistance	*Dyspnea;* ↑temperature; absent or diminished breath sounds over affected area, asymmetrical chest expansion, ↑ respirations and pulse rate; tracheal shift to affected side when severe; anxiety and restlessness	1. *Position:* unaffected side 2. Turn, cough, and deep breathe; encourage use of inspirometer hourly while awake 3. *Postural drainage* 4. Nebulization 5. *Force* fluids if not contraindicated
Pneumonia—see *Atelectasis* for etiology	Rapid, shallow, painful respirations; crackles; diminished or absent breath sounds; asymmetrical lung expansion; chills and fever, productive cough, rust-colored sputum; and circumoral and nailbed cyanosis	1. *Position of comfort*—semi-Fowler's to high Fowler's 2. *Force* fluids to 3000 mL/day 3. Provide humidification of air and oxygen therapy 4. Oropharyngeal suction prn 5. Assist during coughing 6. Administer *antibiotics* and *analgesics* as ordered 7. *Diet:* high calorie, as tolerated 8. Cautious disposal of secretions; proper oral hygiene 9. Respiratory treatments as ordered
Pleuritis—see *Atelectasis* for etiology	Knifelike chest pain on inspiration; intercostal tenderness; splinting of chest by client; rapid, shallow respirations; pleural friction rub; ↑ temperature; malaise	1. *Position: affected* side to splint the chest 2. Manually splint client's chest during cough 3. Administer *analgesics* as ordered
Hemothorax—chest surgery, gunshot or knife wounds, and multiple fractures of chest wall	Chest pain; increased respiratory rate; dyspnea, decreased or absent breath sounds; decreased blood pressure; tachycardia, and mediastinal shift may occur (heart, trachea, and esophagus great vessels are pushed toward unaffected side)	1. Observe vital signs closely for signs of shock and respiratory distress 2. Assist with thoracentesis (needle aspiration of fluid) 3. Assist with insertion of chest tube to closed-chest drainage (see care of water-sealed drainage system)

(Continued on following page)

Condition and Etiology ◆	Assessment: Signs and Symptoms ◆	Nursing Care Plan/ Implementation
Pneumothorax, closed or tension—thoracentesis (needle nicks the lung), rupture of alveoli or bronchi due to accidental injury, and chronic obstructive lung disease	Marked dyspnea, sudden sharp chest pain, subcutaneous emphysema (air in chest wall tissue); cyanosis; tracheal shift to unaffected side; hyperresonance on percussion, decreased or absent breath sounds; increased respiratory rate, tachycardia; asymmetrical chest expansion, feeling of pressure within chest; *mediastinal shift*—severe dyspnea and cyanosis, deviation of larynx and trachea toward unaffected side, deviation either medially or laterally of apex of heart, decreased blood pressure; distended neck veins; increased pulse and respirations	1. Remain with client—keep as calm and quiet as possible; **STAT** chest x-ray 2. *Position:* high-Fowler's (sitting) 3. Notify physician through another nurse, and have thoracentesis equipment brought to bedside 4. Administer oxygen as necessary 5. Take vital signs to evaluate respiratory and cardiac function 6. Assist with thoracentesis 7. Assist with chest tube insertion and maintenance of closed-chest drainage

Circulatory Complications —Shock, Thrombophlebitis, Pulmonary Embolism, and Disseminated Intravascular Coagulation (DIC)

Shock—hemorrhage, sepsis, decreased cardiac contractility (myocardial infarction, cardiac failure, tamponade), drug sensitivities, transfusion reactions, pulmonary embolism, and emotional reaction to pain or deep fear	Dizziness; fainting; restlessness; anxiety; ↓ LOC *BP:* ↓or falling *Pulse:* weak, thready *Respirations:* ↑, shallow *Skin:* pale, cool, clammy, cyanotic, ↓ temperature; Oliguria CVP <5 cm H_2O; Thirst	1. *Position:* foot of bed raised 20 degrees, knees straight, trunk horizontal, head slightly elevated; *avoid* Trendelenburg's position 2. Administer blood transfusions, plasma expanders, and intravenous infusions as ordered; medications specific to type of shock. 3. Check: vital signs, CVP, temperature 4. Insert urinary catheter to monitor hourly urine output 5. Administer oxygen as ordered
Deep vein thrombosis (thrombophlebitis)—injury to vein wall by tight leg straps or leg holders during gynecological surgery; hemoconcentration due to dehydration or fluid loss; stasis of blood in extremities due to postoperative circulatory depression; prolonged immobility; placement of catheters (PICC line, femoral line) that impede venous flow	Calf pain or cramping in affected extremity, redness and swelling (the left leg is affected more frequently than the right); slight fever, chills; *Homans'* sign and tenderness over the anteromedian surface of thigh; decreased pulse in affected extremity due to swelling and venous congestion	1. Maintain complete bedrest, *avoiding positions* that restrict venous return 2. Apply elastic stockings to prevent swelling and pooling of venous blood 3. Apply warm, moist soaks to area as ordered 4. Administer *anticoagulants* as ordered 5. Use bed cradle over affected limb 6. Provide active and passive ROM exercises in unaffected limb
Pulmonary embolism—obstruction of a pulmonary artery by a foreign body in bloodstream, usually a blood clot that has been dislodged from its original site *Disseminated Intravascular Coagulation* (DIC) (see **p. 506**).	*Sudden*, severe stabbing chest pain; *severe* dyspnea; cyanosis; *rapid* pulse; anxiety and apprehension; pupillary dilation: *profuse* diaphoresis; *loss of* consciousness	1. Administer oxygen and inhalants while client *is sitting upright* 2. Maintain bedrest and frequent reassurance 3. Administer heparin sodium, as ordered 4. Administer *analgesics,* such as morphine SO_4, to reduce pain and apprehension

Wound Complications—Infection, Dehiscence, and Evisceration

Wound infection—*obesity or undernutrition,* particularly protein and vitamin deficiencies; *decreased* antibody production in aged; *decreased* phagocytosis in newborn; metabolic disorder, such as diabetes mellitus, Cushing's syndrome, malignancies, and shock; breakdown in aseptic technique	Redness, tenderness, and heat in area of incision; wound drainage; ↑temperature; ↑ pulse rate.	1. Assist in cleansing and irrigation of wound and insertion of a drain 2. Give *antibiotics* as ordered; observe responses

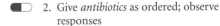

(Continued on following page)

Adult

TABLE 7.26 Postoperative Complications *(Continued)*

Condition and Etiology	◆ Assessment: Signs and Symptoms	◆ Nursing Care Plan/ Implementation
Wound dehiscence and evisceration—obesity and undernutrition, particularly protein and vitamin C deficiencies; immunosuppression; metabolic disorders, cancer; liver disease; common site is midline abdominal incision, frequently about 7 days postoperatively; precipitating factors include: abdominal distention, vomiting, coughing, hiccups, and uncontrolled motor activity	Slow parting of wound edges with a gush of pinkish serous drainage; or rapid parting with coils of intestines escaping onto the abdominal wall; the latter accompanied by pain and often by vomiting. Client reports "giving" sensation.	1. *Position:* bedrest, low Fowler's or horizontal position 2. Notify physician **STAT** 3. Cover exposed coils of intestines with sterile towels or dressing and keep moist with sterile normal saline 4. Monitor vital signs frequently 5. Remain with client; reassure that physician is coming 6. Prepare for physician's arrival; set up IV, suction equipment, and nasogastric tube; obtain sterile gown, mask, gloves, towels, and warmed normal saline. 7. Notify surgery that client will be returning to operating room

Urinary Complications —Retention and Infections

Urinary retention—obstruction in bladder or urethra; neurological disease; mechanical trauma as in childbirth or gynecological surgery; psychological conditioning that inhibits voiding in bed; prolonged bedrest; pain with lower abdominal surgery; epidural narcotics	Inability to void within 8 hr post-surgery, despite adequate fluid replacement; palpable bladder, frequent voiding of small amounts of urine or dribbling; suprapubic pain	1. Assist client to stand, or use bedside commode if not contraindicated 2. Provide privacy 3. Reduce tension, provide support 4. Use warm bedpan 5. Run tap water 6. Place client's feet in warm water 7. Pour warm water over perineum 8. Catheterize if conservative measures fail
Urinary tract infections—urinary retention, bladder distention, repeated or prolonged catheterization	*Urinary:* burning and frequency *Pain:* low back or flank Pyuria, hematuria; ↑temperature, chills; anorexia; positive urine culture	1. *Push fluids* to 3000 mL daily, unless contraindicated 2. *Avoid* stimulants such as caffeine 3. Give *antibiotics*, sulfonamides, or acidifying agents as ordered 4. Give perianal care after each bowel movement

Gastrointestinal Complications—Gastric Distention, Paralytic Ileus, and Intestinal Obstruction

Gastric distention—depressed gastric motility due to sympathoadrenal stress response; idiosyncrasy to drugs: emotions, pain, shock; fluid and electrolyte imbalances	Feeling of fullness, hiccups, overflow vomiting of dark, foul-smelling liquid; severe retention leads to decreased blood pressure (due to pressure on vagus nerve) and other symptoms of shock syndrome	1. Report signs to physician **immediately** 2. Insert or assist in insertion of NG tube; attach to intermittent suction 3. Irrigate NG tube with *saline* (water will deplete electrolytes and result in metabolic alkalosis) 4. Administer IV infusions with electrolytes as ordered
Paralytic ileus—see *Gastric distention*	Greatly decreased or absent bowel sounds, failure of either gas or feces to be passed by rectum; nausea and vomiting; abdominal tenderness and distention; fever; dehydration	1. Notify physician 2. Insert or assist with insertion of NG tube; attach to low, intermittent suction 3. Insert rectal tube 4. Administer IV infusion with electrolytes as ordered 5. Irrigate nasogastric tube with saline 6. Assist with insertion of Miller-Abbott tube if indicated 7. Administer medications to increase peristalsis as ordered

(Continued on following page)

Adult

Condition and Etiology	◆ Assessment: Signs and Symptoms	◆ Nursing Care Plan/ Implementation
Intestinal obstruction—due to poorly functioning anastomosis, hernia, adhesions, fecal impaction	Severe, colicky abdominal pains, mild to severe abdominal distention, nausea and vomiting, anorexia and malaise; fever; lack of bowel movement; electrolyte imbalance; highpitched tinkling bowel sounds	1. Assist with insertion of nasoenteric tube and attach to intermittent suction 2. Maintain IV infusions with electrolytes 3. Encourage nasal breathing to *avoid* air swallowing 4. Check abdomen for distention and bowel sounds every 2 hr 5. Encourage verbalization 6. Plan rest periods for client 7. Administer oral hygiene frequently

Transfusion Reactions—Allergic, Febrile, and Hemolytic

Allergic and febrile reactions—unidentified antigen or antigens in donor blood or transfusion equipment; previous reaction to transfusions; small thrombi; bacteria; lysed red blood cells	Fever to 103°F, may have *sudden* onset; chills; itching; erythema; urticaria; nausea, vomiting; dyspnea and wheezing, occasionally	1. **Stop** transfusion and notify physician 2. Administer *antihistamines*, as ordered 3. Send **STAT** urine to lab for analysis 4. Institute *cooling* measures if indicated 5. Maintain *strict* input and output records 6. Send remaining blood to lab for analysis, and order recipient blood sample for analysis
Hemolytic reaction—infusion of incompatible blood (less common, more serious)	*Early:* chills and fever; throbbing headache, feeling of burning in face; hypotension; tachycardia; chest, back, or flank pain; nausea, vomiting; feeling of doom; *later:* spontaneous and diffuse bleeding; icterus; oliguria; anuria; hemoglobinuria	1. **Stop infusion immediately;** take vital signs and notify physician 2. Send client blood sample and unused blood to lab for analysis 3. Send **STAT** urine to lab 4. Save *all* urine for observation of discoloration 5. Administer parenteral infusions to combat shock, as ordered 6. Administer medications as ordered—*diuretics, sodium bicarbonate, hydrocortisone,* and *vasopressors*

Emotional Complications

Emotional disturbances—grief associated with loss of body part or loss of body image; previous emotional problems; decreased sensory and perceptual input; sensory overload; fear and pain; decreased resistance to stress as a result of age, exhaustion, or debilitation	Restlessness, insomnia, depression, hallucinations, delusions, agitation, suicidal thoughts	1. Report symptoms to physician 2. Encourage verbalization of feelings; give realistic assurance 3. Orient to time and place as necessary 4. Provide safety measures, such as side rails 5. Keep room lit, to reduce incidence of visual hallucinations 6. Administer *tranquilizers* as ordered. 7. Use restraints as a *last* resort

proper ventilation, staying with client and encouraging verbalization.

d. Reduce incidence of pain: change position frequently; support dependent extremities with pillows, sandbags, and footboards; keep bedding dry and straight.

e. Give *analgesics* or *tranquilizers* as ordered; assure client that they will help.

f. Observe for desired and untoward effects of medication.

3. Goal: *promote adequate nutrition and fluid and electrolyte balance.*

a. Parenteral fluids, as ordered.

b. Monitor blood pressure, I&O to assess adequate, deficient, or excessive extracellular fluid volume.

c. *Diet: liquid* when nausea and vomiting stop and bowel sounds are established; progress as ordered.

4. Goal: *assist client with elimination.*

a. Encourage voiding within 8 to 10 hr after surgery.

(1) Allow client to stand or use commode, if not contraindicated.

(2) Run tap water or soak feet in warm water to promote micturition.

(3) Catheterization if bladder is distended and conservative treatments have failed.

b. Maintain accurate I&O records.

c. Expect bowel function to return in 2 to 3 days.

5. Goal: *facilitate wound healing and prevent infection.*

a. Incision care: *avoid* pressure to enhance venous drainage and prevent edema.

b. *Elevate* injured extremities to reduce swelling and promote venous return.

c. Support or splint incision when coughing.

d. Check dressings q2h for drainage.

e. Change dressings on draining wounds prn; *aseptic technique;* protective ointments to reduce skin irritation may be ordered.

f. Carefully observe wound suction (e.g., *Jackson-Pratt*), if applied, for kinking or twisting of the tubes.

6. Goal: *promote comfort and rest.*

a. Recognize factors that may cause restlessness—fear, anxiety, pain, oxygen lack, wet dressings.

b. *Comfort measures: analgesics* or *barbiturates;* apply oxygen as indicated; change positions; encourage deep breathing; massage back to reduce restlessness.

c. Allow rest periods between care—group activities.

d. Give *antiemetic* for relief of nausea and vomiting, as ordered.

e. Vigorous oral hygiene (brushing) to prevent "surgical mumps" or parotitis from preop atropine or general anesthesia.

7. Goal: *encourage early movement and ambulation to prevent complications of immobilization.*

a. Turn or reposition q2h.

b. ROM: passive and active exercises.

c. Encourage leg exercises.

d. Use preventive treatments—antiembolic stockings, graduated compression stockings, or external pneumatic compression sleeves:

(1) With compression stockings, highest pressure (100%) at ankles, lowest pressure (40%) at midthigh.

(2) Compression sleeves, three chambers sequentially inflated-deflated to stimulate venous return.

e. Assist with standing or use of commode if allowed.

f. Encourage resumption of personal care as soon as possible.

g. Assist with ambulation in room as soon as allowed. *Avoid* prolonged chair sitting because it enhances venous pooling and may predispose to thrombophlebitis. *Elevate* legs when chair sitting.

◆ **E. Evaluation/outcome criteria:**

1. Incision heals without infection.

2. No complications (e.g., atelectasis, pneumonia, thrombophlebitis).

3. Normal bowel and bladder functions resume.

4. Carries out activities of daily living, self-care.

5. Accepts possible limitations: dietary, activity, body image (e.g., no depression, complies with treatment regimen).

NUTRITION

I. General nutritional deficiencies

◆ **A.** Assessment:

1. *Subjective data:*

a. Mental irritability or confusion.

b. History of poor dietary intake.

c. History of lack of adequate resources to provide adequate nutrition.

d. Lack of knowledge about proper diet, food selection, or preparation.

e. History of eating disorders.

f. Paresthesia (burning and tingling): hands and feet.

2. *Objective data:*

a. *Appearance:* listless; *posture:* sagging shoulders, sunken chest, poor gait.

b. *Muscle:* weakness, fatigue, wasted appearance.

c. *GI:* indigestion, vomiting, enlarged liver, spleen.

d. *Cardiovascular:* tachycardia on minimal exertion; bradycardia at rest; enlarged heart, elevated BP.

e. *Hair:* brittle, dry, thin, sparse; lack of natural shine; color changes; can be easily plucked out.

f. *Skin:* dryness (xerosis), scaly, dyspigmentation, petechiae, lack of fat under skin.

g. *Mouth:*

(1) *Teeth:* missing, abnormally placed, caries.

(2) *Gums:* bleed easily, receding.

(3) *Tongue:* swollen, sore.

(4) *Lips:* red, swollen, angular fissures at corners.

h. *Eyes:* pale conjunctiva, corneal changes.

i. *Nails:* brittle, ridged.

j. *Nervous system:* abnormal reflexes.

k. Lab data: blood: *decreased* albumin, iron-binding capacity, lymphocyte, hemoglobin, and hematocrit.

l. Anthropometric measurements document nutritional deficiencies.

◆ **B. Analysis/nursing diagnosis:**

1. *Altered nutrition, less than body requirements,* related to poor dietary intake.

2. *Knowledge deficit* (learning need) related to nutritional requirements.

3. *Altered health maintenance* related to inability to provide own nutritional care.

4. *Ineffective individual coping* related to eating disorders.

5. *Ineffective family coping, disabling,* related to inadequate resources or knowledge to provide appropriate family nutrition.

TABLE 7.27	Essential Nutrients and Potential Deficiencies	
Nutrient	**Function**	**Deficiency Leads to**
Calcium	Aids in formation and maintenance of bones and teeth; permits healthy nerve functioning and normal blood clotting	↑Neuromuscular irritability, impaired blood clotting
Phosphorus	Bone building	Rickets
Magnesium	Cellular metabolism of carbohydrates and protein;	↓Cellular metabolism of carbohydrates and protein; tetany
Sodium	Fluid and electrolyte balance; acid-base balance; electro-chemical impulses of nerves and muscles	Fluid and electrolyte imbalance; ↓ muscle contraction
Potassium	Osmotic pressure and water balance	Fluid and electrolyte imbalance; ↓ cardiac and skeletal muscular contractility
Chloride	Fluid and electrolyte balance; acid-base balance; digestion	Fluid imbalances; alkalosis
Iron	Hemoglobin formation; cellular oxidation	Anemia; ↑ risk of infection
Iodine	Synthesis of thyroid hormone; overall body metabolism	Goiter
Zinc	Constituent of cell enzyme system; CO_2 carrier in RBC	↓Metabolism of protein and carbohydrates; delayed wound healing; ↑ risk of infection
Vitamin A	Collagen synthesis	Poor healing; scaly skin
Vitamin C	Capillary integrity	Poor healing; bruising
Vitamin K	Coagulation	Bruising and hemorrhage
Pyridoxine and thiamine	Antibody, RBC, and WBC formation	↑Risk of infection; anemia
Protein	Wound repair; clotting; WBC production; phagocytosis	Poor healing; edema
Fats	Cellular energy; cell membrane integrity	Impaired tissue repair
Carbohydrates	Cellular energy; spare protein	Interference with healing

◆ **C. Nursing care plan/implementation:**
  1. Goal: *prevent complications of specific deficiency.*
    a. Identify etiology of nutritional deficiency.
    b. Recognize signs of nutritional deficiencies (**Table 7.27**).
    c. Identify foods high in deficient nutrient (see **Unit 9**).
    d. Evaluate economic resources to purchase appropriate foods.
    e. Identify community resources for assistance.
    f. Monitor progress for potential additional illnesses.
  2. Goal: *health teaching.*
    a. Effects of nutritional deficiencies on health.
    b. Foods to include in diet to avoid deficits.

◆ **D. Evaluation/outcome criteria:**
  1. Complications do not occur.
  2. Client gains weight.
  3. Client selects appropriate foods to alleviate deficiency.

II. **Celiac disease** (gluten enteropathy, nontropical sprue): immune to gluten, causing impaired absorption and digestion of nutrients through the small bowel. Affects adults and children and is characterized by inability to digest and use sugars, starches, and fats.
  A. **Pathophysiology:** intolerance to the gliadin fraction of grains causing degeneration of the epithelial surface of the intestine, atrophy of the intestinal villi, and impaired absorption of essential nutrients.

B. **Risk factors:**
  1. Possible genetic or familial factors.
  2. Hypersensitivity response.
  3. History of childhood celiac disease.

◆ **C. Assessment:**
  1. *Subjective data:* family history.
  2. *Objective data:*
    a. Loss: weight, fat deposits, musculature.
    b. Anemia.
    c. Vitamin deficiencies.
    d. Abdomen distended with flatus.
    e. *Stools:* diarrhea, foul smelling, bulky, fatty, float in commode.
    f. Skin condition known as *dermatitis herpetiformis.*
    g. History of acute attacks of fluid and electrolyte imbalances.
     h. *Diagnostic tests:* stool for fat; barium enema; antibody tests, including endomyosial (EMA); blood studies of: iron, folate, proteins, minerals, and clotting factors; small bowel biopsy.
    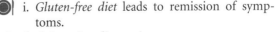 i. *Gluten-free diet* leads to remission of symptoms.

◆ **D. Analysis/nursing diagnosis:**
  1. *Altered nutrition, less than body requirements,* related to inability to digest and use sugars, starches, and fats.
  2. *Diarrhea* related to intestinal response to gluten in diet.

3. *Fluid volume deficit* related to loss through excessive diarrhea.
4. *Knowledge deficit* (learning need) related to dietary restrictions to control symptoms.

◆ **E. Nursing care plan/implementation:**
  1. Goal: *prevent weight loss.*
  🍽 a. *Diet:* high in calories, protein, vitamins, and minerals, and gluten free.
        (1) *Avoid:* wheat, rye, oats, barley.
        (2) All other foods permitted.
     b. Daily weights to monitor weight changes.
  2. Goal: *health teaching.*
     a. Nature of disease.
     b. Dietary restrictions and allowances.
     c. Complications of noncompliance.

◆ **F. Evaluation/outcome criteria:**
  1. No further weight loss.
  2. Normal stools.
  3. Fluid/electrolyte balance obtained and maintained.

III. Hepatitis: inflammation of the liver.
  A. Pathophysiology:
    1. Infection with *hepatitis A* (formerly called infectious hepatitis), *hepatitis B* (formerly called serum hepatitis), *hepatitis C* (single-stranded RNV virus of the *Flaviviridae* family; usually asymptomatic), *delta hepatitis* (infection caused by a defective RNA virus that requires HBV to multiply), or *hepatitis E* (major etiological agent of the enterically transmitted non-A, non-B hepatitis worldwide) → inflammation, necrosis, and regeneration of liver parenchyma. Hepatocellular injury impairs clearance of urobilinogen → elevated urinary urobilinogen; and, as injury increases → conjugated bilirubin not reaching the intestines → decreased urine and fecal urobilinogen → increased serum bilirubin → jaundice.
    2. Failure of liver to detoxify products → increased toxic products of protein metabolism → gastritis and duodenitis.

  B. Risk factors:
    1. Exposure to virus.
    2. Exposure to carriers of virus.
    3. Exposure to hepatotoxins such as dry-cleaning agents.
    4. Nonimmunized.

◆ **C. Assessment:**
  1. *Subjective data:*
     a. Anorexia, nausea.
     b. Malaise, dull ache in right upper quadrant, abdominal pain.
     c. Repugnance to: food, cigarette smoke, strong odors, alcohol.
     d. Headache.
  2. *Objective data:*
     a. Fever.
     b. Liver: enlarged (hepatomegaly), tender, smooth.

  c. *Skin:* icterus in sclera of eyes, jaundice; rash; pruritus; petechiae, bruises.
  d. Urine: normal, dark.
  e. Stool: normal, clay colored, loose.
  f. Vomiting, weight loss.
  g. Lymph nodes: enlarged.
  h. Lab data:
     (1) Blood—leukocytosis.
     (2) *Increased* AST (SGOT), ALT (SGPT), and bilirubin levels, alkaline phosphatase.
     (3) Urine—*increased* urobilinogen.
  i. See **Table 7.28** for comparison of hepatitis A, B, C, and D.

◆ **D. Analysis/nursing diagnosis:**
  1. *Pain* related to inflammation of liver.
  2. *Impaired skin integrity* related to pruritus.
  3. *Activity intolerance* related to fatigue.
  4. *Risk for infection* to others related to incubation/infectious period.
  5. *Altered nutrition, less than body requirements,* related to repugnance of food.
  6. *Social isolation* related to isolation precautions.

◆ **E. Nursing care plan/implementation:**
  1. Goal: *prevent spread of infection to others.*
     a. Isolation according to type
        (1) *Hepatitis A:*
           (a) *Contact* precautions (**Table 7.29**).
           (b) Private room preferred.
           (c) Gown/gloves for direct contact with feces.
           (d) Handwashing when in direct contact with feces.
        (2) *Hepatitis B: blood and body fluid* precautions.
           (a) *Needle/dressing* precautions.
           (b) Private room not necessary.
           (c) Gown: only if enteric precautions also necessary.
           (d) Handwashing: use gloves when in direct contact with blood.
        (3) *Hepatitis C: blood and body fluid precautions*—same as hepatitis B, except when in countries with fecal-oral form, then use hepatitis A precautions also.
        (4) *Delta:* same as hepatitis B.
     b. Passive immunity for contacts.
        (1) *Hepatitis A:* hepatitis A vaccine (Havrix, VAQTA), immune serum globulin (ISG), administered before and after exposure.
        (2) *Hepatitis B:* hepatitis B immune globulin (HBIG) (Recombivax HB, Energix-B) or ISG.
        (3) *Hepatitis C:* prophylaxis not as effective; IG may be given.
        (4) *Delta:* same as for hepatitis B.
     c. Goal: *promote healing.*
        🍽 (1) *Diet* as tolerated:
           (a) NPO with parenteral infusions, when in acute stage.

TABLE 7.28	Etiology, Incidence, Epidemiological, and Clinical Comparison of Hepatitis A, Hepatitis B, Hepatitis C, and Delta Hepatitis			
	Hepatitis A	**Hepatitis B**	**Hepatitis C**	**Delta Hepatitis**
Incubation	2 to 6 wk	4 wk to 6 mo	Variable: 14 to 160 days; average, 50 days	Same as hepatitis B
Communicable	Until 7 to 9 days after jaundice occurs	Several months—as long as virus present in blood	As long as virus present in blood	As long as virus present in blood
Transmission	Fecal-oral; blood; sexual	Parenteral; sexual; perinatal	Percutaneous, via contaminated blood, parenteral drug abuse; some fecal-oral forms; sexual; perinatal	Parenteral; blood
Sources	Crowding; contaminated food, milk, or water	Contaminated needles, syringes, surgical instruments	Persons who have received 15 or more blood transfusions; IV drug users; persons traveling to contaminated areas	Contaminated needles, syringes
Portal of entry	GI tract; asymptomatic carriers	Integumentary: blood plasma or transfusions	Blood	Integumentary: blood
HB antigen	Not present	Present	Not present	Present as with hepatitis B
Incidence	Sporadic epidemics; increased in children <15	Increased in ages 15 to 29, particularly in heroin addiction; occupational hazard for laboratory workers, nurses, physicians	All age groups; higher in adults because of exposure to risk factors	Same as hepatitis B
Immunity	*Preexposure:* immune globulin, 0.02 mL/kg *Postexposure:* within 2 wk of exposure, as above	*Preexposure:* hepatitis B vaccine *Postexposure:* immune globulin with high amounts of anti-HBs (HBIG); hepatitis B vaccine	None; immune globulin may be given	None
Prevention	Handwashing, use of gloves; hepatitis A vaccine	Care when handling products contaminated by blood, use of gloves; hepatitis B vaccine	Same as hepatitis B	Same as hepatitis B
Severity	Mild	Mild to moderate	Mild to moderate	Moderate to severe
Fever	Common	Uncommon	Uncommon	Uncommon
Nausea/vomiting	Common	Common	Common	Common

TABLE 7.29	Contact Precautions

1. Private room if the client's hygiene is poor. In general clients with the same infection *may share* a room.
2. Masks are *not* indicated.
3. Growns are indicated if soiling is likely.
4. Gloves are indicated for touching infective material.
5. Hands must be washed before and after touching the client or potentially contaminated articles.
6. Contaminated articles should be discarded or bagged and labeled.

    (b) *High* protein, *high* carbohydrate, *low* fat, offered in frequent small meals.
    (c) Push fluids, if not contraindicated; I&O.
  (2) Medications:
    (a) *Antiviral* for clients with persistently elevated ALT levels.
    (b) Interferon for initial treatment of hepatitis C.
  d. Goal: *monitor for worsening of disease process, failure to respond to prescribed treatment.*
    (1) Observe urine—dark due to presence of bile and stool, clay-colored.
    (2) Observe sclera, lab tests for increasing jaundice.

(3) Mental confusion, unusual somnolence may indicate decreased liver function.

(4) Weigh daily—increase indicates fluid retention and possible ascites.

e. Goal: *health teaching.*

(1) Diet and fluid intake to promote liver regeneration.

(2) Importance of rest and limited activity to reduce metabolic workload of liver.

(3) Personal hygiene practices to prevent contamination.

(4) *Avoid:* alcohol, blood donations, and contact with communicable infections.

(5) Follow-up case referral; may take 6 mo for full recovery.

(6) Teach contacts about available immunizations.

2. Goal: *promote comfort.*

a. Bedrest to combat fatigue and reduce metabolic needs until hepatomegaly subsides; *semi-Fowler's* or *supine* positioning.

b. Oral hygiene q1 to 2h to decrease nausea.

c. ROM exercises to maintain muscle strength.

d. *Measures to reduce pruritus:*

(1) Mild, oil-based lotion to reduce itching.

(2) Nails cut short, cotton gloves, long-sleeved clothing to prevent skin injury from scratching.

(3) Environment: cool and dry.

(4) Cool wet soaks to skin.

(5) Diversional activities.

(6) Medications as ordered:

(a) *Emollients* to relieve dry skin.

(b) *Topical corticosteroids* to reduce inflammation.

(c) *Antihistamines* to reduce itch.

(d) *Tranquilizers and sedatives* to allow rest and prevent exhaustion.

◆ **F. Evaluation/outcome criteria:**

1. Tolerates food; nausea and vomiting decreased.

2. Signs of infection/inflammation absent.

3. No complications, hemorrhage, liver damage, ascites.

4. No jaundice noted.

IV. Pancreatitis: inflammatory disease of the pancreas that may result in autodigestion of the pancreas by its own enzymes.

A. Pathophysiology: proteolytic enzymes within the pancreas are activated by endotoxins, exotoxins, ischemia, anoxia, or trauma. Pancreatic enzymes begin process of autodigestion of pancreas and surrounding tissues; also activate other enzymes that digest cellular membranes. Autodigestion leads to edema, hemorrhage, vascular damage, coagulation necrosis, and fat necrosis.

B. Risk factors:

1. Obesity.

2. Alcoholism, alcohol consumption.

3. Biliary tract disease.

4. Abdominal trauma.

5. Surgery.

6. Drugs.

7. Metabolic disease.

8. Intestinal disease.

9. Obstruction of the pancreatic ducts.

10. Infections.

11. Carcinoma.

12. Adenoma.

13. Hypercalcemia.

◆ **C. Assessment:**

1. *Subjective data:*

a. *Pain:*

(1) Sudden onset; severe, widespread, constant, and incapacitating.

(2) Location—epigastrium, right upper quadrant (RUQ) and left upper quadrant (LUQ) of abdomen; radiates to back, flanks, and substernal area.

b. Nausea.

c. History of risk factors.

d. Dyspnea.

2. *Objective data:*

a. *Elevated:* temperature, pulse, respirations, BP (unless in shock).

b. *Decreased* breath sounds related to atelectasis/pleural effusion.

c. *Increased* crackles, cyanosis.

d. Hemorrhage, shock.

e. Vomiting.

f. Fluid and electrolyte imbalances, dehydration.

g. *Decreased* bowel sounds; abdominal tenderness with guarding.

h. *Stools:* bulky, pale, foul smelling, steatorrhea (excessive fat in stools).

i. *Skin:* pale, moist, cold; may be jaundiced.

j. Muscle rigidity.

k. Supine position leads to increased pain.

l. Fluid accumulation in the abdomen.

m. Lab data:

(1) *Elevated:*

(a) Amylase, serum, and urine.

(b) Serum lipase, AST (SGOT).

(c) Alkaline phosphatase.

(d) Bilirubin, glucose; serum and urine.

(e) Urine protein, WBC.

(f) Leukocytes.

(g) BUN.

(h) LDH (liver function, lactate dehydrogenase).

(2) *Decreased:*

(a) Serum calcium.

(b) Protein.

n. Ultrasound for gallstones, CAT scan.

◆ **D. Analysis/nursing diagnosis:**

1. *Altered nutrition, less than body requirements,* related to nausea and vomiting.

2. *Pain* related to inflammatory and autodigestive processes of pancreas.

3. *Fluid volume deficit* related to inflammation, decreased intake, and vomiting.
4. *Ineffective breathing pattern* related to pain and pleural effusion.
5. *Knowledge deficit* (learning need) related to risk factors and disease management.

◆ **E. Nursing care plan/implementation:**

1. Goal: *control pain.*
   a. Medications: *analgesics*—meperidine (*not* morphine or codeine due to spasmodic effect).
   b. *Position:* sitting with knees flexed.
2. Goal: *rest injured pancreas.*
   a. NPO.
   b. NG tube to low suction.
   c. Medications:
      (1) *Antiulcers.*
      (2) *Antibiotics.*
      (3) *Antiemetics.*
      (4) *Antispasmodics.*
      (5) *Anticholinergics.*
      (6) *Histamine-2 receptors* (cimetidine).
3. Goal: *prevent fluid and electrolyte imbalance.*
   a. Monitor: vitals, CVP.
   b. IVs, fluids, blood, albumin, plasma.
4. Goal: *prevent respiratory and metabolic complications.*
   a. Cough, deep breathe, change position.
   b. Monitor: blood sugar as ordered.
   c. Monitor calcium levels: *Chvostek's* and *Trousseau's sign* positive when calcium deficit exists (see **XVI. Thyroidectomy, p. 643,** for description of tests).
5. Goal: *provide adequate nutrition.*
   a. *Low fat diet.*
   b. Bland, small, frequent meals.
   c. Vitamin supplements.
   d. *Avoid* alcohol.
6. Goal: *prevent complications.*
   a. Monitor for signs of:

   > (1) Peritonitis.
   > (2) Perforation.
   > (3) Respiratory complications.
   > (4) Hypotension, shock.
   > (5) DIC.
   > (6) ARDS.
   > (7) Hemorrhage from ulcers, varices.
   > (8) Anemia.
   > (9) Encephalopathy.

7. Goal: *health teaching.*
   a. Food selections for low fat, bland diet.
   b. Necessity of vitamin therapy.
   c. Importance of avoiding alcohol.
   d. Signs and symptoms of recurrence.
   e. Importance of rest, to prevent relapse.
   f. Desired effects and side effects of prescribed medications:
      (1) *Narcotics* for pain.
      (2) *Antiemetics* for nausea and vomiting.

      (3) *Pancreatic hormone and enzymes* to replace enzymes not reaching duodenum.

◆ **F. Evaluation/outcome criteria:**

1. Pain is relieved.
2. No complications (e.g., peritonitis, respiratory).
3. States dietary allowances and restrictions.
4. Takes medications as ordered; states purposes, side effects.

V. Cirrhosis: chronic inflammation and fibrosis (irreversible scarring) of the liver in which some liver cells (hepatocytes) undergo necrosis and others undergo proliferative regeneration.

A. Pathophysiology: progressive destruction of hepatic cells → loss of normal metabolic function of the liver and formation of scar tissue. Regeneration and proliferation of fibrous tissue → obstruction of the portal vein → increased portal hypertension, ascites, liver failure, and eventual death.

B. Risk factors:

1. Alcohol abuse most common cause.
2. Nutritional deficiency with decreased protein intake.
3. Hepatotoxins.
4. Virus.
5. Hepatitis B and C.

◆ **C. Assessment:**

1. *Subjective data:*
   a. Chronic feeling of malaise.
   b. Anorexia, nausea.
   c. Abdominal pain.
   d. Pruritus.
2. *Objective data:*
   a. *GI:*
      (1) Malnutrition, weight loss.
      (2) Vomiting.
      (3) Flatulence.
      (4) Ascites.
      (5) Enlarged liver and spleen.
      (6) Glossitis.
      (7) Fetid breath (sweet, musty odor).
   b. *Blood*—coagulation defects, possible esophageal varices, portal hypertension, bleeding from gums and injection sites.
   c. *Skin and hair*—edema, jaundice, spider angioma (telangiectasias); palmar erythema, decreased pubic and axillary hair.
   d. *Reproductive*—menstrual abnormalities, gynecomastia, testicular atrophy, impotence.
   e. *Neurological deficits*—memory loss, hepatic coma, decreased level of consciousness: flapping tremor, grimacing.

   f. Lab data:
      (1) *Decreased:* albumin, potassium, magnesium, blood urea nitrogen (BUN).
      (2) *Elevated:* prothrombin time, globulins, ammonia, AST (SGOT), bromsulphalein (BSP), alkaline phosphate, uric acid, blood sugar.

Adult

g. *Diagnostic tests*
   (1) Celiac angiography, hepatoportography
   (2) Liver biopsy
   (3) Paracentesis

◆ **D. Analysis/nursing diagnosis:**
1. *Altered nutrition, less than body requirements,* related to decreased intake, nausea, and vomiting.
2. *Risk for injury* related to decreased prothrombin production.
3. *Activity intolerance* related to fatigue.
4. *Fatigue* related to anorexia and nutritional deficiencies.
5. *Self-esteem disturbance* related to physical body changes.
6. *Risk for impaired skin integrity* related to pruritus.

◆ **E. Nursing care plan/implementation:**
1. Goal: *provide for special safety needs.*
   a. Monitor vitals (including neurological) frequently for hemorrhage from esophageal varices (may have *Sengstaken-Blakemore* or *Linton* tube inserted).
   b. Prepare client for *LeVeen shunt* surgery for portal hypertension as needed.
   c. Assist with *paracentesis* performed for ascites; monitor vitals to prevent shock during procedure.
2. Goal: *relieve discomfort caused by complications.*
   a. *Position: semi-Fowler's* or *Fowler's* to decrease pressure on diaphragm due to ascites.
   b. Deep breathing q2h to prevent respiratory complications.
   c. Skin care, topical medications to relieve pruritus; nail care to decrease possibility of further skin injury.
   d. Frequent oral hygiene related to nausea, vomiting, and fetid breath.
3. Goal: *improve fluid and electrolyte balance.*
   a. IV fluids and vitamins.
   b. I&O, hourly urines during acute attacks.
   c. Daily: girths, weights to monitor fluid balance.
   d. *Diuretics* as ordered to decrease edema.
   e. May receive *serum albumin* to promote adequate vascular volume, prevent azotemia and encephalopathy, and promote diuresis (observe carefully, because albumin could escape quickly through cell walls and cause increase in ascites).
4. Goal: *promote optimum nutrition within dietary restrictions.*
   a. NPO during acute episodes.
   b. Small, frequent meals when able to eat.
   c. *Low protein* (to decrease the amount of nitrogenous materials in the intestines) and *sodium* (to decrease fluid retention).
   d. *Moderate carbohydrate* (to meet energy demands) and *fat* (to make diet more palatable to clients who are anorexic).
5. Goal: *provide emotional support.*

a. Quiet environment during acute episodes to decrease external stimuli.
b. Refer to *community agencies* for assistance for client (e.g., Alcoholics Anonymous; for family, Al-Anon/Alateen).
6. Goal: *health teaching.*
   a. *Avoid* alcohol, exposure to infections.
   b. Dietary allowances, restrictions (see **Unit 9,** Sodium-restricted diet, **p. 722,** and Purine-restricted diet, **p. 722**).
   c. Drugs: names, purposes.
   d. Signs, symptoms of disease; complications.
   e. Stress-management techniques.

◆ **F. Evaluation/outcome criteria:**
1. No complications.
2. Nutritional status improves; lists dietary restrictions.
3. No alcohol consumption.
4. Lists signs and symptoms of progression of disease and complications.
5. Complies with discharge plan, becomes involved with an alcohol treatment program.

VI. Esophageal varices: life-threatening hemorrhage from tortuous dilated, thin-walled veins in submucosa of lower esophagus. May rupture when chemically or mechanically irritated, or when pressure is increased because of sneezing, coughing, use of the Valsalva maneuver, or excessive exercise.

A. Pathophysiology: portal hypertension related to cirrhosis of the liver → distended branches of the azygos vein and inferior vena cava where they join the smaller vessels of the esophagus.

B. Risk factors for hemorrhage:
1. Exertion that increases abdominal pressure.
2. Trauma from ingestion of coarse foods.
3. Acid pepsin erosion.

◆ **C. Assessment:**
1. *Subjective data:*
   a. Fear.
   b. Dysphagia.
   c. History: alcohol ingestion, liver dysfunction.
2. *Objective data:*
   a. Hematemesis.
   b. Hemorrhage: sudden, often fatal.
   c. *Decreased* BP; *increased* pulse, respirations.
   d. Melena (occult blood in stool).
   e. Diagnostic endoscopy.

◆ **D. Analysis/nursing diagnosis:**
1. *Fluid volume deficit* related to blood loss.
2. *Risk for injury* related to hemorrhage.
3. *Fear* related to massive blood loss.
4. *Ineffective individual coping* related to complications of cirrhosis.

◆ **E. Nursing care plan/implementation:**
1. Goal: *provide safety measures related to hemorrhage.*
   a. Recognize signs of shock; vitals q15min.
   b. Assist with insertion of *Sengstaken-Blakemore*

(or Minnesota) or *Linton tube* (tube is large and uncomfortable for client during insertion); explain procedure briefly to decrease fear and attempt to gain client's cooperation.

▶ c. While tube is in place, observe for respiratory distress; if present, *deflate the balloon by releasing pressure; do not cut the tube.*

d. Deflate the balloon as ordered to prevent necrosis.

▶ e. NG tube to low gastric suction; monitor for amount of bright-red blood; irrigate only as ordered using tepid, *not* iced, solutions.

f. Vitamin K as ordered to control bleeding.

2. Goal: *promote fluid balance.*

a. IV fluids, expanders.

b. Fresh blood as ordered to avoid increased ammonia; aids in coagulation.

3. Goal: *prevent complications of hepatic coma.*

a. *Saline cathartics* as ordered to remove old blood from GI tract.

b. *Antibiotics* as ordered to prevent infection.

c. Reduce portal hypertension; give propranolol (Inderal), vasopressin (Pitressin).

4. Goal: *provide emotional support.*

a. Stay with client.

b. Calm atmosphere.

5. Goal: *health teaching.*

a. Explain use of tube to client and family.

b. Bland diet instructions.

c. Recognize signs of bleeding.

d. *Avoid* straining at stool.

e. *Avoid* aspirin because of increased bleeding tendency.

◆ F. **Evaluation/outcome criteria:**

1. Survives acute bleeding episode.

2. Further episodes prevented by avoiding irritants, especially alcohol.

3. Improves nutritional status.

4. Recognizes symptoms of complications, e.g., bleeding.

5. Demonstrates knowledge of medications by avoiding aspirin.

VII. **Diaphragmatic (hiatal) hernia:** protrusion of part of stomach through diaphragm and into thoracic cavity **(Figure 7.8).** *Types:* sliding (most common); paraesophageal "rolling."

A. **Pathophysiology:** weakening of the musculature of the diaphragm, aggravated by increased intra-abdominal pressure → protrusion of the abdominal organs through the esophageal hiatus → reflux of gastric contents → esophagitis.

B. **Risk factors:**

1. Congenital abnormality.

2. Penetrating wound.

3. Age (middle-aged or elderly).

4. Women more than men.

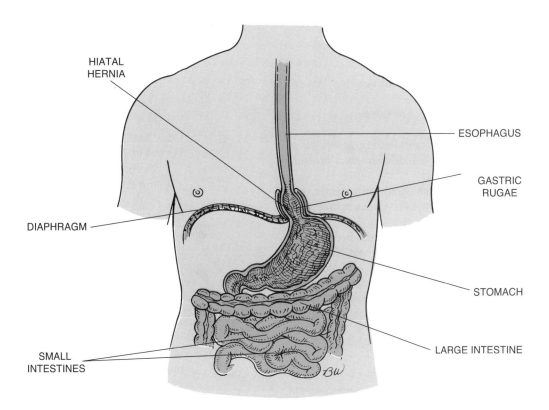

FIGURE 7.8   Hiatal hernia. (From Venes, D [ed]: Taber's Cyclopedic Medical Dictionary, ed. 20. FA Davis, Philadelphia, 2005.)

5. Obesity.
6. Ascites.
7. Pregnancy.
8. History of constipation.

◆ **C. Assessment:**
1. *Subjective data:*
   a. Pressure: substernal.
   b. *Pain:* epigastric, burning.
   c. Eructation, heartburn after eating.
   d. Dysphagia.
   e. Symptoms aggravated when recumbent.
2. *Objective data:*
   a. Cough, dyspnea.
   b. Tachycardia, palpitations.
   c. *Bleeding:* hematemesis, melena, signs of anemia due to gastroesophageal irritation, ulceration, and bleeding.
   d. *Diagnostic tests:*
      (1) Chest x-rays, showing protrusion of abdominal organs into thoracic cavity.
      (2) Barium swallow (upper GI series) to show presence of hernia.
      (3) Endoscopy
   e. Symptoms parallel those of gastroesophageal reflux disease (GERD).

◆ **D. Analysis/nursing diagnosis:**
1. *Pain* related to irritation of lining of GI tract.
2. *Altered nutrition, less than body requirements,* related to dysphagia.
3. *Sleep pattern disturbance* related to increase in symptoms when recumbent.
4. *Risk for aspiration* related to reflux of gastric contents.
5. *Activity intolerance* related to dyspnea.
6. *Anxiety* related to palpitations.

◆ **E. Nursing care plan/implementation:**
1. *Presurgical:*
   a. Goal: *promote relief of symptoms.*
      (1) *Diet:*
         (a) Small, frequent feedings of *soft, bland* foods, to reduce abdominal pressure and reflux.
         (b) Fluid when swallowing solids may push food into stomach; *hot* fluid may work best.
         (c) *Avoid* eating 2 hr before bedtime.
         (d) *High* protein, *low* fat foods to decrease heartburn.
      (2) *Positioning: head elevated* to increase movement of food into stomach. Symptoms may decrease if head of bed at home is elevated on 8-inch blocks.
      (3) Weight reduction to decrease abdominal pressure.
      (4) Medications as ordered:
         (a) 30 mL *antacid* 1 hr *after* meals and at bedtime.
         (b) *Avoid* anticholinergic drugs, which decrease gastric emptying.

2. *Postsurgical:*
   a. Goal: *provide for postoperative safety needs.*
      (1) Respiratory: deep breathing, coughing, splint incision area.
      ▶ (2) *Nasogastric (NG) tube:* check patency.
         (a) Drainage: should be small amount.
         (b) Color: dark brown 6 to 12 hr after surgery, changing to greenish yellow.
         (c) Do *not* disturb tube placement to *avoid* traction on suture line.
      (3) *Position:* initially head of bed elevated slightly, then *semi-Fowler's;* turn side to side frequently, to prevent pressure on diaphragm.
      ▶ (4) Maintain closed chest drainage if indicated (see **Table 11.11**).
      (5) Check for return of bowel sounds.
   b. Goal: *promote comfort and maintain nutrition.*
      (1) IVs for hydration and electrolytes.
      ▶ (2) Initiate feeding through *gastrostomy* tube if present.

   > (a) Usually attached to intermittent, low suction after surgery.
   > (b) Aspirate gastric contents before feeding—delay if 75 mL or more is present; report these findings to physician.
   > (c) Feed in *high Fowler's* or sitting position; keep head elevated for 30 min after eating.
   > (d) Warm feeding to room temperature; dilute with H_2O if too thick.
   > (e) Give 50 mL H_2O before feeding; 200 to 500 mL feeding by gravity over 10 to 15 min; follow with 50 mL H_2O.
   > (f) Give frequent mouth care.

   c. Goal: *health teaching.*
      (1) *Avoid* constricting clothing and activities that increase intra-abdominal pressure (e.g., lifting, bending, straining at stool).
      (2) Weight reduction.
      (3) Dietary needs: small, frequent, soft, bland meals.
      (4) Chew thoroughly
      (5) Upright position for at least 1 hr after meals.

◆ **F. Evaluation/outcome criteria:**
1. Obtains relief from symptoms; is comfortable.
2. Receives adequate, balanced nutrition.
3. Describes dietary changes, recommended positioning, and activity limitations to prevent recurrence.

VIII. Gastroesophageal reflux disease (GERD): inappropriate relaxation of the lower esophageal sphincter (LES) in response to unknown stimulus.

A. **Pathophysiology:** gastric volume or intraabdominal pressure elevated, or LES tone decreased→ frequent episodes of acid reflux→ breakdown of mucosal barrier→esophageal inflammation, hyperemia, and erosion→ fibrotic tissue formation → esophageal stricture→ impaired swallowing.

B. **Risk factors:**
1. Hiatal hernia.
2. Diet—foods that lower pressure of LES (fatty foods, chocolate, cola, coffee, tea).
3. Smoking.
4. Drugs (calcium channel blockers, NSAIDs, theophylline).
5. Elevated intra-abdominal pressure (obesity, pregnancy, heavy lifting).

C. **Assessment:**
1. *Subjective data:*
   a. Heartburn (pyrosis)—substernal or retrosternal; may mimic angina; 20 min to 2 hr after eating.
   b. Regurgitation—sour or bitter taste not associated with belching or nausea.
   c. Dysphagia or odynophagia (difficult or painful swallowing)—severe cases.
   d. Belching, feeling bloated.
   e. Nocturnal cough.
2. *Objective data:*
   a. Hoarseness, wheezing.
   b. *Diagnostic tests:* 24 hr pH monitoring; barium swallow with fluoroscopy; endoscopy.

D. **Analysis/nursing diagnosis:**
1. *Pain* related to acid reflux and esophageal inflammation.
2. *Knowledge deficit* (learning need) related to modifications needed to control reflux.

E. **Nursing care plan/implementation:**
1. Goal: *promote comfort and reduce reflux episodes.*
   a. Medications as ordered:
      (1) *Antacids* to neutralize gastric acid.
      (2) *Histamine (H_2) receptor antagonists* (cimetidine, ranitidine, famotidine) to reduce gastric acid secretion and support tissue healing.
      (3) *Proton pump inhibitor* (omeprazole [Prilosec]) to inhibit gastric enzymes and suppress gastric acid secretion.
   b. *Diet: avoid* strong stimulants of acid secretion (caffeine, alcohol); *avoid* foods that reduce LES competence (fatty foods, onions, tomato-based foods); *increase* protein; *restrict* spicy, acidic foods until healing occurs.
   c. Activity: *avoid* heavy lifting, straining, constrictive clothing, bending over.
   d. *Position: elevate head* of bed 6 to 12 inches for sleeping. Reflux more likely on right side.
2. Goal: *health teaching.*
   a. Weight reduction if indicated.
   b. Smoking cessation.
   c. Diet modification: *avoid* overeating—eat 4 to 6 small meals.
   d. Medication administration.
   e. Potential complications if uncontrolled (hemorrhage, aspiration).

F. **Evaluation/outcome criteria:**
1. No heartburn reported.
2. Changes diet as instructed.
3. No complications of continued reflux.

IX. **Peptic ulcer disease:** circumscribed loss of mucosa, submucosa, or muscle layer of the gastrointestinal tract caused by a decreased resistance of gastric mucosa to acid-pepsin injury. *Peptic ulcer disease* is a chronic disease and may occur in the distal esophagus, stomach, upper duodenum, or jejunum. *Gastric ulcers,* located on the lesser curvature of the stomach, are larger and deeper than duodenal ulcers and tend to become *malignant. Duodenal ulcers* are located on the first part of the duodenum and are more common than gastric ulcers. *Esophageal ulcers* occur in the esophagus. *Stress ulcers,* an acute problem, occur after a major insult to the body.

A. **Pathology:** failure of the body to regenerate mucous epithelium at a sufficient rate to counterbalance the damage to tissue during the breakdown of protein; decrease in the quantity and quality of the mucus; poor local mucosal blood flow, along with individual susceptibility to ulceration. A *peptic ulcer* is a hole in the lining of the stomach, duodenum, or esophagus. This hole occurs when the lining of these organs is corroded by the acidic digestive juices secreted by the stomach cells. Excess acid is still considered to be significant in ulcer formation. The leading cause of ulcer disease is currently believed to be infection of the stomach by *Helicobacter pylori (H. pylori).* Another major cause of ulcers is chronic use of nonsteroidal antiinflammatory drugs (NSAIDs). Cigarette smoking is also an important cause of ulcers.

B. **Risk factors:**
1. *Gastric ulcers.*
   a. Infection with *H. pylori.*
   b. Decreased resistance to acid-pepsin injury.
   c. Increased histamine release → inflammatory reaction.
   d. Ulcerogenic drugs (aggravate preexisting conditions).
   e. Cigarette smoking.
   f. Increased alcohol and caffeine use (aggravates preexisting conditions).
   g. Gastric ulcer is thought to be a risk for gastric cancer.
   h. Difficulty coping with stressful situations.
2. *Duodenal ulcers.*
   a. Infection with *H. pylori.*
   b. Elevated gastric acid secretory rate.
   c. Elevated gastric acid levels postprandially (after eating).

d. Increased rate of gastric emptying→ increased amount of acid in duodenum→ irritation and breakdown of duodenal mucosa.

e. Ulcerogenic medication use (aggravates pre-existing conditions).

f. Cigarette smoking.

g. Alcohol and caffeine use (aggravates pre-existing condition).

h. Difficulty coping with stressful situations.

3. *Stress ulcers.*

a. Severe trauma or major illness.

b. Severe burns *(Curling's ulcer);* develop in 72 hr with majority of persons with burns over more than 35% of the body surface.

c. Head injuries or intracranial disease *(Cushing's ulcer).*

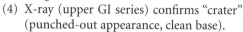 d. Medications in large doses: corticosteroids, salicylates, ibuprofen, indomethacin, phenyl-butazone (Butazolidin).

e. Shock.

f. Sepsis.

◆ **C. Assessment:**

1. *Subjective data:*

a. *Gastric ulcers.*

(1) *Pain:*

(a) *Type:* gnawing, aching, burning.

(b) *Location:* epigastric, left of midline, localized.

(c) *Occurrence:* periodic pain, often 2 hr after eating.

(d) *Relief: antacids;* may be aggravated, *not* relieved, by food.

(e) Some clients report no discomfort at all.

(2) Weakness.

(3) History of risk factors as above.

b. *Duodenal ulcers.*

(1) *Pain:*

(a) *Type:* gnawing, aching, burning, hungerlike, boring.

(b) *Location:* right epigastric, localized; steady pain near midline of back may indicate perforation.

(c) *Occurrence:* 1 to 3 hr after eating, worse at end of day or during the night; initial attack occurs spring or fall; history of remissions and exacerbations.

(d) *Relief:* food, *antacids,* or both.

(e) Some clients report no discomfort at all.

(2) Nausea.

(3) History of risk factors (see **IX. B.**).

c. *Stress ulcers.*

(1) *Pain:* often painless until serious complication (hemorrhage, perforation) occurs.

(2) History of risk factors as above.

2. *Objective data.*

a. *Gastric ulcer.*

(1) Vomiting blood (hematemesis).

(2) Melena (tarry stools).

(3) Weight loss.

(4) X-ray (upper GI series) confirms "crater" (punched-out appearance, clean base).

(5) Endoscopy confirms presence of ulcer; biopsy for cytology.

(6) Monitor for blood loss: CBC, stool for occult blood.

(7) Orthostatic hypotension.

(8) *Lab data:* positive for *H. pylori.*

b. *Duodenal ulcer.*

(1) Eructation.

(2) Vomiting blood (hematemesis).

(3) Regurgitation of sour liquid into back of mouth.

(4) Constipation.

(5) X-ray (upper GI series) confirms ulcer craters and niches, as well as outlet deformities: round or oval funnel-like lesion extending into musculature.

(6) Endoscopy for direct visualization.

(7) Monitor for blood loss: CBC, stool for occult blood.

(8) Orthostatic hypotension.

(9) *Lab data:* positive for *H. pylori.*

c. *Stress ulcer.*

(1) GI bleeding.

(2) Multiple, superficial erosions affecting large area of gastric mucosa.

◆ **D. Analysis/nursing diagnosis** (all types):

1. *Pain* related to erosion of gastric lining.

2. *Ineffective individual coping* related to inability to change lifestyle.

3. *Altered nutrition, less than body requirements,* related to inadequate intake.

4. *Knowledge deficit* (learning need) regarding preventive measures.

5. *Risk for injury* related to possible hemorrhage or perforation.

◆ **E. Nursing care plan/implementation** (all types):

1. Goal: *promote comfort.*

a. Medications as ordered to decrease pain (see E. Goal: *health teaching*); *sedatives* to decrease anxiety.

b. Prepare for *diagnostic tests.*

(1) X-rays; upper GI series (barium swallow); lower GI (barium enema).

(2) Endoscopy.

(3) Gastric analysis, to determine amount of hydrochloric acid in GI tract.

2. Goal: *prevent/recognize signs of complications.*

a. Monitor vitals for shock.

b. Check stool for occult blood/hemorrhage.

c. Palpate abdomen for perforation (rigid, boardlike); arterial bleeding.

3. Goal: *provide emotional support.*

a. Stress-management techniques.

b. Restful environment.

 c. Prepare for surgery, if necessary.

4. Goal: *health teaching.*
   a. Medications:
      (1) *Antibiotics.* Sometimes antibiotics work best if given in combination with Prilosec, H$_2$ blockers, or Pepto-Bismol. *Caution:* use of antibiotic treatment can cause allergic reactions, diarrhea, and severe antibiotic-induced colitis.
         (a) Tetracycline.
         (b) Amoxicillin.
         (c) Metronidazole (Flagyl).
         (d) Clarithromycin (Biaxin).
      (2) *Histamine antagonists: given with meals/ bedtime* to block the action of histamine-stimulated gastric secretions (basal and stimulated); inhibit pepsin secretion and reduce the volume of gastric secretions.
         (a) Cimetidine (Tagamet) inhibits gastrin release; can be given PO, IV, or IM; *cannot* be given within 1 hr of antacid therapy.
         (b) Ranitidine (Zantac) has greater reduction of acid secretion, longer duration, less frequent administration (bid vs. qid), and fewer side effects than cimetidine.
         (c) Nizatidine (Axid).
         (d) Famotidine (Pepcid).
      (3) *Proton pump inhibitors* (gastric acid inhibitors): superior in treating esophageal ulcers; equal to other H$_2$ receptors for gastric and duodenal ulcers.
         (a) Omeprazole (Prilosec).
         (b) Lansoprazole (Prevacid).
         (c) Pantoprazole.
      (4) *Antiulcers: give 1 to 3 hr after meals and at bedtime* to decrease pain by lowering acidity; monitor for:
         (a) Diarrhea (seen most often with magnesium carbonate and magnesium oxide [Maalox, Mylanta]).
         (b) Constipation (seen most often with calcium carbonate [Tums] or aluminum hydroxide [Amphojel]).
         (c) Electrolyte imbalance (seen with systemic antacid, soda bicarbonate).
         (d) Best 1 to 3 hr *after meals.*
         (e) Liquids more effective than tablets; if taking tablets, chew slowly.
      (5) *Sucralfate* (Carafate) and misoprostol (Cytotec): *given 1 hr before meals and at bedtime.*
         (a) Locally active topical agent that forms a protective coat on mucosa, prevents further digestive action of both acid and pepsin.
         (b) Must *not* be given within 30 min of antacids.

      (6) *Anticholinergic*—when used, given *before* meals to decrease gastric acid secretion and delay gastric emptying.
      (7) Important: *avoid aspirin* (could increase bleeding possibility).
   b. *Diet:*
      (1) Change diet only to relieve symptoms; diet may not influence ulcer formation.
      (2) *Avoid* foods that increase acidity—caffeine and alcohol in moderation.
      (3) *Plan:*
         (a) Small, frequent meals (to prevent exacerbations of symptoms related to an empty stomach).
         (b) Weight control.
   c. Complications—signs and symptoms:
      (1) Gastric ulcers may be premalignant.
      (2) Perforation.
      (3) Hemorrhage.
      (4) Obstruction.
   d. *Lifestyle changes:*
      (1) Decrease:
         (a) Smoking.
         (b) Noise.
         (c) Rush.
         (d) Confusion.
      (2) Increase:
         (a) Communication.
         (b) Mental/physical rest.
         (c) Compliance with medical regimen.

◆ **F. Evaluation/outcome criteria:**
   1. *Avoids* foods/liquids that cause irritation.
   2. Takes prescribed medications.
   3. Pain decreases.
   4. No complications.
   5. States signs and symptoms of complications.
   6. Participates in stress-reduction activities.
   7. Stops smoking.

X. Gastric surgery: peformed when ulcer medical regimen is unsuccessful, ulcer is determined to be precancerous, or complications are present.
   A. Types:
      1. *Subtotal gastrectomy:* removal of a portion of the stomach.
      2. *Total gastrectomy:* removal of the entire stomach.
      3. *Antrectomy:* removal of entire antrum (lower) portion of the stomach.
      4. *Pyloroplasty:* repair of the pyloric opening of the stomach.
      5. *Vagotomy:* interruption of the impulses carried by the vagus nerve, which results in reduction of gastric secretions and decreased physical activity of the stomach (being done less often).
      6. Combination of vagotomy and gastrectomy.
   ◆ **B. Analysis/nursing diagnosis:**
      1. *Pain* related to surgical incision.

Adult

2. *Ineffective breathing pattern* related to high surgical incision.
3. *Risk for trauma* related to possible complications postgastrectomy.
4. *Knowledge deficit* (learning need) regarding medication regimen and factors that aggravate condition.
5. *Fear* related to possible precancerous lesion.
6. *Ineffective individual coping* related to adjustments in lifestyle needed to lessen symptoms.

◆ **C. Nursing care plan/implementation:**
  1. Goal: *promote comfort in the postoperative period.*
    a. *Analgesics:* to relieve pain and allow client to cough, deep breathe to prevent pulmonary complications.
    b. *Position: semi-Fowler's* to aid in breathing.
  2. Goal: *promote wound healing.*
    a. Keep dressings dry.
    b. NG tube to low intermittent suction (Levin) or low continuous suction (Salem-sump).
      (1) Check drainage from NG tube; normally bloody first 2 to 3 hr postsurgery, then brown to dark green.
      (2) Excessive bright-red blood drainage: take vital signs; report vital signs, color and volume of drainage to MD **immediately.**
      (3) Irrigate gently with saline in amount ordered; do **not** irrigate against resistance; may not be done in early postoperative period.
      (4) Tape securely to face, but prevent obstructed vision.
      (5) Frequent mouth and nostril care.
  3. Goal: *promote adequate nutrition and hydration.*
    a. Administer parenteral fluids as ordered.
    b. Accurate I&O.
    c. Check bowel sounds, at least q4h; NPO 1 to 3 days; bowel sounds normally return 21 to 36 hr; oral fluids as ordered when bowel sounds present—usually 30 mL, then *small* feedings, then *bland* liquids to soft diet.
    d. Observe for nausea and vomiting due to suture line edema, food intake (too much, too fast).
  4. Goal: *prevent complications.*
    a. Check dressing q4h for bleeding.
    b. *Vitamin B$_{12}$* and iron replacement as indicated to avoid pernicious anemia and iron deficiency anemia.
    c. *Avoid* dumping syndrome.

◆ **D. Evaluation/outcome criteria:**
  1. Hemorrhage, dumping syndrome avoided.
  2. Healing begins.
  3. Adjust lifestyle to prevent recurrence/marginal ulcer.

XI. Dumping syndrome: hypoglycemic-type episode; occurs postoperativly after gastric resection (may also occur after vagotomy, antrectomy, or gastroenterostomy), when food and fluids that are more hyperos-

molar than the jejunal secretions pass *quickly* into jejunum, producing fluid shifts from bloodstream to jejunum. This is a mild problem for about 20% of clients and will disappear in a few months to a year. Symptoms cause serious problem for about 7% of clients. This discomfort may occur during a meal or up to 30 min after the meal and last from 20 to 60 min. The reaction is greatest after the ingestion of sugar.

◆ **A. Assessment:**
  1. *Subjective data:*
    a. Feeling of fullness, weakness, faintness.
    b. Palpitations.
    c. Nausea.
    d. Discomfort during or after eating.
  2. *Objective data:*
    a. Diaphoresis.
    b. Diarrhea.
    c. Fainting.
    d. Symptoms of hypoglycemia.

◆ **B. Analysis/nursing diagnosis:**
  1. *Altered nutrition, more than body requirements,* related to body's inability to properly digest high carbohydrate, high sodium foods.
  2. *Diarrhea* related to food passing into jejunum too quickly.
  3. *Risk for injury* related to hypoglycemia.
  4. *Knowledge deficit* (learning need) related to dietary restrictions.

◆ **C. Nursing care plan/implementation:**
  1. Goal: *health teaching.*
    a. *Include:*
      (1) *Increased fat, protein* to delay emptying.
      (2) Rest after meals.
      (3) Small, frequent meals.
      (4) Fluids *between* meals.
    b. *Avoid:*
      (1) Foods high in *salt, carbohydrate.*
      (2) Large meals.
      (3) Stress at mealtime.
      (4) Fluids at mealtime.

◆ **D. Evaluation/outcome criteria:**
  1. No complications.
  2. Client heals.
  3. No further ulcers.
  4. Incorporates health teaching into lifestyle and prevents syndrome.

XII. Total parenteral nutrition (TPN): nutrition through a central venous line to clients who are in a catabolic state; are malnourished and cannot tolerate food by mouth or enteral nutrition; are in negative nitrogen balance; or have conditions that interfere with protein ingestion, digestion, and absorption (e.g., Crohn's disease, major burns, and side effects of radiation therapy of abdomen). Least desirable route for nutrition.

A. Types of solutions:
  1. Hydrolyzed proteins (Hyprotein, Amigen).
  2. Synthetic amino acids (Freamine).
  3. Usual components:

a. 3% to 8% amino acid.

b. 10% to 25% glucose.

c. Multivitamins.

d. Electrolytes.

4. Supplements that can be added:

a. Fructose.

b. Alcohol.

c. Minerals: iron, copper, calcium.

d. Trace elements: iodine, zinc, magnesium.

e. Vitamins: A, B, C.

f. Androgen hormone therapy.

g. Insulin.

h. Heparin.

i. Fats (lipid or fat emulsions) with prolonged use. Lipid emulsions are *contraindicated* if client has allergy to eggs or who are on ↑ lipid-containing medications like propofol (Diprivan).

B. Administration:

1. Dosage varies with clinical condition; 1 to 2 L over 24 hr at a constant IV drip rate. If TPN is discontinued, the rate must be tapered over 4 to 8 hr to avoid fluid, electrolyte abnormalities.

2. Solution prepared under laminar flow hood (usually in pharmacy); solution must be *refrigerated;* when refrigerated, expires in *24* hr; once removed from refrigerator, expires in *12* hr.

3. Incompatible with most medications; check with pharmacy. Give in a dedicated TPN line. Do **not** inject IV push meds into TPN line.

4. Route: *Must* be given via central line catheter—double- or triple-lumen catheter or infusion port of PA catheter inserted by physician into internal jugular or subclavian vein. More commonly given via peripherally inserted central catheter (PICC line), inserted by specially trained IV nurses into brachial or cephalic veins. Placement must be confirmed by x-ray before beginning infusion. Catheter tip in superior vena cava or right atrium.

5. Management of PICC line:

a. Always wash hands before handling.

b. Do *not* take BP in PICC arm.

c. *No* needle sticks near or above PICC. If possible draw blood from opposite arm.

d. *Avoid* excessive shoulder use; if sent home with PICC, cautious use of backpacks, playing basketball, shoveling, weight lifting.

e. Cover PICC arm before bathing/showering.

f. If dressing becomes wet, soiled, or loose, change as soon as possible.

g. If catheter breaks, secure with tape and call care provider.

h. If sudden chest pain, SOB, or gurgling sensation heard near ear with catheter breakage, clamp or pinch catheter, have client lie on left side with head down. Call MD.

6. *Side effects:*

a. Hyperosmolar coma.

b. Hyperglycemia >130 mg/dL.

c. Septicemia.

d. Thrombosis/sclerosis of vein.

e. Air embolus.

f. Pneumothorax.

◆ **C. Analysis/nursing diagnosis:**

1. *Fluid volume excess, potential,* related to inability to tolerate amount and consistency of solution.

2. *Fluid volume deficit* related to state of malnutrition.

3. *Risk for injury* related to possible complications.

4. *Altered nutrition, more or less than body requirements,* related to ability to tolerate parenteral nutrition.

◆ **D. Nursing care plan/implementation:**

1. Goal: *prevent infection.*

a. Dressing change:

(1) Strict *aseptic* technique.

(2) Nurse and client wear mask during dressing change.

(3) Cleanse skin with solution as ordered:

(a) Acetone to defat the skin, destroy the bacterial wall.

(b) Iodine 1% solution as *antiseptic* agent.

(4) Dressing changed q48 to 72h; transparent polyurethane dressings may be changed weekly.

(5) Mark with nurse's initials, date and time of change.

(6) Air occlusive dressing.

b. Attach final filter on tubing setup, to prevent air embolism.

c. Solution: change q24h to prevent infection.

d. Culture wound and catheter tip if signs of infection appear.

e. Monitor temperature q4h.

f. Use lumen line for feeding *only* (not for CVP or medications).

2. Goal: *prevent fluid and electrolyte imbalance.*

a. Daily weights.

b. I&O.

c. Blood glucose q6h for 24 hrs using glucometer; may need insulin coverage. If normal range, change to daily.

d. Monitor Chem 20 electrolytes biweekly initially.

e. Infusion pump to maintain constant infusion rate.

3. Goal: *prevent complications.*

a. Warm TPN solution to room temperature to prevent chills.

b. Monitor for signs of complications (**Table 7.30**).

(1) Infiltration.

(2) Thrombophlebitis.

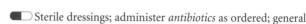

TABLE 7.30	Complications Associated with Total Parenteral Nutrition

Problem	◆ Nursing Interventions
Infection Local infection (pain, redness, edema) Generalized, systemic infection (elevated temperature, WBC)	Sterile dressings; administer *antibiotics* as ordered; general comfort measures
Arterial Puncture Artery is punctured instead of vein Physician aspirates bright-red blood that is pulsating strongly	Needle is withdrawn and pressure is applied
Air Embolus Air enters venous system during catheter insertion or tubing changes; or catheter/tubing pull apart Chest pain, dizziness, cyanosis, confusion	STAT ABGs, chest x-ray, ECG Connect catheter to sterile syringes, and aspirate air Clean catheter tip, connect to new tubing *Place client on left side with head lowered* (left Trendelenburg prevents air from going into pulmonary artery) *Prevention: have client perform Valsalva maneuver or use plastic-coated clamp on catheter at insertion or tubing changes*
Catheter Embolus Catheter must be checked for placement by x-ray and observed when removed to be sure it is intact	Careful observation of catheter Monitor for signs of distress
Pneumothorax If need punctures pleura, client reports dyspnea, chest pain	May seal off or may need chest tubes

(3) Fever.

(4) Hyperglycemia.

(5) Fluid and electrolyte imbalance.

  c. Have client perform *Valsalva maneuver* or apply a plastic-coated clamp when changing tubing to prevent air embolism.

  d. Tape tubings together to prevent accidental separation.

◆ **E. Evaluation/outcome criteria:**

1. No signs of infection.

2. Blood sugar < 130 mg/dL.

3. Electrolytes within normal limits.

4. Wounds begin to heal.

5. Weight: no further loss, begins to gain.

XIII. Diabetes: heterogeneous group of diseases involving the disruption of the metabolism of carbohydrates, fats, and protein. If uncontrolled, serious vascular and neurological changes occur.

  A. Types:

1. *Type 1:* formerly called *insulin-dependent diabetes mellitus (IDDM);* and also formerly called "juvenile-onset diabetes." Insulin is needed to prevent ketosis; onset usually in youth but may occur in adulthood; prone to ketosis, unstable diabetes.

2. *Type 2:* formerly called *non–insulin-dependent diabetes mellitus (NIDDM);* and also *formerly* called "maturity-onset diabetes" or "adult-onset diabetes." May be controlled with diet and oral hypoglycemics or insulin; client less apt to

have ketosis, except in presence of infection. May be further classified as *obese type 2* or *nonobese type 2.*

3. *Type 3: gestational diabetes mellitus (GDM):* glucose intolerance during pregnancy in women who were not known to have diabetes before pregnancy; will be reclassified after birth; may need to be treated or may return to prepregnancy state and need no treatment.

4. *Type 4:* diabetes secondary to another condition, such as pancreatic disease, other hormonal imbalances, or drug therapy such as receiving glucocorticoids.

  B. Pathophysiology:

1. *Type 1*—absolute deficiency of insulin due to destruction of pancreatic beta cells by the interaction of genetic, immunological, hereditary, or environmental factors.

2. *Type 2*—relative deficiency of insulin due to:

  a. An islet cell defect resulting in a slowed or delayed response in the release of insulin to a glucose load; or

  b. Reduction in the number of insulin receptors from continuously elevated insulin levels; or

  c. A postreceptor defect; or

  d. A major peripheral resistance to insulin induced by hyperglycemia. These factors lead to deprivation of insulin-dependent cells → a marked decrease in the cellular rate of glucose uptake, and therefore elevated blood glucose.

Adult

C. Risk factors:
1. Obesity.
2. Family history of diabetes.
3. Age 45 or older.
4. Women whose babies at birth weighed more than 9 lb.
5. History of autoimmune disease.
6. Members of high-risk ethnic group (African-American, Latino, or Native American).
7. History of gestational diabetes mellitus.
8. Hypertension.
9. Elevated HDL.

◆ **D. Assessment:**
1. *Subjective data:*
   a. *Eyes:* blurry vision.
   b. *Skin:* pruritus vulvae.
   c. *Neuromuscular:* paresthesia, peripheral neuropathy, lethargy, weakness, fatigue, increased irritability.
   d. *GI:* polydipsia (increased thirst).
   e. *Reproductive:* impotence.
2. *Objective data:*
   a. *Genitourinary:* polyuria, glycosuria, nocturia (nocturnal enuresis in children).
   b. *Vital signs:*
      (1) *Pulse* and *temperature:* normal or elevated.
      (2) *BP:* normal or decreased, unless complications present.
      (3) *Respirations: increased* rate and depth (*Kussmaul's* respirations).
   c. *GI:*
      (1) Polyphagia, dehydration.
      (2) Weight loss, failure to gain weight.
      (3) Acetone breath.
   d. *Skin:* cuts heal slowly; frequent infections, foot ulcers, vaginitis.
   e. *Neuromuscular:* loss of strength, peripheral neuropathy.

   f. Lab data:
      (1) *Elevated:*
         (a) Blood sugar >126 mg/dL fasting or 200 mg/dL 1 to 2 hr after eating.
         (b) Glucose tolerance test.
         (c) Glycosuria (>170 mg/100 mL).
         (d) Potassium (>5) and chloride (>145).
         (e) Hemoglobin A_{1c} >7%.
      (2) *Decreased:*
         (a) pH (<7.4).
         (b) $Paco_2$ (<32).

   g. Long-term pathological considerations:
      (1) *Cataract formation and retinopathy:* thickened capillary basement membrane, changes in vascularization and hemorrhage, due to chronic hyperglycemia.
      (2) *Nephropathy:* due to glomerulosclerosis, arteriosclerosis of renal artery and pyelonephritis, progressive uremia.
      (3) *Neuropathy:* due to reduced tissue perfu-

sion; affecting motor, sensory, voluntary, and autonomic functions.
      (4) *Arteriosclerosis:* due to lesions of the intimal wall.
      (5) *Cardiac:* angina, coronary insufficiency, myocardial infarction.
      (6) *Vascular changes:* occlusions, intermittent claudication, loss of peripheral pulses, arteriosclerosis.

◆ **E. Analysis/nursing diagnosis:**
1. *Altered nutrition, less than body requirements,* related to inability to metabolize nutrients and weight loss.
2. *Altered nutrition, more than body requirements,* related to excessive glucose intake.
3. *Risk for injury* related to complications of uncontrolled diabetes.
4. *Body image disturbance* related to long-term illness.
5. *Knowledge deficit* (learning need) related to management of long-term illness and potential complications.
6. *Ineffective individual coping* related to inability to follow diet/medication regimen.
7. *Sexual dysfunction* related to impotence from diabetes and treatment.

◆ **F. Nursing care plan/implementation:**
1. Goal: *obtain and maintain normal sugar balance.*
   a. Monitor: vital signs; blood glucose before meals, at bedtime, and as symptoms demand (urine testing for glucose levels is not as accurate as capillary blood testing).
   b. Medications:
      (1) *Oral hypoglycemics:*
         (a) Sulfonylureas; tolbutamide (Orinase), chlorpropamide (Diabenese), tolazamide (Tolinase), acetohexamide (Dymelor), glimepiride (Amaryl), glyburide (DiaBeta and Micronase), and glipizide (Glucocotrol).
         (b) Others: metformin (Glucophage) increases body's sensitivity to insulin. Acarbose (Precose) inhibits cells of the small intestine from absorbing complex carbohydrates.
      (2) *Insulin* (biosynthetic human insulin): *bolus insulin*—released in response to meals; *basal insulin*—released between meals, at nighttime.
         (a) Rapid-acting bolus analogue of human insulin (Lispro, Aspart).
         (b) Short acting bolus (crystalline, regular) (Humulin R).
         (c) Intermediate acting basal (Lente and NPH).
         (d) Slow acting (protamine zinc).
         (e) Long, extended acting basal (Ultralente).
         (f) Long acting basal analogue (Glargine).

(3) Methods of administration:
  (a) Subcutaneous injection.
  (b) Prefilled injectable insulin pens (Novopen and Novolin).
  (c) Continuous subcutaneous insulin infusion therapy (insulin pumps).

c. *Diet*, as ordered.
  (1) Carbohydrate, 50% to 60%; protein, 20%; fats, 30% (saturated fats limited to 10%, unsaturated fats, 90%).
  (2) Calorie reduction in adults who are obese; enough calories to promote normal growth and development for children or adults who are not obese.
  (3) Limit refined sugars.
  (4) Add vitamins, minerals as needed for well-balanced diet.

d. Monitor for signs of *acute* (hypoglycemia, ketoacidosis) or *chronic* (circulatory compromise, neuropathy, nephropathy, retinopathy) complications.

2. Goal: *health teaching:*
  a. *Diet:* foods allowed, restricted, substitutions.
  b. Medications: administration techniques, importance of using room-temperature insulin and rotating injection sites to prevent tissue damage.
  c. Desired and side effects of prescribed insulin type; onset, peak, and duration of action of prescribed insulin.
  d. Blood glucose testing techniques.
  e. Signs of complications (**Table 7.31**).
  f. Importance of health maintenance:
    (1) Infection prevention, especially foot and nail care.
    (2) Routine checkups.
    (3) Maintain stable balance of glucose by carefully monitoring glucose level and making necessary adjustments in diet and activity level; seeking medical attention when unable to maintain balance; regular exercise program.

◆ G. **Evaluation/outcome criteria:**
  1. Optimal blood-glucose levels achieved.
  2. Ideal weight maintained.
  3. Adequate hydration.
  4. Carries out self-care activities: blood testing, foot care, exchange diets, medication administration, exercise.
  5. Recognizes and treats hyperglycemic or hypoglycemic reactions.
  6. Seeks medical assistance appropriately.

XIV. **Nonketotic hyperglycemic hyperosmolar coma (NKHHC):** profound hyperglycemia and dehydration without ketosis or ketoacidosis; seen in non–insulin-dependent diabetes; brought on by infection or illness. This condition may lead to impaired consciousness and seizures. The client is *critically ill.* Mortality rate is over 50%.

A. **Pathophysiology:** hyperglycemia greater than 1000 mg/dL, causes osmotic diuresis, depletion of extracellular fluid, and hyperosmolarity related to infection or another stressor as the precipitating factor. Client unable to replace fluid deficits with oral intake.

B. **Risk factors:**
  1. Old age.
  2. History of non–insulin-dependent diabetes.
  3. Infections: pneumonia, pyelonephritis, pancreatitis, gram-negative infections.
  4. Kidney failure: uremia and peritoneal dialysis or hemodialysis.
  5. Shock:
    a. Lactic acidosis related to bicarbonate deficit.
    b. Myocardial infarction.
  6. Hemorrhage:
    a. GI.
    b. Subdural.
    c. Arterial thrombosis.
  7. Medications:
    a. Diuretics.
    b. Glucocorticoids.
  8. Tube feedings.

◆ C. **Assessment:**
  1. *Subjective data:*
    a. Confusion.
    b. Lethargy.
  2. *Objective data:*
    a. Nystagmus.
    b. Dehydration.
    c. Aphasia.
    d. Nuchal rigidity.
    e. Hyperreflexia.

  f. Lab data:
    (1) Blood-glucose level 1000 mg/dL.
    (2) Serum sodium and chloride—normal to *elevated.*
    (3) BUN >60 mg/dL (higher than in ketoacidosis because of more severe gluconeogenesis and dehydration).
    (4) Arterial pH—slightly *depressed.*

◆ D. **Analysis/nursing diagnosis:**
  1. *Risk for injury* related to hyperglycemia.
  2. *Altered renal peripheral tissue perfusion* related to vascular collapse.
  3. *Ineffective airway clearance* related to coma.

◆ E. **Nursing care plan/implementation:**
  1. Goal: *promote fluid and electrolyte balance.*
    a. IVs: fluids and electrolytes, sodium chloride solution used initially to combat dehydration. Rate of infusion will be determined by: BP assessment, cardiovascular status, balance between fluid input and output, and lab values.
    b. Monitor I&O because of the high volume of fluid replaced in the critical stage of this condition.

TABLE 7.31	Comparison of Diabetic Complications	
	Hypoglycemia	**Ketoacidosis**
Pathophysiology	Major metabolic complication when too little food or too large dose of insulin or hypo-glycemic agents administered; interferes with oxygen consumption of nervous tissue	Major metabolic complication in which there is insufficient insulin for metabolism of carbohydrates, fats, and proteins; seen most frequently with clients who are insulin dependent; precipitated in the person with known diabetes by stressors (such as infection, trauma, major illness) that increase insulin needs
Risk factors	Too little food Emotional or added stress Vomiting or diarrhea Added exercise	Insufficient insulin or oral hypoglycemics Noncompliance with dietary instructions Major illness/infections Therapy with steroid administration Trauma, surgery Elevated blood sugar >200 mg/dL
◆ **Assessment**	**Behavioral change:** *Subjective data*—nervous, irritable, anxious, confused, disoriented *Objective data*—abrupt mood changes, psychosis **Visual:** *Subjective data*—blurred vision, diplopia *Objective data*—dilated pupils **Skin:** *Objective data*—diaphoresis, **pale**, cool, clammy, goose bumps (piloerection), tenting **Vitals.** *Objective data*–palpitations **Gastrointestinal:** *Subjective data*—hunger, nausea *Objective data*—diarrhea, vomiting **Neurological:** *Subjective data*—headache; lips/tongue: tingling, numbness *Objective data*—fainting, yawning; speech: inco-herent; convulsions; coma **Musculoskeletal:** *Subjective data*—weak, fatigue *Objective data*—trembling Blood sugar: <80 mg/dL	**Behavioral change:** *Subjective data*—irritable, confused *Objective data*—drowsy **Visual:** *Objective data*—eyeballs: soft, sunken **Skin:** *Objective data*—loss of turgor, flushed face, pruritus vulvae **Vitals:** *Objective data*— tachycardia; thready; respirations: *Kussmaul's;* BP: hypovolemic shock **Gastrointestinal:** *Subjective data*—increased thirst and hunger, abdominal pain, nausea *Objective data*—vomiting, diarrhea, dry mucous membrane; lips, tongue: red, parched; breath: fruity **Neurological:** *Subjective data*—headache; irritability; confusion; lethargy, weakness **Musculoskeletal** *Subjective data,*—fatigue; general malaise **Renal:** *Objective data*—polyuria Blood sugar: >130 mg/dL
◆ **Analysis/nursing diagnosis**	*Risk for injury* related to deficit of needed glucose *Knowledge deficit* (learning need) related to proper dietary intake or proper insulin dosage *Altered nutrition, less than body requirements,* related to glucose deficiency	*Risk for injury* related to glucose imbalance *Knowledge deficit* (learning need) related to proper balance of diet and insulin dosage
◆ **Nursing care plan/ implementation**	Goal: *provide adequate glucose to reverse hypo-glycemia:* administer simple sugar STAT, PO or IV, glucose paste absorbed in mucous membrane; monitor blood sugar levels; iden-tify events leading to complication Goal: *health teaching:* how to prevent further episodes (see Diabetes, *Health teaching,* **p. 574**); importance of careful monitoring of balance between glucose levels and insulin dosage	Goal: *promote normal balance of food and insulin:* **regular** insulin as ordered; IV saline, as ordered; bicarbonate and electrolyte replacements, as ordered; potassium replace-ments once therapy begins and urine output is adequate Goal: *health teaching:* diet instructions, desired effects and side effects of prescribed insulin or hypoglycemic agent (onset, peak, and duration of action); importance of recognizing signs of imbalance
◆ **Evaluation/outcome criteria**	Adheres to diet and correct insulin dosage Adjusts dosage when activity is increased Glucose level 80–120 mg/dL	Accepts prescribed diet Takes medication (correct dose and time) Serious complications avoided Glucose level 80–120 mg/dL

Adult

c. Administer nursing care for the problem that precipitated this serious condition.

d. *Diet:* Food by mouth when client is able.

2. Goal: *prevent complications.*

a. Administer *regular* insulin (initial dose usually 5 to 15 U) and food, as ordered.

b. Uncontrolled condition leads to: cardiovascular disease, renal failure, blindness, and diabetic gangrene.

◆ F. **Evaluation/outcome criteria:**

1. Blood sugar returns to normal level of 80 to 120 mg/dL.

2. Client is alert to time, place, and person.

3. Primary medical problem resolved.

4. Client recognizes and reports signs of imbalance.

XV. **Cholecystitis/cholelithiasis:** inflammation of gallbladder due to bacterial infection, presence of cholelithiasis (stones, cholesterol, calcium, or bile in the gallbladder), or choledocholithiasis (stone in the common bile duct) and/or obstruction. *Acute* cholecystitis is abrupt in onset, but the client usually has a history of several attacks of fatty-food intolerance. Client with *chronic* cholecystitis has a history of several attacks of moderate severity and has usually learned to avoid fatty foods to decrease symptoms.

A. **Pathophysiology:** calculi from increased concentration of bile salts, pigments, or cholesterol due to metabolic or hemolytic disorders, biliary stasis → precipitation of salts into stones, or inflammation causing bile constituents to become altered.

B. **Risk factors:**

1. Womanhood.
2. Obesity.
3. Pregnancy or previous pregnancies.
4. Use of birth control pills or hormone replacement therapy.
5. High fat, low fiber diets.
6. Rapid weight loss.
7. History of Crohn's disease.
8. Genetics.
9. Age: increased risk over 40.
10. Certain drugs to lower lipids; clofibrate (Atromid-S).
11. Other diseases: cirrhosis of liver.

◆ C. **Assessment:**

1. *Subjective data:*
   a. *Pain:*
      (1) *Type*—severe colic, radiating to the back under the scapula and to the right shoulder.
      (2) Positive *Murphy's sign*—a sign of gallbladder disease consisting of pain on taking a deep breath when pressure is placed over the location of the gallbladder.
      (3) *Location*—right upper quadrant, epigastric area, flank (**Figure 7.9**).
      (4) *Duration*—spasm of duct attempting to dislodge stone lasts until dislodged or

relieved by medication, or sometimes by vomiting.

b. *GI*—anorexia, nausea, feeling of fullness, indigestion, intolerance of fatty foods.

2. *Objective data:*
   a. *GI*—belching, vomiting, clay-colored stools.
   b. *Vital signs*—*increased* pulse, fever.
   c. *Skin*—chills, jaundice.
   d. *Urine*—dark amber.

   e. Lab data—*elevated:*
      (1) WBC.
      (2) Alkaline phosphatase.
      (3) Serum amylase, lipase.
      (4) AST (SGOT).
      (5) Bilirubin.

   f. *Diagnostic studies:*
      (1) Ultrasound.
      (2) Cholangiography.
      (3) Computed tomography (CT) scan.
      (4) Endoscopic retrograde cholangiopancreatography (ERCP).

◆ D. **Analysis/nursing diagnosis:**

1. *Pain* related to obstruction of bile duct due to cholelithiasis.
2. *Altered nutrition, more than body requirements,* related to ingestion of fatty foods.
3. *Altered nutrition,* less than body requirements, related to hesitancy to eat due to anorexia and nausea.
4. *Risk for fluid volume deficit* related to episodes of vomiting.
5. *Knowledge deficit* (learning need) related to dietary restrictions.

◆ E. **Nursing care plan/implementation:**

1. Nonsurgical interventions:
   a. Goal: *promote comfort.*
      (1) Medications as ordered: meperidine, *antibiotics, antispasmodics, electrolytes.*
      (2) *Avoid* morphine due to spasmodic effect.
      ▶ (3) NG tube to low suction.
      (4) *Diet: fat free* when able to tolerate food.
      (5) Lithotripsy: gallstones fragmented by shock waves
      (6) Oral dissolution therapy: ursodeoxycholic acid (ursodiol [Actigall]).
   b. Goal: *health teaching:*
      (1) Signs, symptoms, and complications of disease.
      (2) Fat free diet.
      (3) Desired effects and side effects of prescribed medications.
      (4) Prepare for possible removal of gallbladder (cholecystectomy) if conservative treatment unsuccessful.

2. Surgical interventions:
   a. *Preoperative*—Goal: *prevent injury* (see **I. Preoperative preparation, p. 546**).
   b. *Postoperative*—Goal: *promote comfort* (see also **III. Postoperative experience, p. 553**).

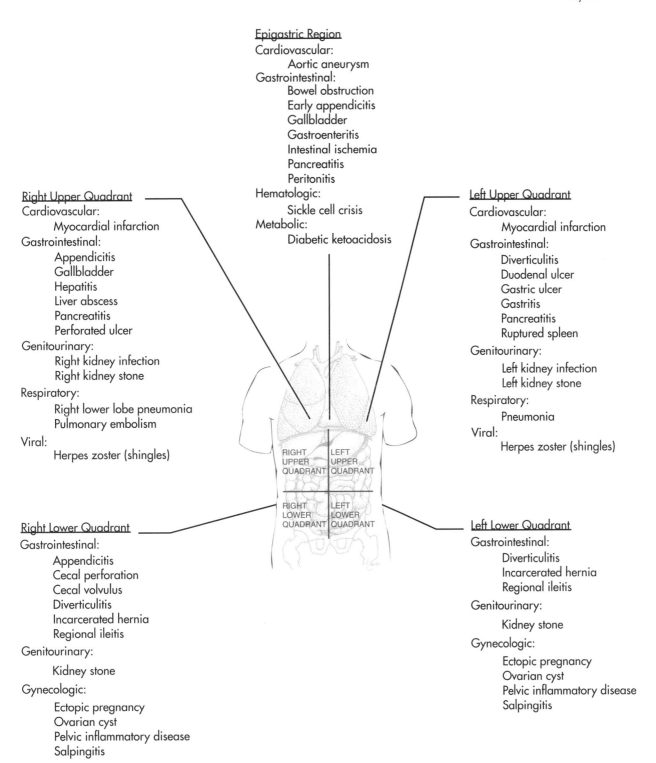

Epigastric Region
Cardiovascular:
 Aortic aneurysm
Gastrointestinal:
 Bowel obstruction
 Early appendicitis
 Gallbladder
 Gastroenteritis
 Intestinal ischemia
 Pancreatitis
 Peritonitis
Hematologic:
 Sickle cell crisis
Metabolic:
 Diabetic ketoacidosis

Right Upper Quadrant
Cardiovascular:
 Myocardial infarction
Gastrointestinal:
 Appendicitis
 Gallbladder
 Hepatitis
 Liver abscess
 Pancreatitis
 Perforated ulcer
Genitourinary:
 Right kidney infection
 Right kidney stone
Respiratory:
 Right lower lobe pneumonia
 Pulmonary embolism
Viral:
 Herpes zoster (shingles)

Left Upper Quadrant
Cardiovascular:
 Myocardial infarction
Gastrointestinal:
 Diverticulitis
 Duodenal ulcer
 Gastric ulcer
 Gastritis
 Pancreatitis
 Ruptured spleen
Genitourinary:
 Left kidney infection
 Left kidney stone
Respiratory:
 Pneumonia
Viral:
 Herpes zoster (shingles)

Right Lower Quadrant
Gastrointestinal:
 Appendicitis
 Cecal perforation
 Cecal volvulus
 Diverticulitis
 Incarcerated hernia
 Regional ileitis
Genitourinary:
 Kidney stone
Gynecologic:
 Ectopic pregnancy
 Ovarian cyst
 Pelvic inflammatory disease
 Salpingitis

Left Lower Quadrant
Gastrointestinal:
 Diverticulitis
 Incarcerated hernia
 Regional ileitis
Genitourinary:
 Kidney stone
Gynecologic:
 Ectopic pregnancy
 Ovarian cyst
 Pelvic inflammatory disease
 Salpingitis

FIGURE 7.9   Abdominal pain by location. (Modified from Caroline, NL: Emergency Care in the Streets, ed. 5. Boston, Little, Brown, 1995, p 641; and from Venes, D [ed]: Taber's Cyclopedic Medical Dictionary, ed. 20. FA Davis, Philadelphia, 2005.)

Adult

(1) *Laparoscopic laser cholecystectomy*—tiny incisions/puncture wounds; gallbladder is removed using a video-guided system with a camera; client is discharged that day or next day, able to resume normal diet and work activities in a few days.

(2) *Endoscopic retrograde cholangiopancreatography (ERCP)* with papillotomy—removes stones from bile duct. No incision; done under sedation, not anesthesia.

(3) *Open-incision cholecystectomy.*

▶ (a) Promote tube drainage:

> (i) NG tube to low suction.
> (ii) *T-tube* to closed-gravity drainage, to preserve patency of edematous common duct and ensure bile drainage; usual amount 500–1000 mL/24 hr; dark brown drainage.
> (iii) Provide enough tubing to allow turning without tension.
> (iv) Empty and record bile drainage q8h.

(b) *Position: low Fowler's* to *semi-Fowler's* to facilitate T-tube drainage.

(c) Dressing: dry to protect skin (because bile excoriates skin).

▶ (d) Clamp T-tube as ordered.

(i) Observe for abdominal distention, pain, nausea, chills, or fever.
(ii) Unclamp tube and notify MD if symptoms appear.

c. Goal: *prevent complications.*

(1) IV fluids with vitamins.
(2) Cough, turn, and deep breathe with open incision, particularly with removal of gallbladder (prone to respiratory complication because of high incision).
(3) Early ambulation to prevent vascular complications and aid in expelling flatus.
(4) Monitor for jaundice: skin, sclera, urine, stools.
(5) Monitor for signs of hemorrhage, infection.

d. Goal: *health teaching.*

(1) *Diet:* fat free for 6 wk.
(2) Signs of complications of food intolerance, pain, infection, hemorrhage.

◆ **F. Evaluation/outcome criteria:**
1. No complications.
2. Able to tolerate food.
3. Plans follow-up care.
4. Possible weight reduction.

XVI. Obesity—more calories consumed than expended leading to fat accumulation. Most common nutritional/metabolic disease in the United States.

A. Definition: *Women*—more than 45% above ideal body weight. *Men*—more than 35% above ideal body weight. Determined by body mass index (BMI) formula: divide weight in kilograms by height in meters squared (or divide weight in pounds by height in inches squared and multiply by 703).

$$\frac{\text{Wt (lb)} \times 703}{\text{Ht (in}^2)} \quad \text{or:} \quad \frac{\text{Wt (kg)} \times 703}{\text{Ht (m}^2)}$$

B. Risk factors:
1. Genetics (e.g., ↓ BMR), hormonal.
2. Environmental (e.g., ↓ physical activity).
3. Diet (e.g., ↑ fat, calories).
4. Some medications (e.g., TCAs, insulin, sulfonylurea agents).

C. Comorbidity:
1. Cardiovascular disease; hypertension.
2. Type 2 diabetes.
3. Gallbladder disease.
4. Arthritis.
5. Cancer (colorectal, breast, prostate).
6. Stroke.
7. Emotional distress.
8. Surgical risk.

◆ **D. Assessment:**
1. *Overweight*—BMI 25.0 to 29.9 kg/m².
2. *Obese*—BMI ≥30.0 kg/m².
3. *Morbid obesity*—BMI >40 kg/m².

◆ **E. Analysis/nursing diagnosis:**
1. *Altered nutrition, more than body requirements,* related to genetics, environmental, or dietary factors.
2. *Chronic low self-esteem/body image disturbance* related to view of self in contrast to societal values; control, sex, and love issues (see also **Unit 6, Body Image Disturbance, p. 359**).
3. *Activity intolerance* related to imbalance between oxygen supply and demand, and to sedentary lifestyle.

◆ **F. Nursing care plan/implementation**—Goal: *decrease weight, initially 10% from baseline.*
1. Modify eating pattern (quality vs. quantity); ↓ portion size; modify composition: ↓ calories, fat and CHO; ↓ daily kcal by 500–1000.
2. Increase activity—moderate activity 30 min. daily.
3. Behavioral therapy—change eating behaviors; motivation and readiness to lose weight.
4. Weight-loss drugs in combination with lifestyle changes.
5. Surgery—gastric stapling, bariatric (Roux-en-Y).

◆ **G. Evaluation/outcome criteria:**
1. Weight loss of 1 to 2 lbs/wk for 6 months.
2. Reduction in Kcal by 500 to 1000/day.
3. Increased daily physical activity.
4. Expressed commitment to lose weight.

Adult

ELIMINATION

Conditions Affecting Bowel Elimination

I. **Appendicitis:** obstruction of appendiceal lumen and subsequent bacterial invasion of appendiceal wall; **acute emergency.**
  A. **Pathophysiology:** when obstruction is partial or mild, inflammation begins in mucosa with slight appendiceal swelling, accompanied by periumbilical pain. As the inflammatory process escalates and/or obstruction becomes more complete, the appendix becomes more swollen, the lumen fills with pus, and mucosal ulceration begins. When inflammation extends to the peritoneal surface, pain is referred to the right lower abdominal quadrant. *Danger:* rigidity over the entire abdomen is usually indicative of ruptured appendix; the client is then prone to peritonitis.
  B. **Risk factors:**
    1. Men more than women.
    2. Most frequently seen between age 10 and 30 yr.
  ◆ C. **Assessment:**
    1. *Subjective data:*
      a. *Pain:* generalized, then right lower quadrant at McBurney's point, with rebound tenderness.
      b. Anorexia, nausea.
    2. *Objective data:*
      a. *Vital signs: elevated temperature,* shallow respirations.
      b. Either diarrhea or constipation.
      c. Vomiting, fetid breath odor.
      d. Splinting of abdominal muscles, flexion of knees onto abdomen.

      e. Lab data:
        (1) WBC *elevated* (>10,000).
        (2) Neutrophil count *elevated* (>75%).

      f. *Diagnostic studies:*
        (1) Ultrasound.
        (2) CT scan.
  ◆ D. **Analysis/nursing diagnosis:**
    1. *Pain* related to inflammation of appendix.
    2. *Risk for trauma* related to ruptured appendix.
    3. *Knowledge deficit* (learning need) related to possible surgery.
  ◆ E. **Nursing care plan/implementation:**
    1. Goal: *promote comfort.*
      a. *Preoperative:*
        (1) Explain procedures.
        (2) Assist with diagnostic workup.
      b. *Postoperative:*
        (1) Relieve pain related to surgical incision.
        ▶ (2) Prevent infection: wound care, dressing technique.
         (3) Prevent dehydration: IVs, I&O, fluids to solids by mouth as tolerated.
        (4) Promote ambulation to prevent postoperative complications.
  ◆ F. **Evaluation/outcome criteria:**
    1. No infection.
    2. Tolerates fluid; bowel sounds return.
    3. Heals with no complications.

II. **Hernia:** protrusion of the intestine through a weak portion of the abdominal wall.
  A. **Types:**
    1. *Reducible:* visceral contents return to their normal position, either spontaneously or by manipulation.
    2. *Irreducible, or incarcerated:* contents cannot be returned to normal position.
    3. *Strangulated:* blood supply to the structure within the hernia sac becomes occluded (usually a loop of bowel).
    4. Most common hernias: umbilical, femoral, inguinal, incisional, and hiatal.
  B. **Pathophysiology:** weakness in the wall may be either congenital or acquired. Herniation occurs when there is an increase in intraabdominal pressure from: coughing, lifting, crying, straining, obesity, or pregnancy.
  ◆ C. **Assessment:**
    1. *Subjective data:*
      a. Pain, discomfort.
      b. History of feeling a lump.
    2. *Objective data:*
      a. Soft lump, especially when straining or coughing.
      b. Sometimes alteration in normal bowel pattern.
      c. Swelling.
  ◆ D. **Analysis/nursing diagnosis:**
    1. *Activity intol*erance related to pain and discomfort.
    2. *Risk for trauma* related to lack of circulation to affected area of bowel.
    3. *Pain* related to protrusion of intestine into hernia sac.
  ◆ E. **Nursing care plan/implementation:**
    1. Goal: *prevent postoperative complications.*
      ▶ a. Monitor bowel sounds.
      b. Prevent postoperative scrotal swelling with inguinal hernia by applying ice and support to scrotum.
    2. Goal: *health teaching.*
      a. Prevent recurrence with correct body mechanics.
      b. Gradual increase in exercise.
  ◆ F. **Evaluation/outcome criteria:** healing occurs with no further hernia recurrence.

III. **Diverticulosis:** a *diverticulum* is a small pouch or sac composed of mucous membrane that has protruded through the muscular wall of the intestine. The presence of several of these is called *diverticulosis.* Inflammation of the diverticula is called *diverticulitis.*

A. Pathophysiology: weakening in a localized area of muscular wall of the colon (especially the sigmoid colon), accompanied by increased intraluminal pressure.

B. Risk factors:
1. Diverticulosis:
   a. Age: seldom before 35 yr; 60% incidence in older adults.
   b. History of constipation.
   c. Diet history: low in vegetable fiber, high in carbohydrate.
2. Diverticulitis: highest incidence between ages 50 and 60 yr.

C. Assessment:
1. *Subjective data: pain:* cramplike; left lower quadrant of abdomen.
2. *Objective data:*
   a. Constipation or diarrhea, flatulence.
   b. Fever.
   c. Rectal bleeding.
   d. *Diagnostic procedures:*
      (1) Palpation reveals tender colonic mass.
      (2) Barium enema (done only in absence of inflammation) reveals presence of diverticula.
      (3) Sigmoidoscopy/colonoscopy.

D. Analysis/nursing diagnosis:
1. *Constipation* related to dietary intake.
2. *Pain* related to inflammatory process of intestines.
3. *Risk for fluid volume deficit* related to episodes of diarrhea or bleeding.
4. *Risk for injury* related to bleeding.
5. *Knowledge deficit* (learning need) related to prevention of constipation.

E. Nursing care plan/implementation:
1. Goal: *bowel rest during acute episodes.*
   a. *Diet: soft, liquid.*
   b. Fluids, IVs if oral intake not adequate.
   c. Medications:
      (1) *Antibiotics:* ciprofloxacin (Cipro), metronidazole (Flagyl), cephalexin (Keflex), doxycycline (Vibramycin).
      (2) *Antispasmodics:* chlordiazepoxide (Librax), dicyclomine (Bentyl), Donnatal, hyoscyamine (Levsin).
   d. Monitor stools for signs of bleeding.
2. Goal: *promote normal bowel elimination.*
   a. *Diet:* bland, *high* in vegetable fiber if no inflammation.
      (1) *Include:* fruits, vegetables, whole-grain cereal, unprocessed bran.
      (2) *Avoid:* foods difficult to digest (corn, nuts).
   b. *Bulk-forming* agents as ordered: methylcellulose, psyllium.
   c. Monitor: abdominal distention, acute bowel symptoms.
3. Goal: *health teaching.*
   a. Methods to avoid constipation.

   b. Foods to include/avoid in diet.
   c. Relaxation techniques.
   d. Signs and symptoms of complications of chronic inflammation: abscess, obstruction, fistulas, perforation, or hemorrhage.

F. Evaluation/outcome criteria:
1. Inflammation decreases.
2. Bowel movements return to normal.
3. Pain decreases.
4. No perforation, fistulas, or abscesses noted.

IV. Ulcerative colitis: inflammation of mucosa and submucosa of the large intestine. Inflammation leads to ulceration with bleeding. Involved areas are continuous. Disease is characterized by remissions and exacerbations.

A. Pathophysiology: Currently believed to be an autoimmune disease. The body's immune system is called on to attack the inner lining of the large intestine, causing inflammation and ulceration. Edema and hyperemia of colonic mucous membrane → superficial bleeding with increased peristalsis, shallow ulcerations, abscesses; bowel wall thins and shortens and becomes at risk for perforation. Increased rate of flow of liquid ileal contents → decreased water absorption and diarrhea.

B. Risk factors:
1. Highest occurrence in young adults (age 20 to 40 yr).
2. Genetic predisposition: higher in whites, Jews.
3. Autoimmune response.
4. Infections.
5. More common in urban areas (upper-middle incomes and higher educational levels).
6. Nonsmokers/ex-smokers.
7. Genetic, inherited, or familial tendencies.
8. Chronic ulcerative colitis is a risk factor for colon cancer.

C. Assessment:
1. *Subjective data:*
   a. Urgency to defecate, particularly when standing.
   b. Loss of appetite, nausea.
   c. Colic-like abdominal pain.
   d. History of intolerance to dairy products.
   e. Emotional depression.
2. *Objective data:*
   a. *Diarrhea:* 10 to 20 stools/day; can be chronic or intermittent, episodic or continual; stools contain blood, mucus, and pus.
   b. Weight loss and malnutrition, dehydration.
   c. Fever.
   d. Rectal bleeding.
   e. Lab data: *decreased:* RBC, potassium, sodium, calcium, bicarbonate related to excessive diarrhea.
   f. Lymphadenitis.
   g. *Diagnostic tests:*

(1) Sigmoidoscopy/colonoscopy for visualization of lesions.

(2) Barium enema.

◆ **D. Analysis/nursing diagnosis:**

1. *Diarrhea* related to increased flow rate of ileal contents.

2. *Self-esteem disturbance* related to progression of disease and increased number and odor of stools.

3. *Pain* (acute) related to inflammatory process.

4. *Fluid volume deficit* related to frequent episodes of diarrhea.

5. *Knowledge deficit* (learning need) related to methods to control symptoms.

6. *Social isolation* related to continual diarrhea episodes.

◆ **E. Nursing care plan/implementation:**

1. Goal: *prevent disease progression and complications.*

a. Administer medications:

(1) *Salicylates:* sulfasalazine (Azulfidine), olsalazine (Dipentum), mesalamine (Asacol, Pentasa). All given PO in high doses. Mesalamine (Rowasa) is given in enema or suppository form.

(2) *Corticosteroids:* prednisone, PO or IV. Hydrocortisone (Cortenema) is given by enema.

(3) *Immunosuppressants:* azathioprine (Imuran), and 6-mercaptopurone (Purinethol), cyclosporine (Sandimmune), and methotrexate (Rheumatrex).

(4) *Nicotine.*

(5) *Sedatives and tranquilizers to produce rest and comfort.*

(6) *Absorbents:* kaolin/pectin (Kaopectate).

(7) *Anticholinergics* and *antispasmotics to relieve cramping and diarrhea:* atropine sulfate, phenobarbital, diphenoxylate/atropine sulfate (Lomotil).

(8) *Anti-infective* agents *to relieve bacterial overgrowth in bowel* and *limit secondary infections:* metronidazole (Flagyl).

(9) *Potassium supplements to relieve deficiencies* related to excessive diarrhea.

(10) *Calcium folate and vitamin B_{12}* when malabsorption is present.

2. Goal: *reduce psychological stress.*

a. Provide quiet environment.

b. Encourage verbalization of concerns.

3. Goal: *health teaching.*

a. *Diet:*

(1) *Avoid:* coarse-residue, high fiber foods (e.g., raw fruits and vegetables), whole milk, cold beverages (because of inflammation).

(2) *Include:* bland, *high* protein, *high* vitamin, *high* mineral, *high* calorie foods.

(3) Parenteral hyperalimentation for severely ill.

(4) Force fluids by mouth.

b. Monitor for colon cancer, especially 8 to 10 years after incidence.

4. Goal: *prepare for surgery if medical regimen unsuccessful.*

a. Possible surgical procedures:

(1) Permanent ileostomy *(J pouch).*

(2) Continent ileostomy *(Kock pouch).*

(3) Total colectomy, anastomosis with rectum.

(4) Total colectomy, anastomosis with anal sphincter.

◆ **F. Evaluation/outcome criteria:**

1. Fluid balance is obtained and maintained.

2. Alterations in lifestyle are managed.

3. Stress-management techniques are successful.

4. Complications such as fistulas, obstruction, perforation, and peritonitis are avoided.

5. Client is prepared for surgery if medical regimen is unsuccessful or complications develop.

V. **Crohn's disease:** a chronic inflammatory disease causing ulcerations in the small and large intestines. The immune system seems to react to a variety of substances and/or bacteria in the intestines, causing inflammation, ulceration, and bowel injury. Called Crohn's *colitis* when only large intestine is involved; Crohn's *enteritis* when only small intestine is involved; *terminal ileitis* when lowest part of small intestine is involved; Crohn's *enterocolitis* or *ileocolitis* when both small and large intestines are involved.

A. **Pathophysiology:** *one of two conditions called "inflammatory bowel disease"* (ulcerative colitis is the other) that affects all layers of the ileum, the colon, or both, causing patchy, shallow, longitudinal mucosal ulcers; possible correlation with autoimmune disease and adenocarcinoma of the bowel. Small, scattered shallow crater-like areas cause scarring and stiffness of the bowel → bowel becomes narrow → obstruction, then pain, nausea, and vomiting.

B. **Risk factors:**

1. Age: 15 to 20, 55 to 60 yr.

2. Whites, especially Jewish.

3. Familial predisposition.

4. Possible virus involvement.

5. Possible psychosomatic involvement.

6. Possible hormonal or dietary influences.

◆ C. **Assessment** (see **IV. Ulcerative colitis, p. 580,** for analysis/nursing diagnosis, nursing care plan/implementation, and evaluation/outcome criteria):

1. *Subjective data:*

a. Abdominal pain.

b. Anorexia.

c. Nausea.

d. Malaise.

e. History of isolated, intermittent, or recurrent attacks.

2. *Objective data:*

a. Diarrhea.

b. Weight loss, vomiting.

c. Fever, signs of infection.

Adult

d. Fluid/electrolyte imbalances.
e. Malnutrition, malabsorption.
f. Occult blood in feces.

VI. Intestinal obstruction: blockage in movement of intestinal contents through small or large intestine.

A. Pathophysiology:
1. *Mechanical causes*—physical impediments to passage of intestinal contents (e.g., adhesions, hernias, neoplasms, inflammatory bowel disease, foreign bodies, fecal impactions, congenital or radiational strictures, intussusception, or volvulus).
2. *Paralytic causes*—passageway remains open, but peristalsis ceases (e.g., after abdominal surgery, abdominal trauma, hypokalemia, myocardial infarction, pneumonia, spinal injuries, peritonitis, or vascular insufficiency).

B. Assessment:
1. *Subjective data: pain* related to:
   a. *Proximal loop obstruction:* upper abdominal, sharp, cramping, intermittent pain.
   b. *Distal loop obstruction:* poorly localized, cramping pain.
2. *Objective data:*
   a. Bowel sounds: initially loud, high pitched; then when smooth muscle atony occurs, bowel sound absent.
   b. Increased peristalsis above level of obstruction in attempt to move intestinal contents through the obstructed area.
   c. Obstipation (no passage of gas or stool through obstructed portion of bowel; no reabsorption of fluids).
   d. Distention.
   e. Vomiting:
      (1) *Proximal loop obstruction:* profuse nonfecal vomiting.
      (2) *Distal loop obstruction:* less frequent fecal-type vomiting.
   f. Urinary output: *decreased.*
   g. Temperature: *elevated;* pulse: *tachycardia;* BP: *hypotension* → shock if untreated.
   h. Dehydration, hemoconcentration, hypovolemia.

   i. Lab data:
      (1) Leukocytosis.
      (2) *Decreased:* sodium (<138), potassium (<3.5).
      (3) *Increased:* bicarbonate (>26 mEq/L), BUN (>18 mg/dL).
      (4) *pH:* If obstruction is at gastric outlet, pH will be *elevated,* indicating *metabolic alkalosis;* if obstruction is distal duodenal or proximal jejunal, the pH will *drop* and *metabolic acidosis* occurs.

C. Analysis/nursing diagnosis:
1. *Fluid volume deficit* related to vomiting.
2. *Pain* related to increased peristalsis above the level of obstruction.

3. *Altered nutrition, less than body requirements,* related to vomiting.
4. *Risk for trauma* related to potential perforation.

◆ **D. Nursing care plan/implementation:**
1. Goal: *obtain and maintain fluid balance.*
   ▶ a. Nursing care of client with nasogastric tube (see **Table 11.11**).
      (1) *Miller-Abbott tube:* dual lumen, balloon inflated with air after insertion. *Caution:* do *not* tape tube to face until tube reaches point of obstruction.
      (2) *Cantor tube:* has mercury in distal sac, which helps move tube to point of obstruction. *Caution:* do *not* tape tube to face until tube reaches point of obstruction.
   b. Nothing by mouth, IV therapy, strict I&O.
   ▶ c. Take daily weights (early morning), monitor CVP for hydration status.
   ▶ d. Monitor abdominal girth for signs of distention and urinary output for signs of retention or shock.
2. Goal: *relieve pain and nausea.*
   a. Medications as ordered:
      (1) *Analgesics, antiemetics.*
      (2) If problem is paralytic: medical treatment includes neostigmine *to stimulate peristalsis.*
   b. Observe for bowel sounds, flatus (tape intestinal tube to face once peristalsis begins).
   c. Skin and frequent mouth care.
3. Goal: *prevent respiratory complications.*
   a. Encourage coughing and deep breathing.
   b. *Semi-Fowler's* or position of comfort.
4. Goal: *postoperative nursing care* (if treated surgically) (see **Postoperative experience p. 553**).

◆ **E. Evaluation/outcome criteria:**
1. Fluid balance obtained and maintained.
2. Shock prevented.
3. Obstruction resolved.
4. Pain decreased.
5. Fluids tolerated by mouth.
6. Complications such as perforation and peritonitis avoided.

VII. Fecal diversion—*stomas:* performed because of disease or trauma; may be temporary or permanent.

A. Types (Table 7.32).
1. *Temporary*—fecal stream rerouted to allow GI tract to heal or to provide outlet for stool when obstructed.
2. *Permanent*—intestine cannot be reconnected. Rectum and anal sphincter removed (abdominal perineal resection). Often performed for cancer of the colon and/or rectum.
3. *Continent ileostomy*—pouch is created inside the wall of the intestine. The pouch serves as a reservoir similar to a rectum. The pouch is emptied on a regular basis with a small tube.
4. *Ileoanal anastomosis (J pouch, S reservoir or ileoperistaltic reservoir)*—the large intestine is

TABLE 7.32	Comparison of Ileostomy and Colostomy	
	Ileostomy	**Colostomy**
Procedure	Surgical formation of a fistula, or stoma, between the abdominal wall and *ileum*: continent ileostomy (*Kock* pouch) may be constructed	Surgical formation of an artificial opening between the surface of the abdominal wall and *colon* *Single barrel*—only one loop of bowel is opened to the abdominal surface *Double barrel*—two loops of bowel, a proximal and distal portion, are open to the abdominal wall; feces will be expelled from the proximal loop, mucus will be expelled from the distal loop; client may expel some excreta from rectum as well
Reasons performed	Unresponsive ulcerative colitis: complications of ulcerative colitis (e.g., hemorrhage, carcinoma [suspected])	*Single barrel:* colon or rectal cancer *Double barrel:* relieve obstruction
Results	Permanent stoma	*Single barrel:* permanent stoma *Double barrel:* temporary stoma
Discharge	Green liquid, nonodorous	Consistency of feces dependent on diet and portion of the bowel used as the stoma; from brown odorous liquid to normal stool consistency
Nursing care	See **VII. Fecal diversion, p. 582**	See **Tables 11.12, Emptying Colostomy Appliance,** and **11.13, Changing Colostomy Appliance**

removed and the small intestine is inserted into the rectum and attached just above the anus. The muscles of the rectum remain intact and the normal route of stool elimination is maintained.

◆ **B. Analysis/nursing diagnosis:**
1. *Bowel incontinence* related to lack of sphincter in newly formed stoma.
2. *Altered health maintenance* related to knowledge of ostomy care.
3. *Body image disturbance* related to stoma.
4. *Fear* related to medical condition requiring stoma.
5. *Fluid volume deficit* related to increased output through stoma.

◆ **C. Nursing care plan/implementation:**
1. *Preoperative period:*
   a. Goal: *prepare bowel for surgery.*
   (1) Administer neomycin as ordered to *reduce* colonic bacteria.
   (2) Administer cathartics, enemas as ordered to *cleanse* the bowel of feces.
   (3) Administer *low residue* or *liquid diet* as ordered.
   b. Goal: *relieve anxiety and assist in adjustment to surgery.*
   (1) Provide accurate, brief, and reassuring explanations of procedures; allow time for questions.
   (2) Referral: have enterostomal nurse visit to discuss ostomy management and placement of stoma appliance.
   (3) Referral: offer opportunity for a visit with an Ostomy Association Visitor.

   c. Goal: *health teaching.*
   (1) Determine knowledge of surgery and potential impact.
   (2) Begin teaching regarding ostomy.
2. *Postoperative period:*
   a. Goal: *maintain fluid balance.*
   (1) Monitor I&O because large volume of fluid is lost through stoma.
   (2) Administer IV fluids as ordered.
   (3) Monitor losses through NG tube.
   b. Goal: *prevent other postoperative complications.*
   (1) Monitor for signs of intestinal obstruction.
   ▶ (2) Maintain sterility when changing dressings; *avoid* fecal contamination of incision.
   (3) Observe appearance of stoma: rosy pink, raised (**Figure 7.10**).

   ▶ c. Goal: *initiate ostomy care.*
   (1) *Protect skin around stoma:* use commercial preparation to toughen skin and use protective barrier wafer (Stomahesive) or paste (Karaya or substitute) to keep drainage (which can cause excoriation) off the skin.
   (2) *Keep skin around stoma clean and dry;* empty appliance frequently. Check for drainage in appliance at least twice during each shift. If drainage present (diarrhea-type stool):
   (a) Unclip bottom of bag.

(Continued on following page)

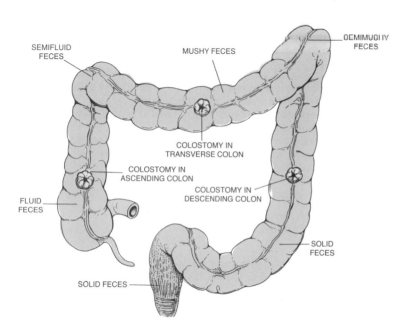

SEMIFLUID FECES

MUSHY FECES

SEMIMUSHY FECES

COLOSTOMY IN TRANSVERSE COLON

COLOSTOMY IN ASCENDING COLON

COLOSTOMY IN DESCENDING COLON

FLUID FECES

SOLID FECES

SOLID FECES

FIGURE 7.10 Colostomy sites. (From Venes, D [ed]: Taber's Cyclopedic Medical Dictionary, ed 20. FA Davis, Philadelphia, 2005.)

(b) Drain into bedpan.

(c) Use a squeeze-type bottle filled with warm water to rinse inside of appliance.

(d) Clean clamp, if soiled.

(e) Put a few drops of deodorant in appliance if not odorproof.

(f) Fasten bottom of appliance securely (fold bag over clamp two or three times before closing).

(g) Check for leakage under appliance every 2 to 4 hr.

(3) *Change appliance* when drainage leaks around seal, or approximately every 2 to 3 days. Initially, size of stoma will be large due to edema. Pouch opening should be slightly larger than stoma so it will not constrict. Stoma will need to be measured for each change until swelling subsides to ensure appropriate fit.

(a) Gather equipment: gloves, skin prep packet, colostomy appliance measured to fit stoma properly (use stoma measuring guide), skin barrier, warm water and soap, face cloth/towel, plastic bag for disposal of old equipment.

(b) Remove old appliance carefully, pulling from area with least drainage to area with most drainage.

(c) Wash skin area (*not* stoma) with soap and water. Be careful *not to:* irritate skin, put soap on stoma, irritate stoma; do *not* put anything dry onto stoma. *Remember:* bowel is very fragile; working near bowel

increases peristalsis so that feces and flatulence may be expelled.

(d) Observe skin area for potential breakdown.

(e) Use packet of skin prep on the skin around the stoma. Do *not* put this solution onto stoma, because it will cause irritation. Allow skin prep solution to dry on skin before applying colostomy appliance.

(f) Apply skin barrier you have measured and cut to size.

(g) Put appliance on so that bottom of appliance is easily accessible for emptying (e.g., if client is *out* of bed most of the time, put the bottom facing the feet; if client is *in* bed most of the time, have bottom face the side). Picture frame the adhesive portion of the appliance with 1-inch tape.

(h) Put a few drops of deodorant in appliance if not odorproof.

(i) Use clamp to fasten bottom of appliance.

(j) Talk to client (or communicate in best way possible during and after procedure). *This is a very difficult alteration in body image.*

(k) Good handwashing technique.

(4) Use deodorizing drops in appliance and provide adequate room ventilation to decrease odors. *Caution:* deodorizing drops must be safe for mucous membranes. *No* pinholes in pouch.

(5) If continent ileostomy, a *Kock pouch,* has

been constructed, the client does not have to wear an external pouch. The stool is stored intra-abdominally. The client drains the pouch several times daily, when there is a feeling of fullness, using a catheter. The stoma is flat and on the right side of the abdomen.

    d. Goal: *promote psychological comfort.*
      (1) Support client and family—accept feelings and behavior.
      (2) Recognize that such a procedure may initiate the grieving process.
    e. Goal: *health teaching.*
      (1) Self-care management skills related to ostomy appliance, skin care, and irrigation, if indicated (**Table 7.33**).
      (2) *Diet:* adjustments to control character of feces; *avoid* foods that increase flatulence.
      (3) Signs of complications of infection, obstruction, or electrolyte imbalance.
      (4) Community referral for follow-up care.

◆ **D. Evaluation/outcome criteria:**
    1. Demonstrates self-care skill for independent living.
    2. Makes dietary adjustments.
    3. Ostomy functions well.
    4. Adjusts to alteration in bowel elimination pattern.

VIII. Hemorrhoids: enlarged vein/veins in mucous membrane of rectum. Hemorrhoids can be internal or external. Bleeding internal hemorrhoids can be painful and are best treated by: rubber band ligation, injection sclerotherapy, infrared coagulation, or surgery (scalpel, cautery, or laser). Laser surgery is usually done as an outpatient and causes minimal discomfort. High fiber diets can minimize constipation and prevent hemorrhoids.

    A. Pathophysiology: venous congestion and interference with venous return from hemorrhoidal veins → increase in pelvic pressure, swelling, and distortion.

TABLE 7.33	▶ **Colostomy Irrigation**[*]

1. Assemble all equipment for irrigation and appliance change.
2. Remove and discard old pouch.
3. Clean the peristomal skin.
4. Apply the irrigating sleeve; place in toilet or bedpan.
5. Fill container with 500 to 1000 mL of warm water, *never* more than 1000 mL. Clear air from tubing. Insert lubricated tubing 2 to 4 inches into stoma. Do *not* force. Hold container about 18 inches above stoma. Infuse gently over 7 to 10 min.
6. Allow stool to empty into toilet. Evacuation usually occurs in 20 to 25 min.
7. If no return after irrigation, ambulate, gently massage abdomen, or give client a warm drink.
8. Once complete, remove the sleeve, and follow guidelines for applying appliance.

[*]Colostomy irrigation is seldom used with newer colostomies.

B. Risk factors:
    1. Straining to expel constipated stool.
    2. Pregnancy.
    3. Intraabdominal or pelvic masses.
    4. Interference with portal circulation.
    5. Prolonged standing or sitting.
    6. History of low fiber, high carbohydrate diet, which contributes to constipation.
    7. Family history of hemorrhoids.
    8. Enlarged prostate.

◆ **C. Assessment:**
    1. *Subjective data:* discomfort, anal pruritus, pain.
    2. *Objective data:*
      a. Bleeding, especially on defecation.
      b. Narrowing of stool.
      c. Grapelike clusters around anus (pink, red, or blue).
      d. *Diagnostic test:*
        (1) Visualization for external hemorrhoids.
        (2) Digital exam or proctoscopy for internal hemorrhoids.

◆ **D. Analysis/nursing diagnosis:**
    1. *Pain* related to defecation.
    2. *Constipation* related to dietary habits and pain at time of defecation.
    3. *Knowledge deficit* (learning need) related to foods to prevent constipation.

◆ **E. Nursing care plan/implementation:**
    1. Goal: *reduce anal discomfort.*
      a. Sitz baths, as ordered; perineal care to prevent infection.
    ▶ b. Hot or cold compresses as ordered to reduce inflammation and pruritus.
      c. Topical medications as ordered:
        (1) *Antiinflammatory:* hydrocortisone cream (Anusol).
        (2) *Astringents:* witch hazel–impregnated pads.
        (3) *Topical anesthetics:* pramoxine (Procto-Foam); dibucaine (Nupercainal).
      d. *Bulk laxatives:* psyllium (Metamucil), Konsyl, polycarbophil (FiberCon).
    2. Goal: *prevent complications related to surgery.*
      a. Encourage postoperative ambulation.
      b. *Pain* relief until packing removed.
      c. Monitor for: bleeding, infection, pulmonary emboli, phlebitis.
      d. Facilitate bowel evacuation: stool softeners, laxatives, suppositories, oil enemas as ordered.
      e. Monitor for: syncope/vertigo during first postoperative bowel movement.
      f. *Diet:*
        (1) *Low* residue (postoperative)—until healing has begun.
        (2) *High* fiber to prevent constipation after healing.
      g. Increase fluid intake.
    3. Goal: *health teaching*—methods to avoid constipation.

◆ **F. Evaluation/outcome criteria:**
1. No complications.
2. Client has bowel movement.
3. Incorporates knowledge of correct foods into lifestyle.

Conditions Affecting Urinary Elimination

I. Pyelonephritis (PN): acute or chronic inflammation due to bacterial infection of the parenchyma and renal pelvis; 95% of cases caused by gram-negative enteric bacilli *(Escherichia coli)*; occurs more frequently in women.

A. Pathophysiology: inflammation of renal medulla or lining of the renal pelvis → nephron destruction; hypertrophy of nephrons needed to maintain urine output → impaired sodium reabsorption (salt wasting); inability to concentrate urine; progressive renal failure; hypertension (two-thirds of all cases).

B. Risk factors:
1. Urinary obstruction (tumors, prostate).
2. Cystitis.
3. Neurogenic bladder.
4. Pregnancy.
5. Catheterization, cystoscopy.

◆ **C. Assessment:**
1. *Subjective data:*
   a. *Pain:* flank—one or both sides; back; dysuria; headache.
   b. *Loss of appetite;* weight loss.
   c. *Night sweats;* chills.
   d. *Urination:* frequency, urgency.
2. *Objective data:*
   a. Fever; shaking chills.
   b. Lab data:
      (1) *Blood*—polymorphonuclear leukocytosis >11,000/mm³.
      (2) *Urine*—leukocytosis, hematuria, white blood cell casts, proteinuria (<3 g in 24 hr), positive cultures; specific gravity—normal *or increased* with acute PN, *decreased* with chronic PN; cloudy; foul smelling.
   c. Intravenous pyelogram (IVP)—may manifest structural changes.

◆ **D. Analysis/nursing diagnosis:**
1. *Altered urinary elimination* related to kidney disease.
2. *Pain* related to dysuria and kidney damage.
3. *Hyperthermia* related to inflammation.
4. *Risk for fluid volume excess* related to renal failure.

◆ **E. Nursing care plan/implementation:**
1. Goal: *combat infection, prevent recurrence, alleviate symptoms.*
   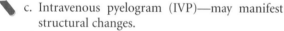 a. Medications:
      (1) *Antibiotics, urinary antiseptics,* and/or sulfonamides appropriate for causative organism; also reduce pain.

(2) *Analgesics* for pain—phenazopyridine (Pyridium); stronger if calculi present.
(3) *Antipyretics* for fever—acetaminophen (Tylenol).
   b. *Fluids:* 1500–2000 mL/day to flush kidneys, relieve dysuria, reduce fever, prevent dehydration.
   c. Observe hydration status: I&O (output minimum 1500 mL/24 hr); daily weight; urine—check each voiding for protein, blood, specific gravity; vital signs q4h to monitor for hypertension, tachycardia; skin turgor.
   d. *Hygiene:* meticulous perineal care; cleanse with soap and water; antibiotic ointment may be used around urinary meatus with retention catheter.
   e. Cooling measures: tepid sponging.
   f. *Diet:* sufficient calories and protein to prevent malnutrition; sodium supplement as ordered. *Acid-ash* to prevent renal calculus.
2. Goal: *promote physical and emotional rest.*
   a. Activity: bedrest or as tolerated—depends on whether anemia or fever is present; encourage activities of daily living as tolerated.
   b. Emotional support: encourage expression of fears (possible renal failure, dialysis); provide diversional activities; include family in care; answer questions.
3. Goal: *health teaching.*
   a. Medications: take regularly to maintain blood level; side effects.
   b. *Personal care:* perineal hygiene; *avoid* urethral contamination (by wiping perineum front to back); *avoid* tub baths.
   c. Possible recurrence with pregnancy.
   d. Monitoring daily weight.

◆ **F. Evaluation/outcome criteria:**
1. Normal renal function (minimum 1500 mL urine/24 hr).
2. Blood pressure within normal range.
3. No recurrence of symptoms.
4. Laboratory findings within normal limits.

II. Acute glomerulonephritis (see **Unit 5, p. 309**).

III. Acute renal failure (ARF): broadly defined as rapid onset of oliguria accompanied by a rising BUN and serum creatinine; usually reversible.

A. Pathophysiology: acute renal ischemia → tubular necrosis → decreased urine output. *Oliguric phase* (<400 mL/24 hr)—waste products are retained → metabolic acidosis → water and electrolyte imbalances → anemia. *Recovery phase*—diuresis → dilute urine → rapid depletion of sodium, chloride, and water → dehydration.

B. Types and risk factors:
1. *Prerenal*—due to factors *outside* of kidney; usually circulatory collapse—cardiovascular disorders, hypovolemia, peripheral vasodilation, renovascular obstruction, severe vasoconstriction.

2. *Intrarenal*—parenchymal disease from ischemia or *nephrotoxic damage;* nephrotoxic agents—poisons, such as lead (carbon tetrachloride); heavy metals (mercury); antibiotics (gentamicin); incompatible blood transfusion; alcohol myopathies; obstetric complications; acute renal disease—acute glomerulonephritis, acute pyelonephritis.

3. *Postrenal*—obstruction in *collecting system:* renal or bladder calculi; tumors of bladder, prostate, or renal pelvis; gynecological or urological surgery in which ureters are accidentally ligated.

◆ **C. Assessment:**

1. *Subjective data:*

   a. Sudden decrease or cessation of urine output (<400 mL/24 hr).

   b. Anorexia, nausea, vomiting from azotemia.

   c. Sudden weight gain from fluid accumulation.

   d. Headache.

2. *Objective data:*

   a. *Vital signs* (vary according to cause and severity):

      (1) *BP*—usually *elevated.*

      (2) *Pulse*—tachycardia, irregularities.

      (3) *Respirations*—*increased* rate, depth, crackles.

   b. *Neurological:* decreasing mentation, unresponsive to verbal or painful stimuli, psychoses, convulsions.

   c. *Halitosis;* cracked mucous membranes; uremic odor.

   d. *Skin:* dry, rashes, purpura, itchy, pale.

   e. Lab data:

      (1) Blood: *increased*—potassium, BUN, creatinine, WBC; *decreased*—pH, bicarbonate, hematocrit, hemoglobin.

      (2) Urine: **oliguric renal failure**—*decreased* volume, specific gravity fixed or ↑; *increased*—protein, casts, red and white blood cells, sodium. **Non-oliguric renal failure**—up to 2L/day, ↓ specific gravity, dilute, isomolar.

◆ **D. Analysis/nursing diagnosis:**

1. *Altered urinary elimination* related to kidney malfunction.

2. *Fluid volume excess* related to decreased urine output.

3. *Altered nutrition, less than body requirements,* related to anorexia.

4. *Altered oral mucous membrane* related to stomatitis.

5. *Altered thought processes* related to uremia.

◆ **E. Nursing care plan/implementation:**

1. Goal: *maintain fluid and electrolyte balance and nutrition.*

   a. Monitor: daily weight (should not vary more than ±1 lb); vital signs—include CVP; blood chemistries (BUN 6–20 mg/dL; creatinine 0.6–1.5 mg/dL).

   b. *Fluids:* IV as ordered; blood: plasma, packed cells, electrolyte solutions to replace losses; restricted to 400 mL/24 hr if hypertension present or during oliguric phase to prevent fluid overload.

   c. *Diet,* as tolerated: *high* carbohydrate, *low* protein, may be *low* potassium and *low* sodium; hypertonic glucose (TPN) if oral feedings not tolerated; intravenous L-amino acids and glucose.

   d. Control hyperkalemia: infusions of hypertonic glucose and insulin to force potassium into cells; calcium gluconate (IV) to reduce myocardial irritability from K^+; sodium bicarbonate (IV) to correct acidosis; polystyrene sodium sulfonate (Kayexalate) or other exchange resins, orally or rectally (enema), to remove excess K^+; continuous renal replacement therapy, peritoneal or hemodialysis.

   e. Medications—*diuretics* (mannitol, furosemide [Lasix]) to increase renal blood flow and diuresis.

2. Goal: *use assessment and comfort measures to reduce occurrence of complications.*

   a. *Respiratory:* monitor rate, depth, breath sounds, arterial blood gases; encourage deep breathing, coughing, turning; use incentive spirometer or nebulizer as indicated.

   b. Frequent oral care to prevent stomatitis.

   c. Observe for signs of:

      (1) *Infection*—elevated temperature, localized redness, swelling, heat, or drainage.

      (2) *Bleeding*—stools, gums, venipuncture sites.

3. Goal: *maintain continual emotional support.*

   a. Same caregivers, consistency in procedures.

   b. Give opportunities to express concerns, fears.

   c. Allow family interactions.

4. Goal: *health teaching.*

   a. Preparation for dialysis (indications: uremia, uncontrolled hyperkalemia, or acidosis). **Continuous renal replacement therapy** (CRRT) may be used in ARF with fluid overload or rapidly developing azotemia and metabolic acidosis. Continuous ultrafiltration (8 to 24 hr) of extracellular fluid and uremic toxins. Client's BP powers system. Arterial and venous access required.

   b. Dietary *restrictions: low sodium, fluid restriction.*

   c. Disease process; treatment regimen.

◆ **F. Evaluation/outcome criteria:**

1. Return of kidney function— normal creatinine level (<1.5 mg/dL), urine output.

2. Resumes normal life pattern (about 3 mo after onset).

IV. Chronic renal failure: as a result of progressive destruction of kidney tissue, the kidneys are no longer able to maintain their homeostatic functions; considered irreversible.

Adult

A. **Pathophysiology:** destruction of glomeruli → reduced glomerular filtration rate → retention of metabolic waste products; decreased urine output; severe fluid, electrolyte, acid-base imbalances → uremia. Clinical picture includes:

1. Ammonia in skin and alimentary tract by bacterial interaction with urea → inflammation of mucous membranes.
2. Retention of phosphate → decreased serum calcium → muscle spasms, tetany, and increased parathormone release → demineralization of bone.
3. Failure of tubular mechanisms to regulate blood bicarbonate → metabolic acidosis → hyperventilation.
4. Urea osmotic diuresis → flushing effect on tubules → decreased reabsorption of sodium → sodium depletion.
5. Waste product retention → depressed bone marrow function → decreased circulating RBCs → renal tissue hypoxia → decreased erythropoietin production → further depression of bone marrow → anemia.

B. **Risk factors:**

1. Diabetic retinopathy.
2. Chronic glomerulonephritis.
3. Chronic urinary obstruction, ureteral stricture, calculi, neoplasms.
4. Chronic pyelonephritis.
5. Hypertensive nephrosclerosis.
6. Congenital or acquired renal artery stenosis.
7. Systemic lupus erythematosus.

C. **Assessment:**

1. *Subjective data:* excessive fatigue, weakness.
2. *Objective data:*
   a. Skin: bronze colored, uremic frost.
   b. Ammonia breath.
   c. See also **III. Acute renal failure, p. 586;** symptoms gradual in onset.

D. **Analysis/nursing diagnosis:**

1. In addition to the following, see **III. Acute renal failure, p. 586.**
2. *Fatigue* related to severe anemia.
3. *Risk for impaired skin integrity* related to pruritus.
4. *Ineffective individual coping* related to chronic illness.
5. *Body image disturbance* related to need for dialysis.
6. *Noncompliance* related to denial of illness.

E. **Nursing care plan/implementation:**

1. Goal: *maintain fluid/electrolyte balance and nutrition* (see also **III. Acute renal failure, p. 586**).
   a. *Diet:* *low* sodium; foods *high* in: calcium, vitamin B complex, vitamins C and D, and iron (to reduce edema, replace deficits, and promote absorption of nutrients).
   b. Medications: given to control BP, regulate electrolytes, control fluid volume; supplemental vitamins if deficient; *electrolyte modifier* (aluminum hydroxide [Alu-Cap,

Amphojel]), calcium carbonate to bind phosphate.
   c. I&O; intake should be equivalent to previous daily output to prevent fluid retention.

2. Goal: *employ comfort measures that reduce distress and support physical function.*
   a. *Activity:* bedrest; facilitate ventilation; turn, cough, deep breathe q2h; ROM—active and passive, to prevent thrombi.
   b. *Hygiene:* mouth care to prevent stomatitis and reduce discomfort from mouth ulcers; perineal care.
   c. *Skin care:* soothing lotions to reduce pruritus.
   d. Encourage communication of concerns.

3. Goal: *health teaching.*
   a. *Dietary restrictions:* *no* added salt when cooking; change cooking water in vegetables during process to *decrease* potassium; read food labels to *avoid* Na$^+$ and K$^+$; *protein restriction* according to BUN/creatinine ratio (10:1).
   b. Importance of daily weight: same scale, time, clothing.
   c. Prepare for dialysis; transplantation.

F. **Evaluation/outcome criteria:**

1. Acceptance of chronic illness (no indication of indiscretions, destructive behavior, suicidal tendency).
2. Compliance with dietary restriction—no signs of protein excess (e.g., nausea, vomiting) or fluid/sodium excess (e.g., edema, weight gain).

V. **Dialysis:** diffusion of solute through a semipermeable membrane that separates two solutions; direction of diffusion depends on concentration of solute in each solution; rate and efficiency depend on concentration gradient, temperature of solution, pore size of membrane, and molecular size; two methods available (**Table 7.34**).

A. **Indications:** acute poisonings; acute or chronic renal failure; hepatic coma; metabolic acidosis; extensive burns with azotemia.

B. **Goals:**

1. *Reduce level of nitrogenous waste.*
2. *Correct acidosis, reverse electrolyte imbalances, remove excess fluid.*

C. *Hemodialysis:* circulation of client's blood through a compartment formed of a semipermeable membrane (polysulfone, polyacrylonitrile) surrounded by dialysate fluid.

1. Types of venous access for hemodialysis:
   a. External shunt (**Figure 7.11**).
      (1) Cannula is placed in a large vein and a large artery that approximate each other.
      (2) External shunts, which provide easy and painless access to bloodstream, are prone to infection and clotting and cause erosion of the skin around the insertion area.
         (a) Daily cleansing and application of a sterile dressing.

TABLE 7.34	Comparison of Hemodialysis and Peritoneal Dialysis	
	Hemodialysis	Peritoneal Dialysis
Process	Rapid—uses either external AV shunt (acute renal failure) or internal AV fistula (chronic renal failure); typical treatment is 3 to 4 hr, 3 days/wk; also used for barbiturate overdoses to remove toxic agent quickly	**Intermittent**—up to 36 hr for hospitalized clients; outpatient 4 to 8 hr, 5 to 6 times per week; dwell time 30 to 45 min for manual dialysis or 10 to 20 min for automatic cycler; either rigid stylet catheter or surgically inserted soft catheter; advantage for clients who cannot tolerate rapid fluid and electrolyte changes
		Continuous—two methods: (1) four cycles in 24 hr; dwell time is 4 to 5 hr during the day and 8 to 12 hr overnight; no need for machinery, electricity, or water source; surgically inserted soft catheter; closely resembles normal renal function; (2) automated cycler infuses and removes dialysate; generally done while client sleeps; built-in alarms for client safety.
Vascular access	Required	Not necessary; therefore suitable for clients with vascular problems
Heparinization	Required: systemic or regional	Little or no heparin necessary; therefore suitable for clients with bleeding problems
Complications (other than fluid and electrolyte imbalances, which are common to all)	Dialysis dysequilibrium syndrome (preventable) Mechanical dysfunctions of dialyzer	Peritonitis Hypoalbuminemia Bowel or bladder perforation Plugged or dislodged catheter

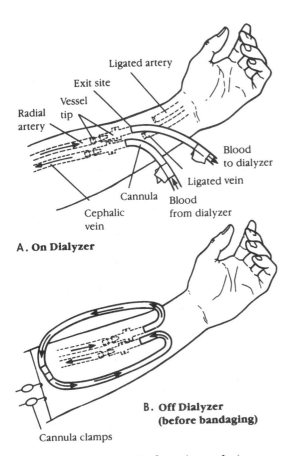

A. On Dialyzer

B. Off Dialyzer (before bandaging)

FIGURE 7.11   AV shunt (cannulae).

(b) Prevention of physical trauma and avoidance of some activities, such as swimming.

b. Arteriovenous fistulas or graft (**Figure 7.12**).

(1) Large artery and vein are sewn together (anastomosed) below the surface of the skin (fistula) or subcutaneous graft using the saphenous vein, synthetic prosthesis, or bovine xenograft to connect artery and vein.

(2) Purpose is to create one blood vessel for withdrawing and returning blood.

(3) *Advantages:* greater activity range than AV shunt and no protective asepsis.

(4) *Disadvantage:* necessity of two venipunctures with each dialysis.

c. Vein catheterization.

(1) Femoral or subclavian vein access is immediate.

(2) May be short- or long-term duration.

2. **Complications during hemodialysis:**

a. *Dysequilibrium syndrome*—rapid removal of urea from blood → reverse osmosis, with water moving into brain cells → cerebral edema → possible headache, nausea, vomiting, confusion, and convulsions; usually occurs with initial dialysis treatments; shorter dialysis time and slower rate minimizes.

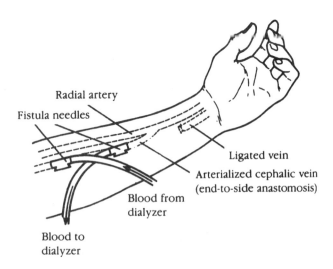

FIGURE 7.12   AV fistula.

b. *Hypotension*—results from excessive ultrafiltration or excessive antihypertensive medications.

c. *Hypertension*—results from volume overload (water and/or sodium), causing *dysequilibrium syndrome* or anxiety.

d. *Transfusion reactions* (see **Unit 11, Table 11.4**).

e. *Arrhythmias*—due to hypotension, fluid overload, or rapid removal of potassium.

f. *Psychological problems:*
   (1) Clients react in varying ways to dependence on hemodialysis.
   (2) Nurse needs to identify client reactions and defense mechanisms and to employ supportive behaviors (e.g., include client in care; continual repetition and reinforcement); do *not* interpret client's behavior—for example, do *not* say, "You're being hostile" or "You're acting like a child"; answer questions honestly regarding quality and length of life with dialysis and/or transplantation; encourage independence as much as possible.

3. Commonly used medications:
   a. *Antihypertensives* (ACE inhibitors, beta-blockers, diuretics).
   b. *Phosphorous binders* (calcium acetate, calcium carbonate, Renagel).
   c. *B complex vitamins* with vitamin *C* and *folic acid.*
   d. *Synthetic erythropoietin* (Aranesp, Epogen).
   e. Iron.
   f. Activated vitamin *D*

D. *Intermittent peritoneal dialysis:* involves introduction of a dialysate solution into the abdomen, where the peritoneum acts as the semipermeable membrane between the solution and blood in abdominal vessels. *Procedure:*
   1. Area around umbilicus is prepared and anesthetized with local anesthetic, and a catheter is inserted into the peritoneal cavity through a trocar; the catheter is then sutured into place to prevent displacement.
   2. Warmed dialysate is then allowed to flow into the peritoneal cavity. Inflow time: 5 to 10 min; 2 liters of solution are used in each cycle in the adult; solutions contain glucose, Na^+, Ca^{++}, Mg^{++}, K^+, Cl^-, and lactate or acetate.
   3. When solution bottle is empty, dwell time (exchange time) begins. *Dwell time:* 10 to 20 min; processes of diffusion, osmosis, and filtration begin to move waste products from bloodstream into peritoneal cavity.
   4. Draining of the dialysate begins with the unclamping of the outflow clamp. *Outflow time:* usually 10 min; returns less than 2 liters usually result from incomplete peritoneal emptying; turn side to side to increase return; multiple exchanges in 24 hr depending on client need.

E. *Continuous ambulatory peritoneal dialysis (CAPD):* functions on the same principles as peritoneal dialysis, yet allows greater freedom and independence for clients on dialysis. *Procedure:*
   1. Dialysis solution is infused into peritoneum three times daily and once before bedtime.
   2. *Dwell time*—≥ 4 hr for each daily exchange, and overnight for the fourth (8 to 12 hr).
   3. Indwelling peritoneal catheter is connected to solution bag at all times—serves to fill and drain peritoneum; concealed in cloth pouch, strapped to the body during dwell time; client can move about doing usual activities.

F. *Continuous cycling peritoneal dialysis (CCPD):* same principles as CAPD, except uses an automated system to infuse and remove dialysate; reduces nursing care needs with clients who are hospitalized. Cumbersome equipment inhibits nighttime mobility. *Procedure:*
   1. Long exchanges without an automated cycler during the day and short exchanges with a cycler at night.
   2. *Dwell time*—6 to 8 hr while sleeping.
   3. Automatic alarms to prevent malfunction with home use.

VI. **Kidney transplantation:** placement of a donor kidney (from sibling, parent, cadaver) into the iliac fossa of a recipient and the anastomosis of its ureter to the bladder of the recipient; indicated in end-stage renal disease.

A. *Criteria for recipient:* irreversible kidney function; under 70 yr of age; patent and functional lower urinary tract; and good surgical risk, free of serious cardiovascular complications. *Contraindicated* in those with another life-threatening condition.

B. *Donor selection:*
   1. Sibling or parent—survival rate of kidney is greater; preferred for transplantation.
   2. Cadaver—greater rate of rejection following transplantation, although majority of transplantations are with cadaver kidneys.

C. Bilateral nephrectomy: necessary for clients with rapidly progressive glomerulonephritis, malignant hypertension, or chronic kidney infections; prevents complications in transplanted kidney (see **VII. Nephrectomy** for nursing care, **p. 592**).

◆ **D. Analysis/nursing diagnosis:**
1. *Altered urinary elimination* related to kidney failure.
2. *Fear* related to potential transplant rejection.
3. *Risk for infection* related to immunosuppression.
4. *Body image disturbance* related to immunosuppression.

◆ **E. Nursing care plan/implementation:**
1. *Preoperative:*
   a. Goal: *promote physical and emotional adjustment.*
      (1) Informed consent.
      (2) Lab work completed—histocompatibility, CBC, urinalysis, blood type and cross-match.
      (3) Skin preparation.
   b. Goal: *encourage expression of feelings:* origin of donor, fear of complications, rejection.
   c. Goal: *minimize risk of organ rejection:* give medications: begin *immunosuppression* (azathioprine, corticosteroids, cyclosporine); *antibiotics* if ordered.
   d. Goal: *health teaching.*
      (1) Nature of surgery; placement of kidney.
      (2) Postoperative expectations: deep breathing, coughing, turning, early ambulation; reverse isolation.
      (3) Medications: *immunosuppressive* therapy: purpose, effect.
2. *Postoperative:*
   a. Goal: *promote uncomplicated recovery of recipient.*
      (1) Vital signs; CVP; I&O—urine output usually immediate with living donor; with cadaver kidney may not work for a week or more and dialysis will be needed within 24 to 48 hr. Report<100 mL/hr **immediately.**
      (2) *Isolation:* strict *reverse* isolation with immunosuppression; wear face mask when out of room.
      (3) *Position:* back to *nonoperative* side; *semi-Fowler's* to promote gas exchange.
      (4) Indwelling catheter care: *strict* asepsis; characteristics of urine—report gross hematuria, heavy sediment; clots; perineal care; bladder spasms may occur after removal of catheter.
      (5) Activity: ambulate 24 hr after surgery; *avoid* prolonged sitting.
      (6) Weigh daily.
      (7) Medications: *immunosuppressives; analgesics* as ordered (pain decreases significantly after 24 hr).
      (8) Drains: irrigate *only* on physician order; *meticulous* catheter care.

(9) *Diet:* regular after return of bowel sounds; liberal amounts of protein; *restrict* fluids, sodium, potassium *only if* oliguric.
   b. Goal: *observe for signs of rejection*—most dangerous complication. Three classifications:
      (1) **Hyperacute**—occurs within 5 to 10 min up to 48 hr after transplantation (rare).
      (2) **Acute**—most common 7 to 14 days; varies depending on living (1 wk to 6 mo) or cadaver (1 wk to 2 yr) donor.
      (3) **Chronic**—occurs several months to years.
   ◆ **Assessment:**
      (a) *Subjective data:*
         (i) Lethargy, anorexia.
         (ii) Tenderness over graft site.
      (b) *Objective data:*
         (i) Lab data: **Urine** *decreased*—output, creatinine clearance, sodium; *increased*—protein. **Blood:** *increased*—BUN, creatinine.
         (ii) Rapid weight gain; more than 3 lb/day.
         (iii) *Vital signs:* BP, temperature—*elevated.*
   c. Goal: *maintain immunosuppressive therapy.*
      (1) Azathioprine *(Imuran)*—an antimetabolite that interferes with cellular division. *Side effects:*
         (a) Gastrointestinal bleeding (give PO form with food).
         (b) Bone marrow depression; leukopenia; anemia.
         (c) Development of malignant neoplasms.
         (d) Infection.
         (e) Liver damage.
      (2) Prednisone—believed to affect lymphocyte production by inhibiting nucleic acid synthesis: antiinflammatory action helps prevent tissue damage if rejection occurs. *Side effects:*
         (a) Stress ulcer with bleeding (give with food).
         (b) *Decreased* glucose tolerance (hyperglycemia).
         (c) Muscle weakness.
         (d) Osteoporosis.
         (e) Moon facies.
         (f) Acne and striae.
         (g) Depression and hallucinations.
      (3) Cyclosporine (Neoral, Sandimmune)—polypeptide antibiotic used to prevent rejection of kidney, liver, or heart allografts; PO dose given with *room temperature chocolate milk or orange juice* in a glass dispenser. *Side effects:*
         (a) Nephrotoxicity (*increased* BUN, creatinine).
         (b) Hypertension.

Adult

(c) Tremor.

(d) Hirsutism, gingival hyperplasia.

(e) *GI*—nausea, vomiting, anorexia, diarrhea, abdominal pain.

(f) Infections—pneumonia, septicemia, abscesses, wound.

 (4) Additional drugs may include cyclophosphamide (Cytoxan), antithymocyte (ATG), antilymphocyte globulin, muromonab-CD3 (OKT3), tacrolimus (Prograf), and mycophenolate mofetil (CellCept).

d. Goal: *health teaching.*

(1) Signs of rejection (see Goal b).

(2) Drugs: side effects of immunosuppression (see Goal c).

(3) *Self-care activities:* temperature, blood pressure, I&O, urine specimen collection.

(4) Avoidance of infection.

(5) See also goals of care, under **Postoperative experience, p. 553.**

◆ **F. Evaluation/outcome criteria:**

1. No signs of rejection (e.g., no weight gain, oliguria).

2. No depression.

3. Client resumes role responsibilities.

VII. Nephrectomy (radical or partial): removal of kidney through flank, retroperitoneal, abdominal, thoracic, or thoracic-abdominal approach; indicated with malignant tumors, severe trauma, or under certain conditions before renal transplantation (see **VI. Kidney transplantation, p. 590**).

◆ **A. Analysis/nursing diagnosis:**

1. *Pain* related to surgical incision.

2. *Risk for infection* related to wound contamination.

3. *Risk for fluid volume excess.*

4. *Risk for aspiration* related to vomiting.

5. *Constipation* related to paralytic ileus.

6. *Anxiety* related to possible loss of function in remaining kidney.

7. *Dysfunctional grieving* related to perceived loss.

◆ **B. Nursing care plan/implementation:**

1. *Preoperative:* Goal: *optimize physical and psychological functioning* (see **I. Preoperative preparation, p. 546**).

2. *Postoperative:* Goal: *promote comfort and prevent complications.*

a. Observe for signs of:

(1) *Paralytic ileus*—abdominal distention, absent bowel sounds, vomiting (common complication following renal surgery).

(2) *Hemorrhage.*

b. Fluid balance: daily weight—maintain within 2% of preoperative level.

◆ **C. Evaluation/outcome criteria:**

1. No complications (e.g., hemorrhage, paralytic ileus, wound infection).

2. Acceptance of loss of kidney.

VIII. Renal calculi (urolithiasis): formation of calculi (stones) in renal calyces or pelvis that pass to lower regions of urinary tract—ureters, bladder, or urethra; occurs after age 30, with greatest incidence in *men,* particularly over age 50.

A. Pathophysiology: organic crystals form (most consist of calcium salts or magnesium—ammonium phosphate (struvite) → obstruction, infection; increased backward pressure in kidney → hydronephrosis → atrophy, fibrosis of renal tubules.

B. Risk factors (in over 50% of cases, cause is idiopathic):

1. Urinary tract infection.

2. Urinary stasis—obstruction.

3. Metabolic factors—excessive intake of vitamin D or C, calcium carbonate.

◆ **C. Assessment** (depends on size, shape, location of stone):

1. *Subjective data:*

a. *Pain:* occasional, dull, in loin or back when stones are in calyces or renal pelvis; *excruciating* in flank area (renal colic), radiating to groin when stones are ureteral.

b. Nausea associated with pain.

2. *Objective data:*

a. Pallor, sweating, syncope, shock, and vomiting due to pain.

b. Palpable kidney mass with hydronephrosis.

c. Fever and pyuria with infection.

d. Lab data:

(1) Urinalysis: abnormal—pH (acidic or alkaline); RBCs (injury); WBCs (infection); *increased*—specific gravity; casts; crystals; other organic substances, depending on type of stone (i.e., calcium, struvite, uric acid or cystine); *positive* culture.

(2) Blood: *increased* calcium, phosphorus, total protein, alkaline phosphatase, creatinine, uric acid, BUN.

e. *Diagnostic tests:*

(1) IVP: reveals nonopaque stones, degree of obstruction.

(2) X-ray; radiopaque stones seen.

(3) Ultrasound may also be used.

◆ **D. Analysis/nursing diagnosis:**

1. *Pain* related to passage of stone.

2. *Altered urinary elimination* related to potential obstruction.

3. *Urinary retention* related to obstruction of urethra.

◆ **E. Nursing care plan/implementation:**

1. Goal: *reduce pain and prevent complications.*

a. Medication: *narcotics, antiemetics, antibiotics.*

b. Fluids: 3 to 4 L/day; IVs if nauseated, vomiting.

c. Activity: ambulate to promote passage of stone, except bed rest during acute attack (colic).

d. Reduce spasms: warm soaks to affected flank.

e. Observe for signs of:

(1) *Obstruction*—decreased urinary output, increased flank pain.

(2) *Passage of stone* (90% will pass <5 mm size)—cessation of pain; filter urine with gauze.

f. Monitor: hydration status—I&O, daily weight; vital signs—particularly temperature for sign of infection; urine—color, odor.

2. Goal: *health teaching.*

a. Importance of *fluids:* minimum 3000 mL/day; 2 glasses during night.

b. *Diet:* modify according to stone type (see **Unit 9**).

(1) *Calcium oxalate and calcium phosphate stones—low* calcium, phosphorus and oxalate (e.g., *avoid* tea, cocoa, cola, beans, spinach, acidic fruits).

(2) *Magnesium-ammonium phosphate—low* phosphorus.

(3) *Uric acid stones—low* purine.

(4) *Cystine stones—low* protein.

c. *Acid-ash diet* with calcium oxalate and calcium phosphate stones, magnesium and ammonium phosphate (struvite) stones.

d. *Alkaline-ash diet* with uric acid and cystine stones (see **Common Therapeutic Diets** in **Unit 9, p. 721**).

e. Signs of urinary infection: dysuria, frequency, hematuria; seek immediate treatment.

f. Prepare for removal if indicated; 20% of stones require additional treatment: *cytoscopy* for small stones; *cystolitholapaxy* for soft stones; *lithotripsy* or *surgical removal* (nephroscopic, pyelolithotomy, or nephrolithotomy).

◆ F. **Evaluation/outcome criteria:**

1. Relief from pain.

2. No signs of urinary obstruction (e.g., increased flank pain, decreased urine output).

3. No recurrence of lithiasis (adheres to diet and fluid regimen).

IX. **Lithotripsy.** *Laser lithotripsy*—newer treatment using laser and a ureteroscope; constant water irrigation because of heat. *Extracorporeal shock wave*—a noninvasive mechanical procedure used to break up renal calculi so they can pass spontaneously, in most cases. The trunk of the client is submerged in distilled water. In addition to being strapped to a frame, the client may also receive *sedation* and *analgesia* for pain from sound waves. The procedure takes 30 to 45 min, and remaining still is important. An underwater electrode generates shock waves that fragment the stone so it can be excreted in the urine a few days after the procedure. A degree of renal colic may occur, requiring *narcotics* for up to 3 days. **Nursing measures** should encourage ambulation and promote diuresis through *forcing* fluids. *Percutaneous lithotripsy*—nephrostomy tract above kidney region; nephroscope used to retrieve calculi. Urinary drainage from incision for 3 to 4 days is normal. May be required for large fragments remaining after extracorporeal lithotripsy. **Nursing measures** include: dressing changes to prevent infection and prevent skin breakdown, and administration of *antibiotics* and *narcotics* for pain.

X. **Benign prostatic hyperplasia** (**BPH**): bladder outlet obstruction resulting from an enlargement of the prostate gland.

A. **Pathophysiology:** prostate enlarges, bulges upward, blocks flow of urine from bladder into urethra → obstruction → hydroureter, hydronephrosis.

B. **Risk factors:**

1. Changes in estrogen and androgen levels.

2. Men >50.

◆ C. **Assessment:**

1. *Subjective data—urination:*

a. Difficulty starting stream.

b. Smaller, less forceful.

c. Dribbling.

d. Frequency.

e. Urgency.

f. Nocturia.

g. Retention (incomplete emptying).

h. Inability to void after ingestion of alcohol or exposure to cold.

2. *Objective data:*

▶ a. Catheterization for residual urine: 25 to 50 mL after voiding.

b. Enlarged prostate on rectal exam.

c. Lab data:

(1) Urine—*increased* RBC, WBC.

(2) Blood—*increased* creatinine, PSA.

◆ D. **Analysis/nursing diagnosis:**

1. *Urinary retention* related to incomplete emptying.

2. *Altered urinary elimination* related to obstruction.

3. *Urinary incontinence* related to urgency, pressure.

4. *Anxiety* related to potential surgery.

5. *Body image disturbance* related to threat to masculine identity.

◆ E. **Nursing care plan/implementation:**

1. Goal: *relieve urinary retention.*

▶ a. Catheterization: release maximum of 1000 mL initially; *avoid* bladder decompression, which results in hypotension, bladder spasms, ruptured blood vessels in bladder; empty 200 mL every 5 min.

▶ b. Patency: irrigate intermittently or continually, as ordered.

c. *Fluids:* minimum 2000 mL/24 hr.

2. Goal: *health teaching.*

a. Preparation for surgery (cystostomy, prostatectomy):

(1) Expectations—indwelling catheter (will feel urge to void).

(2) *Avoid* pulling on catheter (this increases bleeding and clots).

(3) Bladder spasms common 24 to 48 hr after surgery, particularly with transurethral resection and suprapubic approaches.

(4) Threatening nature of procedure (possibility of impotence with perineal prostatectomy).

b. See also **I. Preoperative preparation, p. 546.**

XI. Prostatectomy: surgical procedure to relieve urinary retention and frequency caused by benign prostatic hyperplasia or cancer of the prostate.

A. Types

1. *Transurethral resection (TUR)*—removal of obstructive prostatic tissue surrounding urethra by an electrical wire (resectoscope) introduced through the urethra; hypertrophy may recur, and TUR repeated; little risk of impotence. Laser also being used.

2. *Suprapubic*—low midline incision is made directly over the bladder; bladder is opened and large mass of prostatic tissue is removed through incision in urethral mucosa.

3. *Retropubic*—removal of hypertrophied prostatic tissue high in pelvic area through a low abdominal incision; bladder is not opened; client may remain potent.

4. *Perineal*—removal of prostatic tissue low in pelvic area is accomplished through an incision made between the scrotum and the rectum; usually results in impotency and incontinence.

◆ **B. Nursing care plan/implementation:**

1. *Preoperative* (see **X. Prostatic hyperplasia, p. 593**).

2. *Postoperative:*

a. Goal: *promote optimal bladder function and comfort.*

(1) Urinary drainage: sterile closed-gravity system—maintain external traction as ordered.

(2) Reinforce purposes, sensations to expect.

▶ (3) Bladder irrigation to control bleeding, keep clots from forming.

▶ (4) Suprapubic catheter care (suprapubic prostatectomy)—closed-gravity drainage system; observe character, amount, flow of drainage.

(5) *After removal:*

(a) Observe for urinary drainage q4h for 24 hr.

(b) Skin care.

(c) Report excessive drainage to physician.

(6) Dressings: keep dry, clean; reinforce if necessary (may need to change suprapubic dressing if urinary drainage); notify physician of *excessive bleeding.*

(7) Observe for signs of:

(a) *Bladder distention*—distinct mound over pubis, slow drip in collecting bottle; irrigate catheter as ordered.

(b) *Increased bleeding*—expect and report frank bleeding (if *venous* bleeding, increase traction on catheter); if bright red drainage, and clots (*arterial* bleeding), may need surgical control; cool, clammy, pale skin and increased pulse rate indicate *shock.*

b. Goal: *assist in rehabilitation.* Emotional support: *fears* of incontinence, loss of masculine identity, impotence.

c. Goal: *health teaching.*

(1) Expectations: mild incontinence, dribbling for a while (several months) after surgery; need to void as soon as urge is felt; *push fluids.*

(2) Exercises: perineal (Kegel) 1 to 2 days after surgery—buttocks are tightened for a count of ten, 20 to 50 times daily.

(3) *Avoid:*

(a) Long auto trips, vigorous exercise, heavy lifting (anything heavier than 10 lb), and sexual intercourse for about 3 wk or until medical permission, because they may increase tendency to bleed.

(b) Alcoholic beverages for 1 mo, because this may cause burning on urination; caffeine, because it causes diuresis.

(c) Tub baths, because of increase chance of infection.

(4) Medications: *stool softeners* or mild *cathartics* to decrease straining.

◆ **C. Evaluation/outcome criteria:**

1. Relief of symptoms.

2. No complications (e.g., hemorrhage, impotence).

XII. Urinary diversion. *Incontinent*—ileal conduit: anastomosis of ureters to a small portion of the ileum; stoma is called urostomy; urine flow is constant; requires external collection device. *Continent*—Kock pouch, Indiana pouch: segment of small bowel or colon is used to create a pouch; holds urine without leakage; requires self-catheterization.

A. Indications:

1. Congenital anomalies of bladder.

2. Neurogenic bladder.

3. Mechanical obstruction to urine flow (e.g., bladder cancer).

4. Chronic progressive pyelonephritis.

5. Trauma to lower urinary tract.

◆ **B. Analysis/nursing diagnosis:**

1. *Altered urinary elimination* related to surgical diversion.

2. *Risk for impaired skin integrity* related to leakage of urine.
3. *Risk for infection* related to contamination of stoma.
4. *Constipation* related to absence of peristalsis.
5. *Body image disturbance* related to stoma.

◆ **C. Nursing care plan/implementation:**
1. *Preoperative:* optimal bowel and stoma site preparation.
    a. *Diet:* low residue 2 days followed by clear liquids for 24 hr.
    b. Medications:
      (1) Neomycin (for bowel sterilization).
      (2) Cathartics (GoLYTELY), enemas.
    c. Site selection: appliance faceplate (incontinent diversion) must bond securely; *avoid* areas of pressure from clothing (waistline); usual site is right or left lower abdominal quadrant.
    d. See also **I. Preoperative preparation, p. 546.**
2. *Postoperative:*
    a. Goal: *prevent complications and promote comfort.*
      (1) Observe for signs of:
        (a) *Paralytic ileus* (common complication)—keep NG tube patent.
        (b) *Stoma necrosis*—dusky or cyanotic color (**emergency** situation).
      (2) Skin care: check for leakage around ostomy bag.
      (3) Urinary drainage—stents or catheter in stoma; blood in urine in immediate postoperative period; mucus normal.
      (4) See **III. Postoperative experience, p. 553.**
    b. Goal: *health teaching.*
      (1) Self-care activities:

> (a) *Peristomal skin care*—prevent irritation, breakdown; proper cleansing— soap and water; adhesive remover, if needed.
> (b) *Appliance application and emptying;* pouch opening 2 to 3 mm larger than stoma; do *not* remove each day; change appliance every 3 to 5 days or when leaking.
> (c) *Odor control*—dilute urine, hygiene, acid-ash diet; *avoid* asparagus, tomatoes.
> (d) *Use of night drainage system if necessary* for uninterrupted sleep.

      (2) Signs *of complications:* change in urine color, clarity, quantity, smell; stomal color change (normal is bright pink or red).

◆ **D. Evaluation/outcome criteria:**
1. Acceptance of new body image.
2. Regains independence.
3. Demonstrates confidence in management of self-care activities.

SENSORY/PERCEPTUAL FUNCTIONS

I. Laryngectomy with radical neck dissection: removal of entire larynx, lymph nodes, submandibular salivary gland, sternomastoid muscle, spinal accessory nerves, and jugular vein for cancer of the larynx that extends beyond the vocal cords. Permanent tracheostomy; new methods of speech will have to be learned.

Partial laryngectomy: removal of lesion on larynx. Client will be able to speak after operation, but quality of voice may be altered.

◆ **A. Assessment:**
1. *Subjective data:*
    a. Feeling of lump in throat.
    b. *Pain:* Adam's apple; may radiate to ear.
    c. Dysphagia.
2. *Objective data:*
    a. Hoarseness: persistent (longer than 2 weeks), progressive.
    b. Lymphadenopathy: cervical.
    c. Breath odor: foul.

◆ **B. Analysis/nursing diagnosis:**
1. *Impaired verbal communication* related to removal of larynx.
2. *Body image disturbance* related to radical neck dissection.
3. *Ineffective airway clearance* related to copious amounts of mucus.
4. *Fear* related to diagnosis of cancer.
5. *Impaired swallowing* related to edema.
6. *Impaired social interaction* related to altered speech.

◆ **C. Nursing care plan/implementation:**
1. *Preoperative care:*
    a. Goal: *provide emotional support and optimal physical preparation.*
      (1) Encourage verbalization of fears; answer all questions honestly, particularly about having no voice after surgery.
      (2) Referral: visit from person with laryngectomy (contact New Voice Club, Lost Chord, or International Association of Laryngectomees).
    b. Goal: *health teaching.*
      (1) Prepare for tracheostomy.
      (2) Other means to speak (esophageal "burp" speech, tracheoesophageal prosthesis or electronic artificial larynx).
2. *Postoperative care:*
    a. Goal: *maintain patent airway and prevent aspiration.*
      (1) *Position:* semi-Fowler's (elevate 30 to 45 degrees), preventing forward flexion of neck to reduce edema and keep airway open.
      (2) Observe for hypoxia:
        (a) *Early signs:* increased respiratory and pulse rates, apprehension, restlessness.

Adult

(b) *Late signs:* dyspnea, cyanosis; swallowing difficulties—client should chew food well and swallow with water.

> (3) *Laryngectomy* tube care:
> (a) Observe for stridor (coarse, high-pitched inspiratory sound)—**report immediately.**
> (b) Have extra laryngectomy tube at bedside.
> ▶ (c) Suction with sterile equipment; 2 to 3 mL of sterile saline into stoma may be used to loosen secretions.

b. Goal: *promote optimal physical and psychological function.*
(1) Frequent mouth care.
(2) *Wound:* exposed site; note color and amount of drainage.
▶ (3) *Tubes:* closed drainage system *(Hemovac, Jackson-Pratt)* **(Figure 7.13);** expect <100 up to 300 mL of serosanguineous drainage first postoperative day; drainage should decrease daily; observe patency.
(4) Pain management—consider impact of impaired communication on assessment.
(5) Post-drainage system removal—observe: skin flaps down, adherent to underlying tissue.
(6) Use surgical *asepsis.*
(7) Answer call bell *immediately;* use preestablished means of communication.
(8) Reexplain all procedures while giving care.
(9) Support head when lifting.

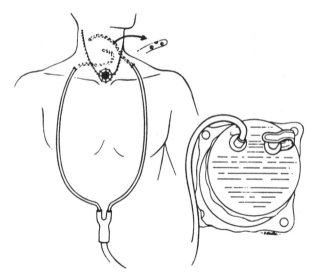

FIGURE 7.13   Closed drainage system for constant suction. Suction is maintained by a plastic container. The container serves as both suction source and receptacle for blood. It is emptied as required, and drainage tubes are left in the neck for approximately 3 days. (From De Weese, DD: Saunders' Textbook of Otolaryngology. Mosby, St. Louis, 1987.)

c. Goal: *health teaching.*
(1) Referral: speech rehabilitation as soon as esophageal suture is healed.
(a) Information on laryngeal speech (International Association of Laryngectomees, American Cancer Society, American Speech and Hearing Association).
(b) *Esophageal speech* best learned in speech clinic—learn to burp column of air needed for speech; new voice sounds are natural but hoarse.

> ▶ (2) *Stoma* care:
> (a) Cover with scarf or shirt made of a porous material (material substitutes for nasal passage—warms and filters out particles).
> (b) Use source of humidification ("mister" or commercial humidifier).
> (c) *Caution* while bathing or showering, to decrease likelihood of aspiration.
> (d) Swimming *not* recommended.
> (e) Procedure for suctioning if cough ineffective.

(3) Simple ROM of neck; how to support head.
(4) Possible *contraindications:* use of talcum powder, tissues.

◆ **D. Evaluation/outcome criteria:**
1. No surgical complications (e.g., no airway obstruction, infection, hemorrhage).
2. Learns alternative speech 30 to 60 days after surgery.
3. Demonstrates proper stoma care.
4. Resumes productive lifestyle (work, family).
5. Normal response to change in body image (e.g., anger, grief, denial).

II. **Aphasia:** impaired ability to understand or use commonly accepted words or symbols; interferes with ability to speak, write, or read; language center—usually left hemisphere (85% of population). *Dysarthria* is motor impairment—inability to articulate words.
A. **Types and pathophysiology:**
1. *Receptive (sensory)*—lesion usually Wernicke's area of temporal lobe; difficulty understanding spoken word (*auditory* aphasia) or written word (*visual* aphasia).
2. *Expressive (motor)*—difficulty expressing thoughts in speech or writing (*motor* aphasia); understands written and spoken words. Three types: *anomic*—fluent speech, but unable to name objects, qualities, and conditions; *fluent*—articulate and grammatically correct, but no content or meaning; *nonfluent*—unable to select, organize, and initiate speech (involves Broca's area of brain); may affect writing.
B. **Risk factors:**
1. Vascular disease of the brain (brain attack).
2. Alzheimer's disease (degeneration).
3. Tumor.
4. Trauma.

◆ **C. Analysis/nursing diagnosis:**
1. *Impaired verbal communication* related to cerebral cortex disorder.
2. *Powerlessness* related to inability to express needs/concerns.
3. *Impaired social interaction* related to difficulty communicating.

◆ **D. Nursing care plan/implementation:** Goal: *assist with communication:* client does best when rested; small improvements will occur up to 1 year after injury (age is a factor). *Strategies: Nonfluent*—allow time to respond; support efforts to speak; acknowledge frustration of client—anticipate needs when appropriate; use picture board or flashcards, pointing, to encourage communication; assess efforts to communicate with open-ended questions. *Fluent*—face the client, speak slowly and distinctly, not loudly; use gestures, repeat instructions as needed; involve family in techniques to improve communication; acknowledge frustration.

◆ **E. Evaluation/outcome criteria:**
1. Communication reestablished.
2. Minimal frustration exhibited.
3. Participates in speech therapy.

III. **Meniere's disease:** chronic, recurrent disorder of inner ear; attacks of vertigo, tinnitus, and vestibular dysfunction; lasts 30 min to full day; usually no pain or loss of consciousness.

A. Pathophysiology: associated with excessive dilation of cochlear duct (unilateral) from overproduction or decreased absorption of endolymph (endolymphatic hydrops) → progressive sensorineural loss.

B. Risk factors:
1. Emotional or endocrine disturbance (diabetes mellitus).
2. Spasms of internal auditory artery.
3. Head trauma.
4. Allergic reaction.
5. High salt intake.
6. Smoking.
7. Ear infections.

◆ **C. Assessment:**
1. *Subjective data:*
   a. Tinnitus (constant or intermittent).
   b. Headache; feeling of fullness or pressure in affected ear.
   c. True vertigo: sudden attacks; room appears to spin.
   d. Depression; irritability; withdrawal.
   e. Nausea with sudden head motion.
2. *Objective data:*
   a. Impaired hearing, especially *low* tones.
   b. Change in gait; lack of coordination.
   c. Vomiting with sudden head motion.
   d. Nystagmus—during attacks.
   e. *Diagnostic test:* caloric (cold water in ear canal)—may precipitate attack; audiometry—loss of hearing.

◆ **D. Analysis/nursing diagnosis:**
1. *Risk for injury* related to vertigo, lack of coordination.
2. *Auditory sensory/perceptual alteration* related to progressive hearing loss.
3. *Anxiety* related to uncertainty of treatment.
4. *Risk for activity intolerance* related to sudden onset of vertigo.
5. *Sleep pattern disturbance* related to tinnitus.
6. *Ineffective individual coping* related to chronic disorder.

◆ **E. Nursing care plan/implementation:**
1. Goal: *provide safety and comfort during attacks.*
   a. Activity: bedrest during attack; side rails up; lower to chair or floor if attack occurs while standing; assist with ambulation (sudden dizziness common).
   b. *Position:* recumbent; *affected ear uppermost* usually.
   c. Identify prodromal symptoms (aura, ear pressure, increased tinnitus).
2. Goal: *minimize occurrence of attacks.*
   a. Give medications as ordered:
      (1) *Anticholinergics* (oral or transdermal scopolamine, atropine, glycopyrrolate [Robinul]) to minimize GI symptoms.
      (2) *Antihistamines* (dimenhydrinate [Dramamine], diphenhydramine HCl [Benadryl]) to sedate vestibular system.
      (3) *Antiemetics and antivertigo agents* (diazepam [Valium], meclizine HCl [Antivert]).
      (4) *Diuretics* may help (hydrochlorothiazide) to decrease endolymphatic fluid.
   b. *Diet: low* sodium (<2 g/day).
   c. *Avoid* precipitating stimuli: bright, glaring lights; noise; sudden jarring; turning head or eyes (stand in front of client when talking).
3. Goal: *health teaching.*
   a. *No* smoking (causes vasospasm) or alcoholic beverages (fluid retention, contraindicated with medications).
   b. Management of symptoms: play radio to mask tinnitus, particularly at night.
   c. Keep medication available at all times.
   d. Prepare for surgery if indicated (labyrinthectomy if hearing gone; or vestibular neurectomy to relieve vertigo and preserve hearing).

◆ **F. Evaluation/outcome criteria:**
1. Decreased frequency of attacks.
2. Complies with treatment regimen and restrictions (e.g., low sodium diet, no smoking).
3. Hearing preserved.

IV. **Otosclerosis:** disease of the bone of otic capsule; insidious, progressive deafness; most common cause of conductive deafness; cause unknown.

A. Pathophysiology: formation of new spongy bone in labyrinth → fixation of stapes → prevention of sound transmission through ossicles to inner ear fluids.

Adult

B. **Risk factors:**
1. Heredity.
2. Women, puberty to 45 yr.
3. Pregnancy.

◆ C. **Assessment:**
1. *Subjective data:*
   a. Difficulty hearing—gradual loss in both ears.
2. *Diagnostic tests:*
   a. *Rinne* (tuning fork placed over mastoid bone)—*reduced* sound conduction by air and intensified by bone.
   b. *Weber* (tuning fork placed on top of head)—*increased* sound conduction to affected ear.
   c. *Audiometry—diminished* hearing ability.

◆ D. **Analysis/nursing diagnosis:**
1. *Auditory sensory/perceptual alteration* related to hearing loss.
2. *Body image disturbance* related to hearing aid.
3. *Ineffective individual coping* related to grief reaction to loss.
4. *Impaired social interaction* related to hearing loss.

E. **Nursing care plan/implementation, evaluation/outcome criteria** (see **V. Stapedectomy,** following).

V. **Stapedectomy:** removal of the stapes and replacing it with a prosthesis (steel wire, Teflon piston, or polyethylene); treatment for deafness due to otosclerosis, which fixes the stapes, preventing it from oscillating and transmitting vibrations to the fluids in the inner ear.

◆ A. **Analysis/nursing diagnosis:**
1. *Sensory/perceptual alteration* related to edema and ear packing.
2. See **The Perioperative Experience, p. 546,** for diagnoses relating to surgery.

◆ B. **Nursing care plan/implementation:**
1. *Preoperative* health teaching.
   a. Important to keep head in position ordered by physician postoperatively.
   b. *Caution:* sneezing, blowing nose (keep mouth open), vomiting, coughing—all of which increase pressure in eustachian tubes (blow one side gently).
   c. Breathing exercises.
2. *Postoperative:*
   a. Goal: *promote physical and psychological equilibrium.*
      (1) *Position:* as ordered by physician—varies according to preference.
      (2) Activity: assist with ambulation; *avoid* rapid turning, which might increase vertigo.
      (3) Dressings: check frequently; may change cotton pledget in outer ear.
       (4) Give medications as ordered:
         (a) *Antiemetics.*
         (b) *Analgesics.*
         (c) *Antibiotics.*
      (5) Reassurance: reduction in hearing is normal; hearing may not immediately improve after surgery.

   b. Goal: *health teaching.*
      (1) Ear care: keep covered outdoors; keep outer ear plug clean, dry, and changed.
      (2) *Avoid:*
         (a) Water in ear for 6 wk:
            (i) Use barrier when washing hair.
            (ii) Use two pieces of cotton; saturate outer piece with petroleum jelly.
         (b) Pressure or vibration from loud noise, flying, or heavy lifting until advised by MD.

◆ C. **Evaluation/outcome criteria:**
1. Hearing improves—evaluate 1 mo postoperatively (may require hearing aid).
2. Returns to work (usually 2 wk after surgery).
3. Continues medical supervision.

VI. **Deafness:** (1) *Hard of hearing*—slight or moderate hearing loss that is serviceable for activities of daily living. (2) *Deaf*—hearing is nonfunctional for activities of daily living.

A. **Risk factors:**
1. *Conductive* hearing losses (transmission deafness):
   a. Impacted cerumen (wax).
   b. Foreign body in external auditory canal.
   c. Defects (thickening, scarring) of eardrum.
   d. Otosclerosis of ossicles.
2. *Sensorineural* hearing losses (perceptive or nerve deafness):
   a. Arteriosclerosis.
   b. Infectious diseases (mumps, measles, meningitis).
   c. Drug toxicities (quinine, streptomycin, neomycin SO_4).
   d. Tumors.
   e. Head traumas.
   f. High-intensity noises.
3. *Central* deafness:
   a. Tumors.
   b. Stroke (brain attack).
4. *Noise-induced or occupational noise* hearing loss:
   a. Blast injury.
   b. Firearms.
   c. Loud music.
5. *Aging* (presbycusis).

◆ B. **Assessment**—*objective data:*
1. Facial expression: inattentive or strained.
2. Speech: excessive loudness or softness.
3. Frequent need to clarify content of conversation or inappropriate responses.
4. Tilting of head while listening.
5. Lack of response when others speak.
6. Audiological exams:
   a. Pure tone air conduction.
   b. Bone conduction test.
   c. Speech reception threshold.
   d. Word recognition.

◆ C. **Analysis/nursing diagnosis:**
1. *Auditory/sensory/perceptual alteration* related to loss of hearing.
2. *Impaired social interaction* related to deafness.

◆ D. **Nursing care plan/implementation:**
1. Goal: *maximize hearing ability and provide emotional support.*

   a. Gain person's attention before speaking; *avoid* startling.
   b. Provide adequate lighting so person can see who is speaking.
   c. Look at the person when speaking.
   d. Use nonverbal cues to enhance communication, e.g., writing, hand gestures, pointing.
   e. Speak slowly, distinctly; do *not* shout (excessive loudness distorts voice).
   f. If person does not understand, use different words; write it down.
   g. Use alternative communication system:
      (1) Speech (lip) reading.
      (2) Sign language.
      (3) Hearing aid.
      (4) Paper and pencil.
      (5) Flash cards.
   h. Supportive, nonstressful environment; alert staff to client's hearing impairment.

2. Goal: *health teaching.*
   a. Prepare for evaluative studies—audiogram.
   b. Referral: appropriate community resources: National Association of Hearing and Speech Agencies for *counseling services;* National Association for the Deaf to assist with *employment, education, legislation;* Alexander Graham Bell Association for the Deaf, Inc., serves as *information* center for those working with the client with hearing aid impairments; American Hearing Society provides educational information, employment services, *social clubs.*
   c. See **Table 11.16** for care of hearing aids.
   d. Safety precautions: when crossing street, driving.

◆ E. **Evaluation/outcome criteria:**
1. Method of communication established.
2. Achieves independence (use of Dogs for Deaf, special telephones, visual signals).
3. Copes with lifestyle changes (minimal depression, anger, hostility).

VII. **Glaucoma** (acute and chronic): increased intraocular pressure; second most common cause of blindness.

A. **Pathophysiology:**
1. *Acute (closed-angle)*—impaired passage of aqueous humor into the circular canal of Schlemm due to closure of the angle between the cornea and the iris. **Medical emergency;** *requires surgery.*
2. *Chronic (open-angle)*—degenerative changes in trabecular meshwork; local obstruction of aque-

ous humor between the anterior chamber and the canal. *Most common; treated with medication* (*miotics, carbonic anhydrase inhibitors*).
3. *Secondary*—in some cases neovascularization (new vessels) may form; blocks passage of aqueous humor (uveitis, trauma, drugs, diabetes, retinal vein occlusion).
4. Untreated: imbalance between rate of secretion of intraocular fluids and rate of absorption of aqueous humor → increased intraocular pressures → decreased peripheral vision → corneal edema → halos and blurring of vision → blindness.

B. **Risk factors**—unknown, but associated with:
1. Emotional disturbances.
2. Hereditary factors.
3. Allergies.
4. Vasomotor disturbances.

◆ C. **Assessment:**
1. *Subjective data:*
   a. *Acute (closed-angle):*
      (1) Pain: severe, in and around eyes.
      (2) Rainbow halos around lights.
      (3) Blurring of vision.
      (4) Nausea, vomiting.
   b. *Chronic (open-angle):*
      (1) Eyes tire easily.
      (2) Loss of peripheral vision.
      (3) Dull, morning headache.
2. *Objective data:*
   a. Corneal edema.
   b. Decreased peripheral vision.
   c. Increased cupping of optic disc.
    d. Tonometry—pressures >22 mm Hg
   e. Pupils: dilated.
   f. Redness of eye.

◆ D. **Analysis/nursing diagnosis:**
1. *Visual sensory/perceptual alterations* related to increased intraocular pressure.
2. *Pain* related to sudden increase in intraocular pressure.
3. *Risk for injury* related to blindness.
4. *Impaired physical mobility* related to impaired vision.

◆ E. **Nursing care plan/implementation:**
1. Goal: *reduce intraocular pressure.*
   a. Activity: bedrest.
   b. *Position:* semi-Fowler's.
   c. Medications as ordered:
      (1) *Miotics* (pilocarpine, carbachol); may not be effective with intraocular pressure (IOP) >40 mm Hg.
      (2) *Carbonic anhydrase inhibitors* (acetazolamide [Diamox]).
      (3) *Anticholinesterase* (demecarium bromide [Humorsol]) to facilitate outflow of aqueous humor.
      (4) *Ophthalmic beta-blockers* (timolol) to decrease IOP.

2. Goal: *provide emotional support.*
   a. Place personal objects within field of vision.
   b. Assist with activities.
   c. Encourage verbalization of concerns, fears of blindness, loss of independence.
3. Goal: *health teaching.*
   a. *Prevent* increased IOP by *avoiding:*
      (1) Anger, excitement, worry.
      (2) Constrictive clothing.
      (3) Heavy lifting.
      (4) Excessive *fluid* intake.
      (5) Atropine or other mydriatics that cause dilation.
      (6) Straining at stool.
      (7) Eye strain.
   b. Relaxation techniques; stress management if indicated.
   c. Prepare for surgical intervention, if ordered: laser trabeculoplasty, trabeculectomy (filtering), laser peripheral iridotomy.
   d. Medications: purpose, dosage, frequency; ▶ *eyedrop installation*—(1) wash hands; (2) head back, expose conjunctiva of lower lid, instill in center *without* touching eyelashes or eye; (3) close eyes gently, apply slight pressure to corner of eye to decrease systemic absorption; (4) wait at least 2 minutes before instilling a second eyedrop medication; have extra bottle in case of breakage or loss.
   e. Activity: moderate exercise—walking.
   f. Safety measures: eye protection (shield or glasses); MedicAlert band or tag; *avoid* driving 1 to 2 hr after instilling miotics.
   g. Community resources as necessary.

◆ **F. Evaluation/outcome criteria:**
   1. Eyesight preserved if possible.
   2. Intraocular pressure lowered (<22 mm Hg).
   3. Continues medical supervision for life—reports reappearance of symptoms immediately.

VIII. **Cataract:** developmental or degenerative opacification of the crystalline lens.
   A. Risk factors:
      1. Aging (most common).
      2. Trauma (x-rays, infrared or possibly ultraviolet exposure).
      3. Systemic disease (diabetes).
      4. Congenital defect.
      5. Drug effects (corticosteroids).
   ◆ **B. Assessment:**
      1. *Subjective data*—vision: blurring, loss of acuity (see best in low-lit conditions); distortion; diplopia; photophobia.
      2. *Objective data:*
         a. Blindness: unilateral or bilateral (particularly in congenital cataracts).
         b. Loss of red reflex; gray or cloudy white opacity of lens.

◆ **C. Analysis/nursing diagnosis:**
   1. *Visual sensory/perceptual alterations* related to opacity of lens.
   2. *Risk for injury* related to accidents.
   3. *Social isolation* related to impaired vision.

IX. **Cataract removal:** removal of opacified lens because of loss of vision; extracapsular cataract extraction followed by intraocular lens (IOL) insertion is procedure of choice.
   ◆ **A. Nursing care plan/implementation:**
      1. *Preoperative:*
         a. Goal: *prepare for surgery* (ambulatory center). *Antibiotic* drops or ointment, *mydriatic* eyedrops as ordered; note dilation of pupils; *avoid* glaring lights; usually done under local anesthetic with sedation.
         b. Goal: *health teaching.* Postoperative expectations: do *not* rub, touch, or squeeze eyes shut after surgery; eye patches will be on; assistance will be given for needs; overnight hospitalization not required unless complications occur; mild iritis usually occurs.
      2. *Postoperative:*
         a. Goal: *reduce stress on the sutures and prevent hemorrhage.*
            (1) Activity: ambulate as ordered, usually soon after surgery; generally discharged few hours after surgery.
            (2) *Position: flat* or *low Fowler's;* on *back* or turn to *nonoperative* side 3 to 4 wk, because turning to operative side increases pressure.
            (3) *Avoid* activities that increase IOP: straining at stool, vomiting, coughing, brushing teeth, brushing hair, shaving, lifting objects over 20 lb, *bending,* or *stooping;* wear glasses or shaded lens during day, eyeshield at night.
            (4) Provide mouthwash, hair care, personal items within easy reach, "step-in" slippers to *avoid* bending over.
         b. Goal: *promote psychological well-being.* With elderly, frequent contacts to prevent sensory deprivation.
         c. Goal: *health teaching.*
            (1) If intraocular lens not inserted, prescriptive glasses may be used (cataract glasses); explain about magnification, perceptual distortion, blind areas in peripheral vision; guide through activities with glasses; need to look through central portion of lens and turn head to side when looking to the side to decrease distortion.
            (2) Eye care: instillation of eyedrops (mydriatics and carbonic anhydrase inhibitors) to prevent glaucoma and adhesions if IOL not inserted; with IOL, steroid-antibiotic use (see **Glaucoma,**

E.3.d., p. 600, for correct technique); eye shield at night to prevent injury for 1 mo.

   (3) Signs/symptoms of *infection* (redness, pain, edema, drainage); iris *prolapse* (bulging or pear-shaped pupil); *hemorrhage* (sharp eye pain, half-moon of blood).

   (4) *Avoid:* heavy lifting; potential eye trauma.

◆ **B. Evaluation/outcome criteria:**

  1. Vision restored.

  2. No complications (e.g., severe eye pain, hemorrhage).

  3. Performs self-care activities (e.g., instills eyedrops).

  4. Returns for follow-up ophthalmology care—recognizes symptoms requiring immediate attention.

X. Retinal detachment: separation of neural retina from underlying retinal pigment epithelium.

  A. Risk factors:

    1. Trauma.

    2. Degeneration.

◆ **B. Assessment:**

    1. *Subjective data:*

      a. Flashes of light before eyes.

      b. Vision: blurred, sooty (*sudden* onset); sensation of floating particles; blank areas of vision.

    2. *Objective data*—ophthalmic exam: retina is grayish in area of tear; bright red, horseshoe-shaped tear; B-scan ultrasonography.

◆ **C. Analysis/nursing diagnosis:**

    1. *Visual sensory/perceptual alteration* related to blurred vision.

    2. *Anxiety* related to potential loss of vision.

    3. *Risk for injury* related to blindness.

◆ **D. Nursing care plan/implementation:**

    1. *Preoperative:*

      a. Goal: *reduce anxiety and prevent further detachment.*

        (1) Encourage verbalization of feelings; answer all questions; reinforce physician's explanation of surgical procedures.

        (2) Activity: *bedrest;* eyes usually covered to promote rest and maintain normal position of retina; side rails up.

        (3) *Position:* according to location of retinal tear; involved area of eye should be in a *dependent* position.

        (4) Give medications as ordered: *cycloplegic* or *mydriatics* to dilate pupils widely and decrease intraocular movement.

        (5) Relaxing diversion: conversation, music.

      b. Goal: *health teaching.* Prepare for surgical intervention (often combination used):

        (1) *Cryopexy* or *cryotherapy*—supercooled probe is applied to the sclera, causing a scar, which pulls the choroid and retina together.

        (2) *Laser photocoagulation*—a beam of intense light from a carbon arc is directed through the dilated pupil onto the retina; seals hole if retina not detached.

        (3) *Scleral buckling*—the sclera is resected or shortened to enhance the contact between the choroid and retina; frequently combined with cryopexy.

        (4) *Banding or encirclement*—silicone band or strap is placed under the extraocular muscles around the globe.

        (5) *Pneumatic retinopexy*—instillation of expandable gas or oil to tamponade tear.

    2. *Postoperative:*

      a. Goal: *reduce intraocular stress and prevent hemorrhage.*

        (1) *Position: flat* or *low Fowler's;* sandbags may be used to position head; turn to nonoperative side if allowed, retinal tear dependent; special positions may be: *prone, side-lying,* or *sitting with face down* on table if gas or oil bubble injected; position may be restricted 4 to 8 days.

        (2) Activity: bedrest; decrease intraocular pressure by *not* stooping or bending and *avoiding* prone position.

        (3) Give medications as ordered:

          (a) *Cycloplegics* (atropine).

          (b) *Antibiotics.*

          (c) *Corticosteroids* to reduce eye movements and inflammation and prevent infection.

        (4) ROM—isometric, passive; elastic stockings to avoid thrombus related to immobility.

      b. Goal: *support coping mechanisms.*

        (1) Plan all care with client.

        (2) Encourage verbalization of feelings, fears.

        (3) Encourage family interaction.

        (4) Diversional activities.

      c. Goal: *health teaching.*

        (1) Eye care: eye patch or shield at night for about 2 wk to prevent touching eye while asleep; dark glasses; *avoid* rubbing, squeezing eyes.

        (2) Limitations: *no* reading, needlework for 3 wk, *no* physical exertion for 6 wk; OK to watch TV, walk, except with bubble restrictions.

        (3) Medications: dosage, frequency, purpose, side effects: *avoid* nonprescription medications.

        (4) **Signs of redetachment:** flashes of light, increase in "floaters," blurred vision, acute eye pain.

◆ **E. Evaluation/outcome criteria:**

    1. Vision restored.

    2. No further detachment—recognizes signs and symptoms.

    3. No injury occurs—accepts limitations.

XI. Blindness: legally defined as vision less than 20/200 with the use of corrective lenses, or a visual field of no greater than 20 degrees; greatest incidence after 65 yr.

A. Risk factors:

1. Glaucoma.
2. Cataracts.
3. Macular degeneration.
4. Diabetic retinopathy.
5. Atherosclerosis.
6. Trauma.

◆ **B. Analysis/nursing diagnosis:**

1. *Visual sensory/perceptual alteration* related to blindness.
2. *Impaired social interaction* related to loss of sight.
3. *Risk for injury* related to visual impairment.
4. *Self-care deficit* related to visual loss.

◆ **C. Nursing care plan/implementation:**

1. Goal: *promote independence and provide emotional support.*
   a. Familiarize with surroundings; encourage use of touch.
   b. Establish communication lines; answer questions.
   c. Deal with feelings of loss, overprotectiveness by family members.
   d. Provide diversional activities: radio, CDs, talking books, tapes.
   e. Encourage self-care activities; allow voicing of frustrations when activity is not done to satisfaction (spilling or misplacing something), to decrease anger and discouragement.
2. Goal: *facilitate activities of daily living.*
   a. *Eating:*
      (1) Establish routine placement for tableware, e.g., plate, glass.
      (2) Help person mentally visualize the plate as a clock or compass (e.g., "3 o'clock" or "east").
      (3) Take person's hand and guide the fingertips to establish spatial relationship.
   b. *Walking:*
      (1) Have person hold your forearm: walk a half step in front.
      (2) Tell the person when approaching stairs, curb, incline.
   c. *Talking:*
      (1) Speak when approaching person; tell them before you touch them.
      (2) Tell them who you are and what you will be doing.
      (3) *Do not avoid* words such as "see" or discussing the appearance of things.
3. Goal: *health teaching.*
   a. Accident prevention in the home.
   b. Referral: *community resources:*
      (1) Voluntary agencies:
         (a) American Foundation for the Blind—provides catalogs of devices for visually handicapped.
         (b) National Society for the Prevention of Blindness—comprehensive educational programs and research.
         (c) Recording for the Blind, Inc.—provides recorded educational books on free loan.
         (d) Lion's Club.
         (e) Catholic charities.
         (f) Salvation Army.
      (2) Government agencies:
         (a) Social and Rehabilitation Service—counseling and placement services.
         (b) Veterans Administration—screening and pensions.
         (c) State Welfare Department, Division for the Blind—vocational.

◆ **D. Evaluation/outcome criteria:**

1. Acceptance of disability—participates in self-care activities, remains socially involved.
2. Regains independence with rehabilitation.

XII. Traumatic injuries to the brain

A. Primary trauma:

1. *Concussion*—transient disorder due to injury in which there is brief loss of consciousness due to paralysis of neuronal function; recovery is usually total.
2. *Contusion*—structural alteration of brain tissue characterized by extravasation of blood cells (bruising); injury may occur on side of impact or on opposite side (when cranial contents shift forcibly within the skull with impact).
3. *Laceration*—tearing of brain tissue or blood vessels due to a sharp bone fragment or object or tearing force.
4. *Fracture*—linear (may result in epidural bleed); comminuted or depressed (may tear dura and result in CSF leak); basilar (most serious). Basilar skull fracture may result in meningitis or brain abscess; bleeding from nose or ears; CSF present in drainage; bruising over mastoid process (*Battle's sign*) and periorbital ecchymosis (raccoon eyes).

B. Secondary trauma (response to primary trauma):

1. *Hematomas:*
   a. *Subdural*—blood from ruptured or torn vein collects between arachnoid and dura; may be acute, subacute, or chronic.
   b. *Extradural* (epidural)—blood clot located between dura mater and inner surface of skull; most often from tearing of middle meningeal artery; **emergency** condition.
2. *Increased intracranial pressure* (see **XIII. Increased intracranial pressure, p. 604**).

C. Mechanisms of injury:

1. Deformation (blow to the head).
2. Acceleration-deceleration (coup-contracoup)—forward and rebounding motion.
3. Rotation (tension, stretching, shearing force).

D. Pathophysiology of impaired CNS functioning:

1. Depressed neuronal activity in reticular activating system→depressed *consciousness* (**Table 7.35**).

TABLE 7.35	Levels of Consciousness
Stage	**Characteristics**
Alertness	Aware of time and place
Automatism	Aware of time and place but demonstrates abnormality of mood (euphoria to irritability)
Confusion	Inability to think and speak in coherent manner; responds to verbal requests but is unaware of time and place
Delirium	Restlessness and violent activity; may not comply with verbal instructions
Stupor	Quiet and uncommunicative; may appear conscious—sits or lies with glazed look; unable to respond to verbal instructions; bladder and rectal incontinence may occur
Semicoma	Unresponsive to verbal instructions but responds to vigorous or painful stimuli
Coma	Unresponsive to vigorous or painful stimuli

TABLE 7.36	Glasgow Coma Scale
Best eye-opening response	Purposeful and spontaneous: To voice To pain No response Untestable
Best verbal response	Oriented Disoriented Inappropriate words Incomprehensible sounds No response Untestable
Best motor response	Obeys commands Localizes pain Withdraws to pain Flexion to pain Extension to pain No response Untestable

2. Depressed neuronal functioning in lower brain stem and spinal cord → depression of reflex activity → decreased eye movements, unequal pupils → decreased response to light stimuli → widely dilated and fixed *pupils.*

3. Depression of respiratory center→altered respiratory pattern → decreased rate→*respiratory arrest.*

◆ **E. Risk factors:** accidents—automobile, industrial and home, motorcycle, military.

◆ **F. Assessment:**
   1. *Objective data:*
      a. Headache.
      b. Dizziness, loss of balance.
      c. Double vision.
      d. Nausea.
   2. *Objective data:*
      a. Laceration or abrasion around face or head; profuse bleeding from scalp (highly vascular, poor vasoconstrictive abilities).
      b. Drainage from ears or nose (serosanguineous).
      c. Projectile vomiting, hematemesis.
      d. Vital signs indicating increased intracranial pressure (see **XIII. Increased intracranial pressure, p. 604**).
      e. Neurological exam:
         (1) *Altered level of consciousness;* a numerical assessment, such as the Glasgow Coma Scale (**Table 7.36**), may be used. The lower the score, the poorer the prognosis, generally.
         (2) *Pupils*—equal, round, react to light; *or* unequal, dilated, unresponsive to light.
         (3) *Extremities*—paresis or paralysis.
         (4) *Reflexes*—hypotonia or hypertonia; *Babinski* present (flaring of great toe when sole is stroked).

◆ **G. Analysis/nursing diagnosis:**
   1. *Altered thought processes* related to brain trauma.
   2. *Sensory/perceptual alteration* related to depressed neuronal activity.
   3. *Risk for injury* related to impaired CNS functioning.
   4. *Risk for aspiration* related to respiratory depression.
   5. *Self-care deficit* related to altered level of consciousness.
   6. *Ineffective breathing pattern* related to CNS trauma.

◆ **H. Nursing care plan/implementation:**
   1. Goal: *sustain vital functions and minimize or prevent complications.*
      a. Patent airway: endotracheal tube or tracheostomy may be ordered.
      b. Oxygen: as ordered (hypoxia increases cerebral edema).
      c. *Position: semiprone* or *prone* (coma position) with head level to prevent aspiration *(keep off back);* turn side to side to prevent stasis in lungs.
      d. Vital signs as ordered.
      e. *Neurological check:* pupils, level of consciousness, muscle strength; report changes.
      f. Seizure precautions: padded side rails.
      g. Medications as ordered:
         (1) *Steroids* (dexamethasone [Decadron]).
         (2) *Anticonvulsants* (phenytoin [Dilantin], phenobarbital).
         (3) *Analgesics* (**morphine contraindicated**).
      h. Cooling measures or hypothermia to reduce elevated temperature.
      i. Assist with *diagnostic tests:*
         (1) Lumbar puncture (**contraindicated** with increased intracranial pressure).
         (2) Electroencephalogram (EEG).

Adult

j. *Diet:* NPO for 24 hr, progressing to clear liquids if awake.

k. Fluids: IVs; nasogastric *tube feedings;* I&O.

l. Monitor blood chemistries: sodium imbalance common with head injuries.

2. Goal: *provide emotional support and use comfort measures.*

   a. *Comfort:* skin care, oral hygiene; sheepskins; wrinkle-free linen.

   b. Eyes: lubricate q4h with artificial tears if periocular edema present.

   c. ROM—passive, active; physical therapy as tolerated.

   d. *Avoid* restraints.

   e. Encourage verbalization of concerns about changes in body image, limitations.

   f. Encourage family communication.

◆ **I. Evaluation/outcome criteria:**

1. Alert, oriented—no residual effects (e.g., cognitive processes intact).

2. No signs of increased intracranial pressure (e.g., decreased respirations, increased systolic pressure with widening pulse pressure, bradycardia).

3. No paralysis—regains motor/sensory function.

4. Resumes self-care activities.

XIII. Increased intracranial pressure (ICP): intracranial hypertension associated with altered states of consciousness.

A. Pathophysiology: increases in intracranial blood volume, cerebrospinal fluid, or brain tissue mass→ increased intracranial pressure→impaired neural impulse transmission→cellular anoxia, atrophy.

B. Risk factors:

1. Congenital anomalies (hydrocephalus).

2. Space-occupying lesions (abscesses or tumors).

3. Trauma (hematomas or skull fractures).

4. Circulatory problems (aneurysms, emboli).

5. Inflammation (meningitis, encephalitis).

◆ **C. Assessment:**

1. *Subjective data:*

   a. Headache (early, but nonspecific symptom).

   b. Nausea.

   c. Visual disturbance (diplopia).

2. *Objective data:*

   a. Changes in level of consciousness (*early* sign).

   b. Pupillary changes—unequal (**emergency—notify MD, indicates herniation**), dilated, and unresponsive to light (*late* sign).

   c. *Vital signs*—changes are variable.

      (1) *Blood pressure*—gradual or rapid elevation, widened pulse pressure.

      (2) *Pulse*—bradycardia, tachycardia; significant sign is *slowing of pulse as blood pressure rises.*

      (3) *Respirations*—pattern changes (*Cheyne-Stokes,* apneusis, *Biot's*), deep and sonorous; hiccups.

      (4) *Temperature*—moderate elevation.

d. Projectile vomiting (more common in children).

e. *Diagnostic test:* Head CT—structural changes.

◆ **D. Analysis/nursing diagnosis:**

1. *Altered cerebral tissue perfusion* related to increased intracranial pressure.

2. *Altered thought processes* related to cerebral anoxia.

3. *Ineffective breathing pattern* related to compression of respiratory center.

4. *Risk for aspiration* related to unconsciousness.

5. *Self-care deficit* related to altered level of consciousness.

6. *Impaired physical mobility* related to abnormal motor responses.

◆ **E. Nursing care plan/implementation:** *promote adequate oxygenation and limit further impairment.*

1. *Vital signs:* report changes **immediately.**

2. Patent airway; keep alkalotic, to prevent increased intracranial pressure from elevated CO_2; hyperventilate if necessary.

3. Give medications as ordered:

   a. *Hyperosmolar diuretics* (mannitol, urea) to reduce brain swelling.

   b. *Steroids* (dexamethasone [Decadron]) for antiinflammatory action.

   c. *Antacids* or H_2 antagonist to prevent stress ulcer.

4. *Position:* head of bed *elevated* 30 degrees.

5. Fluids: *restrict;* strict I&O.

6. Cooling measures to reduce temperature, because fever increases ICP.

7. Prepare for surgical intervention (see **XIV. Craniotomy,** following).

◆ **F. Evaluation/outcome criteria:**

1. No irreversible brain damage—regains consciousness.

2. Resumes self-care activities.

XIV. Craniotomy: excision of a part of the skull (burr hole to several centimeters) for exploratory purpose and biopsy; to remove neoplasms, evacuate hematomas or excess fluid, control hemorrhage, repair skull fractures, remove scar tissue, repair or excise aneurysms, and drain abscesses; produces minimal neurological deficit.

◆ **A. Analysis/nursing diagnosis:**

1. *Altered cerebral tissue perfusion* related to edema.

2. *Altered thought processes* related to disorientation.

3. *Self-care deficit* related to continued neurological impairment.

4. Also see nursing diagnosis for **XII.** Traumatic injuries to the brain, **XIII.** Increased intracranial pressure, and **The Perioperative Experience, p. 546.**

◆ **B. Nursing care plan/implementation:**

1. *Preoperative:*

   a. Goal: *obtain baseline measures.*

(1) Vital signs.

(2) Level of consciousness.

(3) Mental, emotional status.

(4) Pupillary reactions.

(5) Motor strength and functioning.

b. Goal: *provide psychological support:* listen; give accurate, brief explanations.

c. Goal: *prepare for surgery.*

(1) Cut hair; shave scalp (usually done in surgery); save hair if client/family desire.

(2) Cover scalp with clean towel.

▶ (3) Insert indwelling Foley catheter as ordered.

2. *Postoperative:*

a. Goal: *prevent complications and limit further impairment.*

(1) *Vital signs (indications of complications):*

(a) **Decreased blood pressure**—*shock.*

(b) **Widened pulse pressure**—*increased ICP.*

(c) **Respiratory failure**—*compression* of medullary *respiratory* centers.

(d) **Hyperthermia**—disturbance of heat-regulating mechanism; *infection.*

(2) Neurological:

(a) Pupils—ipsilateral dilation *(increased ICP),* visual disturbances.

(b) Altered level of consciousness.

(c) Altered cognitive or emotional status—disorientation common.

(d) Motor function and strength—hypertonia, hypotonia, seizures.

(3) Blood gases, to monitor adequacy of ventilation.

(4) Dressings: check frequently; *aseptic* technique; reinforce as necessary.

(5) Observe for:

(a) CSF leakage (glucose-positive drainage from nose, mouth, ears)—***report immediately.***

(b) Periorbital edema—apply light ice compresses as necessary—remove crusts from eyelids; instill lubricant eyedrops.

▶ (6) Check integrity of seventh cranial nerve (facial)—incomplete closure of eyelids.

(7) *Position:*

(a) *Supratentorial surgery* (cerebrum)—*semi-Fowler's* (30-degree elevation); may *not* lie on operative side.

(b) *Infratentorial* (brain stem, cerebellum)—*flat* in bed (prone); may turn to either side but *not* onto back.

(8) Fluids and food: NPO initially; tube feeding until alert and intact gag, swallow, and cough reflexes present. Aspiration risk.

(9) Medications as ordered:

(a) *Osmotic diuretics* (mannitol).

(b) *Corticosteroids* (dexamethasone [Decadron]).

(c) *Mild analgesics* (do *not* mask neurological or respiratory depression).

(d) *Stool softeners* to prevent constipation and straining.

(10) Orient frequently to person, time, place—to reduce restlessness, confusion.

(11) Side rails up for safety.

(12) *Avoid* restraints (may increase agitation and ICP).

(13) Ice bags to head to reduce headache.

(14) Activity: assist with ambulation.

b. Goal: *provide optimal supportive care.*

(1) Cover scalp once dressings are removed (scarves, wigs).

(2) Deal realistically with neurological deficits—facilitate acceptance, adjustment, independence.

c. Goal: *health teaching.*

(1) Prepare for physical, occupational, or speech therapy, as needed.

(2) Activities of daily living.

◆ **C. Evaluation/outcome criteria:**

1. Regains consciousness—is alert, oriented.

2. Resumes self-care activities within limits of neurological deficits.

XV. Epilepsy: seizure disorder characterized by sudden transient aberration of brain function; associated with motor, sensory, autonomic, or psychic disturbances.

A. Seizure: involuntary muscular contraction and disturbances of consciousness from abnormal electrical activity.

B. Risk factors:

1. Brain injury.

2. Infection (meningitis, encephalitis).

3. Water and electrolyte disturbances.

4. Hypoglycemia.

5. Tumors.

6. Vascular disorders (hypoxia or hypocapnia).

C. Generalized seizures:

1. *Tonic-clonic* (grand mal) seizures:

a. **Pathophysiology:** increased excitability of a neuron→possible activation of adjacent neurons→synchronous discharge of impulses→vigorous involuntary sustained muscle spasms (*tonic* contractions). Onset of neuronal fatigue→intermittent muscle spasms (*clonic* contractions)→cessation of muscle spasms→fatigue.

◆ b. **Assessment:**

(1) *Subjective data*—aura: flash of light; peculiar smell, sound; feelings of fear; euphoria.

(2) *Objective data:*

(a) *Convulsive stage*—tonic and clonic muscle spasms, loss of consciousness, breath holding, frothing at mouth, biting of tongue, urinary or fecal incontinence; lasts 2–5 min.

(b) *Postconvulsion*—headache, fatigue (postictal sleep), malaise, vomiting, sore muscles, choking on secretions, aspiration.

2. *Absence* (petit mal) seizures:
   a. **Pathophysiology:** unknown etiology, momentary loss of consciousness (10 to 20 sec); usually no recollection of seizure; resumes previously performed action.
   b. **Assessment**—*objective data:*
      (1) Fixation of gaze; blank facial expression.
      (2) Flickering of eyelids.
      (3) Jerking of facial muscle or arm.

3. *Minor motor* seizures:
   a. *Myoclonic*—involuntary "lightning-like" jerking contraction of major muscles; may throw person to the floor; no loss of consciousness.
   b. *Atonic*—brief, total loss of muscle tone; person falls to the floor; loss of consciousness (common in children).

D. Partial (focal) seizures:
1. *Partial motor:* arises from region in motor cortex (posterior frontal lobe); most commonly begins in upper extremities, spreading to face and lower extremity (*jacksonian march*); noting progression is important in identifying area of cortex involved.
2. *Partial sensory:* sensory symptoms occur with partial seizure activity; varies with region in brain; transient.
3. *Partial complex* (psychomotor): arises out of anterior temporal lobe; frequently begins with an aura; characteristic feature is automatism (e.g., lip smacking, chewing, patting body, picking at clothes); lasts from 2 to 3 min to 15 min; do *not* restrain.

E. Analysis/nursing diagnosis:
1. *Risk for injury* related to convulsive disorder.
2. *Anxiety* related to sudden loss of consciousness.
3. *Self-esteem disturbance* related to chronic illness.
4. *Impaired social interaction* related to self-consciousness.

F. Nursing care plan/implementation (generalized seizures):
1. Goal: *prevent injury during seizure.*
   a. Do *not* force jaw open during convulsion.
   b. Do *not* restrict limbs—protect from injury; place something soft under head (towel, jacket, hands).
   c. Loosen constrictive clothing.
   d. Note: time, level of consciousness, type and duration of seizure.
2. Goal: *postseizure care:*
   a. *Turn on side* to drain saliva and facilitate breathing.
   b. Suction as necessary.

c. Orient to time and place.
d. Oral hygiene if tongue or check injured.
e. Check vital signs, pupils, level of consciousness.
f. Notify physician; medication may need adjusting.

3. Goal: *prevent or reduce recurrences of seizure activity.*
   a. Encourage client to identify precipitating factors.
   b. Moderation in diet and exercise.
   c. Medications as ordered: phenytoin (Dilantin); phenobarbital; carbamazepine (Tegretol); primidone (Mysoline); valproate (Depacon).

4. Goal: *health teaching.*
   a. Medications:
      (1) Actions, side effects (apathy, ataxia, hyperplasia of gums).
      (2) Complications with sudden withdrawal (*status epilepticus*—continuous seizure activity; give diazepam per order, O_2).
   b. Attitude toward life and treatment; adhere to medication program.
   c. Clarify misconceptions, fears—especially about insanity, bad genes.
   d. Maintain activities, interests—expect *no* driving until seizure free for period of time specified by state Department of Motor Vehicles.
   e. *Avoid:* stress; lack of sleep; emotional upset; alcohol.
   f. Relaxation techniques; stress-management techniques.
   g. Use MedicAlert band or tag.
   h. Refer to appropriate community resources.

G. Evaluation outcome criteria:
1. Avoids precipitating stimuli—achieves seizure control.
2. Complies with medication regimen.
3. Retains independence.

XVI. Transient ischemic attacks (TIAs): temporary, complete, or relatively complete cessation of cerebral blood flow to a localized area of brain, producing symptoms (2 to 30 min) ranging from weakness ("drop attacks") and numbness to monocular blindness; an important precursor to stroke. Surgical intervention includes *carotid endarterectomy;* most common postoperative cranial nerve damage causes vocal cord paralysis or difficulty managing saliva and tongue deviation (cranial nerves VII, X, XI, XII); usually temporary; stroke may also occur.

XVII. Stroke (CVA, brain attack): neurologic changes caused by interruption of blood supply to a part of the brain. **Ischemic stroke**—commonly due to thrombosis or embolism; thrombotic strokes more common. **Hemorrhagic stroke**—rupture of cerebral vessel, causing bleeding into the brain tissue; most common after age 50.

A. Pathophysiology: reduced or interrupted blood flow → interruption of nerve impulses down corticospinal tract → decreased or absent voluntary movement on one side of the body (fine movements are more affected than coarse movements); later, autonomous reflex activity → spasticity and rigidity of muscles.

B. Risk factors:
1. Hypertension (modifiable risk factor).
2. Prior ischemic episodes (TIAs).
3. Cardiovascular disease; atrial fibrillation.
4. Oral contraceptives.
5. Emotional stress.
6. Family history.
7. Advancing age.
8. Diabetes mellitus.

◆ **C. Assessment:**
1. *Subjective data:*
   a. Weakness: sudden or gradual loss of movement of extremities on one side.
   b. Difficulty forming words.
   c. Difficulty swallowing (dysphagia).
   d. Nausea, vomiting.
   e. History of TIAs.
2. *Objective data:*
   a. *Vital signs:*
      (1) *BP—elevated* with thrombosis, normal with embolism. *Widened* pulse pressure with large ischemic strokes or hemorrhage.
      (2) *Temperature—elevated.*
      (3) *Pulse—*normal, slow.
      (4) *Respirations—*tachypnea, altered pattern; deep; sonorous.

      (5) CT scan of head—negative if no hemorrhage, indicates ischemic stroke.
   b. Neurological (vary by type and location of stroke):
      (1) Altered level of consciousness; progression to coma with hemorrhage.
      (2) Pupils—unequal; vision—homonymous hemianopia.
      (3) Ptosis of eyelid, drooping mouth.
      (4) Paresis or paralysis (hemiplegia).
      (5) Loss of sensation and reflexes.
      (6) Incontinence of urine or feces.
      (7) Aphasia (see **p. 596**).

◆ **D. Analysis/nursing diagnosis:**
1. *Impaired physical mobility* related to hemiplegia.
2. *Impaired swallowing* related to paralysis.
3. *Impaired verbal communication* related to aphasia.
4. *Risk for aspiration* related to unconsciousness.
5. *Sensory/perceptual alterations* related to altered cerebral blood flow, visual field blindness.
6. *Altered thought processes* related to cerebral edema.
7. *Self-care deficit* related to paresis or paralysis.

8. *Body image disturbance* related to hemiplegia.
9. *Total incontinence* related to interruption of normal nerve transmission.
10. *Impaired social interaction* related to aphasia or neurological deficit.
11. *Risk for impaired skin integrity* related to immobility.
12. *Unilateral neglect* related to cerebral damage.

◆ **E. Nursing care plan/implementation (also see Clinical Pathway 7.3: Stroke):**
1. Goal: *reduce cerebral anoxia.*
   a. Patent airway:
      ▶ (1) Oxygen therapy as ordered; suctioning to prevent aspiration.
      (2) Turn, cough, deep breathe q2h due to high incidence of aspiration pneumonia.
   b. Activity: bedrest, progressing to out of bed as tolerated.
   ◪ c. *Position:*
      (1) Maximize ventilation.
      (2) Support with pillows when on side; use hand rolls and arm slings as ordered.
2. Goal: *promote cerebrovascular function and maintain cerebral perfusion.*
   a. Vital signs; neurological checks.
   ⬤▬ b. Medications as ordered:
      (1) **Ischemic stroke—***thrombolytic agents* (recombinant tissue plasminogen activator or rt-PA) within 3 hr of onset of stroke; *antihypertensives* only if BP >185 mm Hg systolic or 105 mm Hg diastolic; *mannitol* to decrease ICP; heparin **only** if risk for cardiogenic emboli; *antiplatelet agents* (aspirin, ticlopidine, clopidogrel) to decrease risk for thrombus formation.
      (2) **Hemorrhagic stroke—***antihypertensives* for systolic pressure >160 mm Hg; **never** treat with rt-PA; *mannitol* to decrease ICP.
   c. *Fluids:* IVs to prevent hemoconcentration; I&O; weigh daily. Nutritional support as indicated.
   d. ROM exercises to prevent contractures, muscle atrophy; deep vein thrombosis prophylaxis; early referral to PT.
   e. Skin care and position changes to prevent decubiti.
3. Goal: *provide for emotional relaxation.*
   a. Identify grief reaction to changes in body image. Early referral to OT if indicated.
   b. Encourage expression of feelings, concerns. Early referral to speech therapy if indicated.
4. Goal: *client safety.*
   a. Identify existence of *homonymous hemianopia* (visual field blindness) and *agnosia* (disturbance in sensory information).

Instructions:
Circle variances and document on opposite side

DATE	ED	Day 1	Day 2
Discharge Planning		☐ Evaluation of home situation ☐ Contact SW (social work)	☐ Discharge planning started ☐ SW evaluation
Consultations/ Referrals	☐ Evaluate for tPA ☐ Neurology consult ☐ PMD / House staff notified ☐ tPA consent ☐ Neurosurgery consult	☐ Neurology consult ☐ Dietary screen ☐ PT eval ☐ OT eval ☐ Speech/swallow eval	Complete day one evals: ☐ PT ☐ OT ☐ Speech/swallow ☐ Dietary eval
Diagnostic Tests/ Screening	☐ PT, INR ☐ C×R ☐ PTT ☐ CT scan ☐ Electrolytes ☐ BUN ☐ CBC ☐ Creatinine ☐ EKG ☐ Dip Stick UA ☐ Type and screen ☐ Glucose	☐ PT, INR ☐ PTT ☐ CBC ☐ Carotid ultrasound ☐ Echocardiogram+/− bubbles ☐ Hypercoag. Panel ☐ MRI/A	☐ PT, INR ☐ PTT
Treatments/ Medications	☐ Suction ☐ IV fluids _____ ☐ O₂ ☐ tPA ☐ Blood pressure control medications ☐ Heparin IV/SQ ☐ LMWH SQ ☐ Aspirin/Antiplatelets	☐ Suction ☐ Respiratory therapy ☐ IV fluids_____ ☐ Warfarin ☐ Heparin IV/SQ ☐ LMWH SQ ☐ Aspirin/Antiplatelets ☐ Stool softener ☐ Other	☐ Suction ☐ Respiratory therapy ☐ IV to saline lock ☐ Warfarin ☐ Heparin IV/SQ ☐ LMWH SQ ☐ Aspirin/Antiplatelets ☐ Stool softener ☐ Other
Diet/ Nutrition	☐ NPO	Diet (check one): ☐ NPO ☐ Other _____ Feeding (check one): ☐ Oral self ☐ Feeding tube ☐ Oral assisted feed ☐ Supplements	Diet (check one): ☐ NPO ☐ Other _____ Feeding (check one): ☐ Oral self ☐ Feeding tube ☐ Oral assisted feed ☐ Supplements
Activity	☐ Bedrest	☐ Bedrest ☐ Other _____	☐ Physical therapy ☐ Speech therapy ☐ Occupational therapy

Nursing Assessment/ Intervention	☐ VS as per ED routine
	☐ I & O
	☐ Baseline neuro exam
	☐ Glasgow Coma Score
	☐ Cardiac monitor
	☐ Weight _____
		A E P
		VS as per unit routine ☐ ☐ ☐
		I&O ☐ ☐ ☐
		O₂ sat above 92% ☐ ☐ ☐
		Cardiac monitor ☐ ☐ ☐
		Saline lock ☐ ☐ ☐
		Neuro assessment q____hr ☐ ☐ ☐
		TEDs, SCD ☐ ☐ ☐
		Bleeding precautions ☐ ☐ ☐
		Aspirations precautions ☐ ☐ ☐
		Falls precautions ☐ ☐ ☐
		Regular apical pulse, peripheral
		  pulses palpable and equal ☐ ☐ ☐
		Abdomen soft nontender, bowel
		  sounds present ☐ ☐ ☐
		Voiding adequate amounts,
		  urine clear yellow to amber ☐ ☐ ☐
		Foley draining adequate
		  amounts, clear urine ☐ ☐ ☐
		Weight _____
			A E P
			VS as per unit routine ☐ ☐ ☐
			I&O ☐ ☐ ☐
			O₂ sat. above 92% ☐ ☐ ☐
			Cardiac monitor ☐ ☐ ☐
			Saline lock ☐ ☐ ☐
			Neuro assessment q____hr ☐ ☐ ☐
			TEDs, SCD ☐ ☐ ☐
			Bleeding precautions ☐ ☐ ☐
			Aspirations precautions ☐ ☐ ☐
			Falls precautions ☐ ☐ ☐
			Regular apical pulse, peripheral
			  pulses palpable and equal ☐ ☐ ☐
			Abdomen soft nontender, bowel
			  sounds present ☐ ☐ ☐
			Voiding adequate amounts, urine clear
			  yellow to amber, consider PVR ☐ ☐ ☐
			Foley draining adequate amounts,
			  clear urine ☐ ☐ ☐
			Weight _____

Knowledge Deficit Patient/Family Teaching	☐ Client/family teaching regarding current status, immediate plan ☐ Give client/family health matter copy of client pathway portion ☐ Pastoral support	☐ Include client/family in plan of care ☐ Begin assessment of client/family knowledge of stroke ☐ Stroke risk factors discussed	☐ Update plan of care ☐ PT/OT to start teaching client/family: ☐ Mobility ☐ Safety ☐ Transfers ☐ Assistive devices ☐ Discharge goals ☐ SW to discuss D/C options ☐ Client/family able to identify risk factors

(Continued on following page)

Adult

Source: UCSF Healthcare, San Francisco, Calif. With permission from Jane E. Hirsch, RN, MS, Vice President, Nursing and Patient Care Services.
Modified Rankin Scale Bonita and Beaglehole, Stroke 1988; 10:1487–1500
Grade I - No deficit; Grade II - Functionally insignificant impairments of movements, but with control movements through full range
Grade III - Presence of muscle contraction and movement against gravity or resistance, but limited range and not controlled; Grade IV - Little or no active movements

/ /	/ /	/ /
Day 3	**Day 4/Discharge**	**Discharge Outcomes**
□ D/C plan identified □ Transportation needs identified	□ D/C plan in place □ Transportation arranged	□ D/C Home □ D/C SNF □ D/C Rehab.
□ Interdisciplinary form for SNF or Rehab. initiated □ Home care liaison referral	□ Complete referral for SNF or Rehab. □ Home care arranged	F/U MD appointment made F/U with appropriate home care services arranged □ Refer to stroke support group
□ PT, INR □ PTT □ If Foley d/c'd UA with micro □ BUN □ Creatinine	□ If Foley d/c'd UA with micro □ PT, INR □ PTT □ BUN □ Creatinine	
□ Suction □ Respiratory therapy □ Saline lock □ Warfarin □ Aspirin / Antiplatelets □ Stool softener □ LMWH SQ □ Laxative □ Other	□ Suction □ Respiratory therapy □ Saline lock □ Warfarin □ Aspirin / Antiplatelets □ Stool softener □ LMWH SQ □ Laxative □ Other	□ INR therapeutic □ D/C medications teaching complete □ LMWH administration teaching complete with patient or family □ Coumadin teaching complete □ FU with primary care MD arranged □ Next blood draw for INR arranged □ D/C Rx given to patient/family
Diet (check one): advance as tol: □ NPO □ Other _____ Feeding (check one): □ Oral self □ Feeding tube □ Oral assisted feed □ Supplements	Diet (check one): advance as tol: □ NPO □ Other _____ Feeding (check one): □ Oral self □ Feeding tube □ Oral assisted feed □ Supplements □ Feeding plan for home identified	□ Nutritional needs met at home □ Client tolerates self feeds or □ Family able to assist with feeds □ Feeding tube in place □ Home referral complete □ Feeding/nutrition teaching complete
□ Physical therapy: advance as tol. □ Speech therapy □ Occupational therapy: advance as tol.	□ Physical therapy: advance as tol. □ Speech therapy □ Occupational therapy: advance as tol.	□ Assistive devices equipment given □ Delivery arranged □ Told where to obtain □ Home safety addressed □ Mobility, ADL, and communications needs addressed
A E P VS as per unit routine □ □ □ I&O □ □ □ O₂ sat above 92% □ □ □ Cardiac monitor □ □ □ Saline lock □ □ □ Neuro assessment q____hr □ □ □ TEDs, SCD □ □ □ Bleeding precautions □ □ □ Aspirations precautions □ □ □ Falls precautions □ □ □ Regular apical pulse, peripheral pulses palpable and equal □ □ □ Abdomen soft nontender, bowel sounds present □ □ □ Voiding adequate amounts, urine clear yellow to amber, consider PVR □ □ □ Foley draining adequate amounts, clear urine □ □ □ Weight _____	A E P VS as per unit routine □ □ □ I&O □ □ □ O₂ sat above 92% □ □ □ Cardiac monitor □ □ □ Saline lock □ □ □ Neuro assessment q____hr □ □ □ TEDs, SCD □ □ □ Bleeding precautions □ □ □ Aspirations precautions □ □ □ Falls precautions □ □ □ Regular apical pulse, peripheral pulses palpable and equal □ □ □ Abdomen soft nontender, bowel sounds present □ □ □ Voiding adequate amounts, urine clear yellow to amber, consider PVR □ □ □ Foley draining adequate amounts, clear urine □ □ □ Weight _____	□ Negative for DVT □ Skin intact/alterations addressed □ BM within last 24 hr □ Afebrile □ Neurologically stable
□ Update plan of care □ Warfarin teaching started, appropriate teaching material given □ Feeding/nutrition teaching initiated □ PT teaching □ OT teaching □ Client/family states ways to modify risk factors	□ Update plan of care □ Warfarin teaching started, appropriate teaching material given □ Feeding/nutrition teaching □ PT teaching □ OT teaching □ Client/family states ways to modify risk factors	Client/family able to verbalize instructions on: □ D/C □ D/C medications □ Precautions □ Activity □ F/U services □ MD appointment

b. Use side rails and assist as needed.

c. Remind to walk slowly, take adequate rest periods, ensure good lighting, look where client is going.

5. Goal: *health teaching.*

a. Exercise routines.

b. Diet: self-feeding, but assist as needed.

c. Resumption of self-care activities.

d. Use of supportive devices; transfer techniques.

e. Involvement of family in rehab activities.

◆ **F. Evaluation/outcome criteria:**

1. No complications (e.g., pneumonia).

2. Regains functional independence—resumes self-care activities.

3. Return of control over body functions (e.g., bowel, bladder, speech).

XVIII. Bacterial meningitis (see **Unit 5, p. 313**).

XIX. Encephalitis (also includes aseptic meningitis): inflammation of the brain and its coverings due to direct viral invasion, which usually results in a lengthy coma.

A. Pathophysiology: brain tissue injury→release of enzymes that increase vascular dilation, capillary permeability→edema formation→increased intracranial pressure→depression of CNS function.

B. Risk factors:

1. Arboviruses.

2. Enteroviruses (poliovirus, echovirus).

3. Herpesvirus.

4. Varicella-zoster (chickenpox).

5. Postinfection complication (measles, mumps, smallpox).

◆ **C. Assessment:**

1. *Subjective data:*

a. Headache—severe.

b. Fever—*sudden.*

c. Nausea, vomiting.

d. Sensitivity to light (photophobia).

e. Difficulty concentrating.

2. *Objective data:*

a. Altered level of consciousness.

b. Nuchal rigidity.

c. Tremors; facial weakness.

d. Nystagmus.

e. Elevated temperature.

f. *Diagnostic test:* lumbar puncture—fluid cloudy; *increased* neutrophils, protein.

g. Lab data: blood—slight to moderate leukocytosis (about 14,000).

◆ **D. Analysis/nursing diagnosis:**

1. *Self-care deficit* related to altered level of consciousness.

2. *Risk for injury* related to coma.

3. *Sensory/perceptual alteration* related to brain tissue injury.

4. *Altered thought processes* related to increased intracranial pressure.

◆ **E. Nursing care plan/implementation:**

1. Goal: *support physical and emotional relaxation.*

a. Vital signs; neurological signs as ordered.

b. Seizure precautions.

c. *Position:* to maintain patent airway; prevent contractures; ROM.

d. Medications as ordered:

(1) *Analgesics* for headache and neck pain.

(2) *Antipyretics* for fever.

(3) *Antivirals.*

(4) *Anticonvulsants* for seizures.

(5) *Antibiotics* for infection in aseptic meningitis.

(6) *Osmotic diuretics* (mannitol) to reduce cerebral edema.

(7) *Corticosteroids* for inflammation.

e. No isolation.

2. Goal: *health teaching:* self-care activities with residual motor and speech deficits; physical therapy.

◆ **F. Evaluation/outcome criteria:**

1. Regains consciousness; is alert, oriented.

2. Performs self-care activities with minimal assistance.

COMFORT, REST, ACTIVITY, AND MOBILITY

I. Pain—the "fifth vital sign" in the care of clients; a complex subjective sensation; unpleasant sensory and emotional experience associated with real or potential tissue damage. *Pain* is considered to be whatever the person experiencing it says it is, existing whenever he or she says it does.

A. Classifications:

1. *Acute pain:* lasts typically less than 1 mo; characterized by: tachycardia, tachypnea, increased BP, diaphoresis, dilated pupils. Responsive to analgesics.

2. *Chronic pain:* persists or is recurring for longer than 3 mo; often characterized by: lassitude, sleep disturbance, decreased appetite, weight loss, diminished libido, constipation, depression. Rarely responsive to analgesics.

3. *Somatogenic* (organic/physiological):

a. *Nociceptive:* somatic or visceral pain–sensations, normal pain transmission, such as aching or pressure (e.g., cancer pain, chronic joint and bone pain).

b. *Neuropathic:* aberrant processes in peripheral and/or central nervous system; part of a defined neurological problem; sensations such as sharp, burning, shooting pain (e.g.,

TABLE 7.37	Required Pain Assessment on Admission for Clients Who Are Hospitalized

Do you have pain now? Have you had pain in the recent past? If "yes" to either question, the following data are obtained:

- Pain intensity (use a scale appropriate for the client population)
- Location (ask client to mark on diagram or point to the site)
- Quality, patterns of radiation, character (use client's own words)
- Onset, duration, variations, and patterns
- Alleviating and aggravating factors
- Present pain management regimen and effectiveness
- Pain management history (medication history, barriers to reporting pain and using analgesics, manner of expressing pain)
- Effects of pain (impact on daily life, function, sleep, appetite, relationships with others, emotions, concentration)
- Client's pain goal (pain intensity and goals related to function, activities, quality of life)
- Physical examination/observation of site(s) of pain

Joint Commission on Accreditation of Healthcare Organizations, Oakbrook Terrace, Ill., 1999. (www.jcaho.org)

nerve compression, polyneuropathy, central pain of stroke, phantom pain after amputation).
 4. *Psychogenic* (without organic pathology sufficient to explain pain).
 B. **Components of pain experience**—pain related to:
  1. *Stimuli*—sources: chemical, ischemic, mechanical trauma, extremes of heat/cold.
  2. *Perception*—viewed with fear by children, can be altered by level of consciousness, interpreted and influenced by previous and current experience, is more severe when alone at night or immobilized.
  3. *Response*—variations in physiological, cultural, and learned responses; anxiety is created; pain seen as justified punishment; pain used as means for attention-getting.
 ◆ C. **Assessment:**
  1. *Subjective data* (**Table 7.37**):
   a. *Site*—medial, lateral, proximal, distal.
   b. *Strength:*
    (1) Certain tissues are more sensitive.
    (2) Change in intensity.
    (3) Based on expectations.
    (4) Affected by distraction or concentration, state of consciousness.
    (5) Described as: slight, medium, severe, excruciating.
   c. *Quality*—aching, burning, crushing, dull, piercing, shifting, throbbing, tingling.
   d. *Antecedent factors*—physical exertion, eating, extreme temperatures, physical and emotional stressors (e.g., fear).

   e. *Previous experience*—influences reaction to pain.
   f. *Behavioral clues*—demanding, worried, irritable, restless, difficult to distract, sleepless.
  2. *Objective data:*
   a. *Verbal clues*—moaning, groaning, crying.
   b. *Nonverbal clues*—clenching teeth, grimacing; splinting of body parts, body position, knees drawn up, involuntary reflex movements; tossing/turning, rhythmic rubbing movements; voice pitch and speed; eyes shut.
   c. *Physical clues*—breathing irregularities, abdominal distention; skin color changes, skin temperature changes; excessive salivation, perspiration.
   d. *Time/duration*—onset duration, recurrence, interval, last occurrence.
 ◆ D. **Analysis/nursing diagnosis:**
  1. *Pain,* acute or chronic, related to specific client condition.
  2. *Activity intolerance* related to discomfort.
  3. *Sleep pattern disturbance* related to pain.
  4. *Fatigue* related to state of discomfort or emotional stress.
  5. *Ineffective individual coping* related to chronic pain.
 ◆ E. **Nursing care plan/implementation:**
  1. Goal: *provide relief of pain.*
   a. Assess level of pain; ask client to rate on scale of 0 to 10 (0 = no pain; 10 = worst pain) or smile/sad faces. Use age-, condition-, and language-appropriate scale (**Table 7.38**).
  ▶ b. Determine cause and try nursing *comfort* measures *before* giving drugs:
    (1) *Environmental factors:* noise, light, odors, motion.
    (2) *Physiological needs:* elimination, hunger, thirst, fatigue, circulatory impairment, muscle tension, ventilation, pressure on nerves.
    (3) *Emotional:* fear of unknown, helplessness, loneliness (especially at night).

TABLE 7.38	Format for Assessing Pain

FIRST, assess the pain:

Frequency	Is it intermittent or constant?
Intensity	What is the quality of the pain? Sharp or dull? Throbbing? Squeezing?
Radiation	Does the pain move to other parts of the body?
Severity	On a scale of 1 to 10, how bad is the pain?
Timing	When did the pain begin? How long does it last? Does anything make it worse or take the pain away? What precedes the pain?

Adult

c. *Relieve:* anger, anxiety, boredom, loneliness.

d. *Report* **sudden, severe, new** pain, pain **not** relieved by medications or comfort measures; pain associated with **casts** or **traction.**

e. *Remove pain stimulus:*
- (1) Administer pain medication—*nonopioids:* NSAIDs—ketorolac (Toradol); *opioids:* first-line analgesics include morphine, hydromorphone, fentanyl, oxycodone, hydrocodone (see **Table 10.9**); *adjuvants:* local anesthetics, sedatives, muscle relaxants; give at appropriate time intervals; do *not* withhold due to overestimated danger of addiction.
- (2) *Avoid* cold (to reduce immediate tissue reaction to trauma).
- (3) Apply heat (to relieve ischemia).
- (4) Change activity (e.g., restrict activity in cardiac pain).
- (5) Change, loosen dressing.
- (6) Comfort (e.g., smooth wrinkled sheets, change wet dressing).
- (7) Give food (e.g., for ulcer).
- (8) Decrease stimulation (e.g. ↓ bright lights, noise, temperature).

f. *Reduce pain-receptor reaction.*
- (1) Ointment (use as coating).
- (2) Local anesthetics.
- (3) Padding (of bony prominences).

g. Assist with medical/surgical interventions to *block pain-impulse transmission:*
- (1) Injection of local anesthetic into nerve (e.g., dental).
- (2) Cordotomy—sever anterolateral spinal cord nerve tracts.
- (3) Electrical stimulation—transcutaneous (skin surface), percutaneous (peripheral nerve).
- (4) Peripheral nerve implant—electrode to major sensory nerve.
- (5) Dorsal column stimulator—electrode to dorsal column.

h. *Minimize barriers to effective pain management:*
- (1) Achieve "balanced analgesia"; around-the-clock administration of NSAIDs or acetaminophen if possible, continuous infusion, client-controlled analgesia (PCA); combination therapy (opioids, nonopioids, adjuvants).
- (2) Accept client and family report of pain.
- (3) Discuss fear of addiction with client/family (incidence <1% when opioids taken for pain relief).
- (4) Discuss fear of respiratory depression with staff; preventable; related to sedation.

i. *Document response to pain-relief measures.*

2. Goal: *use **nonpharmacological methods to reduce pain.***
- a. *Distraction,* e.g., TV (cerebral cortical activity blocks impulses from thalamus).
- b. *Aromatherapy*—assists in relaxation.
- c. *Hypnosis*—assess appropriateness for use for psychogenic pain and for anesthesia; needs to be open to suggestion.
- d. *Acupuncture*—assess emotional readiness and belief in it.

3. Goal: *alter interpretation and response to pain.*
- a. Administer *narcotics*—result: no longer sees pain as disturbing.
- b. Administer *hypnotics*—result: changes perception and decreases reaction.
- c. Help client obtain interpersonal satisfaction from ways other than attention received when in pain.

4. Goal: *promote client control of pain and analgesia: patient-controlled analgesia (PCA),* an analgesia administration system designed to maintain optimal serum analgesia levels; safely delivers intermittent bolus doses of a narcotic analgesic; preset to maximum hourly dose.
- a. *Advantages:* decreased client anxiety; improved pulmonary function; fewer side effects.
- b. *Limitations:* requires an indwelling intravenous line; analgesia targets central pain, may not relieve peripheral discomfort; cost of PCA unit.

5. Goal: *health teaching.*
- a. Explain causes of pain and how to describe pain.
- b. Explain that it is acceptable to admit existence of pain.
- c. Relaxation exercises.
- d. Biofeedback methods of pain perception and control.
- e. Proper medication administration (PCA, continuous around-the-clock dosing), when necessary, for self-care.

◆ **F. Evaluation/outcome criteria:**
1. Verbalizes comfort; awareness of pain decreased.
2. Knows source of pain; how to reduce stimulus and perception.
3. Uses alternative measures for pain relief.
4. Able to cope with pain, e.g., remains active, relaxed appearance; verbal and nonverbal clues of pain absent.

II. Immobility: impaired physical mobility or limitation of physical movement may be accompanied by a number of complications that can involve any or all of the major systems of the body. Regardless of the cause of immobilization, there are a number of conditions that arise primarily as a complication of immobility. These are discussed in **Table 7.39.**

TABLE 7.39   Complications of Immobilization

Disorder	Pathophysiology	Assessment	Analysis/ Nursing Diagnosis	Nursing Care Plan/ Implementation	Evaluation/ Outcome Criteria
Orthostatic hypotension	A decrease in BP >30/15 caused by failure of vasomotor responses to compensate for change from a recumbent to an upright position	*Subjective data:* weakness; dizziness *Objective data:* decreased BP >30/15 measured 2 min after moving from a supine to a sitting or standing position; loss of muscle tone and strength; client may faint	*Decreased cardiac output* related to orthostatic hypotension *Risk for injury* related to vertigo *Activity intolerance* related to dizziness	*Prevent trauma resulting from sudden decrease in BP* 1. Change position gradually 2. Elastic stockings 3. Leg exercises 4. Dangle before getting up 5. Tilt table 6. Sitting and lying BP 7. Monitor side effects of drugs *Health teaching* 1. Explain signs and symptoms to client 2. Encourage client to dangle before standing 3. Encourage slow movement from sitting to standing 4. Exercises to maintain muscle tone	Client tolerates increased activity No trauma occurs BP remains within normal limits
Cardiac overload	When the body is recumbent, some of the total blood volume that would be in the legs as a result of gravity is redistributed to other parts of the body, thereby increasing the circulating volume and increasing the workload of the heart; heart rate, which is decreased because blood is prevented from entering the thoracic vessels by pressure from the Valsalva maneuver, increases when normal breathing resumes	*Subjective data:* fear; apprehension *Objective data:* Valsalva maneuver (pressure against the closed glottis when breath is held) 10–20 times/hr, when trying to move in bed; tachycardia; decreased exercise tolerance	*Risk for injury* related to increased workload of heart *Activity intolerance* related to increased workload of heart *Fear* related to tachycardia	*Prevent injury and further ischemic damage to cardiac tissue by decreasing workload of heart* 1. Out of bed in chair when possible 2. *Semi-recumbent* position when in bed; pillows between legs when side-lying 3. Exercises: passive and active ROM, isometric 4. Encourage participation in self-care 5. Turn every 2 hr, dangle 6. *Avoid* Valsalva, fatigue 7. Minimize constipation 8. Encourage slow, deep breathing when moving in bed *Health teaching* 1. Exhale while turning; do *not* hold breath 2. Measures to conserve energy	No complications noted Client tolerates increased activity Heart rate within normal limit
Thrombus formation	Mass of blood constituents formed in the heart or blood vessels due to pooling of blood from lack of activity; increased viscosity related to dehydration or possible external pressure	*Subjective data:* discomfort over involved vessel *Objective data:* increased RBC; venous stasis; hypercoagulability	*Altered peripheral tissue perfusion* related to obstructed vessel *Risk for injury* related to emboli	*Prevent injury by reducing risk factors and venous stasis* 1. *Position:* change q1–2h 2. Do *not* gatch bed (causes pressure against leg vessels) 3. *Increase* fluid intake 4. Monitor coagulation lab values 5. *Medications: anticoagulation* therapy, as prescribed for clients at risk (immobilized, trauma, low pelvic surgery) 6. Ambulate as soon as possible	No thromboemboli *Note:* If *Homans'* sign present (discomfort behind knee on forced dorsiflexion of the foot) see *nursing care for client with thromboemboli,* **pp. 510, 555**

(Continued on following page)

Adult

TABLE 7.39 Complications of Immobilization *(Continued)*

Disorder	Pathophysiology	Assessment	Analysis/Nursing Diagnosis	Nursing Care Plan/Implementation	Evaluation/Outcome Criteria
				Health teaching 1. How to recognize signs of thrombophlebiti/thromboemboli 2. Leg exercise program to strengthen muscles for improved tone, to prevent pooling of blood in vessels 3. Precautions necessary when on anticoagulation therapy 4. Side effects of anticoagulation therapy (bleeding from gums, body fluids, obvious bleeding)	
Respiratory congestion related to decreased respiratory movements	Decreased thoracic movement due to: restriction against bed or chair, lack of position change, restrictive clothing or binders/bandages, or abdominal distention	*Subjective data:* dyspnea; pain. *Objective data:* trauma; immobilization of thorax or abdomen, due to position in bed; inability to cough or deep breathe; abdominal distention	*Ineffective breathing pattern* related to splinting to reduce pain. *Ineffective airway clearance* related to retained secretions. *Impaired physical mobility* related to trauma	*Prevent complications related to respiratory status* 1. Maintain a clear airway, assist with ventilation prn 2. Remove or minimize causes of dyspnea 3. Conserve client's energy (periods of rest and activity—client able to cough more effectively when rested) 4. Incentive spirometry *Promote comfort* 1. Maintain hydration and nutrition 2. Position: change q2h; out of bed in chair when possible (chest expansion greater when sitting in chair) *Health teaching* 1. Methods to allay anxieties precipitated by dyspnea 2. Effective breathing and coughing exercises	No respiratory complications or excess secretions noted
Respiratory congestion related to pooled secretions	Inability of cilia to move normal secretions out of bronchial tree due to: ineffective coughing, lack of thoracic expansion, or effects of medications	*Subjective data:* dyspnea; pain. *Objective data:* dehydration; drugs—anticholinergic, CNS depressants, anesthesia; inadequate coughing; stationary position	*Ineffective airway clearance* related to pooled secretions. *Impaired gas exchange* related to ineffective coughing	*Prevent atelectasis, infection, stasis of air, and secretions in lungs* 1. Maintain patent airway; cough; suction; change position 2. See nursing care plan for *Respiratory congestion related to decreased respiratory movements* (see above) *Health teaching* 1. Effective coughing techniques 2. Importance of adequate hydration	No respiratory complications. Client coughs and removes secretions
Oxygen/carbon dioxide imbalance	Imbalance in oxygen and carbon dioxide levels related to pulmonary congestion, ineffective breathing patterns, trauma, or effects of medications	*Subjective data:* confusion, irritable, restless, dyspnea. *Objective data:* hypoxia, hypercapnia, cyanosis	*Impaired gas exchange* related to immobilization	*Promote improved respirations* 1. Change position frequently 2. Increase humidification 3. Monitor side effects of administered medication, especially narcotics, barbiturates 4. See nursing care plan for *Respiratory congestion related to decreased respiratory movements* above	No respiratory complications. Respiratory rate and depth are adequate for maintaining balance of oxygen and carbon dioxide

Malnutrition of adult who is immobilized	Assessment	Nursing diagnosis	Nursing care plan/implementation	Evaluation/outcome criteria
Lack of adequate dietary intake to maintain healthy tissue related to lack of food; lack of knowledge about food; problems with ingestion, digestion, or absorption; or psychosocial factors that influence client's motivation to eat	*Subjective data:* anorexia, nausea; diet history validating lack of adequate nutritional intake; mental irritability *Objective data:* 1. Recent weight loss of >10% 2. *Decreased:* healing ability, GI motility, absorption, secretion of digestive enzymes 3. *Appearance:* listlessness, muscle weakness; posture—sagging shoulders, sunken chest 4. Anthropometric data (measurement of size, weight, and body proportions): <85% of standard 5. *Cardiovascular:* tachycardia (> 100 beats/min) on minimal exertion; bradycardia at rest 6. *Hair:* brittle, dry, thin 7. *Skin:* dry, scaly 8. Lack of financial resources: sociocultural influences 9. *Decreased blood values:* serum albumin, iron-binding capacity, lymphocyte levels, hematocrit, and hemoglobin	*Altered nutrition, less than body requirements,* related to decreased appetite *Knowledge deficit* (learning need) related to nutrition requirements	*Improved nutritional intake* to maintain basal metabolism requirements and replace losses from catabolism 1. Provide balanced or prescribed diet, *soft or ground food* if cannot chew or is edentulous 2. *Increase fluid intake* 3. Attain/maintain normal weight 4. Feed, assist with feeding, or place foods within client's reach *Promote comfort* 1. Mouth care; to facilitate mastication of food→ improved digestion and absorption 2. Relieve constipation (see nursing care plan for **Constipation, p. 616**) 3. Observe for stomatitis, bleeding, changes in skin texture, color 4. Medications: monitor nausea and vomiting side effects of prescribed medications; administer *antiemetics* as ordered to control nausea and vomiting 5. Ambulate to alleviate flatulence and distention 6. Alleviate pain and discomfort by: distractions, increased social interactions, pleasant environment, backrubs, and administration of prn pain medications, as ordered *Health teaching* 1. Diet and elimination 2. See **Unit 9** for foods *high in protein and carbohydrate*	No complications Client obtains/maintains normal weight No tissue breakdown

(Continued on following page)

Adult

TABLE 7.39 Complications of Immobilization (*Continued*)

Disorder	Pathophysiology	Assessment	Analysis/ Nursing Diagnosis	Nursing Care Plan/ Implementation	Evaluation/ Outcome Criteria
Constipation	Waste material in the bowel is too hard to pass easily; or bowel movements are so infrequent that client has discomfort	*Subjective data:* discomfort, pain, distress, and pressure in the rectum; reported decrease in normal elimination pattern *Objective data:* immobilization; hardformed stool, possible palpable impaction; decreased bowel sounds; bowel elimination less frequent than usual	*Constipation* related to decreased water and fiber intake *Knowledge deficit* (learning need) related to dietary and exercise requirements to prevent constipation	*Promote normal pattern of bowel elimination* 1. Administer: *stool softeners* or *bulk cathartics* as ordered; oil retention, soap suds enemas as ordered 2. Encourage change of position and activity as tolerated 3. Provide *high-bulk diet* 4. *Increase fluid* intake 5. Provide for privacy 6. Encourage regular time for evacuation *Health teaching* 1. Dietary instructions regarding *increased fiber* 2. Exercise program as tolerated 3. *Increase fluids*	Client has normal bowel elimination pattern No impactions Increases fluid and fiber in diet
Osteoporosis	Metabolic bone disorder in which there is a generalized loss of bone density due to an imbalance between formation and bone resorption; immobilization can cause calcium losses of 200–300 mg/day *Risk factors:* women, family history; postmenopause, thin and/or small frame, anorexia or bulimia, diet low in calcium; use of corticosteroids and anticonvulsants; inactive lifestyle; cigarette smoking, excessive use of alcohol	*Subjective data:* backache *Objective data:* demineralization of bone seen on x-ray; kyphosis; spontaneous fracture of bone (hip, spine, wrist); collapsed vertebrae; loss of height; stooped posture	*Pain* related to bone fractures or body structural changes	*Prevent injury related to decreased bone strength* 1. *Position:* correct body alignment, firm mattress 2. Encourage self-care activities: plan maximum activity allowed by physical condition; muscle exercises against resistance as tolerated 3. Rest/activity pattern: encourage ROM exercise; *avoid fatigue* 4. *Weight-bearing* positions, tilt table 5. *Diet:* high protein, *high vitamin D, calcium* rich 6. *Increase fluids* to prevent renal calculi (calcium from bones could cause kidney stones) *Health teaching* 1. Dietary instructions: foods to include for high protein, high Vitamin D, high calcium diet 2. Exercise program 3. Sign and symptoms of renal calculi 4. *Avoid* smoking, alcohol	No fractures No renal calculi Incorporates dietary improvements in daily menu selection Participates in exercise program on a regular basis Regular bone density tests (1 to 2 years for ages 40–65+)
Contractures	Abnormal shortening of muscle tissue, rendering the muscle highly resistant to stretching; related to lack of active or passive ROM, or improper support and positioning of joints affected by arthritis or injury	*Subjective data:* pain *Objective data:* muscles—fixed, shortened, decreased tone; resistance of muscles to stretch; decreased ROM in affected limb	*Impaired physical mobility* related to muscle weakness and contractures *Pain* related to injury *Self-care deficit* related to immobility	*Prevent deformities* 1. Active or passive ROM 2. *Positioning:* functional, correct alignment 3. Footboard to prevent footdrop 4. *Avoid* knee gatch *Health teaching* 1. Importance of ROM 2. Correct anatomical positions	ROM maintained No deformities noted

| Skin breakdown | Presence of risk factors that could lead to skin breakdown, such as immobility, inadequate nutrition, lack of position changes | Subjective data: fatigue; pain; inability to turn on own. Objective data: interruption of skin integrity, especially over ears, occiput, heels, sacrum, scrotum, elbows, trochanter, ischium, scapula; immobilization; malnutrition | Impaired skin integrity related to lack of frequent position change | Prevent skin breakdown
1. Change position q1 to 2h and prn, out of bed when possible
2. Protect from infection
3. Increase dietary intake: protein, carbohydrates
4. Increase fluids
Assess for/reduce contributing factors known to cause decubitus ulcers: incontinence, stationary position, malnutrition, obesity, sensory deficits, emotional disturbances, paralysis
Promote healing
1. Wash gently, pat dry—to avoid skin abrasion
2. Clean, dry, wrinkle-free bedlinens and pads
3. Massage skin with lotion that does not contain alcohol (alcohol dries skin)
4. Protect with: wafer barrier, alternating mattress, sheepskin pads, protectors, flotation devices
5. No "doughnuts" or rubber rings (interfere with circulation of tissue within center of ring) | No skin breakdown |
| **Urinary stasis** | Immobility leads to inability to completely empty the bladder, which increases risk for urinary tract infection and renal calculi | Subjective data: pain, due to infection or renal calculi. Objective data: difficulty in urinating due to position or lack of privacy; infection related to catheter insertion or stasis of urine; hematuria | Altered urinary elimination related to inability to empty bladder | Prevent urinary infections, stasis, and renal calculi
1. Increase activity as allowed
2. Check for distended bladder
3. Increase fluids, I&O
4. Diet: acid ash to increase acidity, thereby preventing infection
5. Avoid catheterization; use intermittent catheterization instead of Foley whenever possible or Credé maneuver to empty bladder (manual exertion of pressure on the bladder to force urine out)
6. Bladder training | No urinary infections or evidence of renal calculi; bladder emptied, no urinary stasis |

Adult

A. **Types of immobility:**
1. *Physical*—physical restriction due to limitation in movement or physiological processes (e.g., breathing).
2. *Intellectual*—lack of action due to lack of knowledge (e.g., mental retardation, brain damage).
3. *Emotional*—immobilized when highly stressed (e.g., after loss of loved person or diagnosis of terminal illness).
4. *Social*—decreased social interaction due to separation from family when hospitalized or when alone, as in old age.

B. **Risk factors:**
1. Pain, trauma, injury.
2. Loss of body function or body part.
3. Chronic disease.
4. Emotional, mental illness; neglect.
5. Malnutrition.
6. Bedrest, traction, surgery, medications.

◆ C. **Assessment:**
1. *Subjective data: psychological/social effects* of immobility:
   a. Decreased motivation to learn; decreased retention.
   b. Decreased problem-solving abilities.
   c. Diminished drives; decreased hunger.
   d. Changes in body image, self-concept.
   e. Exaggerated emotional reactions, inappropriate to situation or person; aggression, apathy, withdrawal.
   f. Deterioration of time perception.
   g. Fear, anxiety, feelings of worthlessness related to change in role activities, e.g., when no longer employed.
2. *Objective data: physical effects* of immobility:
   a. *Cardiovascular.*
      (1) Orthostatic hypotension.
      (2) Increased cardiac load.
      (3) Thrombus formation.
   b. *Gastrointestinal.*
      (1) Anorexia.
      (2) Diarrhea.
      (3) Constipation.
   c. *Metabolic.*
      (1) Tissue atrophy and protein catabolism.
      (2) BMR reduced.
      (3) Fluid/electrolyte imbalances.
   d. *Musculoskeletal.*
      (1) Demineralization (osteoporosis).
      (2) Contractures and atrophy.
      (3) Skin breakdown.
   e. *Respiratory.*
      (1) Decreased respiratory movement.
      (2) Accumulation of secretions in respiratory tract.
      (3) O_2/CO_2 level imbalance.
   f. *Urinary.*
      (1) Calculi.
      (2) Bladder distention, stasis.
      (3) Infection.
      (4) Frequency.

◆ D. **Analysis/nursing diagnosis:**
1. *Impaired physical mobility* related to specific client condition.
2. *Impaired skin integrity* related to physical immobilization.
3. *Urinary retention* related to incomplete emptying of bladder.
4. *Constipation* related to inactivity.
5. *Risk for disuse syndrome* related to lack of range of motion.
6. *Bathing/hygiene self-care deficit* related to musculoskeletal impairment.
7. *Sensory/perceptual alteration* related to complications of immobility.
8. *Body image disturbance* related to physical limitations.

◆ E. **Nursing care plan/implementation:**
1. Goal: *prevent physical, psychological hazards.*
   a. Apply nursing measures to promote venous flow, muscle strength, endurance, joint mobility, skin integrity.
   b. Assess and counteract *psychological* impact of immobility (e.g., feelings of helplessness, hopelessness, powerlessness).
   c. Help maintain accurate sensory processing to prevent and lessen *sensory disturbances.*
   d. Help adapt to *altered body image* due to increased dependency, sensory deprivation, and changes in status and power that accompany immobility.
   e. Offer counseling when sexual expression is impaired.
2. Goal: *health teaching:* how to prevent physical problems related to immobility (e.g., anticonstipation diet, range of motion, skin care); teach activities while immobile that encourage independence and provide sensory stimulation.

◆ F. **Evaluation/outcome criteria:**
1. Minimal contractures, skin breakdown, muscle atrophy or loss of strength.
2. Interest in self and environment; positive self-image.
3. Returns to optimal level of physical activity.

III. **Fractures:** disruptions in the continuity of bone as the result of trauma or various disease processes, such as *Cushing's* syndrome or osteoporosis, that weaken the bone structure.

A. **Types (Figure 7.14):**
1. *Open or compound*—fractured bone extends *through skin* and mucous membranes; increased potential for infection.
2. *Closed or simple*—fractured bone *does not* protrude through skin.
3. *Complete*—fracture extends through *entire bone,* disrupting the periosteum on both sides of the bone, producing two or more fragments.
4. *Incomplete*—fracture extends *only part way* through bone; bone continuity is not totally interrupted.
5. *Greenstick* or *willow-hickory stick*—fracture of *one*

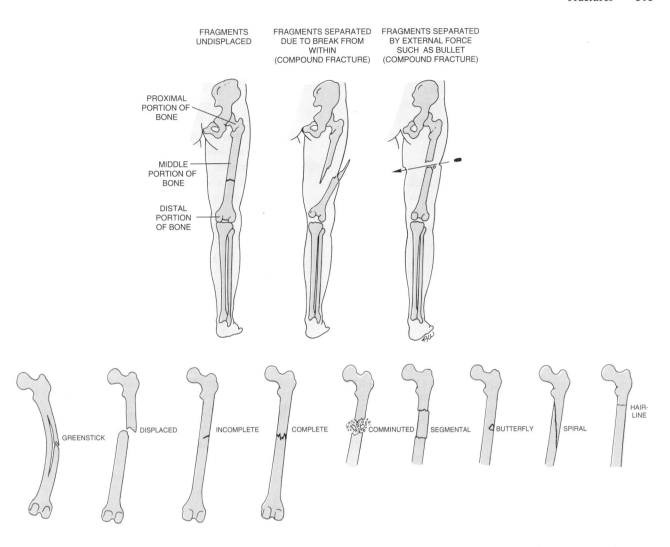

FIGURE 7.14   Types of fractures and terminology. (From Venes, D [ed]: Taber's Cyclopedic Medical Dictionary, ed. 20. FA Davis, Philadelphia, 2005.)

side of bone; *other side merely bends;* usually seen only in children.

6. *Impacted or telescoped*—fracture in which bone fragments are *forcibly driven into* other or adjacent bone structures.

7. *Comminuted*—fracture having *more than one* fracture line and with bone fragment broken into *several pieces.*

8. *Depressed*—fracture in which bone or bone fragments are driven *inward,* as in skull or facial fractures.

9. See also **VI. Total hip replacement, p. 627.**

B. **Methods used to reduce/immobilize fractures:** reduction or setting of the bone—restores bone alignment as nearly as possible.

1. *Closed reduction*—manual traction or manipulation. Usually done under anesthesia to reduce pain and muscle spasm. Maintenance of reduction and immobilization is accomplished by casting (fiberglass or plaster of Paris).

2. *Open reduction*—operative procedure utilized

to achieve bone alignment; pins, wire, nails, or rods may be used to secure bone fragments in position; prosthetic implants may also be used.

3. *Traction reduction*—force is applied in two directions: to obtain alignment, and to reduce or eliminate muscle spasm. Used for fractures of long bones. May be:

a. Continuous—used with fractures or dislocations of bones or joints.

b. Intermittent—used to reduce flexion contractures or lessen pain and muscle spasm.

c. Applied as follows:

(1) *Skin*—traction applied to skin by using a commercial foam-rubber *Buck's* traction splint or by using adhesive, plastic, or a moleskin strip bound to the extremity by elastic bandage; exerts indirect traction on bone or muscles (e.g., *Bryant's, Buck's* extension, head, pelvic, *Russell's*) (**Figure 7.15, parts *A* through *E*).**

(2) *Skeletal*—direct traction applied to bone using pins (*Steinmann*), wires (*Kirchner*). Pin is inserted through the bone in or close to the involved area and usually protrudes through skin on both sides of the extremity. Skeletal traction for fractured vertebrae accomplished with tongs (e.g., *Crutchfield* tongs, *Gardner-Wells* tongs) (see **Figure 7.15, parts F through H**).

d. Specific types of traction:

(1) *Cervical*—direct traction applied to cervical vertebrae using a head halter or *Crutchfield, Gardner-Wells,* or *Vinke* tongs that are inserted into the skull (see **Fig. 7.15, parts C and G**). Traction is increased with weights until vertebrae move into position and alignment is regained. After reduction is obtained, weights are decreased to the amount needed to maintain reduction. *Weight amount is prescribed by physician.*

(2) *Balanced suspension*—countertraction produced by a force other than client's body weight; extremity is suspended in a traction apparatus that maintains the line of traction despite changes in the client's position (e.g., *Russell's* leg traction, *Thomas'* splint with *Pearson's* attachment) (see **Figure 7.15, parts E and F**).

(3) *Running*—traction that exerts a pull in one plane; countertraction is supplied by the weight of the client's body or can be increased through use of weights and pulleys in the opposite direction (e.g., *Buck's* extension, *Russell's* traction) (see **Figure 7.15, parts B through E**).

(4) *Halo*—an apparatus that employs both a plastic and metal frame; molded frame extends from the axilla to iliac crest and houses a metal frame. The struts of the frame extend to skull and attach to round metal (halo) device. The halo is attached to skull by four pins—two located anterolaterally and two located posterolaterally. They are inserted into external cortex of the cranium (see **Figure 7.15, part H**). Used to immobilize the cervical spine following spinal fusion, give some correction to scoliosis before spinal fusion, and immobilize nondisplaced fracture of spine.

4. *Immobilization*—maintains reduction and promotes healing of bone fragments. Achieved by:

a. *External fixation:*

(1) Casts—types:

(a) *Spica*—applied to immobilize hip or shoulder joints.

(b) Body cast—applied to trunk.

(c) Arm or leg cast—joints above and below site included in cast.

(2) Splints, continuous traction.

(3) External fixation devices (*Charnley*)—multiple pins/rods through limb above and below fracture site, attached to external metal supports. Client able to become ambulatory.

b. *Internal fixation*—pins, wires, nails, rods (see **Total hip replacement, p. 627**, and **Total knee replacement, p. 632**).

◆ **C. Assessment:**

1. *Subjective data:*

a. Pain, tenderness.

b. Tingling, numbness.

c. Nausea.

d. History of traumatic event.

e. Muscle spasm.

2. *Objective data:*

a. Function: abnormal or lost.

b. Deformities.

c. Ecchymosis, increased heat over injured part.

d. Localized edema.

e. Crepitation (grating sensations heard or felt as bone fragments rub against each other).

f. Signs of shock.

g. Indicators of anxiety.

 h. X-ray: *fracture*—positive interruption of bone; *dislocation*—abnormal position of bone.

◆ **D. Analysis/nursing diagnosis:**

1. *Pain* related to interruption in bone.

2. *Impaired physical mobility* related to fracture/treatment modality.

3. *Risk for injury* related to complications of fractures.

4. *Knowledge deficit* (learning need) regarding cast care, crutch walking, traction.

5. *Constipation* related to immobilization.

6. *Risk for impaired skin integrity* related to immobility or friction from materials used to immobilize the fracture during healing.

◆ **E. Nursing care plan/implementation:**

1. Goal: *promote healing and prevent complications of fractures* (**Table 7.40**).

a. *Diet:* high protein, iron, vitamins, to improve tissue repair; *moderate* carbohydrates to prevent weight gain; *no* increase in calcium, to prevent kidney stones (decalcification and demineralization occur when client is immobilized).

(1) Encourage *increased fluid intake,* to prevent kidney stones.

(2) Prevent or correct constipation through *increasing bulk foods, fruits, and fruit juices,* or using prescribed *stool softeners, laxatives,* or *cathartics* as necessary.

b. Provide activities to reduce perceptual deprivation—reading, handcrafts, music, special interests/hobbies that can be done while maintaining correct position for healing.

2. Goal: *prevent injury or trauma in relation to:*

SKIN

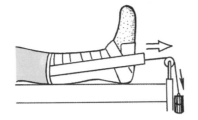

A. Bryant's traction

B. Buck's traction

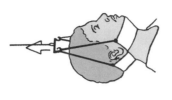

C. Head halter traction

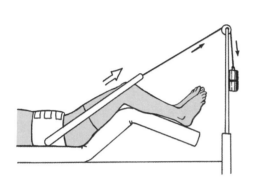

D. Pelvic traction

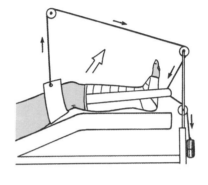

E. Russell's traction

SKELETAL

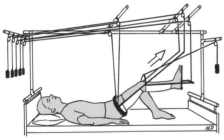

F. Balanced suspension traction

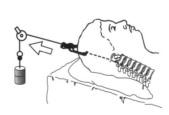

G. Crutchfield tongs

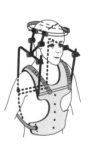

H. Halo vest

FIGURE 7.15   Types of skin and skeletal traction.

a. *Fracture care:*
   (1) Maintain affected part in optimum alignment.
   (2) Maintain skin integrity; check all bony prominences for evidence of pressure q4h and prn, depending on amount of pressure.
   (3) Monitor: circulation in, sensation of, and motion of (CSM) affected part q15min for first 4 hr; q1h until 24 hr; q4h and prn, depending on amount of edema (**Table 7.41**).

   (4) Maintain mobility in unaffected limb and unaffected joints of affected limb by active and passive ROM; prevent footdrop by using ankle-top sneakers.

b. *Skin traction:*
   (1) Maintain correct alignment:
      (a) If tape or moleskin is used, shave extremity and apply benzoin to improve adherence of strip and reduce itching.
      (b) Check apparatus for slippage, bunching; replace prn.

Adult

TABLE 7.40 Complications of Fractures

Complication	Assessment	Analysis/Nursing Diagnosis	Nursing Care Plan/Implementation	Evaluation/Outcome Criteria
Shock (see p. 504) **Thrombophlebitis** (see **p. 510, 555**) **Fat emboli:** serious, potentially life-threatening complication in which pressure changes in interior of fracture force molecules of fat from marrow into systemic circulation; may cause problems in respiratory or nervous system; seen most frequently on *third day* after multiple fractures, fractures of long bones, or comminuted fracture	*Subjective data:* dyspnea, severe chest pain; confusion, agitation; decrease in level of consciousness; numbness; feeling faint; history of diabetes, obesity *Objective data:* cyanosis; pupillary changes; muscle twitching; petechiae—chest, buccal cavity, axilla, conjunctiva, soft palate; extremities—pallor, cold; shock; vomiting	*Risk for injury* related to fat emboli *Altered tissue perfusion* related to fat emboli	1. *Position:* high-Fowler's to relieve respiratory symptoms 2. Administer oxygen **STAT,** to relieve anoxia and reduce surface tension of fat globules 3. Institute respiratory support measures, as ordered—IPPB, respiratory assistive devices: **be prepared for CPR** in event of respiratory failure 4. Monitor vital signs, cardiac monitor, q15min during acute episode and prn (shock/cardiac failure possible) 5. Obtain baseline data and monitor level of consciousness, neurological signs q15min during acute episode and prn (neurological involvement possible) 6. Administer parenteral fluids, as ordered: IV alcohol, blood and fluid replacements 7. Administer medications as ordered: *corticosteroids; digitalis; aminophylline; heparin* sodium 8. **DO NOT RUB ANY LEG CRAMPS, BUT REPORT IMMEDIATELY**	Client alert Pain relieved Respiratory, cardiac, and neurological systems have no permanent damage
Nerve compression: pressure on nerve in affected area from edema, dislocation of bone, or immobilization apparatus; if pressure not relieved, permanent paralysis can result	*Subjective data:* discomfort, pain, referred pain; burning, tingling, "stinging sensation"; numbness, altered sensation, inability to distinguish touch *Objective data:* limited movement; muscle weakness; paralysis; reflexes—diminished, irritable, or absent; color changes related to impaired circulation	*Pain* related to pressure on nerve *Potential for physical injury* related to pressure on nerve *Impaired tissue perfusion* related to impaired circulation *Impaired physical mobility* related to joint contracture, numbness	1. Monitor for potential signs q1h for first 48 hr; neurovascular assessment q12h and prn as condition indicates (circulation, sensation, and motion *[CSM]*) 2. *Elevate* affected limb; *flex* hand or foot of affected extremity; passive and active ROM exercises 3. **Be prepared to cut cast or remove constrictions if signs of impairment exist** 4. Begin active ROM exercises to unaffected extremities 5. Use footboard to prevent footdrop 6. Encourage use of trapeze if applicable 7. Isometric exercises, as ordered 8. Ambulation, weight bearing as ordered, support casts	Sensation, motor function are normal No complications noted
Avascular necrosis/circulatory impairment: interference with normal circulation to affected area due to interruption of blood vessel, pressure on the vessel from dislocation, edema, or immobilization devices; results of impaired circulation lead to discomfort and, if not corrected, necrosis of tissue and bone due to lack of oxygen supply	*Subjective data:* tenderness; pain, especially on passive motion *Objective data:* edema, swelling in affected area; decreased color, temperature, mobility; bleeding from wound	*Risk for altered peripheral tissue perfusion* related to vessel damage	1. Monitor for potential signs q1h for first 48 hr; blanching, coolness, edema; palpate pulse above and below injury; report absent pulse or major discrepancies **STAT** 2. *Elevate* affected limb to decrease edema 3. Report to physician if signs persist 4. Be prepared to assist with bivalving of casts, or cut cast to relieve pressure 5. Monitor size of drainage stains on casts; measure accurately and report if size increases	Circulation adequate to limb, to prevent tissue damage

	Assessment	Nursing Diagnosis	Nursing Interventions	Desired Outcomes/Evaluation Criteria
Infection	*Subjective data:* pain *Objective data: elevated* temperature and pulse: erythema—discoloration of surrounding skin; edema—*sudden,* local induration; drainage—thin, watery, foul-smelling exudate; crepitus (may be indicative of **gas gangrene**); with cast—warm area, foul smell	*Risk for injury* related to tissue destruction *Altered peripheral tissue perfusion* related to swelling	1. Monitor vital signs, drainage 2. Ensure client has had prophylactic tetanus toxoid 3. May have prophylactic **antibiotics** ordered if wound was contaminated at time of injury 4. Instruct client *not* to touch open wound or pin sites or put anything inside cast (could interrupt skin integrity and become potential source of infection)	No infection or heals with no serious complications
Delayed union/nonunion: failure of bone to heal within normal time related to lack of use, inadequate circulation, other complicating medical conditions such as diabetes or poor nutrition	*Subjective data:* pain *Objective data:* lack of callus formation on x-ray: poor alignment	*Risk for injury* related to poor healing of bone fracture *Impaired physical mobility* related to lower-limb fractures *Dressing/grooming bathing/hygiene, self-care deficit* related to upper-limb fracture	1. Maintain immobilization and alignment of affected limb 2. Maintain adequate nutrition 3. *Avoid* trauma to affected limb 4. Monitor for circulatory or infection complication 5. Dietary instructions regarding foods containing *calcium* and *protein* necessary for bone healing	Bone heals No complications noted Pain decreased Ambulation and self-care return to preinjury status
Skin breakdown (related to cast)	*Subjective data:* pain *Objective data:* temperature and pulse *elevated;* erythema—cast edges, exposed distal portion of limb, limb area within cast; drainage and foul odor from break in skin (may be under cast and stain through or exit at ends of cast); crepitus (crackling sound could indicate **gas gangrene**); *hyperactive reflexes*	*Impaired skin integrity* related to cast trauma	1. If open wound: verify tetanus administration; monitor site through cast window, change dressing daily and prn 2. Apply lotion or cornstarch to exposed skin (*no* powder) 3. Petal tape edges of cast to reduce irritation 4. Inspect skin for irritation, edema, odor, drainage—q2h initially, then q3h 5. Instruct client *not* to place any object under cast because skin abrasions may lead to decubitus ulcers 6. Promote drying of cast by leaving it uncovered and exposed to air for 48 hr; use *no* plastic 7. Prevent indenting casts with fingertips or hard surface: place on pillows; use palms of hands when positioning affected limb 8. *Avoid* excessive padding of Thomas splint in groin area—padding traps moisture, may lead to skin breakdown	No skin breakdown
Duodenal distress (with spica cast): *spica cast* incorporates the trunk and affected limb and can cause respiratory or abdominal distress when edema is present under the cast or cast is too tight to allow for normal body functions	*Subjective data:* anorexia, nausea, abdominal pain *Objective data:* duodenal distress, vomiting, distention, cast too tight	*Ineffective breathing* related to pressure from cast *Pain* related to abdominal distress from pressure *Fear* related to cast constriction	1. Place on firm mattress; use bed boards if necessary to reduce muscle spasm 2. Maintain warmth by covering uncasted areas 3. *Avoid* turning for first 8 hr; when turning: use enough personnel to logroll; do *not* use bar between legs as turning device; support chest with pillows 4. Monitor for signs of respiratory distress: increased respirations, apprehension 5. Monitor for signs of duodenal distress: vomiting, distention; *if these signs occur:* place in *prone* position; have cast bivalved; may need NG tube; monitor for fluid imbalance 6. Protect cast with nonabsorbent material during elimination	Complications avoided or detected early enough to prevent serious damage

TABLE 7.41 ☼ Assessing Injured Limb: CSM

C Circulation
Is it warm to touch?
Are both limbs equal in size?
Are peripheral pulses present?
Is there adequate capillary refill?

S Sensation
Does the client feel pain?
Can the client distinguish different sensations (e.g., painful stimuli vs. soft touch)?
Is the client aware of the position of the limb?

M Motion
Can the client move extremities that are not immobilized?
Can the client do this independently?
Can the client do this on command?

(2) Prevent tissue injury:
    (a) Check all bony prominences for evidence of pressure: q15min for first 4 hr; q1h until 24 hr, q4h and prn, depending on amount of edema.
    (b) Nonadhesive traction may be removed q8h to check skin (e.g., *Bryant's*).
▶ c. *Skeletal traction:*
    (1) Maintain affected part in optimum alignment:
        (a) Ropes on pulleys.
        (b) Weights hang free.
        (c) *Elevate* head of bed as prescribed.
        (d) Check knots routinely.
    (2) Maintain skin integrity:
        (a) Frequent skin care.
        (b) Keep bed linens free of crumbs and wrinkles.
    (3) Prevent infection: special skin care to pin insertion site tid. Keep area around pins clean and dry. Use prescribed solution for cleansing.
    (4) Monitor circulation in, sensation of, and motion of affected part (see **E.2.a. Fracture care, p. 621**, and **Table 7.41**).
    (5) Maintain mobility in unaffected limb and unaffected joints; prevent footdrop of affected limb.
▶ d. *Running traction* (see **Fig. 7.15, pp. 620; 621**):
    (1) Keep well centered in bed.
    (2) *Elevate head of bed only* to point of countertraction.
    (3) *No* turning from side to side—will cause rubbing of bony fragments.
    (4) Check distal circulation frequently.
    (5) Frequent back care to prevent skin breakdown.
    (6) Fracture bed pan for toileting.
    (7) *Avoid* excessive padding of splints in groin area to prevent tissue trauma.
▶ e. *Balanced suspension traction* (see **Fig. 7.15, part F, p. 621**):
    (1) Maintain alignment and countertraction:

        (a) Ropes on pulleys.
        (b) Weights hang free.
        (c) *Elevate* head of bed as prescribed.
        (d) Check knots routinely.
    (2) May move client, but turn only slightly (*no more than 30 degrees* to *unaffected* side).
    (3) Heel of affected leg must remain *free* of the bed.
    (4) *20-degree angle* between thigh and bed.
    (5) Check for pressure from sling to popliteal area.
    (6) Provide foot support to prevent footdrop.
    (7) Maintain *abduction* of extremity.
    (8) Check for signs of infection at pin insertion sites; cleanse tid as ordered.
    (9) If tape or moleskin is used, shave extremity and apply benzoin to improve adherence of strip and reduce itching.
▶ f. *Cervical traction* (see **Fig. 7.15, pp. 620; 621**):
    (1) May be placed on specialized bed (e.g., *Stryker frame*).
    (2) *Position:* maintain body alignment.
    (3) Keep tongs free from bed, and keep weights hanging freely to allow traction to function properly.
▶ g. *Halo traction:*
    (1) Several times a day, check screws to the head and screws that hold the upper portion of the frame, to determine correct position.
    (2) Pin sites cleansed tid with *bacteriostatic* solution to prevent infection.
    (3) Monitor for signs of infection.
    (4) *Position* as any other client in body cast, except *no* pressure to rest on halo—pillows may be placed under abdomen and chest when client is prone.
    (5) Institute ROM exercises to prevent contractures.
    (6) Turn frequently to prevent development of pressure areas.
    (7) Allow client to verbalize about having screws placed in skull.
    (8) Postapplication nursing care same as pin insertion for other traction.
▶ h. *External fixation devices:*
    (1) Pin care same as for skeletal traction.
    (2) Teach clothing adjustment.
    (3) Teach to adjust for size of apparatus.
▶ i. *Internal fixation devices:*
    (1) Monitor for signs of infection/allergic reaction to materials used for maintenance of reduction (drainage, pain, increased temperature).
    (2) Position as ordered to prevent dislocation.
▶ j. *Casts:*
    (1) Support drying cast on *firm pillow; avoid* finger imprints on cast.
    (2) *Elevate* limb to reduce edema.
    (3) Prevent complications of fractures as listed.

(4) Closely monitor *circulation* (blanching, swelling, decreased temperature); *sensation* (absence of feeling; pain or burning); and *motion* (inability to move digits of affected limb).

(5) **Be prepared to notify MD or cut cast if circulatory impairment occurs.**

(6) Protect skin integrity: *avoid* pressure of edges of cast; petal prn.

(7) Monitor for signs of infection if skin integrity impaired.

3. Goal: *provide care related to ambulation with crutches.*

▶ a. Teach appropriate gate (**Table 7.42**)

▶ b. Measure crutches correctly (see also **Table 7.43**).

> (1) Subtract 16 inches from total height; top of crutch should be 2 inches below the axilla.
> (2) Complete extension of the elbows should be possible *without* pressure of axilla bar into the axilla.
> (3) Handgrip should be adjusted so that complete wrist extension is possible.
> (4) Instruct in correct body alignment:
>   (a) Head erect.
>   (b) Back straight.
>   (c) Chest forward.
>   (d) Feet 6 to 8 inches apart, wide base for support.

4. Goal: *provide safety measures related to possible complications following fracture* (see **Table 7.40**).

5. Goal: *health teaching.*

a. Explain and show apparatus before application, if possible.

b. Pin care at least once daily to prevent granulation and cellulitis.

c. Correct position for rest/sleep and prevention of injury with halo traction—*no* pressure on halo.

d. Purpose of cast: to immobilize, to support body tissues, to prevent or correct deformities.

e. Teach signs and symptoms of *complications* to report related to cast care (i.e., numbness, odor, crack/break in cast; extremity cold, bluish).

▶ f. Isometric exercises for use with affected joint.

▶ g. *Safety measures with crutches:*

> (1) Weight bearing on hands, *not* axilla.
> (2) Position crutches 4 inches to side and 4 inches to front.
> (3) Use short strides, looking ahead, not at feet.
> (4) Prevent injury: if client begins to fall, throw crutches to side to prevent falling on them; body should be relaxed.
> (5) Check for environmental hazards: rugs, water spills.

TABLE 7.42	**Teaching Crutch Walking**

A. When only *one* leg can bear weight:
1. *Swing-to-gait:* crutches forward; swing body to crutches.
  a. Move both crutches forward.
  b. Move both legs to meet the crutches.
  c. Continue pattern.
2. *Swing-through-gait:* crutches forward; swing body through crutches.
  a. Move both crutches forward.
  b. Move both legs farther ahead than crutches.
  c. Continue pattern.
3. *Three-point gait:* crutches and affected extremity forward; swing forward, placing nonaffected foot ahead of or between crutches.
  a. Both crutches and affected limb move at same time.
  b. Move both crutches and affected leg (e.g., left) ahead 6 inches.
  c. Move unaffected leg (e.g., right) to same place as left and crutches.
  d. Continue pattern.

B. When *both* legs can move separately and bear some weight:
1. *Four-point gait:* right crutch forward, left foot forward; swing weight to right side while bringing left crutch forward, then right foot forward; gait simulates normal walking.
  a. Move right crutch forward 4 to 6 inches.
  b. Move left foot forward same distance as right crutch.
  c. Move left crutch forward ahead of left foot.
  d. Move right foot forward to meet right crutch.
  e. Continue pattern.
2. *Two-point gait:* same as four-point gait but faster; one crutch and opposite leg moving forward at same time.
  a. Opposite crutch and limb move together.
  b. Move right crutch and left leg ahead 6 inches.
  c. Move left crutch and right leg ahead.
  d. Continue pattern.

C. When client is *unable* to walk: *tripod gait:* crutches forward at a wide distance; drag legs to point just behind crutches, balance, and repeat.

◆ **F. Evaluation/outcome criteria:**

1. No injury or complications related to apparatus or immobilization (e.g., infection, tissue injury, altered circulation/sensation, dislocation).

2. Bone remains in correct alignment and begins to heal.

3. Demonstrates elevated limb position to relieve edema with casted extremity.

4. Lists complications related to circulation or neurological impairment and infection.

TABLE 7.43	▶ **Measuring Crutches Correctly**

1. Have client lie on a flat surface. Measure from anterior fold of axilla to 4 inches lateral to heel.
2. Have client stand. Measure from 1 to 2 inches below axilla to 2 inches in front of and 6 inches to the side of the foot.
3. Hand placement on bar of crutch: have client stand upright, support body weight with hand on bar (*not* putting weight on axilla). Elbow flexion should be *30 degrees.*
4. Slightly pad the shoulder rests of the crutches for general comfort.
5. Make sure there are nonskid rubber tips on the crutches.

5. Begins to use affected part.
6. Demonstrates correct technique for ambulation with crutches—no pressure on axilla, uses strength of arms and wrists.
7. No falls while using crutches.

IV. **Compartment syndrome:** an accumulation of fluid in the muscle compartment, resulting in an increase in pressure that reduces blood flow to the tissues. Can lead to neuromuscular deficit, amputation, and death.

A. **Pathophysiology:** inability of the fascia surrounding the muscle group to expand to accommodate the increased volume of fluid→compartment pressure increases→venous flow impaired→arterial flow continues, increasing capillary pressure→fluid pushed into the extravascular space→ intracompartment pressure further increased→prolonged or severe ischemia→muscle and nerve cells destroyed, contracture, loss of function, necrotic tissue, infection, release of potassium, hydrogen, and myoglobin into bloodstream.

B. **Risk factors:**
1. Fractures.
2. Burns.
3. Crushing injuries.
4. Restrictive bandages.
5. Cast.
6. Prolonged lithotomy positioning.
7. Ischemic injury (arterial or venous injury).

◆ C. **Assessment:**
1. *Subjective data:*
   a. Severe, unrelenting pain, unrelieved by narcotics and associated with passive stretching of muscle.
   b. Paresthesias.
2. *Objective data:*
   a. Edema; tense skin over limb.
   b. Paralysis.
   c. Decreased or absent peripheral pulses.
   d. Poor capillary refill.
   e. Limb temperature change (colder).
   f. Ankle-arm pressure index (API) *decreased;* 0.4 indicates ischemia (see **Unit 11, Doppler ultrasonography, p. 791**).
   g. Urine output—*decreased* (developing acute tubular necrosis); reddish-brown color.

◆ D. **Analysis/nursing diagnosis:**
1. *Pain* related to tissue swelling and ischemia.
2. *Risk for injury* related to neuromuscular deficits.
3. *Impaired physical mobility* related to contracture and loss of function.
4. *Risk for infection* related to tissue necrosis.
5. *Altered urinary elimination* related to acute tubular necrosis from myoglobin accumulation.
6. *Body image disturbance* related to limb disfigurement.

◆ E. **Nursing care plan/implementation:**
1. Goal: *recognizes early indications of ischemia.*
   ▶ a. Assess *neurovascular* status frequently (q1h): skin temperature, capillary refill, peripheral pulses, mobility, and sensation.
   b. Listen to client complaints; report suspected complications.
   c. Report nonrelief of pain with narcotics.
   d. Recognize unrelenting pain with passive muscle stretching.
2. Goal: *prevent complications.*
   ◢ a. *Elevate* injured extremity initially; if ischemia suspected, keep extremity at *heart level* to prevent compensatory increase in blood flow.
   b. *Avoid* tight bandages, splints, or casts.
   c. Monitor intravenous infusion for signs of infiltration.
   d. Prepare client for fasciotomy (incision of skin and fascia to release tight compartment).

◆ F. **Evaluation/outcome criteria:**
1. Relief from pain; normal perfusion restored.
2. Neurovascular status within normal limits.
3. Retains function of limb; no contractures or infection.
4. Compartment pressure returns to normal (<20 mm Hg).
5. No systemic complications (e.g., normal cardiac and renal function, acid-base balance within normal limits).

V. **Osteoarthritis:** joint disorder characterized by degeneration of articular cartilage and formation of bony outgrowths at edges of weight-bearing joints.

A. **Pathophysiology:** excessive friction combined with risk factors → thinning of articular cartilage, narrowing of joint space, and loss of joint stability; cartilage erodes, producing shallow pits on articular surface and exposing bone in joint space. Bone responds by becoming denser and harder.

B. **Risk factors:**
1. Aging (>50).
2. Rheumatoid arthritis.
3. Arteriosclerosis.
4. Obesity.
5. Trauma.
6. Family history.

◆ C. **Assessment:**
1. *Subjective data:*
   a. Pain; tender joints.
   b. Fatigability, malaise.
   c. Anorexia.
   d. Cold intolerance.
   e. Extremities: numb, tingling.
2. *Objective data:*
   a. *Joints:*
      (1) Enlarged.
      (2) Stiff, limited movement.
      (3) Swelling, redness, and heat around affected joint.
      (4) Shiny stretched skin over and around joint.
      (5) Subcutaneous nodules.
   b. Weight loss.
   c. Fever.
   d. Crepitation (creaking or grating of joints).
   e. Deformities, contractures.
   f. Cold, clammy extremities.

g. Lab data: *decreased* Hgb, *elevated* WBC.

h. *Diagnostic tests:* x-ray, thermography, arthroscopy.

◆ **D. Analysis/nursing diagnosis:**

1. *Pain* related to friction of bones in joints.
2. *Bathing/hygiene self-care deficit* related to decreased mobility of involved joints.
3. *Risk for injury* related to fatigability.
4. *Impaired physical mobility* related to stiff, limited movement.
5. *Impaired home maintenance management* related to contractures.

◆ **E. Nursing care plan/implementation:**

1. Goal: *promote comfort: reduce pain, spasms, inflammation, swelling.*
   a. Medications as prescribed.
      (1) *Nonsteroidal antiinflammatory agents:* aspirin (Ecotrin), acetaminophen (Tylenol), ibuprofen (Motrin), indomethacin (Indocin), corticosteroids, nabumetone (Relafen), naproxen (Naprosyn).
      (2) *Antimalarials:* chloroquine (Aralen), hydroxychloroquine (Plaquenil), to relieve symptoms.
   b. Heat to reduce muscle spasms, stiffness.
   c. Cold to reduce swelling and pain.
   d. Prevent contractures:
      (1) Exercise.
      (2) Bedrest on firm mattress during attacks.
      (3) Splints to maintain proper alignment.
   e. *Elevate* extremity to reduce swelling.
   f. Rest.
   g. Assistive devices to decrease weight bearing of affected joints (canes, walkers).
2. Goal: *health teaching to promote independence.*
   a. Encourage self-care with assistive devices for activities of daily living (ADL).
   b. Activity, as tolerated, with ambulation-assistive devices.

c. Scheduled rest periods.
d. Correct body posture and body mechanics.
3. Goal: *provide for emotional needs.*
   a. Accept feelings of frustration regarding long-term debilitating disorder.
   b. Provide diversional activities appropriate for age and physical condition to promote comfort and satisfaction.

◆ **F. Evaluation/outcome criteria:**

1. Remains independent as long as possible.
2. No contractures.
3. States comfort has increased.
4. Uses methods that are successful in pain control.

VI. Total hip replacement: femoral head and acetabulum are replaced by a prosthesis, which is cemented into the bone with plastic cement. Performed to replace a joint with limited and painful function due to bony alkalosis and deformity, caused by degenerative joint disease or when vascular supply to femoral head is compromised from a fracture. *Goal of the surgery:* restore or improve mobilization of hip joint and prevent complications of extended immobilization.

A. Risk factors:

1. Rheumatoid arthritis.
2. Osteoarthritis.
3. Complications of femoral neck fractures—avascular necrosis and malunion (**Table 7.44**).
4. Congenital hip disease.

◆ **B. Analysis/nursing diagnosis:**

1. *Risk for injury* related to implant surgery.
2. *Knowledge deficit* (learning need) regarding joint replacement surgery.
3. *Impaired physical mobility* related to major hip surgery.
4. *Pain* related to surgical incision.
5. *Risk for impaired skin integrity* related to immobility.

◆ **C. Nursing care plan/implementation** (also see **Clinical Pathway 7.4: Primary Hip Arthroplasty**):

TABLE 7.44	**Fractures of the Hip**			
Risk	**Types**	◆ **Assessment**		**Surgical Intervention**
Osteoporosis Age >60 Women (White) While postmenopausal Immobility/ sedentary lifestyle	Intracapsular (femoral neck; within hip joint and capsule)	Slight trauma Pain: groin and hip Lateral rotation, shortening of leg, minimal deformity		Total hip replacement
	Extracapsular (outside hip joint; also called intertrochanteric)	Direct trauma Severe pain External rotation, shortening of leg, obvious deformity		Internal fixation with nail (open reduction) Possible total hip replacement
	Subtrochanteric (below lesser trochanter)	Direct trauma Leg pain near fracture site External rotation, shortening of leg, deformity Presence of hematoma		Internal fixation with nail (open reduction) Closed reduction

Adult

PCA-	Patient-Controlled Analgesia	AES-	Antiembolism Stockings	Y-	Yes
SCDs-	Sequential Compression Device	MSW-	Medical Social Worker	N-	No
		D/C-	Discontinue		

CLINICAL PATHWAY 7.4: Primary Hip Arthroplasty

Circle items not completed, and document exceptions.
Review circled items daily. Date circled items when completed. Items with boxes are for non-nursing discipline.

HEALTH CARE ACTIVITIES/PHYSICIAN ORDER REQUIRED

	DOS Date	/ /	/ /
	THA	Day 1	Day 2
• Milestones		• Patient dangles and stands first time with physical therapy Y N	
1. Discharge Planning	Admission nursing assessment completed		☐ MSW interview and collaborates with Home Care Liaison Interdisciplinary team collaborates with MSW regarding discharge goal ☐ MSW assess services, equipment, transportation and possible placement
2. MD Consult/Activity			☐ D/C wound drains ☐ Dressing changed to light dressing
3. Diagnostic Tests		CBC P.T. (if on warfarin)	CBC P.T. (if on warfarin)
4. Treatments Instrumentation	Balanced suspension/ abduction pillow Foley AES, SCDs Wound drains O$_2$ via nasal prongs I&O	Balanced suspension/ abduction pillow Foley AES, SCDs Wound drains O$_2$ via nasal prongs I&O	D/C Balanced suspension Abduction pillow D/C Foley AES, SCDs D/C O$_2$ I&O
5. Diet and Nutrition	Diet as tolerated	Diet as tolerated	Diet as tolerated
6. Medications a. Antibiotics b. Pain Management c. Anticoagulation d. Bowel Regimen e. IV	IV antibiotics PCA with basal or parenteral analgesics Anticoagulation IV continuous	IV antibiotics PCA with basal or parenteral analgesics Anticoagulation IV continuous	D/C antibiotics D/C basal, continue self-dose PCA or parenteral analgesics and begin oral analgesics ATC ×24 Anticoagulation Bowel intervention IV continuous
7. Activity/position	Bedrest with operated leg in balanced suspension/abduction pillow Reposition as needed Adjust balanced suspension/ abduction pillow prn	☐ PT: evaluation instruction isometrics, precautions, PT program • **Dangle (stand if client tolerates)** Complete bath/partial bath Adjust balanced suspension/ abduction pillow prn	☐ PT: advances activity as tol. incl. transfers, ADLs and gait ☐ PT: adv. exercises as tol. Partial bath, OOB to chair, toilet Adjust abduction pillow prn
8. Nursing Assessment ◆ CSM= circulation, sensation, movement	VS every 4 hr with O$_2$ sats CSM every 4 hr Systems assessment every 8 hr	VS every 4 hr with O$_2$ sats CSM every 4 hr Systems assessment every 8 hr	VS every 8 hr CSM every 4 hr Systems assessment every 8 hr
9. Client Teaching	Orientation to room, call light and nursing care Begin teaching to include: 1. PCA/analgesic instruction 2. Positioning, THA precautions 3. Protocol for advancing diet 4. Purpose of anticoagulation, AES, SCDs 5. ICS, C + DB 6. Pain scale, 0–10	Reinforce teaching for. 1. PCA 2. Positioning, THA precautions, ROM 3. Advancing diet 4. Anticoagulation, AES, SCDs 5. ICS, C + DB 6. Reinforce pain scale ☐ PT: Post-op exercise instruction	Teach ATC PO pain management Teach sx hip dislocation Balance diet to include iron & fiber Reinforce teaching for: 1. THA precautions 2. Advancing diet 3. Anticoagulation, AES, SCDs 4. ICS, C + DB

Adult

/ /	/ /	/ /	Discharge Outcomes
Day 3	**Day 4**	**Day 5**	
Final post discharge destination made and transportation initiated **Y N**		• **Client is discharged Y N** • **Client independent in and out of bed Y N**	
• **Initiate home care referral form or Interfacility Transfer form**	☐ MSW confirm transportation ☐ Home care referral made by Home Care Liaison	Give clinic appointment Prescriptions for discharge meds • **Discharge client**	Client/caregiver receives discharge resources: 1. Supplies 2. Equipment 3. Home care or other d/c arrangements
		☐ Dressing change	
P.T. (if on warfarin)	Duplex scan D/C hip x-rays PT (if on warfarin) Platelet Count (enoxaparin)	PT (if on warfarin)	Correct prosthetic placement by x-ray confirmation Urine clear
Abduction pillow AES, D/C SCDs Monitor drsg for drainage, change prn D/C I&O	Abduction pillow AES Monitor drsg for drainage. Change prn	Abduction pillow AES	Wound healing with minimum redness or drainage
Diet as tolerated	Diet as tolerated	Diet as tolerated	Tolerates normal diet
D/C PCA or parenteral analgesics Continue oral analgesics ATC ×24 Anticoagulation HL IV	Discharge planning for: Analgesics Anticoagulation Oral analgesics prn Anticoagulation Bowel intervention HL IV	Discharged on: Oral analgesics prn Appropriate anticoagulation Oral analgesics prn Anticoagulation D/C HL	Pain under control by self report on oral analgesics Normal circulation to extremities Abdomen soft, reports GI comfort
☐ PT: advances activity as tol. incl. transfers, ADLs and gait ☐ PT: adv. exercises as tol. ☐ PT: assess and order equip Self bath with help Adjust abduction pillow prn Assist with progressive gait	☐ PT: advances activity as tol. incl. transfers, ADLs and gait ☐ PT: adv. exercises as tol. ☐ PT: Stair climbing Self bath with help Adjust abduction pillow prn Assist with progressive gait	• **In/out of bed independently** ☐ PT: advances activity as tol. incl. transfers, ADLs and gait ☐ PT: adv. exercises as tol. ☐ PT: Stair climbing Self bath with help Adjust abduction pillow prn Assist with progressive gait	Follows THA precautions and uses assistive devices correctly Independent in/out of bed
VS every 8 hrs CSM every 4 hrs Systems assessment every 8 hrs	VS every 8 hrs CSM every 4 hrs Systems assessment every 8 hrs	VS every 8 hrs CSM every 4 hrs Systems assessment every 8 hrs	Temp < 38 for 24 hours prior to D/C CSM status same as prior to surgery or improved All systems returned to baseline
Bacteremia teaching, "Protecting Your Joint From Infection" given. Review S+Sx of infection Reinforce teaching for: 1. THA precaution 2. Anticoagulation, AES Teach ATC vs prn pain management	Anticoagulation teaching $S+S_x$ thrombophlebitis. Watch ADL videotape Reinforce teaching for: 1. THA precautions 2. Anticoagulation, AES 3. Prn pain medication management	Review staple/wound care Give "Care of your wound" handout Reinforce teaching for: 1. THA precautions 2. Anticoagulation, AES Discharge medication teaching	Able to verbalize $S+S_x$: wound infection, thrombophlebitis, bacteremia, hip and wound precautions, diet high in *iron* and *fiber*, indications and side effects of discharge medications 🍽

Adult

(Continued on following page)

CLINICAL PATHWAY 7.4: Primary Hip Arthroplasty *(Continued)*

	DOS Date / /	/ /	/ /
	THA	**Day 1**	**Day 2**
10. Comfort	Verbalizes acceptable level of pain at_____ and able to cooperate with activities Uses PCA/analgesic appropriately	Verbalizes acceptable level of pain at_____ and able to cooperate with activities Uses PCA/analgesic appropriately	Verbalizes acceptable level of pain at _____ and able to cooperate with activities Uses PCA appropriately without basal rate and takes PO pain meds appropriately
11. Physical Mobility	Uses overhead trapeze appropriately Maintains operated leg in balanced suspension with THA precautions/abduction pillow in place Tolerates balanced suspension/abduction pillow Follows THA positioning guidelines	Uses overhead trapeze appropriately Dangles with assist, stands if tol. Tolerates balanced suspension/abduction pillow Follows THA precautions	Up to chair 30 min BID and amb. in room Stands with PT assist and progress ambulation Uses walker or crutches approp. Maintains THA precautions with abduction pillow
12. Bowel and Bladder Function	Urine output > 30 cc/hour Bowel sounds present Abdomen soft, nondistended Tolerates diet	Urine output > 30 cc/hour Bowel sounds present Abdomen soft, nondistended Tolerates diet	Urine output > 30 cc/hour Bowel sounds present + flatus Abdomen soft, nondistended. Has bowel movement
13. Self Care Ability		Verbalizes understanding of care needs Assists staff as able Uses bedpan with max assist	Washes face, arms, and chest with set up Uses bedpan with moderate assist
14. Skin Integrity	Skin intact Dressing dry and intact PURV _____	Skin intact Dressing dry and intact	Skin intact Dressing dry and intact
15. Safety Falls Assessment *If score ≥ 6 follow orthopedic standardized NCP or individualize *Intervention Guideline for client at risk for fall.		65 or older .... 1 Mental status limitations ..... 5 History of falls .... 5 Mobility limitations .... 4 Elimination problems .... 2 Medications .... 1 TOTAL SCORE .... _____*	65 or older .... 1 Mental status limitations .... 5 History of falls .... 5 Mobility limitations .... 4 Elimination problems .... 2 Medications .... 1 TOTAL SCORE .... _____*

1. *Preoperative:*
   a. Goal: *prevent deep vein thrombosis or pulmonary emboli.*
      (1) Antiembolic stockings.
      (2) *Increase* fluid intake.
   b. Goal: *prevent infection: antibiotics* as ordered, given prophylactically (Cefazolin).
   c. Goal: *health teaching.*
      (1) *Isometric exercises*—gluteal, abdominal, and quadricep setting; dorsiflexion and plantarflexion of the feet.
      (2) Use of trapeze.
      (3) Explain position of operative leg and hip postoperatively to prevent *adduction* and flexion.
      (4) Transfer techniques—bed to chair and chair to crutches; dangle at bedside first time out of bed.
      (5) Assist client with skin scrubs with antibacterial soap.

2. *Postoperative:*
   a. Goal: *prevent respiratory complications.*
      (1) Turn, cough, and deep breathe.
      (2) Incentive spirometry.
   b. Goal: *prevent complications of shock or infection.*

/ /	/ /	/ /	Discharge Outcomes
Day 3	**Day 4**	**Day 5**	
Verbalizes acceptable level of pain at _____ and able to cooperate with activities Reports pain relief with non-pharmacological methods (i.e. turning, positioning, relaxation, etc.) Tolerates ATC PO pain meds	Verbalizes acceptable level of pain at _____ and able to cooperate with activities Requests PO prn pain meds approp.	Verbalizes acceptable level of pain at _____ and able to cooperate with activities Able to verbalize understanding of indications and side effects of D/C meds Requests prn PO pain meds approp.	Pain controlled by self report on oral analgesics
Ambulates with PT assistance in hall Tolerates 30 min in chair TID Able to get in and out of bed with moderate assist Uses walker or crutches approp.	Increases walking distance with PT or Nsg Assist in hall Uses walker or crutches approp. Able to get in and out of bed with minimal assist	Increases walking distance with PT or Nsg Assist in hall Uses walker or crutches approp. Able to get in and out of bed with minimal assist	Independent/min assist in and out of bed Verbalizes understanding of hip precautions No dislocation of prosthesis
Maintains THA precautions	Maintains THA precautions	Maintains THA precautions	
Voids spontaneously Bowel sounds present + flatus Abdomen soft, nondistended	Voids spontaneously Bowel sounds present + flatus Has bowel movement	Voids spontaneously Bowel pattern same as preop status	Voids spontaneously Bowel pattern normal
Washes areas in reach Uses bedpan with minimal assist Uses bathroom with mod. assist	Washes areas in reach Uses bathroom with minimal assist	Bathes self Independent/min assist to bathroom with assistive devices	Able to bathe self/bathe with setup Independent/min assist to bathroom with assistive devices
Skin intact Dressing dry and intact PURV _____	Skin intact Dressing dry and intact	Skin intact Dressing dry and intact PURV _____	Skin intact Incision well approximated without redness or drainage
65 or older .... 1 Mental status limitations ..... 5 History of falls .... 5 Mobility limitations .... 4 Elimination problems .... 2 Medications 1	65 or older .... 1 Mental status limitations ..... 5 History of falls .... 5 Mobility limitations .... 4 Elimination problems .... 2 Medications 1	65 or older .... 1 Mental status limitations ...... 5 History of falls .... 5 Mobility limitations .... 4 Elimination problems .... 2 Medications 1	
TOTAL SCORE .... _____*	TOTAL SCORE .... _____*	TOTAL SCORE .... _____*	

Source: UCSF Healthcare, San Francisco, Calif. With permission from Jane E. Hirsch, RN, MS, Vice President, Nursing and Patient Care Services.

▶ (1) Check dressings for drainage q1h for first 4 hr; then q4h and prn; may have Hemovac or other drainage tubes inserted in wound to keep dressing dry.

(2) Monitor I&O and vital signs hourly for 4 hr, then q4h and prn.

c. Goal: *prevent contractures, muscle atrophy:* initiate exercises as soon as allowed: isometric quadriceps, dorsiflexion and plantarflexion of foot, and flexion and extension of the ankle—sequential compression device while in bed.

d. Goal: *promote early ambulation and movement.*

(1) Use trapeze.

(2) Transfer technique (pivot on unaffected leg); crutches/walker.

(3) Initiate progressive ambulation as ordered; ensure *maximum extension* of leg when walking.

(4) Administer *anticoagulation* therapy as ordered (warfarin immediately postop) to prevent deep vein thrombosis and pulmonary emboli.

(5) Recognize early side effects of medications and report appropriately.

e. Goal: *prevent constipation.*

(1) *Increase* fluid intake.

(2) Use fracture bed pan.

Adult

f. Goal: *prevent dislocation of prosthesis.*

(1) Maintain *abduction* of the affected joint (prevent external rotation); *elevate* head of bed, turn according to physician's order. When turning to unaffected side, turn with abduction pillow between legs to maintain abduction.

(2) *Buck's extension* or *Russell's traction* may be applied (temporary skin traction).

(3) Plaster booties with an abduction bar may be used.

(4) *Wedge Charnley* (triangle-shaped) pillow to *maintain abduction* between knees and lower legs.

(5) Provide periods throughout day when client lies flat in bed to *prevent hip flexion* and strengthen hip muscles.

(6) Report signs of dislocation: *anteriorly*—knee flexes, leg turns outward, leg looks longer than other, femur head may be felt in groin area; *posteriorly*—leg turns inward, appears shorter than other, greater trochanter elevated.

g. Goal: *promote comfort.*

(1) Initiate skin care; monitor pressure points for redness; back care q2h.

(2) Alternating pressure mattress; sheepskin when sitting in chair.

h. Goal: *health teaching.*

(1) Exercise program with written list of activity restrictions.

(2) Methods to *prevent* hip adduction.

(3) *Avoid* sitting for more than 1 hr: stand, stretch, and walk frequently to *prevent* hip flexion contractures.

(4) Advise *not to exceed 90 degrees of hip flexion* (dislocation can occur, particularly with posterior incisions); *avoid* low chairs.

(5) Teach alternative methods of usual self-care activities to prevent hip dislocation (e.g., *avoid*: bending from waist to tie shoes, sitting up straight in a low chair, using a low toilet seat).

(6) *Avoid* crossing legs, driving a car for 6 wk.

(7) Wear support hose for 6 wk to enhance venous return and avoid thrombus formation.

◆ D. **Evaluation/outcome criteria:**

1. Participates in postoperative nursing care plan to prevent complications.

2. Reports pain has decreased.

3. Ambulates with assistive devices.

4. Complications of immobility avoided.

5. Able to resume self-care activities.

VII. **Total knee replacement:** both sides of the joint are replaced by metal or plastic implants.

◆ A. **Analysis** (see **VI. Total hip replacement, p. 627**).

◆ B. **Nursing plan/implementation:**

1. See **VI. Total hip replacement, p. 627.**

2. Goal: *achieve active flexion beyond 70 degrees.*

a. *Immediately postop:* may have continuous passive motion (CPM) device for flexion/extension of affected knee. Maximum flexion *110 degrees.*

b. Monitor drainage in *Hemovac* (q15 min for first 4 hr, q1h until 24 hr; q4h and prn while Hemovac in place).

c. Analgesics as ordered for pain.

d. While dressings are still on: quadriceps-setting exercises for approximately 5 days (consult with physical therapist for specific instructions).

e. After dressings removed: active flexion exercises.

f. *Avoid* pressure on heel.

◆ C. **Evaluation/outcome criteria:**

1. No complications of infection, hemorrhage noted.

2. ROM of knee increases with exercises.

VIII. **Amputation:** surgical removal of a limb as a result of trauma or circulatory impairment (gangrene). The amount of tissue amputated is determined by the severity of disease or trauma and the ability of the remaining tissue to heal.

A. **Risk factors:**

1. Atherosclerosis obliterans.

2. Uncontrolled diabetes mellitus.

3. Malignancy.

4. Extensive and intractable infection.

5. Result of severe trauma.

◆ B. **Assessment** *(preoperative):*

1. *Subjective data:* pain in affected part.

2. *Objective data:*

a. Soft-tissue damage.

b. Partial or complete severance of a body part.

c. Lack of peripheral pulses.

d. Skin color changes, pallor → cyanosis → gangrene.

e. Infection, hemorrhage, or shock.

◆ C. **Analysis/nursing diagnosis:**

1. *Impaired physical mobility* related to lower-limb amputation.

2. *Body image disturbance* related to loss of body part.

3. *Pain* related to interruption of nerve pathways.

4. *Anxiety* related to potential change in lifestyle.

5. *Knowledge deficit* (learning need) related to rehabilitation goals.

◆ D. **Nursing care plan/implementation:**

1. Goal: *prepare for surgery, physically and emotionally.*

a. Validate that client and family are aware that amputation of body part is planned.

b. Validate that informed consent is signed.

c. Allow time for grieving.

▶ d. If time allows, prepare client for postoperative phase (e.g., teach arm-strengthening exercises if lower limb is to be amputated; teach alternative methods of ambulation).

e. Provide time to discuss feelings.

f. Prepare surgical site to decrease possibility of infection (e.g., shave, scrub as ordered).

g. Discuss postoperative expectations.

2. Goal: *promote healing postoperatively.*

▶ a. Monitor *respiratory status* q1 to 4h and prn: rate, depth of respiration; auscultate for signs of congestion; and question client about chest pain (*pulmonary emboli* common complication).

b. Monitor for hemorrhage; keep tourniquet at bedside.

c. Medicate for pain as ordered—client may have phantom limb pain.

d. Support stump on pillow for first 24 hr; **remove pillow** after 24 hr to prevent contracture.

e. *Position: turn client on to stomach* to prevent hip contracture.

▶ f. ROM exercises for joint above amputation to prevent joint immobilization; strengthening exercises for arms, nonaffected limbs, abdominal muscles.

▶ g. *Stump care:*
(1) Early postoperative dressings changed prn.
(2) As incision heals, bandage is applied in cone shape to prepare stump for prosthesis.
(3) Inspect for blisters, redness, abrasions.
(4) Remove stump sock daily and prn.

h. Assist in rehabilitation program.

◆ E. **Evaluation/outcome criteria:**
1. Begins rehabilitation program.
2. No hemorrhage, infection.
3. Adjusts to altered body image.

IX. **Gout:** disorder of purine metabolism; genetic disease believed to be transmitted by a dominant gene, characterized by recurrent attacks of acute pain and swelling of one joint (usually the great toe).

A. **Pathophysiology:** urate crystals and infiltrating leukocytes appear to damage the intracellular phagolysosomes, resulting in leakage of lysomal enzymes into the synovial fluid, causing tissue damage and joint inflammation.

B. **Risk factors:**
1. Men.
2. Age (>50).
3. Genetic/familial tendency.
4. Prolonged hyperuricemia (elevated serum uric acid).
5. Obesity.
6. Moderate to heavy alcohol intake.

7. Hypertension.
8. Abnormal kidney function.

◆ C. **Assessment:**
1. *Subjective data:*
a. *Pain:* excruciating
b. Fatigue
c. Anorexia.
2. *Objective data:*
a. *Joint:* erythema (redness), hot, swollen, difficult to move; skin stretched and shiny over joint.
b. Subcutaneous nodules, tophi (deposits of urate) on hands and feet.
c. Weight loss.
d. Fever.
e. Sensory changes, with cold intolerance.
f. Lab data:
(1) Serum uric acid: *increased significantly* (6.5/100 mL in women, 7.5/100 mL in men) in chronic gout; only *slightly increased* in acute gout.
(2) WBC: 12,000 to 15,000/μL.
(3) Erythrocyte sedimentation rate: >20 mm.
(4) 24 hr urinary uric acid: slightly *elevated.*
(5) Proteinuria (chronic gout).
(6) Azotemia (presence of nitrogen-containing compounds in blood) in chronic gout.
g. *Diagnostic tests:* arthrocentesis, x-rays.

◆ D. **Analysis/nursing diagnosis:**
1. *Pain* related to inflammation and swelling of affected joint.
2. *Impaired physical mobility* related to pain.
3. *Knowledge deficit* (learning need) related to diet restrictions and increased fluid needs.
4. *Altered urinary elimination* related to kidney damage.

◆ E. **Nursing care plan/implementation:**
1. Goal: *decrease discomfort.*
a. Administer antigout medications as ordered:
(1) Treatment of *acute* attacks: colchicine, phenylbutazone (Butazolidin), indomethacin (Indocin), allopurinol (Zyloprim), naproxen (Naprosyn), corticosteroids (prednisone).
(2) *Preventive therapy:* probenecid (Benemid), sulfinpyrazone (Anturane). These drugs are *not* used during acute attacks.
b. Absolute rest of affected joint→gradual increase in activities, to prevent complications of immobilization; at the same time, rest for comfort.
2. Goal: *prevent kidney damage.*
a. *Increase* fluid intake to 2000 to 3000 mL/day.
b. Monitor urinary output.
3. Goal: *health teaching.*
a. Need for *low purine diet* during acute attack (see **VII. Purine-restricted diet, Common Therapeutic Diets, Unit 9, p. 722**).

Adult

b. Importance of *increased fluid in diet.*

c. Signs and symptoms of increased progression of disease.

d. Dosage and side effects of prescribed medications.

◆ **F. Evaluation/outcome criteria:**

1. Swelling decreased.
2. Discomfort alleviated.
3. Mobility returned to status before attack.
4. Lab values return to normal.

X. Herniated/ruptured disk (ruptured nucleus pulposus): strain or injury to a weakened cartilage between vertebrae can result in herniation of the nucleus, causing pressure on nerve roots in spinal canal, pain, and disability.

A. Pathophysiology: pulpy substance of disk interior (nucleus pulposus) bulges or ruptures through the outer annulus fibrosus → irritation and pressure on nerve endings in the spinal ligaments → muscle spasm and distortion of the joints of vertebral arches.

B. Risk factors:

1. Strain as result of poor body mechanics.
2. Trauma.
3. History of back injuries.
4. Degenerative disk (spondylosis).

◆ **C. Assessment:**

1. *Lumbar injuries* (90% of herniations):
   a. *Subjective data:*
      (1) *Pain:* low back, radiating to buttocks, posterior thigh, and calf; relieved by recumbency; aggravated by sneezing, coughing, and flexion; sciatic pain continues even when back pain subsides.
      (2) Numbness, tingling.
   b. *Objective data:*
      (1) Muscle weakness—leg and foot.
      (2) Inability to flex leg.
      (3) Sensory loss, leg and foot.
      (4) Alterations in posture: leans to side, unable to stand up straight.
      (5) Edema: leg and foot.
      (6) Positive *Lasègue's sign:* straight leg raising with hip flexed and knee extended will produce sciatic pain.
2. *Cervical injuries* (10% of herniations):
   a. *Subjective data:*
      (1) *Pain*—upper extremities, radiating to hands and fingers; aggravated by coughing, sneezing, and straining.
      (2) Tingling, burning sensation in upper extremities and back of neck.
   b. *Objective data:*
      (1) Upper extremities: weakness and atrophy.
      (2) Neck: restricted movement.
      (3) *Diagnostic tests* for both lumbar and cervical injuries.

(a) Spine x-rays.
(b) CT scan.
(c) MRI.
(d) Myelography (less preferred than CAT scan or MRI).
(e) Electromyography.
► (f) *Neurological* exam: special attention to *sensory* status, including pain, touch, and temperature identification; and to *motor* status, including strength, gait, and reflexes.

◆ **D. Analysis/nursing diagnosis:**

1. *Pain* related to pressure on nerve roots.
2. *Fear* related to disease progression and/or potential surgery.
3. *Knowledge deficit* (learning need) related to correct body mechanics.
4. *Impaired physical mobility* related to continued pain.
5. *Sleep pattern disturbance* related to difficulty finding comfortable position.

◆ **E. Nursing care plan/implementation:**

1. Goal: *relieve pain and promote comfort.*
   a. Bedrest with bedboard.
   b. *Position—avoid* twisting.
      (1) *Lumbar disk: William's* (*head elevated* 30 degrees, knee gatch *elevated* to flatten the lumbosacral curve). Can be duplicated at home with pillow placement.
      (2) *Cervical: low Fowler's.*
   c. Medications as ordered:
      (1) *Analgesics.*
      (2) *Muscle relaxants.*
      (3) *Antiinflammatory.*
      (4) *Stool softeners.*
   d. Moist heat.
   e. Fracture bedpan.
   f. Gradual increase in activity.
   g. Brace application for support.
   h. Traction application prn for comfort.
   i. Prepare for surgery if medical regimen unsuccessful.
2. Goal: *health teaching.*
   a. Correct body mechanics, keep back straight.
   b. Exercise program as symptoms decrease.

◆ **F. Evaluation/outcome criteria:**

1. Reports pain decreased.
2. Mobility increased, normal body posture attained.

XI. Laminectomy: excision of dorsal arch of vertebrae with or without spinal fusion of two or more vertebrae with a bone graft from iliac crest, to stabilize spine (see **Clinical Pathway 7.5: Posterior Spinal Fusion**):

◆ **A. Analysis/nursing diagnosis:**

1. *Pain* related to edema of surgical procedure.
2. *Impaired physical mobility* related to pain and discomfort resulting from surgery.

◆ **B. Nursing care plan/implementation:**
1. Goal: *relieve anxiety.*
   a. Answer questions, explain routines.
   b. See **The Perioperative Experience, p. 546.**
2. Goal: *prevent injury postoperatively.*
   a. Monitor vital signs:
      (1) *Neurological* signs, e.g., check sensation and motor strength of limbs.
      (2) *Respiratory* status (risk for **respiratory depression** with cervical laminectomy).
   b. Monitor I&O (**urinary retention** common, especially with cervical laminectomy); may need catheterization. Encourage *fluids.*
   c. Monitor bowel sounds (**paralytic ileus** common with lumbar laminectomy).
   d. Monitor dressing for possible bleeding.
   e. Bed *position* as ordered:
      (1) *For lumbar laminectomy: head of bed flat;* supine with slight flexion of legs; with pillow between knees for turning and side-lying position.
      (2) *For cervical laminectomy: head of bed elevated,* neck immobilized with collar or sandbags.
   f. Encourage deep breathing to prevent respiratory complications. Use of inspirometer q1hr when awake.
   g. Prevent strain or flexion at surgical site: *log-rolling* with spinal fusion.
   h. Some surgical interventions that require small incisions (microsurgery) have no specific postoperative positions.
3. Goal: *promote comfort.*
   a. Administer *analgesics* if sciatic-type pain continues after lumbar surgery (arm pain after cervical surgery), due to edema from trauma of surgery.
4. Goal: *prepare for early discharge.*
   a. Clients having microsurgery for repair of herniated disk will usually be discharged from the hospital 1 day postoperative; teaching regarding allowed and restricted activities must be done early.
5. Goal: *health teaching.*
   a. How to *turn and move* from side to side in one motion, *sit up,* and *get out of bed without twisting spine*; to get out of bed: raise head of bed while in side-lying position, then put feet over edge of bed, and stand.
   b. Proper positioning and *ambulation* techniques.
   c. Correct posture, *body mechanics,* activities to prevent further injury; increase activities according to tolerance.
   d. Referral: physiotherapy; encourage compliance for full rehabilitation.

◆ **C. Evaluation/outcome criteria:**
1. No respiratory, bowel, or bladder complications noted.
   a. Lung sounds clear.
   b. Bowel sounds present; able to pass gas and feces.
   c. Urinary output adequate.
2. Regains mobility.
3. Comfort level increases: reports leg and back pain decreased.
4. Demonstrates protective positioning and ambulation techniques.

XII. **Spinal cord injuries:** trauma from hyperextension, hyperflexion, axial compression, lateral flexion, or shearing of the spine.
   A. Types:
   1. *C-1 and C-2 injury level*—resulting deficit:
      a. Phrenic nerve involvement.
      b. Diaphragmatic paralysis.
      c. Respiratory difficulties (require permanent ventilatory support).
      d. Possible quadriplegia.
      e. Possible death.
   2. *C-4 through T-1 injury level*—resulting deficit: possible quadriplegia.
   3. *Thoracic-lumbar injury level*—resulting deficit: possible paraplegia.
   B. Pathophysiology: trauma → vertebral dislocation or fractures → cord trauma, compression, or severance of the cord.
   C. Risk factors:
   1. Motor vehicle accidents.
   2. Diving, surfing, contact sports.
   3. Falls.
   4. Gunshot wounds.
◆ **D. Assessment:**
   1. *Subjective data:*
      a. Pain *at* the level of injury.
      b. Numbness/weakness, loss of sensation *below* level of injury.
      c. Psychological distress related to severity of injury and its effects.
   2. *Objective data:*
      a. Symptoms depend on extent of injury to spinal cord/spinal nerves.
      b. Paralysis: motor, sphincter.
         (1) Initially a period of *flaccid paralysis* and loss of reflexes, called *spinal* or *neural shock.*
         (2) *Incomplete injuries* may lead to loss of voluntary movement and sensory deficits below injury level (symptoms vary depending on injury).
         (3) *Complete injury* leads to loss of function and all voluntary movement below level of injury.
      c. Respiratory distress.
      d. Alterations in temperature control.
      e. Alterations in bowel and bladder function.

Adult

Circle items not completed or not within normal limits, and document exceptions. Review circled items daily.
Date circled items when completed. Items with boxes are for non-nursing discipline charting.

Name._____

	Pre Admit	Day of Surgery	/ / Day 1	/ / Day 2
PCA: *Patient Controlled Analgesia* SCDs- *Sequential Compression Device* AES- *Antiembolism Stockings* MSW- *Medical Social Worker* D/C- *Discontinue* Y- *Yes* N- *No*				
Milestones				• **Stands 5 minutes** Y N
1. Discharge Planning	Spine Service Nurse/ Case Manager assesses home situation and collaborates with MSW			☐ MSW interview and collaborates with Home Care Liaison Interdisciplinary Team collaborates with MSW regarding discharge goal ☐ MSW assess services, equipment, transportation and possible placement
2. MD/Consult/Activity	Pain management consult as indicated	☐ PT requisition	☐ Pain management Pharmacy consult	☐ D/C drain
3. Diagnostic Tests			CBC	CBC

4. Treatments/ Instrumentation		Intake + Output
		AES, SCDs
		Foley
		O₂ via nasal prongs
		Assess wound
		Wound drain
		  Type _____
		  Site _____
		Describe drainage
		_____
			Intake + Output
			AES, SCDs
			Foley
			O₂ via nasal prongs
			Assess wound
			Wound drain
			  Type _____
			  Site _____
			Describe drainage
			_____
				Intake + Output
				AES, SCDs
				Foley
				O₂ via nasal prongs
				Assess wound
				Wound drain
				  Type _____
				  Site _____
				Describe drainage _____

5. Diet/Nutrition	NPO after midnight day before surgery	NPO	NPO	Ice chips, 30 cc/hr if bowel sounds

6. Medications
  a) Routine
  b) Pain Management
  c) Bowel Regimen
  d) IV (Intravenous) HL (saline lock)
	Discontinue non-steroidal anti-inflammatory drugs 2 weeks before surgery
	Continue analgesics as ordered and evaluate analgesic use
	Fleets enema evening before surgery
		IV Antibiotic
		
		PCA with Basal
		
		IV continuous
			IV Antibiotic
			
			PCA with Basal
			
			IV continuous
				D/C IV Antibiotic (48 hr.) post surgery)
				PCA with Basal
				
				Bowel intervention
				Suppository
				IV continuous

7. Activity/ Mobility		Bedrest Logroll q 2 hours	Bedrest Logroll q 2 hours	Bedrest Logroll q 2 hours Dangle 2–3 times • **Stands 5 minutes** Notify orthotist if able to stand
8. Physical Therapy (PT) Occupational Therapy (OT)	Physical therapy instructions Occupational therapy instructions		☐ PT evaluation Instruction supine exercises Dangle if ordered	☐ PT advance exercises as tolerated. Dangle, stand if tolerated. Instruct body mechanics, self care mobilization exercises ☐ OT Evaluation as needed
9. Assessment **VS = T, R, P, BP** **CSM = Circulation Sensation Movement** **GI = Bowel sounds** **Pulmonary = Auscultate lung fields**	VS Q 4° hours	VS Q 4° hours CSM q 4 hours GI/GU q 4 hours Pulmonary q 4 hours O₂ sat. q 4 hours Neurological: Q shift Cardiovascular: Q shift Musculoskeletal: Q shift Skin assessment: Q shift Psychosocial/Behavioral Assessment: Q shift	VS Q 4 hours CSM q 4 hours GI/GU q 4 hours Pulmonary q 4 hours O₂ sat. q 4 hours Neurological: Q shift Cardiovascular: Q shift Musculoskeletal: Q shift Skin assessment: Q shift Psychosocial/Behavioral Assessment: Q shift	VS QID CSM QID GI/GU q 8 hours Pulmonary q 4 hours O₂ sat. q 4 hours Neurological: Q shift Cardiovascular: Q shift Musculoskeletal: Q shift Skin assessment: Q shift Psychosocial/Behavioral Assessment: Q shift

HEALTH CARE TEAM ACTIVITIES—PHYSICIAN ORDER REQUIRED

Adult

	/ /	/ /	/ /	/ /	/ /	Discharge Outcomes
Day 3	**Day 4**	**Day 5**	**Day 6**	**Day 7**	Date———
	· **Brace molded Y N**			· **Discharge Y N**	
	☐ Home Care Liaison assesses equipment and transport needs Start Home Care referral	☐ Home Care Liaison starts Home Care Referral Continue Home Care Referral/insurance info	☐ Home Care Liaison confirms transport and equipment needs	Give clinic appointment and prescriptions for discharge meds · Discharge client	Client is discharged
☐ Change dressing Apply light dressing or steri strips open to air	☐ Brace molded by orthotist	☐ Brace returned and fitted	☐ Brace adjusted if needed	☐ Dressing change ☐ PDP completed ☐ Prescriptions written	Brace fits property
CBC, UA, C + S, if fever or urine cloudy			Full spine x-ray (in brace if ordered)		Spine alignment confirmed per x-ray
Intake + Output AES, SCDs D/C Foley D/C O$_2$ Assess wound	D/C Intake + Output AES, SCDs Assess wound	AES; discontinue SCDs when ambulating independently Assess wound	Wears AES Assess wound	Discontinue AES on discharge	
Clear liquids, if flatus passed	Advance diet Type of diet ——— % taken B_ L_ D_	Advance diet Type of diet ——— % taken B_ L_ D_	Advance diet Type of diet ——— % taken B_ L_ D_	Advance diet Type of diet ——— % taken B_ L_ D_	Client tolerates diet
Begin PO medications + FESO$_4$, MVI, DOSS PCA, no Basal Begin PO medications around the clock for 24 hours Bowel intervention IV continuous	PO medications Discontinue PCA PO pain medications, prn Bowel intervention HL IV	PO medications PO pain medications, prn Bowel intervention DC IV	PO medications PO pain medications, prn Bowel intervention	PO medications PO pain medications, prn Bowel intervention	Pain under control by self report on oral analgesics Abdomen soft Reports GI comfort
Dangle 2–3 times. Logroll · **Stand in AM 8–10 minutes for brace mold** Chair 30 minutes maximum	Stand, sit in chair for meals Progress activity per MD order	Sit in chair for meals Progress activity Wear brace as ordered	Sit in chair for meals Progress to independence or goal Wear brace as ordered	Progress to independence or goal Wear brace as ordered	Independent in/out of bed and ambulates with/without assistive device
☐ PT advance activity as tolerated including transfers and gait ☐ OT: Increase independent lower extremities with bed mobility, standing tolerance and precautions.	☐ PT advance activity as tolerated including transfers, gait and home exercise program. ☐ OT: Independent in lower extremities self care. Independent with caregiver transfer training.	☐ PT advance to stairs ☐ OT Don/Doff brace with assistance Independent in transfer activities (car, toilet, chair, shower chair)	☐ PT/OT: Order equipment as needed Review progression of activity after discharge		Client meets physical therapy D/C criteria
VS BID CSM BID GI/GU BID Pulmonary BID Discontinue O$_2$ sat. Neurological Q shift Cardiovascular Q shift Musculoskeletal Q shift Skin assessment Q shift Psychosocial/Behavioral Assessment Q shift	VS BID CSM BID GI/GU BID Pulmonary BID Neurological Q shift Cardiovascular Q shift Musculoskeletal Q shift Skin assessment Q shift Psychosocial/Behavioral Assessment Q shift	VS BID CSM BID GI/GU BID Pulmonary BID Neurological Q shift Cardiovascular Q shift Musculoskeletal Q shift Skin assessment Q shift Psychosocial/Behavioral Assessment Q shift	VS BID CSM BID GI/GU BID Pulmonary BID Neurological Q shift Cardiovascular Q shift Musculoskeletal Q shift Skin assessment Q shift Psychosocial/Behavioral Assessment Q shift	VS BID CSM BID GI/GU BID Pulmonary BID Neurological Q shift Cardiovascular Q shift Musculoskeletal Q shift Skin assessment Q shift Psychosocial/Behavioral Assessment Q shift	Temp < 38 for 24 hours prior to D/C; CSM status same as prior to surgery or improved; All systems returned to baseline Coping appropriately; communicates needs and concerns

Adult

637

	Pre Admit	Day of Surgery	Day 1 / /	Day 2 / /
10. IV Access IV WNL: No erythema, drainage, tenderness or swelling. Document time for IV assessment / interventions		insert date / WNL / erythema / drainage / tender / swelling / site care / tubing change / line D/C DOS TYPE SITE TYPE SITE TYPE SITE	insert date / WNL / erythema / drainage / tender / swelling / site care / tubing change / line D/C DAY 1 TYPE SITE TYPE SITE TYPE SITE	insert date / WNL / erythema / drainage / tender / swelling / site care / tubing change / line D/C DAY 2 TYPE SITE TYPE SITE TYPE SITE
11. Client Teaching ICS-Incentive Spirometer TCDB-turn, cough, deep breathe	Client teaching re: D/C options, post hospitalization destination options, purpose of invasive lines/tubes, ICU stay, PCA use, diet advancement Give clinical pathway client version	Teach PCA and ICS, logroll, positioning, T,C,DB Confirm client has received client version of clinical pathway	Review PCA, ICS, logroll, positioning, T,C,DB Reinforce PT bed exercises and activity progress Review client version of clinical pathway	Explain brace molding procedure Review dangling Teach anxiety reduction strategies Evaluate client for *Bridge to Home* protocol Give *Bridge to Home* pamphlet if appropriate Review client version of clinical pathway
12. Pain Relief		Verbalize acceptable level of pain at _____ Uses PCA appropriately	Verbalizes acceptable level of pain at _____ and able to cooperate with activities Uses PCA appropriately	Verbalizes acceptable level of pain at _____ and able to cooperate with activities Uses PCA appropriately
13. Physical Mobility		Logrolls and repositions with maximal assistance	Logrolls with moderate–maximal assistance Participates in PT exercises and activity progression	Logrolls with mod-max assist Dangles 2 times, maximal assistance Stands 5 minutes
14. Tissue Perfusion		CSM status at baseline	CSM status at baseline	CSM status at baseline
15. Respiratory Function		Cooperates with C.T. & DB Uses ICS, O$_2$ sat > 94% Respiratory system WNL	C.T. & DB Uses ICS q 1 hour volume _____ O$_2$ sat. > 94% Respiratory system WNL	C.T. & DB Uses ICS q2-hours volume _____ O$_2$ sat. > 94% Respiratory system WNL
16. Skin Integrity		WNL: skin warm, dry and intact Normal color and turgor PURV_____	WNL: skin warm, dry and intact Normal color and turgor	WNL: skin warm, dry and intact Normal color and turgor
17. Anxiety		Receives information about postop care	Receives information about postop activities and procedures Participates in care Exhibits mild to severe anxiety	Receives information about activities Participates in care Begins to use functional coping mechanisms Verbalizes fears and concerns
18. Bowel and Bladder Function		Urine output > 30 cc/hour Bowel sounds minimal or absent Abdomen soft, nontender	Urine output > 30 cc/hour Bowel sounds minimal or absent Abdomen soft, nontender	Urine output > 30 cc/hour Bowel sounds present Abdomen soft, nontender Passing flatus or has a bowel movement
19. Musculoskeletal Neurological Cardiovascular Sysems Function		Systems WNL	Systems WNL	Systems WNL
20. Self Care Ability			Verbalizes understanding of care needs, assists staff as able	Washes face, arms and chest
21. Safety Falls Assessment *Follow orthopedic standardized NCP		65 or older 1 Mental status limitations 5 History of falls 5 Mobility limitations 4 Elimination problems 2 Medications 1 TOTAL SCORE ___*	65 or older 1 Mental status limitations 5 History of falls 5 Mobility limitations 4 Elimination problems 2 Medications 1 TOTAL SCORE ___*	65 or older 1 Mental status limitations 5 History of falls 5 Mobility limitations 4 Elimination problems 2 Medications 1 TOTAL SCORE ___*

CLIENT OUTCOME

Adult

Day 3	Day 4	Day 5	Day 6	Day 7	Date———
(grid: insert date, WNL, erythema, drainage, tender, swelling, site care, tubing change, line D/C — TYPE/SITE ×3)	(grid ×3)	(grid ×3)	(grid ×3)	(grid ×3)	
Give "After Spine Surgery" booklet. Reinforce anxiety reduction strategies Start *Bridge to Home* program Review client version of clinical pathway	Review brace molding Reinforce PT body mechanics *Bridge to Home* Program Review client version of clinical pathway	Review "After Spine Surgery" booklet with client and family Reinforce relaxation techniques and deep breathing *Bridge to Home* Program Reinforce brace Don/ Doff Technique Review client version of clinical pathway	Reinforce PT instructions *Bridge to Home* Program Review client version of clinical pathway	Instruct discharge medications/ follow-up appointments and give prescriptions Give certificate for completion of *Bridge to Home* Program Review client version of clinical pathway	Able to verbalize S+S$_x$ of wound infection, brace and skin care, activity progression, limitations, medications, when to call physician
Verbalizes pain at acceptable level Uses PCA appropriately w/o basal + takes PO pain medication around the clock	Verbalizes pain at acceptable level on PO prn pain medication	Pain at acceptable level with PO medication prn	Pain at acceptable level with PO medication prn	Pain at acceptable level with PO medication prn	Pain at acceptable level with PO medication prn
Logrolls minimal–moderate assistance Dangles 2 times, moderate assistance Stands 8–10 minutes for brace mold	Gets in/out of bed moderate assistance Sits in chair for meals 1–2 times Walks in room, moderate-maximal	Gets in/out of bed minimal assistance Sits in chair 2–3 times Walks in hall, moderate assistance 3 times Wearing brace as ordered Reports need for adjustment of brace	Gets in/out of bed Sits in chair 2–3 times Walks in hall minimal assistance 3 times	Gets in/out of bed independently Sits in chair 2–3 times Walks independently 3 times Reports brace correctly fitting	Independent in/out of bed Walking on level and up/down stairs or reached goal Client/family demonstrate on/off brace technique
CSM status at baseline	CSM status at baseline	CSM status at baseline	CSM status at baseline	CSM status at baseline	CSM status at baseline
C.T. & DB Uses ICS q 2° volume ____ O$_2$ sat.> 94% on room air Respiratory system WNL	Uses ICS independently volume ____ Respiratory system WNL	Uses ICS independently volume ____ Respiratory system WNL	Uses ICS independently; volume ____ Respiratory system WNL	Respiratory system WNL	Respiratory system WNL
WNL: skin warm, dry and intact Normal color and turgor PURV ____	WNL: skin warm dry and intact Normal color and turgor	WNL: skin warm, dry and intact. Normal color and turgor	WNL: skin warm, dry and intact Normal color and turgor PURV ____	WNL: skin warm, dry and intact Normal color and turgor	Skin clean, dry, and intact Wound well–approximated without redness/swelling
Receives and verbalizes understanding of information booklet Participates in care Anxiety reduction strategies Able to group requests Exhibits decreased anxiety	Verbalizes understanding of information Participates in care Able to use anxiety reduction strategies	Verbalizes understanding of information Participates in care Able to make decisions	Discusses plans for going home Participates in care Makes decisions	Verbalizes ability to manage at home Participates in care Makes decisions	Verbalizes ability to manage at home and/or with continuing care arrangements
Voiding without difficulty Bowel sounds present Abdomen nontender Passing flatus or has a bowel movement	Voiding without difficulty Bowel sounds present Abdomen nontender Passing flatus or has a bowel movement	Voiding Bowel sounds present Abdomen nontender Passing flatus or has a bowel movement	Voiding Bowel sounds present Abdomen nontender Passing flatus, and has a bowel movement	Voiding Bowel sounds present Abdomen nontender Passing flatus, or has a bowel movement	Voiding Had BM during hospitalization
Systems WNL	Systems WNL	Systems WNL	Systems WNL	Systems WNL	Systems WNL
Washes areas in reach Feeds self	Washes areas in reach Feeds self	Bathes self with minimal assistance	Bathes and toilets self with minimal assistance	Independent in self care or reaches goal	Independent in self care or reaches goal
65 or older 1 Mental status limitations 5 History of falls 5 Mobility limitations 4 Elimination problems 2 Medications _ 1 TOTAL SCORE ____*	65 or older 1 Mental status limitations 5 History of falls 5 Mobility limitations 4 Elimination problems 2 Medications _ 1 TOTAL SCORE ____*	65 or older 1 Mental status limitations 5 History of falls 5 Mobility limitations 4 Elimination problems 2 Medications 1 TOTAL SCORE ____*	65 or older 1 Mental status limitations 5 History of falls 5 Mobility limitations 4 Elimination problems 2 Medications 1 TOTAL SCORE ____*	65 or older 1 Mental status limitations 5 History of falls 5 Mobility limitations 4 Elimination problems 2 Medications 1 TOTAL SCORE ____*	No falls

Adult

639

f. Involved muscles become spastic and hyper-reflexic within days or weeks.

◆ **E. Analysis/nursing diagnosis:**
1. *Ineffective breathing pattern* related to high-level injury.
2. *Impaired physical mobility* related to injuries affecting lower limbs.
3. *Fear* related to uncertain future health status.
4. *Anxiety* related to loss of control over own activities of daily living.
5. *Bathing/hygiene self-care deficit* related to injuries above T-1.
6. *Impaired home maintenance management* related to possible quadriplegia and paraplegia.
7. *Risk for altered body temperature* related to absence of sweating below level of injury.
8. *Risk for injury* related to equipment necessary for daily activities.
9. *Tactile sensory/perceptual alterations* related to injury level.
10. *Body image disturbance* related to permanent change in physical status.

◆ **F. Nursing care plan/implementation:**
1. Goal: *maintain patent airway.*
   ▶ a. Suction, cough, tracheostomy care, prn.
   ▶ b. Oxygen, ventilator care.
   c. Monitor blood gas levels.
2. Goal: *prevent further damage.*
   a. Immobilize spine.
   b. Firm mattress, *Stryker frame, Foster frame, CircO-electric* bed, traction, braces (see **III. Fractures, p. 619**).
   c. Skeletal traction via tongs: *Crutchfield, Gardner-Wells* (see **III. Fractures, p. 620**).
   d. *Halo* traction (see **III. Fractures, p. 620**).
3. Goal: *relieve edema: antiinflammatory* medications, *corticosteroids.*
4. Goal: *relieve discomfort: analgesics, sedatives, muscle relaxants.*
5. Goal: *promote comfort:*
   a. Maintain fluid intake: PO/IV, I&O.
   b. Increase nutritional intake.
   c. Prevent contractures and decubiti.
   d. Assist client to deal with psychosocial issues (e.g., role changes).
   e. Begin rehabilitation plan.
6. Goal: *prevent complications.*
   a. Monitor for *spinal shock* during *initial* phase of injury (see **XIII. Spinal shock, p. 640**).
   b. Monitor for *hyperreflexia* with severed spinal cord injuries (see **XIV. Autonomic hyper-reflexia, p. 641**).
7. Goal: *health teaching.*
   a. Self-care techniques for highest level of independence; include significant others in teaching.
   b. How to use ambulation assistive devices (battery-operated wheelchair controlled by mouthpiece or hand controls, depending on level of paralysis).

c. Identify community resources for follow-up care and career counseling.
d. Signs and symptoms of autonomic hyper-reflexia (see **XIV. p. 641**).
e. Methods to prevent skin breakdown, infections of respiratory, urinary tract.
f. Bowel, bladder program.

◆ **G. Evaluation/outcome criteria:**
1. Complications avoided.
2. Accomplishes self-care to greatest level for injury.
3. Participates in rehabilitation plan.
4. Grieves over loss and begins to integrate self into society.

XIII. Spinal shock: temporary flaccid paralysis and areflexia following a severe injury to the spinal cord.
A. Pathophysiology: squeezing or shearing of the spinal cord due to fractures or dislocation of vertebrae; interruption of sensory tracts; loss of conscious sensation; interruption of motor tracts; loss of voluntary movement; loss of facilitation; loss of reflex activity; loss of muscle tone; loss of stretch reflexes, leading to bowel and bladder retention. If injury between *T-1 and L-2*, leads to loss of sympathetic tone and *decrease* in *blood pressure. Afferent* impulses are unable to ascend from below the injured site to the brain, and *efferent* impulses are unable to descend to points below the site.

B. Risk factors:
1. Automobile/motorcycle accidents.
2. Athletic accidents (e.g., diving in shallow water).
3. Gunshot wounds.

◆ **C. Assessment:**
1. *Subjective data:*
   a. Loss of sensation below level of injury.
   b. Inability to move extremities.
   c. Pain at level of injury.
2. *Objective data:*
   a. *Neurological* exam:
      (1) *Absent:* pinprick, pressure, and vibratory sensations below level of injury; reflexes below level of injury.
      (2) Muscles: flaccid.
   b. *Vital signs:*
      (1) *BP decreased* (loss of vasomotor tone below level of injury).
      (2) *Bradycardia.*
      (3) *Elevated temperature.*
      (4) *Respirations:* may be *depressed*; possible respiratory failure if diaphragm involved.
   c. Absence of sweating below level of injury.
   d. Urinary retention.
   e. Abdominal distention: retention of feces, paralytic ileus.
   f. Skin: cold, clammy.

◆ **D. Analysis/nursing diagnosis:**
1. *Decreased cardiac output* related to loss of vasomotor tone below level of injury.

2. *Ineffective breathing pattern* related to injuries involving diaphragm.
3. Impaired *physical mobility* related to loss of voluntary movement of limbs.
4. *Urinary retention* related to loss of stretch reflexes.
5. *Fear* related to serious physical condition.
6. *Risk for injury* related to potential organ damage if shock continues.

◆ **E. Nursing care plan/implementation:**
   1. Goal: *prevent injury related to shock.*
   ▶ a. Maintain patent airway: intubation and mechanical ventilation may be necessary with cervical spinal injuries due to involvement of diaphragm.
      b. Monitor vital signs; *profound hypotension* and *bradycardia* are **most dangerous** *aspects* of spinal shock.
   ⬭ c. Administer blood/IV fluids as ordered.
      d. Nutrition and hydration:
         (1) NPO in *acute* stage: maintain nutrition by IV infusions as ordered.
      🍽 (2) When allowed to eat: *high protein, high calorie, high vitamin diet.*
   ▨ e. Maintain proper *position* to prevent further injury.
         (1) Backboard is necessary to transport from place of injury.
         (2) Support head in neutral alignment and prevent flexion.
         (3) Skeletal traction will be applied once diagnosis is made.
   ▶ f. Monitor urinary output q1h; may have Foley catheter while in shock; later, intermittent catheterization will be used as needed.
   ⬭▶ g. Relieve bowel distention; use lubricant containing *anesthetic,* as necessary, when checking for or removing impaction.

◆ **F. Evaluation/outcome criteria:**
   1. Complications are avoided.
   2. Body functions are maintained.

XIV. **Autonomic dysreflexia** (autonomic hyperreflexia): a group of symptoms in which many spinal cord autonomic responses are activated simultaneously. This may occur when cord lesions are *above the sixth thoracic* vertebra; it is *most commonly* seen with *cervical* and *high thoracic* cord injuries; may occur up to 6 yr after injury.
   A. Pathophysiology: pathological reflex condition, which is an acute **medical emergency** characterized by extreme hypertension and exaggerated autonomic responses to stimuli.
   B. Risk factors:
      1. Distention of bladder or rectum.
      2. Stimulation of skin, e.g., decubitus ulcers, wrinkled clothing.
      3. Stimulation of pain receptors.
   ◆ **C. Assessment:**
      1. *Subjective data:*

   a. Severe, pounding headache.
   b. Blurred vision; sees spots in front of eyes.
   c. Nausea.
   d. Restlessness.
   e. Feels flushed.
2. *Objective data:*
   a. *Severe hypertension* (systolic BP may reach 300 mm Hg).
   b. *Bradycardia* (30 to 40/min); fever.
   c. Profuse diaphoresis, *above* level of injury.
   d. Flushing of skin *above* level of injury.
   e. Pale skin *below* level of injury.
   f. Pilomotor spasm (goose flesh); chills.
   g. Nasal congestion.
   h. Distended bladder, bowel.
   i. Skin breakdown.
   j. Seizures.

◆ **D. Analysis/nursing diagnosis:**
   1. *Dysreflexia* related to high spinal cord injury.
   2. *Risk for injury* related to complications of hypertension, stroke.
   3. *Visual sensory/perceptual alteration* related to blurred vision.
   4. *Urinary retention* related to inability to empty bladder due to spinal injury.
   5. *Constipation* related to inability to establish successful bowel training program.
   6. *Impaired skin integrity* related to immobility.

◆ **E. Nursing plan/implementation:**
   1. Goal: *decrease symptoms to prevent serious side effects.*
   ▨ a. *Elevate head of bed;* this lowers BP in persons with high spinal cord injuries.
      b. Identify and correct source of stimulation if possible; notify physician.
      c. Monitor vital signs (BP) q15min and prn; uncontrolled hypertension can lead to stroke, blindness, death.
   ⬭ d. Give medications as ordered: nitrates, nifedipine (Procardia), or hydralazine (Apresoline).
   ▶ 2. Goal: *maintain patency of catheter.*
      a. Monitor output; *palpate* for distended bladder.
      b. Check for tubing kinks; *irrigate* catheter prn.
      c. Insert new catheter **immediately** if blocked. Do *not* Credé (see **Table 7.39, p. 617**) or tap the bladder; it could exacerbate the response.
      d. Culture if infection suspected.
   3. Goal: *promote regular bowel elimination.*
   ▶ a. Bowel training program.
   ⬭ b. Administer *suppository/enemas/laxatives* as ordered and prn.
   ⬭ c. When checking for and removing impaction, first use *anesthetic ointment* (e.g., dibucaine [Nupercainal] ointment) to decrease irritation.
   4. Goal: *prevent decubitus ulcers.*
      a. Meticulous skin care.
   ▨ b. *Position change* q1 to 2h.

c. Flotation pads, alternating pressure mattress on bed and wheelchair.
    5. Goal: *health teaching.*
        a. How to recognize risk factors that could initiate this condition.
        b. Methods to prevent situations that increase risk (e.g., bowel program, bladder program, skin care, position change schedule).
◆ **F. Evaluation/outcome criteria:**
    1. BP remains within normal limits.
    2. No complications occur.

XV. Hyperthyroidism (also called *thyrotoxicosis; Graves' disease*): spectrum of symptoms of accelerated metabolism caused by excessive amounts of circulating thyroid hormone. *Graves' disease* is most common cause of hyperthyroidism. The three components of *Graves' disease* are: (1) *hyperthyroidism*, (2) *ophthalmopathy* (protrusion of the eyes), and (3) *skin lesions* (dermopathy). *Graves' disease* is triggered by: stress, smoking, radiation of the neck, some medications (interleukin-2), and infections. *Treatment* of hyperthyroidism is accomplished by antithyroid medications, radioactive iodine administration (capsule given once), or surgery. Clients may need to take supplemental thyroid hormone (levothyroxine) after treatment.

A. Pathophysiology: diffuse hyperplasia of thyroid gland → overproduction of thyroid hormone and increased blood serum levels. Hormone stimulates mitochondria to increase energy for cellular activities and heat production. As metabolic rate increases, fat reserves are utilized, despite increased appetite and food intake. Cardiac output is increased to meet increased tissue metabolic needs, and peripheral vasodilation occurs in response to increased heat production. Neuromuscular hyperactivity → accentuation of reflexes, anxiety, and increased alimentary tract mobility. *Graves' disease* is caused by stimulation of the gland by immunoglobulins of the IgG class.

B. Risk factors:
    1. Possible autoimmune response resulting in increase of a gamma globulin called *long-acting thyroid stimulator* (LATS).
    2. Occurs in third and fourth decade.
    3. Affects women more than men.
    4. Emotional trauma, infection, increased stress.
    5. Overdose of medications used to treat hypothyroidism.
    6. Use of certain weight-loss products.
    7. Radiation of neck.
◆ **C. Assessment:**
    1. *Subjective data:*
        a. Nervousness, mood swings.
        b. Palpitations.
        c. Heat intolerance.
        d. Dyspnea.
        e. Weakness.

    2. *Objective data:*
        a. *Eyes:* exophthalmos, characteristic stare, lid lag.
        b. *Skin:*
            (1) Warm, moist, velvety.
            (2) Increased sweating; increased melanin pigmentation.
            (3) Pretibial edema with thickened skin and hyperpigmentation.
        c. *Weight:* loss of weight *despite* increased appetite.
        d. *Muscle:* weakness, tremors, hyperkinesia.
        e. *Vital signs:* BP—*increased* systolic pressure, *widened pulse pressure*; tachycardia.
        f. *Goiter:* thyroid gland noticeable and palpable.
        g. *Gynecological:* abnormal menstruation.
        h. GI: frequent bowel movements.
        i. Activity pattern: overactivity leads to fatigue, which leads to depression, which stimulates client into overactivity, and pattern continues. *Danger:* total exhaustion.

        j. Lab data:
            (1) *Elevated:* serum T_4 (>11 µg/100 mL), free T_4 or free T_4 index, T_3 level (>35%) and free T_3 level.
            (2) *Elevated:* thyroid uptake of radioiodine (RAIU).
            (3) *Elevated:* metabolic rate (BMR).
            (4) *Decreased:* WBC caused by *decreased* granulocytosis (<4500).

◆ **D. Analysis/nursing diagnosis:**
    1. *Altered nutrition, less than body requirements*, related to elevated basal metabolic rate.
    2. *Risk for injury* related to exophthalmos and tremors.
    3. *Activity intolerance* related to fatigue from overactivity.
    4. *Fatigue* related to overactivity.
    5. *Anxiety* related to tachycardia.
    6. *Sleep pattern disturbance* related to excessive amounts of circulating thyroid hormone.
◆ **E. Nursing care plan/implementation:**
    1. Goal: *protect from stress:* private room, restrict visitors, quiet environment.
    2. Goal: *promote physical and emotional equilibrium.*
        a. Environment: quiet, cool, well ventilated.
        b. Eye care:
            (1) Sunglasses to protect from photophobia, dust, wind.
            (2) Protective drops (methylcellulose) to soothe exposed cornea.
        c. Diet:
            (1) *High:* calorie, protein, vitamin B.
            (2) 6 meals/day, as needed.
            (3) Weigh daily.
            (4) *Avoid* stimulants (coffee, tea, colas, tobacco).

3. Goal: *prevent complications.*
   a. Medications as ordered:
      (1) Propylthiouracil to block thyroid synthesis; hyperthyroidism returns when therapy is stopped.
      (2) Methimazole (Tapazole) to inhibit synthesis of thyroid hormone.
      (3) Iodine preparations: used in combination with other medications when hyperthyroidism not well controlled; saturated solution of potassium iodide (SSKI) or *Lugol's* solution; more palatable if diluted with water, milk, or juice; give through a *straw* to prevent staining teeth. Takes 2 to 4 wk before results are evident.
      (4) Propranolol (Inderal), atenolol (Tenormin), metoprolol (Lopressor) given to counteract the increased metabolic effect of thyroid hormones, but do not alter their levels. Relieve the symptoms of tachycardia, tremors, and anxiety.
   b. Monitor for *thyroid storm (crisis)*—**medical emergency:** acute episode of thyroid overactivity caused when increased amounts of thyroid hormone are released into the bloodstream and metabolism is markedly increased.

   (1) **Risk factors** for thyroid storm: client with uncontrolled hyperthyroidism (usually *Graves' disease*) who undergoes severe sudden stress, such as:
      (a) Infection.
      (b) Surgery.
      (c) Beginning labor to give birth.
      (d) Taking inadequate antithyroid medications before thyroidectomy.
   (2) **Assessment:**
      (a) *Subjective data*—thyroid storm:
         (i) Apprehension.
         (ii) Restlessness.
      (b) *Objective data*—thyroid storm:
         (i) *Vital signs: elevated* temperature (106°F), hypotension, *extreme* tachycardia.
         (ii) Marked respiratory distress, pulmonary edema.
         (iii) Weakness and delirium.
         (iv) **If untreated, client could die of heart failure.**
   (3) Medications—thyroid storm:
      (a) Propylthiouracil or methimazole (Tapazole) *to decrease synthesis of thyroid hormone.*
      (b) Sodium iodide IV; Lugol solution orally *to facilitate thyroid hormone synthesis.*
      (c) Propranolol (Inderal) *to slow heart rate.*
      (d) Aspirin *to decrease temperature.*
      (e) Steroids *to combat crisis.*
      (f) Diuretics, digitalis *to treat heart failure.*

4. Goal: *health teaching.*
   a. Stress-reduction techniques.
   b. Importance of medications, their desired effects and side effects.
   c. Methods to protect eyes from environmental damage.
   d. Signs and symptoms of thyroid storm (see **E. 3. b.**).
5. Goal: *prepare for additional treatment as needed.*
   a. *Radioactive iodine therapy:* ¹³¹I, a radioactive isotope of iodine to decrease thyroid activity.
      (1) ¹³¹I dissolved in water and given by mouth.
      (2) Hospitalization necessary only when large dose is administered.

      (3) *Minimal precautions* needed for usual dose.
         (a) Sleep alone for several nights.
         (b) Flush toilet several times after use.

      (4) Effectiveness of therapy seen in 2 to 3 wk; single dose controls 90% of clients.
      (5) Monitor for signs of hypothyroidism.
   b. Surgery (see **XVI. Thyroidectomy,** following).

F. Evaluation/outcome criteria:
   1. Complications avoided.
   2. Compliance with medical regimen.
   3. No further weight loss.
   4. Able to obtain adequate sleep.

XVI. Thyroidectomy: partial removal of thyroid gland (for hyperthyroidism) or total removal (for malignancy of thyroid).
   A. Risk factor: unsuccessful medical treatment of hyperthyroidism.
   B. Analysis/nursing diagnosis:
      1. *Risk for injury* related to possible trauma to parathyroid gland during surgery.
      2. *Ineffective breathing pattern* related to neck incision.
      3. *Pain* related to surgical incision.
      4. *Altered nutrition, less than body requirements,* related to difficulty in swallowing because of neck incision.
      5. *Impaired verbal communication* related to possible trauma to nerve during surgery.
      6. *Risk for altered body temperature* related to thyroid storm.
   C. Nursing care plan/implementation: *Prepare for surgery* (see **I. Preoperative preparation, p. 546**). *Postoperative:*
      1. Goal: *promote physical and emotional equilibrium.*

Adult

a. *Position: semi-Fowler's* to reduce edema.

b. *Immobilize* head with pillows/sandbags.

c. Support head during position changes to *avoid* stress on sutures, *prevent flexion* or *hyperextension* of neck.

2. Goal: *prevent complications of hypocalcemia and tetany,* due to accidental trauma to parathyroid gland during surgery; signs of tetany indicate necessity of *calcium gluconate IV.*

   a. Check *Chvostek's sign*—tapping face in front of ear produces spasm of facial muscles.

   b. Check *Trousseau's sign*—compression of upper arm (usually with BP cuff) elicits carpal (wrist) spasm.

   c. Monitor for *respiratory distress* (due to laryngeal nerve injury, edema, bleeding); keep tracheostomy set/suction equipment at bedside.

   d. Monitor for elevated temperature, indicative of *thyroid storm* (see **Objective assessment data for thyroid storm**).

   e. Monitor vital signs, check dressing and beneath head, shoulders for bleeding q1h and prn for 24 hr; *hemorrhage* is possible complication; if swallowing is difficult, loosen dressing. If client still complains of tightness when dressing is loosened, look for further signs of hemorrhage.

   f. Check voice postoperatively as soon as responsive after anesthesia and every hour (assess for possible *laryngeal nerve damage*); crowing voice sound indicates laryngeal nerves on both sides have been injured; *respiratory distress possible from swelling.*

      (1) *Avoid* unnecessary talking to lessen hoarseness.

      (2) Provide alternative means of communication.

3. Goal: *promote comfort measures.*

   a. *Narcotics* as ordered.

   b. Offer iced fluids.

   c. Ambulation and *soft diet,* as tolerated.

4. Goal: *health teaching.*

   a. How to support neck to prevent pressure on suture line: place both hands behind neck when moving head or coughing.

   b. Signs of hypothyroidism; needs supplemental thyroid hormone if total thyroidectomy.

   c. Signs and symptoms of hemorrhage and respiratory distress.

   d. Importance of adequate rest and nutritious diet.

   e. Importance of voice rest in early recuperative period.

D. **Evaluation/outcome criteria:**

1. No respiratory distress, hemorrhage, laryngeal damage, tetany.

2. Preoperative symptoms relieved.

3. Normal range of neck motion obtained.

4. States signs and symptoms of possible complications.

XVII. **Hypothyroidism (myxedema):** deficiency of circulating thyroid hormone; often a final consequence of *Hashimoto's thyroiditis* and *Graves' disease.*

A. **Pathophysiology:** atrophy, destruction of gland by endogenous antibodies or inadequate pituitary thyrotropin production → insidious slowing of body processes, personality changes, and generalized, interstitial nonpitting (mucinous) edema—myxedema; pronounced involvement in systems with high protein turnover (e.g., cardiac, GI, reproductive, hematopoietic).

B. **Risk factors:**

1. Total thyroidectomy; inadequate replacement therapy.

2. Inherited autosomal recessive gene coding for disorder.

3. Hypophyseal failure.

4. Dietary iodine deficiencies.

5. Irradiation of thyroid gland.

6. Overtreatment of hyperthyroidism.

7. Chronic lymphocytic thyroiditis.

8. Postpartum thyroiditis.

9. Viral thyroiditis.

10. Medications, such as amiodarone HCl (Cordarone), used to treat abnormal heart rhythms.

C. **Assessment:**

1. *Subjective data:*

   a. Weakness, fatigue, lethargy.

   b. Headache.

   c. Slow memory, psychotic behavior.

   d. Loss of interest in sexual activity.

2. *Objective data:*

   a. Depressed basal metabolism rate (BMR).

   b. Cardiomegaly, bradycardia, hypotension, anemia.

   c. Menorrhagia, amenorrhea, infertility.

   d. Dry skin, brittle nails, coarse hair, hair loss.

   e. Slow speech, hoarseness, thickened tongue.

   f. Weight gain: edema, generalized interstitial; peripheral nonpitting; periorbital puffiness.

   g. Intolerance to cold.

   h. Hypersensitive to narcotics and barbiturates.

   i. *Lab data:*

      (1) *Elevated:* thyroid-releasing hormone (TRH), thyroid-stimulating hormone (TSH), cholesterol (>220 mg/dL), lipids (>850 mg/dL), protein (>8g/dL).

      (2) *Normal-low:* serum thyroxine (T_4), serum triiodothyrinine (T_3).

      (3) *Decreased:* radioactive iodine uptake (RAIU).

D. Analysis/nursing diagnosis:
1. *Risk for injury* related to hypersensitivity to drugs.
2. *Altered nutrition, more than body requirements,* related to decreased BMR.
3. *Activity intolerance* related to fatigue.
4. *Constipation* related to decreased peristalsis.
5. *Decreased cardiac output* related to hypotension and bradycardia.
6. *Risk for impaired skin integrity* related to dry skin and edema.
7. *Social isolation* related to lethargy.

E. Nursing care plan/implementation:
1. Goal: *provide for comfort and safety.*
   a. Monitor for infection or trauma; may precipitate *myxedema coma,* which is manifested by: unresponsiveness, bradycardia, hypoventilation, hypothermia, and hypotension.
   b. Provide warmth; prevent heat loss and vascular collapse.
   c. Administer thyroid medications as ordered: levothyroxine (Synthroid)—most common drug used; liothyronine sodium (Cytomel); dosage adjusted according to symptoms.
2. Goal: *health teaching.*
   a. *Diet: low* calorie, *high* protein.
   b. Signs and symptoms of hypothyroidism and hyperthyrodism.
   c. Lifelong medications, dosage, desired effects and side effects.
   d. Medication dosage adjustment: *take one-third to one-half the usual dose of narcotics and barbiturates.*
   e. Stress-management techniques.
   f. Exercise program.

F. Evaluation/outcome criteria:
1. No complications noted. Most common complications: atherosclerotic coronary heart disease, acute organic psychosis, and myxedema coma.
2. Dietary instructions followed.
3. Medication regimen followed.
4. Thyroid hormone balance obtained and maintained.

XVIII. Cushing's disease: an endogenous overproduction of adrenocorticotropic hormone (ACTH) that can be caused by pituitary-dependent adenomas. **Cushing's syndrome:** condition marked by chronic excessive circulating cortisol with or without pituitary involvement. One of the most common causes of Cushing's syndrome is the administration of cortisone-like medications for treatment of a variety of conditions.

A. Pathophysiology:
1. Excess glucocorticoid production, leading to:
   a. *Increased* gluconeogenesis→raised serum-glucose levels→glucose in urine, increased fat deposits in face and trunk.
   b. *Decreased* amino acids → protein deficiencies, muscle wasting, poor antibody response, and lack of collagen.

B. Risk factors:
1. Adrenal hyperplasia.
2. Excessive hypothalamic stimulation.
3. Tumors: adrenal, hypophyseal, pituitary, bronchogenic, or gallbladder.
4. Excessive steroid therapy.

C. Assessment:
1. *Subjective data:*
   a. Headache, backache.
   b. Weakness, decreased work capacity.
   c. Mood swings.
2. *Objective data:*
   a. Hypertension, weight gain, pitting edema.
   b. Characteristic fat deposits, truncal and cervical obesity (*buffalo hump*).
   c. Pendulous abdomen, purple striae, easy bruising.
   d. Moon face, acne.
   e. Hyperpigmentation.
   f. Impotence.
   g. Virilization in women: hirsutism, breast atrophy, and amenorrhea.
   h. Pathological fractures, reduced height.
   i. Slow wound healing.
   j. Lab data:
      (1) Urine: *elevated* 17-ketosteroids (>12 mg/24 hr) and glucose (>120 mg/dL).
      (2) Plasma: *elevated* 17-hydroxycorticosteroids, cortisol (>10 μg/dL). Cortisol *does not decrease during the day* as it should.
      (3) Serum: *elevated*—glucose, RBC, WBC; *diminished*—potassium, chlorides, eosinophils, lymphocytes.
   k. X-rays and scans to determine tumors/metastasis.

D. Analysis/nursing diagnosis:
1. *Body image disturbance* related to changes in physical appearance.
2. *Activity intolerance* related to backache and weakness.
3. *Risk for injury* related to infection and bleeding.
4. *Knowledge deficit* (learning need) related to management of disease.
5. *Pain* related to headache.

E. Nursing care plan/implementation.
1. Goal: *promote comfort.*
   a. Assist with preparation of diagnostic work-up.
   b. Explain procedures.
   c. Protect from trauma.

2. Goal: *prevent complications;* monitor for:

a. Fluid balance—I&O, daily weights.

b. Glucose metabolism—blood, urine for sugar and acetone.

c. Hypertension—vital signs.

d. Infection—skin care, urinary tract; check temperature.

e. Mood swings—observe behavior.

3. Goal: *health teaching.*

a. *Diet:* increased protein, potassium; *decreased* calories, sodium.

b. Medications:

(1) *Cytotoxic agents:* aminoglutethimide (Cytadren), trilostane (Modrastane), mitotane (Lysodren)—decrease cortisol production.

(2) *Replacement hormones* as needed.

c. Signs and symptoms of progression of disease as noted in assessment.

d. Preparation for adrenalectomy if medical regimen unsuccessful.

◆ F. **Evaluation/outcome criteria:**

1. Symptoms controlled by medication.

2. No complications—adrenal steroids within normal limits.

3. If adrenalectomy necessary (see **XX. Adrenalectomy**).

XIX. **Pheochromocytoma:** a rare, typically benign neuroendocrine tumor of the adrenal medulla. Appears to have a familial basis; common in middle age—rare after 60 yrs.

A. **Pathophysiology:** catecholamine-secreting tumor → ↑ epinephrine and norepinephrine (paroxysm) → hypertensive retinopathy and nephropathy, myocarditis → cerebral hemorrhage and cardiac failure.

B. **Risk factors for paroxysm:**

1. Voiding.

2. Smoking.

3. Drugs (i.e., histamine, anesthesia, atropine, steroids, fentanyl).

4. Bending, straining, exercising (displacing abdominal organs) → ↑ abdominal pressure.

◆ C. **Assessment:**

1. *Subjective data*

a. Apprehension.

b. Pounding headache.

c. Nausea.

d. Pain with vomiting.

e. Visual disturbances.

f. Palpitations.

g. Heat intolerance.

2. *Objective data*

a. Hypertension: rapid onset, abrupt cessation; postural hypotension.

b. Profuse diaphoresis with acute attack.

c. Pulse: rapid, dysrhythmia.

d. Pupils: dilated.

e. Extremities: cold, tremors.

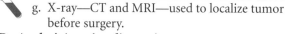

f. Lab data:

(1) Hyperglycemia, glycosuria.

(2) ↑Urinary catecholamines: single-voided, 2 to 4 hr specimen and 24-hr urine, >14 mg/100 mL.

(3) Direct assay of catecholamines—epinephrine >0.2 mg/L; norepinephrine 0.5 mg/L.

(4) ↑BMR.

g. X-ray—CT and MRI—used to localize tumor before surgery.

◆ D. **Analysis/nursing diagnosis:**

1. *Anxiety* related to excessive physiological stimulation of sympathetic nervous system.

2. *Fluid volume deficit* related to excessive gastric losses, hypermetabolic state, diaphoresis.

3. *Risk for decreased cardiac output* related to excessive secretions of catecholamines as evidenced by hypertension.

4. *Risk for injury* related to excessive release of epinephrine and norepinephrine.

5. *Altered nutrition, greater than body requirements,* related to elevated glucose.

◆ E. **Nursing care plan/implementation:**

1. Goal: *prevent paroxysmal hypertension.*

a. Rest: reduce stress, ↓ environmental stimulation.

b. Give *sedatives, alpha-adrenergic blocker* (phenoxybenzamine) for hypertension and *anti-dysrhythmics* as ordered.

c. *Diet:* high vitamin, *high* calorie, mineral, calcium; *restrict* caffeine.

d. Monitor VS (especially BP in sitting and supine positions).

2. Goal: *prepare for surgical removal of tumor* (see **XX. Adrenalectomy**).

◆ F. **Evaluation/outcome criteria:**

1. No paroxysmal hypertension.

2. See **XX. Adrenalectomy.**

XX. **Adrenalectomy:** surgical removal of adrenal glands because of tumors or uncontrolled overactivity; also bilateral adrenalectomy may be performed to control metastatic breast or prostate cancer.

A. **Risk factors:**

1. Pheochromocytoma.

2. Adrenal hyperplasia.

3. Cushing's syndrome.

4. Metastasis of prostate or breast cancer.

5. Adrenal cortex or medulla tumors.

◆ B. **Assessment:**

1. *Objective data:* validated evidence of:

a. Benign lesion (unilateral adrenalectomy) or malignant tumor (bilateral adrenalectomy).

b. Adrenal hyperfunction that cannot be managed medically.

c. Bilateral excision for metastasis of breast and sometimes metastasis of prostate cancer.

C. **Analysis/nursing diagnosis:**
1. *Knowledge deficit* (learning need) related to planned surgery.
2. *Risk for physical injury* related to hormone imbalance.
3. *Risk for decreased cardiac output* related to possible hypotensive state resulting from surgery.
4. *Risk for infection* related to decreased normal resistance.
5. *Altered health maintenance* related to need for self-administration of steroid medications, orally or by injection.

D. **Nursing care plan/implementation:**
1. Goal: *preoperative: reduce risk of postoperative complications.*
   a. Prescribed *steroid* therapy, given 1 wk before surgery, is gradually decreased; will be given again postoperatively.
   b. *Antihypertensive* drugs are *discontinued* because surgery may result in severe hypotension.
   c. *Sedation* as ordered.
   d. General preoperative measures (see **p. 546**).
2. Goal: *postoperative: promote hormonal balance.*
   a. Administer *hydrocortisone* parenteral therapy as ordered; rate indicated by fluid and electrolyte balance, blood sugar, and blood pressure.
   b. Monitor for signs of *addisonian (adrenal) crisis* (see **p. 648**).
3. Goal: *prevent postoperative complications.*
   a. Monitor vital signs until stability is regained; if on *vasopressor* drugs such as metaraminol (Aramine):
      (1) Maintain flow rate as ordered.
      (2) Monitor BP q5 to 15 min, notify physician of significant elevations in BP (dose needs to be *decreased*) or drop in BP (dose needs to be *increased*). *Note:* readings that are normotensive for some may be hypotensive for clients who have been hypertensive.
   b. NPO—attach *nasogastric tube* to intermittent suction; abdominal distention is common side effect of this surgery.
   c. Respiratory care:

   > (1) Turn, cough, and deep breathe.
   > (2) Splint flank incision when coughing.
   > (3) Administer *narcotics* to reduce pain and allow client to cough; flank incision is close to diaphragm, making coughing very painful.
   > (4) Auscultate breath sounds q2hr; decreased or absent sounds could indicate *pneumothorax*.
   > (5) Sudden chest pain and dyspnea should be reported ***immediately*** (*spontaneous pneumothorax*).

   d. *Position: flat* or *semi*-Fowler's.
   e. Mouth care.
   f. Monitor dressings for bleeding; reinforce prn.
   g. Ambulation, as ordered.
      (1) Check BP q15min when ambulation is first attempted.
      (2) Place elastic stockings on lower extremities to enhance stability of vascular system.
   h. *Diet*—once NG tube removed, diet as tolerated.
4. Goal: *health teaching.*

   a. *Signs and symptoms of adrenal crisis:*
      (1) Pulse: rapid, weak, or thready.
      (2) Temperature: elevated.
      (3) Severe weakness and hypotension.
      (4) Headache.
      (5) Convulsions, coma.

   b. Importance of maintaining steroid therapy schedule to ensure therapeutic serum level.
   c. Weigh daily.
   d. Monitor blood-glucose levels daily.
   e. Report undesirable side effects of steroid therapy or adrenal crisis to physician.
   f. *Avoid* persons with infections, due to decreased resistance.
   g. Daily schedule: include adequate rest, moderate exercise, good nutrition.

E. **Evaluation/outcome criteria:**
1. Adrenal crisis avoided.
   a. Vitals within normal limits.
   b. No neurological deficits noted.
2. Healing progresses: no signs of infection or wound complications.
3. Adjusts to alterations in physical status.
   a. Complies with medication regimen.
   b. Avoids infections.
   c. Incorporates good nutrition, periods of rest and activity into daily schedule.

XXI. **Addison's disease:** chronic primary adrenal corticotropic insufficiency. A hormonal (endocrine) disorder involving destruction of the adrenal glands, which then are unable to produce sufficient adrenal hormones (cortisol) necessary for the normal body functions.

A. **Pathophysiology:**
1. Atrophy of adrenal gland is most common cause of adrenal insufficiency; manifested by *decreased* adrenal cortical secretions.
   a. Deficiency in mineralocorticoid secretion *(aldosterone)*→increased sodium excretion→dehydration→hypotension→decreased cardiac output and resulting decrease in heart size.
   b. Deficiency in glucocorticoid secretion *(cortisol)*→decrease in gluconeogenesis→ hypogly-

Adult

cemia and liver glycogen deficiency, emotional disturbances, diminished resistance to stress. Cortisol deficiency→failure to inhibit anterior pituitary secretion of ACTH and melanocyte-stimulating hormone→increased levels of ACTH and hyperpigmentation.

    c. Deficiency in androgen hormone → less axillary and pubic hair in women (testes supply adequate sex hormone in men, so no symptoms are produced).

B. Risk factors:
1. Autoimmune processes.
2. Infection.
3. Malignancy.
4. Vascular obstruction.
5. Bleeding.
6. Environmental hazards.
7. Congenital defects.
8. Bilateral adrenalectomy.
9. Tuberculosis.

◆ **C. Assessment:**
1. *Subjective data:*
   a. Muscle weakness, fatigue, lethargy.
   b. Dizziness, fainting.
   c. Nausea, food idiosyncrasies, anorexia.
   d. Abdominal pain/cramps.
2. *Objective data:*
   a. *Vital signs: decreased BP,* orthostatic hypotension, *widened* pulse pressure.
   b. Pulse—*increased,* collapsing, irregular.
   c. Temperature—*subnormal.*
   d. Vomiting, diarrhea, and weight loss.
   e. Tremors.
   f. Skin: poor turgor, excessive pigmentation (*bronze tone*).
   g. Lab data:
      (1) Blood:
         (a) *Decreased:* sodium (<135 mEq/L); glucose (<60 mg/dL), chloride (<98 mEq/L), bicarbonate (<23 mEq/L).
         (b) *Increased:* hematocrit, potassium (>5 mEq/L).
      (2) Urine: *decreased* (or absent) 17-ketosteroids, 17-hydroxycorticosteroids (<5 mg/24 hr).
    h. *Diagnostic tests:*
      (1) CT scan, MRI.
      (2) ACTH stimulation test (cortisol levels are measured *before* and *after* administration of synthetic ACTH).

◆ **D. Analysis/nursing diagnosis:**
1. *Fluid volume deficit* related to decreased sodium.
2. *Altered renal tissue perfusion* related to hypotension.
3. *Decreased cardiac output* related to aldosterone deficiency.
4. *Risk for infection* related to cortisol deficiency.
5. *Activity intolerance* related to muscle weakness and fatigue.

6. *Altered nutrition, less than body requirements,* related to nausea, anorexia, and vomiting.

◆ **E. Nursing care plan/implementation:**
1. Goal: *decrease stress.*
   a. Environment: quiet, nondemanding schedule.
   b. Anticipate events for which extra resources will be necessary.
2. Goal: *promote adequate nutrition.*
   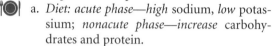 a. *Diet: acute phase—high* sodium, *low* potassium; *nonacute phase—increase* carbohydrates and protein.
   b. *Fluids: force,* to balance fluid losses; monitor I&O, daily weights.
   c. Administer lifelong exogenous replacement therapy as ordered:
      (1) *Glucocorticoids*—prednisone, hydrocortisone.
      (2) *Mineralocorticoids*—fludrocortisone (Florinef).
3. Goal: *health teaching.*
   a. Take medications *with* food or milk.
   b. May need antacid therapy to prevent GI disturbances.
   c. Side effects of steroid therapy.
   d. *Avoid* stress; may need adjustment in medication dosage when stress is increased.
   e. Signs and symptoms of *addisonian (adrenal) crisis:* very serious condition characterized by severe hypotension, shock, coma, and vasomotor collapse related to strenuous activity, infection, stress, omission of prescribed medications. **If untreated, could quickly lead to death.**
4. Goal: *prevent serious complications if addisonian crisis evident.*
   a. Complete bedrest; *avoid* stimuli.
   b. High dose of hydrocortisone IV or cortisone IM.
   c. Treat shock—IV saline.
   d. I&O, vital signs q15min to 1 hr or prn until crisis passes.

◆ **F. Evaluation/outcome criteria:**
1. No complications occur.
2. Medication regimen followed, is adequate for client's needs.
3. Adequate nutrition and fluid balance obtained.

XXII. Multiple sclerosis: progressive neurological disease, common in northern climates, characterized by demyelination of brain and spinal cord leading to degenerative neurological function; chronic remitting and relapsing disease; cause unknown. Visual problems are often the first indication of multiple sclerosis. Classifications of multiple sclerosis: relapsing-remitting, primary-progressive, secondary-progressive, and progressive-relapsing. Exacerbations aggravated by fatigue, chilling, and emotional distress.

A. Pathophysiology: multiple foci (patches) of nerve degeneration throughout brain, spinal cord, optic nerve, and cerebrum cause nerve impulses to be interrupted (blocked) or distorted (slowed). Researchers suggest that in genetically susceptible people, the disease results from an abnormal autoimmune response to some agent, perhaps a virus or environmental trigger.

B. Risk factors:
1. Northern climate.
2. Onset age: 20 to 40 yr.
3. Two to three times more common in women than men.

◆ **C. Assessment:**
1. *Subjective data:*
   a. Extremities: weak, numb, decreased sensation.
   b. Emotional: instability, apathy, irritability, mood swings, fatigue.
   c. Eyes: diplopia (double vision), spots before eyes (scotomas), potential blindness.
   d. Difficulty in swallowing.
   e. Pain.
2. *Objective data:*
   a. Nystagmus (involuntary rhythmic movements of eyeball) and decreased visual acuity.
   b. Inappropriate outbursts of laughing or crying (sometimes related to ingestion of hot food).
   c. Disorders of speech.
   d. Susceptible to infections.
   e. Tremors to severe muscle spasms and contractures.
   f. Changes in muscular coordination; *gait:* ataxic, spastic.
   g. Changes in bowel habits (e.g., constipation).
   h. Urinary frequency and urgency.
   i. Incontinence (urine and feces).
   j. Sexual dysfunction.
   k. Cognitive changes/depression.
   l. *Lab tests:* cerebrospinal fluid has presence of gamma globulin IgG.
   m. *Diagnostic tests:*
      (1) Neurological examination.
      (2) Positive *Lhermitte's* sign (electric shock–like sensation along spine on flexion of the head).
      (3) Positive *Babinski* reflex.
      (4) MRI detects plaques.

◆ **D. Analysis/nursing diagnosis:**
1. *Impaired physical mobility* related to changes in muscular coordination.
2. *Self-esteem disturbance* related to chronic, debilitating disease.
3. *Altered health maintenance* related to spasms and contractures.
4. *Risk for impaired skin integrity* related to contractures.
5. *Constipation* related to immobility.
6. *Impaired swallowing* related to tremors.
7. *Visual sensory/perceptual alteration* related to nystagmus and decreased visual acuity.

◆ **E. Nursing care plan/implementation:**
1. Goal: *maintain normal routine as long as possible.*
   a. Maintain mobility—encourage walking as tolerated; active and passive ROM; splints to decrease spasticity.
   b. *Avoid* fatigue, infections.
   c. Frequent position changes to prevent skin breakdown and contractures; *position at night: prone,* to minimize flexor spasms of knees and hips.
   d. Bowel/bladder training program to minimize incontinence.
   e. *Avoid* stressful situations.
2. Goal: *decrease symptoms*—medications as ordered:
   a. Methylprednisolone (high dose, IV) plus sodium succinate, followed by gradual tapering of steroids to treat at *initial* diagnosis.
   b. Methylprednisolone (Solu-Medrol), prednisone (Deltasone), and dexamethasone (Decadron) used to treat *acute relapses.*
   c. Methotrexate (Rheumatrex) (low dose) used *to delay progression of impairment.*
   d. Interferon β-1ᵦ (Betaseron) reduces *number* of lesions and *frequency of relapses.*
   e. Glatiramer (Copaxone) *to reduce number of relapses.*
   f. Baclofen (Lioresal) for *alleviating spasticity* 5 mg three times daily, increased by 5 mg every 3 days; not to exceed 80 mg/day (20 mg four times daily). Optimal effect between 40 and 80 mg; sudden withdrawal of medication may cause *hallucinations* and *rebound spasticity.*
   g. Diazepam (Valium), dantrolene (Dantrium) to relieve *muscle spasm.*
   h. Carbamazepine (Tegretol) or amitriptyline HCl (Elavil) for *dysesthesias* or *neuralgia.*
   i. Ciprofloxacin (Cipro) to treat *bladder dysfunction.*
   j. Psyllium hydrophilic mucilloid (Metamucil) to treat *bowel dysfunction.*
   k. Phenytoin (Dilantin) to treat *sensory symptoms.*
   l. Analgesics to treat *pain.*
3. Goal: *health teaching to prevent complications.*
   a. Signs and symptoms of disease; measures to prevent exacerbations.
   b. Teach to monitor respiratory status to prevent infections.
   c. Referral: importance of *physical therapy* to prevent contractures.
   d. Referral: possible counseling or community support group for assistance in accepting long-term condition.
   e. Teach special skin care to prevent decubitus ulcers.
   f. Teach use of assistive devices to maintain independence.
4. Goal: *provide psychosocial support.*

Adult

a. Answer questions of client and family members.

b. Provide referrals to appropriate agencies.

c. Monitor for signs of suicide (higher incidence of suicide in clients with MS than the general population).

d. Encourage communication.

◆ **F. Evaluation/outcome criteria:**

1. Establishes daily routine; adjusts to altered lifestyle.

2. Injuries prevented; no falls.

3. Urinary and bowel routines established; incontinence decreased.

4. Infections avoided.

5. Symptoms minimized by medications.

XXIII. Myasthenia gravis: Chronic neuromuscular disease characterized by weakness and easy fatigability of facial, oculomotor, pharyngeal, and respiratory muscles. The muscle weakness increases during periods of activity and improves after periods of rest.

A. Pathophysiology: inadequate acetylcholine or excessive or altered cholinesterase, leading to impaired transmission of nerve impulses to muscles at myoneural junction.

B. Risk factors:

1. Possible autoimmune reaction.

2. Thymus tumor.

3. Young women and older men, but can occur at any age.

◆ **C. Assessment:**

1. *Subjective data:*

a. Diplopia (double vision).

b. Severe generalized fatigue.

2. *Objective data:*

a. Muscle weakness: hands and arms affected first.

b. Ptosis (drooping of eyelids), expressionless facies.

c. Hypersensitivity to narcotics, barbiturates, tranquilizers.

d. Abnormal speech pattern, with high-pitched nasal voice.

e. Difficulty chewing/swallowing food.

f. Decreased ability to cough and deep breathe, vital capacity.

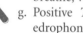 g. Positive *Tensilon test* (administration of edrophonium chloride, 10 mg IV, produces relief of symptoms within 30 sec).

h. Positive *Prostigmin test* (1.5 mg subcutaneous neostigmine methylsulfate, produces relief of symptoms within 15 min; increased muscle strength within 30 min).

◆ **D. Analysis/nursing diagnosis:**

1. *Ineffective breathing pattern* related to weakness.

2. *Risk for injury* related to muscle weakness.

3. *Activity intolerance* related to severe fatigue.

4. *Bathing/dressing self-care deficit* related to progressive disease.

5. *Impaired physical mobility* related to decrease in strength.

6. *Anxiety* related to physical symptoms and disease progression.

7. *Knowledge deficit* (learning need) related to medication administration and expected effectiveness.

◆ **E. Nursing care plan/implementation:**

1. Goal: *promote comfort.*

a. Passive and active ROM, as tolerated, to increase strength.

b. Mouth care: before and after meals.

c. *Diet:* as tolerated, *soft,* pureed, or *tube* feedings.

d. Skin care to prevent decubiti.

e. Eye care: remove crusts; patch affected eye prn.

f. Monitor respiratory status—suction airway prn.

2. Goal: *decrease symptoms.*

a. Administer medications as ordered:

(1) Anticholinesterase (neostigmine [Prostigmin], pyridostigmine [Mestinon]) to elevate concentration of acetylcholine at myoneural junction.

(2) Give *before* meals to aid in chewing, *with* milk or food to *decrease GI symptoms*; may be given parenterally.

3. Goal: *prevent complications.*

a. Respiratory assistance if breathing pattern not adequate.

b. Monitor for choking/increased oral secretion.

c. **Avoid:** narcotics, barbiturates, tranquilizers.

4. Goal: *promote increased self-concept.*

a. Encourage independence when appropriate.

b. Encourage communication; provide alternative methods when speech pattern impaired.

5. Goal: *health teaching.*

a. Medication information:

(1) Adjust dosage to maintain muscle strength.

(2) Medication must be taken at prescribed time to avoid:

(a) *Myasthenic crisis* (too little medication).

(b) *Cholinergic crisis* (too much medication).

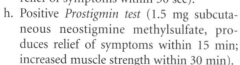 b. *Signs and symptoms of crisis:* dyspnea, severe muscle weakness, respiratory distress, difficulty in swallowing.

c. Importance of *avoiding upper respiratory infections.*

d. Determine methods to conserve energy, to maintain independence as long as possible, while avoiding overexertion.

e. *Refer* to Myasthenia Gravis Foundation and other *community agencies* for assistance in reintegration into the community and plans for follow-up care.

◆ **F. Evaluation/outcome criteria:**

1. Independence maintained as long as possible.

2. Respiratory arrest avoided.

3. Infection avoided.

4. Medication regimen followed and crisis avoided.

XXIV. **Parkinson's disease:** progressive disease of the brain occurring generally in later life; characterized by stiffness of muscles and by tremors.

A. **Pathophysiology:** depigmentation of the substantia nigra of basal ganglia→decreased dopamine (neurotransmitter necessary for proper muscle movement)→decreased and slowed voluntary movement, masklike facies, and difficulty initiating ambulation. Decreased inhibitions of alpha-motoneurons → increased muscle tone → rigidity of both flexor and extensor muscles and tremors at rest.

B. **Risk factors:**

1. Age >40; most often 50 to 60 yr.

2. Affects men and women equally.

3. Cause unknown; possibly connected to arteriosclerosis or viral infection.

4. Drug-induced parkinsonian syndromes have been linked to:

a. Phenothiazines.

b. Reserpine (Serpasil).

c. Butyrophenones (haloperidol).

◆ C. **Assessment:**

1. *Subjective data:*

a. Insomnia.

b. Depression.

c. Defects in judgment related to emotional instability; dementia (memory loss).

2. *Objective data:*

a. Limbs, shoulders: stiff, offer resistance to passive ROM.

b. Loss of coordination, muscular weakness with rigidity.

c. Shuffling gait: difficulty in initiating, then propulsive, trunk bent forward.

d. Tremors: pill-rolling of fingers, to-and-fro head movements.

e. Loss of postural reflexes.

f. Weight loss, constipation.

g. Difficulty in maintaining social interactions because of impaired speech, lack of facial affect, drooling.

h. Facies: wide-eyed, decreased eye blinking, decreased facial expression.

i. Akinesia (abnormal absence of movement).

j. Excessive salivation, drooling.

k. Speech: slowed, slurred.

l. Judgment defective (e.g., poor decision making); intelligence intact.

m. Heat intolerance.

◆ D. **Analysis/nursing diagnosis:**

1. *Impaired physical mobility* related to loss of coordination.

2. *Altered health maintenance* related to defective judgment.

3. *Risk for injury* related to altered gait.

4. *Dressing/grooming self-care deficit* related to muscular rigidity.

5. *Sleep pattern disturbance* related to insomnia.

6. *Body image disturbance* related to tremors and drooling.

7. *Social isolation* related to altered physical appearance.

8. *Altered nutrition, less than body requirements,* related to lack of appetite.

9. *Impaired swallowing* related to excessive drooling.

10. *Constipation* related to dietary changes.

◆ E. **Nursing care plan/implementation:**

1. Goal: *promote maintenance of daily activities.*

a. ROM exercises, skin care, physical therapy.

b. Encourage ambulation; discourage sitting for long periods.

c. Assist with meals—*high protein, high calorie; soft diet;* small, frequent feedings; encourage increased fluids.

d. Encourage compliance with medication regimen:

(1) *Dopamine agonists:*

(a) Levodopa: given in increasing doses until symptoms are relieved; given *with food* to decrease GI symptoms. *Side effects:* nausea, vomiting, anorexia, postural hypotension, mental changes, cardiac arrhythmias. Levodopa (L-Dopa) helps *restore dopamine deficiency* in striated muscles: 500 to 1000 mg/day in divided doses; increase by 100 to 750 mg/day every 3 to 7 days until response reached; usual maintenance dose should *not* exceed 18 g/day.

(b) Carbidopa-levodopa (Sinemet): 25/250 mg/day in 3 to 4 divided doses. Limits the metabolism of levodopa peripherally and provides more levodopa for the brain.

(2) *Anticholinergics:* effective in *lessening muscle rigidity.*

(a) Benztropine mesylate (Cogentin): 0.5–6 mg/day in 1 to 2 divided doses.

(b) Biperiden (Akineton): 2 mg 3 to 4 times daily, *not* to exceed 16 mg/day.

(c) Trihexyphenidyl (Artane): 1 to 2 mg/day; increased by 2 mg every 3 to 5 days; usual maintenance dose: 5 to 15 mg/day in 3 to 4 divided doses.

(3) *Antihistamines:* have mild central anticholinergic properties.

2. Goal: *protect from injury.*

a. Monitor BP, side effects of medications (e.g., orthostatic hypotension).

b. Monitor for GI disturbances.

c. *Avoid* pyridoxine (vitamin B_6): it cancels effect of levodopa.

d. Levodopa *contraindicated* with:

Adult

(1) Glaucoma (causes increased intraocular pressure).
(2) Monoamine oxidase (MAO) inhibitors (causes possible hypertensive crisis).
3. Goal: *health teaching.*
  a. Teach client and family about medications: dosage range, side effects, not discontinuing medications abruptly.
  b. Exercise program to maintain ROM and normal body posture; also to get adequate rest to prevent fatigue.
  c. *Dietary adjustment and precautions* regarding cutting food in small pieces to prevent choking, taking fluid with food for easier swallowing.
  d. Importance of adding *roughage* to *diet* to prevent constipation.
  e. Assist client and family to adjust to this chronic debilitating illness.

◆ **F. Evaluation/outcome criteria:**
1. Activity level maintained.
2. Symptoms relieved by medications; no drug interactions.
3. Complications avoided.

XXV. **Amyotrophic lateral sclerosis** (ALS; Lou Gehrig's disease): progressive degeneration of motor neurons within the brain, spinal cord, or both, leading to death within 2 to 7 years, usually from infection (pneumonia) or consequences of respiratory or bulbar paralysis. There are three types of ALS: classic sporadic, familial, and Mariana Islands (Guam).
  A. Pathophysiology: myelin sheaths destroyed, replaced by scar tissue; involves lateral tracts of spinal cord, eventually medulla and ventral tracts.
  B. Risk factors:
  1. Affects men more than women.
  2. Usually in middle age.
  3. Viral infection possible causal agent.
  4. Possible familial or genetic component.

◆ **C. Assessment:**
  1. *Subjective data:*
    a. Early symptoms: fatigue, awkwardness.
    b. Dysphagia, dysarthria; speech slurred—may sound drunk.
    c. Alert, no sensory loss.
  2. *Objective data:*
    a. Symptoms depend on which motor neurons affected.
    b. Decreased fine finger movement.
    c. Progressive muscular weakness, atrophy, especially lower limbs at onset of disease; later, arms, hands, and shoulders.
    d. Spasticity of flexor muscles; one side of body becomes more involved than other.
    e. Progressive respiratory difficulties → diaphragmatic paralysis.
    f. Progressive disability of upper and lower extremities.
    g. Fasciculations (muscle twitching visible under skin).
    h. *Diagnostic tests:*
      (1) Electromyography (EMG).
      (2) Nerve conduction velocities (NCV).

◆ **D. Analysis/nursing diagnosis:**
1. *Ineffective airway clearance* related to difficulty in coughing.
2. *Ineffective breathing pattern* related to progressive respiratory difficulties and eventually respiratory paralysis.
3. *Altered health maintenance* related to inability to perform self-care activities.
4. *Impaired physical mobility* related to progressive muscular weakness.
5. *Self-care deficits: bathing/hygiene and dressing/grooming*
6. *Powerlessness* related to lifestyle of progressive physical helplessness.
7. *Impaired swallowing* related to disease progression.

◆ **E. Nursing care plan/implementation:**
1. Goal: *maintain independence as long as possible.*
  a. Assistance with ADL; splints, prosthetic devices to support weak limbs and maintain mobility.
  b. Skin care to prevent decubiti.
  c. *Soft/liquid diet* to aid in swallowing, prevent choking; suction prn; *head of bed elevated* when eating.
  d. Respiratory assistance as needed; ventilators as disease progresses and diaphragm becomes involved.
  e. Arrange long-term care arrangements if home maintenance no longer feasible.
  f. Emotional support, when client is alert; continue involving client in decisions regarding care.
  g. Medications: riluzolet (Rilutek); has some effect in reducing disease progression; other drugs offer temporary relief of symptoms.
2. Goal: *health teaching.*
  a. Skin care to prevent decubitus ulcer.
  b. Explain ramifications of disease so client and family can make decisions regarding future care, whether client will remain at home as disease progresses or enter a long-term care facility.
  c. How to use suction apparatus to clear airway.
  d. Care of nasogastric or gastrostomy feeding tube.

◆ **F. Evaluation/outcome criteria:**
1. Obtains physical and emotional support.
2. Complications avoided in early stage of disease.
3. Remains in control of ADL as long as possible.
4. Skin breakdown avoided.
5. Peaceful death.

XXVI. Guillain-Barré syndrome: an uncommon, acquired autoimmune disease resulting in demyelination of the cranial and peripheral nerves and a *progressive ascending* paralysis that is usually reversible; develops in hours or up to 10 days. Also known as **acute inflammatory polyradiculoneuropathy**; incidence 1.6/100,000. Client is often completely paralyzed, yet sensation and mentation remain intact.

A. Pathophysiology: macrophages attack normal myelin of the peripheral nerves → demyelination and blocked conduction of impulses to muscles → progressive symmetrical and bilateral muscle weakness from distal lower extremities to proximal upper extremities, trunk, and neck.

B. Risk factors:
1. Viral infection 1 to 3 weeks before paralysis in 50% of cases.
2. Gastroenteritis.
3. Immunizations.
4. May be linked to cytomegalovirus and Epstein-Barr virus.

◆ **C. Assessment:**
1. *Subjective data:*
   a. Pain, tingling in legs and back (paresthesias).
   b. Reports falling.
   c. Dyspnea.
2. *Objective data:*
   a. Footdrop; unable to walk.
   b. Gradual, progressive facial weakness; dysphagia; dysarthria.
   c. Flaccid paralysis; absent superficial and deep tendon reflexes (DTR).
   d. Respiratory muscle paralysis → respiratory failure.
   e. Postural hypotension; arterial hypertension, heart block, tachycardia.
   f. Lab data: ↑ CSF protein.

   g. *Diagnostic tests*: lumbar puncture; electrophysiologic studies (*EEG:* abnormal; *EMG:* slowed neural conduction).

◆ **D. Analysis/nursing diagnosis:**
1. *Impaired physical mobility* related to progressive muscular weakness.
2. *Ineffective breathing pattern* related to progressive respiratory difficulties and eventual respiratory paralysis.
3. *Anxiety* related to disease progression.
4. *Self-care deficits: bathing/hygiene and dressing/grooming.*

◆ **E. Nursing care plan/implementation:**
1. Goal: *prevent complications during recovery from paralysis.*
   ▶ a. Respiratory:
      (1) Observe for signs of failure: ↓ forced vital capacity, oximetry.
      (2) Prepare for mechanical ventilation if needed.
      (3) Trach care and ventilator weaning as indicated.
   b. Prepare for IV plasma exchanges.
      (1) 2 to 3 hours daily over 4 to 5 days; 200 to 250 mL/kg body weight of albumin exchanged.
      (2) *Monitor* for: hypotension, arrhythmias, vascular access problems.
   c. IV immune globulin also may be given. Complications include: hypotension, dyspnea, fever, transient hematuria.
2. Goal: *monitor for signs of autoimmune dysfunction.*
   a. Acute periods of ↑ BP alternating with ↓ BP.
   b. Arrhythmias: give *antiarrhythmic* meds.
3. Goal: *prevent tachycardia.*
   a. Med: propranolol.
   b. ECG monitoring (continuous) to detect alteration in cardiac rate and pattern.
4. Goal: *assess cranial nerve function.*
   a. Check *gag* and *swallowing* reflex.
   b. Check ability to clear secretions.
   c. Check *voice.*
5. Goal: *maintain adequate ventilation.*
   a. Monitor respiratory rate and depth.
   b. Perform serial vital capacities and ABGs.
   c. Observe for ventilatory insufficiency.
   d. Prevent pneumonia, atelectasis.
6. Goal (in acute phase): *check for progression of muscular weakness*—check individual muscle groups q2h.
7. Goal: *maintain nutrition.*
   a. NG tube—balanced liquid diet; mouth care.
   b. Check gag and swallowing reflex before starting soft, pureed foods.
8. Goal: *prevent injury and complications.*
   a. *Eye* care: artificial tears or ointment, due to lack of blinking or poor eyelid closure.
   b. *Mobility:*
      (1) ROM.
      (2) Prevent DVT, contractures: use splints, high-top sneakers, foot boards, heel and elbow protectors.
      (3) Anti-embolic stockings.
   c. *Elimination:*
      (1) Observe for urinary retention and constipation.
      (2) *Avoid* enemas if possible (prevent further autonomic response).
9. Goal: *support communication.*
   a. Develop two methods:
      (1) To indicate immediate needs.
      (2) For basic conversation.

◆ **F. Evaluation/outcome criteria:**
1. Complete reversal of paralysis.
2. Complications avoided: maintains respiratory function, able to swallow, no complications from immobility.
3. After onset and plateau period, recovery may take 3 to 12 months.

CANCER

I. The client with cancer: Cancer is a multisystem stressor. Regardless of the specific type of cancer, certain aspects of the disease and of nursing care are the same. The following principles apply universally and should be referred to when studying individual kinds of cancer.

A. Pathophysiology: result of altered cellular mechanisms. Several theories about causation, but current thinking is multiple causation. Alterations result in a progressive, uncontrolled multiplication of cells, with selective ability to invade and metastasize.

B. Risk factors:
1. Heredity (e.g., retinoblastoma).
2. Familial susceptibility (e.g., breast).
3. Acquired diseases (e.g., ulcerative colitis).
4. Virus (e.g., Burkitt's tumor).
5. Environmental factors:
   a. Tobacco.
   b. Alcohol.
   c. Radiation.
   d. Occupational hazards.
   e. Drugs (e.g., immunosuppressive, cytotoxic).
   f. Asbestos.
6. Age.
7. Air pollution.
8. Diet (e.g., high animal protein).]
9. Chronic irritation.
10. Precancerous lesions (e.g., gastric ulcers).
11. Stress.

◆ **C. Assessment:**
1. Specific symptoms depend on the anatomical and functional characteristics of the organ or structure involved.
2. *Mechanical effects:*
   a. *Pressure*—tumors growing in confined areas such as bone produce pain early, whereas tumors growing in expandable areas such as the abdomen may be undetected for some time.
   b. *Obstruction*—tumors that compress tubular structures such as the esophagus, bronchi, or lymph channels may cause symptoms such as swallowing difficulties, shortness of breath, edema. Symptoms depend on location of tumor and on the particular organ or structure receiving pressure.
   c. *Interruptions of blood supply*—compression of blood vessels or diversion of blood supply may cause necrosis or ulceration or may precipitate hemorrhage.
3. *Systemic effects:*
   a. Anorexia, weakness, weight loss.
   b. Metabolic disturbances—*malabsorption syndrome.*
   c. Fluid and electrolyte imbalances.
   d. Hormonal imbalances—increased antidiuretic hormone (ADH), adrenocorticotropic hormone (ACTH), thyrotropin (TSH), or parathyroid hormone (PTH).

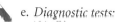

e. *Diagnostic tests:*
   (1) *Biopsy*—excision of part of tumor mass.
   (2) *Needle biopsy*—aspiration of cells from subcutaneous masses or organs such as liver.
   (3) *Exfoliative cytology*—scraping of any endothelium (cervix, mucous membranes, skin) and applying to slide.
   (4) *X-rays*—detect tumor growth in GI, respiratory, and renal systems.
   (5) *Endoscopy*—visualization of body cavity through endoscope.
   (6) *Computed tomography (CT)*—visualization of a body part whereby layers of tissue can be seen utilizing the very narrow beams of this type of x-ray equipment.
   (7) *Magnetic resonance imaging (MRI)*—a scanning device using a magnetic field for visualization.

f. Lab data:
   (1) *Blood and urine tests*—refer to **Appendix A** for normal values.
   (2) *Alkaline phosphatase*—greatly *increased* in osteogenic carcinoma (>92 U/L).
   (3) *Calcium—elevated* in multiple myeloma bone metastases (>10.5 mg/dL).
   (4) *Sodium—decreased* in bronchogenic carcinoma (<135 mEq/L).
   (5) *Potassium—decreased* in extensive liver carcinoma (<3.5 mEq/L).
   (6) *Serum gastrin*—measures gastric secretions. *Decreased* in gastric carcinoma. Normal value 0 to 180 ng/L.
   (7) *Neutrophilic leukocytosis*—tumors.
   (8) *Eosinophilic leukocytosis*—brain tumors, Hodgkin's disease.
   (9) *Lymphocytosis*—chronic lymphocytic anemia.

◆ **D. Analysis/nursing diagnosis:**
1. *Pain* related to diagnostic procedures, pressure, obstruction, interruption of blood supply, or potential side effects of drugs.
2. *Anxiety* related to fear of diagnosis or disease progression, treatment, and its known or expected side effects.
3. *Altered nutrition, less than body requirements,* related to anorexia.
4. *Risk for injury* related to radioactive contamination of excreta.
5. *Body image disturbance* related to loss of body parts, change in appearance as a result of therapy.
6. *Powerlessness* related to diagnosis and own perception of its meaning.
7. *Self-esteem disturbance* related to impact of cancer diagnosis.
8. *Risk for infection* related to immunosuppression from radiation and chemotherapy.
9. *Altered urinary elimination* related to dehydration.
10. *Risk for injury* related to normal tissue damage from radiation source.

11. *Fluid volume deficit* related to nausea and vomiting.
12. *Diarrhea* related to radiation of bowel.
13. *Constipation* related to dehydration.

◆ **E. Nursing care plan/implementation—general care** of the client with cancer:

1. Goal: *promote psychosocial comfort* (see also **Unit 6.**)
   a. Assist with diagnostic workup by providing psychological support and information about specific disease, diagnostic tests, diagnosis, and treatment options.
   b. Reduce anxiety by listening, making *referrals* for special problems (peer support groups, self-help groups such as Reach to Recovery), supplying information, or correcting misinformation, as appropriate.
   ▶ c. Stress-management techniques (see **Orientation, Unit 1**).
   d. Nursing management related to client who is depressed (see **Unit 6**).

2. Goal: *minimize effects of complications.*
   a. Anorexia/anemia:
      (1) *Decrease anemia* by:
         (a) Providing well-balanced, *iron-rich, small, frequent* meals.
         (b) Administering supplemental vitamins and iron as ordered.
         (c) Administering packed red blood cells as ordered.
      ▶ (d) Maintaining hyperalimentation as ordered.
         (e) Monitoring red blood cell count.
      (2) *Enhance nutrition* by providing nutritional supplements and a *diet high in protein;* necessary because of increased metabolism related to metastatic process. *Consult* with dietitian for suggestions of best food for individual client.
   b. Hemorrhage: monitor platelet count and maintain platelet infusions as ordered. Teach client to monitor for any signs of bleeding.
   c. Infection: observe for signs of sepsis (changes in vital signs, temperature of skin, mentation, urinary output or pain); monitor laboratory values (WBCs); administer *antibiotics* as ordered.
   ▶ d. Pain and discomfort: alleviate by frequent position changes, diversions, conversations, guided imagery, relaxation, back rubs, and *narcotics* as ordered.
   e. Assist in adjusting to altered body image by encouraging expression of fears and concerns. Do *not* ignore client's questions, and give honest answers; be available.
   f. Fatigue. Encourage periods of rest and a decrease in daily exertion.

3. Goal: *general health teaching.*
   a. Self-care skills to maintain independence (e.g., client who has a colostomy should know how to manage the colostomy before going home).
   b. Importance of follow-up care and routine physical examinations to monitor for general health and possible signs of further disease.
   c. Dietary instructions, adjustments necessary to maintain nutrition during and after treatment.
   d. Health maintenance programs: teach hazards of the use of tobacco and alcohol. *Avoid* high fat, low roughage diet.
   e. Risk factors: family history, stress, age, diet, occupation, environment.
   f. Access to information: clients should have telephone numbers where questions can be answered and symptoms reported 24 hours a day.

F. General surgical intervention: surgery may be *diagnostic, curative* (when the lesion is localized or with minimal metastases to the lymph nodes), *palliative* (to decrease symptomatology), or *reconstructive.* (see also **The Perioperative Experience, p. 546,** and specific types of cancer, following.)

◆ 1. **Nursing care plan/implementation**—*preoperative:*
   a. Goal: *prevent respiratory complications.*
      (1) Coughing and deep-breathing techniques.
      (2) *No smoking for 1 wk before surgery.*
   b. Goal: *counteract nutritional deficiencies.*
      (1) *Diet:*
         (a) *High* protein, *high* carbohydrate for tissue repair.
         (b) Vitamin and mineral supplements.
         (c) Hyperalimentation as ordered.
      (2) Blood transfusions may be needed if counts are low.
   c. Goal: *reduce apprehension.*
      (1) Clarify postoperative expectations.
      (2) Explain care of ostomies or tubes.
      (3) Answer client's questions honestly.

2. *Postoperative:*
   a. Goal: *prevent complications.*
      (1) Monitor respiratory status and hemodynamic status.
   ▶ (2) Wound care; active and passive exercises as allowed; respiratory hygiene; coughing, deep breathing, and turning; fluids (see **III. Postoperative experience, p. 553**).
   b. Goal: *alleviate pain and discomfort.*
      (1) Encourage early ambulation, depending on surgical procedure.
      (2) Administer prescribed medications as needed.
      (3) Administer *stool softeners* and enemas as ordered.
   c. Goal: *health teaching.*
      (1) Involve client, significant others, and family members in rehabilitation program.
      (2) Prepare for further therapies, such as radiation or chemotherapy.

(3) Referral: *support groups,* as appropriate: Reach to Recovery, Ostomy Associates, Laryngectomy Association.

(4) Develop skills to deal with disease progression if cure not realistic or metastasis evident (see **J. Palliative care, p. 660**).

G. Chemotherapy: used as single treatment or in combination with surgery and radiation, for early or advanced diseases. Used to cure, increase survival time, or decrease specific life-threatening complications. Antineoplastic agents' primary mode of action involves interfering with the supply and utilization of building blocks of nucleic acids, as well as interfering with intact molecules of DNA or RNA, which are needed for replication and cell growth. *Bone marrow, hair follicles,* and the *gastrointestinal tract are three areas of the body* in *which cells are actively dividing;* this is why most side effects are related to these areas of the body. Most often antineoplastic agents are used in combination.

1. *Types: alkylating* agents, *antimetabolites, antitumor antibiotics, antimiotic* agents, *plant alkaloids, enzymes, hormones,* and *biotherapy.* (e.g., BCG, interferon) (see **Table 10.8**).
2. *Major problem:* lacks specificity, thus affecting normal as well as malignant cells.
3. *Major side effects:* bone marrow depression, stomatitis, nausea and vomiting, gastrointestinal ulcerations, diarrhea, and alopecia (**Table 7.45**).

| TABLE 7.45 | Common Side Effects of Chemotherapeutic Agents |

	Nausea and Vomiting	Mucositis	Diarrhea	Skin Reactions	Lung	Neurological
Alkylating Agents						
Busulfan	0	+	0	Hyperpigmentation	0	0
Carboplatin	+	0	0	0	0	0
Cisplatin	+	0	0	Alopecia	0	+
Chlorambucil	0	0	0	0	+	0
Cyclophosphamide	+	0	0	0	+	0
DTIC	+	0	0	0	0	0
Ifosfamide	+	0	0	Alopecia	0	Encephalopathy
Mechlorethamine	+	+	+	Alopecia, rash	0	0
Melphalan	0	0	0	0	0	0
Antimetabolites						
Cytosine arabinoside	0	0	+	0	+	0
Fludarabine	+	0	0	0	0	0
5-Fluorouracil	0	+	+	Phlebitis	0	Cerebellar
Hydroxyurea	0	0	0	Skin atrophy	0	0
Methotrexate	+	+	+	Dermatitis	+	0
with leucovorin	+	+	+	Dermatitis	+	0
2-Deoxycoformycin	+	0	0	Erythema	0	Lethargy, coma
6-Mercaptopurine	+	0	0	Rash	0	0
Thioguanine	+	+	0	0	0	0
2-Chlorodexyadeonosine	+	0	0	0	0	0
Antitumor Antibiotics						
Bleomycin	0	0	0	Erythema	+	0
Dactinomycin	+	+	0	Alopecia, rash	0	0
Daunorubicin	+	+	+	Alopecia, vesicant	0	0
Doxorubicin	+	+	+	Alopecia, vesicant	0	0
Idarubicin	+	+	+	Alopecia, vesicant	0	0
Mitomycin C	+	+	0	Vesicant	+	0
Mitoxantrone	+	+	+	Alopecia, vesicant	0	0
Nitrosoureas						
Carmustine (BCNU)	+	0	0	0	+	0
Lomustine (CCNU)	+	0	0	0	0	0
Streptozocin	+	0	0	0	0	0
Thiotepa	+	+	+	Alopecia, rash	0	0
Plant Alkaloids						
Etoposide (VP-16)	0	0	0	0	0	0
Vinblastine	+	+	0	Alopecia, vesicant	0	+
Vincristine	0	0	0	Vesicant	0	+ Neuropathy
Taxol	+	0	0	Alopecia	0	Neuropathy

+, present; 0, absent.

Adapted from Ewald G, McKenzie C: Manual of Medical Therapeutics. Little, Brown, Boston.

Adult

4. *Routes of administration:* oral, intramuscular, intravenous (*Hickman or Groshong catheter*), subclavian lines, porta caths, peripheral, intra-arterial (may have infusion pump for continuous or intermittent flow rate), intracavity (e.g., bladder through cystoscopy). (see next column for information about administration of IV chemotherapeutic agents.)

◆ 5. **Nursing care plan/implementation:**

    a. Goal: *assist with treatment of specific side effects.*

      (1) *Nausea and vomiting—antiemetic* drugs (e.g., prochloroperazine, Zofran) as ordered and scheduled; small, frequent, *high calorie, high potassium, high protein* meals; chopped or blended foods for ease in swallowing; include milk and milk products when tolerated for *increased calcium;* carbonated drinks; frequent mouth care; *antacid* therapy as ordered; rest after meals; *avoid* food odors during preparation of meals; pleasant environment during meals; appropriate distractions; IV therapy; *nasogastric* tube for control of severe nausea or as route for *tube feeding* if unable to take food by mouth; *hyperalimentation.*

      (2) *Diarrhea—low residue diet; increased potassium; increased* fluids; atropine SO_4 – diphenoxylate HCl (Lomotil) or kaolin-pectin (Kaopectate) as ordered; *avoid* hot or cold foods/liquids.

      (3) *Stomatitis* (painful mouth)—soft toothbrushes or sponges (toothettes); mouth care q2 to q4; viscous lidocaine HCl (Xylocaine) as ordered before meals. Oral salt and soda mouth rinses; *avoid* commercial mouthwashes that contain high level of alcohol, which could be very irritating to mucous membranes. *Avoid* hot foods/liquids; include *bland* foods at cool temperatures; remove dentures if sores are under dentures; moisten lips with lubricant.

      (4) *Skin care*—monitor: wounds that do not heal, infections (client receives frequent sticks for blood tests and therapy); *avoid* sunlight; use sunblock, especially if receiving doxorubicin (Adriamycin).

      (5) *Alopecia*—be gentle when combing or lightly brushing hair; use wigs, night caps, scarves; provide frequent linen changes. Advise client to have hair cut short before treatment with drugs known to cause alopecia (bleomycin, cyclosphosphamide, dactinomycin, daunorubicin hydrochloride, doxorubicin hydrochloride, 5-fluorouracil, ICRF-159, hydroxyurea, methotrexate, mitomycin, VP 16–213, vincristine). Other techniques

may be used, depending on client's age and protocol in clinical agency.

      (6) *Extravasation*—infiltration of chemotherapeutic agents into surrounding tissues. Document and treat according to agency protocols for administered drug.

    b. Goal: *health teaching.*

      (1) Orient client and family to purpose of proposed drug regimen and anticipated side effects.

      (2) Advise that frequent checks on hematological status will be necessary (client will receive frequent IV sticks, lab tests).

      (3) Advise client/family on increased risk for infection (*avoid* uncontrolled crowds and individuals with upper respiratory tract infections or childhood diseases).

      (4) Monitor injection site for signs of extravasation (infiltration); site must be changed if leakage suspected, and guidelines to neutralize must be followed according to drug protocol.

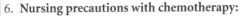

6. **Nursing precautions with chemotherapy:**

    a. Nurse should wear gloves and mask when preparing chemotherapy drugs for administration. Mixing of drug into IV bag done under laminar flow hood.

    b. Drugs are toxic substances, and nurses must take every precaution to handle them with care.

    c. When expelling air bubbles from syringes, care must be taken that the drugs are not sprayed into the atmosphere.

    d. Contaminated needles and syringes should be disposed of intact (to prevent aerosol generation) in plastic-lined box according to environmental standards. Disposable equipment should be used whenever possible.

    e. If skin becomes contaminated with a drug, wash under running water.

    f. Nurses should know the half-life and excretion route of the drugs being administered and take the special precautions necessary. For example, while the drug is actively being excreted, use gloves when touching client, stool, urine, dressings, vomitus, etc.

    g. If the nurse is in the early phase of pregnancy, she should seek specific information about risks to her unborn child before caring for the client receiving chemotherapeutic agents.

H. Radiation therapy: used in high doses to kill cancer cells, or palliatively for pain relief. *Side effects of radiation therapy* depend on site of therapy (side effects are also variable in each individual): nausea, vomiting, stomatitis, esophagitis (*Candida*), dry mouth, diarrhea, depression of bone marrow, suppression of immune response, decreased life span, and sterility.

Adult

1. **External radiation:** cobalt or linear accelerator machine.
   a. *Procedure:* daily treatments, Monday through Friday, for prescribed number of times according to size and location of tumor (length of treatment schedule is usually 4 to 6 wk). Client remains alone in room during treatment. (Nurse, therapist, family members cannot stay in room with client due to radiation exposure during treatment.) Client instructed to lie still so exactly same area is irradiated each treatment. Marks (tattoos or via permanent-ink markers) are made on skin to delineate area of treatment; marks must *not* be removed during entire treatment course.
   b. **Nursing care plan/implementation:**
      (1) Goal: *prevent tissue breakdown.*
         (a) Do *not* wash off site-identification marks (tattoos cannot be removed); dosage area is carefully calculated and must be exact for each treatment.
         (b) Assess skin daily and teach client to do same (most radiation therapy is done on outpatient basis, so client needs skills to manage independently).
         (c) Keep skin dry; cornstarch usually the only topical application allowed; 100% aloe (no alcohol) for redness.
         (d) *Contraindications:*
            (i) Talcum powders, due to potential radiation dosage alteration.
            (ii) Lotions, due to increased moistening of skin.
            (iii) Products containing alcohol, due to increased dryness.
         (e) Reduce skin friction by *avoiding* constricting bedclothes or clothing, and by using electric shaver.
         (f) Dress areas of skin breakdown with nonadherent dressing and paper tape.
      (2) Goal: *decrease side effects of therapy.*
         ▶ (a) Provide meticulous oral hygiene.
         (b) If diarrhea occurs, may need IV infusions, *antidiarrheal* medications; monitor bowel movements (possible adhesions from surgery and radiation treatments).
         (c) Monitor vital signs, particularly respiratory function, and BP (sloughing of tissue puts client at *risk for hemorrhage*).
         (d) Monitor hematological status—bone marrow depression can cause *fatal toxicosis and sepsis.*
         (e) Institute *reverse isolation* as necessary to prevent infections (reverse isolation usually instituted if less than 50% neutrophils).

      (3) Goal: *health teaching.*
         (a) Instruct client to *avoid*:
            (i) Strong sunlight; must wear sunblock lotion, protective clothing over radiation site.
            (ii) Extremes in temperature to the area (hot-water bottles, ice caps, spas).
            (iii) Synthetic, nonporous clothes or tight constrictive clothing over area.
            (iv) Eating 2 to 3 hr before treatment and 2 hr after, to decrease nausea; give small, frequent meals *high* in protein and carbohydrates and *low* in residue.
            (v) Strong alcohol-base mouthwash; use daily salt and soda mouthwash.
            (vi) Fatigue, an overwhelming problem. Need to pace themselves, nap; may need someone to drive them to therapy; can continue with usual activities as tolerated.
            (vii) Crowds and persons with upper respiratory infections or any other infections.
         (b) Provide appropriate birth control information for clients of childbearing age.

2. **Internal radiation: sealed** (radium, iridium, cesium):
   a. Used for localized masses (e.g., mouth, cervix, breast, testes). Due to exposure from radiation source, precautions must be taken while it is in place. Health-care personnel and family must adhere to *principles of time, distance, and shielding to decrease exposure* (*shortest* amount of time possible, stay as *far away* as possible from the source of radiation, and wear *protective* lead apron, gloves). If source of radiation accidentally falls out, it should be picked up only with *forceps.* Radiation officer should be notified **immediately.** Client should be in *private* room, and bed should be in the center of the room, if possible, to protect others. Unless the walls are lead lined, radiation will penetrate them; placing the bed in *center of room* will decrease exposure. Once the source of radiation has been removed, there is no exposure from client, excretions, or linens.
   b. **Nursing care plan/implementation:**
      (1) Goal: *assist with cervical radium implantation* (cervical radium is used here as the most common example of internal radiation source).
         ▶ (a) *Before insertion*—give douche, enema, perineal prep; insert Foley, as ordered.

(b) *After implantation*—check position of applicator q24h.

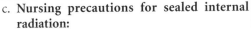

    (i) Keep client on bedrest in *flat position* to *avoid* displacing applicator (may turn to side for eating).

    (ii) Notify physician if temperature elevates, nausea and/or vomiting occur (indicates *radiation reaction or infection*).

    (iii) *After removal* of implant (48 to 144 hr)—bathe, douche, and remove catheter as ordered.

(2) Goal: *health teaching.*

    (a) Explain that nursing care will be limited to essential activities in postinsertion period.

    (b) Signs and symptoms of complications so client can notify staff if something unusual happens (bleeding, radiation source falls out, fever, etc.).

◆ **c. Nursing precautions for sealed internal radiation:**

   (1) **Never handle radium directly**—if applicators should accidentally be removed, pick up applicator by strings with long-handled forceps and **notify radiation officer.**

   (2) Linen must remain in client's room and *not* be sent to laundry until source of radiation has been accounted for and returned to its container.

   (3) **Time, distance,** and **shielding** are factors that increase or decrease potential effects on personnel. Need to minimize exposure of nursing staff, client's family, and other health professionals. Nurses who may be pregnant should *not* care for clients with radiation because of possible damage to the fetus from radiation exposure. Children under 16 should *not* be allowed to visit while internal radiation is in use.

3. **Internal radiation: unsealed** (radioisotope/radionuclide)

   a. Source of radiation is given orally or intravenously or instilled into a cavity as a liquid.

◆ b. **Nursing care plan/implementation:** Goal: *reduce radiation exposure of others.*

   (1) *Isolate* client and tag room with radioactivity symbol.

   (2) *Rotate* personnel to avoid overexposure *(principles of time, distance, and shielding).* Staff should use good hand-washing technique. Client should be in a room with running water. (Nurse who may be pregnant should *not* care for client while radiation source still active.)

(3) Encourage family to maintain telephone contact or use intercom, to decrease exposure to others.

(4) Plan independent diversional activities.

◆ c. *Specific nursing precautions* (post in chart, on client's door).

   (1) *Radioactive iodine* (^{131}I): half-life 8.1 days; excreted in urine, saliva, perspiration, vomitus, feces.

    (a) Wear gloves and isolation gowns when handling client, *excreta,* or dressings directly.

    (b) Collect paper plates, eating utensils, dressings, and linen in impermeable bags; label and dispose according to agency protocol.

    (c) Collect excreta in shielded container and send to lab daily to monitor excretion rate and disposal.

   (2) *Radioactive phosphorus* (^{32}P): half-life 14 days; injected into cavity or given IV or orally.

    (a) If injected into cavity, turn client q 10 to 15 min for 2 hr to ensure distribution.

    (b) No radiation hazard unless leakage from instillation site or from client's *excreta,* which are collected in *lead-lined containers* and brought to the radioisotope laboratory for disposal. Linen is collected in container, marked *radioactive,* and brought to the radioisotope lab for special handling.

    (c) Seepage will stain linens *blue;* wear gloves when handling contaminated linens, dressings. Excreta disposed of as in (b).

   (3) *Radioactive gold* (^{198}Au): half-life 2.7 days; usually injected into pleural or abdominal cavity.

    (a) May seep from instillation site or drainage tubes in cavity; stains *purple.*

    (b) Turn client q15min for 2 hr, as in (2)(a).

    (c) Same precautions regarding handling excreta as in (1)(a) and (2)(b).

4. **Precautions for nurses:**

   a. Use *principles of time, distance,* and *shielding* when caring for clients who are having active radiation therapy treatments.

   b. Nurses who may be pregnant should *not* accept an assignment caring for clients who have active radiation in place.

   c. *Always* use gloves, gowns to protect skin and clothing.

   d. Wear detection badge to determine exposure to energy source.

Adult

I. Immunotherapy: it has been hypothesized that clinical malignancy may occur as a result of failure of the immunological surveillance system of the body to fight off cancer cells as they develop. The goal of immunotherapy is to immunize clients against their own tumors.

1. *Nonspecific* immunotherapy—encourages a host-immune response by use of an unrelated agent. Bacille Calmette-Guérin (BCG) vaccine and *Corynebacterium parvum* are the two agents used for this type of immunotherapy.

2. *Specific* immunotherapy—uses substances that are antigenically related to the tumor that stimulate a specific host-immune response.

3. *Side effects*—malaise, chills, nausea, vomiting, diarrhea; local reaction at site of injection, such as pruritus, scabbing.

◆ 4. **Nursing care plan/implementation:**

   a. Goal: *decrease discomfort associated with side effects of therapy.*

      (1) Identify measures to lessen symptoms of side effects (see **E. Nursing care plan/implementation—general care** of the client with cancer, **p. 655**).

      (2) Know type of immunotherapy being used, adverse and desirable effects of therapy.

      (3) Administer fluids, encourage rest.

      (4) Administer *acetaminophen* as ordered to decrease flulike symptoms.

      (5) Administer *antiemetics* as ordered for nausea.

      (6) Monitor for respiratory distress.

      (7) Administer *analgesics* as ordered for pain.

   b. Goal: *health teaching.*

      (1) Comfort measures to decrease side effects of therapy.

      (2) Expected and side effects of therapy.

      (3) Investigational nature of therapy.

      (4) Care of site of administration.

      (5) Answer questions honestly.

J. Palliative care: when treatment has been ineffective in control of the disease, the nurse must plan palliative, terminal care. Cure is not possible for such clients in an advanced phase of malignancy. Symptoms increase in severity; clients and family have many special problems.

1. General problems of clients with terminal cancer:

   a. *Cachexia:* progressive weakness, wasting, and weight loss.

   b. *Anemia:* leukopenia, thrombocytopenia, hemorrhage.

   c. *Gastrointestinal disturbances:* anorexia, constipation.

   d. *Tissue breakdown* leading to decubiti, seeping wounds.

   e. *Urine:* retention, incontinence, renal calculi, tumor obstruction of ureters.

   f. *Hypercalcemia* occurs in 10% to 30% of clients.

   g. *Pain* due to tumor growth, obstruction, vertebral compression, or secondarily to complications (e.g., decubiti, stiffened joints, stomatitis). Also neuropathy, due to prolonged use of neurotoxic chemotherapeutic agents such as vincristine.

   h. *Fatigue:* major and debilitating problem.

◆ 2. **Nursing care plan/implementation:**

   a. Goal: *make client as comfortable as possible;* involve nursing staff, family, support personnel, clergy, volunteers, support groups. Hospice is **very** valuable program.

      (1) *Nutrition:* obtain nutritional consultation; *high calorie, high protein diet;* small, frequent meals; blenderized or strained; commercial nutritional supplements (Ensure, Vivonex, Sustacal).

      (2) Prevent tissue breakdown and vascular complications: frequent turning, massage, air mattress, active and passive ROM exercises.

      (3) *GI tract* disturbances: observe for toxic reactions to therapy, particularly vomiting and diarrhea; administer medications: *antiemetics, antidiarrheal* agents as ordered.

      (4) Relieve pain.

         (a) Use supportive measures such as massage, relaxation techniques, guided imagery; and drugs for *pain* relief: administer codeine, fentanyl, aspirin–oxycodone HCl (Percodan), pentazocine (Talwin), morphine, methadone, as ordered.

         (b) Methods of administration: oral, injected, rectal, analgesic patches, or pumps (IV or SC).

         (c) Monitor for side effects of narcotics: depressed respiratory status, constipation, anorexia.

   b. Goal: *assist client to maintain self-esteem and identity.*

      (1) Encourage self-care.

      (2) Spend time with client; isolation is a great fear for the client who is dying.

   c. Goal: *assist client with psychological adjustment*—see nursing care for clients who are grieving, clients who are dying (see **Unit 6**).

◆ **K. Evaluation/outcome criteria:**

1. Tolerates treatment modality—complications of surgery are avoided or minimized; tolerates chemotherapy; completes radiation therapy.

2. Side effects of treatment are managed by effective nursing care and health teaching.

3. Maintains good nutritional status.

4. Uses effective coping mechanisms or seeks appropriate assistance to deal with psychosocial concerns.

5. Makes choices for follow-up care based on accurate information.

6. Finds methods to control pain and minimize discomfort.
7. Participates in decisions regarding continuation of therapy (living will, health-care proxy, DNR decisions).
8. Dignity maintained until death and during dying.

II. Lung cancer

A. **Pathophysiology:** *squamous cell carcinoma:* undifferentiated, pleomorphic in appearance; accounts for 45% to 60% of all lung cancer; *small-cell (oat-cell) carcinoma:* small, dark cells located between cells of mucosal surfaces; characterized by early metastasis and poor prognosis; *large-cell (giant-cell) carcinoma:* located in the peripheral areas of the lung, has poor prognosis; *adenocarcinoma:* found in men and women; not necessarily related to smoking.

B. **Risk factors:**
1. Heavy cigarette smoking, 20 yr smoking history.
2. Exposure to certain industrial substances, such as asbestos.
3. Increased incidence in women during the last decade of life.

C. **Annual incidence:** 178,100 new cases; 160,400 estimated deaths.

◆ D. **Assessment:**
1. *Subjective data:*
   a. Dyspnea.
   b. *Pain:* on swallowing; dull and poorly localized chest pain, referred to shoulders.
   c. Anorexia.
   d. History of cigarette smoking over a period of years; recurrent respiratory infections with chills and fever, especially pneumonia or bronchitis.
2. *Objective data:*
   a. Wheezing; dry to productive persistent cough; hemoptysis, hoarseness.
   b. Weight loss.
   c. Positive diagnosis: cytology report of cells from bronchoscopy.
   d. Chest pain.
   e. Signs of metastasis.

◆ E. **Analysis/nursing diagnosis:**
1. *Ineffective breathing pattern* related to pain.
2. *Impaired gas exchange* related to tumor growth.
3. *Pain* related to disease progression.
4. *Fear* related to uncertain future.
5. *Powerlessness* related to inability to control symptoms.
6. *Knowledge deficit* (learning need) related to disease and treatment.

◆ F. **Nursing care plan/implementation:**
1. Goal: *make client aware of diagnosis and treatment options.*
   a. Allow time to talk and to discuss diagnosis.
   b. Client makes informed decision regarding treatment.
2. Goal: *prevent complications related to surgery* for client who is diagnosed early and for whom surgery is an option: wedge or segmental resec-

tion, laser therapy, lobectomy, or pneumonectomy are usual procedures.
   a. See **Nursing care plan/implementation for the client having thoracic surgery, p. 537.**
   b. Monitor vital signs, including accurate respiratory assessment for *respiratory congestion, blood loss, infection.*
   c. Assist client to deep breathe, cough, change position.
3. Goal: *assist client to cope with alternative therapies* when surgery is deemed not possible.
   a. *Radiation:* megavoltage x-ray, cobalt—usual form of radiation (see **Nursing care plan/ implementation for the client having radiation therapy, pp. 658, 659**).
   b. *Chemotherapy:*
      (1) Cisplatin and VP-16 with irradiation has become standard form of induction chemotherapy. Cyclophosphamide (Cytoxan), doxorubicin (Adriamycin), CCNU, methotrexate, vincristine sulfate (Oncovin) are the other drugs given for lung cancer.
      (2) See **Nursing care plan/implementation for the client having chemotherapy, p. 657.**
4. Goal: *health teaching.*
   a. Encourage client to stop smoking to offer best possible air exchange.
   b. Encourage *high protein, high calorie diet* to counteract weight loss.
   c. *Force fluids,* to liquefy secretions so they can be expectorated.
   d. Encourage adequate rest and activity to prevent problems of immobility.
   e. Desired effects and side effects of medications prescribed for therapy and pain relief.
   f. Coping mechanisms for maximal comfort and advanced disease (see **J. Palliative care, p. 660**).

◆ G. **Evaluation/outcome criteria:**
1. Copes with disease and treatment.
2. Side effects of treatment are minimized by proper nursing management.
3. Acid-base balance is maintained by careful management of respiratory problems.
4. Client is aware of the seriousness of the disease.

III. Colon and rectal cancer

A. **Risk factors:**
1. Men, middle age, personal or family history of colon and rectal cancer, personal or family history of polyps in the rectum or colon, ulcerative colitis.
2. Diet high in beef and low in fiber.
3. *Gardner's syndrome* (multiple colonic adenomatous polyps, osteomas of the mandible or skull, multiple epidermoid cysts, or soft-tissue tumors of the skin).

B. **Annual incidence:** 131,200 new cases, 56,600 estimated deaths.

◆ C. **Assessment:**
1. *Subjective data:*

Adult

a. Change in bowel habits.
b. Anorexia.
c. Weakness.
d. Abdominal cramping or vague discomfort with or without pain.
e. Chills.

2. *Objective data:*
a. Diarrhea (pencil-like or ribbon-shaped feces) or constipation.
b. Weight loss.
c. Rectal bleeding; anemia.
d. Fever.
e. Digital exam reveals palpable mass if lesion is in ascending or descending colon.
f. Signs of intestinal obstruction: constipation, distention, pain, vomiting, fecal oozing.
g. *Diagnostic tests:*
   (1) Digital examination.
   (2) Slides of stool specimen, for occult blood.
   (3) Proctoscopy.
   (4) Sigmoidoscopy, colonoscopy.
   (5) Barium enema.

h. Lab data: occult blood, blood serotonin *increased,* carcinoembryonic antigen (CEA); *positive* radioimmunoassay of serum or plasma indicates presence of carcinoma or adenocarcinoma of colon; positive result after resection indicates return of tumor.

◆ **D. Analysis/nursing diagnosis:**
1. *Constipation or diarrhea* related to presence of mass.
2. *Altered health maintenance* related to care of stoma.
3. *Sexual dysfunction* related to possible nerve damage during radical surgery.
4. *Body image disturbance* related to colostomy.

◆ **E. Nursing care plan/implementation** (see also **E. Nursing care plan/implementation—general care of the client with cancer, p. 655**):
1. *Radiation:* to reduce tumor or for palliation.
2. *Chemotherapy:* to reduce tumor mass and metastatic lesions.
   a. *Antitumor antibiotics*—mitomycin C, doxorubicin hydrochloride (Adriamycin).
   b. *Alkylating agents*—methyl-CCNU.
   c. *Antimetabolites*—5-fluorouracil (5-FU).
   d. *Steroids* and *analgesics* for symptomatic relief.
3. Prepare client for surgery (colostomy) if necessary.

◆ **F. Evaluation/outcome criteria:**
1. Return of peristalsis and formed stool following resection and anastomosis.
2. Adjusts to alteration in bowel elimination route following abdominoperineal resection (e.g., no depression, resumes lifestyle).
3. Demonstrates self-care skills with colostomy.
4. Makes dietary adjustments that affect elimination as indicated.

5. Identifies alternative methods of expressing sexuality, if needed.

IV. Breast cancer
A. Risk factors:
1. Women > age 50.
2. Family history of breast cancer.
3. Never bore children, or bore first child after age 30.
4. Had breast cancer in other breast.
5. Menarche before age 11.
6. Menopause after age 50.
7. Exposure to endogenous estrogens.
8. Exposure to ionizing radiation.
9. High alcohol and fat intake may increase risk.

B. Annual incidence: 181,600 new cases; 44,190 estimated deaths.

◆ **C. Assessment:**
1. *Subjective data:*
   a. Burning, itching of nipple.
   b. Reported painless lump.
2. *Objective data:*
   a. Firm, nontender lump or mass.
   b. Asymmetry of breast.
   c. Nipple—retraction, discharge.
   d. Alteration in breast skin—redness, dimpling, ulceration.
   e. Palpation reveals lump.
   f. *Diagnostic tests:* mammography, needle biopsy, core biopsy, excisional biopsy—level of estrogen-receptor protein predicts response to hormonal manipulation of metastatic disease and may represent a prognostic indicator for primary cancer; carcinoembryonic antigen (CEA) useful with metastatic disease of the breast.

◆ **D. Analysis/nursing diagnosis:**
1. *Risk for injury* related to surgical intervention.
2. *Body image disturbance* related to effects of surgery, radiation, or chemotherapy.
3. *Altered sexuality patterns* related to loss of breast.

◆ **E. Nursing care plan/implementation** (see also **E. Nursing care plan/implementation—general care of the client with cancer, p. 655**):
1. Goal: *assist through treatment protocol.*
   a. *Radiation*—primary treatment modality; adjunctive, external, or implantation to primary lesion site or nodes.
   b. *Chemotherapy* usually given in combinations.
      (1) *Cytotoxic* agents to destroy tumor and control metastasis.
      (2) *Alkylating* agents: cyclophosphamide (Cytoxan).
      (3) *Antitumor antibiotics:* doxorubicin (Adriamycin).
      (4) *Antimetabolites:* fluorouracil (5-FU); methotrexate (Amethopterine, MTX).
      (5) *Plant alkaloids:* vincristine sulfate (Oncovin).
      (6) *Hormones* to control metastasis, provide palliation: androgens, fluoxymesterone

(Halotestin), testosterone (Teslac), diethylstilbesterol (estrogen).

(7) *Antiestrogens:* tamoxifen (Nolvadex) may be used after initial treatment.

(8) *Cortisols:* cortisone, prednisolone (Delta-Cortef), prednisolone acetate (Meticortelone), prednisone (Deltasone, Delta).

c. *Surgery.*

(1) *Preoperative:*

(a) Goal: *prepare for surgery—types:*

(i) *Lumpectomy* (with or without radiation)—used when lesion is small; section of breast is removed with clear margin around lesion (often accompanied by radiation therapy and then radium interstitial implant).

(ii) *Simple mastectomy*—breast removed, no alteration in nodes.

(iii) *Modified radical mastectomy*—breast, some axillary nodes, subcutaneous tissue removed; pectoralis minor muscle removed.

(iv) *Radical mastectomy*—breast, axillary nodes, and pectoralis major and minor muscles removed.

(v) Reconstructive surgery—done at time of initial mastectomy or (most often) later, when other adjuvant therapy has been completed.

(b) Goal: *promote comfort.*

(i) Allow client and family to express fears, feelings.

(ii) Provide correct information about diagnostic tests, operative procedure, postoperative expectations.

(iii) Client may be hospitalized for 24 hours or less. Have telephone number available for questions. Make appropriate community referrals.

(2) *Postoperative:*

(a) Goal: *facilitate healing.*

(i) Observe pressure dressings for bleeding; will appear under axilla and toward the back.

(ii) Report if dressing becomes saturated; reinforce dressing as need; monitor drainage from Hemovac or suction pump.

(iii) *Position:* semi-Fowler's to facilitate venous and lymphatic drainage; use pillows to *elevate affected* arm *above right atrium,* to prevent edema if nodes removed.

(b) Goal: *prevent complications.*

(i) Monitor vital signs for shock.

(ii) Use gloves when emptying drainage.

(iii) Maintain joint mobility—flexion and extension of fingers, elbow, shoulder.

(iv) ROM as ordered to prevent ankylosis.

(v) If skin graft done, check donor site and limit exercises.

(c) Goal: *facilitate rehabilitation.*

(i) Encourage client, significant others, and family to look at incision.

(ii) Involve client in incisional care, as tolerated.

(iii) *Refer* to Reach to Recovery program of the American Cancer Society

(iv) Exercise program, hydrotherapy for clients who are postmastectomy, to reduce lymphedema.

(d) Goal: *health teaching.*

(i) How to avoid injury to affected area; how to prevent lymphedema.

(ii) Exercises to gain full ROM.

(iii) Availability of prosthesis, reconstructive surgery.

(iv) Correct breast self-examination (BSE) technique (client is at risk for breast cancer in remaining breast) **(Figure 7.16).** Best time for exam: *women who are premenopausal,* seventh day of cycle; *women who are postmenopausal,* same day each month.

◆ **F. Evaluation/outcome criteria:**

1. Identifies feelings regarding loss.

2. Demonstrates postmastectomy exercises.

3. Gives rationale for avoiding fatigue and avoiding constricting garments on affected arm; necessity for avoiding injury (cuts, bruises, burns) while carrying out activities of daily living.

4. Describes signs and symptoms of infection.

5. Demonstrates correct BSE technique.

V. Uterine cancer (endometrial): originates from epithelial tissues of the endometrium; second only to cervical cancer as cause of pelvic cancer. Slow growing; metastasizes late; responsive to therapy with early diagnosis; Pap test not as effective—more effective to have endometrial tissue sample **(Table 7.46** and **Table 7.47). Table 7.48** discusses cervical cancer.

A. Risk factors:

1. History of infertility (nulliparity).

2. Failure of ovulation.

3. Prolonged estrogen therapy.

4. Obesity.

5. Menopause after age 52.

6. Diabetes.

B. Annual incidence: 37,400 new cases; 6400 estimated deaths.

◆ **C. Assessment:**

1. *Subjective data:*

a. History of risk factor(s).

b. Pain (late symptom).

2. *Objective data:*

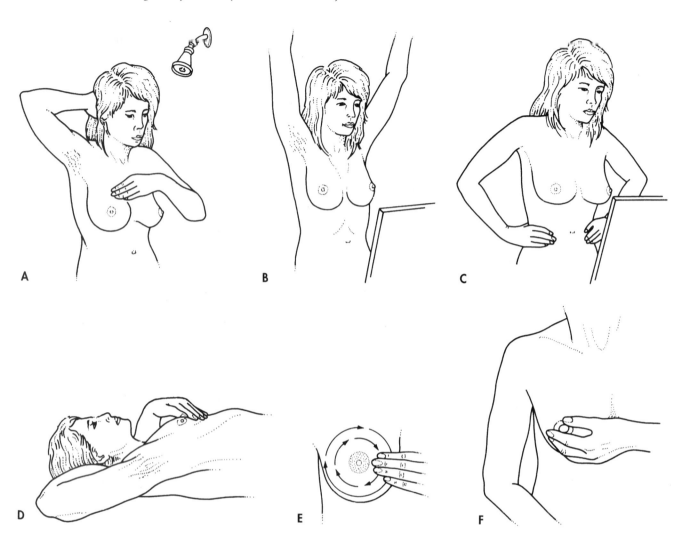

FIGURE 7.16   Breast self-examination. *(A)* Examine breasts during bath or shower because flat fingers glide easily over wet skin. Use right hand to examine left breast and vice versa. *(B)* Sit or stand before a mirror. Inspect breasts with hands at sides, then raised overhead. Look for changes in contour or dimpling of skin. *(C)* Place hands on hips and press down firmly to flex chest muscles. *(D)* Lie down with one hand under head and pillow or folded towel under that scapula. *(E)* Palpate that breast with the other hand using concentric circle method. It usually takes three circles to cover all breast tissue. Include the tail of the breast and the axilla. Repeat with other breast. *(F)* End in a sitting position. Palpate the areola areas of both breasts, and inspect and squeeze nipples to check for discharge.

TABLE 7.46	**Papanicolaou-Smear Classes**
Class	**Recommended Actions**
I Normal	
II Atypical cells, nonmalignant	Treat vaginal infections; repeat Pap smears
III Suspicious cells	Biopsy; dilation and curettage
IV Abnormal cells; suspicious of malignancy	Biopsy: dilation and curettage, conization
V Malignant cells present	See **Table 7.47**

TABLE 7.47	**Uterine Cancer: Recommended Treatment, by Stage of Invasion**
Stage of Invasion	**Recommended Treatment**
0 (In situ) Atypical hyperplasia	Cryosurgery, conization
I Uterus is of normal size	Hysterectomy
II Uterus slightly enlarged, but tumor is undifferentiated	Radiation implant, x-ray; hysterectomy 4–6 wk postradiation
III Uterus enlarged, tumor extends outside uterus	Radiation implant, total hysterectomy 4–6 wk postradiation
IV Advanced metastatic disease	Radiation, chemotherapy; progestin therapy to reduce pulmonary lesions

TABLE 7.48	International System of Staging for Cervical Carcinoma		
Stage	Location	Prognosis	Treatment
0	In situ	Highly curable	Conization
I	Cervix	Cure rate decreases as stage progresse	Radiation
II	Cervix to upper vagina		Radiation
III	Cervix to pelvic wall or lower third of vagina		Surgeries:
			1. Panhysterectomy, wide vaginal excision with removal of lymph nodes; ileal conduit
IV	Cervix to true pelvis, bladder, or rectum		2. Pelvic exenteration: a. Anterior: removal of vagina and bladder; ileal conduit b. Posterior: removal of rectum and vagina; colostomy c. Total: both anterior and posterior 3. Chemotherapy

a. Obese.
b. Abnormal cells obtained from aspiration of endocervix or endometrial washings.
c. Postmenopausal uterine bleeding.
d. Abnormal menses; intermenstrual or unusual discharge.

D. **Analysis/nursing diagnosis:**
1. *Pain* related to surgery.
2. *Risk for injury* related to surgery.
3. *Body image disturbance* related to loss of uterus.

E. **Nursing care plan/implementation** (see also **care of the client with cancer, p. 655**):
1. Goal: *assist client through treatment protocol.*
   a. *Radiation*—external, internal, or both with client who is a poor surgical risk.
   b. *Chemotherapy*—to reduce tumors and produce remission of metastasis. Antineoplastic drugs: dacarbazine (DTIC), doxorubicin (Adriamycin), medroxyprogesterone acetate (Provera), megestrol acetate (Megace).
2. Goal: *prepare client for surgery—types:*
   a. *Subtotal hysterectomy:* removal of the uterus; cervical stump remains.
   b. *Total hysterectomy:* removal of entire uterus, including cervix (abdominally [approximately 70%] or vaginally).
   c. *Total hysterectomy with bilateral salpingo-oophorectomy:* removal of entire uterus, fallopian tubes, and ovaries.
3. Goal: *reduce anxiety and depression:* allow for expression of feelings, concerns about feminity, role, relationships.
4. Goal: *prevent postoperative complications.*
   a. Catheter care—temporary bladder atony may be present as a result of edema or nerve trauma, especially when vaginal approach is used.
   b. Observe for abdominal distention and hemorrhage:
      (1) Auscultate for bowel sounds.
      (2) Measure abdominal girth.
      (3) Use rectal tube to decrease flatus.
   c. *Decrease pelvic congestion* and prevent venous stasis.
      (1) *Avoid* high-Fowler's position.
      (2) Antiembolic stockings as ordered.
      (3) Institute passive leg exercises.
      (4) Apply abdominal support as ordered.
      (5) Encourage early ambulation.
5. Goal: *support coping mechanisms* to prevent psychosocial response of depression: allow for verbalization of feelings.
6. Goal: *health teaching* to prevent complication of hemorrhage, infection, thromboemboli.
   a. *Avoid:*
      (1) Douching or coitus until advised by physician.
      (2) Strenuous activity and work for 2 mo.
      (3) Sitting for long time and wearing constrictive clothing, which tend to increase pelvic congestion.
   b. Explain hormonal replacement if applicable; correct dosage, desired and side effects of prescribed medications.
   c. Explain:
      (1) Menstruation will no longer occur.
      (2) Importance of reporting symptoms, e.g., fever, increased or bloody vaginal discharge, and hot flashes.

F. **Evaluation/outcome criteria:**
1. Adjusts to altered body image.
2. No complications—hemorrhage, shock, infection, thrombophlebitis.

VI. **Prostate cancer:** malignant neoplasm, usually adenocarcinoma; most common cause of cancer in men.
   A. **Risk factors:**
   1. Men > age 50.
   2. Familial history.
   3. Geographic distribution, environmental (e.g., industrial exposure to cadmium).
   4. Hormonal factors (testosterone).
   5. Diet (high fat).

B. **Annual incidence:** 185,000 new cases; 40,000 estimated deaths.

◆ C. **Assessment:**

1. *Subjective data:*
   a. Difficulty in starting urinary stream (hesitancy); urgency.
   b. Pain due to metastasis in lower back, hip, legs; perianal or rectal discomfort.
   c. Symptoms of cystitis; frequency, urgency.

2. *Objective data:*
   a. Urinary: smaller, less forceful stream; terminal dribbling; frequency, nocturia; *retention* (inability to void after ingestion of alcohol or exposure to cold).
   b. *Diagnostic tests:* digital rectal examination (DRE); transrectal ultrasonography (TRUS). Needle biopsy or tissue specimen reveals positive cancer cells.

   c. Lab data: *increased:*
      (1) Prostate-specific antigen (PSA)—over 4 ng/mL.
      (2) Urine RBCs (hematuria).
      (3) Gleason score for prostate cancer grading system (range: 2 to 10).

◆ D. **Analysis/nursing diagnosis:**

1. *Altered urinary elimination* related to incontinence.
2. *Altered sexuality pattern* related to nerve damage and erectile dysfunction.
3. *Anxiety* related to diagnosis.
4. *Pain* related to metastasis to bone.

◆ E. **Nursing care plan/implementation** (see also **care of the client with cancer, p. 655**):

1. Goal: *assist client through decisions about treatment protocol* (varies by stage: 0 to IV).
   a. *Radiation*—alone or in conjunction with surgery. Types: external beam radiation, 3-D conformal (focal), radioactive seed implants (brachytherapy).
   b. *Surgery*—cryosurgery; radical retropubic prostatectomy (see **p. 594**).
   c. Other options: hormones (*luteinizing hormone–releasing hormone agonists* [Lupron, Zoladex, Casodex, Nilandron]), *antiandrogen* (flutamide [Eulexin]); drugs in conjunction with orchiectomy, to limit production of androgens *(androgen deprivation therapy).*
   d. **Watchful waiting**—recommended with small contained tumor; older men; where surgery is contraindicated for other serious health problems.

◆ F. **Evaluation/outcome criteria** (see **Prostatectomy, p. 594**).

VII. **Bladder cancer:** bladder is most common site of urinary tract cancer.

   A. **Risk factors:**
   1. Contact with certain dyes.
   2. Cigarette smoking.
   3. Excessive coffee intake.

4. Prolonged use of analgesics with phenacetin.
5. Three times more common in men.

B. **Annual incidence:** 54,500 new cases; 12,100 estimated deaths.

◆ C. **Assessment:**

1. *Subjective data:*
   a. Frequency, urgency.
   b. *Pain:* flank, pelvic; dysuria.

2. *Objective data:*
   a. Painless hematuria (initially).
   b. *Diagnostic tests:*
      (1) Cystoscopy, intravenous pyelogram *(IVP)*—mass or obstruction.
      (2) Bladder biopsy, urine cytology—malignant cells.

   c. Lab data: urinalysis—*increased* RBC ($>4.8/$ μL—men, $>4.3/$ μL—women); erythrocytes (>30 mg/dL).

◆ D. **Analysis/nursing diagnosis:**

1. *Risk for injury* related to surgical intervention.
2. *Altered urinary elimination* related to surgery.

◆ E. **Nursing care plan/implementation** (see also **care of the client with cancer, p. 655**):

1. Goal: *assist client through treatment protocol.*
   a. *Radiation:* cobalt, radioisotopes, radon seeds; often before surgery to slow tumor growth.
   b. *Chemotherapy:*
      (1) *Antitumor antibiotics:* doxorubicin hydrochloride (Adriamycin), mitomycin.
      (2) *Antimetabolites:* 5-fluorouracil (5-FU).
      (3) *Alkylating* agents: thiotepa.
      (4) *Sedatives, antispasmodics.*

2. Goal: *prepare client for surgery*—types:
   a. *Transurethral fulguration or excision:* used for small tumors with minimal tissue involvement.
   b. *Segmental resection:* up to half the bladder may be resected.
   c. *Cystectomy with urinary diversion:* complete removal of the bladder; performed when disease appears curable.

3. Goal: *assist with acceptance of diagnosis and treatment.*

4. Goal: *prevent complication during postoperative period.*
   a. *Transurethral fulguration or excision:*
      (1) Monitor for clots, bleeding, spasms.
      ▶ (2) Maintain patency of Foley catheter.
   b. *Urinary diversion with stoma:*
      (1) Protect skin, ensure proper fit of appliance—because constantly wet with urine (see also **ileal conduit, p. 594** and **ostomies and stoma care, pp. 583–585**).
      (2) Prevent infection by increasing *acidity* of urine and increasing *fluid* intake.
      (3) *Health teaching.*
         (a) Self-care of stoma and appliance.
         (b) Expected and side effects of medications.

(c) Importance of follow-up visits for early detection of metastasis.

◆ **F. Evaluation/outcome criteria:**
1. Accepts treatment plan.
2. Uses prescribed measures to decrease side effects of surgery, radiation, chemotherapy.
3. Plans follow-up visits for further evaluation.
4. Maintains dignity.

VIII. Laryngeal cancer
   A. Risk factors:
   1. Eight times more common in men.
   2. Occurs most often after age 60.
   3. Cigarette smoking.
   4. Alcohol.
   5. Chronic laryngitis, vocal abuse.
   6. Family predisposition to cancer.
   B. Annual incidence: 10,900 new cases; 4230 estimated deaths.
◆ **C. Assessment:**
   1. *Subjective data:*
      a. Dysphagia—pain in areas of Adam's apple; radiates to ear.
      b. Dyspnea.
   2. *Objective data:*
      a. Persistent hoarseness.
      b. Cough and hemoptysis.
      c. Enlarged cervical nodes.
      d. General debility and weight loss.
      e. Foul breath.

f. Diagnosis made by history, laryngoscopy with biopsy and microscopic study of cells.

◆ **D. Analysis/nursing diagnosis:**
1. *Impaired verbal communication* related to removal of larynx.
2. *Body image disturbance* related to radical surgery.
3. *Ineffective airway clearance* related to increased secretions through tracheostomy.

◆ **E. Nursing care plan/implementation** (see also **care of the client with cancer, p. 655**): treatment primarily surgical (see **Laryngectomy, p. 595**); radiation therapy may also be indicated.

◆ **F. Evaluation/outcome criteria** (see **Laryngectomy, p. 595**).

IX. Additional types of cancer (Table 7.49).

EMERGENCY NURSING PROCEDURES

I. Purpose—to initiate assessment and intervention procedures that will speed total care of the client toward a successful outcome.

II. Emergency nursing procedures for adults are detailed in **Table 7.50.**

III. Legal issues (see **Unit 3**).

Testicular self-examination

To help detect abnormalities early, every male should examine his testes once a month. Instruct the client to follow this procedure:

1 If possible, take a warm bath or shower before beginning; the scrotum, which tends to contract when cold, will be relaxed, making the testes easier to examine.

2 With one hand, lift the penis and check the scrotum (the sac containing the testes) for any change in shape, size, or color. The left side of the scrotum normally hangs slightly lower than the right.

3 Next, check the testes for lumps and masses. Locate the crescent-shaped structure at the back of each testis. This is the epididymis, which should feel soft.

4 Use the thumb and first two fingers of your left hand to squeeze the spermatic cord gently; it extends upward from the epididymis, above the left testis. Then repeat on the right side, using your right hand. Check for lumps and masses by palpating along the entire length of the cord.

5 Next, examine each testis. To do so, place the index and middle fingers on its underside and the thumb on top, then gently roll the testis between the thumb and fingers. A normal testis is egg-shaped, rubbery-firm, and movable within the scrotum; it should feel smooth, with no lumps. Both testes should be the same size.

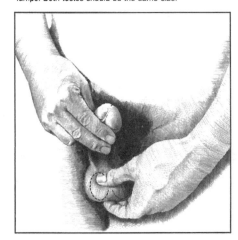

6 Promptly report any lumps, masses, or changes to the physician.

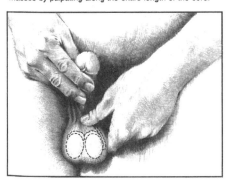

FIGURE 7.17 Testicular self-examination. (From Morton, PG: Health Assessment in Nursing. FA Davis, Philadelphia, 1993, p 451.)

TABLE 7.49 Selected Cancer Problems

	◆ Assessment			
	Subjective Data	**Objective Data**	**Risk Factors**	**Annual Incidence**	**Specific Treatment**
GASTROINTESTINAL TRACT					
Oral cancer	Difficulty chewing, swallowing, moving tongue or jaws; history of heavy smoking, alcohol use, or chewing tobacco	Sore that bleeds and does not heal; persistent red or white patch; diagnosis by biopsy; early detection: dental checks	Heavy smoking and drinking, user of chewing tobacco, men > age 40 (affects twice as many men as women)	30,750 new cases; 8440 estimated deaths	*Surgery*, with reconstructive surgery useful for cure and palliatively (see care of client with cancer having surgery, **pp. 655–656**) *Radiation* using simulated computer localization to avoid destruction of normal tissue (see care of client having radiation therapy, **pp. 657–659**)
Esophageal cancer	Dysphagia—difficulty in swallowing; discomfort described as: lump in throat, pressure in chest, pain; fatigue, lethargy, apathy; depression; anorexia	Weight loss; regurgitation, vomiting; diagnostic tests—*barium swallow,* esophagoscopy, biopsy	Over age 50, alcoholism, use of tobacco; increasing risk in nonwhite women, in people with achalasia (inability to relax lower esophagus with swallowing) or hiatal hernias	12,500 new cases; 12,200 estimated deaths	*Surgery:* resection with anastomosis, or removal with gastrostomy *Radiation:* best form of therapy *Chemotherapy:* antineoplastic drugs *ineffective;* medications to reduce symptoms of pain, discomfort, and anxiety (see nursing care plan/implementation for client with cancer, **p. 655;** having radiation therapy, **pp. 657–659;** having chemotherapy, **p. 656;** having surgery, **p. 655**)
Stomach cancer	Vague feeling of fullness, pressure, or epigastric pain following ingestion of food; anorexia, nausea, meat intolerance; malaise	Eructation, regurgitation, vomiting; melena, hematemesis, anemia; jaundice, diarrhea, ascites; big belly, upper gastric area; often palpable mass	Men, lower socioeconomic classes, colder climates, early exposure to dietary carcinogens, blood group A, pernicious anemia, atrophic achlorhydric gastritis	22,400 new cases; 14,000 estimated deaths	*Surgery:* gastrectomy (see gastric surgery, **p. 569,** for nursing care). *Radiation: not* as useful because dosage needed would cause side effects unlikely to be tolerated by client *Chemotherapy* alone or in conjunction with surgery: antitumor antibiotics, antimetabolites, nitrosoureas, hematics (see nursing care plan for client having chemotherapy, **p. 656**)

Type	Incidence	Causes/Risk factors	Assessment	Diagnostic findings	Treatment
Pancreatic cancer	27,600 new cases; 28,100 estimated deaths	Excessive use of alcohol; exposure to dry-cleaning chemicals, gasoline; coffee and decaffeinated coffee; possibly diabetes and chronic pancreatitis	Anorexia, nausea; pain in upper abdomen, radiating to back; dyspnea	Jaundice, vomiting, weight loss; determination of solid mass in area of pancreas by *computed tomography* and *ultrasound*; tissue identification by thin-needle *percutaneous biopsy*	*Surgery:* removal (must then have supplemental *pancreatic enzymes*; some clients become diabetic, type 1) or bypass to relieve obstruction (see nursing care plan/implementation for client with diabetes, **pp. 573–574**) *Chemotherapy:* pain relief, antiemetics, insulin, pancrelipase, 5-fluorouracil (5-FU), Cytoxan, cyclophosphamide (5-FU), Cytoxan, carmustine (BCNU), methotrexate, vincristine, mitomycin-C (see nursing care plan/implementation for client having chemotherapy, **p. 657**) *Radiation:* intraoperative high dose to pancreatic tumors with external high beam; palliative radiation therapy for pain (see nursing care plan/implementation for client having radiation therapy, **pp. 658–659**; see nursing care plan/implementation for client with cancer, **p. 655**)
SKIN Skin cancer: basal cell	900,000 new cases; 7300 estimated deaths; 44,200 of those are malignant melanoma	Exposure to sun, coal tar, pitch, arsenic compounds, creosote, radium; fair complexion	Reported painless lesion	Scaly plaques, papules that ulcerate; pale, waxy, pearly nodule or red, sharply outlined patch; unusual skin condition, change in size or color, or other darkly pigmented growth or mole	*Surgery:* electrodesiccation (dehydration of tissue by use of needle electrode); cryosurgery (destruction of tissue by application of extreme cold) (see care of cancer client, **p. 655**) *Radiation therapy* (see care of client having radiation therapy, **pp. 658–659**) *Prevention: avoid* sun from 10 A.M. to 3 P.M.; use protective clothing, sunblock lotion

(Continued on following page)

Adult

TABLE 7.49 Selected Cancer Problems *(Continued)*

◆ **Assessment**

	Subjective Data	Objective Data	Risk Factors	Annual Incidence	Specific Treatment
NERVOUS SYSTEM Brain	*Headache:* steady, intermittent, severe (may be intensified by physical activity); nausea; lethargy, easy fatigability; forgetfulness, disorientation, impaired judgment; visual disturbances; blackouts	Vomiting, may be projectile; sight loss, auditory changes; signs of increased intracranial pressure; seizures; paresthesia; behavior changes. *diagnostic studies*—CT scan, arteriography, cytology of cerebrospinal fluid	None known for primary tumors; brain is common site for metastasis	17,600 new cases (brain and spinal cord); 13,200 estimated deaths	*Surgery:* craniotomy with excision of lesion; ventricular shunt to allow for drainage of fluid (see nursing care plan/implementation for craniotomy, **pp. 604–605;** see nursing care plan/implementation for client with cancer, **p. 655**) *Radiation:* cobalt (local or entire CNS); total brain radiation causes alopecia, which may be permanent (see nursing care plan/implementation for client having radiation therapy, **pp. 657–659**); could be used alone, with surgery, or with chemotherapy *Chemotherapy:* antineoplastic alkylating agents: nitrosoureas (cross blood-brain barrier to reduce tumor)—carmustine (BCNU), lomustine (CCNU), semustine (methyl-CCNU); cerebral diuretics to reduce edema; anticonvulsants; analgesics; sedatives (see nursing care plan/implementation for client having chemotherapy, **p. 657**)
ENDOCRINE Thyroid cancer	Painless nodule; dysphagia; difficulty breathing	Enlarged thyroid, thyroid nodule; palpable thyroid, lymph nodes; hoarseness; hypofunctional nodule seen on *isotopic imaging scanning; needle biopsy for cytology studies*	Radiation exposure in childhood	18,100 new cases; 1200 estimated deaths	*Surgery:* total thyroidectomy, possible radical neck dissection (see Thyroidectomy, **pp. 643–644**) *Radiation:* external, or with radioactive iodine (^{131}I) (see care of client having radiation therapy, **pp. 657–659**) *Chemotherapy:* chlorambucil, doxorubicin, vincristine (Leukeran, Adriamycin, Oncovin, respectively) (see care of client having chemotherapy, **p. 657**)

				Staging and treatment:
Hodgkin's disease	Fatigue; generalized pruritus; anorexia	Painless enlargement of lymph nodes, especially in cervical area; fever, night sweats; hepatosplenomegaly; anemia; peak age of incidence, 15 to 35; *diagnostic tests—* biopsy shows presence of *Reed-Sternberg cells; x-rays, scans, laparotomy*	For young adults from 15 to 35 yr old, not clearly defined, some relationship to socioeconomic status; men-women ratio is 1.5:1; increased frequency among White persons	7500 new cases; 1300 estimated deaths	*Stage I*—involvement of a single node or a single node region; excision of lesion, and total nodal radiation (see care of client having radiation therapy, **pp. 657–659**) *Stage II*—involvement of two or more lymph node regions on same side of diaphragm; excision of lesion and radiation (see care of client having radiation therapy, **pp. 657–659**) *Stage III*—involvement of lymph node regions on both sides of the diaphragm, which may include the spleen; combination of radiation and chemotherapy *Stage IV*—involvement of one or more extralymphatic organs or tissues, with or without lymphatic involvement; treated with chemotherapy alone, radiation therapy alone, or both Presence or absence of symptoms of night sweats, significant fever, and weight loss; treated with *chemotherapy*, MOPP — Mustargen (mechlorethamine HCl, alkylating agent), Oncovin (vincristine, plant alkaloid), procarbazine (antineoplastic); prednisone (corticosteroid) (see care of client having chemotherapy, **p. 657**)
Non-Hodgkin's lymphoma	Night sweats	Nontender lymphadenopathy, enlarged liver and spleen, weight loss, fever	Age 50 to 60 yr	53,600 new cases; 23,800 estimated deaths	Stage I—rarely observed, but remission possible with radiation therapy Stage II—radiation therapy Stage III and IV— combination chemotherapy, with or without radiation therapy

(Continued on following page)

Adult

671

TABLE 7.49	Selected Cancer Problems (Continued)

	◆ Assessment				
	Subjective Data	Objective Data	Risk Factors	Annual Incidence	Specific Treatment
Multiple myeloma	Weakness; history of frequent infections, especially pneumonias; severe bone pain on motion; neurological symptoms, paralysis	Fractures of long bones; deformity of: sternum, ribs, vertebrae, pelvis; hepatosplenomegaly; anemia and bleeding tendencies *Elevated uric acid*	Exposure to ionizing radiation; middle-aged or older women	13,200 new cases; 11,400 estimated deaths	*Surgery:* relieve spinal cord compression; orthopedic procedures to relieve or support bone problems (see nursing care plan/implementation for clients with internal fixation for fractures, **p. 624**; client with spinal cord injuries when paralysis occurs, **p. 639**) *Radiation:* for some lesions (see nursing care plan/implementation for clients having radiation therapy, **pp. 657–659**) ⬤ *Chemotherapy:* alkylating agents; antitumor antibiotics; plant alkaloids; hormones—melphalan and prednisone (see nursing care plan/implementation for clients having chemotherapy, **p. 657**)
URINARY ORGANS Kidney cancer	Fatigue; abdominal or flank pain; night sweats	Painless, gross hematuria; firm, nontender, palpable kidney; weight loss; FUO; testicular enlargement. *Complications:* hypertension; *nephrotic syndrome;* metastasis to lung, brain, liver, bones (e.g., scapula or pelvis); vena cava involvement *Lab and diagnostic tests:* CAT scans (chest, abdomen, pelvis) with contrast; MRI; bone scan; urinalysis—presence of red cells and albumin; CBC—*decrease* in red cells and leukocytes, *reduction* in serum albumin, *elevation* of alpha globulin and calcium	More common among men than women, Whites than Blacks; lymphoma; smoking; exposure to chemicals used in leather manufacturing; radiation exposure; possible familial influence; common site of metastasis from lung	30,000 new cases; 1900 estimated deaths	*Surgery:* stereotactic surgery; gamma knife (for brain metastasis); nephrectomy (see pre/postoperative nursing care, **p. 592**) *Radiation:* irradiation of *metastatic* sites when tumor is radiosensitive (see nursing care plan/implementation for client having radiation therapy, **pp. 657–659**) ⬤ *Chemotherapy:* plant alkaloids—vincristine (Oncovin); antitumor antibiotics—dactinomycin (Actinomycin D), doxorubicin (*Adriamycin*), gemcitabine (*Gemzar*); alkylating agents—cyclophosphamide (Cytoxan); IL-2; interferon alpha. (see nursing care plan/implementation for client having chemotherapy, **p. 657**) *Clinical trials:* Avastin, bone marrow transplant, Bay 43

GENITAL ORGANS

Testicular cancer

Aching or dragging sensation in groin, usually painless

Gynecomastia; enlargement, swelling, lump, hardening of testes; young adult men early diagnosis—monthly testicular self-exam (see **Fig 7.17, p. 667**)

Second most common malignancy among men age 25 to 40 yr; possibly exposure to chemical carcinogens; trauma, orchitis; gonadal dysgenesis; cryptorchidism (undescended testicles)

7400 new cases; 300 estimated deaths; 95% to 100% 5 yr survival rate for early-detected nonmetastasized lesions

Surgery: orchiectomy (see nursing care plan/ implementation for the preop and postop client, **pp. 546–547, 550–551, 553–558**)

Radiation: see nursing care plan/implementation for client having radiation therapy, **pp. 657–659**

Chemotherapy: cisplatin, bleomycin, etoposide, steroids (see nursing care plan/implementation for client having chemotherapy, **p. 657**)

Cervical cancer

Vague pelvic or low back discomfort, pressure, or pain

Intermenstrual, postcoital, or postmenopausal bleeding, vaginal discharge—serosanguineous and malodorous hypermenorrhea; abdominal distention with urinary frequency; abnormal Pap test (see **Table 7.46**); recommended guidelines by American Cancer Society: *Pap test* annually; after three consecutive normal test, MD may recommend less frequent testing; pelvic/uterine exam every 3 yr

Early age at first intercourse; multiple sex partners; low socioeconomic status; exposure to herpesvirus 2

14,500 new cases; 6400 estimated deaths

Staging (see **Table 7.48**)
Stage 0—carcinoma in situ; no distinct tumor observable; stage may last for 8 to 10 yr; cure rate 100% following treatment of wedge or cone resection of cervix during childbearing years, or simple hysterectomy
Stage I—malignant cells infiltrate cervical mucosa; lesion bleeds easily; cure rate 80% with treatment of hysterectomy
Stage II—neoplasm spreads through cervical muscular layers, involves upper third of vaginal mucosa; cure rate 50% with treatment of radical hysterectomy
Stage III—neoplasm involves lower third of vagina; cure rate 25% with pelvic exenteration
Stage IV—involves metastasis to bladder, rectum, and surrounding tissues; considered incurable

Radiation: external or internal or both, in conjunction with surgery or alone, depending on stage of disease or condition of client (see nursing care plan/implementation for client having radiation therapy, **pp. 657–659**)

Chemotherapy: progestin, antineoplastics, megestrol (Megace), medroxyprogesterone (Curretab, Provera); alkylating agents—dacarbazine (DTIC)

TABLE 7.50	Nursing Care of the Adult in Medical and Surgical Emergencies		
Condition	◆ Assessment: Signs and Symptoms	▶ Prehospitalization Nursing Care	▶ In-hospital Nursing Care
Cardiovascular Emergencies			
Myocardial infarction—ischemia and necrosis of cardiac muscle secondary to insufficient or obstructed coronary blood flow	*Prehospital:* Chest pain: viselike choking, unrelieved by rest or nitroglycerin *Skin:* ashen, cold, clammy *Vital signs:* pulse—rapid, weak, thready; increased rate and depth of respirations; dyspnea *Behavior:* restless, anxious *In hospital:* *C/V:* blood pressure and pulse pressure *decreased* *Heart sounds:* soft; S₃ may be present *Respirations:* fine basilar crackles *Lab:* ECG consistent with tissue necrosis (Q waves) and injury (ST-segment elevation); serum enzymes elevated (CPK-MB, troponin)	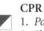1. If coronary suspected, call physician, paramedic service, or emergency ambulance 2. Calm and reassure client that help is coming 3. Place in *semi-Fowler's* position 4. Keep client warm but not hot	1. Rapidly assess hemodynamic and respiratory status 2. Place on cardiac monitor to determine treatment 3. Place on O₂ 4. Start IV as ordered—usually 5% D/W per microdrip to establish lifeline for emergency drug treatment 5. Relieve pain—morphine SO₄ IV as needed, aspirin, nitroglycerin 6. Draw blood for electrolytes, enzymes, as ordered 7. Take 12-lead ECG 8. Once client is stable, transfer to CCU
Cardiac arrest—cardiac standstill or ventricular fibrillation secondary to rapid administration or overdose of anesthetics or narcotic drugs, obstruction of the respiratory tract (mucus, vomitus, foreign body), acute anxiety, cardiac disease, dehydration, shock, electric shock, or emboli	Cyanosis, gasping *Respirations:* rapid, shallow, absent *Pulse:* weak, thready, >120 beats/min, absent Muscle twitching *Pupils:* dilated *Skin:* cold, clammy Loss of consciousness	**CPR** 1. *Position:* flat on back 2. Shake vigorously—establish unresponsiveness 3. Call for help: 9-1-1. If second rescuer present, send for help/get AED (automated external defibrillator); use within 5 min 4. Tilt head back (chin lift) 5. Check for breathing—*listen* at mouth, *look* at chest, *feel* with cheek *No breathing:* 1. Kneel close to head; place hand on forehead, bringing lower jaw forward and opening airway 2. Pinch nostrils shut and blow two full breaths into client's mouth 3. Lips must form airtight seal 4. Watch chest for adequate expansion; clear throat if indicated 5. Check pulse—if present, breathe into mouth every 5 sec	1. If monitored, note rhythm; call for help and note time 2. **Immediate** countershock if rhythm is ventricular fibrillation or ventricular tachycardia 3. If countershock unsuccessful, begin CPR, as in prehospital care 4. Assess breathing

(Continued on following page)

Condition	◆ Assessment: Signs and Symptoms	▶ Prehospitalization Nursing Care	▶ In-hospital Nursing Care
		No heartbeat: *One- or two-person lay CPR rescuers:* 80 chest compressions per minute, with two rescue breaths between every 15 compressions (no difference in ratio for one or two persons); with EMS responders: 5 compressions to one breath Check pulse at neck after 1 min and every few minutes thereafter Check pupils to determine effectiveness of CPR—should begin to constrict *Provide early defibrillation* with automated external defibrillator (AED) within 5 min of arrest if indicated *If heartbeat returns:* assist respiration and monitor pulse; continue CPR until help arrives	*Two-person rescue* *First person:* begins CPR as described in prehospital care *Second person:* 1. Pages arrest team 2. Brings defibrillator to bedside and countershocks, if indicated by rhythm; defibrillate within 3 min of arrest if indicated 3. Brings emergency cart to bedside 4. Suctions airway, if indicated due to vomitus or secretions 5. Bags client with 100% O_2 6. Assists with intubation when arrest team arrives 7. Establishes intravenous line if one is not available
Shock—cellular hypoxia and impairment of cellular function secondary to: trauma, hemorrhage, fright, dehydration, cardiac insufficiency, allergic reactions, septicemia, impairment of nervous system, poisons	**Early shock** *Sensorium:* conscious, apprehensive, and restless; some slurring of speech *Pupils:* dull but reactive to light *Pulse:* rate <140/min; amplitude full to mildy decreased *Blood pressure:* normal to slightly decreased *Neck veins:* normal to slightly flat in supine position; may be full in septic shock or grossly distended in cardiogenic shock *Skin:* cool, clammy, pale *Respirations:* rapid, shallow *GI:* nausea, vomiting, thirst *Renal:* urine output 20 to 40 mL/hr	1. Check breathing—clear airway if necessary; if no breathing, give artificial respirations; if breathing is irregular or labored, raise head and shoulders 2. Control bleeding by placing pressure on the wound or at pressure points (proximal artery) 3. Make comfortable and reassure 4. Cover lightly to prevent heat loss, but do *not* bundle up 5. If neck or spine injury is suspected—do *not* move, unless victim in danger of more injury **If client unconscious or has wounds of the lower face and jaw**— place on *side* to promote drainage of fluids; position client on *back* unless otherwise indicated	1. Check vital signs rapidly—pulse, pupils, respirations 2. Check airway; clear if necessary; draw ABGs; Po_2 should be maintained above 60 mm Hg; elevated Pco_2 indicates need for intubation and ventilatory assistance 3. Control gross bleeding 4. Prepare for insertion of intravenous line and central lines—if abdominal injuries present 5. Peripheral line should be placed in upper extremity if fluids being lost in abdomen 1. Draw blood for specimens: Hgb, Hct, CBC, glucose, CO_2, sodium amylase, BUN, K^+; type and crossmatch, blood gases, CPK-MB, troponin, prothrombin times 2. Prepare infusion of crystalloid replacement—NS usual choice; may include Ringer's lactate or half-normal saline

(Continued on following page)

Adult

TABLE 7.50 Nursing Care of the Adult in Medical and Surgical Emergencies *(Continued)*

Condition	◆ Assessment: Signs and Symptoms	▶ Prehospitalization Nursing Care	▶ In-hospital Nursing Care
	Severe or late shock *Sensoriun:* confused. disoriented, apathetic, unresponsive; slow, slurred speech, often incoherent *Pupils:* dilating, dilated, slow or nonreactive to light *Pulse:* rate >150 beats/min, thready, weak *Blood pressure:* 80 mm Hg or unobtainable *Neck veins:* flat in a supine position—no filling; full to distended in septic *or* cardiogenic shock *Skin:* cold, clammy, mottled; circumoral cyanosis, dusky, cyanotic *Eyes:* sunken—vacant expression *Renal:* urine output <20 mL/hr	1. *Raise* feet 6 to 8 inches unless client has head or chest injuries; if victim becomes less comfortable, lower feet 2. If client complains of thirst, do *not* give fluids unless client is more than 6 hr away from professional medical help; under **no** conditions give water to clients who are unconscious, having seizures or vomiting, appearing to need general anesthetic, or with a stomach, chest, or skull injury 3. Be calm and confident; reassure client help is on the way	1. Assess and intervene as for early shock; then obtain information as to onset and past history. **Treat underlying cause STAT.** 2. Catheterize and monitor client urine output as ordered 3. Take 12-lead ECG 4. Insert nasogastric tube and assess aspirate for volume, color, and blood; save specimen if poison or drug overdose suspected 5. If *CVP low* (<12)—infuse 200 to 300 mL over 5 to 10 min If *CVP rises* sharply, fluid restriction necessary; if remains low, hypovolemia present 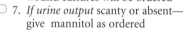 6. *If client febrile*—blood cultures and wound cultures will be ordered 7. *If urine output* scanty or absent— give mannitol as ordered 8. *If systolic BP*<90 mm Hg, give vasopressors (Levophed, vasopressin)
Respiratory Emergencies			
Choking—obstruction of airway secondary to aspiration of a foreign object	Gasping, wheezing; looks panicky, but can still breathe, talk, cough *Cough:* weak, ineffective; breathing sounds like high-pitched crowing; *Color*—white, gray, blue Difficulty speaking; clutches throat	Do not interfere if coughing; do *not* slap on back; watch closely; call for assistance **▶** *Victim standing/sitting and conscious:* Perform *obstructive airway maneuver* (formerly called Heimlich maneuver): stand behind victim, wrap arms around waist, place fist against abdomen, and with your other hand, press it into the victim's abdomen with a quick upward thrust until the obstruction is relieved or the victim becomes unconscious	As in prehospital care
		Victim lying down: Roll the victim onto his or her back; straddle the victim's thighs; place heel of hand in the middle of abdomen; place other hand on top of the first; stiffen arms and deliver 6 to 10 abdominal thrusts	As in prehospital care
		Unconscious victim: *Lay rescuers*—proceed to CPR. No abdominal thrusts or blind finger sweeps	As in prehospital care; when probing mouth for foreign object, turn *head to side*, unless client has neck injury; in event of neck injury, *raise* the arm opposite you and roll the head and shoulders as a unit, so that head ends up supported on the arm

(Continued on following page)

Condition	◆ Assessment: Signs and Symptoms	▶ Prehospitalization Nursing Care	▶ In-hospital Nursing Care
Respiratory Emergencies (cont'd)		*EMS responders* —Try to ventilate; if unsuccessful, deliver abdominal thrusts using technique described for obstructive airway; probe mouth for foreign objects; keep repeating above procedure until ventilation occurs; as victim becomes more deprived of air, muscles will relax and maneuvers that were previously unsuccessful will begin to work; when successful in removing obstruction, give two breaths; check pulse; start CPR if indicated On ***obese or pregnant*** victims—use chest thrusts instead of abdominal thrusts ***You are victim and alone:*** Place your two fists for abdominal thrusts; bend over back of chair, sink, etc. and exert hard, repeated pressure on abdomen to force object up; push fingers down your throat to encourage regurgitation	
Acute respiratory failure— sudden onset of an abnormally low PaO_2 (<60 mm Hg) or high Pco_2 (>60 mm Hg) secondary to: lung disease or trauma, peripheral or central nervous system depression, cardiac failure, severe obesity, airway obstruction, environmental abnormality	*Hypoxia* *Sensorium:* acute apprehension *Respiration:* dyspnea; shallow, rapid respirations *Skin:* circumoral cyanosis; pale, dusky skin and nailbeds *C/V:* slight hypertension and tachycardia, or hypotension and bradycardia *Hypercapnia* *Sensorium:* decreasing mentation; headache *Skin:* flushed, warm, moist *C/V:* hypertension; tachycardia	If you suspect respiratory distress, call physician; calm and reassure client; place in a chair or *semisitting* position; keep warm but not hot; phone for ambulance; *if respirations cease* or client becomes unconscious: clear airway and commence respiratory resuscitation; check pulse: initiate CPR if necessary; continue resuscitation until help arrives	Check client's ability to speak; maintain airway by placing in *high Fowler's position*; check vital signs: BP, pulse rate and rhythm, temperature, skin color, rate and depth of respirations; place on O_2, pulse oximetry, **STAT** ABG *Prepare for intubation if:* 1. Client has flail chest 2. Client is comatose without gag reflex 3. Has respiratory arrest; open airway, Ambubag with 100% O_2 via face mask until intubation 4. $Paco_2$ > 55 mm Hg 5. Pao_2 < 60 mm Hg 6. F_iO_2 > 50 % using nasal cannula, catheter, or mask 7. Respiratory rate > 36 *After intubation:* 1. Check bilateral lung sounds 2. Observe for symmetrical lung expansion 3. Maintain humidified oxygen at lowest F_iO_2 possible to achieve Pao_2 of 60 mm Hg 4. Monitor exhaled CO_2 with caprometer.

Adult

(Continued on following page)

	◆ **Assessment: Signs**	▶ **Prehospitalization**	▶ **In-hospital**
Condition	**and Symptoms**	**Nursing Care**	**Nursing Care**
			Improve ventilation (decrease Pco₂) by:
			1. Frequent suctioning—oral and above cuff of ET tube
			2. IPPB indicated if tidal volume decreases
			3. Administer *drugs* as ordered: sympathomimetics, xanthines, antibiotics, and steroids
			4. Monitor: arterial blood gases, electrolytes, Hct, Hgb, and WBC
			5. Bronchoscopy may be indicated for thick, tenacious secretions
			Do not:
			1. Administer sedatives
			2. Correct acid-base problems without monitoring electrolytes
			3. Overcorrect Paco₂
			4. Leave client alone while oxygen therapy is initiated. Once client is stable, transfer to ICU
Near-drowning— asphyxiation or partial asphyxiation due to immersion or submersion in a fluid or liquid medium	*Conscious victim:* Acute anxiety, panic; increased rate of respirations Pale, dusky skin	*Conscious victim:* 1. Try to talk victim out of panic so can find footing and way to shore 2. Utilize devices such as poles, rings, clothing to extend to victim; do *not* let victim who is panicked grab you; do *not* attempt swimming rescue unless specially trained 3. If you suspect head or neck injury—handle carefully, floating victim back to shore with body and head as straight as possible; do *not* turn head or bend back	*Nonsymptomatic near-drowning victim:* 1. Draw blood for arterial blood gases with client breathing room air 2. PA and lateral chest x-ray 3. Auscultate lungs 4. Admit to hospital for further evaluation if: a. Pao₂ < 80 mm Hg b. pH < 7.35 c. Pulmonary infiltrates present, or auscultation reveals crackles d. Victim inhaled fluids containing: choline, hydrocarbons, sewage, or hypotonic or fresh water
	Unconscious victim: Shallow or no respirations Weak or no pulse	*Unconscious victim:* 1. *If victim not breathing:* as soon as you have firm support, begin mouth-to-mouth resuscitation 2. Tilt head back, bring jaw forward, pinch nostril shut, give two quick breaths	
		On shore: 1. Check breathing 2. Lay victim flat on back; cover and keep warm 3. Calm and reassure victim 4. Do *not* give food or water 5. Get to medical assistance as soon as possible 6. *If unconscious and not breathing:* begin sequence for CPR; compress water from abdomen *only* if interfering with ventilation attempts 7. *If airway obstructed:* reposition head; attempt to ventilate; *if EMS responder:* perform 6 to 10 abdominal thrusts; sweep mouth deeply; attempt to ventilate; repeat until successful	*Symptomatic near-drowning victim:* 1. Provide basic or advanced cardiac life support 2. Provide clear airway and adequate ventilation by: a. Suctioning airway b. Inserting artificial airway and attaching it to ventilator as indicated c. Inserting nasogastric tube to suction to minimize aspiration of vomitus 3. Monitor ECG continuously 4. Start IV infusion 5% D/W at keep-open rate for *fresh water near-drowning;* 5% D/NS in *salt water near-drowning*

(Continued on following page)

Adult

Condition	◆ Assessment: Signs and Symptoms	▶ Prehospitalization Nursing Care	▶ In-hospital Nursing Care

		8. Once ventilation established, check pulse; *if absent*, begin chest compressions as in CPR, one-person or two-person rescue
		9. Continue CPR until victim revives or help arrives
		10. If victim revives, cover and keep warm; reassure victim help is on the way
		11. Rescue personnel can further assist emergency department personnel by:
		  a. Documenting prehospital resuscitation methods used
		  b. Immobilizing victims suspected of cervical spine injuries
		  c. Using a sterile container to take a sample of immersion fluid
		  d. Taking on-scene arterial blood gas sample for later analysis
			5. Assist with insertion of *CVP* and *PA (pulmonary artery) catheter* to guide subsequent infusion rates
			6. Administer drugs as ordered: anticonvulsants; steroids, antibiotics, stimulants, antiarrhythmics
			7. Provide rewarming if hypothermia present
			8. Insert *Foley* to assess kidney function because fresh water near-drowning causes renal tubular necrosis due to RBC hemolysis
			9. Transfer to ICU when stabilized

Systemic Injuries

| *Multiple traumas* | *Sensorium:* alert; disoriented, stuporous, comatose
Respirations: increased rate, depth; shallow; asymmetrical; paradoxical breathing; mediastinal shift; gasping, blowing
C/V: signs of shock (see **pp. 504–505**)
Abdomen: contusions; pain; abrasions; open wounds; rigidity; increasing distention
Skeletal system: pain; swelling; deformity; inappropriate or no movement
Neurological: pupils round, equal, react to light; ipsilateral dilation and unresponsive; fixed and dilated bilaterally
Bilateral movement and sensation in all extremities
Progressive contralateral weakness
Loss of voluntary motor function | 1. Do *not* move client unless you must, to prevent further injury; send for help
2. Check breathing—give mouth-to-mouth resuscitation if indicated
3. Check for bleeding
4. Control bleeding by applying pressure on wound or on pressure points (artery proximal to wound)
5. Use tourniquet *only* if above pressure techniques fail to stop severe bleeding
6. Check for shock (pulse, pupils, skin color) and other injuries
7. Fractures: keep open-fracture area clean
8. Do *not* try to set bone
9. If client must be moved—splint broken bones with splints that extend past the limb joints; tie splints on snugly but not so tight as to cut off circulation
10. Check peripheral pulses
11. If head or back injury suspected—keep body *straight;* move only with help | 1. Assess vital functions; ECG monitoring, continuous pulse oximetry
2. Establish airway; ventilate with Ambubag, ventilator
3. Draw arterial blood gases
4. Control bleeding
5. Prepare infusions of blood, crystalloids
6. Assess for other injuries: head injuries—suspect cervical neck injury with all head injuries
7. Place sandbags to immobilize head and neck
8. Do *mini-neurological exam:* level of consciousness, pupils, bilateral movement, and sensation
9. Get history—time of injury; any loss of consciousness; any drug ingestion
10. Stop bleeding on or about head
11. Apply ice to contusions and hematomas
12. Check for bleeding from nose, pharynx, ears
13. Check for cerebrospinal fluid from ears or nose
14. Assist with spinal tap if ordered
15. Keep accurate I&O
16. Protect from injury if restless, seizures; orient to time, place, person |

(Continued on following page)

Adult

TABLE 7.50	Nursing Care of the Adult in Medical and Surgical Emergencies *(Continued)*		
Condition	◆ **Assessment: Signs and Symptoms**	▶ **Prehospitalization Nursing Care**	▶ **In-hospital Nursing Care**
	See *Sensorium* p. 679 for level of consciousness	12. Reassure client that help is on the way	17. Administer steroids, diuretics, as ordered
			18. *Check for signs of increasing intracranial pressure:* slowing pulse and respiration, widened pulse pressure, decreasing mentation
Spinal injuries			1. Assess and support vital functions as above
			2. Immobilize—no flexion or extension allowed
			3. *If in respiratory distress*—nasotracheal intubation or tracheostomy to *avoid* hyperextending neck
			4. *Check for level of injury and function*, asking client to: a. Lift elbow to shoulder height (C-5) b. Bend elbow (C-6) c. Straighten elbow (C-7) d. Grip your hand (C-8-T-1) e. Lift leg (L-3) f. Straighten knee (L-4, L-5) g. Wiggle toes (L-5) h. Push toes down (S-1)
			5. *If client is comatose:* a. Rub sternum with knuckles b. If all extremities move, severe injury unlikely c. If one side moves and other does not, potential hemiplegia d. If arms move and legs do not, lower spinal cord injury
			6. Administer steroids as ordered
			7. Assist with application of skull tongs—*Vinke* or *Crutchfield*
			8. Maintain IV infusions
			9. Insert *Foley* as indicated
			10. Assist with dressing of open wounds
Chest injuries			1. Note color and pattern of respirations, position of trachea
			2. Auscultate lungs and palpate chest for: crepitus, pain, tenderness, and position of trachea
			3. Place gauze soaked in petroleum jelly, if available, over open pneumothorax (sucking chest wound) to seal hole and decrease respiratory distress
			4. Assist with tracheostomy if indicated
			5. Prepare for insertion of chest tubes if pneumothorax or hemothorax present
Abdominal injuries			1. Observe for rigidity
			2. Check for hematuria
			3. Auscultate for bowel sounds
			4. Assist with paracentesis to confirm bleeding in abdominal cavity
			5. Prepare for exploratory laparotomy
			6. Insert nasogastric tube—to detect presence of upper GI bleeding
			7. Monitor vital signs
			If organs protruding: 1. *Flex* client's knees 2. Cover intestines with sterile towel soaked in saline 3. Do *not* attempt to replace organs
Fractures			1. Administer tetanus toxoid as ordered
			2. Observe for pain, peripheral pulses, pallor, loss of sensation and/or movement
			3. Assist with wound cleansing, casting, x-rays, reduction
			4. Prepare for surgery if indicated
			5. Monitor vital signs

(Continued on following page)

Adult

Condition	◆ Assessment: Signs and Symptoms	▶ Prehospitalization Nursing Care	▶ In-hospital Nursing Care
Burns—tissue trauma secondary to scalding fluid or flame, chemicals, or electricity	*Superficial (first degree):* Erythema and tenderness Usually sunburn	Relieve pain by applying cold, wet towel or cold water (*not* iced)	1. Cleanse thoroughly with mild detergent and water 2. Apply gauze or sterile towel 3. Administer sedatives and narcotics as ordered 4. Arrange for follow-up care, or prepare for admission if burn ambulatory care impractical

	Partial thickness (second degree): Swelling, blisters; moisture due to escaping plasma	1. Douse with cold water until pain relieved
		2. Blot skin dry and cover with clean towel
		3. Do *not*: break blisters, remove pieces of skin, or apply antiseptic ointments
		 4. If arm or leg burned, keep *elevated*
		
		┌─────────────────────────────┐
		5. Seek medical attention if *second-degree* burns:
		  a. Cover 10% of body surface
		  b. Involve hands, feet, or face
		└─────────────────────────────┘
			1. Check tetanus immunization status
			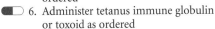 2. Administer sedatives or narcotics as ordered
			3. Assess respiratory and hemodynamic status; oxygen or ventilatory assist as indicated, intravenous infusions as ordered to combat shock
			4. Remove all clothing from burn area
			5. Using *aseptic technique*, cleanse burns as indicated

	Full thickness (third degree): White, charred areas	1. Do *not* remove charred clothing
		2. Cover burned area with clean towel, sheet
		 3. *Elevate* burned extremities
		4. Apply cold pack to hand, face, or feet
		5. Sit client up with face or chest wound to assist respirations
		6. Maintain airway
		7. Observe for shock
		
		┌─────────────────────────────┐
		8. Do *not*:
		  a. Put ice water on burns or immerse wounds in ice water—may increase shock
		  b. Apply ointments
		└─────────────────────────────┘
		9. Calm and reassure victim
		10. Get medical help promptly
		11. *If* client conscious, not vomiting, and medical assistance is more than 6 hr away: may give sips of weak solution of salt, soda, and water
			1. Do *not* break blebs or attempt debridement
			2. Assist with application of dressings as ordered
			3. Maintain frequent checks of vital signs, urine output
			4. Provide psychological support—explain procedures, orient, etc.
			5. Assist with application of splints as ordered
			6. Administer tetanus immune globulin or toxoid as ordered
			7. Assist with transfer to hospital unit

	Fourth degree: Black *Chemical burns*	Same as full thickness. 1. Flush with copious amounts of water 2. Get rid of clothing over burned area	1. Flush with copious amounts of water 2. Administer sedation or narcotics as ordered
	Burns of the eye: Acid	1. Flush eye with water for at least 15 min 2. Pour water from inside to outside of eye to *avoid contaminating unaffected eye* 3. Cover—seek medical attention **at once**	1. Irrigate with water: *never* use neutralizing solution 2. Instill 0.5% tetracaine as ordered 3. Apply patch

(Continued on following page)

Adult

TABLE 7.50	Nursing Care of the Adult in Medical and Surgical Emergencies *(Continued)*

Condition	◆ Assessment: Signs and Symptoms	▶ Prehospitalization Nursing Care	▶ In-hospital Nursing Care
	Alkali (laundry detergent or cleaning solvent)	1. Do *not* allow client to rub eye 2. Flush eye with water for at least 30 min 3. Cover—seek medical attention **at once**	As above for acid
Abdominal Emergencies			
Aortic aneurysm—rupture or dissection	Primarily men > age 60 Sudden onset of excruciating pain: abdominal, lumbosacral, groin, or rectal Orthopnea, dyspnea Fainting, hypotension; if dissecting, marked hypertension may be present Palpable, tender, pulsating mass in umbilical area Femoral pulse present; dorsalis pedis—weak or absent	1. Notify physician 2. Lay client flat, or raise head if in respiratory distress 3. Cover to keep warm but *not* hot 4. Institute shock measures as above 5. Calm; reassure that help is on the way.	1. Assess respiratory and hemodynamic status 2. Institute shock measures (see **pp. 675–676**) if indicated 3. Evaluate and compare peripheral pulses 4. Assist with x-rays 5. Assist with emergency preoperative treatment

Blunt injuries—*spleen*	Left upper quadrant pain, tenderness and moderate rigidity; left shoulder pain (*Kehr's sign*)
	Hypotension; weak, thready pulse; increased respirations (shock)
		1. Lay client *flat*
		2. Institute shock measures (see **pp. 675–676**)
			1. Assess respiratory and hemodynamic status
			  a. Maintain airway and ventilation as indicated
			  b. Institute infusions of colloid or crystalloids as ordered
			  c. Insert both CVP and arterial monitoring lines
			  d. Insert *Foley* catheter
			2. Prepare for splenectomy

Eye and Ear Emergencies			
Chemical burns	*See Burns* **p. 681**	*See Burns*	*See Burns*
Blunt injuries secondary to flying missiles (e.g., balls, striking face against car dashboard)	Decreased visual acuity, diplopia, blood in anterior chamber Pain, conjunctiva reddened, edema of eyelids	1. Prevent victim from rubbing eye 2. Cover with patch to protect eye 3. Seek medical help **immediately**	1. Test visual acuity of each eye using *Snellen* or *Jaeger* chart 2. Assist with *fluorescein* administration—to facilitate identifying breaks in cornea
Sharp ocular trauma—secondary to small or larger foreign bodies	Reports feeling as if something were hitting eye Pain, tearing, reddened conjunctiva Blurring of vision Foreign object may be visible	1. Keep victim from rubbing eye 2. Cover very lightly—do *not* apply pressure	1. Check visual acuity in both eyes 2. Check pupils 3. Instill 1% tetracaine HCl as ordered to relieve pain 4. Administer antibiotic drops or ointment as ordered 5. Apply eye patch 6. Provide instructions for subsequent care and follow-up

Foreign bodies in ears—beans, peas, candy, foxtails, insects	Decreased hearing; pulling, poking at ear and ear canal; buzzing, discomfort	1. Do *not* attempt to remove object
		2. Seek medical assistance
			1. Inspect ear canal
			2. Assist with sedating (especially children)—restraint may be necessary
			3. Assist with procedures to remove object:
			  a. Forceps or curved probe for *foxtails, irregularly shaped* objects
			  b. 10F or 12F catheter with tip cut squarely off and attached to suction to remove *round* object
			4. Irrigate external auditory canal to flush out *insects*, materials that do not absorb water; do *not* irrigate if danger of perforation

Questions

Select the one answer that is best for each question, unless otherwise directed.

1. Nursing preparations for a gastroscopy procedure include:
   1. Holding the client NPO for 24 hours before the procedure.
   2. Having an operative or procedure consent form signed.
   3. Reassuring the client that gastroscopy is not an uncomfortable procedure, though he or she will need to lie quietly.
   4. Removing dentures and administering pain medication before the procedure.
2. Which nursing action is the *first* priority during a generalized tonic-clonic seizure episode?
   1. Observe and record all events that occur before, during, and after the seizure.
   2. Maintain a patent airway by turning the head to the side.
   3. Protect the client from injury.
   4. Monitor vital signs, with special attention directed to respiratory status.
3. Which assessment finding indicates circulatory constriction in the client with a newly applied long leg cast?
   1. Tingling and numbness of toes.
   2. Inability to move toes.
   3. Blanching or cyanosis of toes.
   4. Complaints of pressure or tightness of the cast.
4. Paralytic ileus is described by the nurse as:
   1. Edema of the intestinal mucosa.
   2. Acute dilation of the colon.
   3. Absent, diminished, or uncoordinated autonomic stimulation of peristalsis.
   4. High, tinkling bowel sounds over the area of obstruction.
5. The nurse's best explanation of the basic emotional issue underlying or contributing to the development of ulcers would be:
   1. Anxiety neurosis.
   2. Dependence-independence conflict.
   3. Repressed anger and hostility.
   4. Compulsive time orientation.
6. With severe diarrhea, electrolytes as well as fluids are lost. Which of the following would be observed in a client experiencing hypokalemia?
   Select all that apply.
   1. Muscle spasms
   2. Apathy
   3. Muscle weakness
   4. Thirst
   5. GI disturbance
7. Fluid intake for clients suffering from dumping syndrome should be:
   1. Between meals.
   2. Only with meals.
   3. Any time they want.
   4. Restricted to 1200 mL/day.

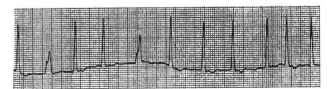

8. The correct interpretation of the above arrhythmia is:
   1. Sinus rhythm with multifocal premature ventricular contractions (PVCs).
   2. Atrial fibrillation with unifocal PVCs.
   3. Sinus tachycardia with unifocal PVCs.
   4. Second-degree atrioventricular block with unifocal PVCs.

9. The nurse explains to a client that a vagotomy is done in conjunction with a subtotal gastrectomy because the function of the vagus nerve is to:
   1. Stimulate increased gastric motility.
   2. Decrease gastric motility, thereby preventing the movement of HCl out of the stomach.
   3. Stimulate both increased gastric secretion and gastric motility.
   4. Stimulate decreased gastric secretion, thereby increasing nausea and vomiting.
10. In planning care for a client with hyperkalemia, the nurse knows that the treatment of choice to reduce hyperkalemia is:
    1. Morphine sulfate.
    2. Sodium polystyrene sulfonate (Kayexalate).
    3. Insulin and 50% glucose solution.
    4. Synthetic aldosterone.

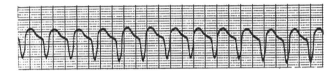

11. The nurse knows that the arrhythmia shown above, if untreated, will most likely cause:
    1. Ventricular fibrillation.
    2. A sudden increase in blood pressure.
    3. Chest pain from a myocardial infarction (MI).
    4. No observable change in the client.
12. The nurse tells a client who is postoperative after a gastrectomy that dumping syndrome is a significant problem for:
    1. 70%–80% of clients having gastrectomies.
    2. 50% of clients having gastrectomies.
    3. 25% of clients having gastrectomies.
    4. 5%–10% of clients having gastrectomies.
13. The nurse knows that, in contrast to clients with hypothyroidism, women with hyperthyroidism have increased:
    1. Serum cholesterol.
    2. Basal metabolic rate and serum T_3 and T_4.
    3. Serum thyroid-stimulating hormone (TSH).
    4. Menstrual volume.
14. Hyponatremia may develop in clients with burns due to:
    1. Displacement of sodium in edema fluids and loss through denuded areas of skin.
    2. Increased aldosterone secretion.
    3. Inadequate fluid replacement.
    4. Metabolic acidosis.
15. The nurse tells a client who is postoperative after a gastrectomy that the nasogastric tube will be removed:
    1. According to standard procedures only on the fourth postoperative day.
    2. When bowel sounds are established and the client has passed flatus or stool.
    3. Thirty-six hours after the cessation of bloody drainage.
    4. After 2 days of alternate clamping and unclamping of the tube.
16. A client with burns is to receive fluid replacement therapy. Besides assessing size and depth of the burn, which physical parameters are also important baseline data for fluid replacement therapy?
    1. Age, sex, and vital signs.
    2. Age, weight, vital signs, and skin turgor.
    3. Vital signs, level of mentation, and urine output.
    4. Vital signs and quantity and specific gravity of urine.
17. The nurse must observe for which imbalance with prolonged nasogastric suctioning?
    1. Hypernatremia.
    2. Hyperkalemia.

3. Metabolic alkalosis.

4. Hypoproteinemia.

18. The client who is postoperative after a nephrectomy should be closely observed by the nurse for:
    1. Hemorrhage.
    2. Hyperkalemia.
    3. Respiratory alkalosis and tetany.
    4. Polyuria.

19. Two days postoperatively, a client who has had an ileostomy begins to refuse care and repeatedly says to the staff, "Leave me alone, I just want to sleep." What would be the first nursing action?
    1. Provide accurate, brief, and reassuring explanations of all procedures.
    2. Encourage ambulation in the hall with other clients.
    3. Invite a member of an "ostomy club" to visit the client.
    4. Encourage the client to verbalize his or her feelings, fears, and questions.

20. The mouth care measure that should be used with caution by the nurse when a client has a nasogastric tube is:
    1. Regularly brushing teeth and tongue with soft brush.
    2. Sucking on ice chips to relieve dryness.
    3. Occasionally rinsing mouth with a nonastringent substance and massaging gums.
    4. Application of lemon juice and glycerine swabs to the lips.

21. Two days before discharge following a left nephrectomy, a client expressed renewed concern over the ability to continue many activities with only one kidney. The nurse responds.
    1. "You seem depressed. Actually you are very lucky, since the pathology reports indicate your tumor was encapsulated."
    2. "Lots of people do quite well with only one kidney."
    3. "Would you like me to call the doctor so you two can discuss it?"
    4. "I can understand your concern, but your remaining kidney is sufficient to maintain normal renal functions."

22. On the morning of discharge, a client who had an emergency abdominal hysterectomy is found sitting with her back to the door, staring out the window. She says that she no longer feels like a real woman. The nurse's response should be to:
    1. Ask her if she would like her diazepam (Valium).
    2. Notify the physician.
    3. Ask, "Can you tell me what makes you feel that way?"
    4. Reassure her that this is a common reaction.

23. Which behavior is *least* likely to be included in the nursing assessment of a client with burns during the recovery period?
    1. Anxiety with mild confusion.
    2. Desperation and panic.
    3. Withdrawal and depression.
    4. Dependency and regression.

24. Forty-eight hours after a nephrectomy, a client complains of increasing nausea and abdominal pressure. The nurse's *first* nursing action is to:
    1. Change the client's position to relieve abdominal pressure.
    2. Auscultate bowel sounds.
    3. Insert a rectal tube to relieve flatus.
    4. Administer morphine SO_4, 6 mg, as ordered for the relief of discomfort.

25. Which instruction would be *inappropriate* when teaching a client to use crutches?
    1. Use axilla to help carry weight.
    2. Use short strides to maintain maximum mobility.
    3. Keep feet 6–8 inches apart to provide a wide base for support.
    4. If the client should begin to fall, throw crutches to the side to prevent falling on them.

26. The nurse explains that epileptic seizures or convulsions result from:

1. Excessive exercise with lactic acid accumulation.
2. Excessive, simultaneous, disordered neuronal discharge.
3. Excessive cerebral metabolism, with local K^+ increased.
4. Excessive circulating cerebrospinal fluid increasing cerebral pressures.

27. What nursing action best facilitates the passage of the nasoenteric tube from the stomach through the pylorus and into the duodenum?
    1. Gently advancing the tube 1–4 inches at regular time intervals.
    2. Positioning the client on the right side for 2 hours after insertion.
    3. Maintaining strict bedrest and avoiding all unnecessary movement.
    4. Positioning the client in a flat supine position.

28. During the initial stage of burns, a primary fluid imbalance occurs. The nurse knows that there has been a shift of fluids from:
    1. The cell to the interstitial space.
    2. The interstitial space into the cell.
    3. The interstitial space to the plasma.
    4. The plasma to the interstitial space.

29. Bedrest is ordered for a client with chronic glaucoma during a period of acute distress, because activity tends to increase intraocular pressure. Which activity of daily living should this client be instructed to avoid?
    1. Watching television.
    2. Brushing teeth and hair.
    3. Self-feeding.
    4. Passive range-of-motion exercises.

30. Which sign(s) and/or symptom(s) would be observed in a client with hypoglycemia and pending insulin shock? *Select all that apply.*
    1. Rapid, shallow respirations.
    2. Fetid breath odor.
    3. Irritability.
    4. Confusion.
    5. Clammy skin.
    6. Slurring of words.

31. The nurse will usually ambulate a client postgastrectomy beginning:
    1. The day after surgery.
    2. 3–4 days after surgery.
    3. After 4 days of bedrest.
    4. Immediately after awakening from anesthesia.

32. If "cholinergic crisis" occurs in a client who has myasthenia gravis, all anticholinesterase drugs are withdrawn. To reduce symptoms, which drug should the nurse be prepared to give?
    1. Atropine.
    2. Ephedrine sulfate.
    3. Potassium chloride.
    4. Neostigmine bromide.

33. Client teaching about glaucoma should include a comparison of the two types. Open-angle, or chronic glaucoma differs from closed-angle or acute glaucoma in that:
    1. Open-angle glaucoma occurs less frequently than closed-angle glaucoma.
    2. Open-angle glaucoma's symptomatology includes pain, severe headache, nausea, and vomiting; closed-angle glaucoma has a slow, silent, and generally painless onset.
    3. The obstruction to aqueous flow in open-angle glaucoma generally occurs somewhere in Schlemm's canal or aqueous veins. It does not narrow or close the angle of the anterior chamber, as in closed-angle glaucoma.
    4. Open-angle glaucoma rarely occurs in families; however, there is a hereditary predisposition for closed-angle glaucoma.

34. The adequacy of fluid volume replacement in the early post-burn period is best reflected by:
    1. Blood pressure, pulse rates, and daily weights.
    2. Quantity of urinary output and vital signs.
    3. Hemoglobin and hematocrit levels.
    4. Serum-electrolyte levels and urinary output.
35. Which would the nurse expect to see with the dumping syndrome?
    1. Feeling of hunger.
    2. Constipation.
    3. Increased strength.
    4. Diaphoresis.
36. Fifty-four hours after deep partial-thickness burns of the left leg and thigh, the client's urine output increased from 1000 to 2300 mL/24 hr; serum sodium, 136 mEq/L; serum potassium, 4 mEq/L; and hematocrit, 34%. The client's urinary output and lab studies indicate:
    1. Beginning of the interstitial-to-plasma fluid shift phase of burns.
    2. Kidney failure.
    3. Circulatory overload due to rapid IV infusion rate.
    4. Hyponatremia.
37. The nurse would be correct in saying that two common causes of primary hypothyroidism are:
    1. Destruction of thyroid tissue by radioactive iodine during therapy for hyperthyroidism, and spontaneous atrophy due to autoimmune response.
    2. Spontaneous atrophy due to autoimmune response, and surgical removal of the thyroid gland.
    3. Surgical removal of the thyroid gland, and tumors of the pituitary gland that decrease the amount of circulating thyroxine.
    4. Tumors of the pituitary gland, and/or large doses of antithyroid drugs.
38. Because medications have been increased for a client with myasthenia gravis, it is important that the nurse observe for signs of "cholinergic crisis." These include:
    1. Dilated pupils, profuse diaphoresis, and trembling.
    2. Constricted pupils, hypersalivation, and hypotension.
    3. Dilated pupils, nausea, and tachycardia.
    4. Constricted pupils, dry mucous membranes, and bradycardia.
39. Iron deficiency anemia is best described as:
    1. Hypochromic microcytic.
    2. Hyperchromic macrocytic.
    3. Hyperchromic microcytic.
    4. Hypochromic macrocytic.
40. The nurse should expect that a client's emotional responses to acute rheumatoid arthritis would primarily depend on the client's:
    1. Self-concept, body image, and usual effective coping strategies.
    2. Relationship with the client's mother.
    3. Usual effective or palliative coping strategies only.
    4. Economic status and work history.
41. Because aldosterone is the major mineralocorticoid secreted by the adrenal cortex, which fluid and electrolyte imbalance should the nurse anticipate with decreased secretion of this hormone?
    1. Hyperkalemia.
    2. Hypernatremia.
    3. Hypervolemia.
    4. Hypercalcemia.
42. Which cardinal sign heralds the onset of thyroid storm?
    1. Fever.
    2. Tachycardia.
    3. Hypertension.
    4. Tremulousness.

43. The nurse would recognize drainage of blood from the nasogastric tube after gastrectomy surgery as abnormal if:
    1. It continued for 4–6 hours.
    2. It continued for a period longer than 12 hours.
    3. It turned greenish yellow in less than 24 hours.
    4. It was dark red in the immediate postoperative period.

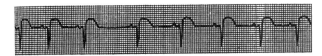

44. The appropriate nursing response to the above arrhythmia would be to:
    1. Administer a bolus of lidocaine, 50 mg IV.
    2. Limit client activity while the arrhythmia is present.
    3. Hold digoxin until atrioventricular node depression reverses.
    4. Do nothing, particularly with no symptoms.
45. Following gastrectomy surgery the nurse must observe for signs of pernicious anemia, which may be a problem after gastrectomy because:
    1. The extrinsic factor is produced in the stomach.
    2. The extrinsic factor is absorbed in the antral portion of the stomach.
    3. The intrinsic factor is produced in the stomach.
    4. Decreased hydrochloric acid production inhibits vitamin B_{12} reabsorption.
46. A client is awaiting surgery for reduction of a fractured right femur. Skeletal traction has been applied. Which nursing diagnosis requires the nurse to function collaboratively to achieve the best outcome for the client?
    1. Risk for impaired skin integrity.
    2. Pain (acute).
    3. Impaired physical mobility.
    4. Risk for fracture deformity.
47. What should be included in the preoperative teaching before a thyroidectomy?
    Select all that apply.
    1. Report hoarseness of voice.
    2. Support the back of the neck when turning.
    2. Flex the neck hourly to avoid contractions.
    4. Keep the neck hyperextended to open airway.
    5. Use the incentive spirometer regularly.
48. Which is most important to include in teaching a client about preventing heat cramps when working outside in hot weather?
    1. Prior history of heat sensitivity.
    2. Need to maintain sodium level in body.
    3. Importance of drinking fluids to stay cool.
    4. Risk of potassium and magnesium loss.
49. The most important information to include when teaching a client who is being discharged on continuous ambulatory peritoneal dialysis (CAPD) would be the need to:
    1. Use sterile technique to prevent infection.
    2. Increase protein in the diet.
    3. Record blood pressure and weight daily.
    4. Wear a medical identification bracelet.
50. A client complaining of severe indigestion while walking in the hall, grabs his chest and falls to the floor. The *first* assessment to make would be to determine:
    1. Unresponsiveness.
    2. Breathing pattern.
    3. Blood pressure.
    4. Presence of a pulse.
51. A client has hypotension, jugular venous distention, and muffled heart sounds on auscultation. The nurse would anticipate that the client's treatment will be directed at:

1. Reversing cardiogenic shock.
2. Improving left ventricular function.
3. Reducing the degree of ventricular hypertrophy.
4. Managing pericardial effusion or tamponade.

52. Which nursing assessment would identify the earliest indication of increasing intracranial pressure?
    1. Temperature over 102°F.
    2. Change in level of consciousness.
    3. Widening pulse pressure.
    4. Unequal pupils.

53. What is the most common reaction to an epidural narcotic for postoperative pain management that a nurse would observe?
    1. Slowing of the respiratory rate.
    2. Increase in the heart rate.
    3. Increased urinary urgency.
    4. Itching.

54. The postoperative priority for a client being transferred from postanesthesia recovery to the surgical floor would be to:
    1. Maintain cardiac output related to blood loss.
    2. Manage pain related to large abdominal incision.
    3. Monitor possible infection related to surgical wound.
    4. Assess risk for activity intolerance.

55. The priority nursing action for a client admitted with a productive cough, weight loss, and a suspected diagnosis of tuberculosis is:
    1. Instruction on preventing disease transmission.
    2. Planning for frequent rest periods.
    3. Recording accurate intake and output.
    4. Reviewing current dietary patterns.

56. The client becomes pulseless with a monitored rhythm of sinus tachycardia following a motor vehicle accident and a fractured right femur. The nurse should prepare for:
    1. Mechanical ventilation and administration of sodium bicarbonate.
    2. CPR and epinephrine IV push.
    3. Atropine IV and intubation with mechanical ventilation.
    4. Isoproterenol (Isuprel) followed by CPR.

57. A person who is diabetic is brought into the emergency department by a friend who found him on the floor unconscious. The first nursing action would be to:
    1. Ask the friend what happened and how long the client was unconscious.
    2. Assess the client for signs of head trauma when he collapsed.
    3. Obtain a blood sugar level and start an IV infusion.
    4. Contact the client's immediate family to come to the hospital.

58. The laboratory findings for a client with polycythemia vera include major and minor criteria. What is the major or defining hematological finding?
    1. Leukocytosis >12,000/mm³.
    2. Thrombocytosis >400,000/mm³.
    3. RBC count >6 million/mm³.
    4. Elevated leukocyte alkaline phosphatase.

59. When ambulating a client who is blind, the nurse should be positioned:
    1. Behind the client, holding the client's elbows.
    2. In front, with the client holding the nurse's arm at elbow.
    3. On the client's side, holding the dominant hand.
    4. On the client's side, holding the nondominant hand.

60. Which problem should the nurse expect following uterine isotope insertion?
    1. Bladder atony.
    2. Constipation.
    3. Foul-smelling vaginal discharge.
    4. Loss of sexual libido.

61. Preoperative nursing measures for a client having a cholecystectomy due to cholelithiasis and cholecystitis include:
    1. Observing for bruising or easy bleeding due to potential prothrombin deficiency.
    2. Informing the client of the purpose of the postoperative Jackson-Pratt drain.
    3. Providing relief for abdominal discomfort by placing a heating pad on the upper abdomen.
    4. Providing a low-carbohydrate diet to stimulate release of glycogen stores in the liver.

62. What is the best single nursing measure of fluid volume status in a client with chronic renal dysfunction?
    1. Skin turgor.
    2. Vital signs.
    3. Daily weights.
    4. Intake and output.

63. When can the nurse expect a client who is receiving NPH insulin at 7:30 A.M. to *most* likely have a hypoglycemic reaction?
    1. Before lunch (10–11 A.M.).
    2. Early afternoon (1–3 A.M.).
    3. Late afternoon (4–7 A.M.).
    4. After supper (8–10 A.M.).

64. The physician has left orders to deflate a client's Sengstaken-Blakemore tube, used to stop esophageal bleeding, for 5 minutes every 12 hours to prevent esophageal erosion. Two hours following the second reinflation, the client suddenly becomes severely dyspneic and dusky. The nurse should:
    1. Call a code blue (cardiac arrest).
    2. Deflate the balloons.
    3. Decrease the traction on the tube where it enters the nose.
    4. Irrigate the tube with ice-cold saline to facilitate movement of the balloons into the stomach.

65. Postoperative coughing and deep breathing may become a nursing problem following cholecystectomy because:
    1. Clients having abdominal surgery are prone to pulmonary complications.
    2. Clients with biliary surgery tend to breathe shallowly to prevent pain and discomfort.
    3. Many people tend to be thoracic breathers rather than diaphragmatic breathers.
    4. Clients with upper-abdominal surgery usually have a nasogastric tube in place, which inhibits deep breathing.

66. Which statement is correct regarding nursing care of a client receiving hyperalimentation?
    1. The client's urine should be tested for glucose and acetone every 8–12 hours.
    2. The hyperalimentation subclavian line may be utilized for CVP readings and/or blood withdrawal.
    3. Occlusive dressings at the catheter insertion site are changed every 48 hours using clean technique.
    4. Records of intake and output and daily weights should be kept.

67. During the procedure to remove an opacified lens, an iridectomy will also be performed. The nurse tells the client that this procedure is done:
    1. To prevent secondary glaucoma from developing in the postoperative period.
    2. To increase pupillary dilatation postoperatively.
    3. To facilitate circulation and postoperative healing.
    4. To prevent corneal scarring during the procedure.

68. Which sign(s) and/or symptom(s) of an acid-base balance may be seen in a client with glomerulonephritis?
    Select all that apply.

1. Tetany.
2. Shallow breathing.
3. Lethargy.
4. Disorientation.
5. Rapid, deep respirations.

69. The preoperative laboratory data of a client recorded a Hgb of 8.5. What is the nurse's *first* responsibility?
    1. To attach the lab report to the chart.
    2. To hang a unit of blood.
    3. To notify the physician immediately.
    4. To chart the report in the nurses' notes.

70. The nurse explains to a client that methyldopa acts to decrease hypertension by:
    1. Dilating peripheral blood vessels and increasing renal flow.
    2. Depleting norepinephrine at postganglionic synapses.
    3. Inhibiting formation of dopamine, a precursor of norepinephrine.
    4. Depressing reticular activating system activity.

71. The client returns to the surgical unit following a bilateral hernia repair. The nurse observes that his scrotum is quite swollen. The *first* nursing action is to:
    1. Notify the surgeon stat.
    2. Elevate the scrotum on a rolled towel and apply ice bags.
    3. Administer prn pain medication.
    4. Encourage vigorous deep breathing and coughing.

72. A client with chest tubes returns to the unit. The *first* nursing measure concerning the closed chest drainage system is:
    1. Milking the tubing to prevent accumulation of fibrin and clots.
    2. Raising the bottle to bed height to accurately assess the meniscus level.
    3. Attaching the chest tubes to the bed linen to ensure that airflow and drainage are unhindered by kinks.
    4. Marking the time and the amount of drainage in the collection bottle.

73. For which complication of thyroidectomy would the nurse monitor?
    1. Hypercalcemia.
    2. Respiratory obstruction.
    3. Elevated serum T_4.
    4. Paralytic ileus.

74. During a postoperative period following a cholecystectomy, the client has a T-tube connected to gravity drainage. The nurse knows that the purpose of the T-tube is to:
    1. Maintain patency of the common bile duct.
    2. Reduce the occurrence of postoperative hemorrhage.
    3. Prevent infection.
    4. Reduce bile flow into the duodenum.

75. A client being admitted for modified radical mastectomy was restless and had the following vital signs: BP, 186/110 mm Hg; pulse, 90 bpm; respirations, 22; and temperature, 98.4°F. A half-hour later the nurse retakes the client's vital signs: BP 132/86 mm Hg; pulse 80 bpm; and respirations 16. The client's initial elevated BP indicated:
    1. She may be an individual who is highly sensitive to sympathetic nervous system stimulation.
    2. She is emotionally labile and will need to be assessed closely in the postoperative period.
    3. She is psychologically unprepared for surgery and a psych consult is in order.
    4. She is denying the possible loss of her breast.

76. A client diagnosed with cirrhosis has been placed on a moderate protein, high carbohydrate, high calorie, low salt diet. Which statement would the nurse select as the best rationale for this diet?
    1. Because the liver may not be able to detoxify proteins, carbohydrates are substituted to meet metabolic and nutritional needs.

2. Proteins are given in sufficient amount to facilitate tissue repair. High carbohydrate diet prevents further weight loss and spares proteins from energy metabolism. Sodium restriction facilitates management of fluid imbalances.
3. High protein foods are harder to digest and also have a high sodium content. Carbohydrates are more palatable and will more quickly correct the client's weight loss.
4. High carbohydrate diets, particularly if they contain adequate fiber, are more likely to decrease dyspepsia and diarrhea. Sodium is always restricted when the client is edematous.

77. The purpose of giving Neomycin before ileostomy surgery is to:
    1. Decrease the incidence of postoperative atelectasis due to decreased depth of respirations.
    2. Increase the effectiveness of the body's immunologic response following surgical trauma.
    3. Reduce the incidence of wound infections by decreasing the number of intestinal organisms.
    4. Prevent postoperative bladder atony due to catheterization.

78. The most important activity a client performs following thoracic surgery is:
    1. Arm exercises to prevent shoulder ankylosis.
    2. Deep breathing and coughing up sputum to prevent airway obstruction.
    3. Leg exercises to prevent thrombophlebitis due to prolonged bedrest.
    4. Deep breathing only to prevent undue suture stress while maintaining ventilation.

79. A client becomes extremely lethargic following administration of meperidine HCl 100 mg IM for pain. What is the most appropriate nursing action?
    1. Give only 50 mg of meperidine next time if pain medication is required.
    2. Administer an oral preparation of meperidine next time instead of the intramuscular preparation.
    3. Consult with physician about decreasing the amount of pain medication ordered.
    4. Try to prolong the time between medication dosages by employing alternative pain relief strategies.

80. Postoperatively, following removal of a cataract, the client should be positioned:
    1. In a semi-Fowler's position.
    2. In a prone position only.
    3. On the back or on the unoperated side.
    4. On the operative side.

81. Paracentesis, a minor surgical procedure, is done at the bedside to remove ascitic fluid. After explaining the procedure to the client, the *next* nursing action would be to:
    1. Position the client in a chair or in high-Fowler's position.
    2. Instruct the client to void.
    3. Take vital signs.
    4. Drape the abdomen with sterile towels.

82. On admission, a client with renal disease is experiencing edema, joint pain, oliguria, muscle cramps, and lethargy. The best explanation for the signs and symptoms is:
    1. Renal ischemia due to increase in circulating toxins and chronic hypertension.
    2. A decrease in the number of functioning nephrons, which further decreases glomerular filtration.
    3. Increased water and salt loss due to flushing effect in the diseased kidney tubules.
    4. Water and salt retention due to insufficient renal blood flow.

83. Which nursing measure(s) will decrease the incidence of hemorrhage following thyroidectomy?
Select all that apply.

1. Frequently checking the dressing.
2. Ice packs to the neck.
3. Semi-Fowler's positioning.
4. Neck flexion to apply incisional pressure.
5. Supine positioning with pillow under the head.

84. One potential complication of an abdominal hysterectomy is abdominal distention. Postoperative nursing measures designed to *avoid* abdominal distention are:
    1. Auscultation of the abdomen for bowel sounds.
    2. Abdominal massage and bed rest.
    3. Insertion of nasogastric and rectal tubes and ambulation, as ordered.
    4. Progression of postoperative diet.

85. Ten hours after bilateral hernia surgery, a male client has not been able to void, despite repeated efforts, including standing to void. He states that he feels like he could void but just can't seem to get his stream started. The nurse should:
    1. Try getting him up in a standing position once again.
    2. Insert a Foley catheter stat.
    3. Run water while he attempts to use the urinal.
    4. Consult with his physician to obtain either a medication or catheterization order.

86. Because ascitic fluids are rich in serum proteins, the client during or following a paracentesis is at greatest risk of experiencing:
    1. Disequilibrium.
    2. Hypotension.
    3. Hypoalbuminuria.
    4. Paralytic ileus.

87. Which activity of daily living must a client avoid to prevent complications upon returning home following cataract removal?
    1. Self-feeding.
    2. Self-dressing.
    3. Adjusting shoelaces.
    4. Ambulating.

88. Nursing measures to eliminate the cause of joint pain from chronic renal failure would include:
    1. Using Amphojel (aluminum hydroxide) to lower the elevated blood phosphate that occurs with renal failure.
    2. Preparing for dialysis to decrease serum-creatinine levels.
    3. Increasing the client's activity level.
    4. Implementing a low purine diet to decrease uric acid level.

89. The nurse explains to a client that urinary retention may be a problem after spinal anesthesia because:
    1. Conduction of autonomic nervous system impulses as well as central nervous system impulses is inhibited.
    2. Sensation and motor responses are decreased.
    3. Clients tend to secrete less ADH with spinal anesthesia than they do with general anesthesia.
    4. Vasomotor depression, which occurs with spinal anesthesia, reduces the glomerular filtration rate.

90. During discharge teaching with a client following abdominal hysterectomy, the nurse should include the following instruction:
    1. Avoid sitting for long period of time.
    2. Evacuate bowels daily.
    4. Restrict sexual activity for 6 months after hysterectomy.
    5. Avoid all household chores for 2 months.

91. The nurse would explain to a client that elevation of the foot of the bed after vein-stripping surgery is done to:
    1. Decrease pain.
    2. Aid venous return.
    3. Increase blood supply to feet.
    4. Make the client more comfortable.

92. Which goals would be described as the highest nursing priority to a client recovering from ileostomy surgery?
    1. Relief of pain to promote rest and relaxation.
    2. Assisting the client with self-care activities.

3. Maintenance of fluid, electrolyte, and nutritional balances.
4. Skin care and control of odors.

93. What ECG changes would the nurse anticipate a client who is in chronic renal failure to demonstrate on assessment, given a potassium level of 6.5 mEq/L?
    1. Peaked T waves.
    2. Flattened T waves.
    3. ST-segment depression.
    4. ST-segment elevation.

94. The nurse can anticipate that the amount of ascitic fluid removed during a paracentesis will generally be:
    1. 500 mL.
    2. 1000 mL.
    3. 2000 mL.
    4. 3000 mL.

95. One week after surgery, a client was fitted with cataract glasses. Which nursing statement would best prepare this client for adjusting to these glasses?
    1. "The cataract lenses magnify objects so that they will seem closer to you than they really are."
    2. "While your central vision may be somewhat distorted, you will be able to see well peripherally."
    3. "These lenses will enable you to see as well as you did before the cataract formed."
    4. "The lenses on these glasses are quite narrow, and therefore you may have some double vision."

96. Upon returning from the recovery room after a thyroidectomy, the client begins to complain of a choking sensation. The immediate nursing action should be to:
    1. Elevate the head to high-Fowler's.
    2. Suggest the client suck on some ice chips.
    3. Assess the wound and dressing for increased swelling, and loosen dressing if necessary.
    4. Call the physician.

97. Four days after admission for cirrhosis of the liver, a client began to bleed from an esophageal varix. The earliest indications of bleeding noted by the nurse would include:
    1. Tachycardia, restlessness, and pallor.
    2. Tachycardia, lethargy, and flushing.
    3. Sudden drop in blood pressure of 10 mm Hg or more.
    4. Increasing combativeness and widening pulse pressure.

98. Objective assessment data indicating circulatory overload in a client who has chronic renal failure would include:
    1. Neck vein distention, apprehension, soft eyeballs.
    2. Periorbital edema, distended neck veins, moist crackles.
    3. Increased blood pressure, flattened neck veins, shock.
    4. Decreased pulse pressure, cool, dry skin, decreased skin turgor.

99. On the fifth postoperative day, a client who has had abdominal surgery complains of a "giving" sensation around the wound when walking about. After assisting the client back in bed, the nurse notes that the dressing covering the incision is saturated with clear, pink drainage. The nurse should suspect:
    1. Late hemorrhage.
    2. Dehiscence.
    3. Infection.
    4. Evisceration.

100. The nurse knows that a Sengstaken-Blakemore tube is primarily used to:
    1. Prevent bleeding by applying pressure to the esophageal varices.
    2. Prevent accumulation of blood in the GI tract, which could precipitate hepatic coma.
    3. Stop bleeding by applying pressure to the cardiac portion of the stomach and against the esophageal varices.
    4. Reduce transfusion requirements.

Answers/Rationales/Tips

1. **(2)** All consent forms must be signed before the procedure. Clients are NPO 6 to 8 hours, not 24 hours (**Answer 1**). Gastroscopy is an uncomfortable procedure; to mislead the client by saying it is not uncomfortable (**Answer 3**) can only increase anxiety and discomfort during the procedure. This procedure involves the passage of a long tube into the stomach, with a lighted, mirrored lens that permits direct visualization of the stomach mucosa. The client must lie quietly during insertion of the tube to prevent perforation of the esophagus. Usually *sedatives, not* pain medications (**Answer 4**), are given before the procedure.

> **TEST-TAKING TIP**—One answer is different from the others. Three of the choices deal with physical preparation.
> **IMP, COM, 4, M/S: Preop, SECE, Management of Care**

2. **(3)** The first priority is to protect the client from injury. Do not restrain the client's arms or legs, but make sure he or she does not hit anything. Protect the head with the nurse's hand, a towel, or a jacket. During the initial tonic phase, the client usually stops breathing for up to a minute. There is no cause for alarm, as spontaneous breathing will, in most clients, return with no harm. In the absence of breathing, airway patency by this position change (**Answer 2**) is *not the first* priority. Muscle contraction will prevent "positioning" of the head. A padded tongue blade, once indicated during a seizure, is also no longer used. **Answers 1** and **4** are appropriate nursing actions *after* the seizure has ended.

> **TEST-TAKING TIP**— The correct choice is broadest, encompassing the other choices. Key word: *first* priority.
> **PL, APP, 2, M/S: GI, PhI, Physiological Adaptation**

3. **(3)** Signs of *circulatory* constriction include blanching (delayed capillary refill) and cyanosis, swelling of the toes, pain that is out of proportion for the type of fracture, and temperature changes. Tingling and numbness (**Answer 1**), loss of movement (**Answer 2**), and constant pain (**Answer 4**) are symptoms associated with constriction or pressure on a *peripheral nerve*.

> **TEST-TAKING TIP**—Requires knowledge of difference between motor, sensory, and circulatory signs/symptoms.
> **AS, ANL, 6, M/S: Vascular, PhI, Reduction of Risk Potential**

4. **(3)** Paralytic ileus is characterized by diminished, absent, or uncoordinated bowel sounds due to inappropriate or absent autonomic nervous system (vagal) stimulation of the intestinal tract. Paralytic ileus may occur due to anesthetic interruption of autonomic outflow or hypokalemia. Edema of the intestinal mucosa (**Answer 1**) is usually found with inflammation or *ulcerative colitis*. Acute dilation of the colon (**Answer 2**) and high, tinkling bowel sounds (**Answer 4**) are associated with *large-bowel* obstruction.

> **TEST-TAKING TIP**—Look for words in the answer that define "paralysis."
> **AN, COM, 8, M/S: GI, PhI, Physiological Adaptation**

KEY TO CODES FOLLOWING RATIONALES:

Nursing process: **AS**, assessment; **AN**, analysis; **PL**, plan; **IMP**, implementation; **EV**, evaluation. *Cognitive level:* **COM**, comprehension; **APP**, application; **ANL**, analysis. *Category of human function:* 1, protective; 2, sensory-perceptual; 3, comfort, rest, activity, and mobility; 4, nutrition; 5, growth and development; 6, fluid-gas transport; 7, psychosocial-cultural; 8, elimination. *Client need:* **SECE**, safe, effective care environment; **HPM**, health promotion/maintenance; **PsI**, psychosocial integrity; **PhI**, physiological integrity. (Client subneed appears after Client need code.) See appendices for full explanation.

5. **(2)** Some authorities believe that the psychosomatic issue contributing to ulcers is an unresolved dependence-independence conflict. This conflict frequently prevents the client from accepting a dependent role, even on a temporary basis. However, the unresolved dependency wish that many of these people have frequently results in irritable, angry behavior when treatments are not exactly on time. Other psychosomatic research has linked anxiety and neurotic behavior (**Answer 1**) with the occurrence of *angina pectoris;* repressed anger and hostility (**Answer 3**) with the development of *rheumatoid arthritis;* and compulsive time orientation (**Answer 4**) (type A personality) with onset of *myocardial infarction.*

> **TEST-TAKING TIP**—Ask which emotional response would most likely stimulate a parasympathetic (stress) response.
> **AN, APP, 7, M/S: GI, PsI, Psychosocial Integrity**

6. **(2, 3, 5)** **Answer 2** is correct because hypokalemia decreases neuromuscular excitability resulting in apathy, lethargy and mental confusion. **Answer 3** is correct because there is decreased muscular function and muscle weakness with hypokalemia. **Answer 5** is correct because a low potassium decreases gastric motility, resulting in vomiting, abdominal distention and flatulence. **Answer 1** is incorrect because potassium deficit leads to decreased muscular function and muscle weakness. **Answer 4** is incorrect because thirst would be seen with dehydration and hyperkalemia.

> **TEST-TAKING TIP**—Know the influences of potassium on tissues and body functioning. Look carefully at each choice. Eliminate the ones that are partially correct.
> **AS, ANL, 6, M/S: F-E, PhI, Physiological Adaptation**

7. **(1)** Clients experiencing dumping syndrome should be advised to ingest liquids between meals rather than with meals (**Answer 2**) or at any time they desire (**Answer 3**). Taking fluids between meals allows for adequate hydration, reduces the amount of bulk ingested with meals, and aids in preventing rapid gastric emptying. Six small meals rather than three large meals, as well as resting after eating, are also measures used to prevent the occurrence of symptoms, which usually disappear over time. There is no need to restrict the quantity of fluids (**Answer 4**), just the timing.

> **TEST-TAKING TIP**—Key point is a *time* factor *(when)*. Decreasing volume *at meal time,* not in general, is the key. Fluid speeds the process.
> **PL, APP, 4, M/S: GI, PhI, Basic Care and Comfort**

8. **(2)** The narrow QRS complexes are normal, within 0.12 second, but there are *no regular P waves* for each QRS. The baseline appears "wavy" and the rhythm is "regularly irregular," which describes atrial fibrillation. The second and fifth QRS complexes are wide and bizarre but alike, indicating a unifocal origin. **Answer 1** is incorrect because there is not one P wave for every QRS, and the multifocal PVCs would look different in configuration. Even though the rate is 100, **Answer 3** is incorrect because the impulse is not originating from the SA node, which is necessary for a sinus rhythm. **Answer 4** is incorrect because atrial fibrillation is more rapid and regular, and though the P waves are difficult to see, they *are* present. Also, the PVCs are unifocal, not multifocal, in origin.

> **TEST-TAKING TIP**—Look for the normal components of an ECG—PQRS. Only one choice has no P waves like the strip.
> **AN, ANL, 6, M/S: Cardiac, PhI, Physiological Adaptation**

9. **(3)** The vagus nerve stimulates an increase in both hydrochloric acid secretion and gastric motility. Vagotomy not only decreases hydrochloric acid secretion but also alters the motil-

Questions

ity of the stomach and intestines; this may result in a sensation of fullness after meals, eructation, and abdominal distention. **Answer 1** is incomplete. **Answers 2** and **4** are the reverse of effects of vagal action.

> **TEST-TAKING TIP**—Look for a choice that would be similar to the problem that led to the gastrectomy. Note that both **Answer 1** and **Answer 3** are correct, but **Answer 3** incorporates **Answer 1**.
> **AN, COM, 4, M/S: GI, PhI, Reduction of Risk Potential**

10. **(3)** Potassium is transported back into the cells along with glucose; therefore the administration of insulin and glucose will facilitate the movement of potassium back into the cell. Sodium polystyrene sulfonate (Kayexalate) (**Answer 2**) is a resin that attacks and binds potassium. It may be given either orally or as an enema; however, its use would *not* be indicated in this case *unless* more conservative means were unsuccessful. Morphine sulfate (**Answer 1**) and synthetic aldosterone (**Answer 4**) are *not* indicated for the management of hyperkalemia.

> **TEST-TAKING TIP**—The "choice" would always be to move K$^+$ back into the cell, not get rid of it through diarrhea (**Answer 2**).
> **PL, COM, 6, PhI, M/S: Metab, PhI, Pharmacological and Parenteral Therapies**

11. **(1)** Ventricular tachycardia occurs most commonly in clients with acute MI and coronary artery disease. Of immediate significance to the client, if untreated, are the hemodynamic dysfunction, a *drop* in blood pressure rather than an increase (**Answer 2**), and the possibility of progressing to ventricular fibrillation. **Answer 3** is incorrect because if pain does result it will be *angina, not MI* pain. **Answer 4** is incorrect because ventricular tachycardia is potentially *life threatening* and requires intervention.

> **TEST-TAKING TIP**—"V-tach" is life-threatening. Look for another life-threatening choice (ventricular fibrillation).
> **AN, ANL, 6, M/S: Cardiac, PhI, Reduction of Risk Potential**

12. **(4)** Although 70% to 80% of clients having subtotal gastrectomies may experience some symptoms of dumping syndrome, it is a significant problem for only a small percentage (5% to 10%). The term *dumping* is used because the symptoms are believed to be due to the rapid emptying of the gastric contents into the small intestine. This produces gastric distention, and some authorities believe that large amounts of extracellular fluid then enter the intestines to dilute the hypertonic stomach contents. The subsequent lowering of the blood volume produces shocklike symptoms, such as weakness, diaphoresis, faintness, and palpitations. **Answers 1, 2,** and **3** are incorrect percentages.

> **TEST-TAKING TIP**—Select the smallest (lowest) percentage because it is *not most* clients who develop a "significant" problem.
> **AN, COM, 4, M/S: GI, PhI, Physiological Adaptation**

13. **(2)** Clients with hyperthyroidism have an increased basal metabolic rate (BMR) and increased T$_3$ and T$_4$. Increased serum cholesterol (**Answer 1**), increased TSH (**Answer 3**), and increased menstrual volume (**Answer 4**) are findings consistent with *hypothyroidism*. Menstruation in hyperthyroidism characteristically is *decreased* in volume. Cycle lengths may be shortened or prolonged, but eventually amenorrhea develops.

> **TEST-TAKING TIP**—Look for an answer with a change in metabolism.
> **AN, APP, 3, M/S: Endocrine, PhI, Physiological Adaptation**

14. **(1)** Hyponatremia, or decreased serum sodium, may develop in clients with burns because sodium tends to move with water into edema fluids and into denuded areas of skin. **Answers 2** and **4** are incorrect because both these mechanisms tend to *increase* sodium reabsorption by the kidney tubules. Inadequate fluid replacement (**Answer 3**) would tend to *mask* hyponatremia because of hemoconcentration.

> **TEST-TAKING TIP**—Look for the only answer that relates to destruction of skin (longest answer *might* be a hint). Also, *hypo*natremia is similar to the word "loss" in the correct option.
> **AN, APP, 6, M/S: Metab., PhI, Physiological Adaptation**

15. **(2)** The nasogastric tube is removed after bowel sounds have been reestablished (generally around the third day) and after the client has passed flatus or stool. **Answers 1** and **3** are incorrect because they do not include the return of bowel sounds. Before removal, the tube is frequently clamped for 2 to 4 hours—*not 2 days* (**Answer 4**)—to test the client's tolerance. Gastric residue is measured after this period. If it is more than 100 mL, the nasogastric tube is left in place. Likewise, if the client experiences any pain, nausea, vomiting, or distention during this period, the tube is left in. If no symptoms occur and there is a minimal amount of gastric residue, the tube is removed.

> **TEST-TAKING TIP**—The "time" depends on the client's bowel sounds. Follow the logic: GI surgery, NG tube→ "bowel sounds" (**Answer 2**). Correct choice is the *only* one without a specific time.
> **EV, APP, 8, M/S: GI, PhI, Basic Care and Comfort**

16. **(2)** Age is important baseline information because IV infusion rates to maintain appropriate quantity and specific gravity of urinary output differ; for example, 10 to 20 mL/hr for infants versus 50 to 70 mL/hr for adults. Weight is significant if the Evans or Brooke formula is used for fluid replacement therapy. Both of these formulas use both the size of the burn and the weight of the client to calculate the amount of fluid to be replaced. Vital signs and skin turgor are both important measures of the degree or extent of hypovolemia. As dehydration develops, skin turgor becomes poor, mucous membranes dry, and the eyeballs feel soft. Likewise, the pulse may become thready and the blood pressure may decrease. Size (weight), as discussed, *not sex* would determine therapy (**Answer 1**). Level of mentation (**Answer 3**) is *less* helpful in this particular situation because of the fear, pain, and acute anxiety experienced by some clients. Quantity and specific gravity of urine output (**Answer 4**) are important in assessing the adequacy of fluid *replacement rather than* as part of the initial *assessment*.

> **TEST-TAKING TIP**—Look for an answer with "body weight."
> **AS, APP, 6, M/S: F-E, PhI, Pharmacological and Parenteral Therapies**

17. **(3)** Removal of gastric secretions incurs the *loss* of sodium, potassium, and hydrochloric acid ions. The loss of these ions may lead not only to metabolic alkalosis (↓H$^+$) but also to *hypo*kalemia. **Answers 1** and **2** are incorrect because hypernatremia and hyperkalemia indicate an *excess* in sodium and potassium ions. Hypoproteinemia (**Answer 4**) occurs with *liver* dysfunctions and is *not* a side effect of nasogastric suctioning.

> **TEST-TAKING TIP**—The key word is *prolonged*. Acid will be lost; therefore, think alkalosis.
> **AN, APP, 4, M/S: Metab., PhI, Physiological Adaptation**

18. **(1)** Hemorrhage may follow nephrectomy because of the difficulty in securing ligatures in the short renal-artery stump.

It may occur on the day of surgery or 8 to 12 days postoperatively, when normal tissue sloughing occurs with healing. Dressing and urine are observed for bright-red bleeding, vital signs are monitored, and the client is continually observed for any other indications of shock. Hyperkalemia (**Answer 2**), tetany (**Answer 3**), and polyuria (**Answer 4**) are *not* common complications after nephrectomy.

> **TEST-TAKING TIP**—After any surgery, bleeding is a potential problem.
> **AS, COM, 6, M/S: Renal, PhI, Reduction of Risk Potential**

19. (**4**) It is important to recognize that the loss of anatomical integrity initiates a grieving process. Allowing the client to express feelings of depression, apathy, or disinterest indicates that such feelings are acceptable and not uncommon. **Answer 1** is always appropriate and should be consistently carried out; however, in the situation depicted it would *follow* the verbalization of feelings. **Answers 2** and **3** are also alternatives the nurse may wish to employ *after* assessing the client's major concerns.

> **TEST-TAKING TIP**—First priority—what is concerning the client? First, *feelings.*
> **IMP, ANL, 7, M/S: Postop, PsI, Psychosocial Integrity**

20. (**2**) The client should be cautioned to limit the number of ice chips he or she sucks on because the nasogastric suction will remove not only the increased water ingested from the melted chips but also essential electrolytes. **Answers 1, 3,** and **4** *are* appropriate mouth care measures for a client who has a nasogastric tube.

> **TEST-TAKING TIP**—One answer is different from the others (teeth, tongue, mouth, gums, lips)—it involves swallowing melted *ice*. Note the key term *with caution.*
> **IMP, APP, 1, M/S: GI, PhI, Basic Care and Comfort**

21. (**4**) Recognizing the client's concern is essential both in maintaining rapport and in keeping the lines of communication open. Having done this, the nurse can then assure the client that one kidney is sufficient to handle renal functions. This statement can then be followed by other discharge instructions, such as the need for adequate fluid intake, avoiding infections, and untoward signs that the client needs to observe for. **Answers 1, 2,** and **3** do not recognize the client's concern or facilitate open communication.

> **TEST-TAKING TIP**—The best answer acknowledges the client's concern. Eliminate "call the doctor" (**Answer 3**) because a nurse *can* discuss the client's concerns. Eliminate **Answers 1** and **2** because they are trite clichés that close off elaboration.
> **IMP, ANL, 7, M/S: Postop, PsI, Psychosocial Integrity**

22. (**3**) It is not uncommon for a client to feel that she will no longer be able to fulfill her role and needs as a woman following a hysterectomy. Verbalization of feelings allows the nurse to assess the client's coping mechanisms and encourages the client to deal with her emotional response. **Answer 3** is an open-ended question that allows the client room to respond. **Answers 1** and **2** avoid the problem initially. **Answer 2** may be appropriate if, after talking to the client, the nurse assesses that her responses represent a more significant or deep-seated problem. **Answer 4** would be appropriate *after* the client has aired her feelings.

> **TEST-TAKING TIP**—Use therapeutic communication—first, explore client's comment. Eliminate MD and meds as initial responses. *First,* focus on *feelings!*
> **IMP, ANL, 7, M/S: Postop, PsI, Psychosocial Integrity**

23. (**2**) Desperation and panic may strike while the injury is occurring but *rarely* occur *during* the recovery period. During the *acute* stage of burn recovery, anxiety is common due to the stress and pain of injury and dressing changes. Anxiety decreases the individual's ability to perceive situations realistically, which may result in an altered mental state (**Answer 1**). During the *intermediate* phase of burn recovery, clients may react to continued pain, changes in body image, and financial stress with various psychological responses, ranging from withdrawal and depression (**Answer 3**) to acting out anger by refusing to cooperate with the medical regimen and by dependency (**Answer 4**).

> **TEST-TAKING TIP**—Note "least likely" in the stem, meaning "which one is incorrect." Also note time period: *during* recovery.
> **AS, APP, 7, M/S: Integ., PsI, Psychosocial Integrity**

24. (**2**) Though nausea may occur following the administration of narcotics, if it is accompanied by the absence of bowel sounds and upper abdominal distention, gastric or small-intestine dilation should be suspected and the nurse's findings reported to the physician. Changing the client's position (**Answer 1**) and insertion of a rectal tube (**Answer 3**) are *not* helpful if peristalsis is not present (bowel sounds). Administering morphine (**Answer 4**) is *not* indicated until the source of the client's discomfort is diagnosed.

> **TEST-TAKING TIP**—Note the *time* of the event following surgery. What functions should return within 48 hours? Only one option deals with *assessment* (auscultate); the other three are implementation responses (change, insert, administer).
> **IMP, ANL, 8, M/S: Postop, PhI, Reduction of Risk Potential**

25. (**1**) In the use of crutches, all weight bearing should be on the hands. Constant pressure in the axilla from weight bearing can lead to damage of the brachial plexus nerves and produce crutch paralysis. **Answers 2, 3,** and **4** *are appropriate* instructions to give to the client preparing for crutch walking.

> **TEST-TAKING TIP**—The best answer is the wrong thing to teach.
> **IMP, APP, 3, M/S: Ortho, PhI, Basic Care and Comfort**

26. (**2**) Epileptic seizures or convulsions are the result of excessive, simultaneous, disordered neuronal discharge in the brain. This dysrhythmic electrical discharge may be focal (jacksonian seizure) or widely dispersed (grand mal seizures). **Answers 3** and **4** are incorrect because theories for the initiation of these convulsions vary from *decreased* (**Answer 3**) intracellular K^+ to *decreased* (**Answer 4**) cerebrospinal fluid to alteration in neuronal defense due to trauma, toxins, or inflammation. Depending on existing potential in the individual, **Answer 1** *may* be a precipitating factor.

> **TEST-TAKING TIP**—Look for the key word: "neuronal."
> **AN, APP, 2, M/S: Neuro, PhI, Physiological Adaptation**

27. (**2**) After the tube has been inserted into the stomach, its movement into the duodenum is first facilitated by having the client lie on the *right* side for 2 hours, then on the back with head *elevated* for 2 hours, and finally on the left side for 2 hours. After the tube has passed the pylorus (this is usually checked by x-ray), *ambulating* the client will help move the tube to the point of obstruction. *After* positioning and ambulation, the physician or the nurse may advance the tube 1 to 4 inches at specified time intervals (**Answer 1**) to provide slack for peristaltic action. Remaining quiet or flat in bed (**Answers 3** and **4**) will *not* facilitate the advancement of the tube either through the pylorus or through the small intestine.

> **TEST-TAKING TIP**—Focus on the two positioning options: right vs. flat supine. Understand the concept of peristalsis and think of the sequence of positioning (right → supine in semi-Fowler's → left).
> **IMP, APP, 8, M/S: GI, PhI, Basic Care and Comfort**

28. **(4)** The hypovolemia that occurs in the initial stage of burns is the result of fluid lost from denuded areas of skin and edema in and around the burned surface area. Edema formation is due to a shift of plasma fluids to the interstitial space. **Answers 1, 2,** and **3** are incorrect because when tissues are burned, a change in the permeability of both tissue and capillary membranes occurs. This change and increased vasodilation result in a shift of excessively large amounts of extracellular fluid (electrolytes and proteins) into the burned area. Most of this fluid loss occurs deep in the wound, where fluid moves into the deeper tissue. Burns of a highly vascular area (muscle, face) are believed to cause more severe fluid volume shifts than comparable burns to other areas of the body.

> **TEST-TAKING TIP**—Where was fluid before the burn? Where would it go after the burn? Note the time period: *initial* stage.
> **AN, COM, 6, M/S: F-E, PhI, Physiological Adaptation**

29. **(2)** Vigorous activities such as brushing the teeth and brushing the hair are generally discouraged during periods of acute distress. These activities tend to increase aqueous production and therefore pressures because they activate sympathetic nervous system stimulation of the vasculature. Quiet activities such as watching TV (**Answer 1**), moderate activities such as reading, self-feeding (**Answer 3**), and passive range-of-motion exercises (**Answer 4**) *are* encouraged.

> **TEST-TAKING TIP**—Look for the activity most likely to increase pressure in the eyes or head. Look for what is *not* OK because the stem says "to avoid." Three activities are quiet, passive; one is active (brushing).
> **IMP, APP, 2, M/S: Eye, PhI, Basic Care and Comfort**

30. **(1, 3, 5, 6)** **Answer 1** is correct because the respiratory rate is rapid in both hypoglycemia and hyperglycemia. However, the depth is shallow. There is no need to blow off carbon dioxide, as with hyperglycemia and ketoacidosis. **Answer 3** is correct because the low blood sugar level affects cerebral function; the client becomes increasingly irritable and apprehensive, eventually lapsing into unresponsiveness if untreated. **Answer 5** is correct because hypoglycemia and insulin shock stimulate epinephrine release and diaphoresis. **Answer 6** is correct because late signs of hypoglycemia and insulin shock mimic alcohol intoxication—slurring of words, combative behavior. **Answer 2** is incorrect because the breath in insulin shock or hypoglycemia is nondescript. Fetid breath is seen in liver failure or with poor oral hygiene. With hyperglycemia, there is a fruity (not fetid) breath odor. **Answer 4** is incorrect because confusion is characteristic of hyperglycemia.

> **TEST-TAKING TIP**—Consider each sign or symptom; ask yourself if too much or too little sugar would produce the change.
> **AS, ANL, 4, M/S: Endocrine, PhI, Physiological Adaptation**

31. **(1)** Clients are ambulated as soon as possible to prevent the complications of bedrest; generally ambulation can begin as soon as 24 hours after surgery. In some instances, such as when the client is severely debilitated or has complications due to ulcer perforation, bedrest may be prolonged, as in **Answers 2** and **3.** If this is the case, the nurse will need to observe closely for signs of complications (atelectasis, thrombophlebitis, etc.) and institute measures to prevent them. The

client is *rarely* if ever gotten up immediately after awakening, as in **Answer 4.**

> **TEST-TAKING TIP**—Look for the best general *timing* to prevent complications and ensure client safety. Key term: "usually," meaning typically (not rarely, or under special circumstances).
> **PL, COM, 3, M/S: Postop, PhI, Basic Care and Comfort**

32. **(1)** In cholinergic crisis, all anticholinesterase drugs are withdrawn, and atropine (an anticholinergic drug) is given in 2 mg doses IV every hour until signs of atropine toxicity develop (dry mouth, blurred vision, tachycardia, rash or flushing of the skin, and elevated temperature). **Answers 2, 3,** and **4** are incorrect because they do *not* act to decrease cholinergic responses. Ephedrine (**Answer 2**) is used in myasthenia gravis to *increase* muscle tone; potassium chloride (**Answer 3**) is used to *increase* serum K^+ because it is believed that adequate serum-potassium levels potentiate the effects of cholinergic drugs; and neostigmine bromide (**Answer 4**) *is* an anticholinesterase that acts to improve cholinergic transmission of impulses at the myoneural junction.

> **TEST-TAKING TIP**—Look for the antidote (an anticholinergic drug) to counteract untoward effects.
> **IMP, COM, 3, M/S: Meds, PhI, Pharmacological and Parenteral Therapies**

33. **(3)** In chronic, or open-angle glaucoma, the obstruction to aqueous outflow is due to degenerative changes in either the trabeculum, Schlemm's canal, or the aqueous veins. Closed-angle glaucoma is characterized by obstruction of aqueous outflow due to narrowing of the angle between the anterior chamber and the root of the iris. The other answers are incorrect because chronic, or open-angle, glaucoma occurs *more frequently* than *closed-angle* (**Answer 1**), is characterized by slow, insidious, painless onset *rather than* the acute symptoms of closed-angle glaucoma (**Answer 2**), and *is* certainly familial, if not hereditary (**Answer 4**). Due to this latter characteristic, family members of clients with open-angle glaucoma should be encouraged to have their intraocular pressure assessed annually, particularly past age 40.

> **TEST-TAKING TIP**—Look for similarity between the condition ("open-angle") and clues in the choice that says "does not close," meaning it is *open*. The question asks how *open* angle is different.
> **AN, COM, 2, M/S: Eye, PhI, Physiological Adaptation**

34. **(2)** Although each of the listed measures *can* be used to assess the adequacy of the fluid replacement, hourly urine outputs and vital signs provide significant information on fluid balance in the acute burn period. Decreased urine output, increased pulse rate, and restlessness are early signs of inadequate fluid replacement. Increase in blood pressure, pulse, respirations, and urine output are early signs of circulatory overload. Changes in daily weights provide accurate data over the *long run* and are extremely important in monitoring fluid volumes in clients on diuretic therapy, such as clients with congestive heart failure or cirrhosis. **Answers 1, 3,** and **4** are *not* the *best* indicators.

> **TEST-TAKING TIP**—Key words: *best* and *early.* Look for indication of adequate volume. Note the two options that include "urinary output," and choose the one that also has *vital* signs that are *vital* to assess ↓fluid volume and overload.
> **EV, ANL, 6, M/S: F-E, PhI, Physiological Adaptation**

35. **(4)** Profuse perspiration, diaphoresis, is one of a group of symptoms that happen 5 to 30 minutes after a high carbohydrate meal or when liquid is taken with the meal. This is caused by entrance of food into the jejunum before it has had

a chance to begin the digestive process. Other symptoms include a feeling of fullness, *not hunger* (**Answer 1**); diarrhea, *not* constipation (**Answer 2**); and weakness, *not* increased strength (**Answer 3**).

> **TEST-TAKING TIP**—Stem asks what would the nurse *see* (objective). Three choices are subjective. Choose the one that is different.
> **EV, COM, 4, M/S: GI, PhI, Physiological Adaptation**

36. (**1**) The diuretic stage of burns occurs 48 to 72 hours after injury. The fluid shift is the opposite of that in the initial stage. Fluids, electrolytes, and proteins may move very rapidly from the interstitial space back into the vascular compartment. Unless renal damage has occurred and there is *no indication* (**Answer 2**), diuresis ensues, due to the increased blood volume and renal blood flow. Serum electrolytes and hematocrit are decreased due to hemodilution. If urine output is insufficient at this time, symptoms of circulatory overload and cardiac failure will occur. There are *no data to support* **Answer 3**. The sodium value is within *normal* limits (**Answer 4**).

> **TEST-TAKING TIP**—Clue: time frame—after the initial phase (54 hours). Think *expected* changes over time in fluid balance (major shifts). Recognize normal serum Na$^+$ value and eliminate **Answer 4**. With *increased output*, you can eliminate **Answers 2 and 3**.
> **AN, ANL, 8, M/S: FE, PhI, Physiological Adaptation**

37. (**1**) The most common cause of hypothyroidism is excess thyroid tissue destruction due to radioactive iodine therapy for hyperthyroidism. Spontaneous hypothyroidism is believed to be due to an autoimmune response. Several studies have revealed a high incidence of antibodies for thyroid antigen in clients with spontaneous atrophy (**Answer 2**). Other, *less common* causes include surgical removal (**Answer 3**), Hashimoto's thyroiditis, overuse of antithyroid drugs (**Answer 4**), and pituitary tumors or insufficiency that decrease the circulating levels of thyroid-stimulating hormone.

> **TEST-TAKING TIP**—Use a process of elimination and keep *two common* causes in mind.
> **AN, COM, 3, M/S: Endocrine, PhI, Physiological Adaptation**

38. (**2**) Signs of "cholinergic crisis" include pupils constricted to less than 2 mm, severe diarrhea, nausea, vomiting, hypersalivation, lacrimation, pallor, and hypotension. Bradycardia may occur but is uncommon. In severe cases, confusion progressing to coma may occur due to blockage of cerebral synapses. **Answers 1** and **3** are symptoms related to increased *adrenergic* discharge. **Answer 4** is only partially correct.

> **TEST-TAKING TIP**—The "eyes" have it! First, decide that *constricted* pupils occur (this means that **Answers 1** and **3** are eliminated). The expected effects of too much medication in this condition would eliminate **Answer 4** (not *dry* mucous membranes, but *hyper*salivation).
> **AS, COM, 2, M/S: Meds, PhI, Pharmacological and Parenteral Therapies**

39. (**1**) Iron deficiency anemia is characterized by a decrease in red blood cell color due to a decrease in iron (hypochromic) and an increase in immature red blood cells (microcytic). **Answer 2** describes the red blood cells in *pernicious anemia*. **Answers 3** and **4** describe *no* particular conditions.

> **TEST-TAKING TIP**—Look for similar meanings in stem and answer—*deficiency* in the stem, and *hypo* and *micro* in the correct option (**Answer 1**).
> **AN, COM, 6, M/S: Blood, PhI, Physiological Adaptation**

40. (**1**) In assessing any client's emotional responses, the nurse should first assess the client's ego strength, body image, and coping abilities for life situations in general. The manner in which the client views himself or herself will greatly affect attitudes toward disease and emotional response. If the client normally denies or represses threatening information or situations, desirable outcomes may be difficult to achieve. Research indicates that social supports are extremely important in maintaining health. The relationship between the client and the client's mother (**Answer 2**) should be assessed. However, if the client has a strong self-image, the issues between mother and adult child should be resolvable either alone or with objective outside help. **Answer 3** is *incomplete*. Economic status and work history (**Answer 4**), depending on their value to the client, *may not* be important determinants of emotional response.

> **TEST-TAKING TIP**—Select the broadest, most inclusive answer that covers them all. When in doubt about the best psychosocial option, choose the "self-image, self-concept" type of answer.
> **AN, APP, 7, M/S: Autoimmune, PsI, Psychosocial Integrity**

41. (**1**) The primary fluid and electrolyte imbalances in Addison's disease are *hypo*natremia, *hypo*volemia, and *hyper*kalemia. These imbalances are caused by *decreased* aldosterone secretion. **Answers 2** and **3** are incorrect because they occur with *excessive* secretion of this hormone. Calcium levels are *not* affected by this condition (**Answer 4**).

> **TEST-TAKING TIP**—Need to know relationship with sodium ($\downarrow$) and potassium ($\uparrow$). Key word is *decreased* aldosterone secretion.
> **EV, COM, 6, M/S: F-E, PhI, Physiological Adaptation**

42. (**1**) Thyroid storm may be precipitated by a number of stresses, such as infection, real or threatened loss of a loved one, or thyroid surgery undertaken before the client was prepared adequately with antithyroid drugs. A change heralding thyroid storm is a fever: the client's temperature may rise as high as 106°F (41°C). **Answers 2, 3,** and **4** *are* symptoms of hyperthyroidism and become *exaggerated* during thyroid storm. Without treatment, the client progresses from delirium to coma; death ensues as the result of heart failure.

> **TEST-TAKING TIP**—Key word is *cardinal*—most important; what you will note *first*.
> **AS, COM, 3, M/S: Endocrine, PhI, Physiological Adaptation**

43. (**2**) Bloody drainage from the nasogastric tube more than 12 hours after surgery should be considered unusual and reported to the surgeon. Prolonged bleeding may be indicative of a slow bleeder, a blood dyscrasia, or problems with incisional closure. Any of these may increase blood loss and lead to shock. **Answers 1, 3,** and **4** are incorrect because they are *normal* findings in the *early* postgastrectomy period.

> **TEST-TAKING TIP**—The key element is a *time* factor, *not* color (i.e., not greenish-yellow, red). Choose an answer indicating the greatest risk to the client (*prolonged bleeding*).
> **EV, ANL, 6, M/S: Postop, PhI, Reduction of Risk Potential**

44. (**4**) Sinus arrhythmias is the most frequent arrhythmia and occurs as a *normal* phenomenon, often related to the respiratory cycle. **Answer 1** is incorrect because lidocaine is used to treat *life-threatening ventricular* arrhythmias. **Answer 2** is incorrect because exercise, which increases the heart rate, will abolish the arrhythmia, so rest or limited activity is *not indicated*. **Answer 3** is incorrect because the arrhythmia originates in the *sinoatrial* node, *not* in the atrioventricular node, and digoxin is the treatment for *atrial arrhythmias*.

TEST-TAKING TIP—Is this ECG pattern OK or not OK? Is it "Oh! Oh!" (i.e., is it a concern or a problem?) or is it "Eh!" (not really a concern)?
EV, APP, 6, M/S: Cardiac, PhI, Reduction of Risk Potential

45. **(3)** Pernicious anemia may occur following subtotal gastrectomy (when large portions of the stomach are removed) due to the loss of tissue that produces the intrinsic factor. Loss of this factor necessitates the parenteral administration of *vitamin B₁₂*— the *extrinsic* factor. **Answer 1** is incorrect because the extrinsic factor is found in *food.* **Answers 2** and **4** are incorrect because it is the *loss of intrinsic* factor that results in the malabsorption of vitamin B₁₂.

TEST-TAKING TIP—Note the pattern in the responses: two extrinsic factors, one intrinsic; choose the one that is different. Need to know reason for expected problem.
EV, APP, 4, M/S: GI, PhI, Physiological Adaptation

46. **(2)** Pain management requires the nurse and physician to collaborate to achieve optimal relief for the client. The use of analgesics for pain requires a physician's order. The nurse assesses the client's response to drug therapy and alerts the MD to needed changes. The nurse may also recommend nondrug interventions to promote client comfort (progressive relaxation, massage). **Answers 1** and **3** are manageable by *independent* nursing actions—careful assessment, ROM, proper positioning. **Answer 4** is *not a nursing diagnosis,* but a medical problem to be corrected by surgery.

TEST-TAKING TIP—The key words in the stem are *best* outcome and *collaboratively.* Although independent nursing actions could be planned for each option, look for the one that requires physician's orders to implement care.
AN, APP, 3, M/S: Ortho, SECE, Management of Care

47. **(2, 5)** **Answer 2** is correct because undue stress on the suture line must be avoided to prevent bleeding. **Answer 5** is correct because any client who has general anesthesia is at risk for atelectasis and pneumonia. Use of the incentive spirometer improves lung expansion. **Answer 1** is incorrect because hoarseness may occur due to irritation of the vocal cords from intubation. The client should be prepared for a possible change, but no reporting is necessary. The voice generally returns to normal. **Answer 3** is incorrect because flexion will stress the incision. The head should remain in a midline position with no pull on the incision. **Answer 4** is incorrect because hyperextension will stress the incision and potentially cause bleeding or injury.

TEST-TAKING TIP—Think prevention of complications: the most immediate concern is integrity of the operative site, and then (with general anesthesia) breathing.
PL, APP, 3, M/S: Preop Teaching, PhI, Reduction of Risk Potential

48. **(2)** Heat cramps occur when fluids are lost through excessive sweating and water is replaced without sodium replacement. A balanced solution or sources of water and sodium should be ingested. Sodium chloride tablets may be taken, but they may cause stomach irritation. If there was a prior history (**Answer 1**) and another admission, there is still a need for client teaching. **Answers 3** and **4** are not incorrect; fluids *are* important for evaporative cooling, and potassium and magnesium *may be* lost, *but* the role of *sodium* is *most important* to prevent future problems.

TEST-TAKING TIP—The stem asks for the *most* important. When all of the options are correct, use a process of elimination to select the one that will make the greatest

difference—prevent harm (**Answer 2**) or incorporates other options.
IMP, APP, 6, M/S: F-E, PhI, Basic Care and Comfort

49. **(1)** Peritonitis is the most serious complication of CAPD. How to maintain aseptic or sterile technique to prevent bacteria from entering the peritoneal cavity is the most important information to teach the client. **Answer 2, 3,** and **4** are also important to teach the client with CAPD *after* the nurse determines that the client will be able to safely perform sterile technique.

TEST-TAKING TIP—This is a "rank order of priority" question. When all of the options are correct, which one prevents the client from the greatest potential risk?
IMP, APP, 8, M/S: Infection, SECE, Safety and Infection Control

50. **(1)** A witnessed or unwitnessed cardiac arrest starts with establishing the state of consciousness of the client. It is important to determine if the client is awake before proceeding with emergency CPR. **Answers 2** and **4** are the *next* steps in initiating CPR. **Answer 3,** although not part of the ABCs of CPR, would be done *after* establishing a pulse.

TEST-TAKING TIP—This is a "rank order of priority" question. Remember "shake and shout," *then* your ABCs.
AS, ANL, 6, M/S: CPR, PhI, Physiological Adaptation

51. **(4)** The client's signs are consistent with an increase in venous pressure. Pericardial effusion or cardiac tamponade impairs the ventricles from adequately filling during diastole. Venous pressure increases and stroke volume decreases. **Answers 1** and **2** would result in signs and symptoms consistent with left-sided heart failure, and difficulty breathing would likely be present. Hypertrophy (**Answer 3**) is *not* reduced, but rather *managed* through drug therapy.

TEST-TAKING TIP—Look for patterns in the options. Three of the choices involve the ventricles—how could you choose just one?
PL, ANL, 6, M/S: CV, PhI, Physiological Adaptation

52. **(2)** As cerebral hypoxia develops, the client becomes restless and drowsy well before any of the characteristic signs and symptoms of increasing intracranial pressure are present. **Answers 1, 3,** and **4** are all consistent with increasing intracranial pressure but occur much *later,* after there has been significant cerebral herniation and distortion of the brain.

TEST-TAKING TIP—The key word in the stem is *early.* A "change" in level of consciousness (could be restlessness or a lack of responsiveness) is almost always the best answer with *neurological* problems. A key word in the best option is *change.*
AN, COM, 2, M/S: Neuro, PhI, Physiological Adaptation

53. **(4)** Frequently clients complain of severe itching from the opioids used with epidural analgesia. Antihistamines and comfort measures are effective for many clients, as well as reduction in the dosage or administering Narcan to control itching without reversing the analgesic effects. Respiratory depression (**Answer 1**) is not a common problem with careful titration of standard dosages. Only when the client becomes sedated does the respiratory function become a concern. **Answers 2** and **3** are *not* expected side effects (however, postural hypotension and constipation are potential problems).

TEST-TAKING TIP—The clue in the stem is "most common." Look for something annoying but not serious. Otherwise epidural analgesia would not be used as often as it is.
EV, COM, 3, M/S: Postop, PhI, Pharmacological and Parenteral Therapies

Answers/Rationales

54. **(1)** Maintaining perfusion is the priority in the early postoperative period. Pain management (**Answer 2**) would also be important; however, it is *not* life threatening. **Answers 3** and **4** are also important, but they are *not actual* problems, although there is risk *potential*.

> **TEST-TAKING TIP**—This is a priority question. Consider the *greatest* risk to the client, meaning the possibility of a life-threatening problem (cardiac).
> **AN, APP, 6, M/S: Postop, PhI, Physiological Adaptation**

55. **(1)** Tuberculosis is an airborne infectious disease. Preventing further spread of the disease would be a priority for care. Covering the mouth when coughing, proper disposal of tissues, and handwashing must be reinforced. **Answers 2, 3,** and **4** are important actions *after* preventing disease transmission.

> **TEST-TAKING TIP**—This is a priority question. Think pre*vention before* treatment.
> **PL, APP, 6, M/S: Infect. Control, SECE, Safety and Infection Control**

56. **(1)** The client is most likely in shock. Bicarbonate is needed with metabolic acidosis, which will develop. The compensatory tachycardia will result in poor oxygenation. Although the question does not indicate difficulty breathing, the client is not being perfused well (pulselessness) and may go into cardiac arrest if emergency treatment is not begun. CPR (**Answers 2** and **4**) would not be done because there *is* a heart rhythm, although perfusion is ineffective. Atropine (**Answer 3**) would not be given because it *increases* heart rate.

> **TEST-TAKING TIP**—Use a process of elimination—CPR is not indicated. Therefore, eliminate **Answers 2** and **4**. Do you give atropine or sodium bicarbonate for shock?
> **PL, APP, 6, M/S: Metab., PhI, Reduction of Risk Potential**

57. **(3)** The first action is to measure the glucose level, start an IV, and prepare to give glucose or insulin. A dangerously low blood sugar level is life-threatening and must be corrected immediately. **Answers 1, 2,** and **4** are not incorrect nursing actions; however, they are *not the first* priority.

> **TEST-TAKING TIP**—The key word is *first*. Only one option takes a direct action to determine the cause of unconsciousness.
> **IMP, ANL, 4, M/S: Metab., PhI, Reduction of Risk Potential**

58. **(3)** Polycythemia vera is a chronic myeloproliferative disorder characterized mainly by erythrocytosis (increased RBC mass). Hemoglobin and hematocrit will be elevated. **Answers 1, 2,** and **4** are also laboratory findings, but they are considered *minor* criteria in this condition.

> **TEST-TAKING TIP**—Know the major physiological abnormality and important diagnostic indicator.
> **AS, COM, 6, M/S: Blood, PhI, Physiological Adaptation**

59. **(2)** The nurse *leading*, without holding, the client is the correct approach. The nurse is the "sight" for the client, and being ahead of the individual who is blind is more secure and safe for the client. **Answers 1, 3,** and **4** all have the nurse holding the client, rather than the client holding onto the nurse.

> **TEST-TAKING TIP**—Look for patterns in the options. Only one has the client being *led* by the nurse.
> **IMP, APP, 3, M/S: Sens.-Percep., PhI, Basic Care and Comfort**

60. **(3)** During treatment (total insertion time varies from 48 to 144 hours), vaginal discharge may become foul-smelling due to tissue destruction; however, perineal care is generally not allowed due to the danger of dislodging the needles. Frequently, clients find this quite distressing. A douche given under low pressure following removal of the applicator helps to reduce this side effect of therapy. Bladder atony (**Answer 1**) is a rare complication; diarrhea, rather than constipation (**Answer 2**), is more likely to occur. Sexual libido (**Answer 4**) following this therapy seems more dependent on the relationship of the partners before therapy than on the therapy itself.

> **TEST-TAKING TIP**—Look for consistency between stem and option; only one option addresses a problem with the immediate area (vagina, uterus).
> **EV, APP, 8, M/S: Radiation, PhI, Physiological Adaptation**

61. **(1)** Fat-soluble vitamins, particularly vitamin K, are poorly absorbed in the absence of bile. This leads to decreased levels of circulating prothrombin, thus reducing normal clotting and increasing the tendency to bleed. Clients will have a T-tube postoperatively, *not* a Jackson-Pratt drain (**Answer 2**). Heating pads (**Answer 3**) are *not* used to relieve the abdominal discomfort of cholelithiasis and cholecystitis since they have little effect on reducing spasms of deeper organs. Instead, antispasmodics are used. A *high* carbohydrate diet, rather than a low carbohydrate one (**Answer 4**), would be given to build up glycogen stores in the liver.

> **TEST-TAKING TIP**—Eliminate the wrong answers: Jackson-Pratt is not used (T-tube is used), heat is not used (medications are used) to decrease spasms, and low carbohydrate is incorrect. (need *high* carbohydrate to build glycogen stores).
> **AS, APP, 6, M/S: GI, PhI, Reduction of Risk Potential**

62. **(3)** The single best measure for assessing fluid volume status is daily weights. Significant water loss must occur before there are changes in skin turgor (**Answer 1**). Similarly, blood pressure (**Answer 2**) may not reflect changes in fluid volume status if the fluid is sequestered in the interstitial spaces (edema formation). Finally, intake and output measures are important (**Answer 4**) but generally do not reflect insensible water losses (water lost per respiration and diaphoresis) and are not always as sensitive to decreases in urine output in chronic renal dysfunction as they are in more acute illnesses.

> **TEST-TAKING TIP**—Key word is "best." Other factors influence status of skin, vital signs, and intake and output besides fluid.
> **AS, APP, 6, M/S: Renal, PhI, Physiological Adaptation**

63. **(3)** The client receiving NPH insulin is most likely to experience a hypoglycemic reaction in the late afternoon. Several factors may be involved, such as increased physical activity or inadequate dietary intake. Clients should be instructed to carry gumdrops or hard candy as a source of quickly absorbed carbohydrates should symptoms occur. **Answers 1, 2,** and **4** are not as likely.

> **TEST-TAKING TIP**—Know that intermediate-acting insulin lasts 8–12 hours.
> **AN, COM, 4, M/S: Meds, PhI, Pharmacological and Parenteral Therapies**

64. **(2)** Symptoms of severe respiratory distress indicate that the tube has dislodged and is obstructing the airway. Reestablishing an airway is the first priority: Deflate the balloons using a syringe. Following deflation, the doctor should be notified to assess the client's condition and determine ongoing medical therapy. A code blue (**Answer 1**) would be called only *after* establishing the airway. Traction on the Sengstaken-Blakemore tube should be increased or decreased (**Answer 3**) *only by* the attending *physician*. Iced saline (**Answer 4**) is no longer used for irrigation during active bleeding, and this problem is respiratory, *not* hemorrhagic.

TEST TAKING TIP   Think of the common, yet most serious, thing that could happen to this special tube. When it was deflated, the position changed. Dyspnea and skin color change represent airway obstruction. Deflate the balloon and assess again.
IMP, ANL, 6, M/S: Resp., PhI, Physiological Adaptation

65. **(2)** Clients having upper-abdominal surgery tend to breathe shallowly after surgery in order to splint incisional discomfort. Consequently, these clients need both assistance and encouragement to breathe deeply and cough. Splinting of the incisional area by the nurse helps, as well as planning deep breathing and particularly coughing times to follow the administration of a pain reliever. **Answers 1** and **3** are correct statements but not the best answers. Clients having abdominal surgery tend to guard against coughing because it increases intra-abdominal pressures and incisional discomfort. Many people do tend to be thoracic breathers and need to be taught abdominal or diaphragmatic breathing in the preoperative period. **Answer 4** is incorrect, because NG tubes do not inhibit deep breathing; rather, they tend to increase oral respirations, which causes drying of the oral mucous membranes.

   TEST-TAKING TIP—Think of where the incision is and consider what organs/function will be most affected due to pain and splinting. Upper abdominal incisions have a significant impact on respiratory function. Look for an answer that explains *why* deep breathing is a problem.
   AN, APP, 6, M/S: Postop, PhI, Physiological Adaptation

66. **(4)** Intake and output records, as well as daily weights, provide important measures of the effectiveness of the treatment and are good monitors of fluid balance. Urine testing (**Answer 1**) is done to detect glycosuria *every 4 to 6 hours,* not 8 to 12 hours. In the event glycosuria occurs, the physician should be notified. The physician may order insulin coverage or a decrease in the flow rate. Blood withdrawal and CVP readings (**Answer 2**) are *contraindicated* because infusion rates must be kept constant to avoid the formation of clots in the catheter. If the catheter insertion site remains dry, dressings are changed every 48 hours utilizing *strict aseptic* technique, *not* just clean technique (**Answer 3**). Gloves and masks are used during the dressing change and while the IV tubing and filter are changed.

   TEST-TAKING TIP—The stem asks for "correct" action. Use the process of elimination. Only one will be right.
   IMP, APP, 6, M/S: GI, PhI, Pharmacological and Parenteral Therapies

67. **(1)** An iridectomy, or removal of a wedge from the iris, is performed with cataract removal to prevent the forward push of the aqueous humor from blocking the canal of Schlemm, which would produce a secondary glaucoma. Iridectomy does *not* affect pupillary dilation (**Answer 2**), facilitate retinal circulation (**Answer 3**), or prevent corneal scarring (**Answer 4**).

   TEST-TAKING TIP—Think about the normal eye structure. What would removing a wedge of iris do?
   IMP, APP, 2, M/S: Eye, PhI, Reduction of Risk Potential

68. **(3, 4, 5)** **Answer 3** is correct because the build-up of CO_2 in metabolic acidosis affects CNS function. **Answer 4** is correct because the build-up of CO_2 in metabolic acidosis affects CNS function. **Answer 5** is correct because the compensatory response for metabolic acidosis is to blow off the excess CO_2 by breathing deeply and rapidly (Kussmaul breathing). **Answer 1** is incorrect because increased neuromuscular irritability is seen with metabolic alkalosis. **Answer 2** is incorrect

because the client would be experiencing metabolic acidosis and a need to blow off CO_2. The breathing would be rapid and deep.

   TEST-TAKING TIP—The primary problem is metabolic—the kidneys are not getting rid of waste—acid. Know the effects of too much acid on the body and how to get rid of the excess acid.
   AN, ANL, 6, M/S: Renal, PhI, Physiological Adaptation

69. **(3)** The initial response would be to notify the physician of the critical hemoglobin (oxygen-carrying protein) level. A hemoglobin of 10 is desirable for the client, decreasing the deleterious risks of general anesthetic and hypovolemic shock. The lab slip is then attached to the chart (**Answer 1**). Most likely a blood transfusion will be ordered before surgery (**Answer 2**), but there is no order yet. The nurse's actions will be charted on the nurse's notes (**Answer 4**), but charting is *not* the *first* priority.

   TEST-TAKING TIP—Know normal values. If no answer involves client comfort or safety, call MD.
   AN, ANL, 6, M/S: Preop, PhI, Reduction of Risk Control

70. **(3)** Methyldopa acts to decrease blood pressure by inhibiting the formation of dopamine, thus decreasing the amount of norepinephrine that is secreted in adrenergic synapses. Decreased adrenergic stimulation results in decreased vasoconstriction, which causes peripheral vascular resistance. **Answer 1** is an example of the effects of hydralazine; **Answer 2**, of guanethidine SO_4; and **Answer 4**, of diazepam.

   TEST-TAKING TIP—Read each choice—look for clues, such as "dopamine" for *dopa.*
   IMP, COM, 6, M/S: Meds, PhI, Pharmacological and Parenteral Therapies

71. **(2)** Postoperative inflammation and edema underlie the frequent occurrence of scrotal swelling after indirect hernia repair. This complication is very painful, and any movement by the client results in discomfort. Elevating the scrotum on rolled towels or providing support with a suspensory helps to reduce edema. Ice bags facilitate pain relief. **Answer 1** is inappropriate because this is not an emergency side effect of surgery. Pain medication (**Answer 3**) may also be administered, but vigorous coughing (**Answer 4**) is contraindicated following herniorrhaphy.

   TEST-TAKING TIP—Look for what the nurse can do to assist with the identified problem. Think of the basic intervention: ice and elevation.
   IMP, ANL, 3, M/S: Postop, PhI, Basic Care and Comfort

72. **(4)** The first nursing measure should be to mark the time and the amount of drainage in the collection bottle to ensure a baseline measurement for further observations. The milking of chest tubes (**Answer 1**) is a matter of debate at this time. Although the process of stripping or milking does assist in the removal of fibrin and clots from the chest tubes, compression of the tubes also increases intrapleural pressures by preventing the movement of air and fluid. Whether the chest tubes are milked or not will depend on institutional or individual physician's policies. **Answer 2** is incorrect because the drainage system is always kept in a dependent position to maintain gravity flow of air and fluids. The nurse's next measure is to secure the tubes to the bed linen (**Answer 3**) to prevent kinking or unnecessary looping of the drainage tubes, which would hinder the flow of air and fluid.

   TEST-TAKING TIP—Think baseline data. Complete assessment first.
   IMP, APP, 6, M/S: Thoracic, PhI, Reduction of Risk Potential

73. **(2)** Respiratory obstruction, hemorrhage, tetany, and laryngeal nerve injury are the major complications following thyroid surgery. *Hypocalcemia,* not hypercalcemia (**Answer 1**), is a complication resulting from damage to the parathyroid glands during surgery. Serum T_4 will be *decreased* or absent, *not* elevated (**Answer 3**), and the client will need replacement therapy because no thyroid hormone is secreted once the total thyroid gland is removed. **Answer 4** is not a good answer. Because the integrity of the gastrointestinal tract is not interrupted during thyroid surgery, paralytic ileus is a *rare* complication.

> **TEST-TAKING TIP**—Think of where this incision is and the first priority—airway.
> **AN, APP, 3, M/S: Postop, PhI, Reduction of Risk Potential**

74. **(1)** The purpose of the T-tube is to maintain the patency of the bile duct after surgery. Localized edema in the surgery area tends to obstruct the outflow of bile, which is continuously being synthesized by the liver. The T-tube does *not directly* prevent postoperative hemorrhage (**Answer 2**) or postoperative wound infection (**Answer 3**). A *secondary* effect of this procedure is that bile flow is directed away from the duodenum (**Answer 4**).

> **TEST-TAKING TIP**—Visualize the T-tube. The horizontal part of the T is inserted into the common bile duct to maintain patency. Drainage comes into the tube from both sides of the horizontal portion of the tube into the vertical part of the T, which is connected to a collection apparatus. The T-tube remains in the duct until the edema subsides, because exploration causes swelling.
> **AN, COM, 4, M/S: Postop, PhI, Reduction of Risk Potential**

75. **(1)** Anxiety, like pain, glucose imbalance, or changes in blood pressure, stimulates discharge of the sympathetic nervous system. In some clients this increased adrenergic discharge results in moderate to severe increases in systolic and diastolic pressures that decrease to normal levels when emotional equilibrium is restored. The client may be emotionally labile (**Answer 2**), but at this time there are insufficient data to make this judgment. She is fearful, but that does not mean she is unprepared for this surgery (**Answer 3**). Should her anxiety remain high, however, the attending physician should be notified. Though the client may be attempting to employ denial (**Answer 4**), her emotional response (restlessness and increased blood pressure) indicates this defense mechanism is ineffective in allaying her present anxieties (**Answer 4**).

> **TEST-TAKING TIP**—When in doubt as to the answer, look for a pattern in the options—three are psychological explanations; choose the one that is different.
> **EV, ANL, 7, M/S: CV, PhI, Physiological Adaptation**

76. **(2)** The diet of a client with cirrhosis should provide ample protein for tissue repair, at least 0.5 g/lb. Some modification occurs *if* serum-ammonia levels are elevated (**Answer 1**). Sufficient carbohydrate intake is needed to sustain weight and prevent proteins from being utilized for energy, *not for the reason* stated in **Answer 3. Answer 4** is partially correct. Salt is restricted to assist in decreasing edema formation. However, the reason for high carbohydrate foods is as discussed above. Fluids may also be restricted to 1000 to 1500 mL/day. Vitamin supplements, particularly fat-soluble vitamins (A, D, and K), are usually prescribed because of decreased bile production and because of the inability of the liver to store them successfully. Initially, if the client has a very poor appetite, liquid protein supplements such as Sustagen may be given. Frequent, small feedings may also increase intake.

> **TEST-TAKING TIP**—How would each dietary restriction or specific allowance relate to the pathophysiology of the disease identified? Clients with cirrhosis often need adequate protein intake. Fluid accumulation is another significant problem to be considered.
> **PL, ANL, 4, M/S: Diet, PhI, Basic Care and Comfort**

77. **(3)** Neomycin is administered preoperatively because it is a poorly absorbed antibiotic and therefore is effective in reducing the number of intestinal organisms that may cause infection of the suture line. Neomycin is not effective in reducing postoperative atelectasis (**Answer 1**). Prevention of atelectasis is dependent on adequate pulmonary hygiene (deep breathing and coughing up of secretions) in the postoperative period. **Answer 2** is correct, but it is not the *best* answer, because the ability of the body to ward off infection is a result of the decrease in intestinal organisms. **Answer 4** is incorrect because bladder atony is generally due to decreased parasympathetic outflow and bladder tone secondary to anesthesia.

> **TEST-TAKING TIP**—Look for an option relating to the *drug action* (i.e., decreased intestinal organisms).
> **AN, COM, 8, M/S: Meds, PhI, Pharmacological and Parenteral Therapies**

78. **(2)** Postoperatively, deep breathing and particularly coughing up of sputum are the most important activities engaged in by the client after chest surgery. These activities reduce bronchotracheal secretions, prevent atelectasis, and promote adequate ventilation. Although **Answers 1** and **3** are also important in preventing postoperative complication, airway integrity is always the *first* priority. **Answer 4** is used for clients having *herniorrhaphies.*

> **TEST-TAKING TIP**—The question is asking for "most important postoperative activity." Priority should focus on prevention of airway complication if appropriate for the location.
> **IMP, APP, 6, M/S: Postop, PhI, Reduction of Risk Potential**

79. **(3)** Although most clients are able to rest more comfortably and even sleep after administration of a narcotic, extreme or prolonged lethargy indicates that the medication dose may be too large. The physician should be consulted for both a change of dose and route of administration (**Answers 1** and **2**). Alternative modes of pain relief can and should be instituted if the clients' discomfort is not severe, but not as a delaying tactic (**Answer 4**) when the issue is the appropriateness of a specific medication dose.

> **TEST-TAKING TIP**—Three options are *not* nursing decisions, once an adverse effect is noted.
> **IMP, ANL, 2, M/S: Meds, PhI, Pharmacological and Parenteral Therapies**

80. **(3)** Postoperatively following removal of a cataract, the client may be placed in a flat or low-Fowler's position on the back or turned to the unoperated side. Turning the client to the operated side (**Answer 4**) or raising the head of the bed (**Answer 1**) increases the stress on the sutures and may lead to hemorrhage. The client may assume a prone position with the head turned to the unoperated side (**Answer 2**), though most clients find a side-lying position more comfortable.

> **TEST-TAKING TIP**—Visualize which position will lower pressure in the head.
> **PL, APP, 2, M/S: Eye, PhI, Reduction of Risk Potential**

81. **(2)** After explaining the procedure to the client, the nurse should then instruct the client to void. This prevents accidental nicking or perforation of the bladder during the procedure. The client is positioned in a chair or in high-Fowler's

position in bed (**Answer 1**), after the vital signs have been taken to establish baseline information (**Answer 3**) and the abdomen is prepared (**Answer 4**).

> **TEST-TAKING TIP**—This question is establishing a priority order. Assume all actions are correct. Instructing the client to void would be the second thing the nurse would do, after procedures have been explained.
> **IMP, ANL, 6, M/S: Preop, PhI, Reduction of Risk Potential**

82. (**2**) Chronic renal failure symptomatology is due to a decrease in the number of functioning nephrons, with resultant decrease in glomerular filtration due to the extension of the disease process. **Answer 1** is incorrect because the cause of the renal failure was likely related to intrarenal damage from acute glomerulonephritis. **Answers 3 and 4** are incorrect because the client has moved from the second stage of chronic kidney disease (renal insufficiency, characterized by water diuresis and mild azotemia) to renal failure, which is characterized by acidosis, marked electrolyte imbalances, fluid retention, anemia, and increases in serum urea, uric acid, and creatinine.

> **TEST-TAKING TIP**—The problem is *within* the kidney (the nephrons), not *to* or *from* the kidney.
> **AN, APP, 8, M/S: Renal, PhI, Physiological Adaptation**

83. (**1, 2, 3**) **Answer 1** is correct because monitoring the dressing frequently for bleeding will prevent the potential of excessive and unrecognized bleeding. Also the sheets under the neck of the client need to be checked. **Answer 2** is correct because ice will reduce hematoma formation and edema. **Answer 3** is correct because a semi-Fowler's position improves gravity drainage from the wound site and facilitates proper positioning of the neck. **Answer 4** is incorrect because neck flexion would stress the suture line and increase the chance of bleeding. **Answer 5** is incorrect because it would be harder for the client to breathe, and placement of a pillow would flex the neck and stress the suture line.

> **TEST-TAKING TIP**—Visualize the incision. Think client comfort, safety and prevention of complications, such as edema and hemorrhage.
> **IMP, APP, 3, M/S: Postop, PhI, Reduction of Risk Potential**

84. (**3**) Manipulation of abdominal contents during surgery produces inhibition of peristalsis for 24 to 48 hours. Measures to avoid potential distention could include insertion of a nasogastric tube before surgery and continuous postsurgical suction until peristalsis returns; rectal tubes can be inserted to remove excess air in the lower colon; and early ambulation promotes return of gastrointestinal functioning. Auscultation of the abdomen for return of bowel sounds (**Answer 1**) will be necessary *when* assessing for the return and degree of peristalsis. Abdominal massage is *not* recommended (**Answer 2**). *When* bowel sounds return, oral intake (**Answer 4**) may be started.

> **TEST-TAKING TIP**—The key word is "avoid."
> **PL, APP, 1, M/S: Postop, PhI, Reduction of Risk Potential**

85. (**4**) If all the secondary measures have been tried and the client's bladder is distended, the physician should be notified if he or she has not left a catheterization order. Occasionally, drugs such as neostigmine bromide (Prostigmin) are ordered to stimulate bladder contractions before resorting to catheterization. **Answer 1** will only tire the client more. Catheters should not be inserted without an order (**Answer 2**), nor should the client be unduly fatigued by continuing to try other measures (**Answer 3**) that most likely were unsuccessful prior to this point in time. The bladder should not be allowed to become overdistended.

> **TEST-TAKING TIP**—All usual activities have been tried. It is time to call the physician.
> **IMP, APP, 8, M/S: GU, PhI, Physiological Adaptation**

86. (**2**) Hypotension and shock can occur during or after paracentesis. Fluid from the vascular compartment shifts into the abdomen to replace fluids that are withdrawn. This complication can be minimized if withdrawal of ascitic fluid is limited to 1000 mL or if lost fluid is replaced by administration of salt-poor albumin. To assess for this complication, vital signs are taken every 15 minutes during the procedure and afterward until stable, then every hour for 4 hours. Disequilibrium (**Answer 1**) occurs with rapid removal of wastes during *renal dialysis*. Hypoalbuminuria (*no protein* in urine) is a *normal* physical finding; therefore **Answer 3** is incorrect. Paralytic ileus (**Answer 4**) is *rarely* a complication of this procedure.

> **TEST-TAKING TIP**—Look for a pattern—only one option would be an *immediate* response.
> **AN, APP, 6, M/S: Vascular, PhI, Reduction of Risk Potential**

87. (**3**) Bending to adjust shoelaces would increase intraocular pressures and should be *avoided* during the early postoperative period; the client who is ambulatory should wear slip-on shoes or slippers to avoid bending or stooping. Other activities to avoid include coughing, brushing the teeth, shaving, and vomiting. Self-feeding (**Answer 1**) *is* encouraged, to help reduce the client's perception of helplessness, though food may need to be cut up for the client to reduce exertion. Self-dressing (**Answer 2**) and ambulation (**Answer 4**) *are* permitted.

> **TEST-TAKING TIP**—Look for an option that increases pressure on the operative site as the activity to *avoid*.
> **IMP, APP, 2, M/S: Eye, PhI, Reduction of Risk Potential**

88. (**4**) Increased circulating levels of uric acid, an end product of purine metabolism, are responsible for the client's gout-like joint discomfort. Thus the diet will exclude foods high in purines (e.g., high protein foods, organ meats). Hyperphosphatemia does occur in the third stage of chronic kidney disease. Normally this would stimulate the parathyroid gland to increase parathormone, thus raising calcium levels and lowering phosphate. However, in chronic renal failure the kidney fails to produce a metabolite of vitamin D, which effectively reduces parathormone activity, lowering serum-calcium levels. Amphojel (an aluminum hydroxide preparation) is given to bind the phosphate excreted in the *bowel* (**Answer 1**). Dialysis is used to decrease the serum-creatinine level, which causes central nervous system *depression* (**Answer 2**), *not* joint pain. Joint pain is usually related to inflammation or trauma *rather than decreased activity* level. Increasing activity (**Answer 3**) might *aggravate* the pain.

> **TEST-TAKING TIP**—Look for a *known* cause of joint pain in answers—increased uric acid, as with gout.
> **AN, ANL, 4, M/S: Metab., PhI, Basic Care and Comfort**

89. (**1**) Urinary retention following spinal anesthesia is due to blockage of autonomic nervous system fibers, which innervate the bladder and sensory perception. **Answer 2,** though correct, is not as complete as **Answer 1.** All clients secrete ADH postoperatively because of the surgical insult. However, ADH reduces the volume of urine (**Answer 3**), as does lowered blood pressure (**Answer 4**), but *neither causes* urinary retention.

> **TEST-TAKING TIP**—Think of the action of spinal anesthesia. The medication used during this type of anesthesia inhibits the conduction of autonomic nervous system impulses and central nervous system impulses. When trying

to figure out what happens, try to think of *why* it should happen.
AN, APP, 8, M/S: Renal, PhI, Physiological Adaptation

90. **(1)** Sitting for long periods of time and wearing constrictive clothing tend to increase pelvic congestion. Daily bowel movements (**Answer 2**) are *not* necessary as long as a normal pattern is achieved. It is important to reinforce the physician's instructions that sexual activity *may be resumed* within a specific period of time, usually 6 to 8 weeks. Six months (**Answer 3**) is *too long*. Paced and gradual ambulation aids in increasing venous return and general strength. Complete avoidance of chores for 2 months (**Answer 4**) is *not* necessary. Lifting of heavy objects, however, may injure the incision site and promote bleeding.

TEST-TAKING TIP—Look for options that will prevent stasis and pooling of blood to prevent complications. Select the option that is not as restrictive as the other three (i.e., "daily" is not necessary; 6 months is too long; "all household chores" is too inclusive). Select the more general answer ("long periods").
IMP, APP, 3, M/S: Postop, PhI, Basic Care and Comfort

91. **(2)** Elevation of the foot of the bed enhances venous return and reduces edema by utilizing the force of gravity. Pain is decreased (**Answer 1**) *as* the edema is reduced. **Answer 3** is incorrect because raising the foot of the bed should not greatly affect arterial blood flow. Reducing edema is what makes the client more comfortable (**Answer 4**).

TEST-TAKING TIP—Visualize the body positions. Would venous stasis be prevented?
IMP, COM, 6, M/S: Vascular, PhI, Reduction of Risk Potential

92. **(3)** Postoperatively the potential for severe fluid and electrolyte imbalances exists for several reasons: (a) the ileostomy drainage contains large amounts of sodium and water, (b) postsurgical diuresis increases both water and potassium excretion, and (c) nasogastric suction further decreases fluid and electrolytes by preventing their normal reabsorption. **Answers 1, 2,** and **4** are also important measures in this client's postoperative care; however, maintenance of fluid and electrolyte balance is *most critical*.

TEST-TAKING TIP—Look for the *most* life-threatening option (a priority question).
PL, APP, 6, M/S: F-E, PhI, Physiological Adaptation

93. **(1)** Increased serum potassium (hyperkalemia) causes the T waves to lose their normal, rounded configuration and become more pointy or peaked (the difference in shape between a mountain and a mound); therefore **Answer 2** is incorrect. ST segments are not significantly affected by this electrolyte imbalance (**Answers 3** and **4**).

TEST-TAKING TIP—Think "mountains" for high K$^+$ and "mounds" for low K$^+$–T-wave changes.
AS, ANL, 6, M/S: Cardiac, PhI, Reduction of Risk Potential

94. **(2)** Hypotension and shock can occur during or after paracentesis. Fluid from the vascular compartment shifts into the abdomen to replace fluids that are withdrawn. This complication can be minimized if withdrawal of ascitic fluid is limited to 1000 mL or if lost fluid is replaced by administration of salt-poor albumin. To assess for this complication, vital signs are taken every 15 minutes during the procedure and afterward until stable, then every hour for 4 hours. **Answers 1, 3,** and **4** are incorrect amounts.

TEST-TAKING TIP—The general rule of thumb is to not remove more than 1000 mL of fluid from anywhere at one time without observation of the client's vital signs.
AN, COM, 6, M/S: F-E, PhI, Physiological Adaptation

95. **(1)** Clients should be informed that the cataract glasses will magnify objects; this not only causes distortions in the shape of an object but also may result in color distortions. The spatial changes that result from these lenses may cause the client to underreach for an object or have difficulty walking and climbing stairs. Peripheral vision is *decreased* (**Answer 2**), so the client needs to be taught to turn the head and utilize the central vision provided by the lenses. **Answers 3** and **4** are incorrect because the magnification created by these lenses (up to 35%) is *not* similar to the size perception before the cataract formed, *nor* do they cause double vision.

TEST-TAKING TIP—Think of the *purpose* of the glasses—magnification.
IMP, APP, 2, M/S: Eye, SECE, Safety and Infection Control

96. **(3)** An immediate response to the choking sensation is assessment of the surgical site by examining under the dressing. If the area appears edematous, loosen the dressing and have someone remain with the client. Elevating the head to a high-Fowler's position (**Answer 1**), though the preferred position for improving ventilation of the lung, will *not* reduce upper-airway obstruction. **Answer 2** is *inappropriate* for this situation and may actually increase the client's distress. Notify the physician (**Answer 4**), who might order the sutures or clips to be removed, *after* assessing the surgical site.

TEST-TAKING TIP—Choose the first step of the nursing process—assess, before implementation.
IMP, ANL, 1, M/S: Wound Care, PhI, Physiological Adaptation

97. **(1)** The earliest clinical signs of bleeding include restlessness, pallor, tachycardia, and cooling of the skin. These symptoms occur as the result of vasoconstriction (increased sympathetic stimulation) in order to maintain venous return and cardiac output. **Answer 2** represents symptoms of *ketoacidosis*. When the vasoconstrictive mechanisms discussed above are *no longer effective*, the blood pressure begins to fall (**Answer 3**). It is essential to identify bleeding early because liver cells are very susceptible to ischemia. **Answer 4** may occur with increases in *intracranial pressure*.

TEST-TAKING TIP—The key word is "earliest." Look for *restlessness*.
AS, ANL, 6, M/S: Blood, PhI, Physiological Adaptation

98. **(2)** Symptoms of circulatory overload result from varying degrees of cardiac decompensation, with blood backing up into the pulmonary (moist crackles) and systemic circuits (neck vein distention, dependent edema, periorbital edema, and hepatomegaly). Symptoms of circulatory *failure* or hypovolemia include apprehension, soft eyeballs, flattened neck veins, shock, decreased pulse pressure, and poor skin turgor (**Answers 1, 3,** and **4**).

TEST-TAKING TIP—Because the question is asking for objective data, eliminate subjective information (apprehension). What would you *see* with fluid volume deficit compared to fluid volume overload? Renal failure means fluids are held in, unable to be excreted.
AS, APP, 6, M/S: Renal, PhI, Physiological Adaptation

99. **(2)** Given the client's complaint and evidence of pink drainage, the nurse should suspect dehiscence. Dehiscence is characterized by a gush of pink serous drainage and a parting

of the wound edges. Dehiscence generally occurs in the fifth to seventh day following surgery, due to increased intra-abdominal pressures from flatus, coughing, retching, or inadequate tissue support. Late hemorrhage (**Answer 1**) would be accompanied by signs of shock such as decreased blood pressure, rapid pulse, and diaphoresis. Wound infection (**Answer 3**) would be characterized by pain, redness, and fever. Evisceration (**Answer 4**) occurs after dehiscence when loops of intestine escape through the opened incision.

> ☼ **TEST-TAKING TIP**—Visualize what the client said about a "giving" sensation, similar to a "splitting" or "moving away" feeling. Know the risks of abdominal surgery. Dehiscence (separation of the wound) comes before evisceration (internal contents protrude through the opened wound), just as a "d" comes before "e" in the alphabet.
> **AN, ANL, 1, M/S: Postop, PhI, Physiological Adaptation**

100. (3) The Sengstaken-Blakemore tube is a triple-lumen tube composed of a catheter that goes to the stomach for suctioning, a lumen that ends in a gastric balloon, and a lumen that ends in an esophageal balloon. The *primary* purpose of this tube is to stop bleeding by applying pressure to the cardiac portion of the stomach and against the esophageal varices. Thus, **Answer 1** is only partially correct. The *secondary* purposes of the tube are (a) to prevent accumulation of blood in the gastrointestinal tract (**Answer 2**), which could precipitate hepatic coma, and (b) to reduce blood transfusion requirements (**Answer 4**).

> **TEST-TAKING TIP**—With two good choices, pick the most comprehensive answer that covers them both. (**Answer 1** is correct but not as complete as **Answer 3**.)
> **PL, APP, 6, M/S: GI, PhI, Reduction of Risk Potential**

The Older Adult

Robyn Nelson

Introduction

This unit is unique in that the primary objective is to present **practical,** concise information of **clinical** relevance for the beginning practitioner that is not covered elsewhere. The focus is on 12 significant problems and concerns associated with the older adult (e.g., *falls, use of restraints, thermoregulation, sleep disturbance, skin breakdown, polypharmacy,* specific types of *hearing changes,* age-related *macular degeneration, incontinence, sexual neglect, caregiver burden,* warning signs of *poor nutrition*).

The unit begins with health assessment of the older adult, system by system, highlighting the most common changes associated with the aging process; it ends with several functional rating scales to assist in management of care in the home or community.

Covered elsewhere in this book are other age-relevant problems and test questions. Refer to **Unit 6** for mental health conditions common in the older adult (e.g., *dementia, Alzheimer's, depression*). **Unit 7** covers common age-relevant *problems related to immobility, bladder and bowel* dysfunction, *hip fracture,* use of *assistive devices,* cardiovascular conditions *(stroke, hypertension), cataracts,* and *glaucoma.* Also covered in **Unit 7** are health problems that have more serious consequences in the older adult, such as *pneumonia* and *osteoporosis. Nutritional needs* of the elderly are included in **Unit 9.**

◆ **I. Health assessment of the older adult** (see also **Unit 7**)
   A. *Skin*
   1. Decrease in elasticity → wrinkles and lines, dryness.
   2. Loss of fullness → sagging.
   3. Generalized loss of adipose and muscle tissue → wasting appearance.
   4. Decrease of adipose tissue on extremities, redistributed to hips and abdomen in middle age.
   5. Bony prominences become visible.
   6. Excessive pigmentation → age spots.
   7. Dry skin and deterioration of nerve fibers and sensory endings → pruritus.
   8. Decreased blood flow → pallor and blotchiness.
   9. Overgrowth of epidermal tissue → lesions (some benign, some premalignant, some malignant).
   B. *Nails:*
   1. Dry, brittle, peeling, ridges.
   2. Increased susceptibility to fungal infections.
   3. Decreased growth rate.
   4. Toenails thick, difficult to cut, ingrown.
   C. *Hair:*
   1. Loss of pigment → graying, white.
   2. Decreased density of hair follicles → thinning of hair.
   3. Decreased blood flow to skin and decreased estrogen production → baldness.
      a. Hair distribution: thin on scalp, axilla, pubic area, upper and lower extremities.
      b. Decreased facial hair in *men.*
   4. Decreased estrogen production → increased facial (chin, upper lip) hair in *women.*
   D. *Eyes:*
   1. Loss of soluble protein with loss of lens transparency → development of *cataracts.*
   2. Decrease in pupil size limits amount of light entering the eye → elderly need more light to see.
   3. Decreased pupil reactivity → decrease in rate of light changes to which a person can readily adapt.
   4. Decreased accommodation to darkness and dim light → diminished night vision.
   5. Loss of orbital fat → sunken appearance.
   6. Blink reflex—slowed.
   7. Eyelids—loose.
   8. Visual acuity—diminished
   9. Peripheral vision—diminished.
   10. Visual fields—diminished (e.g., macular degeneration).
   11. Lens accommodation—decreased; requires corrective lenses.
   12. *Presbyopia*—lens may lose ability to become convex enough to accommodate to nearby objects; starts at age 40 *(farsightedness).*
   13. Color of iris—fades.
   14. Conjunctiva—thins, looks yellow.
   15. Increased intraocular pressure → *glaucoma.*
   16. Previous corrective surgery.
   E. *Ears:*
   1. Changes in cochlea → decrease in average pitch of sound.
   2. Hearing loss—greater in left ear than right; greater in *higher* frequencies than in lower.

3. Tympanic membrane—atrophied, thickened → hearing loss.
4. *Presbycusis*—progressive loss of hearing in old age.
5. Use of hearing devices.
6. Predisposed to wax build-up (cerumen).

F. *Mouth/dental health:*
1. Dental caries.
2. Poor-fitting dentures; no dentures.
3. Cancer of the mouth—increased risk.
4. Decrease in taste buds → inability to taste sweet/salty foods.
5. Olfactory bulb atrophies → decreased ability to smell due to blockage or disease of olfactory receptors in the upper sinus → ↓ awareness of body odor, smoke, fumes, spoiled food.
6. Coating of tongue.

G. *Cardiovascular:*
1. Lack of elasticity of vessels → increased resistance to blood flow; decreased diameter of arteries → *increased blood pressure.*
2. Atherosclerotic and calcium plaques → *thrombosis.*
3. Valves become sclerotic, less pliable → reduced filling and emptying.
4. Diastolic murmurs heard at base of heart.
5. Loss of elasticity, decreased contractility → decreased cardiac output.
6. Changes in the coronary arteries → pooling of blood in systemic veins and shortness of breath → reduced pumping action of the heart.
7. Disturbance of the autonomic nervous system → *dysrhythmias.*
8. Extremities—arteriosclerotic changes → weaker pedal pulses, colder extremities, mottled color; pain with ambulation.

H. *Respiratory:*
1. Efficiency reduced with age.
2. Greater residual air in lungs after expiration.
3. Decreased vital capacity.
4. Weaker expiratory muscles→ decreased capacity to cough → infections of lower respiratory tract.
5. Decreased ciliary activity → stasis of secretions → susceptibility to infections.
6. Oxygen debt in the muscles → dyspnea on exertion (DOE), sleep apnea due to ↓ O_2 to the brain.
7. Reduced chest wall compliance → ↓ expiratory excursion, affecting inspiratory and expiratory volumes.

I. *Breasts:*
1. Atrophy.
2. Cancer risk—increased with age.

J. *Gastrointestinal:*
1. Lack of intrinsic factor → *pernicious anemia.*
2. Gastric motility—decreased → poorer, slower digestion.
3. Esophageal peristalsis—decreased.
4. Hiatal hernia—increased incidence.
5. Digestive enzymes—gradual decrease of ptyalin (which converts *starch*), pepsin and trypsin (which digest *protein*), lipase (*fat*-splitting enzyme).

6. Absorption—decreased.
7. Improper diet → constipation.
8. Decreased thirst sensation → risk for dehydration.
9. Decreased saliva → dysphagia.

K. *Endocrine:*
1. Basal metabolism rate lowered → decreased temperature.
2. Cold intolerance.
3. Women: decreased ovarian function → increased gonadotropins.
4. Decreased renal sensitivity to ADH → unable to concentrate urine as effectively as younger persons.
5. Decreased clearance of blood glucose after meals → elevated postprandial blood glucose.
6. Risk of *diabetes mellitus* increases with age.

L. *Urinary:*
1. Renal function—impaired due to poor perfusion.
2. Filtration—impaired due to reduction in number of functioning nephrons → ↓ in urine concentration.
3. Urgency and frequency: *men*—often due to prostatic hyperplasia; *women*—due to perineal muscle weakness.
4. Nocturia—*both* men and women.
5. Urinary tract infection (e.g., cystitis)—increased incidence.
6. Incontinence—especially with dementia; stress/exercise induced.
7. Retention—due to incomplete bladder emptying.

M. *Musculoskeletal:*
1. Muscle mass—decreased. Loss of lower limb strength.
2. Bony prominences—increased.
3. Demineralization of bone.
4. Narrowing of intervertebral space → shortening of trunk → loss of height.
5. Posture—normal; some kyphosis.
6. Range of motion—limited.
7. *Osteoarthritis*—related to extensive physical activities and joint use.
8. Gait—altered; use of cane or walker.
9. *Osteoporosis* related to menopause, immobilization, elevated levels of cortisone → ↑ fractures.
10. Calcium, phosphorus, and vitamin D decreased.

N. *Neurological:*
1. Voluntary, automatic reflexes—slowed.
2. Sleep pattern—changes.
3. Mental acuity—changes.
4. Sensory interpretation and movement—changes.
5. Pain perception—diminished.
6. Dexterity and agility—lessened.
7. Reaction time—slowed.
8. Memory—past more vivid than recent memory due to loss of neurons from CNS.
9. *Depression.*
10. *Alzheimer's* disease.

O. *Sexuality:*
1. *Women:*

a. Estrogen production—decreased with menopause.
b. Breasts atrophy.
c. Vaginal secretions—reduced lubricants.
d. Sexuality—drive continues; sexual activity declines.

2. *Men:*
a. Testosterone production—decreased.
b. Testes—decrease in size; decreased sperm count.
c. Libido and sexual satisfaction—no changes.

P. *Mental status:* **3 Ds:**
1. *Delirium:* confusion/agitation with time and place disorientation, illusions and/or hallucinations.
2. *Dementia:* cognitive deficits (memory, reasoning, judgment).
3. *Depression:* decreased interest/pleasure in activities.

Q. *Immune system:*
1. Immune response: decreased → ↓ T-cell activity and ↓ in cell-mediated immunity.
2. Increased risk of nosocomial infections (e.g., *Pseudomonas,* staphylococci, enterococci, and fungi), pneumonia, cancer, reactivation of varicella zoster and TB.
3. Atypical inflammatory response; no elevated temperatures or white blood cell counts.

◆ II. **General nursing diagnoses in the older adult**
A. *Risk for loneliness* related to isolation and loss of many friends, family members, and pets due to separation and death.
B. *Self-care deficit* related to inability to complete activities of daily living.
C. *Impaired verbal communication* related to hearing loss.
D. *Fluid volume* deficit related to low fluid intake.
E. *Impaired skin integrity* related to prolonged back-lying position and inability to turn self.
F. *Body image disturbance* related to physical changes associated with the aging process.
G. *Sleep pattern disturbance* related to concern about outcomes of pending diagnostic tests.

III. **Problems associated with the older adult***
A. *Falls:*
◆ 1. **Assessment.** *Risk factors:*
a. Gait changes—prone to trip and stumble; do not pick feet up as high.
b. Postural instability—tendency to lose balance; older adults take steps to correct balance and increase possibility of falling.
c. Impaired muscular control—inability to recover from trip or unexpected step; weaker muscle cushioning and slowed righting reflexes.
d. Deterioration of vision and hearing—impaired ability to avoid obstacles.

e. Loss of short-term memory—prone to trip over forgotten objects.
f. Environmental:
(1) *Home:* unstable furniture and appliances; stairs with poor rails; throw rugs and frayed carpets; poor lighting; low beds and toilets; pets; objects on floor; medications.
(2) *Institutions:* recent admission or transfer; furniture; slick, hard floors; unsupervised activities; meal times; absence of hand rails; inadequate lighting, long hallways.

◆ 2. **Nursing goal/implementation:** reduce risk of falling in the older adult with *fall-prevention measures.*
a. Treat underlying condition (e.g., osteoporosis, muscle weakness, imbalance, pain).
b. Reduce risk factors (e.g., visual problems, orthostasis).
c. Reduce environmental hazards (e.g., provide adequate lighting and night lamps, *avoid* cluttered areas, *no* throw rugs, provide bath and shower support bars).
d. Increase leg range-of-motion (ROM) exercises.
e. Develop an individualized exercise plan.
f. Support adequate nutrition (e.g., calcium intake).

B. *Use of restraints:*
1. *Definition*—any device, material, or equipment attached to the client that cannot be easily removed by the client; restricts free movement; includes leg restraints, arm restraints, hand mitts, soft ties or vests, wheelchair safety bars, "geri-chairs."

◆ 2. **Assessment** of problems resulting from use of restraints:
a. Increased agitation, confusion.
b. Falls.
c. Pressure sores.
d. Bone density loss (demineralization).
e. Immobility hazard.
f. Death from strangulation.

◆ 3. **Nursing goal/implementation:** provide *restraint-free care* with alternatives to restraints:
a. *Physical:* recliners; medications for pain relief; seating adaptations (physical therapy/occupational therapy); chairs with deep seats.
b. *Psychosocial:* encourage expression of feelings, giving time for client response; encourage positive self-concept; offer hope; active listening; increased or decreased sensory stimulation; increased visiting; reality orientation; clocks; animals.
c. *Activity:* structured daily routines; wandering/pacing permitted; physical exercise; night-time activities.
d. *Environmental:* door buzzers; limb bracelet alarms; signs, call bells.

*Source: Cheryl Osborne, EdD, RN, Professor of Nursing, Director of Gerontology, California State University, Sacramento.

Adults

e. *Structural:* exit alarms; increased lighting; enclosed courtyards.

f. *Supervision:* family, nursing; volunteer; security.

g. Sedation.

C. *Thermoregulation*—normal oral temperature for >75 years: 96.9–98.3°F; rectal, 98–99°F. Decreased or absence of increased temperature in infection or dehydration.

1. **Assessment** of causes:

a. Factors affecting the *hypothalmus:* decreased—muscle activity, metabolic rate, food and fluid intake, subcutaneous fat; changes in peripheral blood flow; diseases; medications.

b. *External factors:* environmental temperature; humidity; airflow; type and amount of clothing.

2. **Nursing goal/implementation:** *prevent hypothermia and hyperthermia.*

a. Ensure and monitor adequate fluid and food intake.

b. Maintain constancy in environmental temperature: *avoid* drafts, overheating, prolonged exposure to cold.

c. Monitor ventilation: provide airflow (air conditioners, fans; safe sources of heat).

d. Use layered clothing (remove when warm; add when cold).

D. *Sleep disturbances.*

1. **Nursing goal/implementation:** promote restful sleep and *prevent sleep deprivation* with sleep care strategies:

a. Maintain normal sleep pattern: arrange medications and therapies to minimize sleep interruptions.

b. Encourage daytime activity; discourage daytime naps.

c. Support bedtime routines/rituals: bedtime reading, listening to music, quiet television.

d. Promote comfort: mattress, pillows, wrinkle-free linen, loose bed covering.

e. Promote relaxation: warm milk or soup if not contraindicated, back rub.

f. *Avoid*/minimize stimulation before bedtime: *no* caffeine after dinner, reduce fluid intake before sleep, refrain from smoking.

g. *Avoid*/minimize drugs that negatively influence sleep, such as ranitidine, diltiazem, atenolol, nifedipine.

h. Create a restful environment: turn off lights, reduce or eliminate noise, minimize disruptions for therapy or monitoring.

E. *Skin breakdown.*

1. **Assessment:**

a. *Age-related changes:* slower rate of epidermal proliferation; thinner dermis; *decreased*—dermal blood supply, melanocytes (gray hair), moisture, sweat and sebaceous glands.

b. Predisposing *risk factors:* exposure to ultraviolet rays (sunlight, excessive tanning); adverse medication effects; personal hygiene habits (too frequent bathing); limited activity; heredity.

c. *Functional consequences:* dry skin; skin wrinkles; delayed wound healing; *increased*—susceptibility to burns, injury, infection, altered thermoregulation, skin cancer, cracking nails.

2. **Nursing goal/implementation:** treatment for *pressure sores.*

a. *Stage I*—reddened broken skin: *cover* and *protect* (use sprays, gels, transparent films, transparent occlusive wafers).

b. *Stage II*—blister or partial-thickness skin loss: *cover, protect, hydrate, insulate,* and *absorb* exudate (use transparent films, occlusive wafer dressings, calcium alginate for absorbing exudate; polyurethane foam, moistened gauze dressing).

c. *Stage III*—full-thickness skin loss: *cover, protect, hydrate, insulate, absorb, cleanse, prevent infection,* and *promote granulation* (use occlusive wafer dressings, absorption dressing, calcium alginate, and moistened gauze dressings).

d. *Stage IV*—full-thickness skin loss involving muscle, tendon, and bone: same as stage III except before *promote granulation, dead eschar (tissue) is removed* (use absorption dressing, calcium alginate, and moistened gauze dressings).

F. *Polypharmacy*—concurrent use of several drugs increasing the potential for adverse reactions, drug interactions, and self-medication errors (**Table 8.1**).

1. Reasons for polypharmacy:

a. Lack of communication among multiple health-care providers.

b. Lack of information about over-the-counter drug use.

c. Lack of information about client noncompliance.

d. Use of complementary (alternative, folk medicine) therapies and fear of telling health-care provider.

e. Assumption that once medication is started, it should be continued indefinitely and not changed.

f. Assumption that if there are no early side effects, there will not be any later.

g. Changes in daily habits (smoking, activity, diet/fluid intake).

h. Changes in mental-emotional status that may affect consumption patterns.

i. Changes in health status.

j. Financial limitations (drug substitution).

2. **Nursing goal/implementation:** assist the older adult to use medications safely and try **nonpharmacological interventions** for common health problems.

	Medications That Should *Not*
TABLE 8.1	Be Used by Older Adults

Medication Category	Contraindicated Medications
Antidepressants	Elavil
	Triavil
Cardiovascular	Aldomet
	Catapres
	Cyclospasmol
	Pavabid
	Serpasil
	Trental
Pain and arthritis medications	Bufferin
	Darvocet
	Darvon
	Feldene
	Talwin
Gastrointestinal	Colace
	Dialose-Plus
	Donnatal
	Doxidan
	Mylanta
	Surfak
	Tigan
Tranquilizers and hypnotics	Ativan
	Dalmane
	Halcion
	Librium
	Nembutal
	Restoril
	Valium
	Xanax
Neurological	Artane
	Cogentin

Source: Cheryl Osborne, EdD, RN, Professor of Nursing, Director of Gerontology, California State University, Sacramento.

a. *Constipation:* exercise, relaxation, biofeedback; increase fluid and fiber intake.
b. *Stress incontinence:* pelvic muscle exercises, biofeedback.
c. *Anxiety, depression:* counseling, exercise, meditation, relaxation techniques; touch, music, and pet therapy.
d. *Arthritis:* acupuncture, heat therapy, therapeutic exercise, postural or alignment aids; touch, music, and pet therapy.
e. *Chronic neuromuscular problems:* massage, body work, touch and music therapy.
f. *Sleep problem* (see **D.** Sleep disturbances).
G. *Hearing changes*—external auditory canal atrophies, resulting in thinner walls and increased cerumen buildup; degenerative changes in ossicular joints leading to slower/stiffer movements; loss of hair cells and cochlear neurons in inner ear.
   1. Types:
      a. *Presbycusis*—bilateral loss of **high-pitched** tones; slightly less severe in women than in men.

b. *Impaired pitch discrimination*—after age 55, makes localizing and understanding sounds difficult; impaired ability to understand consonants.
c. *Decline in speech discrimination*—after age 60, speech intelligibility declines; slowing of memory and slowing of mental processes with advancing age may also affect speech, hearing, and understanding.
d. *Diminished vestibular function*—deficits in equilibrium and greater fall risk.
   2. **Nursing goal/implementation:** *improve communication* for person who is hearing-impaired.
      a. *Compensate with other senses*—face listener; make eye contact if culturally acceptable; get person's attention before talking; use touch if culturally appropriate; help with hearing aid; *avoid* walking around room while talking; write down key words if person can read.
      b. *Alter stimulus and behavior*—speak in normal volume of voice or slightly lower, *avoid* shouting; use short sentences; separate important words with pauses; allow more time for communication; have person repeat to show understanding; repeat; teach person to be more assertive about impairment.
      c. *Modify environment*—eliminate or reduce background noise (turn off running water, close doors, lower TV or radio); select areas with sound-absorbing abilities for conversations (carpets, drapes); amplify telephone; allow for adequate light on speaker's face.
H. *Visual impairment.*
   1. *Age-related macular degeneration* (AMD)—leading cause of irreversible and legal blindness for those over 65 yr; blurred far and near vision; loss of central vision; difficulty going up and down steps and stairs; parts of words and letters disappear when reading; straight lines appear to be wavy. Acuity: 20/200 or less.
      a. **Assessment.** *Risk factors:* increased age, women, Caucasian, smoking, UV light exposure, diabetes, diet (low in leafy green vegetables and antioxidants).
      b. *Prevention:* UV light filters, aspirin, vitamins A and B, beta-carotene, zinc.
      c. *Prognosis:* no treatment or cure; laser may prevent spread of AMD in some clients.
      d. **Nursing goal:** assist client to maintain independent functioning.
   2. See **Unit 7** for other causes of visual problems in the older adult, such as stroke, **p. 606;** glaucoma, **p. 599;** cataracts, **p. 600;** and diabetes, **p. 572.**
I. *Loss of urinary control*—neurological mechanism controlling bladder emptying does not work effectively and results in incontinence; a symptom, *not* a diagnosis.
   1. **Assessment.** *Risk factors:*
      a. Immobility.

Adults

b. Cognitive and functional impairments—Parkinson's disease, Alzheimer's disease, multiple sclerosis, alcoholism, stroke, vitamin B deficiency, inability to walk and transfer to toilet.

c. Medications.

d. Institutionalization.

e. Pathological conditions—*men:* hyperplasia leading to infection, incomplete emptying, urgency, and frequency; *women:* weakening of pelvic floor postmenopause, leading to residual urine and infection; atrophy of vaginal and trigonal tissue, leading to frequency, urgency, and incontinence.

f. Childbirth.

2. Incontinence—possible symptom of urinary tract infection, impaction, chronic constipation, dementia, inability to walk and transfer by self to toilet, dehydration.

◆ 3. **Nursing goal/implementation:** *minimize incontinence episodes* and *reduce urinary tract infections.*

a. Regular toileting schedule—every 2 hr, with some exceptions at night; or personalize regimen based on assessment.

b. Modify environment—location of toilet, good lighting, prompt response to calls for assistance, use of Velcro closures on clothing, raised toilet seats with safety bars.

c. Monitor fluid intake; adequate hydration—1–2 L during day; *avoid* alcohol and caffeine and restrict fluids at bedtime.

d. *Avoid* medications contributing to incontinence.

e. *Avoid* use of indwelling catheters if possible.

f. Use usual undergarments; be positive about continence; use absorbent pads to improve perineal hygiene if other measures fail.

g. Treat constipation.

h. Observe for signs of UTI.

J. *Sexual neglect*—many myths exist about sexuality and aging.

1. *Facts* about sexuality in the older adult:

a. Sexual desire can and does exist in advanced age.

b. If in good health, a satisfying sex life can extend into the eighties and beyond; if sexually active in youth and middle age, vigor and interest will be retained into old age.

c. Sexual attractiveness has little to do with age and the appearance of partner.

d. Less than 1% of sudden coronary deaths occur during sexual intercourse; greater anxiety and tension exists if sex is restricted.

e. Vaginal lubrication is decreased because of menopause, but sexual pleasure still exists.

f. Sex may actually be better in later years; partners have an appreciation of intimate sharing and caring.

g. Sexual activity is a good form of exercise and helps maintain flexibility and stamina.

h. Older adults have a strong interest in sexual activity and physical and mental well-being; older adults should be encouraged to continue sexual interests without guilt.

i. Male erections can continue into the eighties and beyond.

◆ 2. **Nursing goal:** assist the client to *reduce barriers* to a satisfying sexual experience.

a. *Barriers* to a satisfying sexual experience:

(1) Loss of sexual responsiveness—*causes:* monotony of a "same old" sexual relationship; mental or physical fatigue; overindulgence in food or drink; preoccupation with career or economic pursuits; physical or mental infirmities of either partner; performance anxiety; lack of privacy.

(2) *Changes with aging*—hormonal; decreased muscle tone and elasticity; prostate hyperplasia; sclerosing arteries and veins; increased time needed for arousal and rearousal; medications (e.g., antihypertensives); surgery (e.g., prostatectomy); response to menopause; availability of a partner.

K. *Caregiver burden*—80%–90% of the care given to adults who are dependent is given by family and friends, especially middle-age women.

1. *Negative* consequences of caregiving:

a. Infringement on privacy.

b. Decreased social contact.

c. Loss of income and assets.

d. Increased family conflict and distress.

e. Little or no time for personal or recreational activities.

f. Increased use of alcohol and psychotropic drugs.

g. Changes in living arrangements (sharing households).

h. Likelihood of decreasing or giving up job responsibilities.

i. Increased risk of clinical depression.

j. Feelings of anger, guilt, anxiety, grief, depression, helplessness, chronic fatigue, emotional exhaustion.

k. Poor health and increased stress-related illness and injuries.

2. *Positive* consequences of caregiving:

a. Family becomes closer.

b. Making a difference in the quality of care.

c. Companionship for adult who is dependent and caregiver.

d. Better understanding of the needs of the adult who is dependent.

e. Feeling useful and worthwhile.

f. Improved relationship between caregiver and adult who is dependent.

3. Impact of hospitalization of older adult on caregiver:

a. Frustration with delays in older adult being admitted.

b. Perception of poor care; complaints about rudeness; upset that call lights and questions are not answered in a timely manner.

c. Lack of involvement in decision making.

d. Lack of preparation for discharge; too much information given too quickly; problems coordinating services (e.g., home visits, needed equipment).

e. Fatigue/stress from going back and forth to hospital.

◆ 4. **Nursing goal/implementation:** assist the caregiver in achieving control and a sense of satisfaction.

a. Strategies to minimize caregiver burden:

(1) Develop and maintain a routine.

(2) Concentrate on the present.

(3) Talk about the reasons for being a caregiver.

(4) Use respite care as needed.

L. *Poor nutrition.*

◆ 1. **Assessment** of warning signs:

a. Disease, illness, or chronic condition that changes eating habits/pattern; also emotional problems: confusion, depression, or sadness.

b. Eating too little or too much, skipping meals, drinking more than 1–2 alcoholic beverages daily.

c. Missing, loose, or rotten teeth, or ill-fitting dentures.

d. Spending less than 25–30 dollars per week on food.

e. Living alone.

f. Taking multiple medications with increased chance for side effects (change in taste, constipation, weakness, drowsiness, diarrhea, nausea).

g. Unplanned weight loss or gain.

h. Problems with self-care (walking, shopping, buying and preparing food).

i. Age >80 (frail elderly).

◆ 2. **Nursing goal:** promote optimal nutritional health for the older adult (see **Unit 9** for additional information on nutrition in the older adult).

◆ 3. **Nursing Implementation:**

a. Encourage fluids during meals.

b. 5–6 small meals/day.

TABLE 8.2	Most Frequent Issues in the Care of the Older Adult
Complication	**Cause**
Loss of functional independence	Immobility, lack of time to perform task, lack of expectations by staff or family
Falling	Postural hypotension, dizziness, medication effects, unfamiliar surroundings
Confusion	Drug effects, unfamiliar environment, sensory deficits
Skin breakdown	Immobility, skin changes with aging, inadequate turning
Incontinence	Cognitive changes, inability to access toilet, need for assistance, loss of sphincter muscle control
Constipation	Drug effects, inactivity, dietary changes, changes in GI motility
Heatstroke	Altered thermoregulation response
Hypothermia	Loss of subcutaneous tissue → decreased insulation
Self-injury	Reduced tactile sensation

Source: Cheryl Osborne, EdD, RN, Professor of Nursing, Director of Gerontology, California State University, Sacramento.

 c. Advise *not* to lie down for one hour after a meal.

d. *Avoid* overuse of salt and sweets.

e. Use alternate seasonings: herbs, garlic, lemon.

M. See **Unit 6** for discussion of *depression, elder abuse,* and causes of *impaired cognition,* such as dementia, Alzheimer's and delirium.

N. See **Unit 7** for discussion of *osteoarthritis* and *Parkinson's.*

IV. **Summary of most frequent issues in the care of the older adult** (Table 8.2).

V. Use the *functional rating scale for the older adult* to rate social resources, economic resources, mental health, physical health, and activities of daily living (**Table 8.3**).

VI. Use the *functional screening examination* to help determine dependent/independent status for planning home care (**Table 8.4**).

TABLE 0.3	Functional Rating Scale for the Older Adult

SOCIAL RESOURCES RATING SCALE

Rate the current social resources of the person being evaluated along the six-point scale presented below. Circle the *one* number that best describes the person's present circumstances.

1. **Excellent social resources.** Social relationships are *very* satisfying and extensive; at least one person would take care of him or her indefinitely.
2. **Good social resources.** Social relationships are *fairly* satisfying and adequate, and at least one person would take care of him or her indefinitely; *or* social relationships are *very satisfying* and *extensive*, and only short-term help is available.
3. **Mildly socially impaired.** Social relationships are *unsatisfactory*, of poor quality, few, but at least one person would take care of him or her indefinitely; *or* social relationships are *fairly* satisfactory, adequate, and only short-term help is available.
4. **Moderately socially impaired.** Social relationships are *unsatisfactory*, of poor quality; few, and only short-term care is available; *or* social relationships are at least adequate or satisfactory; but help would only be available now and then.
5. **Severely socially impaired.** Social relationships are of *poor* quality, few; and help would only be available *now* and *then*; *or* social relationships are at least satisfactory or adequate; but help is *not* even available now and then.
6. **Totally socially impaired.** Social relationships are *unsatisfactory*, of poor quality, few, and help is *not* even available now and then.

ECONOMIC RESOURCES RATING SCALE

Rate the current economic resources of the person being evaluated along the six-point scale presented below. Circle the *one* number that best describes the person's present circumstances.

1. **Economic resources are excellent.** Income is *ample* and person has reserves.
2. **Economic resources are satisfactory.** Income is ample but person has *no* reserves; *or* income is adequate and person has reserves.
3. **Economic resources are mildly impaired.** Income is adequate but person has *no* reserves; *or* income is somewhat *inadequate* but person has reserves.
4. **Economic resources are moderately impaired.** Income is *somewhat* inadequate and person has *no* reserves.
5. **Economic resources are severely impaired.** Income is *totally* inadequate and person *may* or *may not* have reserves.
6. **Economic resources are completely impaired.** Person is *destitute*, completely *without* income or reserves.

MENTAL HEALTH RATING SCALE

Rate the current mental functioning of the person being evaluated along the six-point scale presented below. Circle the *one* number that best describes the person's present functioning.

1. **Outstanding mental health.** Intellectually alert and clearly *enjoying* life. Manages routine and major problems with *ease* and is free from any psychiatric symptoms.
2. **Good mental health.** Handles both routine and major problems *satisfactorily* and is intellectually intact and free of psychiatric symptoms.
3. **Mildly mentally impaired.** Has *mild* psychiatric symptoms and/or mild intellectual impairment. Continues to handle routine, though **not major,** problems satisfactorily.
4. **Moderately mentally impaired.** Has *definite* psychiatric symptoms and/or *moderate* intellectual impairment. Able to make

routine commonsense decisions, but **unable** to handle major problems.
5. **Severely mentally impaired.** Has *severe* psychiatric symptoms and/or severe intellectual impairment that *interferes* with routine judgments and decision making in everyday life.
6. **Completely mentally impaired.** *Grossly* psychotic or *completely* impaired intellectually. Requires either intermittent or constant *supervision* because of clearly abnormal or potentially harmful behavior.

PHYSICAL HEALTH RATING SCALE

Rate the current physical functioning of the person being evaluated along the six-point scale presented below. Circle the *one* number that best describes the person's present functioning.

1. **In excellent physical health.** Engages in *vigorous* physical activity, either *regularly* or at least from time to time.
2. **In good physical health.** *No* significant illnesses or disabilities. Only *routine* medical care such as annual checkups required.
3. **Mildly physically impaired.** Has only *minor* illnesses and/or disabilities that might benefit from medical treatment or corrective measures.
4. **Moderately physically impaired.** Has *one or more* diseases or disabilities that are either *painful* or require *substantial medical treatment*.
5. **Severely physically impaired.** Has one or more illnesses or disabilities that are either *severely painful* or *life-threatening* or require *extensive* medical treatment.
6. **Totally physically impaired.** Confined to *bed* and requires *full-time* medical assistance or nursing care to maintain vital bodily functions.

PERFORMANCE RATING SCALE FOR ACTIVITIES OF DAILY LIVING (ADL)

Rate the current performance of the person being evaluated on the six-point scale presented below. Circle the *one* number that best describes the person's present performance.

1. **Excellent ADL capacity.** Can perform all ADL without assistance and with *ease*.
2. **Good ADL capacity.** Can perform all ADL *without assistance*.
3. **Mildly impaired ADL capacity.** Can perform *all but one to three* ADL. *Some* help is required with one to three, but not necessarily every day. Can get through any single day without help. Is able to prepare own meals.
4. **Moderately impaired ADL capacity.** *Regularly* requires assistance with *at least four ADL* but is able to get through any single day without help; *or regularly* requires help with meal preparation.
5. **Severely impaired ADL capacity.** Requires help *each day* but not necessarily throughout the day or night with *many* ADL.
6. **Completely impaired ADL capacity.** Requires help *throughout* the day and/or night to carry out ADL.

Summary of Ratings:		Projected Outcome
Social resources	_____	>15—Requires help
Economic resources	_____	12–15—Intermediate
Mental health	_____	supports
Physical health	_____	<11—Independent
Activities of daily living	_____	living
Cumulative impairment score (sum of the five ratings)		

Source: Adapted from University of California Davis Medical Center, Alzheimer's Center, Sacramento, Calif.

TABLE 8.4	Functional Screening Examination			
Test Request	**Function Tested**	**Able Normal**	**Limited but Able**	**Unable**
Put both hands together, behind your head	Shoulder external rotation, flexion, abduction; elbow flexion; wrist extension; gross strength (managing clothing, hair combing, washing back)	☐	☐	☐
Put both hands together, behind your back	Shoulder internal rotation, adduction; elbow flexion; gross strength (managing clothing, washing lower back)	☐	☐	☐
Sitting, touch great toe with opposite hand	Back, hip, knee flexion, gross strength, balance (lower extremity dressing and hygiene)	☐	☐	☐
Squeeze my two fingers, each hand	Grasp; approximately 20-lb grasp needed for functional activities (e.g., holding a pan)	☐	☐	☐
Hold paper between thumb and lateral side of index finger (while examiner tries to pull it out)	Pinch; approximately 3-lb grip needed for functional activities (e.g., turning a key)	☐	☐	☐
Show me your medicines	Cognition; knowledge; visual acuity, hand function; compliance; polypharmacy; effective management of health problems; access to health care; support system; finances; polyproviders	☐	☐	☐
Get up from the chair without using your hands, walk 10 ft down hall, turn around, stand with your eyes closed (examiner nudges to determine balance), sit down without using hands	Hip strength; gait, symmetry in posture velocity, step height; balance, ability to withstand sudden changes in position; fall risk; cardiovascular and pulmonary status; transfer ability; motion; fear of falls; judgment and cognition; environmental awareness; need for assistance/equipment; flexibility; endurance; ability to walk and function at home	☐	☐	☐
Take off your shoes and socks	Balance; fine motor skills; dexterity; hearing and receptive language; visual acuity; judgment; registration and attention span; low back flexibility and mobility; weight shifting; safety and adequacy of footware; social support if nails are cut by someone else; pain and comfort on movement	☐	☐	☐
Observe a meal being prepared/eaten	Nutritional intake; intactness of reflexes; use of utensils; hand/oral motor function; sequencing skills, visual acuity; use of utensils and equipment; ability to get needed help; ability to handle food and liquid; ability to compensate for limitations	☐	☐	☐

Summary and conclusions:

_____

_____

_____

_____

_____

_____

_____

_____

_____

Source: Dr. Cheryl Osborne, EdD, RN, Professor of Nursing, Director of Gerontology, California State University, Sacramento.
NOTE: *Totally independent*—total score of 9 in **Able** or **Limited** columns; *dependent* > 1 in **Unable** column.

Adults

Questions

Select the one answer that is best for each question, unless otherwise directed.

1. Which type of caregiver would describe a person who takes a neighbor to a medical appointment and periodically picks up a prescription at the pharmacy?
   1. Primary caregiver.
   2. Crisis caregiver.
   3. Occasional caregiver.
   4. Secondary caregiver.

2. The nurse's knowledge about caregivers in the U.S. guides development of a lesson plan for a caregiver class at the local senior center. What statement is inaccurate and should not be presented in the class?
   1. Caregiving in the U.S. occurs in 1 out of 10 households.
   2. Between 80% and 90% of the care given to older adults who are dependent in the community is given by family and friends.
   3. Caregiving in the U.S. occurs in 1 out of 4 households.
   4. Informal caregivers are unpaid.

3. Based on the primary cause for skin changes in older adults, the initial nursing assessment of an elderly client with dry skin would include:
   1. Presence of age spots.
   2. A diet history.
   3. History of prior sun exposure.
   4. Medications taken as a younger adult.

4. When reading a newspaper, the nurse would expect to see older adults with presbyopia hold the newspaper:
   1. Close to their face.
   2. In their lap.
   3. Directly under the light.
   4. At arm's distance from their face.

5. The nurse knows that elders often have difficulty reading because of an age-related decrease in tear production called "dry eye." The most appropriate intervention for "dry eye" is to:
   1. Encourage use of eye drops.
   2. Encourage reading indoors only.
   3. Empathize with them.
   4. Encourage them to get new eyeware.

6. When working with an elder Latino client who is recovering from a mild MI, the nurse discusses the need for exercise, while keeping in mind that:
   1. The family will encourage an exercise program.
   2. Exercise is seen as inappropriate for Latino elders.
   3. Latino elders usually exercise frequently.
   4. Latino elders usually look forward to physical activity.

7. Nursing interventions should be based on age groupings instead of the aggregate "65+ group." The nurse knows that certain risks can be expected in an 82-year-old. A client in this age group would be referred to as:
   1. An older American.
   2. A young-old American.
   3. A middle-old American.
   4. An old-old American.

8. In conducting a staff education conference on fall reduction for elders, which comment would be appropriate for the nurse to make?
   1. While exercise has been shown to reduce risk factors for falls, such as muscle weakness and abnormal gait, it has not been shown to reduce falls or injuries.
   2. Endurance exercise is generally preferable to strengthening exercise as a fall-reducing strategy.
   3. Balance exercises, such as tai chi, are more effective than endurance exercise as a fall-reducing strategy.
   4. It is important for most elderly persons to undergo cardiac stress testing before beginning an exercise program to prevent falls.

9. An 80-year-old man is admitted to the hospital with a vertebral compression fracture after lifting groceries from a table. Which condition is the most frequent cause of osteoporosis in the over-80 age group?
   1. Glucocorticoid use.
   2. Testosterone deficiency.
   3. Excessive alcohol use.
   4. Idiopathic osteoporosis.

10. Which disease(s) is/are common causes of hospital mortality following surgery for hip fracture in the older adult?
    Select all that apply.
    1. Pneumonia.
    2. Pulmonary embolism.
    3. Pressure ulcer.
    4. Acute delirium.
    5. Myocardial infarction.
    6. Diabetes.

11. The most common cause of falls for an older adult who lives independently is:
    1. Moderate to severe cognitive impairment.
    2. Multiple psychotropic medications.
    3. Tripping over everyday household objects.
    4. Attempting clearly hazardous activities.

12. Which statement(s) about falls in the older adult is/are true?
    Select all that apply.
    1. The majority of older adults fall in their home.
    2. Older adults tend to fall forward, injuring the hands and wrists.
    3. Approximately 10% of falls in the elderly result in serious soft tissue injury or fracture.
    4. Use of psychotropic medications (e.g., benzodiazepines or barbiturates) increases the risk of falls.
    5. Use of alcohol does not appear to increase the risk of falling.

13. When testing the sensory response of a 75-year-old client to dull or sharp objects, which finding would be considered normal? The client is:
    1. Able to identify location of touch correctly but not the type of sensation.
    2. Able to identify type of sensation correctly but not the location.
    3. Able to identify both type and location correctly, but the response is slow.
    4. Unable to identify sensation in any area.

14. The greatest reduction in falls and improved safety for the elderly client with Parkinson's disease would occur with:
    1. Discouraging the client from wearing slippers.
    2. Buying shoes that fit snugly.
    3. Raising the height of toilet seats.
    4. Client holding hands behind back when walking.

Answers/Rationales/Tips

1. **(3)** Occasional caregivers are responsible for infrequent, episodic care. **Answer 1** is incorrect because it refers to the caregiver who is formally identified as the person involved in *managing* the client's care. **Answer 2** is incorrect because it refers to a caregiver who steps into the role when others are not there for a *specific* event. **Answer 4** is incorrect because it refers to the person who is identified as a caregiver if the primary person is *not available* or provides *indirect* care (i.e., financial assistance or respite care for the primary caregiver).

> **TEST-TAKING TIP**—Focus on the word "periodically" = "occasional."
> **AS, COM, 5, M/S: Geriatrics, SECE, Management of Care**

2. **(1)** It is an inaccurate statement. Currently the number of households is 1 out of 4. **Answer 2** is incorrect because it *is* an *accurate* statement according to the current Family Alliance Caregiving and census data. **Answer 3** is incorrect because it *is* an *accurate* statement according to the current Family Alliance Caregiving and census data. **Answer 4** is incorrect according to Family Alliance Caregiving and census data. Formal caregivers *are* paid.

> **TEST-TAKING TIP**—Key concept is "inappropriate/incorrect."
> **IMP, COM, 5, M/S: Geriatrics, HPM, Health Promotion and Maintenance**

3. **(3)** Dry skin is primarily caused by sun exposure experienced during earlier years. **Answer 1** is incorrect because age spots are normal skin changes and not a cause of dry skin. **Answer 2** is incorrect because, although there are dietary effects on skin health, this is not the primary cause of dryness. **Answer 4** is incorrect because although medications are known to affect skin elasticity and sensitivity in older years, the effects of medications taken in earlier years have not been verified.

> **TEST-TAKING TIP**—The question asks for cause of skin change. Is it sun? diet? or meds?
> **AS, COM, 1, M/S: Geriatrics, PhI, Basic Care and Comfort**

4. **(4)** Presbyopia (farsightedness) begins around 40 years and is considered an age-related change in the eye. **Answer 1** is incorrect because this is what someone would do who was nearsighted, not farsighted. **Answer 2** is incorrect because this is how someone might read who was neither near nor farsighted. **Answer 3** is incorrect because this addresses the *amount* of light needed to read, not distance.

> **TEST-TAKING TIP**—Note two contradictory options: close vs far. Picture individuals you know who are elders and how they hold books when reading.
> **AS, COM, 2, M/S: Geriatrics, HPM, Health Promotion and Maintenance**

5. **(1)** A primary symptom and discomfort of "dry eye" is dryness. Eye drops with saline restore and lubricate the eye, and reduce itchiness. **Answer 2** is incorrect because although "dry eye" commonly results in photosensitivity, elders *can* still read outside if they protect their eyes with lubrication and use amber or yellow lenses. **Answer 3** is incorrect because although empathy is a supportive approach, most elders *are* able to continue reading with the use of lubrication. **Answer 4** is incorrect because the condition has already been diagnosed and new glasses will not improve vision.

> 💡 **TEST-TAKING TIP**—Choose a KIS answer! If the eye is *dry*, use *drops*.
> **IMP, APP, 2, M/S: Geriatrics, PhI, Basic Care and Comfort**

KEY TO CODES FOLLOWING RATIONALES:

Nursing process: **AS**, assessment; **AN**, analysis; **PL**, plan; **IMP**, implementation; **EV**, evaluation. *Cognitive level:* **COM**, comprehension; **APP**, application; **ANL**, analysis. *Category of human function:* **1**, protective; **2**, sensory-perceptual; **3**, comfort, rest, activity, and mobility; **4**, nutrition; **5**, growth and development; **6**, fluid-gas transport; **7**, psychosocial-cultural; **8**, elimination. *Client need:* **SECE**, safe, effective care environment; **HPM**, health promotion/maintenance; **PsI**, psychosocial integrity; **PhI**, physiological integrity. (Client subneed appears after Client need code.) See appendices for full explanation.

6. **(2)** The Latino culture does not expect this of their elders. The nurse must therefore focus on the elder and how to encourage the client to do something that may be unusual to do. **Answer 1** is incorrect because the Latino culture does not view exercise as necessary, expected or indicated for their elder population. **Answer 3** is incorrect because the Latino culture does not value exercise for elders. **Answer 4** is incorrect because the Latino culture does not promote exercise in the elder.

> **TEST-TAKING TIP**—Review various cultural beliefs as they relate to health promotion. Select the answer that is different here: 3 are "pro" exercise and 1 is not.
> **IMP, COM, 3, M/S: Cultural Diversity, HPM, Health Promotion and Maintenance**

7. **(3)** A middle-old individual is one between the ages of 75 and 84. **Answer 1** is incorrect because this term is not specific to sub groupings but rather the general 65+ aggregate cohort. **Answer 2** is incorrect because a "young-old" individual is one between the ages of 65 and 74. **Answer 4** is incorrect because an "old-old" individual is one who is 85+ years old.

> **TEST-TAKING TIP**—Memorize year breakdowns to refer to the specific subpopulation and to know what to commonly expect from elders' response to such conditions as chronic diseases, medication reactions, fall prevention, caregiving needs etc.
> **AS, COM, 5, M/S: Geriatrics, HPM, Health Promotion and Maintenance**

8. **(3)** Balance and instability are major causes of falls. An exercise which will improve balance will reduce the incidence of falling. **Answer 1** is incorrect because *certain* types of exercise *will* actually reduce falling, not just improve the risk factors associated with falling. **Answer 2** is incorrect because balance, *not* endurance, is a reason that an older adult may fall. **Answer 4** is incorrect because the type of exercise which will reduce falling is not likely to stress the heart.

> **TEST-TAKING TIP**—Think about why someone falls, besides tripping: you lose your balance.
> **IMP, COM, 3, M/S: Geriatrics, PhI, Basic Care and Comfort**

9. **(4)** The cause of osteoporosis would be considered idiopathic in an 80-year-old man, unlike in a woman following menopause. **Answer 1** is incorrect because glucocorticoids are *not* associated with demineralization of the bone. Muscle wasting would be more common. **Answer 2** is incorrect because osteoporosis is associated with changes in estrogen levels. **Answer 3** is incorrect because excessive alcohol has organic effects, such as cirrhosis, *not* bone demineralization.

> **TEST-TAKING TIP**—The condition seems atypical—idiopathic means the cause is unknown.
> **AS, COM, 3, M/S: Geriatrics, HPM, Health Promotion and Maintenance**

10. **(1, 2, 5, 6)** **Answer 1** is correct because immobility and pain following hip fracture predispose the older adult to pneumonia. **Answer 2** is correct because immobility predisposes the older adult to DVT and possibly pulmonary embolism. **Answer 5** is correct because general anesthesia and surgery are physiologically stressful for older adults who are surgical risks. Cardiac function is reduced with aging and may be challenged by the surgical procedure. **Answer 6** is correct because the stress of surgery may result in a glucose imbalance and therefore a greater risk of ketoacidosis and diabetic coma. **Answer 3** is incorrect because pressure ulcers, while a greater problem in the older adult, are *not* a factor in mortality. **Answer 4** is incorrect because acute delirium is *not*

common postoperatively and would *not* result in death. Confusion, particularly from the effects of anesthesia, would be more likely.

> **TEST-TAKING TIP**—Think about the potential risk of dying for each condition.
> **AN, APP, 1, M/S: Geriatrics, PhI, Reduction of Risk Potential**

11. **(3)** Tripping on furniture, area rugs, and pets are more common causes of falls. **Answer 1** is incorrect because an older adult with severe mental impairment would not be living independently. **Answer 2** is incorrect because older adults are not commonly on multiple psychotropic drugs. **Answer 4** is incorrect because most older adults are cautious and do not commonly perform unsafe tasks.

> **TEST-TAKING TIP**—The question asks for a "common" cause—household hazards would be a risk to all older adults.
> **AN, COM, 1, M/S: Geriatrics, SECE, Safety and Infection Control**

12. **(1, 3, 4)** **Answer 1** is correct because older adults living independently are more likely to fall at home—tripping over a household item. **Answer 3** is correct because the percentage of serious injury or fracture is fortunately only 10%. A hip fracture can result in a loss of independence and even death. **Answer 4** is correct because psychotropic drugs can cause dizziness or affect balance and gait. **Answer 2** is incorrect because older adults tend to fall *back,* landing on their hip or sacrum. **Answer 5** is incorrect because alcohol *does* appear to increase the risk of falling in any age.

> **TEST-TAKING TIP**—Consider how plausible each statement is—true or false.
> **AS, COM, 3, M/S: Geriatrics, PhI, Reduction of Risk Potential**

13. **(3)** The speed (velocity) of nerve impulses decreases with aging, making responses slower. The amount of change varies with individuals, so a *specific* change according to age is *not predictable* (**Answers 1** and **2**). Sensory conduction decreases faster over time compared with motor conduction; some areas are less sensitive (ankle malleolus), but the change is not generalized throughout the body (**Answer 4**).

> **TEST-TAKING TIP**—The key word in the stem is "normal," and the correct choice must apply to all older adults. Choose the most inclusive answer: **Answer 3** includes **Answers 1** and **2**.
> **AS, ANL, 2, M/S: Geriatrics, Sens.-Percep., HPM, Health Promotion and Maintenance**

14. **(3)** Most falls in the elderly, including those with Parkinson's disease, occur in the bathroom. There is a loss of muscle strength in legs with normal aging. Combined with muscle rigidity and postural instability in Parkinson's, the risk for falls is great. **Answers 1** and **2,** *as stated,* are not the most important ways to reduce falls. *Nonskid* soles and proper fit (not necessarily snug) are safety concerns. **Answer 4** improves posture, not necessarily reducing the risk for falling.

> **TEST-TAKING TIP**—*Visualize* each option and how *stability* would be improved.
> **IMP, APP, 3, M/S: Geriatrics, NM, PhI, Basic Care and Comfort**

Review of Nutrition🍽

Sally L. Lagerquist • Janice McMillin • Robyn Nelson • Kathleen Snider

NUTRITION DURING PREGNANCY AND LACTATION

Table 9.1 gives a summary of nutrient needs (maternal and fetal) during pregnancy.

I. **Milk group**—important for calcium, protein of high biological value, and other vitamins and minerals.
   A. *Pregnancy*—three to four servings (four to five for adolescents).
   B. *Lactation*—four to five servings.
   C. *Count as one serving*—1 cup milk; ½ cup undiluted evaporated milk; ¼ cup dry milk; 1¼ cups cottage cheese; 2 cups low fat cottage cheese; 1½ oz cheddar or Swiss cheese; or 1½ cups ice cream.

II. **Meat, poultry, fish, dry beans, nuts, and eggs group—important for protein, iron, and many B vitamins.**
   A. *Pregnancy*—three servings.
   B. *Lactation*—three servings.
   C. *Count as one serving*—½ cup cooked dry beans, 1 egg, or 1½ tbsp peanut butter is equivalent to 1 oz meat; use peanut butter or nuts rarely to *avoid* excessive fat intake; limit eggs to reduce cholesterol intake; trim fat from meat, and remove skin from poultry.

III. **Vegetable and fruit group—vitamins and minerals (especially vitamins A and C) and roughage.**
   A. *Vegetables:*
      1. *Pregnancy*—three to four servings.
      2. *Lactation*—three to five servings.
      3. *Count as one serving*—1 cup raw leafy greens, ½ cup of others.
   B. *Fruits:*
      1. *Pregnancy*—two to four servings.
      2. *Lactation*—two to four servings.
      3. *Count as one serving*—½ medium grapefruit; 1 medium apple, banana, or orange; ¾ cup fruit juice.
   C. *Good sources (vitamin C)*—citrus, cantaloupe, mango, papaya, strawberries, broccoli, and green and red bell peppers.
   D. *Fair sources (vitamin C)*—tomatoes, honeydew melon, asparagus tips, raw cabbage, collards, kale, mustard greens, potatoes (white and sweet), spinach, and turnip greens.
   E. *Good sources (vitamin A)*—dark-green or deep-yellow vegetables and a few fruits (apricots, broccoli, pumpkin, sweet potato, spinach, cantaloupe, carrots, and winter squash).
   F. *Good sources of folic acid*—dark-green *foliage*-type vegetables.

IV. **Bread and cereal group—good for thiamine, iron, niacin, and other vitamins and minerals.**
   A. *Pregnancy*—6 to 11 servings.
   B. *Lactation*—6 to 11 servings.
   C. *Count as one serving*—1 slice bread, 1 oz ready-to-eat cereal, ½–¾ cup cooked cereal, cornmeal, grits, macaroni, noodles, rice, or spaghetti.

V. **Note:** use dark-green leafy and deep-yellow vegetables often; eat dry beans and peas often; count ½ cup cooked dry beans or peas as a serving of vegetables or 1 oz from meat group.

NUTRITIONAL NEEDS OF THE NEWBORN

I. **Calories**—108 kcal/kg/day.

II. **Protein**—2.2 g/kg/day (1 g protein = 1 oz milk).

III. **Fluids**—3.5 oz/kg/day.

IV. **Vitamin D**—400 IU daily for infants who are bottle-fed after week 2.

V. **Fluoride**—0.25 mg daily up to 3 years old when local water supply has less than 0.3 ppm content.

DIETARY REFERENCE INTAKES

Table 9.2

TABLE 9.1	Nutrient Needs During Pregnancy		
Nutrient	**Maternal Need**	**Fetal Need**	**Food Source**
Protein—75 g/day	Maternal tissue growth: uterus, breasts, blood volume, storage	Rapid fetal growth	Milk and milk products; animal meats—muscle, organs; grains, legumes; eggs
Calories—2500/day	Increased BMR	Primary energy source for growth of fetus	Carbohydrates: 4 kcal/g Proteins: 4 kcal/g Fats: 9 kcal/g
Minerals—1200 mg/day (*Calcium* and *phosphorus*)	Increase in maternal Ca^{2+} metabolism	Skeleton and tooth formation	Milk and milk products, especially natural cheese*
Iron—30 mg/day	Increase in RBC mass Prevent anemia Decrease infection risk	Liver storage (especially in third trimester)	Organ meats—liver, animal meat; egg yolk; whole or enriched grains; green leafy vegetables; nuts
Vitamins			
A	Tissue growth	Cell development—tissue and bone growth and tooth bud formation	Butter, cream, fortified margarine; green and yellow vegetables
B	Coenzyme in many metabolic processes	Coenzyme in many metabolic processes	Animal meats, organ meats; milk and cheese; beans, peas, nuts; enriched grains
Folic acid	Meet increased metabolic demands in pregnancy Production of blood products	Meet increased metabolic demands, including production of cell nucleus material Prevent neural tube defects	Liver; deep-green, leafy vegetables; asparagus; avocado
C	Tissue formation and integrity Increase iron absorption	Tissue formation and integrity	Citrus fruits, berries, melons, papaya, kiwi, strawberries; peppers; green, leafy vegetables; broccoli, brussels sprouts, snow pea pods; potatoes
D	Absorption of Ca^{2+}, phosphorus	Mineralization of bone tissue and tooth buds	Fortified milk and margarine
E	Tissue growth; cell wall integrity; RBC integrity	Tissue growth; cell integrity; RBC integrity	Widely distributed: meat, milk, eggs, grains, leafy vegetables, vegetable oils

*Natural cheese contains less lactose; therefore it is a good source for those with lactose intolerance. Tofu (soybean cake) also is high in calcium and contain *no* lactose.

ETHNIC FOOD PATTERNS

Table 9.3 and **Table 9.4**

COMMON VITAMINS AND RELATED DEFICIENCIES

Table 9.5

NUTRITIONAL NEEDS OF THE OLDER ADULT

I. *Calories*—1500–2000 kcal/day to maintain ideal weight; 12% of calories from protein sources; 50%–60% of calories from carbohydrates; 20%–30% of calories from fats.

II. *High fiber*—prevent or alleviate constipation and dependence on laxatives.

III. *Sodium*—3–4 g/day according to cardiac and renal status.

IV. *Fats*—limit to help retard the development of cancer, atherosclerosis, obesity, and other diseases.

V. *Fluids*—6–8 glasses/day.

VI. *Common deficiencies:* calories; calcium; folic acid; iron; thiamine; vitamins A, B_{12}, C, and D; niacin; zinc.

VII. **Factors contributing to food preferences:**
   A. Physical ability to prepare, shop for, and eat food.
   B. Income.
   C. Availability of food if dependent on others.
   D. Food intolerances.

VIII. **Table 9.6 provides interventions for common eating problems in the older adult.**

TABLE 9.2 — Change from Recommended Dietary Allowances (RDA) to Dietary Reference Intakes (DRI)

1989 Recommended Dietary Allowances (RDA)

Age (yrs)	Iron (mg)	Zinc (mg)	Iodine (µg)	Selenium (µg)	Protein (g)	Vitamin A (µg RE)	Vitamin E (mg α-TE)	Vitamin K (µg)	Vitamin C (mg)	Energy (kcal)
Infants										
0.0–0.5	6	5	40	10	13	375	3	5	30	650
0.5–1.0	10	5	50	15	14	375	4	10	35	850
Children										
1–3	10	10	70	20	16	400	6	15	40	1300
4–6	10	10	90	20	24	500	7	20	45	1800
7–10	10	10	120	30	28	700	7	30	45	2000
Boys/Men										
11–14	12	15	150	40	45	1000	10	45	50	2500
15–18	12	15	150	50	59	1000	10	65	60	3300
19–24	10	15	150	70	58	1000	10	70	60	2900
25–50	10	15	150	70	63	1000	10	80	60	2900
51+	10	15	150	70	63	1000	10	80	60	2300
Girls/Women										
11–14	15	12	150	45	46	800	8	45	50	2200
15–18	15	12	150	50	44	800	8	55	60	2200
19–24	15	12	150	55	46	800	8	60	60	2200
25–50	15	12	150	55	50	800	8	65	60	2200
51+	10	12	150	55	50	800	8	65	60	1900
Pregnant	30	15	175	65	60	800	10	65	70	+300
Lactating										
1st 6 mos	15	19	200	75	65	1300	12	65	95	+500
2nd 6 mos	15	16	200	75	62	1200	11	65	90	+500

1997–1998 Dietary Reference Intakes (DRI)

Recommended Dietary Allowances (RDA) and Adequate Intakes (AI)

Age (yrs)	Phosphorus (mg)	Magnesium (mg)	Thiamin (mg)	Riboflavin (mg)	Niacin (mg NE)	Vitamin B6 (mg)	Folate (µg)	Vitamin B12 (µg)	Calcium (mg)	Vitamin D (µg)	Pantothenic Acid (mg)	Biotin (µg)	Choline (mg)	Fluoride (mg)
Infants														
0.0–0.5	100	30	0.2	0.3	2	0.1	65	0.4	210	5	1.7	5	125	0.01
0.5–1.0	275	75	0.3	0.4	4	0.3	80	0.5	270	5	1.8	6	150	0.5
Children														
1–3	460	80	0.5	0.5	6	0.6	150	0.9	500	5	2.0	8	200	0.7
4–8	500	130	0.6	0.6	8	0.6	200	1.2	800	5	3.0	12	250	1.1
Boys/Men														
9–13	1250	240	0.9	0.9	12	1.0	300	1.8	1300	5	4.0	20	375	2.0
14–18	1250	410	1.2	1.3	16	1.3	400	2.4	1300	5	5.0	25	550	3.2
19–30	700	400	1.2	1.3	16	1.3	400	2.4	1000	5	5.0	30	550	3.8
31–50	700	420	1.2	1.3	16	1.3	400	2.4	1000	5	5.0	30	550	3.8
51–70	700	420	1.2	1.3	16	1.7	400	2.4	1200	10	5.0	30	550	3.8
>70	700	420	1.2	1.3	16	1.7	400	2.4	1200	15	5.0	30	550	3.8
Girls/Women														
9–13	1250	240	0.9	0.9	12	1.0	300	1.8	1300	5	4.0	20	375	2.0
14–18	1250	360	1.0	1.0	14	1.2	400	2.4	1300	5	5.0	25	400	2.9
19–30	700	310	1.1	1.1	14	1.3	400	2.4	1000	5	5.0	30	425	3.1
31–50	700	320	1.1	1.1	14	1.3	400	2.4	1000	5	5.0	30	425	3.1
51–70	700	320	1.1	1.1	14	1.5	400	2.4	1200	10	5.0	30	425	3.1
>70	700	320	1.1	1.1	14	1.5	400	2.4	1200	15	5.0	30	425	3.1
Pregnant	*	+40	1.4	1.4	18	1.9	600	2.6	*	*	6.0	30	450	*
Lactating	*	*	1.5	1.6	17	2.0	500	2.8	*	*	7.0	35	550	*

The DRIs are actually a set of four reference values: Estimated Average Requirements (EAR), Recommended Dietary Allowances (RDA), Adequate Intakes (AI), and Tolerable Upper Intake Levels (UL), that have replaced the 1989 Recommended Dietary Allowances (RDAs)

*Use value for women of comparable age.

National Agricultural Library (NAL). Retrieved March 2004 from http://www.nal.usda.gov.

TABLE 9.3	Ethnic Food Patterns	
Ethnic Group	**Cultural Food Patterns**	**Dietary Excesses or Omissions**
Mexican (native)	Basic sources of protein—dried beans, flan, cheese, many meats, fish, eggs Chili peppers and many deep-green and yellow vegetables Fruits include: zapote, guava, papaya, mango, citrus Tortillas (corn, flour); sweet bread; fideo; tacos, burritos, enchiladas	*Limited* meats, milk, and milk products Some are using flour tortillas more than the more nutritious corn tortillas *Excessive* use of lard (manteca), sugar Tendency to boil vegetables for long periods of time
Filipino (Spanish-Chinese influence)	Most meats, eggs, nuts, legumes Many different kinds of vegetables Large amounts of rice and cereals	May *limit* meat, milk, and milk products (the latter may be due to **lactose intolerance**) Tend to prewash rice Tend to fry many foods
Chinese (mostly Cantonese)	Cheese, soybean curd (tofu), many meats, chicken and pigeon eggs, nuts, legumes Many different vegetables, leaves, bamboo sprouts Rice and rice-flour products; wheat, corn, millet seed; green tea Mixtures of fish, pork, and chicken with vegetables—bamboo shoots, broccoli, cabbage, onions, mushrooms, pea pods	Tendency among some immigrants to use *excess* grease in cooking. May be *low* in protein, milk, and milk products (the latter may be due to **lactose intolerance**) Often wash rice before cooking **Large** amounts of soy and oyster sauces, both of which are *high in salt;* MSG (monosodium glutamate)
Puerto Rican	Milk with coffee Pork, poultry, eggs, dried fish; beans (habichuelas) Viandas (starchy vegetables; starchy ripe fruits) Avocados, okra, eggplant, sweet yams Rice, cornmeal	Use *large* amounts of lard for cooking *Limited* use of milk and milk products *Limited* amounts of pork and poultry
African American	Milk with coffee Pork, poultry, eggs *Fruit:* strawberries, watermelon *Vegetables:* turnip, collard, mustard greens; kale, okra, sweet potatoes Cereals (including grits, hominy, cornbread, hot breads) Molasses (dark molasses is especially good source of calcium, iron, vitamins B_1 and B_2, and niacin)	*Limited* use of milk group (**lactose intolerance**) Extensive use of frying, "smothering," simmering for cooking *Large* amounts of fat: salt pork, bacon drippings, lard, gravies May have *limited* use of citrus and enriched breads
Middle Eastern (Greek, Syrian, Armenian)	Yogurt Predominantly lamb, nuts, dried peas, beans, lentils Deep-green leaves and vegetables; dried fruits Dark breads and cracked wheat	Tend to use *excessive* sweeteners, lamb fat, olive oil Tend to fry meats and vegetables *Insufficient* milk and milk products (almost no butter—use olive oil, which has no nutritive value except for calories) *Deficiency* in fresh fruits
Middle European (Polish)	Many milk products Pork, chicken Root vegetables (potatoes), cabbage, fruits Wheat products Sausages, smoked and cured meats, noodles, dumplings, bread, cream with coffee	Tend to use *excessive* sweets and to overcook vegetables *Limited* amounts of fruits (citrus), raw vegetables, and meats
Native American (American Indian—much variation)	If "Americanized," use milk and milk products Variety of meats: game, fowl, fish; nuts, seeds, legumes Variety of vegetables, some wild Variety of fruits, some wild, rose hips; roots Variety of breads, including tortillas, cornmeal, rice	*Nutrition-related problems:* obesity, diabetes, dental problems, iron deficiency anemia; alcoholism *Limited* quantities of high protein foods depending on availability (flocks of game, fowl) and economic situation *Excessive* use of sugar
Italian	Staples are pasta with sauces; bread; eggs; cheese; tomatoes; and vegetables such as artichokes, eggplant, greens, and zucchini Only small amount of meat is used	*Limited* use of whole grains *Insufficient* servings from milk group Tendency to overcook vegetables Enjoy sweets

TABLE 9.4	Hot-Cold Theory of Disease Treatment*				
Hot Diseases or Conditions	**Cold Diseases or Conditions**	**Hot Foods**	**Cold Foods**	**Hot Medicines and Herbs**	**Cold Medicines and Herbs**
Constipation Diarrhea Infections Kidney diseases Liver complaints Skin eruptions Throat (sore) Ulcers Warts	Cancer Common cold Earache Headache Joint pain Malaria Menstrual period Paralysis Pneumonia Rheumatism Stomach cramps Teething Tuberculosis	Beverages, aromatic Cereal grains Cheese Chili peppers Chocolate Coffee Eggs Fruits, temperate zone Goat milk Hard liquor Meats (beef, water fowl, mutton) Oils Onions Peas	Barley water Cod Dairy products Fruits, tropical Honey Meats (goat, fish, chicken) Milk, bottled Raisins Vegetables, fresh	Anise Aspirin Castor oil Cinnamon Cod liver oil Garlic Ginger root Iron preparations Mint Penicillin Tobacco Vitamins	Bicarbonate of soda Linden Milk of magnesia Orange flower water Sage

Adapted from Wilson, HS, and Kneisl, CR: Psychiatric Nursing, ed. 2. Addison-Wesley, Menlo Park, CA (out of print)
*A Latin American, particularly Puerto Rican, approach to treating diseases. A "hot" disease is treated with "cold" treatments (foods, medicines) and vice versa.

TABLE 9.5	Physiological Functions and Deficiency Syndromes of Common Vitamins			
Vitamin	**Chief Functions**	**Results of Deficiency**	**Characteristics**	**Good Sources**
Vitamin A				

Retinol (animal source)
Carotene
Beta carotene
	Essential for maintaining the integrity of epithelial membranes
	Helps maintain resistance to infections
	Necessary for the formation of rhodopsin and prevention of night blindness
	Necessary for proper bone growth
	Facilitates RNA formation from DNA
	Thought to be cancer preventive because of antioxidant properties associated with control of free radical damage to DNA and cell membranes
		Mild:
		Retarded growth
		Increased susceptibility to infection
		Abnormal function of gastrointestinal, genitourinary, and respiratory tracts due to altered epithelial membranes
		Skin dries, shrivels, thickens; sometimes pustule formation
		Night blindness
		Severe:
		Xerophthalmia, a characteristic eye disease, and other local infections
			Fat soluble*
			Not destroyed by ordinary cooking temperatures
			Is destroyed by high temperatures when oxygen is present
			Marked capacity for storage in the liver
			NOTE: Excessive intake of carotene, from which vitamin A is formed, may produce yellow discoloration of the skin *(carotenemia)*; excessive vitamin A intake causes symptoms similar to those of deficiency conditions
				Liver
				Animal fats:
				  Butter
				  Cheese
				  Cream
				  Egg yolk
				  Whole milk
				Fish liver oil
				Liver
				Vegetables:
				  Green leafy, especially escarole, kale, parsley
				  Yellow, especially carrots
				Artificial:
				Concentrates in several forms
				Irradiated fish oils

Vitamin D				
Calciferol Ergocalciferol	Hormone-like regulation of calcium and phosphorus metabolism by promotion of: Gastrointestinal absorption	*Mild:* Interferes with utilization of calcium and phosphorus in bone and tooth formation	Soluble in fats and organic solvents* Relatively stable under refrigeration	Formed in the skin by exposure to sunlight Fortified milk and dairy products

(Continued on following page)

TABLE 9.5 Physiological Functions and Deficiency Syndromes of Common Vitamins *(Continued)*

Vitamin	Chief Functions	Results of Deficiency	Characteristics	Good Sources
Vitamin D—*Cont'd* Cholecalciferol Calcitriol Antirachitic factor	Bone and tooth mineral-ization Renal reabsorption Skeletal reserves Antirachitic	Irritability Weakness *Severe:* Rickets in young children Osteomalacia in adults	Stored in liver Often associated with vitamin A	Egg yolk Fish liver oils Fish having fat distributed through the flesh, salmon, tuna, herring sardines Liver Oysters Artifically prepared forms
Vitamin E Alpha-tocopherol Beta-tocopherol Gamma-tocopherol	Important antioxidant that: Prevents red blood cell hemolysis Protects vitamin A and unsaturated fatty acids from oxidation Promotes cell membrane integrity Improves immune response May protect against cancer	Red blood cell resistance to rupture is decreased, but deficiency seldom occurs except in *premature* infants and people with *chronic fat malabsorption*	Soluble in fat* Stable to heat in absence of oxygen and ultraviolet light Unstable under freez-ing and processing	Vegetable oils Margarine Whole grain or forti-fied cereals Wheat germ Green leafy vegetables
Vitamin K Menadione Phylloquinone Menaquinone	Promotes synthesis of clotting factors	Prolonged clotting time, resulting in bleeding **NOTE:** Seldom occurs in the absence of anticoagu-lant drugs; in addition to food sources, intestinal bacteria manufacture approximately half the body's requirement Fat malabsorption can cause deficiency Synthetic form (menadione) does not depend on fat absorption	Soluble in fat* Stable to heat	Green leafy vegetables Meats Dairy products Intestinal bacteria
Vitamin C Ascorbic acid	Essential to formation of intracellular cement substances in a variety of tissues including skin, dentin, cartilage, and bone matrix Important in healing of wounds and bone frac-tures Prevents scurvy Facilitates absorption of iron Protects folate Antioxidant Promotes capillary permeability	*Mild:* Lowered resistance to infec-tions Joint tenderness Susceptibility to dental caries, pyorrhea, and bleeding gums Delayed wound healing Bruising *Severe:* Hemorrhage Anemia Scurvy **NOTE:** Many drugs affect availability	Soluble in water Easily destroyed by oxidation; heat hastens the process Lost in cooking, particularly if water in which food was cooked is discarded; loss is greater if cooked in iron or copper utensils Quick-frozen foods lose little of their vitamin C Stored in the body to a limited extent	Abundant in most fresh fruits and vegetables, espe-cially citrus fruit and juices, tomato and orange *Artificial:* Ascorbic acid Cevitamic acid

(Continued on following page)

Vitamin	Chief Functions	Results of Deficiency	Characteristics	Good Sources
Thiamine Vitamin B_1	Important role in carbohydrate metabolism Essential for maintenance of normal appetite Essential for normal functioning of nervous tissue Coenzyme for cellular energy production	*Mild:* Loss of appetite Impaired metabolism of starches and sugars Emaciation Irritability *Severe:* Various nervous disorders Loss of coordinating power of muscles Beriberi Paralysis in humans	Soluble in water Not readily destroyed by ordinary cooking temperatures Destroyed by exposure to heat, alkali, or sulfites Not stored in body **NOTE:** Deficiency is often associated with alcoholism	Widely distributed in plant and animal tissues but seldom occurs in high concentration, except in brewer's yeast Enriched or whole grain cereals Pork Peas, beans Nuts *Artificial:* Concentrates from yeast Rice polishings Wheat germ
Riboflavin Vitamin B_2	Important as coenzyme in cellular oxidation Essential to normal growth Participates in light adaptation Vital to protein metabolism Associated with niacin and vitamin B_6 functions	Impaired growth Lassitude and weakness Cheilosis Glossitis Dermatitis Anemia Photophobia Cataracts	Water soluble Alcohol soluble Not destroyed by heat in cooking unless with alkali Unstable in light, especially in presence of alkali	Milk and milk products Enriched foods Whole grain breads and cereals Liver Meats Eggs
Niacin Nicotinic acid Nicotinamide Antipellagra vitamin	As the component of two important enzymes, it is important in glycolysis, tissue respiration, fat synthesis, and cellular energy production Nicotine acid, but not nicotinamide, causes vasodilation and flushing Prevents pellagra	Pellagra Gastrointestinal disturbances Mental disturbances **NOTE:** Associated with alcoholism	Soluble in hot water and alcohol Not destroyed by heat, light, air, or alkali Not destroyed in ordinary cooking	Milk Eggs Meats Legumes Enriched foods Whole grain cereals Nuts **NOTE:** Also formed in the body from dietary tryptophan (amino acid)
Vitamin B_6 Pyridoxine Pyridoxal Pyridoxamine	Used in hemoglobin synthesis Essential for metabolism of tryptophan to niacin Needed for utilization of certain other amino acids	Anemias Depressed immunity Dermatitis around eyes and mouth Neuritis Anorexia, nausea, and vomiting	Soluble in water and alcohol Rapidly inactivated in presence of heat, sunlight, or air	Meats Cereal grains Some fruits Nuts
Folate Folacin Folic acid	Essential for normal functioning of hematopoietic system Important coenzyme for RNA and DNA synthesis Important in fetal development Functions interrelated with those of vitamin B_{12}	Anemia **NOTE:** Neural tube defects (e.g., *spina bifida*) are associated with maternal deficiency; alcohol and contraceptives interfere with absorption	Slightly soluble in water Easily destroyed by heat in presence of acid Decreases when food is stored at room temperature **NOTE:** A large dose may prevent appearance of anemia in a case of pernicious anemia but still permit neurological symptoms to develop	Liver Eggs Fish Green leafy vegetables Asparagus Peas, beans, legumes Nuts, seeds, wheat germ Avocado Some fruits

(Continued on following page)

TABLE 9.5	Physiological Functions and Deficiency Syndromes of Common Vitamins *(Continued)*			
Vitamin	**Chief Functions**	**Results of Deficiency**	**Characteristics**	**Good Sources**
Vitamin B$_{12}$				
Cyanocobalamin Hydroxycobalamin	Necessary for myelin synthesis Essential for normal development of red blood cells Associated with folate metabolism	Pernicious anemia Neurological disorders	Soluble in water or alcohol Unstable in hot alkaline or acid solutions	Found only in animal products (e.g., meats, eggs, dairy products) Most of vitamin B$_{12}$ required by humans is synthesized by intestinal bacteria; can also be recycled

*Vitamins A, D, E, and K are available in water soluble forms and are used in children with cystic fibrosis and celiac disease.
Venes, D (ed): Taber's Cyclopedic Medical Dictionary, ed. 20, FA Davis, Philadelphia, 2005.

TABLE 9.6	Eating Problems of the Older Adult and Ways to Improve Nutrition	
Problem	**Cause**	**Dietary Interventions**

Within the mouth	Impaired taste buds
	Dental caries
	Chewing difficulty due to:
	    Poorly fitting dentures
	    No dentures
	    No saliva
	    Paralysis
	    Metallic taste from medications
		Referral for correction of dental problems
		Mouthwash/oral care before meals
		Food prepared to meet client's needs (chopped, pureed, soft)

In the upper GI tract	Swallowing difficulty Paralysis due to stroke Food causing GI distress	Thickened and jellied liquids Soft, chopped foods Small, frequent meals Presentation important (how food looks on serving plate) *Avoid* expression such as "baby food" (negative connotation)
In the lower GI tract	Constipation Diarrhea Bloating	Add fruits/liquids to restore bowel function (see bowel training) *Avoid* foods that cause diarrhea Plan meals at appropriate times for ease of digestion *Avoid* salt
Psychosocial	Loneliness Meals no longer social event Depression Anorexia	Encourage attendance at meal program if available Arrange group meals/activities when possible Emphasize best nutrition when appetite is at peak (breakfast) Allow time to complete meal Interact with others whenever possible
In the environment	Inability to shop for, prepare, or cook food Impaired vision Lack of resources Difficulty in feeding self Acute or chronic illnesses present (e.g., arthritis, stroke)	Refer to Meals-on-Wheels Encourage family involvement; describe how food is arranged on plate Refer to social services Assess need for assistive devices Assess ability to grasp utensils and guide food to mouth Open packages and milk cartons; butter the bread; cut meat and vegetables

Thomas, CL (ed): Taber's Cyclopedic Medical Dictionary, ed. 18 FA Davis, Philadelphia, 1997.

RELIGIOUS CONSIDERATIONS IN MEAL PLANNING

I. **Orthodox Jews:**
   A. Kosher meat and poultry.
   B. *No* shellfish, eels, or pork products.
   C. Milk and dairy products *cannot* be consumed with meat or poultry; requires separate utensils.
   D. *No* eggs with a blood spot may be eaten. Eggs may be used with either meat or dairy meals.

II. **Conservative and Reform Jews:** dietary practices may vary from religious laws.

III. **Muslims:** *no* pork or alcohol.

IV. **Hindus:** vegetarianism (cows are sacred).

V. **Seventh-day Adventists:**
   A. Vegetarianism is common (lacto-ovo).
   B. *No* shellfish or pork products.
   C. *Avoid* stimulants (coffee, tea, other caffeine sources).
   D. *No* alcohol.

VI. **Mormons (Latter-Day Saints [LDS]):** *no* coffee, tea, or alcohol.

VII. **Catholics:** some still adhere to meatless Fridays and fasting during Lent.

MEDICAL CONDITIONS WITH DIETARY MANAGEMENT

Table 9.7.

SPECIAL DIETS

I. **Low carbohydrate diet**—ketogenic: low carbohydrate, high fat; *dumping syndrome:* low carbohydrate, high fat, high protein.

II. **Gluten-free diet**—elimination of all foods made from oats, barley, wheat, and rye; may have corn and rice. Used for *celiac* disease.

III. **High protein diet**—lean meat, cheese, and green vegetables.
   A. *Nephrotic* syndrome (may also be on low sodium diet).
   B. *Acute leukemia* (combined with high calorie and soft food diets).
   C. *Neoplastic* disease.

IV. **Low protein diet:**
   A. Usually accompanied by high carbohydrate diet and normal fats and calories.
   B. *Renal* failure, uremia, anuria, acute glomerulonephritis.

V. **Low sodium diet:**
   A. *Heart* failure.
   B. *Nephrotic* syndrome.
   C. *Acute glomerulonephritis* (varies with degree of oliguria).

VI. **High phosphorus diet:**
   A. Use when serum phosphorus level is < 2.7 mg/dL due to:
      1. *Insufficient* intake (e.g., malnutrition, starvation)
      2. *Increased* phosphorus excretion due to:
         a. Renal failure.
         b. Hyperparathyroidism.
         c. Malignancy.
         d. Antacids that are aluminum hydroxide–based or magnesium-based.
   B. Sources of phosphorus: beef, chicken, fish, organ meats, pork, nuts, legumes, whole grain breads and cereals, milk, egg, cheese, ice cream, carbonated beverages.

COMMON THERAPEUTIC DIETS

I. **Clear liquid diet**
   A. *Purpose:* relieve thirst and help maintain fluid balance.

TABLE 9.7	Medical Conditions with Dietary Management
Condition	**Recommended Diet**
Celiac sprue	*Avoid* glutens (wheat, buckwheat, rye, oats, barley)
Cholelithiasis	*Avoid* fatty food
Cirrhosis	↓ sodium; limit protein
Diverticulosis	Low residue
Esophagitis	Thick liquids; *avoid* alcohol
Gastroesophageal reflux disease (GERD)	*Avoid:* late meals, chocolate, caffeine, mints
Gout	↓ alcohol, ↓ purine (organ meats, anchovies, sardines, consomme, gravies, fish roes, herring); ↑ fluid
Hyperhomocysteinemia	↑ vitamin B_{12}; ↑ folates
Iron deficiency anemia	Vitamin C with iron supplements
Irritable bowel syndrome (IBS)	↑ fiber, ↓ dairy products
Nephrotic syndrome	↓ sodium
Osteoporosis	↓ alcohol; supplement calcium and vitamin D
Pernicious anemia	Vitamin B_{12} supplements
Renal failure	↓ sodium, potassium, protein, fluids

B. *Use:* postsurgically and following acute vomiting or diarrhea.
C. *Foods allowed:* carbonated beverages; coffee (caffeinated and decaffeinated); tea; fruit-flavored drinks; strained fruit juices; clear, flavored gelatins; broth, consommé; sugar; popsicles; commercially prepared clear liquids; and hard candy.
D. *Foods avoided:* milk and milk products, fruit juices with pulp, and fruit.

II. Full liquid diet

A. *Purpose:* provide an adequately nutritious diet for clients who cannot chew or who are too ill to do so.
B. *Use:* acute infection with fever, gastrointestinal upsets, after surgery as a progression from *clear liquids.*
C. *Foods allowed:* clear liquids, milk drinks, cooked cereals, custards, ice cream, sherbets, eggnog, all strained fruit juices, vegetable juices, creamed vegetable soups, puddings, mashed potatoes, instant breakfast drinks, yogurt, mild cheese sauce or pureed meat, and seasonings.
D. *Foods avoided:* nuts, seeds, coconut, fruit, jam, and marmalade.

III. Soft diet

A. *Purpose:* provide adequate nutrition for those who have trouble chewing.
B. *Use:* clients with no teeth or ill-fitting dentures; transition from full liquid to general diet; and for those who cannot tolerate highly seasoned, fried, or raw foods following acute infections or gastrointestinal disturbances, such as gastric ulcer or cholelithiasis.
C. *Foods allowed:* very tender minced, ground, baked, broiled, roasted, stewed, or creamed beef, lamb, veal, liver, poultry, or fish; crisp bacon or sweetbreads; cooked vegetables; pasta; all fruit juices; soft raw fruits; soft breads and cereals; all desserts that are soft; and cheeses.
D. *Foods avoided:* coarse whole-grain cereals and breads; nuts; raisins; coconut; fruits with small seeds; fried foods; high-fat gravies or sauces; spicy salad dressings; pickled meat, fish, or poultry; strong cheeses; brown or wild rice; raw vegetables, as well as lima beans and corn; spices such as horseradish, mustard, and catsup; and popcorn.

IV. Sodium-restricted diet

A. *Purpose:* reduce sodium content in the tissues and promote excretion of water.
B. *Use:* heart failure, hypertension, renal disease, cirrhosis, toxemia of pregnancy, and cortisone therapy.
C. *Modifications:* mildly restrictive 2 g sodium diet to extremely restricted 200 mg sodium diet.
D. *Foods avoided:* table salt; all commercial soups, including bouillon; gravy, catsup, mustard, meat sauces, and soy sauce; buttermilk, ice cream, and sherbet; sodas; beet greens, carrots, celery, chard, sauerkraut, and spinach; *all canned* vegetables; frozen peas; all baked products containing salt, baking powder, or baking soda; potato chips and popcorn; fresh or canned shellfish; all cheeses; smoked or commercially prepared meats; salted

butter or margarine; bacon; olives; and commercially prepared salad dressings.

V. Renal diet

A. *Purpose:* control protein, potassium, sodium, and fluid levels in body.
B. *Use:* acute and chronic renal failure, hemodialysis.
C. *Foods allowed:* high-biological proteins such as meat, fowl, fish, cheese, and dairy products—range between 20 and 60 mg/day. Potassium is usually limited to 1500 mg/day. Vegetables such as cabbage, cucumber, and peas are lowest in potassium. Sodium is restricted to 500 mg/day. Fluid intake is restricted to the daily urine volume plus 500 mL, which represents insensible water loss. Fluid intake measures water in fruit, vegetables, milk, and meat.
D. *Foods avoided:* cereals, bread, macaroni, noodles, spaghetti, avocados, kidney beans, potato chips, raw fruit, yams, soybeans, nuts, gingerbread, apricots, bananas, figs, grapefruit, oranges, percolated coffee, Coca-Cola, Orange Crush, sport drinks, and breakfast drinks such as Tang or Awake.

VI. High protein, high carbohydrate diet

A. *Purpose:* corrects large protein losses and raises the level of blood albumin. May be modified to include low fat, low sodium, and low cholesterol diets.
B. *Use:* burns, hepatitis, cirrhosis, pregnancy, hyperthyroidism, mononucleosis, protein deficiency due to poor eating habits, geriatric clients with poor food intake, nephritis, nephrosis, and liver and gallbladder disorders.
C. *Foods allowed:* general diet with added protein. In adults, high protein diets usually contain 135–150 g protein.
D. *Foods avoided:* restrictions depend on modifications added to the diet. These modifications are determined by the client's condition.

VII. Purine-restricted diet

A. *Purpose:* designed to reduce intake of uric acid–producing foods.
B. *Use:* high uric acid retention, uric acid renal stones, and gout.
C. *Foods allowed:* general diet plus 2–3 quarts of liquid daily.
D. *Foods avoided:* cheese containing spices or nuts, fried eggs, meat, liver, seafood, lentils, dried peas and beans, broth, bouillon, gravies, oatmeal and whole wheats, pasta, noodles, and alcoholic beverages. *Limited* quantities of meat, fish, and seafood allowed.

VIII. Bland diet

A. *Purpose:* provision of a diet low in fiber, roughage, mechanical irritants, and chemical stimulants.
B. *Use:* gastritis, hyperchlorhydria, functional GI disorders, gastric atony, diarrhea, spastic constipation, biliary indigestion, and hiatus hernia.
C. *Foods allowed:* varied to meet individual needs and food tolerances.

D. *Foods avoided:* fried foods, including eggs, meat, fish, and seafood; cheese with added nuts or spices; commercially prepared luncheon meats; cured meats such as ham; gravies and sauces; raw vegetables; potato skins; fruit juices with pulp; figs; raisins; fresh fruits; whole wheats; rye bread; bran cereals; rich pastries; pies; chocolate; jams with seeds; nuts; seasoned dressings; caffeinated coffee; strong tea; cocoa; alcoholic and carbonated beverages; and pepper.

IX. Low fat, cholesterol-restricted diet

A. *Purpose:* reduce hyperlipidemia, provide dietary treatment for malabsorption syndromes and clients having acute intolerance for fats.

B. *Use:* hyperlipidemia, atherosclerosis, pancreatitis, cystic fibrosis, sprue, gastrectomy, massive resection of the small intestine, and cholecystitis.

C. *Foods allowed:* nonfat milk; low carbohydrate, low fat vegetables; most fruits; breads; pastas; cornmeal; lean meats; unsaturated fats such as corn oil; desserts made without whole milk; and unsweetened carbonated beverages.

D. *Foods avoided:* **remember to avoid the five C's of cholesterol—cookies, cream, cake, coconut, chocolate;** whole milk and whole-milk or *cream* products, avocados, olives, commercially prepared *baked* goods such as donuts and muffins, poultry skin, highly marbled meats, shellfish, fish canned in oil, nuts, *coconut,* commercially prepared meats, butter, ordinary margarines, olive oil, lard, pudding made with whole milk, *ice cream,* candies with *chocolate, cream,* sauces, gravies, and commercially fried foods.

X. Diabetic diet

A. *Purpose:* maintain blood glucose as near normal as possible; prevent or delay onset of diabetic complications.

B. *Use:* diabetes mellitus.

C. *Foods allowed:* choose foods with low *glycemic index;* composed of 45%–55% carbohydrates, 30%–35% fats, and 10%–25% protein. Foods are divided into groups from which exchanges can be made. Coffee, tea, broth, bouillon, spices, and flavorings can be used as desired. Exchange groups include: *milk, vegetables, fruit, starch/bread* (includes starchy vegetables), *meat* (divided into lean, medium fat, and high fat), and *fat* exchanges. The number of exchanges allowed from each group is dependent on the total number of calories allowed. Nonnutritive sweeteners (aspartame) if desired. Nutritive sweeteners (sorbitol) in moderation for those who have controlled diabetes and have normal weight.

D. *Foods avoided:* concentrated sweets or regular soft drinks.

XI. Acid and alkaline ash diet

A. *Purpose:* furnish a well-balanced diet in which the total acid ash is greater than the total alkaline ash each day.

B. *Use:* retard the formation of renal calculi. The type of diet chosen depends on laboratory analysis of the stones.

C. *Acid and alkaline ash food groups:*
1. *Acid ash:* meat, whole grains, eggs, cheese, cranberries, prunes, plums.
2. *Alkaline ash:* milk, vegetables, fruit (except cranberries, prunes, and plums).
3. *Neutral:* sugars, fats, beverages (coffee and tea).

D. *Foods allowed:* all the client wants of the following:
1. Breads: any, preferably whole grain; crackers; rolls.
2. Cereals: any, preferably whole grain.
3. Desserts: angel food or sunshine cake; cookies made without baking powder or soda; cornstarch pudding, cranberry desserts, custards, gelatin desserts, ice cream, sherbet, plum or prune desserts; rice or tapioca pudding.
4. Fats: any, such as butter, margarine, salad dressings, Crisco, Spry, lard, salad oils, olive oil, etc.
5. Fruits: cranberries, plums, prunes.
6. Meat, eggs, cheese: any meat, fish, or fowl, two servings daily; at least one egg daily.
7. Potato substitutes: corn, hominy, lentils, macaroni, noodles, rice, spaghetti, vermicelli.
8. Soup: broth as desired; other soups from foods allowed.
9. Sweets: cranberry or plum jelly; sugar; plain sugar candy.
10. Miscellaneous: cream sauce, gravy, peanut butter, peanuts, popcorn, salt, spices, vinegar, walnuts.

E. *Restricted foods:* no more than the amount allowed each day.
1. Milk: 1 pint daily (may be used in other ways than as beverage).
2. Cream: $1/3$ cup or less daily.
3. Fruits: one serving of fruit daily (in addition to the prunes, plums, and cranberries); certain fruits listed under *Foods avoided* (following) are *not allowed at any time.*
4. Vegetables, including potatoes: two servings daily; certain vegetables listed under *Foods avoided* (following) are *not allowed at any time.*

F. *Foods avoided:*
1. Carbonated beverages, such as ginger ale, cola, root beer.
2. Cakes or cookies made with baking powder or soda.
3. Fruits: dried apricots, bananas, dates, figs, raisins, rhubarb.
4. Vegetables: dried beans, beet greens, dandelion greens, carrots, chard, lima beans.
5. Sweets; chocolate or candies other than those listed under *Foods allowed* (preceding); syrups.
6. Miscellaneous: other nuts, olives, pickles.

XII. High fiber diet
A. *Purpose:* soften stool; exercise digestive tract muscles; speed passage of food through digestive tract to prevent exposure to cancer-causing agents in food; lower blood lipids; prevent sharp rise in blood glucose after eating.
B. *Use:* diabetes, hyperlipidemia, constipation, diverticulosis, anticarcinogenic (colon).
C. *Foods allowed:* recommended intake about 6 g crude fiber daily: all bran cereals; watermelon, prunes, dried peaches, apple with skin; parsnips, peas, brussel sprouts; sunflower seeds.

XIII. Low residue (low fiber) diet
A. *Purpose:* reduce stool bulk and slow transit time.
B. *Use:* bowel inflammation during acute diverticulitis or ulcerative colitis, preparation for bowel surgery, esophageal and intestinal stenosis.
C. *Foods allowed:* eggs; ground or well-cooked tender meat, fish, poultry; milk; mild cheeses; strained fruit juice (except prune); cooked or canned apples, apricots, peaches, pears; ripe bananas; strained vegetable juice; canned, cooked, or strained asparagus, beets, green beans, pumpkin, acorn squash, spinach; white bread; refined cereals (Cream of Wheat).

XIV. Lactose-free diet
A. *Purpose:* decrease symptoms that occur after having milk products: diarrhea, cramps, abdominal pain, increased flatus.
B. *Use:* in lactose intolerance, where there is an inability to tolerate lactose because of absence or deficiency of lactase, an enzyme found in the secretions of the small intestine required for digestion of lactose.
C. *Foods avoided:* milk products.
D. *Foods allowed:* soy-based milk foods; hard cheese, cottage cheese, yogurt (contain inactive lactose enzyme).

ANTICANCER NUTRIENTS AND NONNUTRITIVE COMPOUNDS

I. **Use:** To enhance immune function, promote wellness as an anti-inflammatory agent; to reduce risk of chronic diseases, including cancer.

II. **Source foods:**
A. *Berries.*
1. Rich in: vitamin C, fiber, potassium, phytochemicals (flavonoids).
2. *Effect:*
a. Antioxidants: protect against cell damage.
b. Antiinflammatory.
c. Antiulcerative.
d. Antiviral.
e. May help to inhibit tumor formation in: liver, colon, esophageal, and oral cancer.
3. Servings: daily.

B. *Citrus fruits.*
1. Rich in: vitamin C, folic acid, phytochemicals (e.g., beta carotene, limonoids, monoterpenes, phenols).
2. *Effect:*
a. Inhibit activation of cancer cells; detoxify cancer promoters.
b. Aid protective enzymes.
c. Stimulate cancer-killing immune cells.
d. May reduce risk of: breast, skin, colon cancers.
3. Servings: daily.
C. *Cruciferous vegetable family.*
1. Rich in: antioxidants (e.g., beta carotene and vitamin C); also isothiocyanates; including sulforaphane.
2. Group includes: broccoli, kale, cauliflower, cabbage, bok choy, brussels sprouts.
3. *Effect:*
a. Isothiocyanates: interfere with tumor growth.
b. Neutralize cancer-causing chemicals.
c. Stimulate enzymes (e.g., glutathione *s*-transferase) that inactivate carcinogens.
d. May help reduce risk of hormone-related cancers (e.g., breast, prostate, and thyroid).
e. May help reduce risk of: lung, GI, oral, pharyngeal, and esophageal cancers.
4. Servings: 3 servings/week.
D. *Fatty fish* (salmon, trout, herring, bluefish, sardines).
1. Rich in: omega-3 fatty acids, iron, B vitamins, selenium, vitamin D.
2. *Effect:*
a. Inhibit growth of cancer cells.
b. Stimulate the immune system.
c. Help prevent or reduce muscle wasting.
d. May reduce the risk of cancers of: breast, prostate, endometrium, colon.
3. Servings: twice/week or more often.
E. *Flaxseed.*
1. Rich in: omega-3 fatty acids, lignans, fiber, protein, calcium, potassium, vitamin B, iron.
2. *Effect:*
a. Block tumor growth.
b. Inhibit angiogenesis.
c. Enhance immune system.
d. Antiinflammatory.
3. **Caution:** Not to be used by clients with hormone-sensitive breast cancer and/or if using tamoxifen or other antiestrogenic drugs.
F. *Garlic and onions.*
1. *Effect:*
a. Increase detoxification of enzymes.
b. Stimulate cancer-fighting immune cells.
c. May decrease risk of: prostate, breast, gastric, and colon cancer.
d. May also have antiasthma and cardioprotective effects.
2. Servings: use in any recipe.

G. *Green tea.*
1. Rich in: polyphenols (antioxidants that prevent DNA damage).
2. *Effect:*
   a. Catechins (a type of polyphenol) may help to rid body of carcinogens.
   b. May neutralize cell-damaging free radicals.
   c. Stimulates immune response.
   d. May suppress the growth of cancer cells.
   e. May reduce the risk of: colorectal, prostate, breast, bladder, gastric, esophageal, liver, lung, skin, and head and neck cancers.
3. Servings: 2–4 cups daily.

H. *Herbs and spices.*
1. *Rosemary:* rich in carnosol and ursolic acid with strong antioxidant activity.
2. *Turmeric* and *cumin:* rich in curcumin that may reduce risk of leukemia, skin, and liver cancers.
3. *Chili peppers:* rich in capsaicin that helps to prevent formation of nitrosamines; may reduce risk of colon, gastric and rectal cancers.

I. *Legumes/beans.*
1. Rich in: low fat source of protein and dietary fiber, iron, folic acid, calcium, zinc, phytochemicals (e.g., phytosterols, saponins, phytic acid, isoflavones).
2. *Effect:* prevent DNA damage → provide anticancer activity.
3. Servings: 3–4/week.

J. *Nuts.*
1. Rich in: dietary fiber, vitamin E, healthy fats.
   a. Brazil nuts: high amount of selenium.
   b. Walnuts: high in omega-3 fatty acids.
2. *Effect:* encourage "suicide" of cancer cells.
3. Servings: 2 Brazil nuts daily; 2 tbsp of walnuts daily.

K. *Olive oil* (extra virgin).
1. Rich in: monounsaturated fats, polyphenols.
2. *Effect:*
   a. Inhibit oxidative stress.
   b. Arrest cell proliferation.
   c. Induce cell death (apoptosis).
3. May reduce risk of: breast, prostate, and colorectal cancers.

L. *Vegetables/fruits*—**orange-colored** (carrots, sweet potatoes, winter squash, mangoes, papayas).
1. Rich in: vitamin C, folic acid, other B vitamins, fiber and beta carotene.
2. *Effect:* carotenoids strengthen immune system.
3. May reduce risk of: lung, colorectal, uterine, prostate, and breast cancers.
4. Servings: daily servings of dark orange and green foods.

M. *Soy foods.*
1. Rich in: protein, fiber, calcium, variety of vitamins and minerals; phytoestrogens (e.g., isoflavones, lignans).
2. Dietary sources: soybeans (edamame), tofu, tempeh, miso, soy nuts, soy milk.
3. **Caution:** Those with breast cancer are advised to limit soy consumption to 3–4 servings/week.

4. May reduce risk of cancers: breast, prostate, thyroid, and colon.
5. Servings: 1–2 daily soy servings (10–30 g soy protein and 30–90 mg isoflavones). **Avoid excesses** of more than 200 mg isoflavones daily.

N. *Tomatoes.*
1. Rich in: lycopene, vitamin C, beta carotene, potassium.
2. *Effect:*
   a. Antioxidants that scavenge free radicals.
   b. Reduce tissue damage.
   c. Protect cell membranes.
   d. Prevent formation of nitrosamines.
3. Has been shown to inhibit growth of: prostate, colon, bladder, cervical, stomach, esophageal, and lung cancers.
4. Servings: 4 or more daily.

O. *Whole grains.*
1. Rich in: fiber, vitamins, trace minerals, antioxidants, plant sterols, phytoestrogens, phytases, tocotrienols, lignans, ellagic acid, saponins.
2. Dietary sources: oats, barley, mullet, brown rice, bulgur.
3. *Effect:* may reduce risk of various cancers, as well as hypertension, heart disease, obesity, and diabetes.
4. Servings: ×3 daily.

P. *Yogurt* with live, active cultures.
1. Rich in: protein, calcium, and probiotics.
2. *Effect:*
   a. Boost immunity.
   b. Inhibit cell proliferation.
   c. Induce cell death.
3. May protect against colorectal cancer.

FOOD LIST FOR READY REFERENCE IN MENU PLANNING

I. **High cholesterol foods**—over 50 mg/100 g portion: beef, butter, cheese, egg yolks, shellfish, kidney, liver, pork, veal.

II. **High sodium foods**—over 500 mg/100 g portion: bacon—cured, Canadian; beef—corned, cooked, canned, dried, creamed; biscuits, baking powder; bouillon cubes; bran, added sugar and malt; bran flakes with thiamine; raisins; breads—wheat, French, rye, white, whole wheat; butter, cheese—cheddar, Parmesan, Swiss, pasteurized American; cocoa; cookies, gingersnaps; cornflakes; cornbread; crackers—graham, saltines; margarine; milk—dry, skim; mustard; oat products; olives—green, ripe; peanut butter; pickles, dill; popcorn with oil and salt; salad dressing—blue cheese, Roquefort, French, Thousand Island; sausages—bologna, frankfurters; soy sauce; tomato catsup; tuna in oil.

III. **High potassium foods**—more than 400 mg/100 g portion: almonds; bacon, Canadian; baking powder, low sodium; beans—white, lima; beef, hamburger; fruits, fruit juices; bran with sugar and malt; cake—fruitcake, gingerbread; cashew nuts; chicken, light meat; cocoa; coffee, instant; cookies, gingersnaps; dates; garlic; milk—skim, powdered; peanuts, roasted; peanut butter; peas; pecans; potatoes, boiled in skin; scallops; tea, instant; tomato puree; turkey, light meat; veal; walnuts, black; yeast, brewer's.

IV. **Foods high in B vitamins**
   A. *Thiamine:* pork, dried beans, dried peas, liver, lamb, veal, nuts, peas.
   B. *Riboflavin:* liver, poultry, milk, yogurt, whole-grain cereals, beef, oysters, tongue, fish, cottage cheese, veal.
   C. *Niacin:* liver, fish, poultry, peanut butter, whole grains and enriched breads, lamb, veal, beef, pork.

V. **Foods high in vitamin C:** oranges, strawberries, dark-green leafy vegetables, potatoes, grapefruit, tomato, cabbage, broccoli, melon, liver.

VI. **Foods high in iron, calcium, and residue**
   A. *Iron:* breads—brown, corn, ginger; fish, tuna; poultry; organ meats; whole-grain cereals; shellfish; egg yolk; fruits—apples, berries; dried fruits—dates, prunes, apricots, peaches, raisins; vegetables—dark-green leafy, potatoes, tomatoes, rhubarb, squash; molasses; dried beans and peas; peanut butter; brown sugar; noodles; rice.
   B. *Calcium:* milk—dry, skim, whole, evaporated, buttermilk; cheese—American, Swiss, hard; dark green leafy vegetables—kale, turnip greens, mustard greens, collards; black-eyed peas; tofu; canned fish with bones; figs.
   C. *Residue:* whole-grain cereals—oatmeal, bran, shredded wheat; breads—whole wheat, cracked wheat, rye, bran muffins; vegetables—lettuce, spinach, Swiss chard, raw carrots, raw celery, corn, cauliflower, eggplant, sauerkraut, cabbage; fruits—bananas, figs, apricots, oranges.

VII. **Foods to be used in low protein and low carbohydrate diets**
   A. *Low protein* (these proteins are allowed in various amounts in controlled-protein diets for *renal decompensation*): milk—buttermilk, reconstituted evaporated, low sodium, skim, and powdered; meat—chicken, lamb, turkey, beef (lean), veal; fish—sole, flounder, haddock, perch; cheese—cheddar, American, Swiss, cottage; eggs; fruits—apples, grapes, pears, pineapple; vegetables—cabbage, cucumbers, lettuce, tomatoes; cereals—cornflakes, puffed rice, puffed wheat, farina, rolled oats.
   B. *Low carbohydrate:* all meats; cheese—hard, soft, cottage; eggs; shellfish—oysters, shrimp; fats—bacon, butter, French dressing, salad oil, mayonnaise, margarine; vegetables—asparagus, green beans, beet greens, broccoli, brussels sprouts, cabbage, celery, cauliflower, cucumber, lettuce, green

pepper, spinach, squash, tomatoes; fruits—avocados, strawberries, cantaloupe, lemons, rhubarb.

VIII. **Food guide pyramid**—guide to daily food selection (**Figure 9.1**)
   A. *Fats, oils:* use sparingly.
   B. *Milk group:* two to three servings.
   C. *Meat group:* two to three servings.
   D. *Fruit group:* two to four servings.
   E. *Vegetable group:* three to five servings.
   F. *Bread/cereal group:* 6 to 11 servings.

Questions

Select the one answer that is best for each question, unless otherwise directed.

1. A client who is diabetic states that she is a "peanut butter freak." Which exchange would be equivalent to 2 tbsp peanut butter?
   1. 8 oz whole milk.
   2. 2 tbsp butter.
   3. $^1/_4$ cup cottage cheese.
   4. 2 tbsp cream cheese.
2. A client is placed on an 1800-calorie diabetic diet; a typical lunch would include two meat exchanges, two bread exchanges, one vegetable exchange, one fruit exchange, one fat exchange, and one milk exchange. Given these allowances, which would be inappropriate for this client to consume at a birthday luncheon?
   1. A piece of plain sponge cake.
   2. An 8 oz glass of Coca-Cola.
   3. A taco (tortilla, meat, cheddar cheese, lettuce).
   4. Avocado and orange salad.
3. A client has been placed on a high protein diet. Which food would the nurse suggest this client select?
   1. Rice (1 cup).
   2. Eggnog (8 oz).
   3. Cheddar cheese (1 oz).
   4. Broccoli (1 cup).
4. Which food would the nurse recommend be *avoided* by a client experiencing dumping syndrome?
   1. Liver and bacon.
   2. Orange and avocado salad.
   3. Creamed chicken.
   4. Glazed donuts and coffee.
5. Which food may be more likely to cause discomfort in a client with cholecystitis?
   1. Whole milk.
   2. Cottage cheese.
   3. Whole-grain breads.
   4. Eggs.
6. Small, frequent feedings of which type of diet would the nurse recommend for clients experiencing dumping syndrome?
   1. Low protein, high fat, low carbohydrate diet.
   2. High protein, high fat, high carbohydrate diet.
   3. High protein, high fat, low carbohydrate diet.
   4. Low protein, low fat, high carbohydrate diet.

Answers/Rationales/Tips

1. (**3**) A diabetic diet is most often based on an exchange system. Foodstuffs in this system are divided into six types. Foods from within each list can be substituted for

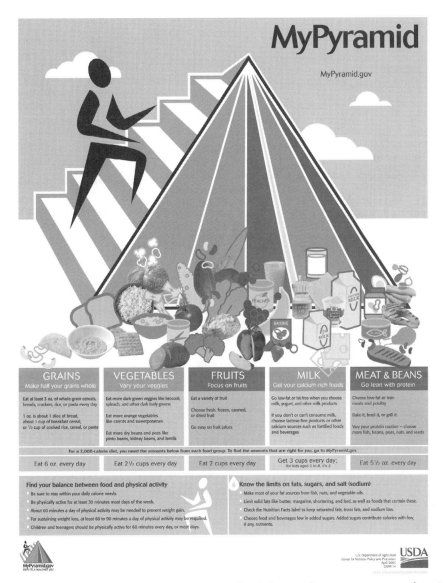

FIGURE 9.1   Food guide pyramid—guide to daily food choices. (U.S. Department of Agriculture.)

another in the same list because they have approximately the same food value. Peanut butter is in the *meat* exchange list, as is cottage cheese, and therefore these can be substituted for one another. Whole milk (**Answer 1**) is on the milk exchange list. Butter and cream cheese (**Answers 2** and **4**) are considered to be fats.

> **TEST-TAKING TIP**—Think "substitute" for a high protein source.
> **IMP, APP, 4, M/S: Endocrine, PhI, Basic Care and Comfort**

KEY TO CODES FOLLOWING RATIONALES:

Nursing process: **AS**, assessment; **AN**, analysis; **PL**, plan; **IMP**, implementation; **EV**, evaluation. *Cognitive level:* **COM**, comprehension; **APP**, application; **ANL**, analysis. *Category of human function:* **1**, protective; **2**, sensory-perceptual; **3**, comfort, rest, activity, and mobility; **4**, nutrition; **5**, growth and development; **6**, fluid-gas transport; **7**, psychosocial-cultural; **8**, elimination. *Client need:* **SECE**, safe, effective care environment; **HPM**, health promotion/maintenance; **PsI**, psychosocial integrity; **PhI**, physiological integrity. (Client subneed appears after Client need code.) See appendices for full explanation.

2. (**2**) All concentrated sweets and regular soft drinks are contraindicated on a diabetic diet. Given the client's food allowances, all these foods (**Answers 1, 3,** and **4**) would be allowed *except* for the Coca-Cola.

> **TEST-TAKING TIP**—Try matching each exchange with the options—one will have *no* match. The question calls for what is *not* OK to eat.
> **PL, ANL, 4, M/S: Endocrine, PhI, Basic Care and Comfort**

3. (**2**) Eggs and milk are two sources of protein with the highest biological values (high-quality proteins). Eggnog (8 oz) contains 15 g protein. Rice (**Answer 1**) contains only 4 g, cheddar cheese (**Answer 3**) contains only 7 g, and broccoli (**Answer 4**) contains only 5 g. Meat, fish, and legumes contain more protein than does eggnog, but their percent of protein utilization is lower, making them almost equal in value to eggnog.

> **TEST-TAKING TIP**—With two possible choices, choose the one with more sources of protein (egg *and* milk).
> **IMP, APP, 4, M/S: Diet, PhI, Basic Care and Comfort**

4. (**4**) Concentrated sugars and carbohydrates should be *avoided* by these clients. Likewise, fluid ingestion with meals or snacks should also be *avoided* to prevent rapid emptying of the stom-

ach. **Answers 1, 2,** and **3** are examples of high protein, high fat, low carbohydrate foods, which *are* appropriate.

> **TEST-TAKING TIP**—Know two things to *avoid* with meals—carbohydrates and fluids.
> **PL, APP, 4, M/S: GI, PhI, Reduction of Risk Potential**

5. **(1)** Whole milk has a *high fat* content, so a client with chole-cystitis is generally advised to switch to low fat or skim milk. Cottage cheese (**Answer 2**), whole-grain breads (**Answer 3**), and eggs (**Answer 4**) *are* allowed in a low fat diet, although eggs may be limited to four per week.

> **TEST-TAKING TIP**—Look for the food that is *not* OK to have. Use a true-false approach option by option to find the item that is high fat and *not* OK to have.
> **IMP, APP, 4, M/S: GI, PhI, Reduction of Risk Potential**

6. **(3)** The symptoms of dumping syndrome are most likely to occur following the ingestion of large amounts of sugars or carbohydrates. Therefore a diet that is high in protein and fats and low in carbohydrates is recommended, to reduce symptomatology and to provide the client with essential energy requirements. **Answers 1** and **4** are incorrect because they do not supply sufficient protein for energy and tissue repair. High protein intake is essential after surgery and most prolonged illnesses for rebuilding tissue. **Answers 2** and **4** are incorrect because they list *high* carbohydrates.

> **TEST-TAKING TIP**—Look for foods that slow the movement of food out of the stomach (e.g., ↓CHO, ↑ fat).
> **PL, APP, 4, M/S: GI, PhI, Basic Care and Comfort**

Review of Pharmacology

Sally L. Lagerquist • Janice McMillin • Robyn Nelson
• Mary St. Jonn Seed • Kathleen Snider

CONVERSIONS AND CALCULATIONS IN MEDICATION ADMINISTRATION

I. **Common metric conversion**
   A. *Weight:*
   1 gram (g) = 1,000,000 micrograms (μg)
   1 milligram (mg) = 1000 micrograms (μg)
   1000 milligrams (mg) = 1 gram (g)
   1 kilogram (kg) = 1000 grams (g)
   B. *Volume:*
   1 liter (L) = 1000 milliliters (mL)
   1 kiloliter (kL) = 1000 liters (L)
   1 milliliter (mL) = 1 cubic centimeter (cc)

II. **Apothecary system** (*Note:* metric is preferred for medication administration.)
   A. *Weight:*
   60 grains (gr) = 1 dram (dr)
   8 drams (dr) = 1 ounce (oz)
   B. *Liquid:*
   60 minims = 1 fluidram (fl dr)
   8 fluidrams (fl dr) = 1 fluidounce (fl oz)
   16 fluidounces (fl oz) = 1 pint (pt)
   2 pints (pt) = 1 quart (qt)
   4 quarts (qt) = 1 gallon (gal)

III. **Equivalent household conversions**
   20 drops (gtt) = 1 milliliter (mL)
   1 teaspoon (tsp) = 5 milliliters (mL)
   1 ounce (oz) = 30 milliliters (mL)
   1 cup (C) = 240 milliliters (mL)
   1 liter (L) = 1000 milliliters (mL)

IV. Determining equivalency from one system to another

Use a proportion. On the left side of the proportion is what you *know* to be an equivalent (e.g., 30 milliliters equals 1 ounce). On the right side of the proportion is what you *need to determine* (e.g., you want to give 1.5 ounces and your medicine cup is in milliliters—you would write "*x*" milliliters equals 1.5 ounces). Rewrite the proportion without using the symbols.

Example:
1 oz. : 30 mL :: x mL : 1.5 oz.
Solve for x
$1x = 30 \times 1.5$
$x = 45$
1.5 ounces equals 45 milliliters (mL)

V. Alternate formula for calculation with like units

$$\frac{D \text{ (Desired Amount)}}{A \text{ (Available Amount)}} \times Q \text{ (Quantity Available)} = x$$

Example: the order is for 50 mg of phenobarbital, which comes in 20 mg per 5 mL.

$$\frac{50 \text{ mg (Desired)}}{20 \text{ mg (Available)}} \times \frac{5 \text{ mL (Quantity)}}{1} = x$$

Solve for x:

$$x = \frac{50}{\cancel{20}\,4} \times \frac{\cancel{5}}{1}$$

$$x = \frac{50 \times 1}{4 \times 1}$$

$$x = \frac{50}{4}$$

$$x = 12.5 \text{ mL}$$

VI. Dimensional analysis for conversion and calculation

Another format for dosage calculation which uses only one equation even when conversion to like units is needed.

Example with like units: penicillin 500 mg comes in 250 mg capsules. You would give ____ capsules.

On the left side of the equation is the drug form you are solving for:
x capsule =

On the right side place the known information in a common fraction with the numerator matching the x quantity (capsule). The amount in each capsule that is known is the denominator (250 mg).

$$x \text{ capsule} = \frac{1 \text{ capsule}}{250 \text{ mg}}$$

Next set up a proportion with the information that matches the denominator (500 mg).

$$x \text{ capsule} = \frac{1 \text{ capsule}}{250 \text{ mg}} \times \frac{500 \text{ mg}}{1}$$

$$x = \frac{1 \times 500}{250}$$

$$x = 2 \text{ capsules}$$

Example with different units: Keflin 400 mg IM q10h. The drug is available in 0.5 g per 2 mL.

$$x \text{ mL} =$$

$$x \text{ mL} = \frac{2 \text{ mL}}{0.5 \text{ g}}$$

Because the available drug is in grams (g), an additional fraction is added for the conversion from grams to milliliters. Remember the numerator of each fraction must match the denominator of the fraction before.

$$x \text{ mL} = \frac{2 \text{ mL}}{0.5 \text{ g}} \times \frac{1 \text{ g}}{1000 \text{ mg}}$$

$$x \text{ mL} = \frac{2 \text{ mL}}{0.5 \text{ g}} \times \frac{1 \text{ g}}{1000 \text{ mg}} \times \frac{400 \text{ mg}}{1}$$

(amount of drug ordered)

Cancel out the like abbreviations on the right side of the equation. If the equation is correct, the only abbreviation remaining on the right side will match the abbreviation on the left side (mL).

$$x \text{ mL} = \frac{2 \text{ mL}}{0.5 \text{ mg}} \times \frac{1 \text{ g}}{1000 \text{ mg}} \times \frac{400 \text{ mg}}{1}$$

Solve for x:

$$x = \frac{2 \times 400}{0.5 \times 1000}$$

$$x = \frac{800}{500}$$

$$x = 1.6 \text{ mL}$$

VII. Determining flow rates for parenteral infusion (see Unit 11, p. 798).

GUIDELINES FOR ADMINISTERING MEDICATIONS TO INFANTS AND CHILDREN

I. Developmental considerations
  A. Be honest. Do *not* bribe or threaten child to obtain cooperation.
  B. When administering medication, do so in the least traumatic manner possible.

C. Describe any sensations child may expect to experience (e.g., "pinch" of needle during IM).
  D. Explain how child can "help" nurse (e.g., "Lie as still as you can").
  E. Tell child that it is OK to cry; provide privacy.
  F. Offer support, praise, and encouragement during and after giving medication.
  G. Allow child opportunity for age-appropriate therapeutic play to work through feelings and experiences, to clarify any misconceptions, and to teach child more effective coping strategies.

II. Safety considerations
  A. Be absolutely sure dose you are giving is both safe (check recommended mg/kg) and accurate (have another nurse check your calculations). Remember: dose should generally be smaller than adult dose.
  B. Check identification band or ask parent or another nurse for child's first and last name.
  C. Restrain child to avoid injury while giving medication; a second person is often required to help hold child.

III. Oral medications
  A. Use syringe without needle to draw up medication.
  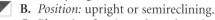 B. *Position:* upright or semireclining.
  C. Place tip of syringe along the side of infant's tongue, and give medication slowly, in small amounts, allowing infant to swallow. Medicine cups can be used for older infants and children. **Never** pinch infant or child's nostrils to force the child to open mouth.
  D. When giving tablets or capsules (that are *not* enteric coated), crush and mix into smallest possible amount of food or liquid to ensure that child takes entire dose. Do *not* mix with essential food or liquid (e.g., milk); select an "optional" food, such as applesauce.

IV. Ophthalmic installations
  A. *Position:* supine or sitting with head extended.
  B. For eye *drops:* hold dropper 1–2 cm above middle of conjunctival sac.
  C. For eye *ointment:* squeeze 2 cm of ointment from tube onto conjunctival sac.
  D. After giving drops or ointment, encourage child to keep eyes closed briefly, to maximize contact with eyes. Child should be asked to look in all directions (with eyes closed) to enhance even distribution of medication.
  E. Whenever possible, administer eye ointments at nap time or bedtime, due to possible blurred vision. Administer eye drops *prior* to ointment (if both are ordered for the same time). Eye drops may "roll off" the slick surface of the eye ointment.

V. Otic installations
  A. *Position:* head to side so that affected ear is uppermost.
  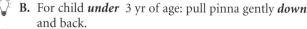 B. For child **under** 3 yr of age: pull pinna gently **down** and back.
  C. For child 3 yr of age and **over:** pull pinna gently **up** and back.

D. After administering ear drops, encourage child to remain with head to side with affected ear uppermost, to maximize contact with entire external canal to reach eardrum. Gentle massage of area in front of ear will facilitate entry of ear drops into canal.

E. If ear drops are kept in refrigerator, allow to warm to room temperature before instilling.

VI. Dermatological installations

A. Remember: young child's skin is more permeable; therefore, there is increased risk for medication absorption and resultant systemic effects; monitor for systemic effects.

B. Apply thin layer of cream or ointment, and confine it to portions of skin where it is essential.

VII. Rectal medications

A. Prepare child emotionally and physically; rectal route is invasive and embarrassing, particularly for children.

B. *Position:* side-lying with upper leg flexed.

C. Lubricate rounded end of suppository and insert past anal sphincter with gloved fingertip (wear double gloves when inserting rectal medication).

D. Remove fingertip but hold child's buttocks gently together until child no longer strains or indicates urge to expel medication.

VIII. Intramuscular medications

A. Because the infant or child is much smaller physically than an adult, the nurse should select a shorter needle, generally 5/8 inch (infant) to 1 inch (child).

B. Preferred injection sites are on the thigh: vastus lateralis (infants); ventrogluteal and dorsal gluteal (child should be walking for at least one year). The deltoid muscle, though small, provides easy access and can be used in children with adequate muscle mass.

C. Usually 1 mL is the maximum volume that should be administered in a single site to infants and children.

D. Because of vast differences in size, muscle mass, and subcutaneous tissue, it is especially important to note bony prominences as landmarks for intramuscular injections.

E. Have a second adult present to help restrain the child.

F. Once the nurse has told the child he or she is to receive an injection, the procedure should be carried out as quickly and skillfully as possible.

COMMON PSYCHOTROPIC DRUGS

I. **Antipsychotics** (also called *neuroleptics, major tranquilizers*)

A. **Typical antipsychotics**

1. **Phenothiazines** (prochlorperazine [Compazine], promazine HCl [Sparine], chlorproma-

zine HCl [Thorazine], thioridazine [Mellaril], trifluoperazine HCl [Stelazine], perphenazine [Trilafon], triflupromazine HCl [Vesprin], fluphenazine enanthate [Prolixin]).

2. **Butyrophenones** (haloperidol [Haldol, Serenace], droperidol fentanyl citrate [Innovar]).

3. **Thiothixenes** (chlorprothixene [Taractan], thiothixene [Navane])—chemically related to phenothiazines, with similar therapeutic effects.

4. **Dibenzoxazepines**—loxapine succinate [Loxitane])

B. **Atypical antipsychotics**

1. Risperidone (Risperdal), olanzapine (Zyprexa), quetiapine (Seroquel), ziprasidone (Geodon).

a. *Use*—incremental increases for first 3 days to manage psychotic symptoms. Effective for both positive and negative symptoms of schizophrenia. Risperadone also available as long-acting injection (Risperdal Consta): IM q2wk in alternate gluteal muscle site; delayed onset of action. *Benefit:* lower incidence of extrapyramidal symptoms.

b. **Assessment**—*side effects:* same as for typical antipsychotics but with higher incidence of weight gain.

2. Clozapine (Clozaril).

a. *Use*—those who do not respond to other neuroleptic antipsychotic drugs; offers relief from schizophrenic symptoms: hallucinations, delusions, flat affect, apathy.

b. **Assessment**—*side effects:*

(1) Most serious is *agranulocytosis* (potentially fatal; reversible if diagnosed within 1–2 wk of onset).

(a) *Symptoms* of agranulocytosis: infection, high fever, chills, sore throat, malaise, ulceration of mucous membranes.

(b) Lab value: Discontinue drug with WBC <2000 μL or granulocyte <1000 μL.

(2) Other side effects: seizures, tachycardia, orthostatic hypotension.

(3) *Caution:* must have weekly blood tests for WBC; do *not* resume clozapine once it is discontinued, due to side effects.

C. **General use of antipsychotic medications**—acute and chronic psychoses; most useful in cases of disorganization of thought or behavior; to decrease panic, fear, hostility, restlessness, aggression, and withdrawal.

D. **General assessment**—*side effects:*

1. *Hypersensitivity* effects:

a. *Blood dyscrasia*—agranulocytosis, leukopenia, granulocytopenia.

b. *Skin reactions*—solar sensitivity, allergic dermatitis, flushing, blue-gray skin.

c. *Obstructive jaundice.*

2. *Extrapyramidal symptoms (EPS)* affecting voluntary movement and skeletal muscles
    a. *Parkinsonism* (also called pseudoparkinsonism)—tremors, cogwheel rigidity, shuffling gait, pill-rolling, masklike facies, salivation, and difficulty starting muscular movement (dyskinesia).
    b. *Dystonia*—limb and neck spasms (torticollis), extensive rigidity of back muscles (opisthotonos), oculogyric crisis, speech and swallowing difficulties, and protrusion of tongue.
    c. *Akathisia*—motor restlessness, pacing, foot tapping, inner tremulousness, and agitation.
    d. **Tardive dyskinesia (TD)**—excessive blinking; vermiform tongue movement; stereotyped, abnormal, involuntary sucking, chewing, licking, and pursing movements of tongue and mouth; grimacing, blinking, frowning, rocking.
       (1) *Cause*—long-term use of high doses of antipsychotic drugs.
       (2) *Predisposing factors*—age, women, organic brain syndrome (OBS); history of electroconvulsive therapy (ECT) or use of tricyclics or anti-Parkinson drugs.
3. *Potentiates* central nervous system depressants.
4. *Orthostatic hypotension* (less with butyrophenones).
5. *Anticholinergic effects* (atropine-like)—dry mouth, stuffy nose, blurred vision, urinary retention, and constipation.
6. Pigment retinopathy—ocular changes (lens and corneal opacity).
7. Photosensitivity.
8. Weight gain (especially true of the atypical antipsychotic medications).

9. *Neuroleptic malignant syndrome (NMS)*
    a. *Description:* a rare complication of antipsychotic drugs, with a rapid progression (1–3 days) and a 20% mortality rate. It is a **serious medical emergency** for which early recognition of symptoms is critical. *Onset:* at start, after change, or dose increase, when used with combination of medications.
    b. **Assessment:**
       (1) ↑**Vital signs: extreme** temperature of 107°F (leading to seizures, diaphoresis, confusion, → stupor, coma), fluctuating BP, *pulse:* irregular, tachycardia.
        (2) Lab values: *increased* creatine phosphokinase (CPK), *increased* potassium, leukocytosis (↑ WBC).
       (3) Renal failure.
       (4) Muscular: parkinsonian rigidity (lead pipe skeletal muscle rigidity) that leads to dyspnea and dysphagia, tremors, dyskinesia.
       (5) *At risk:* clients with organic brain disorders and severe dehydration.
    c. *Medical treatment*
       (1) Discontinue all drugs STAT.
       (2) Institute supportive care.
       (3) Administer Parlodel or Dantrium, dopamine function–enhancing substances (e.g., levodopa, carbidopa, bromocriptine, amantadine).
    d. *Health teaching: avoid* overheating or dehydration.
E. **Antipsychotic agents—comparison of side effects (Table 10.1).**
◆ F. **General nursing care plan/implementation:**

| TABLE 10.1 | Antipsychotic Agents—Comparison of Side Effects |

Classification	Name Generic	Name Trade	Extrapyramidal Symptoms (EPS)	Sedation	Anticholinergic	Orthostatic Hypotension
Typical antipsychotics						
Phenothiazine	Chlorpromazine	Thorazine	3	4	3	4
	Fluphenazine	Prolixin	5	2	2	2
	Perphenazine	Trilafon	4	2	2	2
	Prochlorperazine	Compazine	4	3	2	2
	Promazine	Sparine	3	3	4	3
	Thioridazine	Mellaril	2	4	4	4
	Triflupromazine	Vesprin	3	4	4	3
Butyrophenone	Haloperidol	Haldol	5	1	1	1
Thioxanthene	Thiothixene	Navane	4	2	2	2
Dibenzoxazepine	Loxapine	Loxitane	4	3	2	3
Atypical antipsychotics	Clozapine	Clozaril	1	5	5	4
	Olanzapine	Zyprexa	1	3	2	1
	Quetiapine	Seroquel	1	3	2	1
	Risperidone	Risperdal	1	1	1	3
	Ziprasidone	Geodon	1	2	1	1

1 = very low; 2 = low; 3 = moderate; 4 = high; 5 = very high.

1. Goal: *anticipate and check for side effects.*
   a. Protect the person's skin from *sunburn* when outside.
   b. For *hypotension:* take BP and have person lie down for 30 min, especially after an injection.
   c. Watch for signs of *blood dyscrasia:* sore throat, fever, malaise.
   d. Observe for symptoms of *hypothermic* or *hyperthermic* reaction due to effect on heat-regulating mechanism.
   e. Observe for, withhold drug for, and report early symptoms of: *jaundice* and bile tract obstruction; high fever; upper abdominal pain, nausea, diarrhea; rash; monitor *liver function.*
   f. Relieve excessive *mouth dryness:* mouth rinse, *increase* fluid intake, gum or hard candy.
   g. Relieve gastric irritation, *constipation:* take with and *increase fluids* and *roughage* in diet.
   h. Observe for and report changes in carbohydrate metabolism (glycosuria, weight gain, polyphagia); change diet.
   i. Check blood sugar levels periodically.
2. Goal: *health teaching.*
   a. Dangers of drug potentiation with alcohol or sleeping pills.
   b. Advise about driving or occupations where blurred vision may be a problem.
   c. Caution against abrupt cessation at high doses.
   d. Warn regarding dark urine (sign of jaundice, urinary retention).
   e. Have client with respiratory disorder breathe deeply and cough (drug is a cough depressant).
   f. Need for continuous use of drug and follow-up care.
   g. Prompt reporting of hypersensitivity symptoms: fever, laryngeal edema; abdominal distention (constipation, urinary retention); jaundice; blood dyscrasia.

◆ G. **General evaluation/outcome criteria:**
1. Behavior is less agitated.
2. Knows side effects to observe for, lessen, and/or prevent.
3. Continues to use drug.

II. Antidepressants
A. **Tricyclic antidepressants (TCAs)**—(imipramine HCl [Tofranil], desipramine HCl [Norpramine, Pertofrane], nortriptyline HCl [Pamelor, Aventyl], trimipramine [Surmontil], clomipramine [Anafranil], amitriptyline HCl [Elavil, Endep], amitriptyline HCl/perphenazine [Triavil], protriptyline HCl [Vivactil], doxepin HCl [Sinequan, Adapin]), bupropion (Wellbutrin), trazodone (Desyrel), amoxapine (Asendin)—effective in 2–4 wk.
1. **Use**—elevate mood in depression, increase physical activity and mental alertness; may bring relief of symptoms of depression so that client can attend individual or group therapy; bipolar disorder, depressed; dysthymic disorder; sleep disturbance; agitation.

◆ 2. **Assessment**—*side effects:*
   a. *Behavioral*—activation of latent schizophrenia (hallucinations); hypomania; suicide attempts; mental *confusion.* Withhold drug if observed.
   b. *Central nervous system* (CNS)—*tremors, seizures,* ataxia, jitteriness, irritability.
   c. *Autonomic nervous system* (ANS)—*dry mouth,* nasal congestion, aggravation of glaucoma (blurred vision), constipation, urinary retention, edema, paralysis, *ECG* changes (flattened T waves; **arrhythmia** severe in overdose).

◆ 3. **Nursing care plan/implementation:**
   a. Goal: *assess risk of suicide during initial improvement:* careful, close observation.
   b. Goal: *prevent risk of tachycardia and cardiac arrhythmias and orthostatic hypotension:* use caution with client with cardiovascular disease, hyperthyroidism, having ECT or surgery (gradually discontinue 2–3 days *before* surgery). Monitor BP, pulse twice a day; ECGs, 2–3/wk until dose adjusted.
      (1) *Avoid* long hot showers or baths.
   c. Goal: *observe for signs of urinary retention, constipation:* monitor I&O and *weight gain* (encourage exercise).
      (1) Fiber diet.
      (2) Reduced calories.
   d. Goal: *cautious drug use with glaucoma or history of seizures.* Observe seizure precautions due to lowered seizure threshold.
   e. Goal: *health teaching:*
      (1) Advise against driving car or participating in activities requiring mental alertness, due to *sedative* effects.
      (2) Encourage increased fluid intake and frequent mouth rinsing to combat dry mouth; use candy, ice; take with food.
      (3) *Avoid* smoking, which decreases drug effects.
      (4) *Avoid* use of alcohol and other drugs, due to adverse interactions, especially OTC drugs (e.g., antihistamines).
      (5) Advise of *delay* in desired effect (2–4 wk).
      (6) Instruct gradual discontinuance to *avoid* withdrawal symptoms.

◆ 4. **Evaluation/outcome criteria:** diminished symptoms of agitated depression and anxiety.
B. **Monoamine oxidase inhibitors** (MAOIs) (phenelzine sulfate [Nardil], isocarboxazid [Marplan], tranylcypromine sulfate [Parnate], iproniazid [Marsilid], pargiline HCl [Eutonyl], nialamide [Niamid]).

◆ 1. **Assessment**—*side effects:*
   a. *Behavioral*—may activate latent schizophrenia, mania, excitement.
   b. *CNS*—tremors; **hypertensive crisis** (*avoid:* cheese, colas, caffeine, red wine, beer, yeast, chocolate, chicken liver, and other substances high in *tyramine or pressor amine* (e.g., amphetamines and cold and hay fever medication); *intracerebral hemorrhage; hyperpyrexia.*

c. *ANS—dry mouth,* aggravation of glaucoma, bowel and bladder control problems, edema, paralysis, ECG changes (severe arrhythmia in overdose).

d. *Allergic* hepatocellular jaundice.

◆ 2. **Nursing care plan/implementation:**

 a. Goal: *reduce risk of hypertensive crisis:* diet restrictions of foods high in *tyramine* content.

b. Goal: *observe for urinary retention:* measure I&O.

c. Goal: *health teaching.*

(1) Therapeutic response takes 2–3 wk.

 (2) *Food and alcohol restrictions:* avocado, bananas, raisins, licorice, chocolate, aged cheese, yogurt, sour cream, papaya, figs, over-ripe fruit, sausages, liver, herring, soy sauce, meat tenderizers, red wine, beer, caffeine, cola, yeast, chocolate.

(3) Change position gradually to prevent postural hypotension.

(4) Report any stiff neck, palpitations, chest pain, headaches because of possible hypertensive crises (can be fatal).

(5) Take *no nonprescribed* drugs.

◆ 3. **Evaluation/outcome criteria:**

a. Improvement in sleep, appetite, activity, interest in self and surroundings.

b. Lessening of anxiety and complaints.

C. **Selective serotonin reuptake inhibitors** (SSRIs) (fluoxetine [Prozac], paroxetine [Paxil], sertraline [Zoloft], fluvoxamine [Luvox], citalopram hydrobromide [Celexa]). SSRIs are generally the first line choice because of fewer side effects, do not require blood monitoring, and are safe in overdose.

◆ 1. **Assessment**—*side effects:* CNS stimulation—insomnia, agitation, headache (especially with Prozac); weight loss; sexual dysfunction (men: impotence; women: loss of orgasm, decreased libido). Other side effects are similar to TCAs (dry mouth, sedation, nausea).

◆ 2. **Nursing care plan/implementation:**

a. Goal: *reduce insomnia, agitation:* take early in day; *avoid* alcohol, caffeine; teach relaxation before sleeptime.

b. Goal: *reduce headaches:* give analgesics.

c. Goal: *prevent weight loss:* weigh every day or every other day, same time and scale; do *not* use with clients who are anorexic.

◆ 3. **Evaluation/outcome criteria:**

a. Improvement in mood and hygiene, thought and communication patterns.

b. Has not harmed self.

c. No significant anticholinergic and cardiovascular side effects.

III. **Antianxiety** (also called anxiolytics, minor tranquilizers) (**Table 10.2**)

A. **Antianxiety agents**

1. **Use**—acute alcohol withdrawal, tension, and irrational fears; anxiety disorders, preoperative sedation; has muscle relaxant and anticonvulsant properties.

◆ 2. **Assessment**—*side effects:* hypotension, drowsiness, motor uncoordination, confusion, skin eruptions, edema, menstrual irregularities, constipation, extrapyramidal symptoms, blurred vision, lethargy; increased or decreased libido.

◆ 3. **Nursing care plan/implementation:**

a. Goal: *administer cautiously, because drug may:*

TABLE 10.2	Antianxiety Agents: Comparison	
Drug	**Use**	**Side Effects/Cautions**
Benzodiazepines *Ativan* (Lorazepam) *Librium* (chlordiazepoxide) *Serax* (oxazepam) *Valium* (diazepam) *Tranxene* (clorazepate) *Xanax* (alprazolam) *Klonopin* (clonazepam)	Short-term, for specific stress	Drowsiness Lethal overdose with alcohol High risk for dependency with long-term use; taper gradually over 2–6 wk Symptoms with abrupt withdrawal: irritability, dizziness Do *not* use in pregnancy
Beta-adrenergic Blocker *Inderal* (propranolol hydrochloride)	Stage fright Relief of physical signs of anxiety (tachycardia)	Hypotension Bradycardia No risk of dependence or abuse
Buspirone hydrochloride *BuSpar*	Long-term use	Less sedation; no risk of dependence *Delayed* effect (3 wk); no CNS depression
Diphenylmethane antihistamine *Atarax* (hydroxyzine hydrochloride) *Vistaril* (hydroxyzine pamoate)	Safe for long-term use	No risk of physical dependency or abuse; minimal toxicity May cause drowsiness

Source: Adapted from ©Lagerquist S: Nurse Notes: Psychiatric-Mental Health, Philadelphia, Lippincott.

(1) Be habituating (causing withdrawal convulsions; therefore *gradual withdrawal* necessary).

(2) Potentiate CNS depressants.

(3) Have adverse effect on pregnancy.

(4) Be dangerous for those: with suicidal tendencies or severe psychoses, narrow angle glaucoma, elderly or debilitated.

b. Goal: *reduce* GI effects: crush tablet or take with meals or milk; give *antacids* 1 hr before.

c. Goal: *monitor effects on liver function:*

> Periodic liver function tests and blood counts, especially with upper respiratory infection, hepatic or renal dysfunction.

d. Goal: *reduce* risk of: hypotension, respiratory depression, phlebitis, venous thrombosis.

e. Goal: *health teaching.*

(1) Advise against suddenly stopping drug (withdrawal symptoms begin in 5–7 days).

(2) Talk with physician if plans to be or is pregnant or lactating.

(3) Urge to drink fluids.

(4) *Avoid:* alcohol, OTC drugs (due to potentiation of other CNS depressants), and heavy smoking and caffeine.

(5) Problem with habituation.

4. **Evaluation/outcome criteria:** decreased alcohol withdrawal symptoms or preoperative anxiety; no seizures or confusion; relief of tension, anxiety, skeletal muscle spasm.

IV. Antimanic

A. **Lithium** (Eskalith, Lithane, Lithobid)—effect occurs 1–3 wk after first dose.

1. **Use**—acute manic attack and prevention of recurrence of cyclic manic-depressive episodes of bipolar disorders.

2. **Assessment**—*side effects:* levels from 1.6 to 2.0 mEq/L may cause: blurred vision, tinnitus, tremors, nausea and vomiting, severe diarrhea, polyuria, polydipsia; ataxia. Levels >2 mEq/L may cause: motor weakness, headache, edema, and lethargy; Levels >2.5 mEq/L *may exhibit signs of severe toxicity:* arrhythmias, MI, cardiovascular collapse, oliguria/anuria; *neurological* (twitching, marked drowsiness, slurred speech, dysarthria, athetotic movements, convulsions, delirium, stupor, coma).

a. *Precautions*—cautious use with clients on *diuretics;* with abnormal *electrolytes* (sweating, dehydrated, and clients who are postoperative); with *thyroid* problems, on *low salt diets;* with *heart failure;* with *impaired renal function;* with *pregnancy and lactation;* risk of suicide.

b. *Dosage*—**therapeutic** level 0.8 to 1.6 mEq/L; dose for maintenance 300–1200 mg/day; *toxic* level >2.0 mEq/L; blood sample drawn

 in acute phase 10–14 hr after last dose, taken tid.

3. **Nursing care plan/implementation:**

a. Goal: *anticipate and check for signs and symptoms of toxicity.*

(1) Reduce GI symptoms: take *with meals.*

(2) Check for edema: daily weight, I&O.

 (3) Monitor blood levels >2.0 mEq/L for side effects and signs of *toxicity:* nausea, vomiting, diarrhea, anorexia, ataxia, weakness, drowsiness, fine tremor or muscle twitching, slurred speech.

(4) Monitor results from repeat thyroid and kidney function tests.

(5) Withhold drug and notify MD when 1.5 mEq/L is reached.

(6) Monitor vital signs 2–3 times/day (pulse irregularities, hypotension, arrhythmias).

b. Goal: *report fever, diarrhea, prolonged vomiting immediately.*

 c. Goal: *monitor effect* (therapeutic and toxic) through blood samples taken:

(1) 10–14 hr after last dose.

(2) Every 2–3 days until 1.6 mEq/L is reached.

(3) Once a week while in hospital.

(4) Every 2–3 mo to maintain blood levels <2 mEq/L.

d. Goal: *health teaching.*

(1) Advise client 1–3 wk lag time for effect.

(2) Urge to drink adequate *liquids* (2–3 L/day), ice; strict oral hygiene.

(3) Report: *polyuria* and polydipsia.

 (4) *Diet:* avoid caffeine, crash diets, diet pills, self-prescribed low salt diet, alcohol, antacids, high sodium foods (which increase lithium excretion and reduce drug effect); take *with meals.* Use sugarless candy.

(5) Caution against driving, operating machinery that requires mental alertness until drug is effective.

(6) Warn *not* to change or omit dose.

4. **Evaluation/outcome criteria:**

a. Changed facial affect.

b. Improved posture, ability to concentrate, sleep patterns; mood is stabilized.

c. Assumption of self-care.

d. No signs of lithium toxicity.

V. Antiparkinsonian agents

A. Trihexphenidyl HCl (Artane).

B. Benztropine mesylate (Cogentin).

1. **Use**—counteract drug-induced extrapyramidal reactions.

2. **Assessment:**

a. Trihexyphenidyl HCl

(1) *Side effects*—anticholinergic: *dry mouth, blurred vision,* dizziness, nausea, *constipa-*

tion, drowsiness, *urinary hesitancy or retention; pupil dilation; headache, weakness, tachycardia.*

    (2) *Precautions*—cautious use with: cardiac, liver, or kidney disease or obstructive gastrointestinal-genitourinary disease, BPH, or myasthenia gravis. Do *not* give if glaucoma present.

  b. Benztropine mesylate—*side effects:* same as for trihexyphenidyl HCl *plus:*

    (1) Effect on *body temperature* (hyperpyrexia) may result in life-threatening state (heatstroke).

    (2) *Gastrointestinal (GI) distress.*

    (3) Inability to concentrate, memory difficulties, and mild confusion (often mistaken for senility); *drowsiness.*

    (4) May lead to toxic *psychotic* reactions.

    (5) *Subjective sensations*—light or heavy feelings in legs, numbness and tingling of extremities, *light-headedness* or tightness of head, and giddiness.

◆ 3. **Nursing care plan/implementation:**

  a. Goal: *relieve GI distress* by giving *after* or *with* meals or at bedtime.

  b. Goal: *monitor adverse effects:*

    (1) Hypotension, tachycardia: check pulse, blood pressure; increased temperature; decreased sweating.

    (2) Constipation and fecal impaction: add roughage to *diet.*

    (3) Dry mouth: increase *fluid* intake; encourage frequent mouth rinsing; offer sugarless candy or gum, ice.

    (4) Blurred vision: suggest reading glasses.

    (5) Dizziness: assist with ambulation; use side rails.

    (6) Urinary retention: maintain I&O.

  c. *Health teaching:*

    (1) *Avoid* driving, and limit activities requiring alertness.

    (2) Delayed drug effect (2–3 days).

    (3) Potential abuse due to hallucinogenic effects.

    (4) *Avoid* alcohol and other CNS depressants; *avoid* hot weather.

    (5) Take with food.

    (6) Do *not* stop drug abruptly.

◆ 4. **Evaluation/outcome criteria:**

  a. Less rigidity, drooling, and oculogyric crisis.

  b. Improved gait, balance, posture.

  c. Has not experienced symptoms of hyperthermia.

MIND-ALTERING SUBSTANCES

Major substances used by the public to alter mental states are compared in **Table 10.3.**

ABSORPTION RATES

Table 10.4.

REGIONAL ANALGESIA-ANESTHESIA IN LABOR AND BIRTH

Table 10.5.

COMMON DRUGS

Table 10.6.

FOOD AND FLUID CONSIDERATIONS WITH DRUGS

Table 10.7.

ANTINEOPLASTIC DRUG CLASSIFICATIONS

Table 10.8.

PROPERTIES OF SELECTED ANALGESIC AGENTS

Table 10.9.

EQUIANALGESIC DOSING FOR OPIOID ANALGESICS

Table 10.10.

DIETARY SUPPLEMENTS AND HERBS

Table 10.11.
Table 10.12.

TABLE 10.3 Major Substances Used for Mind Alteration

Official Name	Slang Name	Usual Single Adult Dose/Duration	Legitimate Medical Uses (Present and Projected)	Short-Term Effects	Long-Term Effects
Alcohol—whisky, gin, beer, wine	Booze, hooch, suds, moonshine, firewater, nightcap	1½ oz gin or whiskey, 12 oz beer/2–4 hr	Rare: sometimes used as a sedative (for tension)	CNS depressant; relaxation (sedation); euphoria; drowsiness; impaired judgment, reaction time, coordination, and emotional control; frequent aggressive behavior and driving accidents; loss of inhibitions; slurred speech	Diversion of energy and money from more creative and productive pursuits; habituation; possible obesity with chronic excessive use; irreversible damage to brain and liver; addiction with severe withdrawal illness (DTs) with heavy use; many deaths
Caffeine—coffee, tea, cola, No-Doz, APC	Java, mud, brew	1–2 cups, 1 bottle, 5 mg/2–4 hr	Mild stimulant; treatment of some forms of coma	CNS stimulant; increased alertness; reduction of fatigue	Sometimes insomnia, restlessness, or gastric irritation; habituation
Nicotine (and coal tar)—cigarettes, cigars, pipe tobacco, snuff	Fags, nails, weeds, butts, chaw, cancer sticks	1–2 cigarettes/1–2 hr	None (used as an insecticide)	CNS stimulant; relaxation or distraction	Lung (and other) cancer, heart and blood vessel disease, cough, etc.; higher infant mortality rate; many deaths; habituation; diversion of energy and money; air pollution; fire
SEDATIVES Alcohol—see above					
Barbiturates—amobarbital (Amytal, Tuinal), pentobarbital (Nembutal), secobarbital (Seconal), phenobarbital	Downers Barbs, blue, angel, blue devils, yellow jackets, yellow birds, dolls, red devils, red birds, phennies, goofers, jelly beans, tooies	50–100 mg	Treatment of insomnia and tension Induction of anesthesia As an anticonvulsant	CNS depressants; sleep induction; relaxation (sedation); sometimes euphoria; drowsiness; impaired judgment, reaction time, coordination, and emotional control; relief of anxiety/tension; muscle relaxation	Irritability, weight loss, addiction with severe withdrawal illness (like DTs); diversion of energy and money; habituation, addiction
Glutethimide (Doriden)	Gorilla pills, CBs, D	500 mg			
Chloral hydrate (Noctec)	Peter, Mickey	500 mg			
Meprobamate (Miltown, Equanil)	Dolls, dollies	400 mg/4 hr[a]			

(Continued on following page)

Pharmacology

737

TABLE 10.3   Major Substances Used for Mind Alteration *(Continued)*

Official Name	Slang Name	Usual Single Adult Dose/Duration	Legitimate Medical Uses- (Present and Projected)	Short-Term Effects	Long-Term Effects
STIMULANTS					
Caffeine—see above	Uppers				
Nicotine—see above					
Amphetamines Methamphetamine (Methedrine, Pesoxyn)	Pep pills, wake-ups, Bennies, splash, peaches Water crystal, speed, meth,	2.5–15.0 mg	Treatment of obesity, narcolepsy, fatigue, depression, hyperkinesia	CNS stimulants; increased alertness; reduction of fatigue; loss of appetite; insomnia; often euphoria, agitation	Restlessness, weight loss, toxic psychosis (mainly paranoid); diversion of energy and money; habituation; extreme irritability, toxic psychosis
Dextroamphetamine (Dexedrine)	Dexies, uppers				
	Diet pills	25 mg		*Symptoms of overdose:* hallucinations, convulsions; cardiac, respiratory failure; coma; pulmonary edema	
Phenmetrazine HCl (Preludin) Cocaine	Coke, snow, blow, happy gold dust, toot, lady, flake, crack, cecil, girl, C	Variable/4 hr[a]	Anesthesia of the eye and throat		
TRANQUILIZERS					
Chlordiazepoxide (Librium)	Green and whites, roaches	5–25 mg	Treatment of anxiety, tension, alcoholism, neurosis, psychosis, psychosomatic disorders, and vomiting	Selective CNS depressants; relaxation, relief of anxiety/tension; suppression of hallucinations or delusions, improved functioning	Sometimes drowsiness, dryness of mouth, blurring of vision, skin rash, tremor; occasionally jaundice, agranulocytosis, or death
Phenothiazines Chlorpromazine HCl (Thorazine)		10–50 mg			
Perchlorperazine (Compazine)		5–10 m			
Trifluoperazine HCl (Stelazine)		2–5 mg			
Reserpine (rauwolfia)		0.10–0.25 mg/4–6 h[a]			
Marijuana or cannabis	Pot, grass, Texas tea, weed, stuff, joint, reefers, Mary Jane, MJ, hay, locoweed	Variable–1 cigarette or pipe, or 1 drink or cake (India)/4 hr[a]	Treatment of depression, tension, loss of appetite, high blood pressure, nausea and vomiting from chemotherapy	Relaxation, euphoria, increased appetite; some alteration of time perception; possible impairment of judgment and coordination; mixed CNS depressant-stimulant; lowered inhibitions	Memory impairment; possible diversion of energy and money; habituation; occasional acute panic reactions (with paranoia, delusions, hallucinations)
Hashish[b]	Hash, rope, Sweet Lucy				

ANTIDEPRESSANTS

Drug	Street names	Dose	Medical use	Effects sought	Long-term symptoms
Dibenzazepine (imipramine [Tofranil], amitriptyline HCl [Elavil])		25 mg, 10 mg	Treatment of moderate to severe depression	Relief of depression (elevation of mood), stimulation	Basically the same as tranquilizers above
MAO inhibitors (phenelzine sulfate [Nardil], tranylcypromine sulfate [Parnate])		10 mg, 15 mg/4–6 h[a]			

NARCOTICS (OPIATES, ANALGESICS)

Drug	Street names	Dose	Medical use	Effects sought	Long-term symptoms
Opium	Op, black, poppy, tar, Big O	10–12 "pipes" (Asia)/4 hr[a]	Treatment of severe pain, diarrhea, and cough	CNS depressants; sedation, euphoria, relief of pain, impaired intellectual functioning and coordination	Constipation, loss of appetite and weight, temporary impotency or sterility; habituation, addiction with unpleasant and painful withdrawal illness
Heroin	Horse, H, smack, shit, junk, brown, pcag, TNT	Variable—bag or paper with 5%–10% heroin			
Morphine (Astramorph)	M, white stuff, Miss Emma	10–15 mg			
Codeine	Terp, robo, romo, syrup	15–30 mg	Topical anesthetic		
Aspirin/oxycodone HCl (Percodan)	Perks, Perkies	1 tablet			
Meperidine HCl (Demerol)	Doctors	50–100 mg			
Methadone (Dolophine)	Dollies, done	2.5–40.0 mg			
Cough syrups (Cheracol, Hycodan, Romilar, etc.)		2–4 oz (for euphoria)/4–6 hr[a]			
Dilaudid	DLs, 4s, lords, little D				

HALLUCINOGENS

Drug	Street names	Dose	Medical use	Effects sought	Long-term symptoms
LSD (Lysergic acid diethylamide)	Acid, sugar cube, trip, big D	150 µg/10–12 hr	Experimental study of mind and brain function; enhancement of creativity and problem solving; treatment of alcoholism, mental illness, and reduction of intractable pain in the person who is dying; chemical warfare	Production of visual imagery, increased sensory awareness, anxiety, nausea, impaired coordination; sometimes consciousness expansion	Usually none; sometimes precipitates or intensifies an already existing psychosis (hallucinations); more commonly can produce a panic reaction (extreme hyperactivity)

(Continued on following page)

TABLE 10.3 Major Substances Used for Mind Alteration (Continued)

Official Name	Slang Name	Usual Single Adult Dose/Duration	Legitimate Medical Uses (Present and Projected)	Short-Term Effects	Long-Term Effects
Psilocybin	Magic mushrooms, God's flesh, rooms	25 mg			
STP	Serenity, tranquility, peace	6 mg			
DMT	Businessman's Trip				
Mescaline (peyote)	Cactus, mesc, mescal, half moon, big chief, bad seed	350 mg/12–14 hr			
PCP (Phencyclidine)	Angel dust, hog, rocket fuel				
MDMA	Ecstasy, XTC, Adam				
MISCELLANEOUS					
Glue, gasoline, and solvents		Variable	None except for antihistamines used for allergy and amyl nitrite for fainting	When used for mind alteration generally produces a "high" (euphoria) with impaired coordination and judgment	Variable—some of the substances can seriously damage the liver or kidney, and some produce hallucinations
Amyl nitrite	Pearls, poppers	1–2 ampules			
Antihistamines		25–50 mg			
Nutmeg		Variable/2 hr			
Nonprescription "sedatives" (Compoze)					
Catnip					
Nitrous oxide					

[a]Time given pertains to all drugs listed.

[b]Hashish or charas is a more concentrated form of the active ingredient THC (tetrahydrocannabinol) and is consumed in smaller doses, analogous to vodka–beer ratios.

Copyright © Joel Fort, MD, author of *Alcohol: Our Biggest Drug Problems* (McGraw-Hill) and *The Pleasure Seekers* (Grove Press); founder, The National Center for Solving Special and Health Problem—FORT HELP and the Violence Prevention Program, San Francisco; and formerly Lecturer, School of Criminology, University of California, Berkeley, and Consultant, World Health Organization. Used by permission.

TABLE 10.4	Rates of Absorption by Different Routes

Route of Administration	Time Until Drug Takes Effect*
Topical	Hours to days
Oral	30–90 min
Rectal	5–30 min (unpredictable)
Subcutaneous injection	15–30 min
Intramuscular injection	10–20 min
Sublingual tablet	3–5 min
Inhalation	3 min
Endotracheal	3 min
Intravenous	30–60 sec
Intracardiac	15 sec

*In a healthy person with normal perfusion.

TABLE 10.5	Regional Analgesia-Anesthesia for Labor and Birth

Types	Characteristics	◆ Nursing Implications
Common Agents in 0.5%–1.0% Solution Lidocaine (Xylocaine) Bupivacaine (Marcaine) HCl Tetracaine (Pontocaine) HCl Mepivacaine HCl (Carbocaine) Chloroprocaine HCl (Nesacaine) Ropivucaine (Norapin)	Used with epinephrine (or other vasoconstric-tor drug) to delay absorption, prolong anesthetic effect, and decrease chance of hypotension	*Note any history of allergy;* note response: allergic reaction, hypotension, and lack of wearing off of anesthetic effect; observe for hypertensive crisis if agent combined with epinephrine and oxytocin is also being given
Peripheral Nerve Block Pudendal (5–10 mL each side) anesthetizes lower two-thirds of vagina and perineum	Perineal anesthesia of short duration (30 min); local anesthesia; simple and safe; does not depress neonate; may inhibit bearing-down reflex	To get cooperation, give explanation during procedure
Paracervical (uterosacral) block (5–10 mL given into each side) anesthetizes cervix and upper two-thirds of vagina; *note:* used more for gynecological surgery than for labor	When the cervix is dilated, may be given between 3 and 8 cm by physician when woman is having at least three contractions in 10 min; lasts 45–90 min; can be repeated; can be followed by local, epidural, or other; may cause temporary fetal bradycardia	Explain: especially length and type of needle; take maternal vital signs and FHR; have her void; help position; monitor FHR continuously; monitor contractions; and watch for return of pain
Local infiltration	Useful for perineal repairs	No special nursing care
Epidural lumbar block	Useful during first and second stages; can be given "one shot" or continuously; T-10 to S-5 for vaginal birth; T-8 to S-1 for abdom-inal birth; complete anesthesia for labor and birth	*Hypotension* (with resultant fetal bradycar-dia): (a) turn from supine to lateral, or *elevate* legs, (b) administer humidified oxygen by mask at 8–10 L/min, (c) increase rate of IV fluids (use infusate *without* oxytocin); will need coaching to push and low forceps or vacuum may be required
Subarachnoid spinal Continuous	Useful during first or second stage of labor, or for abdominal surgery	Instruct when to bear down
Low spinal ("saddle," "one shot") block	Same as continuous	Same as continuous
Intrathecal (spinal): morphine, fentanyl, sufentanil	0.5 mg produces marked analgesia for 12–24 hr; onset in 20–30 min Fentanyl and sufentanil produce short-acting analgesia (1 $\frac{1}{2}$–3 $\frac{1}{2}$ hr)	*Side effects:* respiratory depression, pruri-tus, nausea, vomiting, sleepiness, urinary retention; keep *naloxone* 0.4 mg at bedside and respiratory support equipment readily available

TABLE 10.6	Common Drugs		
Drug and Dosage	**Use**	**Action**	◆ **Assessment: Side Effects**

Adrenergics

Alpha and beta agonists

Epinephrine (Adrenalin)—SC or IM 0.1–1 mg in 1:1000 solution; IV—intracardiac 1:10,000 solution; ophthalmic 1:1000–1:50,000 solution	Asystole, bronchospasm, anaphylaxis, glaucoma	Stimulates pacemaker cells; inhibits histamine and mediates bronchial relaxation; ↓ intraocular pressure	Ventricular arrhythmias, fear, anxiety, anginal pain, decreased renal blood flow, burning of eyes, headache

NURSING IMPLICATIONS: Use TB syringe for greater accuracy; massaging injection site hastens action; repeated injections may cause tissue necrosis; *avoid* injection in buttocks because bacteria in area may lead to gas gangrene; may make mucous plugs in lungs more difficult to dislodge

Norepinephrine (Levophed)—IV 8–12 μg/min titrated to desired response	Acute hypotension, cardiogenic shock	Increases rate and strength of heartbeat; increases vasoconstriction	Palpitations, pallor, headache, hypertension; anxiety, insomnia; dilated pupils, nausea, vomiting; glycosuria, tissue sloughing

NURSING IMPLICATIONS: Observe vital signs, mentation, skin temperature, and color (earlobes, lips, nailbeds); tissue necrosis occurs with infiltration; *antidote* is phentolamine 5–10 mg in 10–15 mL normal saline

Beta agonists

Dobutamine (Dobutrex)—IV 1.5–10 μg/kg/min	Acute heart failure	Stimulates cardiac contractile force (positive inotropy); fewer changes in heart rate than dopamine or isoproterenol	Tachycardia, arrhythmias

NURSING IMPLICATIONS: Mix with 5% dextrose; do *not* dilute until ready to use; protect from light; administer with infusion pump; check vital signs constantly; extravasation can produce tissue necrosis; see Norepinephrine

Dopamine (Inotropin)—IV 1–5 μg/kg/min titrated to desired response; gradually increase to 1–4 μg/kg/min increments at 10–30 min intervals; must maintain at 20 μg/kg/min or less	Acute heart failure	↑ Cardiac contractility; ↑ renal blood flow	Ectopic beats; nausea, vomiting; tachycardia, anginal pain, dyspnea, hypotension

NURSING IMPLICATIONS: Monitor vital signs, urine output, and signs of peripheral ischemia; will cause tissue sloughing if infiltration occurs

Isoproterenol (Isuprel)—10–15 mg sublingually; IV 0.5–5.0 μg/min in solution	Cardiogenic shock, heart block, bronchospasm—asthma, emphysema	↑ Cardiac contractility; facilitates AV conduction and pacemaker automaticity	Tachyarrhythmias, hypotension, headache, flushing of skin; nausea; tremor; dizziness

NURSING IMPLICATIONS: Monitor vital signs, ECG; oral inhalation solutions must *not* be injected

Analgesics

(see Table 10.10 for Equianalgesic Dosing)

Acetaminophen (Tylenol, Datril, Panadol)—PO 325–650 mg q4h	Simple fever or pain	Analgesic and antipyretic actions; no antiinflammatory or anticoagulant effects	No remarkable side effects when taken for a short period

NURSING IMPLICATIONS: Consult with physician if no relief after 4 d of therapy

Aspirin (acetylsalicylic acid)—PO or rectal 0.3–0.6 g	Minor aches and pains; fever from colds and influenza; rheumatoid arthritis; anticoagulant therapy	Selectively depresses subcortical levels of CNS	Erosive gastritis with bleeding; coryza, urticaria; nausea, vomiting; tinnitus, impaired hearing, and respiratory alkalosis

NURSING IMPLICATIONS: Administer *with food or after meals*; observe for nasal, oral, or subcutaneous bleeding; push fluids; check *Hct, Hgb, prothrombin times* frequently; *avoid* use in children with flu

(Continued on following page)

Drug and Dosage	Use	Action	◆ Assessment: Side Effects
◆ Butorphanol (Stadol) IM: 1–2 mg IV: 0.5–2 mg	**Obstetric use:** Control pain, especially during labor.	30–40 times more potent than meperidine; onset: 2–15 min; duration; 0.5–2 hr	No excessive sedation. Neonatal respiratory depression less than with meperidine. Pseudo-sinusoidal FHR pattern after administration.

NURSING IMPLICATIONS: Care must be taken that drug is *not* given with meperidine, as it may potentiate effects of meperidine; *avoid* in clients who are opioid-addicted

| Celecoxib (Celebrex)—
PO 100–200 mg bid or 200 mg qd | Arthritis; acute pain; dysmenorrhea | NSAID, antiinflammatory, analgesic, antipyretic; inhibits prostaglandin synthesis | Back pain; peripheral edema; diarrhea; dizziness; rash, rhinitis |

NURSING IMPLICATIONS: Monitor for signs of fluid retention and edema; report *promptly* unexplained wt. gain, rash

| Codeine—PO, IM, or SC 15–60 mg (gr ¼ to 1) | Control pain; may be used during the puerperium | Nonsynthetic narcotic analgesic | Of little use during labor; allergic response; constipation; GI upset |

NURSING IMPLICATIONS: Note response to the medication; less respiratory depression; preferred for client with head injury

| Ecotrin (enteric-coated aspirin) | See Aspirin | See Aspirin | See Aspirin |

NURSING IMPLICATIONS: See Aspirin; do *not* take with milk or dairy

| Etodolac (Lodine)—PO 400–1200 mg/day, 300–400 q6–8h | Management of osteoarthritis; mild to moderate pain | Inhibits prostaglandin synthesis; suppression of inflammation and pain (NSAID) | Dyspepsia; asthma; drowsiness, dizziness; rash, tinnitus, anaphylaxis |

NURSING IMPLICATIONS: Give 30 min *before or* 2 hr *after* meals for rapid effect; may be taken with food to decrease GI irritation

| Fentanyl transdermal (Duragesic)—25–100 μg/hr | Chronic pain; not recommended for postoperative pain

Obstetric use: Short-acting pain control during labor | Binds to opiate receptors in the CNS to alter response and perception of pain | Drowsiness, confusion, weakness; constipation, dry mouth, nausea, vomiting, anorexia; sweating |

NURSING IMPLICATIONS: Apply to upper torso, flat, nonirritated surface; when applying, hold firmly with palm of hand 10–20 sec

| Hydrocodone/Acetaminophen (Vicodin)—PO 5–10 mg q4–6h | Moderate to severe pain

Obstetric use: in postpartum to control pain | Bind to opiate receptors in CNS; alter perception of and response to painful stimuli | Confusion, sedation, hypotension, constipation |

NURSING IMPLICATIONS: Assess: type, location, and intensity of pain before and 1 hr (peak) after giving; prolonged use may lead to physical and psychological dependence; give with *food or milk* to reduce GI irritation

| Hydromorphone (Dilaudid)—PO 2–4 mg q3–6h; IM 1–2 mg q3–6h up to 2–4 mg q4–6h; IV 0.5–1.0 mg q3h | Moderate to severe pain; antitussive | Bind to opiate receptors in the CNS; alter perception and response to pain | Sedation, confusion, hypotension, constipation |

NURSING IMPLICATIONS: Give PO with *food or milk*; give IV 2 mg over 3–5 min; *fluids, bulk,* and laxatives to minimize constipation

| Ibuprofen (Motrin)—300–800 mg oral 3–4/day (not to exceed 3200 mg/day) | Nonsteroid antiinflammatory, antirheumatic used in chronic arthritis pain

Obstetric use: uterine cramping postpartum (not used during pregnancy) | Inhibition of prostaglandin synthesis or release | GI upset, leukopenia; sodium/water retention |

NURSING IMPLICATIONS: Give on *empty stomach* for best result; may mix with food if GI upset severe; teach caution when using other medications

(Continued on following page)

TABLE 10.6	Common Drugs *(Continued)*		
Drug and Dosage	**Use**	**Action**	◆ **Assessment: Side Effects**
Indomethacin (Indocin)—PO 25 mg 3–4/ day; increase to max 200 mg daily in divided doses	Rheumatoid arthritis; bursitis; gouty arthritis Closure of PDA in premature infants and some newborns	Antipyretic/antiinflammatory action; inhibits prostaglandin biosynthesis	GI distress, bleeding; rash; headache; blood dyscrasias; corneal changes
NURSING IMPLICATIONS: Monitor GI side effects; administer *after* meals for best effect or *with* food, milk, or antacids if GI symptoms severe			
Ketorolac (Toradol)—PO, IV 10 mg q4–6h; IM 30–60 mg initially, then 15–30 mg q6h; ophthalmic 1 gtt qid for 1 wk	Short-term management of pain; ocular itching due to allergies (NSAID)	Inhibits prostaglandin synthesis producing peripherally mediated analgesia; antipyretic/ antiinflammatory	Drowsiness, dizziness, dyspnea; prolonged bleeding time; dyspepsia
NURSING IMPLICATIONS: May be given routinely or prn; *advise* dentist or MD before any procedure			
Meperidine HCI (Demerol)— PO or IM 50–100 mg q3–4h	Pain due to trauma or surgery; allay apprehension before surgery	Acts on CNS to produce analgesia, sedation, euphoria, and respiratory depression	Palpitations, bradycardia, hypotension; nausea, vomiting; syncope, sweating, tremors, convulsions
NURSING IMPLICATIONS: Check *respiratory rate* and depth before giving drug; give IM, because subcutaneous administration is painful and can cause local irritation			
	Obstetric use: maternal relaxation may either slow labor or speed up labor	Acts as a uterine irritant; depresses CNS, maternal and fetal; allays apprehension; PO peak action—1–2 hr; IM peak action first hour	Maternal side effects same as above; also can depress fetus
NURSING IMPLICATIONS: Monitor maternal vital signs, contractions, progress of labor, and response to drug; fetal heart rate; if delivery occurs during peak action, prepare to give *narcotic antagonist* to mother or neonate or both			
Morphine SO₄—PO 10–30 mg (Roxanol, MS Contin); SC 8–15 mg; IV 4–10 mg; rectal 10–20 mg	Control pain and relieve fear, apprehension, restlessness, as in pulmonary edema	Depresses CNS reception of pain and ability to interpret stimuli; depresses respiratory center in medulla	Nausea, vomiting; flushing; confusion; urticaria; depressed rate and depth of respirations, decreased blood pressure
NURSING IMPLICATIONS: Check rate and depth of *respirations* before administering drug; observe for gas pains and *abdominal distention;* smaller doses for aged; monitor vital signs; observe for postural hypotension			
	Obstetric use: preeclampsia, eclampsia; uterine dysfunction; pain relief	Increases cerebral blood flow; provides antihypertensive action; CNS depressant	Respiratory and circulatory depression in mother and neonate; may depress contractions
NURSING IMPLICATIONS: Observe for level of sedation, respirations, arousability, and deep-tendon reflex; give *narcotic antagonist* as necessary; check I & O (*urinary retention* possible)			
Nalbuphine (Nubain) IV: 1 mg at 6–10 min intervals	**Obstetric use:** pain relief during labor. *Avoid* in clients who are opioid addicted.	Onset: 2–15 min; duration 1–4 hr	Increased sedation and limited ceiling effect; ceiling effect for neonatal respiratory depression
NURSING IMPLICATIONS: Less nausea and vomiting and sedation if given with PCA. Prophylactic nalbuphine seems unable to prevent pruritus			
Naproxen (Naprosyn)—PO 250–500 mg bid	Mild to moderate pain; dysmenorrhea; rheumatoid arthritis; osteoarthritis (NSAID)	Inhibits prostaglandin synthesis; suppression of inflammation	Headache, drowsiness, dizziness, nausea, dyspepsia, constipation, bleeding
NURSING IMPLICATIONS: Take with a full glass of *water; avoid* exposure to sun			

(Continued on following page)

Drug and Dosage	Use	Action	◆ Assessment: Side Effects
Oxycodone HCl (Percodan, Tylox)—PO 3–20 mg; SC 5 mg	**Postpartum use:** control pain; may be used during puerperium; 5–6 times more potent than codeine	Less potent and addicting than morphine; for moderate pain—episiotomy and "afterpains"; peak action 1 hr	See Morphine SO$_4$

NURSING IMPLICATIONS: Administer per order and observe for effect

Pentazocine (Talwin)—PO 50–100 mg; IM 30–60 mg q3–4h	Relief of moderate to severe pain	Narcotic antagonist, opioid antagonist properties, equivalent to codeine	Repiratory depression, nausea, vomiting, dizziness, light-headedness, seizures

NURSING IMPLICATIONS: Monitor *respirations*, BP; *caution* with client with MI, head injuries, COPD

Antacids (see Antiulcer)

Antiadrenal

Aminoglutethimide (Cytadren)—250 mg q6h	Cushing's	Inhibits enzymatic conversion of cholesterol to pregnenolone, thus reducing synthesis of adrenal glucocorticoids/ mineralocorticoids	Cortical hypofunction, hypotension, hypothyroidism

NURSING IMPLICATIONS: Monitor: vital signs, lab values, disease signs and symptoms; observe frequently during periods of stress

Antianemics

Ferrous sulfate (Feosol, Fer-in-Sol)—adults, PO 300 mg—1.2 g qd; children under 6 yr, PO 75–225 mg qd; 6–12 yr, PO 120—600 mg qd	Iron deficiency anemia; prophylactically during infancy, childhood, pregnancy	Corrects nutritional iron deficiency anemia	Nausea, vomiting, anorexia, constipation, diarrhea; yellow-brown discoloration of eyes, teeth

NURSING IMPLICATIONS: To minimize GI distress, give *with* meals; do *not* give with antacids or tea; liquid form should be taken through straw to prevent *staining* of teeth; causes dark-green/black stool

Antianginals

Atenolol (Tenormin)—PO 50–150 mg daily; IV 5 mg initially, wait 10 min, then another 5 mg	Hypertension: angina; arrhythmias	Blocks (cardiac) beta-adrenergic receptors	Fatigue, weakness, bradycardia, heart failure, pulmonary edema

NURSING IMPLICATIONS: Give 1 mg/min IV; check vital signs; assess for signs of fluid *overload*

Isosorbide dinitrate (Isordil, Isorbid)—sublingual 2.5–10.0 mg q5–10min for 3 doses; PO 5–10 mg initially, 10–40 mg q6h	Acute angina: long-term prophylaxis for angina; heart failure	Produces vasodilation, decreases preload	Headache, dizziness, hypotension, tachycardia

NURSING IMPLICATIONS: *Avoid* eating, drinking, or smoking until sublingual tablets are dissolved; change positions *slowly;* aspirin or acetaminophen for headache. Determine if client is taking drugs for erectile dysfunction—serious drug interaction!

Nitroglycerin—sublingual 0.25–0.6 mg prn; transdermal (patch) 2.5–15.0 mg/day; topical 2–3 inches q8h; IV 10–20 μg/min	Angina pectoris; adjunctive treatment in MI, heart failure, hypertension (IV form)	Directly relaxes smooth muscle, dilating blood vessels; lowers peripheral vascular resistance; increases blood flow	Faintness, throbbing headache; vomiting; flushing, hypotension; visual disturbances

NURSING IMPLICATIONS: Instruct client to sit or lie down when taking drug, to reduce *hypotensive* effect; onset 1–3 min; may take 1–3 doses at 5 min intervals to relieve pain; up to *10/day* may be allowed; if headache occurs, tell client to expel tab as soon as pain relief occurs; keep drug at bedside or on person; watch *expiration* dates—tabs lose potency with exposure to air and humidity; *alcohol* ingestion soon after taking may produce shocklike syndrome from drop in BP; *smoking* causes vasoconstricting effect; causes burning under tongue; may crush between teeth to ↑ absorption

(Continued on following page)

Pharmacology

TABLE 10.6	Common Drugs *(Continued)*		
Drug and Dosage	**Use**	**Action**	◆ **Assessment: Side Effects**
Antiarrhythmics			
(also see Calcium Channel Blockers)			
Amiodarone hydrochloride (Cordarone)—PO 800–1600 mg/d loading dose; 400–600 mg/d maintenance	Life-threatening ventricular arrhythmias; supraventricular arrhythmias (e.g., atrial fibrillation)	Class III antiarrhythmic; antianginal, antiadrenergic	Muscle weakness, fatigue, dizziness, hypotension with IV; corneal microdeposits; anorexia, nausea, vomiting; photosensitivity
NURSING IMPLICATIONS: Monitor VS. Expect possible CNS symptoms 1 wk after beginning drug. Instruct client to protect eyes and skin from sun			
Bretylium (Bretylol)—IV 0.5–10 mg/kg q6h; IM 5–10 mg/kg (max 250 mg in one site)	Ventricular fibrillation; ventricular tachycardia	Inhibits norepinephrine release from sympathetic nerve endings; increased fibrillation threshold	Worsening of arrhythmia; tachycardia and increased BP initially; nausea, vomiting; hypotension later
NURSING IMPLICATIONS: Monitor BP and cardiac status closely; *rotate* IM injection sites; no more than 5 mL/site			
Diphenylhydantoin (Dilantin)—PO 100–200 mg 3–4 times daily; IV loading dose 10–15 mg/kg (not to exceed 50 mg/min), 50–100 mg over 5–10 min	Digitalis toxicity; ventricular ectopy	Depresses pacemaker activity in SA node and Purkinje tissue without slowing conduction velocity	Severe pain if administered in small vein; ataxia, vertigo, nystagmus, seizures, confusion; skin eruptions, hypotension if administered too fast
NURSING IMPLICATIONS: With IV use monitor vital signs; observe for CNS side effects; have O_2 on hand; seizure precautions (padded side rails, nonmetal airway; suction, mouth gag); also see Anticonvulsants			
Lidocaine HCl—IV 50–100 mg; bolus; 1–4 mg/kg/min, IV drip	Ventricular tachycardia; PVCs	Depresses myocardial response to abnormally generated impulses	Drowsiness, dizziness, nervousness, confusion, paresthesias
NURSING IMPLICATIONS: Monitor vital signs; observe for signs of CNS toxicity; monitor ECG for *prolonged PR* interval			
Metoprolol tartrate (Lopressor)—PO 25 mg/d; range 25–300 mg/d	Hypertension; angina; MI	Beta-adrenergic blocker; ↓ CO, ↓ HR	Dizziness, fatigue, insomnia; bradycardia, SOB
NURSING IMPLICATIONS: Monitor: vital signs carefully; I&O, daily wt; check for *rales*. Give with or without food—be consistent			
Procainamide HCl (Pronestyl)—PO, IM 500–1000 mg 4–6 times qd; IV 1 g	Atrial and ventricular arrhythmias; PVCs; overdose of digitalis; general anesthesia	Depresses myocardium; lengthens conduction time between atria and ventricles	Polyarthralgia; fever, chills, urticaria; nausea, vomiting; psychoses; rapid decrease in BP
NURSING IMPLICATIONS: Check pulse rate *before* giving; monitor heart action during IV administration			
Propranolol HCl (Inderal)—0.5–3.0 mg IV push (up to 3 mg); 20—60 mg orally 3–4 times daily	Ventricular ectopy; angina unresponsive to nitrites, paroxysmal atrial tachycardia; hypertension	Beta-adrenergic blocker, ↓ cardiac contractility, ↓ heart rate, ↓ myocardial oxygen requirements	Bradycardia, hypotension, vertigo, paresthesia of hands
NURSING IMPLICATIONS: Instruct client to take pulse *before* each dose; do *not* give to clients with history of asthma or chronic obstructive pulmonary disease, no smoking, because hypertension may occur			
Quinidine SO_4—PO 0.2–0.6 g q2h loading dose; maintenance: 400–1000 mg tid–qid; IV 5–10 mg/kg over 30–60 min	Atrial fibrillation; PAT; ventricular tachycardia; PVCs	Lengthens conduction time in atria and ventricles; blocks vagal stimulation of heart	Nausea, vomiting, diarrhea; vertigo, tremor, headache; abdominal cramps; AV block, cardiac arrest
NURSING IMPLICATIONS: *Count pulse before* giving; report changes in rate, quality, or rhythm; give drug *with food*; monitor BP daily			

(Continued on following page)

Drug and Dosage	Use	Action	◆ Assessment: Side Effects
Antiasthmatics			
Cromolyn sodium—inhale, 1 cap 4 times qd	Perennial bronchial asthma (*not acute* asthma or status asthmaticus)	Inhibits release of bronchoconstrictors—histamine and SRS-A; suppresses allergic response	Cough, hoarseness, wheezing; dry mouth, bitter aftertaste, urticaria; urinary frequency

NURSING IMPLICATIONS: Instruct on use of inhaler—exhale; tilt head back; inhale rapidly, deeply, steadily; remove inhaler exhale—repeat until dose is taken; gargle or drink water after treatment

Anticholelithics			
Ursodeoxycholic (Actigall)	Gallstones	Dissolves gallstones	Diarrhea; *avoid* concurrent use with bile acid sequestrants

NURSING IMPLICATIONS: *Monitor* for pain, GI distress

Anticholinergics (antimuscarinics)			
Atropine, SO_4—0.3–1.2 mg PO, SC, IM, or IV; ophthalmic 0.5–1.0% up to 6 times qd	Peptic ulcer; spasms of GI tract, Stokes-Adams syndrome; control excessive secretions during surgery	Blocks parasympathomimetic effects of acetylcholine on effector organs	Dry mouth, tachycardia, blurred vision, drowsiness, skin flushing; urinary retention; *contraindications:* glaucoma and paralytic ileus

NURSING IMPLICATIONS: Observe for postural *hypotension* in clients who are ambulating; administer cautiously in aged; and monitor vital signs for pulse and respiratory rate changes

Dicyclomine (Bentyl) 10–20 mg 3–4/day	Diverticulosis	Antispasmodic	Blurred vision; constipation; dry eyes, dry mouth

NURSING IMPLICATIONS: Report symptoms listed under side effects, abdominal pain

Glycopyrrolate (Robinul)—PO 1–2 mg bid/tid; IM, IV 4.4 μg/kg (preop); 100–200 μg qid (ulcer)	Inhibit salivation and respiratory secretions; peptic ulcer disease	Inhibits action of acetylcholine (antimuscarinic action)	Tachycardia; dry mouth; urinary hesitancy

NURSING IMPLICATIONS: Give 30–60 min. *before* meals; do *not* give within 1 h of antacids; IM or IV may be given undiluted

Hyoscyamine (Levsinex) 0.125–0.5 mg 3-4/day; or 0.375 mg twice a day in released tablets	Diverticulosis	Manages spasms of irritable bowel syndrome	Constipation; dry mouth, blurred vision

NURSING IMPLICATIONS: *Monitor* for: pain, bleeding, constipation, drug reaction

Propantheline bromide (Pro-Banthine)—PO 15 mg qid; IM or IV 30 mg	Decreases hypertonicity and hypersecretion of GI tract; ulcerative colitis; peptic ulcer	Blocks neural transmission at ganglia of autonomic nervous system and at parasympathetic effector organs	Nausea, gastric fullness, constipation; mydriasis

NURSING IMPLICATIONS: Give *before* meals; observe urinary output to *avoid retention*, particularly in elderly; mouth care to relieve dryness; *contraindicated* with glaucoma

Tincture of belladonna—0.3–0.6 mL tid	Hypermotility of stomach; bowel, biliary, and renal colic; prostatitis	Blocks parasympathomimetic effects of acetylcholine	Dry mouth, thirst; dilated pupils; skin flushing; elevated temperature; delirium

NURSING IMPLICATIONS: Administer 30–60 min *before* meals; observe for side effects; *physostigmine salicylate* is antidote

Tolterodine tartrate (Detrol LA)—PO 2 mg bid; 4 mg SR qd	Overactive bladder	Selective muscarinic urinary bladder receptor antagonist	Dry mouth; back pain; fatigue, weight gain

NURSING IMPLICATIONS: Report eye pain *promptly.* Blurred vision, sensitivity to light, and dry mouth should be reported if bothersome

(Continued on following page)

TABLE 10.8	Common Drugs *(Continued)*		
Drug and Dosage	**Use**	**Action**	◆ **Assessment: Side Effects**
Anticoagulants			
Enoxaparin (Lovenox)—30–40 mg bid SC, 7–10 days; or 1 mg/kg q12h	Deep vein thrombosis; prophylaxis before knee and abdominal surgery	Potentiates inhibitory effect of antithrombin	Bleeding, anemia, thrombocytopenia
NURSING IMPLICATIONS: Observe injection sites for, hematomas, ecchymosis, or inflammation; *ice cube massage* at site, prior to injection may lessen bruising			
Heparin—initial dose: IV 5,000–20,000–40,000 U followed by infusion over 24 hr	Acute thromboembolic emergencies	Prevents thrombin formation	Hematuria, bleeding gums, ecchymosis
NURSING IMPLICATIONS: Observe clotting times—should be 20–30 min; antagonist is *protamine sulfate*			
Warfarin sodium (Coumadin)—initial dose: PO 10–15 mg; maintenance dose: PO 2–10 mg qd	Venous thrombosis; atrial fibrillation with embolization; pulmonary emboli; myocardial infarction	Depresses liver synthesis of prothrombin and factors VII, IX, and X	Minor or major hemorrhage; alopecia; fever; nausea, diarrhea; dermatitis
NURSING IMPLICATIONS: Drug effects last 3–4 days; antagonist is vitamin K; *avoid* foods high in vitamin K; *no* aspirin			
Anticoagulant Antidotes			
Protamine sulfate 1%—IV 10 mg/mL slowly; 1 mg/100 U heparin	Overdose of heparin	Positive electrostatic charge inactivates negatively charged heparin molecules	Excessive coagulation; hypotension, bradycardia, dyspnea
NURSING IMPLICATIONS: Slow IV; no more than 50 mg in 10 min period; monitor VS continuously; check *APTT* for effectiveness			
Vitamin K (Aquamephyton, Konakion)—PO, IM, SC 2.5–25.0 mg; 0.5—1.0 mg in newborns	Warfarin (Coumadin) hypoprothrombinemia; hemorrhagic disease in newborns	Counteracts the inhibitory effects of oral anticoagulants on hepatic synthesis of vitamin K–dependent clotting factors	Flushing, hypotension, allergic reactions; reappearance of clotting problems (high doses)
NURSING IMPLICATIONS: Give IV only if absolutely necessary; dilute with preservative-free 0.9% NaCl, D_5W, or D_5NaCl; protect solution *from light*; repeat injection may cause redness and pain; check *PT* for drug effect			
Anticonvulsants			
Carbamazepine (Tegretol) 200 mg twice/day (range: 600–1200/day in divided doses)	Multiple sclerosis	Decreases synaptic transmission in CNS by affecting sodium channels in neurons	Contraindicated in hypersensitivity, bone marrow depression; drowsiness, ataxia, agranulocytosis, aplastic anemia
NURSING IMPLICATIONS: Monitor: CBC, liver function, ECG. Therapeutic levels should be 6–12 μg/mL; take medication as directed around the clock; use sunscreen due to photosensitivity			
Clonazepam (Klonopin)—PO 1.5 mg in 3 doses initially, 0.5–1.0 mg every third day	Absence seizures (petit mal seizures, myoclonic seizures)	Produces anticonvulsant and sedative effects in the CNS; mechanism unknown	Drowsiness, ataxia, behavioral changes
NURSING IMPLICATIONS: Give with food; evaluate *liver enzymes, CBC,* and *platelets; avoid* abrupt withdrawal—may cause status epilepticus			
Diazepam (Valium)—PO 2–10 mg bid–qid; IM or IV 5–10 mg	All types of seizures **Obstetric use:** eclampsia	Induces calming effect on limbic system, thalamus, and hypothalamus	Drowsiness, ataxia, paradoxical increase in CNS excitability
NURSING IMPLICATIONS: IV may cause phlebitis; give IV injection *slowly*, because respiratory arrest can occur; inject IM *deeply* into tissue			

(Continued on following page)

Drug and Dosage	Use	Action	◆ Assessment: Side Effects
Ethosuximide (Zarontin)—PO 500 mg/day, increase by 250 mg/day until effective	Absence seizures	Depresses motor cortex and reduces CNS sensitivity to convulsive nerve stimul	GI distress: nausea, vomiting, cramps, diarrhea, anorexia; blood dyscrasias

NURSING IMPLICATIONS: Administer *with* meals; 🖊 regular *CBC*; precautions to avoid injury from drowsiness

Magnesium salts 4–5 g by IV infusion	Cirrhosis	Osmotically active in GI tract	Use caution in renal failure; *contraindicated* in: hyper-magnesemia, anuria, heart block

NURSING IMPLICATIONS: *Monitor:* vital signs, seizure precautions, I&O; *respiratory rate must be 16* before administration

Magnesium sulfate—PO 1–5 g/IM or IV 1–4 g loading dose, followed by continuous infusion (2–3 g/hr)	Control seizures in pregnancy, epilepsy; relief of acute constipation; reduces edema, inflammation, and itching of skin; may inhibit preterm contractions	Depresses CNS and smooth, cardiac, and skeletal muscle; promotes osmotic retention of fluid	Flushing, sweating, extreme thirst; complete heart block; dehydration; depressed or absent reflexes, ↓ respirations

NURSING IMPLICATIONS: If given IV, monitor vital signs continuously; I&O; use with caution in clients with *impaired renal* functions; observe mother and newborn for signs of toxicity if given near birth; *antidote:* calcium gluconate

Phenytoin or diphenylhydantoin (Dilantin) SO_4—PO 30–100 mg 3–4 times qd; IM 100–200 mg 3–4 times qd; IV 150–250 mg	Psychomotor epilepsy, convulsive seizures; ventricular arrhythmias	Depresses motor cortex by preventing spread of abnormal electrical impulses	Nervousness, ataxia; gastric distress; nystagmus; slurred speech; hallucinations; gingival hyperplasia

NURSING IMPLICATIONS: Give *with* meals *or* pc; frequent and diligent mouth care; advise client that urine may turn *pink to red-brown;* teach client signs of adverse reactions; mix IV with normal saline (precipitates with D_5W)

Primidone (Mysoline)—PO 100–250 mg, increase over 10 days (not to exceed 2 g/day)	Tonic-clonic, focal, or local seizures	Inhibits abnormal brain electrical activity; dose-dependent CNS depression	Excessive sedation or ataxia, vertigo

NURSING IMPLICATIONS: Careful neurological, cardiovascular, and respiratory assessment; have resuscitation equipment available

Valproic acid (Depakene)—PO 15 mg/kg/day, increase up to 60 mg/kg/day	Absence, tonic-clonic, myoclonic, focal, or local seizures	Inhibits spread of abnormal discharges through brain	Nausea, vomiting, diarrhea (disappear over time); drowsiness or sedation if taken in combination with other anticonvulsants

NURSING IMPLICATIONS: Assess responses; 🧪 monitor blood levels; precautions against excessive sedation; *discourage alcohol* use

Antidiarrheals

Diphenoxylate HCl with atropine sulfate (Lomotil)—PO 5–10 mg tid–qid	Diarrhea	Increases intestinal tone and decreases propulsive peristalsis	Rash; drowsiness, dizziness; depression; abdominal distention; headache, blurred vision; nausea

NURSING IMPLICATIONS: May *potentiate* action of barbiturates, opiates, and other depressants; closely observe clients receiving these drugs, and administer *narcotic antagonists* such as levallorphan tartrate (Lorfan), naloxone HCl (Narcan), and nalorphine HCl (Naline) as ordered; administer cautiously to clients with hepatic dysfunction—may precipitate *hepatic coma*

Kaolin with pectin (Kaopectate)—adults, PO 60–120 mL after each bowel movement (BM); children over 12, PO 60 mL; 6–12 yr, PO 30–60 mL; 3–6 yr, PO 15–30 mL after each BM	Diarrhea	Reported to absorb irritants and soothe	Granuloma of the stomach

NURSING IMPLICATIONS: Do *not* administer for more than 2 days, in presence of fever, or to children younger than 3 yr

(Continued on following page)

Pharmacology

TABLE 10.6	Common Drugs *(Continued)*

Drug and Dosage	Use	Action	◆ Assessment: Side Effects
Paregoric or camphorated opium tincture—5–10 mL q2h, not more than qid	Diarrhea	Acts directly on intestinal smooth muscle to increase tone and decrease propulsive peristalsis	Occasional nausea; prolonged use may produce dependence

NURSING IMPLICATIONS: Contains approximately 1.6 mg morphine or 16 mg opium and is subject to federal narcotic regulations; administer with partial glass of water to facilitate passage into stomach; observe number and consistency of stools—discontinue drug as soon as diarrhea is controlled; keep in tight *light-resistant* bottles

Antiemetics

Drug and Dosage	Use	Action	Assessment: Side Effects
Chlorpromazine (Thorazine)—preop IM 12.5–25.0 g 1–2 hr before; IV 25–50 mg; PO 10–25 mg q4–6h; IM 25–50 mg q3–4h; suppository 50–100 mg q6–8h	Nausea, vomiting, hiccups, preoperative sedation, psychoses	Alters the effects of dopamine in the CNS; anticholinergic, alpha-adrenergic blocking	Sedation, extrapyramidal reactions; dry eyes, blurred vision; hypotension; constipation, dry mouth; photosensitivity

NURSING IMPLICATIONS: Keep *flat* 30 min after IM; change positions slowly; frequent mouth care; may turn urine *pink* to *red-brown*

Drug and Dosage	Use	Action	Assessment: Side Effects
Prochlorperazine dimaleate (Compazine)—5–30 mg qid PO, IM, rectal	Nausea, vomiting, and retching	See Trimethobenzamide HCl	Drowsiness, orthostatic hypotension, palpitations, blurred vision, diplopia, headache

NURSING IMPLICATIONS: Use *cautiously* in children, women who are pregnant, and clients with liver disease

Drug and Dosage	Use	Action	Assessment: Side Effects
Trimethobenzamide HCl (Tigan)—250 mg qid, PO, IM, rectal	Nausea; vomiting	Suppresses chemoreceptors in the trigger zone located in the medulla oblongata	Drowsiness, vertigo; diarrhea, headache, hypotension; jaundice; blurred vision; rigid muscles

NURSING IMPLICATIONS: Give *deep* IM to prevent escape of solution; can cause edema, pain, and burning

Antifungal

Drug and Dosage	Use	Action	Assessment: Side Effects
Amphotericin B (Fungizone)— IV 5 mg/250 mL dextrose over 4–6 hr (to 1 mg/kg body weight)	Severe fungal infections; histoplasmosis	Fungistatic or fungicidal; binds to sterols in fungal cell membrane, altering cell permeability	Febrile reactions; chills, nausea, vomiting; muscle/joint pain; renal damage; hypotension, tachycardia, arrhythmias; hypokalemia

NURSING IMPLICATIONS: Monitor for side effects, thrombophlebitis at IV site; BUN >40; creatinine >3; stop drug because of *nephrotoxicity*

Drug and Dosage	Use	Action	Assessment: Side Effects
Ketoconazole (Nizoral)—oral 200–400 mg daily	Histoplasmosis, systemic fungal infections	Antifungal	Headache, fatigue, dizziness; nausea, vomiting; decreased libido, impotence; gynecomastia, especially in men

NURSING IMPLICATIONS: Administer *with* food; *avoid* concomitant use of antacids, H_2 blockers; advise to report side effects

Drug and Dosage	Use	Action	Assessment: Side Effects
Nystatin (Nilstat, Mycostatin)—PO, rectal, vaginal: 100,000–1,000,000 U 3–4 times qd	Skin, mucous membrane infections *(Candida albicans);* oral thrush, vaginitis; intestinal candidiasis	Fungistatic and fungicidal; binds to sterols in fungal cell membrane	Nausea, vomiting, GI distress, diarrhea

NURSING IMPLICATIONS: *Oral* use—clear mouth of food; keep medication in mouth several minutes before swallowing; *vaginal*—usually requires 2 wk therapy; continue use during menses; consult physician before using antiinfective douches; determine predisposing factors to infection (diabetes, pregnancy, antibiotics, tight-fitting nylon pantyhose)

(Continued on following page)

Drug and Dosage	Use	Action	◆ Assessment: Side Effects

Antigout

Drug and Dosage	Use	Action	Assessment: Side Effects
Allopurinol (Lopurin, Zyloprim)—PO 100 mg initially, 300 mg daily with meals or pc	Primary hyperuricemia, secondary hyperuricemia with cancer therapy	Lowers plasma and urinary uric acid levels; no analgesic, anti-inflammatory, or uricosuric actions	Rash, itching; nausea, vomiting; anemia, drowsiness

NURSING IMPLICATIONS: Report side effects, particularly *rash,* because drug *must be stopped; avoid* driving or other complex tasks until drug effects known; give at least *3000 mL* fluid daily; minimum urine output of *2000 mL/day;* keep urine neutral or *alkaline* with sodium bicarbonate or potassium citrate; use *cautiously* with: liver disease, impaired renal function, history of peptic ulcers, lower GI disease, or bone marrow depression

Colchicine—PO 1.0–1.2 mg acute phase; 0.5–2.0 mg nightly with milk or food; IV 1–2 mg initially	Gouty arthritis, acute gout	Inhibits leukocyte migration and phagocytosis in gouty joints; nonanalgesic, nonuricosuric	Nausea, vomiting, diarrhea, abdominal pain; peripheral neuritis; bone marrow depression (sore throat, bleeding gums, sore mouth); tissue and nerve necrosis with IV use

NURSING IMPLICATIONS: Do *not* dilute IV form with normal saline or 5% dextrose—use sterile water to prevent precipitation; infuse over 3–5 min IV; potentiate drug action with *alkaline ash foods* (milk, most fruits and vegetables)

Probenecid (Benemid)—PO 0.25–0.50 g twice daily pc	Chronic gouty arthritis, no value in acute; adjuvant therapy with penicillin to increase plasma levels	Inhibits renal tubular resorption of uric acid; no analgesic or antiinflammatory activity; competitively inhibits renal tubular secretion of penicillin and many weak organic acids	Headache; nausea, vomiting, anorexia, sore gums; urinary frequency, flushing

NURSING IMPLICATIONS: Give *with* food, milk, or prescribed antacid; 3000 mL/day fluids; *avoid* alcohol, which increases serum urates; do *not* take with aspirin—inhibits action of drug; renal function and hematology should be evaluated frequently; during acute gout, give with colchicine

Antihistamines

Drug and Dosage	Use	Action	Assessment: Side Effects
Astemizole (Hismanal)—PO 10 mg/day	Relief of allergic symptoms (rhinitis, urticaria); less sedating	Blocks the effects of histamine	Drowsiness, headache, fatigue; stimulation; dry mouth; rash; increased appetite (none of these are frequent)

NURSING IMPLICATIONS: Take *1 hr before* or *2 hr after* eating; good oral hygiene; may need to reduce calories

Cetirizine (Zyrtec)—PO 5–10 mg/d; 10 mg qd or bid for urticaria	Seasonal and perennial allergic rhinitis; chronic urticaria	Potent H_1-receptor antagonist	Drowsiness, sedation, headache

NURSING IMPLICATIONS: Sedation more common in older adult. Do **not** take with OTC antihistamines

Chlorpheniramine maleate (Chlor-Trimeton)—PO 2–4 mg tid-qid; SC, IM, or IV 10–20 mg	Asthma; hay fever; serum reactions; anaphylaxis	Inhibits action of histamine	Nausea, gastritis, diarrhea; headache; dryness of mouth and nose; nervousness, irritability

NURSING IMPLICATIONS: IV may drop BP; give slowly; caution client about drowsiness

Diphenhydramine HCl (Benadryl)—PO 25–50 mg tid-qid; IM or IV 10–20 mg	Allergic and pyrogenic reactions; motion sickness; radiation sickness; hay fever; Parkinson's disease	Inhibits action of histamine on receptor cells; decreases action of acetylcholine	Sedation, dizziness, inability to concentrate; headache; anorexia; dermatitis; nausea; diplopia, insomnia

NURSING IMPLICATIONS: *Avoid* use in newborn or preterm infants and clients with glaucoma; supervise ambulation; *caution* against driving or operating mechanical devices; excitation or hallucinations may occur in *children*

(Continued on following page)

Pharmacology

TABLE 10.6	Common Drugs *(Continued)*		
Drug and Dosage	**Use**	**Action**	◆ **Assessment: Side Effects**
Fexofenadine (Allegra)—PO 50 mg bid	Seasonal allergic rhinitis; chronic urticaria	Antagonizes histamine at the H_1-receptor site	Headache, drowsiness, fatigue; dyspepsia; throat irritation
NURSING IMPLICATIONS: Monitor effectiveness. Well tolerated. Consult MD *if breast feeding*			
Loratidine (Claritin)—PO 10 mg qd on empty stomach	Seasonal allergic rhinitis; idiopathic chronic urticaria	Selective peripheral H_1-receptor sites, blocking histamine release	Dizziness; dry mouth, thirst; fatigue; headache
NURSING IMPLICATIONS: Causes significant drowsiness in *older* adult			
Nedocromil (Tilade) inhalation, 2 sprays	Asthma	Prevents the release of histamine from sensitized mast cells	Hypersensitivity, acute asthma attacks; does not relieve (may accelerate) bronchospasm
NURSING IMPLICATIONS: Monitor ✏ pulmonary function; use only as prescribed; if symptoms increase, notify health-care professional; teach proper use of metered-dose inhaler			
Antihyperglycemics			
Alpha-glucosidase inhibitor			
Acarbose (Precose) 25 mg × 3/day; may be increased q4–8wk (range: 50–100 mg × 3/day)	Type 2 diabetes	Alpha-glucosidase inhibitors/oral hypoglycemic	*Overdose signs:* flatulence, diarrhea, abdominal discomfort
NURSING IMPLICATIONS: Observe for side effects of hypoglycemia; take same time each day; do *not* double dose; therapy is long term			
Biguanide			
Metformin (Glucophage) 500 mg 2 × /day; may increase by 500 mg to 2000 mg/day	Type 2 diabetes	Decreases hepatic production of glucose; decreases intestinal absorption of glucose	Lactic acidosis; nausea, vomiting, diarrhea, abdominal bloating
NURSING IMPLICATIONS: Monitor ✏ glucose levels; take medication as directed; dietary compliance; metallic taste resolves spontaneously			
Sulfonylureas			
Acetohexamide (Dymelor)— PO 200–1500 mg qd; 1–2/day; duration 12–24 hr	Oral hypoglycemic; antidiabetic	Lowers blood glucose by stimulating insulin release from beta cells; effective only if pancreas has ability to produce insulin	Hypoglycemia (profuse sweating, hunger, headache, nausea, confusion, ataxia, coma; skin rashes; bone marrow depression, liver toxicity
NURSING IMPLICATIONS: Drug therapy must be combined with diet therapy, weight control, and planned, graded exercise; alcohol intolerance may occur (disulfiram reaction—flushing, pounding headache, sweating, nausea, vomiting); should *not* be taken at bedtime unless specifically ordered (nocturnal hypoglycemia more likely); take at *same time* each day; *contraindicated* in liver disease, renal disease, pregnancy			
Chlorpropamide (Diabinese)— PO 100–500 mg maintenance; not to exceed 750 mg/day; duration 30–60 hr	See Acetohexamide	See Acetohexamide	See Acetohexamide
NURSING IMPLICATIONS: See Acetohexamide			

(Continued on following page)

Drug and Dosage	Use	Action	◆ Assessment: Side Effects
Glimepiride (Amaryl), glipizide (Glucotrol); 1–2 mg once daily; increase slowly up to 8 mg in one dose; 15 mg/day in divided dose	Type 2 diabetes mellitus	Stimulate release of insulin from pancreas	Photosensitivity; hypoglycemia; ingestion of alcohol may induce reaction
NURSING IMPLICATIONS: Observe for signs of hypoglycemia; long-term therapy; *avoid* aspirin, alcohol; follow prescribed diet/exercise program			
Glyburide (Micronase)—PO 2.5–5 mg initially; 1.25–20 mg/day	See Acetohexmide	See Acetohexamide	See Acetohexamide
NURSING IMPLICATIONS: See Acetohexamide			
Tolazamide (Tolinase)—PO 100–500 mg; 1/day; duration 10–14 hr	See Acetohexamide	See Acetohexamide	See Acetohexamide
NURSING IMPLICATIONS: See Acetohexamide			
Tolbutamide (Orinase)—PO 500–3000 mg; 2–3/day; duration 6–12 hr	See Acetohexamide	See Acetohexamide	See Acetohexamide
NURSING IMPLICATIONS: See Acetohexamide			
Insulin—rapid acting Crystalline zinc (Regular) (Humulin R) (clear)—onset 0.5–1.0 hr; peak 2–4 hr; duration 6–8 hr	Poorly controlled diabetes; trauma; surgery, coma	Enhances transmembrane passage of glucose into cells; promotes carbohydrate, fat, and protein metabolism	Hypoglycemia (profuse sweating, nausea, hunger, headache, confusion, ataxia, coma); allergic reaction at injection site
Insulin analogue (Lispro, Aspart)		More rapid absorption and shorter duration	
NURSING IMPLICATIONS: Monitor ⬕ blood and urine for glucose and acetone levels; insulin currently being used can be kept at *room temperature for 1 mo*; refrigerate stock insulin only; rotate injection sites; cold insulin leads to lipodystrophy, reduced absorption, and local reaction; *only* form of insulin that is given IV; need to eat *within 15 min* of insulin analogue injection			
Insulin—intermediate acting basal NPH insulin (isophane insulin suspension) (cloudy)—onset 1–2 hr; peak 5–8 hr; duration 10–20 hr	Clients who can be controlled by one dose per day	See Crystalline zinc (Regular)	See Crystalline zinc (Regular)
NURSING IMPLICATIONS: Gently rotate vial between palms, invert several times to mix; do *not* shake; see Crystalline zinc (Regular)			
Insulin zinc suspension (Lente insulin) (cloudy)—onset 1–3 hr; peak 6–12 hr; duration 18–24 hr	Clients allergic to NPH	See Crystalline zinc (Regular)	See Crystalline zinc (Regular)
NURSING IMPLICATIONS: See Crystalline zinc (Regular)			
Insulin—slow acting Extended insulin zinc suspension (Ultralente, Humulin U)—onset 4–8 hr; peak 12–24 hr; duration 36 hr	Often mixed with Semilente for 24 hr curve	See Crystalline zinc (Regular)	See Crystalline zinc (Regular)

(Continued on following page)

Pharmacology

TABLE 10.6	Common Drugs *(Continued)*			
Drug and Dosage	**Use**	**Action**	◆ **Assessment: Side Effects**

Insulin—long acting basal			
(Glargine) (clear)—onset 1–2 hr; duration 24 hr		Closely imitates pancreas's basal insulin release	Absorbs equally over 24-hr period

NURSING IMPLICATIONS: See Crystalline zinc (Regular); Glargine may cause mild pain at injection site and *cannot be mixed* with other insulins

Antihypertensives			
Captopril (Capoten)—PO 50 mg tid	Hypertension, heart failure	Prevents production of angiotensin II; vasodilation	Hypotension; loss of taste perception; proteinuria; rashes

NURSING IMPLICATIONS: Monitor VS and weight; take 1 hr *before* and 2 hr *after* meals; change positions *slowly*; *avoid* salt and salt substitutes

Clonidine (Catapres)—PO 200–600 µg/day; transdermal 100–300 µg applied every 7 days	Mild to moderate hypertension; also used for epidural pain management	Stimulates alpha-adrenergic receptors in CNS	Drowsiness; dry mouth; postural hypotension

NURSING IMPLICATIONS: Instruct client to take same time each day; *avoid* sudden position changes; *report:* mental depression, swelling of feet, paleness or cold feeling in fingertips or toes, vivid dreams or nightmares

Guanadrel (Hylorel)—PO 5 mg bid (range: 20–75 mg/d)	Moderate to severe hypertension	Prevents release of norepinephrine in response to sympathetic stimulation	Confusion; fainting; fatigue; diarrhea; orthostatic hypotension; dizziness

NURSING IMPLICATIONS: Give with *diuretics* to minimize tolerance and fluid retention; *weigh* twice weekly; less side effects after 8 wk of therapy

Guanfacine hydrochloride (Tenex)—PO 1 mg daily to maximum dose of 3 mg/day	Hypertension, in combination with thiazide-like diuretics	Centrally acting alpha-adrenergic receptor agonist	Drowsiness; weakness; dizziness; dry mouth; constipation; impotence

NURSING IMPLICATIONS: Warn client *not* to drive or perform activities requiring alertness; take at *bedtime* to minimize sedation; monitor BP and pulse

Guanethidine SO$_4$ (Ismelin)—PO 10–50 mg qd in divided doses	Severe to moderately severe hypertension	Blocks norepinephrine at postganglionic synapses	Orthostatic hypotension; diarrhea; inhibition of ejaculation

NURSING IMPLICATIONS: *Postural hypotension* is marked in the morning *accentuated* by hot weather, alcohol, and exercise; teach to rise slowly, with assistance

Hydralazine HCl (Apresoline)—PO 10–50 mg qid	Moderate hypertension	Dilates peripheral blood vessels, increases renal blood flow	Palpitations, tachycardia, angina pectoris, tremors; depression

NURSING IMPLICATIONS: Encourage moderation in exercise and identification of stressful stimuli

	Obstetric use: preeclampsia, eclampsia	Relaxes peripheral blood vessels (opens vascular bed—physiological dehydration)	Headache, heart palpitation; gastric irritation; coronary insufficiency; edema; chills, fever; severe depression

NURSING IMPLICATIONS: Side rails up; must *not* stand without assistance; may be given with diuretics; observe carefully; IM route *only*; monitor BP; IV for severe hypertension and preeclampsia; in pregnancy, must *not* decrease arterial pressure too much or too rapidly; otherwise, will jeopardize uteroplacental perfusion

Lisinopril (Prinivil)—PO 10 mg/d, up to 20–40 mg qd or bid	Hypertension; heart failure; post-MI	Inhibits angiotensin-converting enzyme; alters hemodynamics without reflex tachycardia	Headache, fatigue, hypotension; cough, rash; ↑ BUN and creatinine

NURSING IMPLICATIONS: *Notify MD* if sudden drop in BP with supine positioning 1–5 hrs after initial drug dose. Check BP before dose to determine 24 hr control

(Continued on following page)

Pharmacology

Drug and Dosage	Use	Action	◆ Assessment: Side Effects
Methyldopa (Aldomet)—PO 500 mg–2 g in divided doses	Severe to moderately severe hypertension	Inhibits formation of dopamine, a precursor of norepinephrine	Initial drowsiness, depression with feelings of unreality, edema, jaundice, dry mouth

NURSING IMPLICATIONS: *Contraindicated* in acute and chronic liver disease; encourage not to drive car if drowsy

Minoxidil (Loniten)—PO 5 mg/day (range: 10–40 mg/day)	Severe hypertension; end-stage organ failure	Relaxes vascular smooth muscle	ECG changes; tachycardia; Na^+, water retention; hypertrichosis

NURSING IMPLICATIONS: Depilatory cream may minimize increased hair growth; report resting pulse *increase more than 20 beats/min;* caution client to change positions *slowly*

Phentolamine hydrochloride (Regitine)—PO 50 mg 4–6 doses daily; IV, IM, or local 5–10 mg, diluted in minimum 10 mL normal saline	Prevents dermal necrosis; hypertensive crisis; pheochromocytoma	Blocks alpha-adrenergic receptors	Weakness, dizziness, orthostatic hypotension; nausea, vomiting, abdominal pain

NURSING IMPLICATIONS: When giving parenterally, client should be *supine;* monitor for overdosage (precipitous drop in BP); do *not* give with epinephrine

Prazosin (Minipress)—PO 6–15 mg/d bid or tid	Mild to moderate hypertension	Dilates arteries and veins by blocking postsynaptic alpha$_1$-adrenergic receptors	Dizziness, headache, weakness, palpitations; orthostatic hypotension with first dose

NURSING IMPLICATIONS: Monitor: I&O, VS, and *weight* at beginning of therapy; teach client/family to check BP at least weekly; need to comply with other interventions (wt. reduction, diet, smoking cessation, exercise)

Reserpine (Serpasil)—PO 0.25 mg qd	Mild to moderate hypertension	Depletes catecholamines and decreases peripheral vasoconstriction, heart rate, and BP	Depression; nasal stuffiness; increased gastric secretions; rash, pruritus

NURSING IMPLICATIONS: Watch for signs of *mental depression;* closely monitor pulse rates of clients *also receiving digitalis;* avoid alcohol

	Obstetric use: Pre-eclampsia-eclampsia	CNS-depressant tranquilizer; sedation is major effect; decreases neural transmission to nerves; decreases tone in blood vessels	Low level of toxicity; weight gain; diarrhea; allergic reactions—dry mouth, itching, skin eruptions

NURSING IMPLICATIONS: Side rails up; must *not* stand up without assistance; observe carefully; monitor *BP*

Timolol (Timoptic)—PO 20–40 mg/day; ophthalmic 1 gtt 1–2 times/day	Hypertension, migraine, glaucoma	Blocks stimulation of myocardial (beta$_1$) and pulmonary/vascular (beta$_2$) receptors	Fatigue, weakness; depression; insomnia; peripheral vasoconstriction; diarrhea, nausea, vomiting

NURSING IMPLICATIONS: Check VS and evidence of heart failure; do *not* take if pulse <50; *avoid* OTC cold remedies, coffee, tea, and cola

Metaraminol (Aramine)—2–10 mg IM or 15–100 mg in 500 mL sodium	Adrenalectomy	Elevated systolic and diastolic BP by vasoconstriction	Hypertension, cardiac arrhythmias; may cause hypertensive crisis, if on MAO inhibitors or antidepressants

NURSING IMPLICATIONS: *Monitor* VS frequently (q3–5 min); observe for side effects; have *phentolamine available as antidote*

(Continued on following page)

Pharmacology

TABLE 10.8	Common Drugs *(Continued)*		
Drug and Dosage	**Use**	**Action**	◆ **Assessment: Side Effects**
Antiinfectives			
Amoxicillin (Amoxil)—PO: 250–500 mg q8h; STD: 3 g single dose with probenecid	ENT infections; soft tissue infections (cellulitis); gonorrhea	Broad spectrum; bactericidal	Rash, diarrhea; anaphylaxis
NURSING IMPLICATIONS: Determine allergies to penicillin, cephalosporins. Instruct client to take drug around the clock, and to complete therapy			
Cefazolin (Ancef, Kefzol)—IM or IV 250 mg–1.5 g q6–12 h	*Staphylococcus aureus; Escherichia coli; Klebsiella;* group A and B *Streptococcus; Pneumococcus*	Bactericidal	Allergic reaction; urticaria, rash; abnormal bleeding
NURSING IMPLICATIONS: See Penicillin; may cause *false-positive* lab tests (Coombs, urine glucose); oral probenecid may be taken concurrently to prolong effects of drug			
Cephalexin (Keflex)—PO 1–4 g daily in 2–4 equally divided doses	Infections caused by gram-positive cocci; infections: respiratory, biliary, urinary, bone, septicemia, abdominal; surgical prophylaxis	Bactericidal effects on susceptible organisms, inhibition of bacterial cell wall synthesis	Nausea, vomiting; urticaria; toxic paranoid reactions; dizziness; increased alkaline phosphatase; nephrotoxicity; bone marrow suppression
NURSING IMPLICATIONS: Peak blood levels delayed when given with food; *report:* nausea, flushing, tachycardia, headache; monitor for *nephrotoxicity* and for bleeding			
Cephalothin (Keflin, Seffin)—IM, IV 2–12 g/day in 4–6 equally divided doses	Same as cephalexin, except not recommended for biliary tract infections	Same as Cephalexin	See Cephalexin
NURSING IMPLICATIONS: Same as Cephalexin; pain at site of IM; given in large muscle; rotate sites			
Ciprofloxacin (Cipro)—PO 250–750 mg q12h; IV 200–400 mg q12h; ophthalmic 1–2 gtt q15–30min, then 4–6 times daily	Lower respiratory tract infections; skin, bone, and joint infections; UTI	Inhibits bacterial DNA synthesis	Restlessness; nausea, diarrhea, vomiting, abdominal pain
NURSING IMPLICATIONS: Give PO on an *empty stomach* unless GI irritation occurs, then take with food; 🍽 *do not* take with milk or yogurt; IV over 60 min			
Clarithromycin (Biaxin)—7.5 mg/kg q12h; usual 500 mg q12h	Peptic ulcer	Inhibits protein synthesis of bacterial ribosome	Hypersensitivity to other antibiotics; use with caution in *liver/renal* impairment
NURSING IMPLICATIONS: Take medication around the clock; report signs of superinfection, diarrhea; do *not* take during pregnancy			
Cloxacillin (Tegopen)—PO 250–500 mg q6h	Penicillinase-producing staphylococci infections: respiratory, sinus, and skin	Binds to bacterial cell wall, leading to cell death	Nausea, vomiting, diarrhea; rashes, allergic reactions; seizures (high doses)
NURSING IMPLICATIONS: *Give around the clock* on an *empty* stomach; observe for signs of *superinfection* (black, furry tongue, vaginal itching, loose stools)			
Co-trimoxazole (Bactrim, Septra)—PO 160 mg twice daily or 20 mg/kg/day for *P. carinii* pneumonia	Acute otitis media; urinary tract infection; shigellosis; *P. carinii* pneumonia; prostatitis	Bacteriostatic; anti-infective; antagonizes folic acid production; combination of sulfamethoxazole and trimethoprim	Hypersensitivity; see Sulfisoxazole
NURSING IMPLICATIONS: IV administration can cause phlebitis and *tissue damage* with extravasation			

(Continued on following page)

Drug and Dosage	Use	Action	◆ Assessment: Side Effects
Doxycycline (Vibramycin)—PO 100 mg q12h on day 1; then 100 mg/day × 7 days; IV—200 mg in 1–2 inf. on day 1; then 100–200 mg/day	Chlamydia, other STDs; Lyme disease	Inhibits bacterial protein of the 30S bacterial ribosome	Urticaria, diarrhea; nausea, vomiting; photosensitivity

NURSING IMPLICATIONS: Take prescribed medications as ordered; use sunscreen or protective clothing due to photosensitivity; report signs of superinfection, if original symptoms not improved

Erythromycin—adults, PO 250 mg q6h; children, PO 30–50 mg/kg qd	Pneumonia; pelvic inflammatory disease; intestinal amebiasis; ocular infections; used if allergic to penicillin	Inhibits protein synthesis of microorganism; more effective against gram-positive organisms	Abdominal cramping, distention, diarrhea

NURSING IMPLICATIONS: Be sure culture and sensitivity done *before* treatment; give on *empty* stomach 1 hr before or 3 hr after meals; do *not* crush or chew tabs; do *not* give with fruit juice

Gentamicin (Garamycin)—IM, IV 3–5 mg/kg/day in 3–4 divided doses; topical; skin, eye	Serious gram-negative infections; possible *S. aureus*, uncomplicated urinary infections	Bactericidal effects on susceptible gram-positive and gram-negative organisms and mycobacteria	Serious toxic effects: kidneys, ear; causes muscle weakness/paralysis

NURSING IMPLICATIONS: Monitor ✎ *plasma* levels (peak is 4–10 μg/mL); clients with burns, cystic fibrosis may need higher doses

Metronidazole (Flagyl) 7.5 mg/kg q6h (not to exceed 4 g/day)	Diverticulosis	Disrupts DNA and protein synthesis in susceptible organisms	Cimetidine may decrease metabolism; seizures, dizziness, abdominal pain

NURSING IMPLICATIONS: Administer with *food or milk* to decrease GI symptoms; *avoid* alcohol; has unpleasant metallic taste; *avoid* OTC medication while on this drug

Penicillin—penicillin G, penicillin G potassium, penicillin G procaine, ampicillin 400,000–1.2 mil U q8h × 10 days, or single dose of 2.4 mil U	*Streptococcus; Staphylococcus; Pneumococcus; Gonococcus; Treponema pallidum*	Primarily bactericidal	Dermatitis and delayed or immediate anaphylaxis
	Obstetric use: group B beta strep—prophylaxis	Prophylaxis	

NURSING IMPLICATIONS: Outpatients should be observed for *20 min after injection;* hospitalized clients should be observed at frequent intervals for 20 min after injection

Pentamidine (Pentam)—IV 4 mg/kg once daily; inhale 300 mg via nebulizer	Prevention or treatment of *P. carinii* pneumonia	Appears to disrupt DNA or RNA synthesis to protozoa	Anxiety, headache; bronchospasm, cough; hypotension, arrhythmias; nephrotoxicity; hypoglycemia; leukopenia, thrombocytopenia, anemia, chills

NURSING IMPLICATIONS: Assess for infection and respiratory status; unpleasant metallic taste may occur (not significant)

Sulfisoxazole (Gantrisin), sulfamethizole (Thiosulfil), and sulfisomidine (Elkosin)—PO 2.4 g loading dose, then 1–2 g qid × 7–10 days	Acute, chronic, and recurrent urinary tract infections	Bacteriostatic and bactericidal	Nausea, vomiting; oliguria, anuria; anemia, leukopenia; dizziness; jaundice, skin rashes, and photosensitivity

NURSING IMPLICATIONS: Maintenance of blood levels is important; encourage *fluids* to prevent crystal formation in kidney tubules—push up to 3000 mL/day; *avoid* in later stage of pregnancy and first month of life for newborn (may cause kernicterus)

(Continued on following page)

Pharmacology

TABLE 10.6	Common Drugs *(Continued)*		
Drug and Dosage	**Use**	**Action**	◆ **Assessment: Side Effects**
Tetracyclines—doxycycline hyclate (Vibramycin), oxytetracycline (Terramycin), tetracycline HCl (Sumycin)—PO 250–500 mg q6h; IM 250 mg/day; or IV 250–500 mg q8–12h	Broad-spectrum antibiotic	Primarily bacteriostatic	GI upsets such as diarrhea, nausea, vomiting; sore throat; black, hairy tongue; glossitis; inflammatory lesions in anogenital region
NURSING IMPLICATIONS: *Phototoxic* reactions have been reported; clients should be advised to stay out of direct sunlight; medication should *not* be given with 🍽 milk or snacks, because food interferes with absorption of tetracyclines; do *not* give to women who are pregnant and children under 8 yr			
Trimethoprim (TMP)/sulfamethoxazole (SMZ) (Bactrim)—PO 160 mg TMP or 800 mg SMZ q 12h for 14–21 days; IV 8–10 mg/kg; TMP 40–50 mg/kg; SMZ q6–12h	Bronchitis, *Shigella* enteritis, otitis media, *P. carinii* pneumonia, UTI, traveler's diarrhea	Combination inhibits the metabolism of folic acid in bacteria; bactericidal	Nausea, vomiting; rashes; phlebitis at IV site; aplastic anemia; hepatic necrosis
NURSING IMPLICATIONS: Check IV site frequently; do *not* give IM; give PO on *empty stomach;* take *around the clock; avoid* exposure to sun			

Antiinflammatory

Gastrointestinal

Mesalamine (Asacol, Pentusa, Rowasa)—800 mg × 3/day for 6 wk	Ulcerative colitis	Local-acting antiinflammatory in GI tract	*Contraindicated* if client has allergy to sulfonamides or salicylates; acceleration of symptoms; abdominal pain
NURSING IMPLICATIONS: *Monitor* for: abdominal pain, diarrhea, blood in stools, superinfection; if no improvement notify health-care professional; may need diagnostic studies			
Olsalazine (Dipentum)—see mesalamine—PO 1 g/day in 2 divided doses	See Mesalamine	See Mesalamine	See Mesalamine
NURSING IMPLICATIONS: See Mesalamine			
Sulfasalazine (Azulifidine)— see mesalamine—PO 3–4 g/day in divided doses	See Mesalamine	See Mesalamine	See Mesalamine
NURSING IMPLICATIONS: See Mesalamine			

Glucocorticoids—inhalants

Beclomethasone (Beclovent, Vanceril)—42–50 µg/spray; 2 metered sprays × 3–4/day	Emphysema	Glucocorticoid (inhalation)	Headache, hypersensitivity to fluorocarbon propellant; used with *caution* in diabetes or glaucoma
NURSING IMPLICATIONS: Do *not* exceed 1 mg/day			
Flunisolide (AeroBid) 42–50 µg/spray; 2 metered sprays × 2–4/day	Emphysema	Potent locally acting antiinflammatory and immune modifier	Headache, dysphonia; fungal infections; adrenal suppression with long-term use
NURSING IMPLICATIONS: *Monitor* respiratory status and lung sounds; *assess* clients changing from systemic to inhaled glucocorticoids for signs of *adrenal insufficiency* (anorexia, nausea, weakness, hypotension, hypoglycemia)			
Triaminolone (Azmacort)— See Beclomethasone	Asthma	See Beclomethasone	See Beclomethasone
NURSING IMPLICATIONS: See Beclomethasone			

(Continued on following page)

Drug and Dosage	Use	Action	◆ Assessment: Side Effects
Glucocorticoids—systemic			
Cortisone acetate—PO or IM 20–100 mg qd in single or divided doses	ACTH insufficiency; rheumatoid arthritis; allergies; ulcerative colitis; nephrosis	Antiinflammatory effect of unknown action	Moon facies, hirsutism, thinning of skin, striae; hypertension; menstrual irregularities, delayed healing; psychoses

NURSING IMPLICATIONS: Give oral form pc, with snack at bedtime; give deep IM (*never* deltoid); monitor vital signs; observe for behavior changes; skin care and activity to tolerance; 🍽 *diet*—salt *restricted, high* protein, KCl supplement; protect from injury

Desoxycorticosterone acetate (hydrocortisone)—IM/IV 100–500 mg q2–6h; PO 3–5 mg bid-qid	Addison's disease; burns; surgical shock; adrenal surgery	Promotes reabsorption of sodium; restores plasma volume, BP, and electrolyte balance	Edema, hypertension, pulmonary congestion, hypokalemia

NURSING IMPLICATIONS: 🍽 Salt restriction according to BP readings; *monitor* vital signs; weigh daily

Dexamethasone (Decadron)—PO 0.5–5.0 mg qd; IM or IV 4–20 mg qd	Addison's disease; allergic reactions; leukemia; Hodgkin's disease; iritis; dermatitis; rheumatoid arthritis	Antiinflammatory effect	See Cortisone acetate
	Obstetric use: stimulate surfactant production in client with premature labor		

NURSING IMPLICATIONS: *Contraindicated* in tuberculosis; see Cortisone acetate for nursing care

Methylprednisolone sodium (Solu-Medrol)—IV, IM, 10–40 mg, slowly	Glucocorticoid, corticosteroid	See Dexamethasone	See Dexamethasone

NURSING IMPLICATIONS: See Dexamethasone

Prednisolone (Deltsone)— 5–60 mg/day single or divided dose	Multiple sclerosis	Suppress inflammation and normal immune response	Depression, euphoria; peptic ulceration; thromboembolism

NURSING IMPLICATIONS: *Monitor* for: *Homans' sign*, abdominal pain, vomiting, tarry stools, mental status or mood changes

Prednisone—PO 2.5–15.0 mg qd	Rheumatoid arthritis; cancer therapy	Antiinflammatory effect of unknown action	Insomnia and gastric distress

NURSING IMPLICATIONS: See Cortisone acetate

Antilipemics			
Atorvastatin calcium (Lipitor)—PO 10 mg qd up to 80 mg/d	Reduce: LDL, cholesterol, triglycerides	Increases number of hepatic LDL receptors	Back pain, myalgia; constipation, diarrhea; ↑ liver function tests

NURSING IMPLICATIONS: Assess for: muscle pain, tenderness or weakness—🧪 check CPK level. Use *cautiously* with: antifungals, niacin, erythromycin

Cholestyramine (Questran)— PO 4 g 1–4 times/day	Hypercholesterolemia; pruritus from increased bile	Binds bile acids in GI tract, increased clearance of cholesterol	Nausea, constipation, abdominal discomfort

NURSING IMPLICATIONS: Take *before* meals; do *not* take with other medications; give others 1 hr before or 4–6 hr after

Gemfibrozil (Lopid)—PO 1200 mg/day	Hypercholesterolemia	May inhibit peripheral lipolysis and reduce triglyceride synthesis in liver	GI upset (abdominal pain, epigastric pain, diarrhea, nausea, vomiting); rash; headache, dizziness, blurred vision

NURSING IMPLICATIONS: Use *caution* when driving or doing tasks requiring alertness; take *before* meals

(Continued on following page)

Pharmacology

TABLE 10.6 **Common Drugs** *(Continued)*

Drug and Dosage	Use	Action	◆ Assessment: Side Effects
Niacin (vitamin B$_3$, nicotinic acid)—PO 1.5–6.0 g	Hypercholesterolemia	Decreases liver's production of LDLs and synthesis of triglycerides	GI upset, flushing; pruritus, hyperuricemia, hyperglycemia
NURSING IMPLICATIONS: Take the drug *with* meals; prevent flushing by taking an *aspirin 30 min before*; monitor closely during first year of therapy			
Simvastatin (Zocor)—10–20 mg qd	See Lovastatin	See Lovastatin	See Lovastatin
NURSING IMPLICATIONS: Give once in the *evening* with or without food			
Antineoplastics			
6 mercaptopurine Purinethol)—PO 2.5 mg/kg/day; may increase to 5 mg/kg after 4 wk; maintenance 1.5–2.5 mg/kg/day	Leukemia (ulcerative)	Antineoplastic	Bone marrow depression, severe hepatotoxicity
NURSING IMPLICATIONS: *Monitor:* bleeding, infection, *liver* function tests, skin care, nausea and vomiting			
Methotrexate (Rheumatrex) 15–30 mg/day for 5 days; repeat after 1 wk for 3–5 courses	Leukemia Breast, lung cancer	Interferes with folic acid metabolism, resulting in inhibition of DNA synthesis and cell reproduction	Pulmonary fibrosis; hepatotoxicity; stomatitis, signs and symptoms of chemotherapy side effects
NURSING IMPLICATIONS: Monitor: *liver* function; *assess* respiratory status; see nursing care of clients receiving chemotherapy			
Mitotane (Lysodren) 9–10 g/day in 3–4 divided doses initially; decrease for maintenance	Adrenocortical carcinoma	Affects pituitary disorders	GI complaints; lethargy, somnolence
NURSING IMPLICATIONS: *Monitor:* signs of disease progression, GI abnormalities, abdominal pain			
Antiparkinson Agents			
Benztropine (Cogentin)— 1–2 mg/day (range: 0.5–6 mg/day)	Parkinson's disease	Blocks cholinergic activity in CNS	Blurred vision, dry eyes; constipation; *caution* with antihistamines, phenothiazines
NURSING IMPLICATIONS: Take as directed for best results; monitor for drowsines, dizziness, orthostatic hypotension; good mouth care; use *caution* with OTC drugs, overheating (drug causes a decrease in perspiration)			
Carbidopa/levodopa (Sinemet)—10/100, 25/100, 25/250 carbidopa/levodopa ratio	Parkinson's disease	Levodopa is converted to dopamine in CNS, where it serves as a neurotransmitter	Use with MAO inhibitors may result in hypertensive crisis; some drugs can reverse effects, e.g., phenothiazines, reserpine
NURSING IMPLICATIONS: Rate of dosage increase determined by client response; make accurate observations. May experience "on-off" phenomenon—loss of drug effects and sudden return. Prevent falling from postural hypotension, "leg freezing," instability			
Biperiden (Akineton)—2 mg 3–4 times/ day; *not to exceed* 16 mg/day	Parkinson's disease	Restores natural balance of neurotransmitters in CNS	Same as Benztropine (Cogentin)
NURSING IMPLICATIONS: See Benztropine			
Trihexyphenidyl (Artane)— 1–2 mg daily; usual maintenance dose: 5–15 mg/day in divided dose	Parkinson's disease	Inhibits action of acetylcholine	Dizziness, nervousness, blurred vision, mydriasis
NURSING IMPLICATIONS: Monitor symptoms; *avoid* orthostatic hypotension; mouth care			

(Continued on following page)

Drug and Dosage	Use	Action	◆ Assessment: Side Effects
Antiplatelet			
Clopidogrel (Plavix)—PO 75 mg qd	Reduce risk of atherosclerotic event (MI, stroke)	Inhibits platelet aggregation	Bleeding; neutropenia; reactions similar to aspirin
NURSING IMPLICATIONS: Give once daily without regard to food; *avoid* aspirin, NSAIDs; observe for symptoms of: stroke, peripheral vascular disease, MI			
Dipyridamole (Persantine)—PO 70–100 mg 4 times/day; IV 570 μg/kg	Prevent thromboembolism; surgical graft patency; *diagnostic* agent in myocardial perfusion studies	Decreases platelet aggregation; coronary vasodilator	Headache, dizziness, hypotension; nausea; MI, arrhythmias with IV
NURSING IMPLICATIONS: Take at *evenly* spaced intervals; *avoid* use of alcohol; if no GI irritation, take 1 hr before or 2 hr after meals			
Eptifibatide (Integrilin)—IV 180 μg/kg bolus; 2 μg/kg/min until discharge or up to 72h	Severe chest pain; small heart attacks; unstable angina; before balloon angioplasty	Binds to glycoprotein receptor sites of platelets	Bleeding
NURSING IMPLICATIONS: Minimize any vascular trauma during treatment. Monitor lab tests for indications of bleeding or clotting disorders. **Stop drug immediately** if bleeding occurs			
Ticlopidine (Ticlid)—PO 250 mg bid	Stroke prevention; prevent early restenosis of coronary stents	Inhibits platelet aggregation; prolongs bleeding time	Diarrhea, rashes, bleeding, intracerebral bleeding
NURSING IMPLICATIONS: Give *with* food or immediately *after* eating			
Antituberculous*			
First-line drugs			
Isoniazid—5–10 mg/kg up to 300 mg PO or IM	Tuberculosis	Suppresses or interferes with biosynthesis; bacteriostatic	Peripheral neuritis; hepatitis; hypersensitivity
NURSING IMPLICATIONS: Give pyridoxine (B$_6$) 10 mg as prophylaxis for neuritis; 50–100 mg as treatment			
Ethambutol—15–25 mg/kg PO	See Isoniazid	See Isoniazid	Optic neuritis (reversible with discontinuation of drug; very rare at 15 mg/kg); skin rash
NURSING IMPLICATIONS: Use with *caution* with renal disease or when eye testing is not feasible; used *in combination with* other drug			
Rifamate combination (isoniazid with rifampin) Rifater combination (isoniazid and pyrazinamide with rifampin)—see Rifampin	See Rifampin	See Rifampin	See Rifampin
NURSING IMPLICATIONS: See Rifampin			
Rifampin—10–20 mg/kg PO, 600 mg IV	Tuberculosis, meningitis, *H. influenzae*	Impairs RNA synthesis; bactericidal	Hepatitis, febrile reaction, purpura (rare)
NURSING IMPLICATIONS: *Orange* urine color; *negates* effect of birth control pills			
Streptomycin—15–20 mg/kg up to 1 g IM	Tuberculosis, endocarditis, tularemia	Inhibits protein synthesis; bactericidal	*Eighth cranial* nerve damage, *nephrotoxicity*
NURSING IMPLICATIONS: Use with caution in *older* clients or those with *renal* disease			

* To minimize resistant strains, combination therapy is used long-term.

(Continued on following page)

Pharmacology

TABLE 10.6	Common Drugs *(Continued)*		

Drug and Dosage	Use	Action	◆ Assessment: Side Effects
Pyrazinamide—15–30 mg/kg up to 3 g PO	Tuberculosis	Bactericidal	Hyperuricemia, hepatotoxicity
NURSING IMPLICATIONS: Loss of glycemic control in those with diabetes			

Antiulcer

Drug and Dosage	Use	Action	Assessment: Side Effects
Aluminum hydroxide gel (Amphojel)—PO 5–10 mL q2–4h or 1 hr pc	Gastric acidity; peptic ulcer; phosphatic urinary calculi; ↓ phosphorus level in chronic renal failure	Buffers HCl in gastric juices without interfering with electrolyte balance	Constipation and fecal impaction
NURSING IMPLICATIONS: *Shake well* before administering; encourage *fluids* to prevent impaction and milk–alkali syndrome			
Calcium carbonate (Titralac)—PO 1–2 g taken with H_2O after meals and at bedtime	Peptic ulcer and chronic gastritis	Reduces hyperacidity	Constipation or laxative effect
NURSING IMPLICATIONS: See Aluminum hydroxide gel			
Cimetidine (Tagamet)—PO 300–600 mg q6h (qid); IM, IV 300 mg q6h	Duodenal ulcers, GERD, gastric hypersecretion; peptic acid gastritis, heart burn; esophagitis	Inhibits action of histamine at H_2-receptor site, inhibits gastric acid secretion; neutralizes and absorbs excess acid	Confusion, dizziness; nausea; rash; diarrhea, constipation; hypermagnesemia
NURSING IMPLICATIONS: Give *with* meals or immediately *after; avoid* smoking; *avoid* prolonged administration to clients with renal insufficiency			
Famotidine (Pepcid)—40 mg/day at bedtime or 20 mg twice a day	Peptic ulcer	Inhibits gastric acid secretion by inhibiting histamine at H_2-receptor site	Use with caution: elderly, renal failure; confusion, arrhythmias, agranulocytosis, aplastic anemia
NURSING IMPLICATIONS: Assess for: epigastric pain, blood in stool or emesis; 🧪 monitor lab values to avoid side effects; take medication for full course of treatment; *avoid* self medication with OTC drugs; *avoid* smoking			
Lansoprazole (Prevacid)—15 mg/day; with *H. pylori*: 30 mg twice a day with amoxicillin	Peptic ulcer	Binds to an enzyme in presence of gastric acid; prevents final transport of hydrogen ions into gastric lumen	Hypersensitivity; use with caution in elderly; dose change needed with hepatic impairment
NURSING IMPLICATIONS: *Avoid* alcohol; *report* signs of: GI bleeding, cramping, abdominal pain, vomiting			
Magnesium and aluminum hydroxides (Maalox suspension)—PO 5–30 mL q1–3h pc and hs	Gastric hyperacidity; peptic ulcer; heartburn; reflux esophagitis	Neutralizes and binds gastric acids, heals ulcers	Constipation from aluminum hydroxide; diarrhea from magnesium hydroxide
NURSING IMPLICATIONS: Encourage fluid intake; *contraindicated* for clients who are debilitated or those with renal insufficiency			
Misoprostol (Cytotec) 200 μg 4 times/ day; 800 μg rectally; 25–50 μg vaginally	Peptic ulcer **Obstetric use:** labor induction, to control postpartum hemorrhage	Prostaglandin analogue	Hypersensitivity to prostaglandins; diarrhea; *Avoid* during pregnancy
NURSING IMPLICATIONS: Monitor effectiveness of the drug; report increase in abdominal pain, bleeding			
Nizatidine (Axid) see cimetidine	See Cimetidine	See Cimetidine	See Cimetidine
NURSING IMPLICATIONS: See Cimetidine			

(Continued on following page)

Drug and Dosage	Use	Action	◆ Assessment: Side Effects
Omeprazole (Prilosec) 20 mg once daily	Peptic ulcer GERD	Gastric acid–pump inhibitor	Abdominal pain; *contraindicated:* hypersensitivity

NURSING IMPLICATIONS: May cause drowsiness, dizziness: *Avoid:* alcohol, aspirin, NSAIDs, foods that cause GI irritation

Ranitidine (Zantac)—PO 150 mg bid; IM 50 mg q6–8h; IV 50 mg q6–8h	Duodenal ulcer, gastric ulcer, GERD, gastric hypersecretion	Inhibits action of histamine at H$_2$-receptor site, inhibits gastric acid secretion	Headache, malaise; nausea, constipation, diarrhea

NURSING IMPLICATIONS: Food does *not* affect absorption; give 1 hr *apart* from antacids; *smoking* interferes with action

Sucralfate (Carafate)— PO 1 g qid	Prevention and treatment of duodenal ulcer	Reacts with gastric acid to form a thick paste that adheres to the ulcer surface	Constipation

NURSING IMPLICATIONS: Give 1 hr *before* and *at bedtime;* do *not* crush or chew tablets; take *antacids* 30 min before or 1 hr after sucralfate; 🍽 increase *fluids and dietary* bulk

Antiviral

Acyclovir (Zovirax)—PO 200mg, 3–5 times/day; IV 5 mg/kg q8h over 1 hr; topical 6 times daily for 1 wk	Herpes simplex (1, 2)	Converts to an active cytotoxic metabolite that inhibits viral DNA replication	Headache, nausea, vomiting, diarrhea; *increased* serum BUN and creatinine

NURSING IMPLICATIONS: Measure I&O q8h; ensure adequate *hydration;* assess for common side effects; apply topical with *finger cot* or rubber glove; refer for counseling

Indinavir (Crixivan)—PO 800 mg q8h	HIV; possible prevention in combination therapy	Inhibits action of HIV protease and cleavage of viral polyproteins	Ketoacidosis; kidney stones; hyperglycemia; altered taste; acid regurgitation

NURSING IMPLICATIONS: Give with *water or other liquids* (skim milk, coffee, tea, juice) *1 hr before* or 2 *hr after* meal; 🍽 avoid high fat, high protein meal within 2 hr; with concurrent therapy, may need to take drugs 1 hr apart; capsules are sensitive to moisture—keep desiccant in bottle

Nevirapine (Viramune)—PO 200 mg qd for 2 wk, then bid	HIV; delays disease progression	Binds to the enzyme reverse transcriptase; disrupts DNA sythesis	Rash; *Stevens-Johnson syndrome* (severe erythema multiforme)

NURSING IMPLICATIONS: Give with or without food; drug does not cure AIDS—decreases opportunistic infections

Zidovudine (AZT, Retrovir)— PO 200 mg q4h	AIDS and related disorders	Inhibits HIV replication	Blood disorders, especially anemia and granulocytopenia; headache; nausea; insomnia; myalgia

NURSING IMPLICATIONS: Monitor for signs of opportunistic infection and adverse drug effects; drug must be taken *around the clock;* 🧪 regular blood tests (q2wk)

Blood Viscosity–Reducing Agent

Pentoxifylline (Trental)—PO 400 mg tid	Peripheral vascular disease (intermittent claudication)	Increases flexibility of RBCs; inhibits platelet aggregation	Nausea, vomiting, GI upset; drowsiness; dizziness; headache

NURSING IMPLICATIONS: Give *with* meals to minimize GI irritation; take tablets whole; report persistent GI or CNS side effects

Bronchodilators

Albuterol (Ventolin)—PO 2–6 mg 3–4 times/day; inhale q4–6h or 2 puffs 15 min before exercise	Bronchodilator	Results in accumulation of cyclic adenosine monophosphate (cAMP) at beta-adrenergic receptors	Nervousness, restlessness, tremor, hypertension, nausea

NURSING IMPLICATIONS: Give *with* meals; allow 1 min *between* inhalations; rinse mouth with water *after* inhalation

(Continued on following page)

TABLE 10.6	Common Drugs *(Continued)*		
Drug and Dosage	**Use**	**Action**	◆ **Assessment: Side Effects**
Aminophylline—PO 250 mg bid–qid: rectal 250–500 mg; IV 250–500 mg over 10–20 min	Rapid relief of bronchospasm; asthma; pulmonary edema	Relaxes smooth muscles and increases cardiac contractility; interferes with reabsorption of Na^+ and Cl^- in proximal tubules	Nausea, vomiting; cardiac arrhythmias; intestinal bleeding; insomnia, restlessness; and rectal irritation from suppository
NURSING IMPLICATIONS: Give oral *with* or *after meals;* monitor *vital signs* for changes in BP and pulse; weigh daily; IM injections are painful			
Ephedrine SO_4—PO, SC, or IM 25 mg tid–qid	Asthma: allergies; bradycardia; nasal decongestant	Relaxes hypertonic muscles in bronchioles and GI tract	Wakefulness, nervousness, dizziness, palpitations, hypertension
NURSING IMPLICATIONS: Monitor vital signs; *avoid* giving dose near bedtime; *check urine* output in older adults			
Ipratropium (Atrovent) 1–4 inhalations	Emphysema	Inhibits cholinergic receptors in bronchial smooth muscle	Nasal dryness, epistaxis; fluorocarbon toxicity when used with other inhalants
NURSING IMPLICATIONS: Instruct in proper use of inhaler; do *not* use more than 12 metered doses in 12 hr; if severe bronchospasm occurs, consult physician/nurse practitioner			
Isoproterenol HCl (Isuprel)—inhalation of 1:100 or 1:200 solution	Mild to moderately severe asthma attack; bronchitis; pulmonary emphysema	Relaxes hypertonic bronchioles	Nervousness, tachycardia; hypertension; insomnia
NURSING IMPLICATIONS: Monitor vital signs *before and after* treatment; teach client how to use nebulizer			
Metaproterenol (Alupent) 20 mg 3–4 times/day; inhalation 2–3 metered-dose inhalations	Asthma	Bronchodilation	Nervousness, restlessness, tremor, paradoxical bronchospasm
NURSING IMPLICATIONS: Assess lung sounds, observe for wheezing (paradoxical bronchospasm); observe clients' respiratory signs and symptoms; refer to health-care professional if symptoms persist or shortness of breath continues			
Salmeterol (Serevent)—50 μg twice a day (two inhalations)	Asthma	Produces accumulation of cAMP at beta-adrenergic receptors	Headache, palpitations, abdominal pain; *avoid* use when on beta-adrenergic agents (decreases effectiveness)
NURSING IMPLICATIONS: Assess lung sounds; *monitor* pulmonary function; do *not* use for acute symptoms			
Theophylline—PO 400 mg/day in divided doses; max adult dose: 900 mg divided dose	Treatment/prevention of emphysema, asthma (bronchoconstriction); chronic bronchitis	Bronchodilation	Restlessness; increased respiration, heart rate; palpitations, arrhythmias; nausea, vomiting; increased urine output → dehydration
NURSING IMPLICATIONS: Monitor theophylline levels: 10–20 μg/mL; monitor signs of toxicity; take with 8 oz water or *with* meals to decrease GI symptoms			
Terbutaline (Brethine)—PO 2.5–5.0 mg q6h (*not* to exceed 20 mg/24 hr); SC 0.25 mg, repeat 15–30 min (*not* to exceed 0.5 mg/hr); inhalation—2 puffs (0.2 mg each) q4–6h	Bronchospasm	See Isoproterenol	See Isoproterenol
	Obstetric use: may be used for premature labor; not FDA-approved for use as tocolytic agent, but widely used		If used in pregnancy: maternal and fetal tachycardia
NURSING IMPLICATIONS: See Isoproterenol			

(Continued on following page)

Drug and Dosage	Use	Action	◆ Assessment: Side Effects
Zafirlukast (Accolate)—20 mg twice daily	Asthma	Antagonizes the effects of leukotrienes	Headache, fever, infection, pain

NURSING IMPLICATIONS: *Monitor* lung sounds, respiratory function

Zileuton (Zyflo)— 600 mg qid	Asthma	Enzyme inhibitor	Headache, dizziness; chest pain; increases blood level of theophylline, propranolol, warfarin

NURSING IMPLICATIONS: Assess lung sounds; do *not* discontinue or reduce dosage without consulting health-care professional; not used to treat acute attack

Calcium Channel Blockers

Amlodipine (Norvasc)—PO 5–10 mg qd	Hypertension, angina pectoris, vasospastic angina (Prinzmetal's), muscle cells	Inhibits the transport of calcium into myocardial and vascular smooth muscle	Arrhythmias, peripheral edema, heart failure; photosensitivity; gingival hyperplasia

NURSING IMPLICATIONS: Instruct client to: monitor pulse, report rate <50 beats/min, take with or without food

Diltiaziem (Cardizem)—PO 30–120 mg 3–4 times/day; IV 5–15 mg/hr	Angina, hypertension, atrial arrhythmias	Inhibits excitation-contraction; decreased SA, AV node conduction	Headache, fatigue, arrhythmias, edema, hypotension; constipation; rash

NURSING IMPLICATIONS: May take *with* meals; take pulse; do *not* give drug if pulse <50 beats/min; change positions slowly; may take nitroglycerin sublingually concurrently

Metoprolol (Lopressor)—100 mg/day up to 450 mg/day	Hypertension	Blocks stimulation of myocardial adrenergic receptors (beta$_1$)	*Contraindicated* in: CHF, pulmonary edema; *caution* with renal impairment

NURSING IMPLICATIONS: Monitor vitals, especially BP; prevent *orthostatic hypotension; avoid* self-medication with OTC; may cause drowsiness; medication may increase *sensitivity to cold*

Nicardipine (Cardene)—PO 20–40 mg tid	Angina, hypertension	Calcium channel blocker, inhibits excitation-contraction	Dizziness, light-headedness, headache; peripheral edema; flushing

NURSING IMPLICATIONS: Give on an *empty* stomach; chest pain may occur 30 min after dose (temporary, from *reflex tachycardia*)

Nifedipine (Procardia)—PO 10–30 mg tid (*not* to exceed 180 mg/day); sublingual 10 mg repeated in 15 min	Angina, hypertension **Obstetric use:** may be used for premature labor; not FDA approved for use as tocolytic agent, but widely used	Calcium channel blocker, vasodilation	Dizziness, light-headedness, giddiness, headache, nervousness; nasal congestion; sore throat, dyspnea, cough, wheezing; nausea; flushing, warmth

NURSING IMPLICATIONS: May take *with* meals; make position changes *slowly;* angina may occur 30 min after dose (temporary)

Verapamil (Calan, Isopten)—PO 240–480 mg, 3–4 times/day; IV 75–150 μg/kg over 2min	Angina; supraventricular arrhythmias; essential hypertension	Inhibits calcium movement into smooth-muscle cells; lowers pressure by reducing cardiac contractility	Constipation, AV block, hepatotoxicity

NURSING IMPLICATIONS: Monitor VS and ECG for *bradycardia* and *arrhythmias;* observe for *jaundice, abdominal pain;* 🍽 encourage *fluids* and *bulk-forming* foods

Cardiac Glycosides

Digitoxin—digitalizing dose: PO 200 μg twice/day; IM or IV 200–400 μg; maintenance dose: PO 50–300 μg qd	Heart failure: atrial fibrillation and flutter; supraventricular tachycardia	Increases force of cardiac contractility, slows heart rate, decreases right atrial pressures, promotes diuresis	Arrhythmias; nausea, vomiting; anorexia, malaise; color vision, yellow or blue

NURSING IMPLICATIONS: Hold medication if pulse rate less than *50* or over *120;* 🍽 encourage foods high in *potassium* (e.g., bananas, orange juice); observe for signs of electrolyte depletion, apathy, disorientation, and anorexia

(Continued on following page)

Pharmacology

TABLE 10.6	Common Drugs *(Continued)*		
Drug and Dosage	**Use**	**Action**	◆ **Assessment: Side Effects**
Digoxin (Lanoxin)—digitalizing dose: PO 10–15 μg/kg; IV 0.6–1 mg/kg; maintenance dose: PO 0.125–0.375 mg qd	See Digitoxin	See Digitoxin	See Digitoxin
NURSING IMPLICATIONS: See Digitoxin			
Chemotherapy (see Table 7.45) and Antineoplastics (Table 10.8) Cholinergic			
Bethanechol chloride (Urecholine)—PO 5–30 mg; SC 2.5–5.0 mg	Postoperative abdominal atony and distention; bladder atony with retention; post-surgical or postpartum urinary retention; myasthenia gravis	Increases GI and bladder tone; decreases sphincter tone	Belching, abdominal cramps, diarrhea, nausea, vomiting; incontinence; profuse sweating, salivation; respiratory depression
NURSING IMPLICATIONS: Check *respirations;* have urinal or bedpan close at hand and answer calls quickly; atropine SO_4 is the *antidote* for cholinergic drugs			
Edrophonium (Tensilon)—IV 2 mg; IM 10 mg	Diagnosis of myasthenia gravis; reversal of neuromuscular blockers	Inhibits breakdown of acetylcholine; anticholinesterase, cholinergic	Excess secretions; bronchospasm; bradycardia; abdominal cramps, vomiting, diarrhea; excess salivation; sweating
NURSING IMPLICATIONS: Effects last up to 30 min; give IV *undiluted* with *TB* syringe			
Neostigmine (Prostigmin)—PO 15–30 mg q3–4h; SC, IM 0.25–1 mg	Myasthenia gravis, postoperative bladder distention, urinary retention, reversal of neuromuscular blockers	Inhibits breakdown of acetylcholine; cholinergic	Excess secretions; bronchospasm; bradycardia; abdominal cramps, nausea, vomiting, diarrhea; excess salivation; sweating
NURSING IMPLICATIONS: Take oral form *with* food or milk; with chewing difficulty, take 30 min before eating			
Pilocarpine HCl—1–2 gtt 1%–2% solution up to 6 times/day	Chronic open-angle and acute closed angle glaucoma	Contraction of the sphincter muscle of iris, resulting in miosis	Brow ache, headache, ocular pain, blurring and dimness of vision, allergic conjunctivitis; nausea, vomiting, profuse sweating; bronchoconstriction in clients with bronchial asthma
NURSING IMPLICATIONS: Initially the medication may be irritating; teach proper sterile technique for instilling drops—wipe excess solution to prevent systemic symptoms; discard cloudy solutions			
Physotigmine salicylate (Eserine)—0.1 mL of 0.25%–10% solution: not more than qid; IM, IV 0.5–3 mg	Glaucoma; reverse effects of: tricyclic antidepressants, overdose, toxic effects of atropine and diazepam	Increases concentration of acetylcholine	Sweating; marked miosis, lacrimation; nausea, diarrhea
NURSING IMPLICATIONS: If *brown eyed,* may require stronger solution or more frequent dose			
Pyridostigmine (Mestinon)—PO 60 mg/day × 3 days; IM, IV 2 mg q2–3h Maintenance: 60–150 mg/day	Myasthenia gravis; reversal of neuromuscular blockers	Inhibits breakdown of acetylcholine and prolongs its effects	See Neostigmine
NURSING IMPLICATIONS: See Neostigmine			

(Continued on following page)

Drug and Dosage	Use	Action	◆ Assessment: Side Effects
Central Nervous System Stimulants			
Amphetamine SO$_4$—PO 5–60 mg qd in divided doses	Mild depressive states; narcolepsy; postencephalitic parkinsonism; obesity control; minimal brain dysfunction in children (attention deficit disorder)	Raises BP, decreases sense of fatigue, elevates mood	Restlessness, dizziness, tremors, insomnia; increased libido; suicidal and homicidal tendencies; palpitations; anginal pain

NURSING IMPLICATIONS: Give *before* 4 P.M. to avoid sleep disturbance; dependence on drug may develop; *contraindicated* with: MAO inhibitors, hyperthyroidism, and psychotic states

Methylphenidate hydrochloride (Ritalin)—PO 0.3 mg/kg/day or adults 20–60 mg in divided doses	Childhood hyperactivity; narcolepsy; attention deficit disorder in children	Mild CNS and respiratory stimulation	Anorexia; dizziness, drowsiness, insomnia, nervousness; BP and pulse changes

NURSING IMPLICATIONS: To avoid insomnia take last dose 4–5 hr before bedtime; monitor vital signs; check weight 2–3 times weekly and report weight losses

Decongestants			
Phenylephrine (Neo-Synephrine, Sinex)—SC, IM 2–5 mg q10–15min, *not to exceed* 5 mg; IV 40–60 μg/min; nasal 2–3 gtt or 1–2 sprays q3–4h; ophthalmic 3 gtt/day	Shock, hypotension, decongestant, adjunct to spinal anesthesia, mydriatic	Constricts blood vessels by stimulating alpha-adrenergic receptors	Dizziness, restlessness, dyspnea, tachycardia, arrhythmias; ophthalmological: burning, photophobia, tearing

NURSING IMPLICATIONS: Check for correct concentration; protect eyes from *light sensitivity;* blow nose before using; *rebound congestion* will occur with prolonged use

Pseudoephedrine (Sudafed)—PO 60 mg q4–6h	Nasal congestion, allergies, chronic ear infections	Produces vasoconstriction in respiratory tract and possibly bronchodilation	Nervousness, anxiety, palpitations, anorexia

NURSING IMPLICATIONS: Give at least 2 hr before bedtime to minimize *insomnia*

Electrolyte and Water Balance Agents			
Acetazolamide (Diamox)—PO 250–1000 mg/day; IV 500 mg	Glaucoma; heart failure; convulsive disorders	Weak diuretic; produces acidosis; self-limiting effect; increases bicarbonate excretion	Electrolyte depletion symptomatology—lassitude, apathy, decreased urinary output, mental confusion

NURSING IMPLICATIONS: Weigh daily, I&O; assess edema; give *early* in day to allow sleep at night; observe for side effects; replace electrolytes as ordered

Ethacrynic acid (Edecrin)—PO 50–200 mg qd in divided doses	Pulmonary edema; ascites; edema of heart failure	Inhibits the reabsorption of Na$^+$ in the ascending loop of Henle	Nausea, vomiting, diarrhea; hypokalemia; hypotension; gout; dehydration; deafness; metabolic acidosis

NURSING IMPLICATIONS: Assess for dehydration—skin turgor, neck veins; hypotension; *KCl* supplement

Furosemide (Lasix)—PO 40–80 mg qd in divided doses	Edema and associated heart failure; cirrhosis; renal disease; nephrotic syndrome: hypertension	Inhibits Na$^+$ and Cl$^-$ reabsorption in the loop of Henle	Dermatitis, pruritis; paresthesia; blurring of vision; postural hypotension; nausea, vomiting, diarrhea, dehydration, electrolyte depletion; hearing loss (usually reversible)

NURSING IMPLICATIONS: Assess for weakness, lethargy, leg cramps, anorexia; peak action in 1–2 hr; duration 6–8 hr; do *not* give at bedtime; supplemental *KCl* indicated; may induce *digitalis toxicity*

(Continued on following page)

Pharmacology

TABLE 10.6	Common Drugs *(Continued)*		
Drug and Dosage	**Use**	**Action**	◆ **Assessment: Side Effects**
Hydrochlorothiazide (HydroDIURIL and Esidrix 25–100 mg tid)—PO Diuril 0.5–1.0 qd	Edema; heart failure; Na⁺ retention in steroid therapy; hypertension	Inhibits NaCl and water reabsorption in the distal ascending loop and the distal convoluted tubule of the kidneys	Hypokalemia, nausea, vomiting, diarrhea; dizziness; paresthesias; may exacerbate diabetes
NURSING IMPLICATIONS: Watch for muscle weakness; give well-diluted potassium chloride supplement; *monitor* urine for changes in sugar and acetone			
Mannitol (Osmitrol)—50–100 mg/24 hr as 15%–20% solution	Cerebral edema, oliguria, acute renal failure, drug intoxication	Hypertonic solution that kidney tubules cannot reabsorb, thereby causing obligatory water loss	Diarrhea; water intoxication, thirst, headache
NURSING IMPLICATIONS: Usually Foley catheter required; monitor *cardiac and respiratory* status; a rate of infusion to elicit 30–50 mL urine/hr			
Sevelamer hydrochloride (Renagel)—PO 2 caps or tabs tid	Reduction of serum phosphorus level	Polymer binds intestinal phosphate	Headache; infection; pain; diarrhea, constipation; cough
NURSING IMPLICATIONS: Important to take multivitamin supplement approved by MD. Do **not** take after printed expiration date			
Spironolactone (Aldactone)— PO 25 mg bid–qid	Cirrhosis of liver; when other diuretics are ineffective	Inhibits effects of aldosterone in distal tubules of kidney	Headache; lethargy; diarrhea; ataxia; skin rash; gynecomastia
NURSING IMPLICATIONS: Potassium-sparing drug; do *not* give supplemental KCl; monitor for signs of electrolyte imbalance			
Emetic			
Ipecac syrup—*Adults, elderly adults, children >12 yr:* 15–30 mL followed by 3–4 glasses of water. *Children 1–12 yr:* 15 mL followed by 1–2 glasses of water. *Infants 6 mo–1 yr:* 5–10 mL followed by 1 glass of water	Emergency emetic for poison ingestion	NH₄ ions cause gastric irritation	Violent emesis, tachycardia, decreased BP, dyspnea
NURSING IMPLICATIONS: *Contraindicated* in liver and renal disease; if given for emesis, follow dose with as much *water* as client will drink. Should not be used in the home. Dosage and usage are controversial, as is repetition of dose if vomiting has not occurred in 20–30 min after giving first dose.			
Enzyme			
Pancrelipase (Viokase)— adults, PO 325 mg–1 g qd, during meals; children, PO 300–600 mg tid	Chronic pancreatitis; cystic fibrosis; gastrectomy; pancreatectomy; sprue	Assists in digestion of starch, protein, and fats; decreases nitrogen and fat content of stool	Anorexia, nausea, vomiting, diarrhea; buccal/anal soreness (infants); sneezing; skin rashes; diabetes
NURSING IMPLICATIONS: May be taken with antacid or cimetidine; do *not* crush or chew tabs; *monitor* I&O, weight; be alert for signs of diabetes; children may use sprinkles			
Erectile Dysfunction			
Sildenafil citrate (Viagra)—PO 50 mg 0.5–4hr before sexual activity	Erectile dysfunction	Vasodilation of nitric oxide in the corpus cavernosum of penis	Headache; cardiac arrest with *sudden death;* exfoliative dermatitis
NURSING IMPLICATIONS: 🍽 High fat meal delays drug action. Report to MD: headaches, flushing, chest pain, indigestion, blurred vision, changes in color vision; safety issue if taking nitrates.			

(Continued on following page)

Drug and Dosage	Use	Action	◆ Assessment: Side Effects
Expectorants			
Guaifenesin (Robitussin) — 100–400 mg q4h	Respiratory congestion	Increases expectoration by causing irritation of gastric mucosa; reduces adhesiveness/surface tension of respiratory tract fluid	Low incidence of GI upset; drowsiness
NURSING IMPLICATIONS: Encourage to stop smoking; increase fluid intake; respiratory hygiene			
Terpin hydrate—PO 5–10 mL, q3–4h	Bronchitis; emphysema	Liquefies bronchial secretions	Nausea, vomiting, gastric irritation
NURSING IMPLICATIONS: Give undiluted; push fluids			
Fibrinolytic Agents			
Alteplase, recombinant (Activase, tPA)—IV bolus 100 mg over 90 min: 15 mg bolus given over 1–2 min; then 50 mg over 30 min; then 35 mg over 60 min	Acute MI; under investigation for pulmonary emboli, deep-vein thrombosis, and peripheral artery thrombosis	Promotes conversion of plasminogen to plasmin, which is fibrinolytic	Internal or local bleeding; urticaria; dysrhythmias related to reperfusion; hypotension; nausea, vomiting
NURSING IMPLICATIONS: Assess for signs of reperfusion (relief of chest pain, no ST segment elevation); observe for bleeding; avoid IM injection; do not mix other medications in line			
Streptokinase—IV 1.5 million U diluted to 45 mL infused over 60 min	Lysis of pulmonary or systemic emboli or thrombi; acute MI	Reacts with plasminogen, dissolves fibrin clots	Prolonged coagulation; allergic reactions; mild fever
NURSING IMPLICATIONS: Monitor for signs of excessive bleeding, particularly at injection sites; avoid nonessential handling of client			
Urokinase—IV 4400 IU/kg over 10 min; 1.0–1.8 mL of 5000 IU/mL into catheter	Massive pulmonary emboli, coronary artery thrombi, occluded IV catheter	Directly activates plasminogen	Bleeding, anaphylaxis, rash
NURSING IMPLICATIONS: Vital signs; check q15min for bleeding during first hr; q15–30min for 8 hr; have epinephrine ready			
Fibrinolytic Antidote			
Aminocaproic acid (Amicar)— PO, IV 5 g loading dose; 1 g/hr to 30 g in 24 hr	Management of streptokinase or urokinase overdose.	Inhibits plasminogen activator and antagonizes plasmin.	Hypotension, bradycardia, cardiac arrhythmias
NURSING IMPLICATIONS: Give slowly IV to prevent side effects; not recommended for DIC			
Hematopoietic			
Darbepoetin alfa (ARANESP)—IV/Subcu 0.45 µg/kg once weekly	Treatment of anemia with chronic renal failure	Erythropoiesis-stimulating protein	Peripheral edema; infection; headache, hypertension, hypotension; arrhythmias; nausea, vomiting, diarrhea; myalgia, respiratory infection
NURSING IMPLICATIONS: See Epoetin			
Epoetin alfa (Epogen)—SC/IV 3–500 U/kg/dose 3x/wk	Anemia secondary to chronic kidney failure	Glycoprotein that stimulates RBC production	Headache, hypertension; iron deficiency, clotting of AV fistula
NURSING IMPLICATIONS: Monitor BP closely. Headache is common; report severe or persistent problem			

(Continued on following page)

TABLE 10.6	Common Drugs *(Continued)*		
Drug and Dosage	**Use**	**Action**	◆ **Assessment: Side Effects**

Hormones			
Chlorotrianisene (TACE), estrogen—PO 12–50 mg	Prostatic cancer; menopause	Nonsteroidal synthetic estrogen	Rare after one course of treatment; thromboembolism; impotence and gynecomastia in men

NURSING IMPLICATIONS: Supply client with package insert; *contraindicated* in blood coagulation disorders

Diethylstilbestrol (DES)—PO or IM 0.2–5.0 mg qd; vaginal suppository 0.1–0.5 mg at bedtime	Prostate carcinoma; menopausal symptoms; osteoporosis; pain; mammary carcinoma; atrophic vaginitis	Synthetic nonsteroidal compound with estrogenic effects on pituitary, ovaries, myometrium, endometrium, and other tissues	Anorexia, nausea, vomiting, headache, diarrhea, dizziness, fainting—many side effects with long-term use

NURSING IMPLICATIONS: *Never* give if woman is pregnant—predisposes to vaginal cancer in female offspring at puberty

Estradiol—PO 1–2 mg for replacement therapy; up to 10 mg for cancer qd–tid; cyclic (on 3 wk, off 1 wk)	Menopausal symptoms; osteoporosis; hypogenitalism; sexual infantilism; breast and prostatic carcinoma	Inhibits release of pituitary gonadotropins; promotes growth of female genital tissues	Anorexia, nausea, vomiting, diarrhea, fluid retention; mental depression; headache, thromboembolism; feminization in men

NURSING IMPLICATIONS: Baseline VS; weigh daily; encourage frequent physical checkups to check serum lipids; teach breast self-examination

Medroxyprogesterone (Provera)—PO 2.5–10.0 mg; IM 400–1000 mg weekly	Amenorrhea; functional uterine bleeding; threatened abortion; dysmenorrhea; adjunctive and palliative with renal cancer and endometriosis; PMS	Similar to progesterone, but can be taken orally; thickens uterine decidua	Drowsiness; cyclic menstrual withdrawal bleeding; GI upset; headache; edema; breast congestion

NURSING IMPLICATIONS: Teach client regarding self-administration; breast self-examination for possible breast changes

Menotropins (Pergonal)—IM 1 amp (FSH + LH)/day for 9–12 days (followed by 5000–10,000 U HCG; if ovulation does not occur, repeat with 2 amp)	**Infertility use:** treatment of secondary anovulation; stimulation of spermatogenesis	Human gonadatropic responses; induces ovulation; sperm stimulation	Abortions occur in 25%; failure rate 55%–80% of clients: possible multiple births; ovarian enlargement; gynecomastia in men

NURSING IMPLICATIONS: Assist in collection of urine to assess estrogen levels; counsel regarding couple's need to have daily intercourse from day of HCG injection until ovulation

Progesterone—SC or IM 5–10 mg qd; sublingual 5–10 mg	Amenorrhea; dysmenorrhea; endometriosis; habitual abortion	Converts endometrium into secreting structure; prevents ovulation; stimulates growth of mammary tissue	Nausea, vomiting; dizziness, edema, headache; protein metabolism

NURSING IMPLICATIONS: Give *deep* IM and rotate sites; weigh daily to ascertain fluid retention

Testosterone—PO 5–10 mg qd; IM 25–50 mg 2–3 times/wk; 200–400 mg IM q2–4wk for breast cancer	Hypogonadism; eunuchism; impotence, advanced cancer of breast	Growth of sex organs and appearance of secondary male sex characteristics; counteracts excessive amounts of estrogen	Nausea, dyspepsia; masculinization; hypercalcemia; menstrual irregularities; renal calculi; Na^+, K^+, and H_2O retention

NURSING IMPLICATIONS: Observe for edema; weigh daily; I&O; *push fluids* for clients who are bedridden, to prevent renal calculi

Vasopressin (Pitressin)—IM/SC 5–10 μg bid–qid; IM/SC 2.5–5 μg q2–3d for chronic therapy	Diabetes insipidus	Antidiuretic	Nausea, flatus; tremor; pounding in head; water intoxication

NURSING IMPLICATIONS: *Monitor* fluid balance, vital signs

(Continued on following page)

Drug and Dosage	Use	Action	◆ Assessment: Side Effects
Immune Modifiers			
Glatiramer acetate (Copaxone) —20 mg/day	Multiple sclerosis	Management of relapsing-remitting MS	Allergic reactions; anxiety; chest pain; weight gain; cough

NURSING IMPLICATIONS: Monitor for side effects; new drug to attempt to control signs and symptoms of progressing multiple sclerosis

Interferon β-1b (Betaseron) — 30 μg once a week	Multiple sclerosis	Reduce incidence of relapse	Seizures; GI symptoms; flulike symptoms; neutropenia, injection site reactions

NURSING IMPLICATIONS: Monitor progress of multiple sclerosis; determine if drug is effective in reducing incidence of relapse; provide information about multiple side effects

Immunosuppressant Agents			
Azathioprine (Imuran)— 3–5 mg/kg/day initially; maintenance: 1–3 mg/kg/day	Prevent renal transplant rejection Ulcerative colitis Rheumatoid arthritis	Antagonizes purine metabolism/inhibition of DNA/RNA synthesis	Hypersensitivity; additive myelosuppression with antineoplastics; hepatotoxicity, leukopenia

NURSING IMPLICATIONS: Assess for infection; monitor I & O and *daily weight*

Cyclosporine (Sandimmune)— PO 5–10 mg/kg several hours before surgery; daily for 2 weeks; reduce dosage by 2.5 mg/kg/week to 5–10 mg/kg/day. IV 5–6 mg/kg several hours before surgery daily; switch to PO form as soon as possible	Prevent organ rejection Ulcerative colitis; Rheumatoid arthritis	Inhibits interleukin-2, which is necessary for initiation of T-cell activity	Hypersensitivity; *caution* with alcohol, renal impairment

NURSING IMPLICATIONS: *Monitor:* I&O, daily weight, blood pressure; take as directed (time of day and with food); observe *nephrotoxicity*, gingival hyperplasia; *avoid* self administration of OTC drugs

Muromonab-CD 3 (Orthoclone OKT3)—IV 5 mg/day, 10–14 days	Renal, liver, or cardiac transplant rejection	Immunosuppression of T-cell function	Tremor; dyspnea, shortness of breath, wheezing; chest pain; diarrhea, nausea, vomiting; chills, fever

NURSING IMPLICATIONS: Draw solution into filter; give IV push over <1 min; do *not* give as IV infusion; do *not* mix with other medications

Mycophenolate (CellCept)— PO 1 g bid	Prevent renal transplant rejection	Inhibits purine synthesis; suppresses T and B lymphocytes	Diarrhea; vomiting; leukopenia; sepsis

NURSING IMPLICATIONS: Give initial dose *within* 72 hr of transplant; give on *empty* stomach 1 hr before or 2 hr after meals; do *not* open, crush, or chew capsules; do *not* give with *magnesium or aluminum* antacids

Tracrolimus—PO 0.075–0.15 mg/kg q12h; IV 0.05–0.1 mg/kg/day	Prevent rejection in liver transplant	Inhibits T-lymphocyte activation	Headache, insomnia, tremor; ascites; hypertension; peripheral edema; abdominal pain; rash; hyperglycemia, anemia

NURSING IMPLICATIONS: Give *6 hr after* transplant; oral therapy is preferred because of anaphylaxis with IV; therapy is lifelong

(Continued on following page)

TABLE 10.6	Common Drugs *(Continued)*		

Drug and Dosage	Use	Action	◆ Assessment: Side Effects
Mineralocorticoid Agent			
Fludrocortisone (Florinef)— PO 0.1–0.2 mg qd	Addison's	Causes sodium reabsorption, hydrogen and potassium excretion, and water retention	Heart failure; adrenal suppression, hypertension
NURSING IMPLICATIONS: Do *not* miss dose; therapy is lifelong; high potassium; *report:* weight gain, muscle weakness, cramps, nausea, anorexia, dizziness			
Mucolytic Agent			
Acetylcysteine (Mucomyst)— 1–5 mL of 20% solution or 1–10 mL of 10% solution per nebulizer tid	Emphysema; pneumonia; tracheostomy care; atelectasis; cystic fibrosis. Antidote to acetaminophen overdose, to protect against hepatotoxicity	Lowers viscosity of respiratory secretions by opening disulfide linkages in mucus	Stomatitis, nausea; rhinorrhea; bronchospasm
NURSING IMPLICATIONS: Observe *respiratory rate;* maintain open airway with suctioning as necessary; observe clients with asthma carefully for *increased bronchospasm*; discontinue treatment **immediately** if this occurs; odor disagreeable initially			
Muscle Relaxants			
Baclofen (Lioresal)—5 mg tid up to 10–20 mg 4 times/day maintenance dose	Relief of spasticity of multiple sclerosis, spinal cord injury	Centrally acting skeletal-muscle relaxant; depresses polysynaptic afferent reflex activity at spinal cord level	Pruritis, tinnitus; nausea, vomiting; diarrhea or constipation; drowsiness
NURSING IMPLICATIONS: Administer *with* food if GI symptoms; monitor for safety when ambulating; do *not* discontinue abruptly			
Dantrolene sodium (Dantrium)–25 mg/day–25 mg bid–tid to 100 mg qid max	See Baclofen	See Baclofen	See Baclofen
NURSING IMPLICATIONS: See Baclofen			
Narcotic Antagonist			
Naloxone HCl (Narcan)—IV 0.1–0.2 mg repeated q2–3 min prn up to 0.4–2 mg for narcotic-induced respiratory depression	Reverses respiratory depression due to narcotics	Reverses respiratory depression of morphine SO_4, meperidine HCl, and methadone HCl; does not itself cause respiratory depression, sedation, or analgesia	No common side effects; tachycardia, hypertension; nausea and vomiting with high doses
NURSING IMPLICATIONS: Note time, type of narcotic, dosage received; not useful with CNS depression from other drugs; respiratory depression *may return;* monitor closely			
Sedatives and Hypnotics			
Chlordiazepoxide HCl (Librium)—PO 5–10 mg; IM or IV 50–100 mg	Psychoneuroses; preoperative apprehension; chronic alcoholism; anxiety	CNS depressant resulting in mild sedation; appetite stimulant; anticonvulsant	Ataxia, fatigue; blurred vision, diplopia; lethargy; nightmares; confusion
NURSING IMPLICATIONS: Ensure anxiety relief by allowing client to verbalize feelings; advise client to *avoid* driving and alcoholic beverages			
Chloral hydrate—PO 250 mg tid; hypnotic: PO 0.5–1.0 g; rectal supplement 0.3–0.9 g	Sedation for elderly; delirium tremens; pruritus; mania; barbiturate and alcohol withdrawal	Depresses sensorimotor areas of cerebral cortex	Nausea, vomiting, gastritis; pinpoint pupils; delirium; rash; decreased BP, pulse, respirations, temperature; hepatic damage
NURSING IMPLICATIONS: *Caution:* should not be taken in combination with alcohol; dependency is possible			

(Continued on following page)

Drug and Dosage	Use	Action	◆ Assessment: Side Effects
Diazepam (Valium)—PO 2–10 mg tid–qid; IM or IV 2–10 mg q3–4h	Anxiety disorders; alcohol withdrawal; adjunctive therapy in seizure disorders; status epilepticus; eclamptic seizures; tetanus, preoperative or preprocedural sedation (also see Midazolam)	Induces calming effect on limbic system, thalamus, and hypothalamus	CNS depression—sedation or ataxia (dose related); dry mouth; blurred vision; mydriasis; constipation; urinary retention

NURSING IMPLICATIONS: Do *not* mix with other drugs; IM injection painful; observe for *phlebitis;* monitor response; measures to ensure client safety (e.g., falls); high potential for abuse; *contraindicated* in acute closed-angle glaucoma and porphyria

Flurazepam (Dalmane)—PO >15 yr, 30 mg hs; elderly or debilitated, 15 mg hs	Hypnotic	Fastest acting; see Diazepam	See Diazepam

NURSING IMPLICATIONS: See Diazepam

Hydroxyzine pamoate (Vistaril)—PO 25–100 mg qid	See Chlordiazepoxide (Librium); antiemetic in postoperative conditions; adjunctive therapy **Obstetric use:** prodromal labor	CNS relaxant with sedative effect on limbic system and thalamus Allows relaxation	Drowsiness; headache; itching; dry mouth; tremor

NURSING IMPLICATIONS: Give *deep* IM only; *potentiates* action of: warfarin (Coumadin), narcotics, and barbiturates

Lorazepam (Ativan)—PO 1–2 mg bid–tid (up to 10 mg); 2–4 mg hs; IM 4 mg max; IV 2 mg max	Anxiety disorders; insomnia; alternative to diazepam for status epilepticus; preanesthesia	See Diazepam	See Diazepam

NURSING IMPLICATIONS: See Diazepam

Meprobamate (Equanil, Miltown)—PO 400 mg tid–qid	Anxiety; stress; absence seizures	See Hydroxyzine pamoate (Vistaril)	Voracious appetite; dryness of mouth; ataxia

NURSING IMPLICATIONS: Older clients prone to drowsiness and hypotension; observe for *jaundice*

Midazolam (Versed)—IM 0.05–0.08 mg/kg; IV 0.1–0.15 mg/kg	Preanesthesia; prediagnostic procedures; induction of general anesthesia	Penetrates blood-brain barrier to produce sedation and amnesia	Respiratory depression, apnea; disorientation, behavioral excitement

NURSING IMPLICATIONS: Monitor ventilatory status and oxygenation; prevent injuries from CNS depression; nonirritating to vein

Phenobarbital—sedative, PO 20–30 mg tid; hypnotic, PO 50–100 mg; IV or IM 100–300 mg; butabarbital (Butisol), pentobarbital (Nembutal), secobarbital (Seconal)	Preoperative sedation; emergency control of convulsions; absence seizures	Depresses CNS, promoting drowsiness	Cough, hiccups; restlessness; pain; hangover; CNS and circulatory depression

NURSING IMPLICATIONS: Observe for hypotension during IV administration; put up side rails on bed of older clients; observe for increased tolerance

Promethazine (Phenergan)— IV, IM, PO 25–50 mg	Preoperative sedation; postoperative sedation	Antihistaminic; sedative, antiemetic, anti-motion sickness	Drowsiness; coma; hypotension; hypertension; leukopenia; photosensitivity; irregular respirations; blurred vision; urinary retention; dry mouth, nose, throat

NURSING IMPLICATIONS: Administer PO *with* food, milk; IM *deep* into large muscles, rotate sites; verify compatibility with other drugs; safety concerns due to sedative effect

(Continued on following page)

TABLE 10.6	Common Drugs (Continued)			
Drug and Dosage	**Use**	**Action**		**Assessment: Side Effects**
Zolpidem (Ambien)—PO 5–10 mg h.s., limited to 7–10 days	Short-term treatment of insomnia	Nonbenzodiazepine hypnotic; preserves deep sleep (stages 3 and 4)		Headache on awakening; drowsiness, fatigue; confusion and falls in elderly; myalgia

NURSING IMPLICATIONS: Monitor for: compromised respiratory status, increased depression, cognitive impairment. Onset more rapid on empty stomach. Do **not** breastfeed while taking this med

Serum

Immune globulin—IM 0.02 mL/kg	Hepatitis	Provides passive immunity		Do *not* use if client is hypersensitive

NURSING IMPLICATIONS: Should be administered within *2 wk* of exposure

Thyroid Hormone Inhibitors

Lugol solution—PO 2–6 drops tid 10 days before thyroidectomy	To reduce size, vascularity of thyroid before thyroid surgery; emergency treatment of thyroid storm; or control of hyperthyroid symptoms after radioiodine (^{131}I) therapy	Inhibits thyroid hormone secretion, synthesis		GI distress; stained teeth; increased respiratory secretions; rashes; acne

NURSING IMPLICATIONS: *Dilute in juice,* give through *straw;* bloody diarrhea/vomiting indicates acute poisoning

Propylthiouracil—PO 300–400 mg/day, divided initial dose; 100–150 mg/day maintenance dose; methimazole (Tapazole) 15–60 mg/day initial dose; 5–15 mg/day maintenance dose	Hyperthyroidism; return client to euthyroid state; also used preoperatively	Inhibits functional thyroid hormone synthesis by blocking reactions; responsible for iodide conversion to iodine; inhibition of T_4 conversion to T_3		Blood dyscrasias, hepatotoxicity, hypothyroidism

NURSING IMPLICATIONS: Teach importance of compliance with medication protocol; 🍽 *avoid* iodine-rich foods (seafood, iodized salt); caution when using other drugs

Saturated potassium iodide (SSKI)—300 mg tid–qid	See Lugol's solution	See Lugol's solution		See Lugol solution

NURSING IMPLICATIONS: See Lugol solution

Thyroid Hormone Replacement

Levothyroxine (Levothroid, Synthroid)—PO 0.05–0.10 mg/day; IV 200–500 μg	Hypothyroidism Myxedema coma	Replacement therapy to alleviate symptoms Emergency replacement therapy		Symptoms of hyperthyroidism

NURSING IMPLICATIONS: Teach signs and symptoms of hyperthyroidism, hypothyroidism; monitor bowel activity; teach diet to combat constipation; keep medication in tight light-proof container; 🍽 *avoid foods* that inhibit thyroid secretion (turnips, cabbage, carrots, peaches, peas, strawberries, spinach, radishes)

Liothyronine (Cytomel)—PO 25 μg/day to maintenance dose 25–75 μg	Mild hypothyroidism in adults	Replacement therapy		See Levothyroxine

NURSING IMPLICATIONS: See Levothyroxine

(Continued on following page)

Pharmacology

Drug and Dosage	Use	Action	◆ Assessment: Side Effects
Uterine Contractants			
Ergonovine maleate (Ergotrate)—PO, IM, IV 0.2 mg (gr 1/320)	Postabortal or postpartum hemorrhage; promotes involution after delivery of placenta	Stimulates uterine contractions for 3 hr or more	Nausea, vomiting; occasional transient hypertension, especially if given IV; cramping

NURSING IMPLICATIONS: Store in *cool* place; monitor maternal BP and pulse; *do not use in labor*

Methylergonovine maleate (Methergine)—PO 0.2 mg; IM, IV, 0.2 mg (gr 1/320)	Postpartum hemorrhage, after delivery of placenta	Stimulates stronger and longer contractions than ergonovine maleate (Ergotrate)	Nausea, vomiting; transient hypertension, dizziness, tachycardia; cramping

NURSING IMPLICATIONS: Do *not* give if mother is hypertensive; do *not* use if solution is discolored; *do not use in labor*

Oxytocin (Pitocin, Syntocinon)—IV 2 mL (20 U) in 1000 mL solution; 1 mL IM after delivery	Stimulates rhythmic contractions of uterus	Induces labor; augments contractions; prevents or controls postpartum atony; antidiuretic effect	Tetanic contractions, uterine rupture; cardiac arrhythmias, FHR deceleration

NURSING IMPLICATIONS: *Contraindicated* if cervix is unripe, in CPD, abruptio placentae, and cardiovascular disease; *monitor:* FHR, contractions, maternal BP, pulse, I&O; watch for signs of water intoxication with prolonged IV use; drug of choice in presence of hypertension; *never* use undiluted; DC if tetanic contractions occur; *antidote:* propranolol

Volume Expander			
Albumin—IV 5%, 25% 500 mL as needed	Cirrhosis Nephrotic syndrome	Provides colloidal oncotic pressure, which mobilizes fluid from extracellular back into intravascular space	Hypersensitivity, CHF, hepatic failure

NURSING IMPLICATIONS: Monitor progress of disease; monitor for signs of shock; if fever, tachycardia, or hypotension occur, *stop* treatment and call physician

---

TABLE 10.7	**Food and Fluid Considerations with Drugs**

Key:
1. Take with food or milk
2. Take on empty stomach (1h ac or 2h pc)
3. Don't drink milk or eat dairy products
4. Take with full glass of water
5. Take ½ h before meals
6. Take with or without food

A
Albuterol 1
Allopurinol 1
Aminophylline 1
Amlodipine 6
Amiodarone 1
Amoxicillin 6
Ampicillin 2
Aspirin 1
Augmentin 6
Azo Gantrisin 4, 6

B
Baclofen 1
Bactrim 4, 6
Belladonna 5
Benemid 1, 4
Bisacodyl 3

C
Captopril 2
Cefaclor 6
Cefuroxime axetil 6
Cephalexin 6
Cholestyramine 5
Chlorothiazide 1
Cimetidine 1
Ciprofloxacin 4, 6
Clonazepam 1
Clopidogrel 6
Cloxacillin 2
Co-trimoxazole 4, 6
Cyclosporine 1

D
Demeclocycline 2, 3
Diltiazem 1
Diuril 1
Donnatal 5
Dopar 1
Doxycycline hyclate 3, 6
Dulcolax 3

E
Ecotrin 3
Enalapril 6

Ethosuximide 1
Etodolac 2
Eythromycin stearate 2

F
Famotidine 6
Feldene 1
Ferrous sulfate 3
Flecainide 6
Fluoxetine 6

G
Gantrisin 4, 6
Gemfibrozil 5
Glycopyrrolate 5

H
Hismanyl 2
Hydrocodone/acetaminophen 1
Hydromorphone 1

I
Ibuprofen 1, 2
Ilosone 6
Indinavir 2, 4
Indomethacin 1
Isoniazid 2

K
Keflex 6
Ketoconazole 1
Ketoprofen 1
K-Lor 1

L
Levodopa 1
Librium 1
Lisinopril 6
Lovastatin 1

M
Macrodantin 1
Marax 1
Metronidazole 1
Mexiletine 1
Mycophenolate 2

N
Nafcillin 2
Naproxen 4
Neostigmine 5
Niacin 1
Nicardipine 5
Nitrofurantoin 1

(Continued on following page)

| TABLE 10.7 | Food and Fluid Considerations with Drugs *(Continued)* |

P	Pro-Banthine 5	**S**	Theophylline 1, 4
Parlodel 1	Probenecid 4	Simvastatin 6	Ticlopidine 1
Penicillamine 2		Sinemet 1	Trimethoprim 2
Penicillin G 2	**Q**	Slow-K 1	
Penicillin V 2	Quinidine 1	Sucralfate 2	**V**
Persantine 2		Sulfisoxazole 4, 6	Vasotec 6
Phenylbutazone 1	**R**		
Phenytoin 1	Ranitidine 6	**T**	**Z**
Prednisone 1	Rifampin 2	Tedral 1	Zestril 6
	Robinul 5	Tetracycline 2, 3	

| TABLE 10.8 | Antineoplastic Drug Classifications |

I. Alkylating agents
  A. Alkyl sulfonates
    1. Busulfan (*Myleran*)
  B. Ethylenimines
    1. Thiotepa
  C. Nitrosoureas
    1. Carmustine (BCNU, *BiCNU*)
    2. Lomustine (CCNU, *CeeNu*)
    3. Semustine (methyl-CCNU)
    4. Streptozocin (*Zanosar*, streptozotocin)
  D. Nitrogen mustards
    1. Mechlorethamine hydrochloride (*Mustargen,* HN_2, nitrogen mustard)
    2. Cyclophosphamide (*Cytoxan*)
    3. Chlorambucil (*Leukeran*)
    4. Melphalan (*Alkeran, L-PAM,* L-phenylalanine mustard)
    5. Ifosfamide (*Ifex*)
  E. Triazenes
    1. Dacarbazine (*DTIC-Dome*)

II. Antibiotics
  A. Anthracyclines
    1. Doxorubicin hydrochloride (*Adriamycin*)
    2. Daunorubicin (daunomycin, *Cerubidine*)
    3. Idarubicin (*Idamycin*)
  B. Bleomycins
    1. Bleomycin sulfate (*Blenoxane*)
  C. Dactinomycin (actinomycin D, *Cosmegen*)
  D. Mitomycin (mitomycin C, *Mutamycin*)
  E. Plicamycin (*Mithracin*)

III. Antimetabolites
  A. Folate antagonist
    1. Methotrexate (*Folex, Mexate*)
  B. Purine analogues
    1. Thioguanine (6-TG, 6-thioguanine)
    2. Mercaptopurine (6-MP, *Purinethol*)
    3. Fludarabine (*Fludara*)
    4. Pentostatin (deoxycoformycin, *Nipent*)
    5. Cladribine (2-chloro-deoxyadenosine, *Leustatin*)
  C. Pyrimidine analogues
    1. Cytarabine (cytosine arabinoside, *Cytosar-U*, ara-C)
    2. Fluorouracil (5-FU, 5-fluorouracil)

IV. Cellular growth factors
  A. Filgrastim (*Neupogen*)
  B. Sargramostim (*Leukine, Prokine*)
V. Enzymes
  A. L-Asparaginase (*Elspar*)
VI. Hormonal agents
  A. Androgens/antiandrogens
    1. Flutamide (*Eulexin*)
  B. Estrogens/antiestrogens
    1. Tamoxifen citrate (*Nolvadex*)
    2. Estramustine phosphate sodium (*Emcyt*)
  C. Glucocorticoids
  D. Luteinizing hormone–releasing hormone (LH-RH) antagonists
    1. Buserelin (*Suprefact*)
    2. Leuprolide (*Lupron*)
  E. Octreotide acetate (*Sandostatin*)
VII. Immunomodulating agents
  A. Levamisole (*Ergamisol*)
  B. Interferons
    1. Interferon alfa-2a (*Roferon-A*)
    2. Interferon alfa-2b (*Intron A*)
  C. Interleukins: aldesleukin (interleukin-2, IL-2, *Proleukin*)
VIII. Miscellaneous agents
  A. Carboplatin (*Paraplatin*)
  B. Cisplatin (*cis*-platinum II, *Platinol*)
  C. Hexamethylmelamine (HMM)
  D. Hydroxyurea (*Hydrea*)
  E. Mitotane (o,p′-DDD, *Lysodren*)
  F. Mitoxantrone (*Novantrone*)
  G. Procarbazine (N-methylhydrazine, *Matulane, Natulan*)
IX. Monoclonal antibodies
X. Plant-derived products
  A. Vinca alkaloids
    1. Vincristine (*Oncovin*)
    2. Vinblastine (*Velban*)
  B. Epipodophyllotoxins
    1. Etoposide (*VePesid*)
    2. Teniposide (*Vumon*)
  C. Taxanes: paclitaxel (*Taxol*)

Pharmacology

TABLE 10.9	Properties of Selected Analgesic Agents		
Specific Group	**Analgesic**	**Antipyretic**	**Antiinflammatory**
Nonopioid			
Acetaminophen	*	*	0
Ibuprofen	*	*	*
Naproxen	*	*	*
Fenoprofen	*	*	*
Flurbiprofen	*	*	*
Ketoprofen	*	*	*
Nonsteroidal			
Aspirin	*	*	*
Indomethacin	*	*	*
Sulindac	*	0	*
Meclofenamate	*	0	*
Tolmetin	*	*	*
Diflunisal	*	0	*
Piroxicam	*	*	*
Diclofenac	*	*	*
Etodolac	*	0	*
Nabumetone	*	*	*

* = possesses the property assigned; 0 = lacks the property assigned.

TABLE 10.10	Equianalgesic Dosing for Opioid Analgesics					
	Approximate Equianalgesic Dose		**Recommended Starting Dose (adults > 50 kg body weight)**		**Recommended Starting Dose (children and adults > 50 kg body weight)[a]**	
DRUG	**ORAL**	**PARENTERAL**	**ORAL**	**PARENTERAL**	**ORAL**	**PARENTERAL**
OPIOID AGONIST						
Morphine[b]	30 mg q3–4th (around-the-clock dosing) 60 mg q3–4h (single dose or intermittent dosing)	10 mg q3–4h	30 mg q3–4h	10 mg q3–4h	0.3 mg/kg q3–4h	0.1 mg/kg q3–4h
Codeine[c]	180–200 mg q3–4h	130 mg q3–4h	60 mg q3–4h	60 mg q2h (intramuscular/ subcutaneous)	1 mg/kg q3–4h[d]	Not recommended
Hydrocodone (in Lorcet, Lortab, Vicodin, others)	30 mg q3–4h	Not available	10 mg q3–4h	Not available	0.2 mg/kg q3–4h[d]	Not available
Hydromorphone[b] (Dilaudid)	7.5 mg q3–4h	1.5 mg q3–4h	6 mg q3–4h	1.5 mg q3–4h	0.06 mg/kg q3–4h	0.015 mg/kg q3–4h
Levorphanol (Levo-Dromoran)	4 mg q6–8h	2 mg q6–8h	4 mg q6–8h	2 mg q6–8h	0.04 mg/kg q6–8h	0.02 mg/kg q6–8h
Meperidine (Demerol)	300 mg q2–3h	100 mg q3h	Not recommended	100 mg q3h	Not recommended	0.75 mg/kg q2–3h
Methadone (Dolophine, others)	20 mg q6–8h	10 mg q6–8h	20 mg q6–8h	10 mg q6–8h	0.2 mg/kg q6–8h	0.1 mg/kg q6–8h
Oxycodone (Roxicodone, also in Percocet, Percodan, Tylox, others)	30 mg q3–4h	Not available	10 mg q3–4h	Not available	0.2 mg/kg q3–4h[d]	Not available

(Continued on following page)

TABLE 10.10	Equianalgesic Dosing for Opioid Analgesics *(Continued)*					
	Approximate Equianalgesic Dose		Recommended Starting Dose (adults > 50 kg body weight)		Recommended Starting Dose (children and adults > 50 kg body weight)[a]	
DRUG	**ORAL**	**PARENTERAL**	**ORAL**	**PARENTERAL**	**ORAL**	**PARENTERAL**
Oxymorphone[b] (Numorphan)	Not available	1 mg q3–4hr	Not available	1 mg q3–4h	Not recommended	Not recommended
OPIOID AGONIST-ANTAGONIST AND PARTIAL AGONIST						
Buprenorphine (Buprenex)	Not available	0.3–0.4 mg q6–8h	Not available	0.4 mg q6–8h	Not available	0.004 mg/kg q6–8h
Butorphanol (Stadol)	Not available	2 mg q3–4h	Not available	2 mg q3–4h	Not available	Not recommended
Dezocine (Dalgan)	Not available	10 mg q3–4h	Not available	10 mg q3–4h	Not available	Not recommended
Nalbuphine (Nubain)	Not available	10 mg q3–4h	Not available	10 mg q3–4h	Not available	0.1 mg/kg q3–4h
Pentazocine (Talwin, others)	150 mg q3–4h	60 mg q3–4h	50 mg q4–6h	Not recommended	Not recommended	Not recommended

Adapted from Acute Pain Management Guideline Panel: *Acute Pain Management in Adults: Operative Procedures. Quick Reference Guide for Clinicians.* Agency for Health Care Policy and Research, Public Health and Human Services, Rockville, MD. AHCPR Publication No. 92–0019.

Note: Published tables vary in the suggested doses that are equianalgesic to morphine. Clinical response is the criterion that must be applied for each client; titration to clinical response is necessary. Because there is not complete cross-tolerance among these drugs, it is usually necessary to use a lower than equianalgesic dose when changing drugs and to retitrate to response.

Caution: Recommended doses do not apply to clients with renal or hepatic insufficiency or other conditions affecting drug metabolism and kinetics.

[a]**Caution:** Doses listed for clients with body weight less than 50 kg cannot be used as initial starting doses in babies less than 6 mo of age.

[b]For morphine, hydromorphone, and oxymorphone, *rectal* administration is an alternate route for clients *unable* to take oral medications, but equianalgesic doses may differ from oral and parenteral doses because of pharmacokinetic differences.

[c]**Caution:** Codeine doses *above 65 mg often are not appropriate* because of diminishing incremental analgesia with increasing doses but continually *increasing constipation* and other side effects. Oral doses refer to *combination* with aspirin or acetaminophen.

[d]**Caution:** Doses of aspirin and acetaminophen in combination opioid/NSAID preparations must also be adjusted to the client's body weight.

TABLE 10.11	Dietary Supplements and Herbal Products Used for Psychiatric Conditions		
HERB	**ACTION/USE**	**CAUTION**	**DRUG INTERACTIONS**
DHEA (dehydroepiandros- terone)	▪ Depression ▪ ↓ Fatigue	▪ Hx of PCA or BrCa ▪ Hepatic dysfunction ▪ Diabetes	▪ Antidiabetic agents ▪ Estrogen ▪ Corticosteroids
Ginkgo biloba	▪ ↑ Mental function (e.g., Alzheimer's)	*Contraindication:* ▪ Discontinue 2 weeks before surgery ▪ Blood clotting disorder ▪ Renal failure ▪ Acute infection ▪ ↑ or ↓ BP	▪ Blood-thinning meds (e.g., Coumadin, heparin, NSAIDs, ASA) ▪ Hormonal ▪ MAO inhibitors ▪ Antihypertensives ▪ Caffeine ▪ Decongestants
Ginseng	▪ ↓ Fatigue, stress ▪ ↑ Mental alertness ▪ ↑ Physical endurance	*Contraindicated* with: ▪ Peptic ulcer ▪ Intracranial bleeding ▪ Elderly with CVD ▪ Diabetes	▪ MAO inhibitors ▪ Antihypertensives ▪ Barbiturates ▪ Anticoagulants ▪ Insulin and oral hypo- glycemics ▪ Digoxin

(Continued on following page)

HERB	ACTION/USE	CAUTION	DRUG INTERACTIONS
Kava	<ul><li>↓ Anxiety</li><li>↓ Stress</li><li>↓ Restlessness</li><li>↑ Sleep (↓insomnia)</li><li>↑ Relaxation</li></ul>	<ul><li>Discontinue after 3 months (yellow hair, skin, nails)</li><li>Reaction:</li><li>Euphoria<ul><li>Depression</li><li>Somnolence</li><li>Eye accommodation disturbance</li><li>Muscle weakness</li></ul></li></ul>	<ul><li>Alcohol/CNS depressants</li><li>Barbiturates</li><li>Antipsychotics (e.g., Haldol)</li><li>Antianxiety drugs (Valium, Xanax, Ativan)</li><li>↓ Effects of levodopa (Parkinson's)</li><li>Statins (liver injury)</li></ul>
SAMe (S-adenosyl-methionine)	<ul><li>Depression (not bipolar)</li></ul>	<ul><li>Bleeding</li></ul>	<ul><li>Other antidepressants (MAO inhibitors, TCAs, SSRIs)</li><li>Potentiates St. John's Wort</li></ul>
St. John's Wort	<ul><li>↓ Mild depression</li></ul>	<ul><li>↑ Panic, agitation, confusion</li><li>↑ Skin sensitivity in sun (if also on sulfa, Feldane, Prilosec, Prevacid)</li></ul>	<ul><li>↑ Serotonin level if on antidepressants (e.g., MAO inhibitors, SSRIs, TCAs)</li><li>Reduces effect of:<ul><li>Digoxin</li><li>Immunosuppressants</li><li>Protease inhibitors (HIV)</li><li>Oral contraceptives</li><li>Coumadin</li><li>Theophylline (asthma)</li><li>Antipsychotics (e.g., clozapine)</li><li>Chemotherapy</li></ul></li></ul>
Valerian	<ul><li>Minor tranquilizer</li><li>Anxiety, panic attacks</li><li>Sleep disorders (insomnia)</li></ul>	<ul><li>Lightheadness</li><li>Restless</li><li>Fatigue</li><li>Nausea</li><li>Tremor</li><li>Blurred vision</li></ul>	<ul><li>Potentiates other CNS depressants (e.g., alcohol)</li><li>Benzodiazepines (e.g., Xanax, Valium)</li><li>Anticonvulsants (e.g., Dilantin, phenobarbital)</li><li>Antidepressants (e.g., Elavil, Tofranil, Prozac)</li><li>Avoid taking with substances that cause drowsiness</li></ul>

TABLE 10.12   Herbs and Potential Dangers

HERB	USE	ADVERSE EFFECTS/DRUG INTERACTIONS/CAUTIONS
Aloe	**External:**<ul><li>Heal burns, wounds</li><li>Antiinfective</li><li>Moisturizer</li></ul> **Internal:**<ul><li>Laxative</li><li>General healing</li></ul>	**Adverse effect:**<ul><li>Contact dermatitis</li></ul> **Adverse effect:**<ul><li>Hypokalemia</li></ul> **Caution:**<ul><li>*Avoid* oral use in GI conditions (e.g., inflammation, ulcers, pain of unknown origin)</li></ul>
Arnica	**External:**<ul><li>Inflammation caused by insect bites</li><li>After muscular and joint injuries (e.g., bruises)</li></ul>	**Adverse effect:**<ul><li>Toxic skin reaction</li><li>Avoid use on broken skin</li></ul>
Black cohosh	<ul><li>PMS</li><li>Menopause</li></ul>	**Interaction with:**<ul><li>Oral contraceptives</li><li>Anticoagulants (e.g., Coumadin)</li><li>HRT</li></ul> **Caution with:**<ul><li>Estrogen-sensitive cancers (breast, ovarian)</li><li>Salicylate allergies</li><li>History of thromboembolic disease</li></ul>

(Continued on following page)

TABLE 10.12 Herbs and Potential Dangers *(Continued)*		
HERB	**USE**	**ADVERSE EFFECTS/DRUG INTERACTIONS/CAUTIONS**
Burdock leaf and root	▪ Severe skin problems ▪ Arthritis	**Adverse effect:** ▪ Contaminated with belladonna
Chamomile	**External:** ▪ Topical antiinflammatory agent (for eczema, hemorrhoids, mastitis, leg ulcers) **Internal:** ▪ Indigestion ▪ Antispasmodic (irritable bowel syndrome)	**Caution with:** ▪ Asthma
Echinacea	▪ Immune system stimulant at onset of cold	**Interaction with:** ▪ Immunosuppressants (e.g., cyclosporine) **Caution with:** ▪ Lupus ▪ Multiple sclerosis
Evening primrose oil	▪ Asthma ▪ Diabetic neuropathy ▪ Eczema ▪ Hyperglycemia ▪ Irritable bowel syndrome ▪ Menopause ▪ Multiple sclerosis ▪ Rheumatoid arthritis	**Interaction with:** ▪ Phenothiazines ▪ ASA ▪ NSAIDs ▪ Anticoagulants ▪ Antiplatelet agents ▪ Anticonvulsants **Caution with:** ▪ Peptic ulcer ▪ Intracranial bleeding ▪ Epilepsy ▪ Schizophrenia
Feverfew (see also Appendix P)	▪ Migraines	**Adverse effect:** ▪ Increase bleeding ▪ Spontaneous abortion in early pregnancy **Interaction with:** ▪ Anticoagulants ▪ Antiplatelets ▪ NSAIDs **Caution:** ▪ Do *not* use before or after surgery
Ginger	▪ Antiemetic ▪ Colds, flu ▪ Headaches	**Interaction with:** ▪ Anticoagulants ▪ Antiplatelets ▪ Cardiac glycosides ▪ Hypoglycemic agents **Caution with:** ▪ Diabetes ▪ Gallstones
Goldenseal	Topical treatment of: ▪ Sores ▪ Inflamed mucous membranes	**Interaction with:** ▪ Tretinoins (Retin-A) ▪ Anticoagulants **Adverse effect:** ▪ Causes uterine contractions **Caution with:** ▪ Women who are pregnant ▪ Lactation
Hawthorne	▪ Dementia ▪ CHF ▪ Angina	**Interaction with:** ▪ Ace inhibitors ▪ Anticoagulants ▪ Coronary vasodilators **Caution with:** ▪ Lactation

(Continued on following page)

HERB	USE	ADVERSE EFFECTS/DRUG INTERACTIONS/CAUTIONS
Melaleuca Oil®	■ Topical use for burns ■ Bactericidal ■ Fungicidal	**Adverse effect:** ■ CNS depression ■ Allergic dermatitis
Milk thistle	■ Liver: hepatitis and cirrhosis ■ Gallstones ■ Psoriasis	**Interaction with:** ■ Oral contraceptives **Adverse effect:** ■ Laxative effect
Nettle leaf	■ Kidney, bladder stones ■ UTI	**Caution with:** ■ Pregnancy ■ Lactation
Pennyroyal	**External:** ■ Skin disease **Internal:** ■ Digestive disorders ■ Liver and gallbladder disorders ■ Gout	*Use not recommended because of hepatotoxicity*
Sassafras oil	■ Lice ■ Insect bites	**Adverse effect:** ■ *Carcinogenesis* (e.g., hepatic tumors)
Saw palmetto	■ Anti-androgen therapy ■ BPH	**Interaction with:** ■ HRT ■ Proscar
Senna	■ Catharsis ■ Laxative	**Adverse effect:** ■ Electrolyte imbalance (decrease K^+) **Caution with:** ■ Acute intestinal inflammation (e.g., Crohn's, ulcerative colitis, appendicitis)

Questions

Select the one answer that is best for each question, unless otherwise directed.

1. A client has meperidine, 75 mg every 3–4 hours prn, ordered for postoperative pain. Before administering this narcotic, the nurse should:
   1. Position the client in a semi-Fowler's position to minimize respiratory effects.
   2. Assess the type, location, and intensity of discomfort.
   3. Evaluate whether the pain is real.
   4. Try other measures to relieve discomfort, such as position change.
2. The nurse explains to a client that although salicylates are given to relieve pain in rheumatoid arthritis, they also function as an:
   1. Analgesic.
   2. Antiinflammatory.
   3. Anticholinergic.
   4. Antiadrenergic.
3. Client teaching includes the early side effects of theophylline administration, which are:
   1. Tachycardia and palpitations.
   2. Anorexia, nausea, and vomiting.
   3. Restlessness and tremors.
   4. Headache and insomnia.
4. Based on the peak action of furosemide (Lasix) PO, the nurse will evaluate the drug's effects in:
   1. 30–45 minutes.
   2. 1–2 hours.
   3. 3–4 hours.
   4. 6–8 hours.

5. The nurse knows that the best time to give oral iron preparations is:
   1. With meals, to decrease gastric upset.
   2. 1 hour before eating, to enhance absorption.
   3. 1 hour after eating, to slow absorption.
   4. At bedtime.
6. The nurse administers spironolactone (Aldactone) knowing that it is classified as:
   1. An aldosterone antagonist.
   2. A carbonic anhydrase inhibitor.
   3. A thiazide.
   4. An osmotic diuretic.
7. Which supplement would the nurse not ordinarily administer to the client receiving spironolactone?
   1. Vitamin B_6.
   2. Potassium chloride.
   3. Ascorbic acid.
   4. Calcium carbonate.
8. The primary objective in giving prednisone along with aspirin for acute rheumatoid arthritis is to:
   1. Inhibit the autoimmune factors associated with rheumatoid arthritis.
   2. Prevent further joint destruction.
   3. Decrease inflammation and suppress symptomatology.
   4. Increase glucose levels for tissue repair.
9. The nurse would recognize prednisone toxicity if which of the following occurred?
   1. Tinnitus.
   2. Exfoliative dermatitis.
   3. Glucosuria.
   4. Nausea and vomiting.
10. Propantheline bromide (Pro-Banthine) is given to clients with cholelithiasis and cholecystitis because it:

1. Reduces gastric secretions and intestinal hypermobility.
2. Decreases bile secretion by the liver and gallbladder.
3. Slows the emptying of the stomach, thereby reducing chyme in the duodenum.
4. Inhibits contraction of the gallbladder and the bile duct.

11. The nurse can anticipate side effects of hydrochlorothiazide because it is classified as:
    1. An aldosterone inhibitor.
    2. A carbonic anhydrase inhibitor.
    3. A potassium-sparing drug.
    4. A potassium-wasting drug.

12. Assessment for the side effects of hydrochlorothiazide includes signs of:
    1. Hypernatremia.
    2. Hyperkalemia.
    3. Hypochloremia.
    4. Hypouricemia.

13. A 2-year-old child (diagnosis: meningitis) is to be sedated with phenobarbital, 18 mg PO q6h. The label reads "20 mg per 5 mL." How much phenobarbital should the nurse administer to this child?
    1. 4 mL.
    2. 4.3 mL.
    3. 4.5 mL.
    4. 4.8 mL.

14. A client's CSF culture is positive for *Haemophilus influenzae* meningitis. To protect other members of the client's family who have been exposed to meningitis, the nurse should explain that they may be given:
    1. Amoxicillin/clavulanate potassium (Augmentin).
    2. Sulfisoxazole.
    3. Rifampin.
    4. Immune serum globulin.

15. The nurse is to administer pancreatin to a child with cystic fibrosis. To evaluate the effect of this medication, the nurse should know that the primary purpose of this medication is to increase the absorption of:
    1. Glucose.
    2. Vitamin C.
    3. Sodium chloride.
    4. Fats.

16. Elixir of digoxin (Lanoxin) is available with 0.05 mg of the drug in 1 mL of solution. How much of this elixir should the nurse administer if the physician's order reads "0.125 mg PO bid"?
    1. 2 mL.
    2. 2.25 mL.
    3. 2.5 mL.
    4. 2.75 mL.

17. When a parturient is given epidural (or caudal) anesthesia, the nurse could expect:
    1. Maternal hypotension, low forceps birth, need to remain flat in bed for several hours after birth.
    2. Loss of bearing-down reflex, depression of contractions, maternal hypotension, fetal bradycardia, low forceps birth.
    3. Loss of bearing-down reflex, depression of contractions, maternal hypotension, fetal bradycardia, low forceps birth, postnatal bladder atony, postnatal uterine atony.
    4. Depression of contractions, maternal hypotension.

18. A client is receiving tetracycline preoperatively in preparation for bowel surgery. Which common side effect should the nurse instruct the client to expect with tetracycline?
    1. Urticaria.
    2. Urinary retention.
    3. Jaundice.
    4. Deafness.

19. Some clients who are on phenothiazines are also given benztropine mesylate (Cogentin). The nurse administers this medication in order to:

1. Prevent skin reactions.
2. Increase the effectiveness of the phenothiazines.
3. Decrease motor restlessness.
4. Reduce extrapyramidal side effects.

20. A client has been on IM fluphenazine (Prolixin) for 3 years. This client has recently complained of frequent sore throats and malaise. What potentially serious side effect might these symptoms indicate to the nurse?
    1. Agranulocytosis.
    2. Akathisia.
    3. Dystonia.
    4. Dyskinesia.

21. When nialamide (Niamid) or isocarboxazid (Marplan) is administered, what must the nurse know about the effects of these drugs?
    1. Threshold for seizures is lowered.
    2. Effects are potentiated when taken with other drugs and many common foods.
    3. Muscular contractions are decreased.
    4. Obstructive jaundice commonly occurs.

22. A 9-month-old client has been diagnosed with Hirschsprung's disease. At this time, the child is admitted to the hospital for a temporary colostomy; preoperatively, the doctor orders kanamycin. The nurse caring for this child should know that kanamycin is being given to:
    1. Increase peristalsis.
    2. Decrease amount of GI secretions.
    3. Promote passage of stool and flatus.
    4. Decrease number of intestinal flora.

23. A 22-month-old client is admitted to the pediatric unit for observation following accidental ingestion of 17 children's acetaminophen (Tylenol) caplets. In the first 2–3 days following this child's admission, it is essential that the nurse plan to observe the child closely for signs of:
    1. Hepatic failure.
    2. Renal failure.
    3. Hyperthermia.
    4. Hemorrhage.

24. In an acetaminophen (Tylenol) overdose situation, the nurse should have on hand the antidote to acetaminophen, which is:
    1. Acetylcysteine (Mucomyst).
    2. Potassium chloride.
    3. Aspirin.
    4. Heparin.

25. The doctor orders aminophylline, 100 mg via IV, for a child who is having an acute asthmatic attack. The nurse should know that the main reason the doctor ordered aminophylline is because it is a(n):
    1. Bronchodilator.
    2. Anticholinergic.
    3. Expectorant.
    4. Mucolytic agent.

26. The nurse is to administer 100 mg of aminophylline IV. The ampule contains 500 mg (gr 7$\frac{1}{2}$) of aminophylline in 10 mL of solution. How much solution should the nurse withdraw from the ampule?
    1. 2 mL.
    2. 4 mL.
    3. 6 mL.
    4. 8 mL.

27. While aminophylline is infusing, the nurse should plan to closely monitor the client's:
    1. Level of consciousness.
    2. Blood pressure.
    3. Cardiac rhythm.
    4. Temperature.

28. The nurse should know that, to prevent future asthmatic attacks, a client will most likely receive:

1. Theophylline.
2. Cromolyn sodium.
3. Prednisone.
4. Diphenhydramine.

29. A 15-year-old client is admitted to the hospital with a diagnosis of infectious hepatitis (type A). To protect other members of this client's family who have been exposed to infectious hepatitis, the nurse should explain that they may be given:
    1. Amoxicillin/clavulanate potassium (Augmentin).
    2. Sulfisoxazole.
    3. Rifampin.
    4. Immune globulin.

30. A 17-month-old child has retropharyngeal abscess and is to receive ampicillin four times a day. The child weighs 15 kg (33 lb). The nurses' reference indicates that the correct dosage is 75 mg/kg/day. Which dose should the nurse give to this client at 10 A.M.?
    1. 11 mg.
    2. 28 mg.
    3. 280 mg.
    4. 1125 mg.

31. A 4-year-old client is scheduled for surgery. In preparing this child's preop injections, which size needle should the nurse select to administer this child's IM injection?
    1. 25 G, $5/8$ inch.
    2. 22 G, 1 inch.
    3. 20 G, 1 $1/2$ inch.
    4. 18 G, 1 $1/2$ inch.

32. Meperidine hydrochloride (Demerol) would be preferred over morphine sulfate for a client with a chest tube because Demerol:
    1. Causes less nausea and vomiting.
    2. Reduces anxiety and respiratory rate more effectively.
    3. Causes less smooth muscle spasms.
    4. Causes less respiratory depression.

33. Which client information, documented during an assessment, would be a contraindication to the client receiving verapamil (Calan)?
    1. Epigastric pain and treatment for a peptic ulcer.
    2. Hypertension and angina on exertion.
    3. History of asthma and allergic bronchitis.
    4. Hypotension associated with bradycardia.

34. A transfusion reaction is suspected. The transfusion is stopped and the MD notified. The next appropriate nursing action would be to:
    1. Change all IV tubing to prevent additional infusion of blood cells.
    2. Keep the IV line open with saline until further orders.
    3. Arrange for the laboratory to pick up the remaining unit of blood.
    4. Collect a urine specimen from the client.

35. Magnesium hydroxide (Milk of Magnesia) is the routine laxative order to prevent or correct constipation. For which client would the nurse question the order?
    1. An elderly woman with potential for fecal impaction.
    2. A client with chronic renal failure who is admitted for shunt revision.
    3. A man who is recovering from total knee replacement.
    4. An older man who is being treated for pneumonia.

36. If treatment with thyroid hormone is effective, the nurse should expect:
    1. Diuresis, a decrease in pulse rate, and an increase in blood pressure.
    2. Diuresis, a widening pulse pressure, and an increase in both temperature and respiratory rate.
    3. Increased pulse rate, decreased respiratory rate, and decreased puffiness.
    4. Weight loss, increased diastolic blood pressure, and decreased pulse rate.

37. To correctly instill pilocarpine in a client's eyes, the nurse should gently pull down the lower lid of the eye and instill the drops:
    1. Directly on the central surface of the cornea.
    2. On the inner canthus of the eye.
    3. Into the conjunctival sac.
    4. Directly on the dilated pupil.

38. Nursing implications with diphenylhydantoin given during treatment of status epilepticus include giving the intravenous injection slowly and in small increments to prevent:
    1. Respiratory depression and/or arrest.
    2. Vasodepression and circulatory shock.
    3. Irritation and/or necrosis of the vein and surrounding tissue.
    4. Vasomotor stimulation, with a sudden, malignant increase in blood pressure.

39. A nursing care plan includes observing for the most common client problems arising from the use of pyridostigmine (Mestinon) and neostigmine bromide (Prostigmin), which include:
    1. Gastric distress—nausea, anorexia, diarrhea.
    2. Elimination problems—urinary retention.
    3. Central nervous system excitation—flushing, irritability.
    4. Cardiac arrhythmias—palpitations, PVCs.

40. In order to take full advantage of the effects of pyridostigmine bromide and neostigmine bromide in reducing dysphagia related to myasthenia gravis, how long before meals should the nurse plan to give the medications?
    1. 2 hours.
    2. 60–90 minutes.
    3. 30–45 minutes.
    4. 10–15 minutes.

41. The care plan for a client who is burned includes observing for side effects of mafenide 1% (Sulfamylon), such as:
    1. Severe electrolyte disturbances.
    2. Metabolic acidosis.
    3. Metabolic alkalosis.
    4. Staining of linen.

42. Which nursing intervention can aid in reducing the gastric side effects of pyridostigmine bromide (Mestinon) and neostigmine bromide (Prostigmin)?
    1. Give with milk, soda crackers, or antacids.
    2. Push fluids and encourage ambulation.
    3. Keep room cool and discourage visitors.
    4. Encourage food high in potassium.

Answers/Rationales/Tips

1. **(2)** Before administering any narcotic, the nurse should assess the type, location, and intensity of pain, as well as factors that seem to precipitate or relieve it. Meperidine, like morphine, has hypotensive and respiratory depressant effects. Positioning in anticipation of respiratory changes is *not* indicated (**Answer 1**). Pain and discomfort are subjective symptoms that are *always* real to the client (**Answer 3**). Based on the information gained

KEY TO CODES FOLLOWING RATIONALES:

Nursing process: **AS**, assessment; **AN**, analysis; **PL**, plan; **IMP**, implementation; **EV**, evaluation. *Cognitive level:* **COM**, comprehension; **APP**, application; **ANL**, analysis. *Category of human function:* **1**, protective; **2**, sensory-perceptual; **3**, comfort, rest, activity, and mobility; **4**, nutrition; **5**, growth and development; **6**, fluid-gas transport; **7**, psychosocial-cultural; **8**, elimination. *Client need:* **SECE**, safe, effective care environment; **HPM**, health promotion/maintenance; **PsI**, psychosocial integrity; **PhI**, physiological integrity. (Client Subneed appears after Client need code.) See appendices for full explanation.

in **Answer 2,** it is then possible to decide whether the client needs supportive measures (such as back rub or position change as in **Answer 4**), the bedpan, and/or the administration of a narcotic.

> **TEST-TAKING TIP**—Choose the first step in the nursing process—*assess.*
> **AS, COM, 3, M/S: Meds, PhI, Pharmacological and Parenteral Therapies**

2. **(2)** Salicylates, particularly acetylsalicylic acid (aspirin), are given in divided doses after each meal and at bedtime for their analgesic (reduced pain), antiinflammatory (reduced swelling), and antipyretic (reduced fever) effects. **Answer 1** is incorrect because relief of pain was already described in the question. **Answers 3 and 4** are incorrect because salicylates neither inhibit nor stimulate the autonomic nervous system synapses.

> **TEST-TAKING TIP**—Consider why the drug relieves pain—decreased inflammation.
> **IMP, COM, 3, M/S: Meds, PhI, Pharmacological and Parenteral Therapies**

3. **(2)** Theophylline relaxes bronchial smooth muscles, which helps relieve the wheezing and coughing associated with bronchospasm. Side effects are rare, but the earliest signs of overdose are usually anorexia, nausea, and vomiting. Tachycardia **(Answer 1),** restlessness and tremors **(Answer 3),** headache and insomnia **(Answer 4),** are side effects associated with *bronchodilators.*

> **TEST-TAKING TIP**—Know expected outcomes of drug therapy—desired and untoward effects.
> **IMP, COM, 6, M/S: Meds, PhI, Pharmacological and Parenteral Therapies**

4. **(2)** Furosemide is a rapidly acting diuretic with a peak action in 1–2 hours and a duration of 6–8 hours. The peak time is too rapid for **Answer 1** and too long for **Answers 3 and 4.**

> **TEST-TAKING TIP**—Notice the time overlap—the option that includes both is better. Need to allow for GI absorption before actions.
> **EV, APP, 8, M/S: Meds, PhI, Pharmacological and Parenteral Therapies**

5. **(1)** *Ideally,* oral iron preparations should be taken on an empty stomach **(2).** However, they tend to irritate the gastric mucosa, so they should be administered *with* or *immediately after* meals to ensure client compliance. Thus **Answers 2, 3,** and **4** are *not* the *best* answers. Clients may complain of constipation or loose stools. Stools will change color (dark green to black). Ferrous sulfate is apt to deposit on teeth and gums, so frequent oral hygiene is necessary, and therapy will need to continue even after hemoglobin levels return to normal, to ensure adequate iron stores in the body.

> **TEST-TAKING TIP**—Key word is *best* time. **Answer 1** is better than **Answer 3.** Iron is harsh on the stomach.
> **PL, COM, 4, M/S: Meds, PhI, Pharmacological and Parenteral Therapies**

6. **(1)** Spironolactone (Aldactone) is an aldosterone inhibitor, inhibiting the effects of hyperaldosteronemia, which is common in cirrhosis. This drug safely increases sodium and water excretion but does not cause concomitant losses of potassium as do other diuretics. For this reason, potassium supplements are not generally given to the client. An example of a carbonic anhydrase inhibitor **(Answer 2)** is acetazolamide (Diamox); an example of a thiazide **(Answer 3)** is chlorothiazide (Diuril) or hydrochlorothiazide (HydroDIURIL); and an example of an osmotic diuretic **(Answer 4)** is mannitol.

> **TEST-TAKING TIP**—Look for clues from the stem, such as similarity in words—aldact*one* and aldoster*one.*
> **IMP, COM, 6, M/S: Meds, PhI, Pharmacological and Parenteral Therapies**

7. **(2)** Potassium chloride is not given since the client is on spironolactone (Aldactone), which does *not* cause concomitant *losses* of potassium as do other diuretics. For this reason, potassium supplements are not generally given to the client. Spironolactone would *not* contraindicate the administration of vitamin B$_6$ **(Answer 1)**, ascorbic acid **(Answer 3)**, or calcium gluconate **(Answer 4).**

> **TEST-TAKING TIP**—Know the expected outcome of *potassium*-sparing diuretics. Know drug classifications.
> **PL, APP, 4, M/S: Meds, PhI, Pharmacological and Parenteral Therapies**

8. **(3)** The primary objective in giving corticosteroids is to lessen the symptoms of the disease process. Most clients initially respond well to these drugs; however, as the disease progresses, higher and higher doses are required to relieve symptoms. **Answers 1 and 2** are incorrect because corticosteroids have *no curative* effects, only palliative. Many of the side effects of corticosteroid administration are due to the effects of these drugs on glucose metabolism **(Answer 4)**, such as Cushing-like syndrome.

> **TEST-TAKING TIP**—Look for an option that will improve an "itis"—inflammation.
> **AN, APP, 3, M/S: Meds, PhI, Pharmacological and Parenteral Therapies**

9. **(3)** Side effects of prednisone therapy mimic the manifestations of Cushing's syndrome (moon facies, abnormal fat deposits, purple striae, hyperglycemia with glucosuria, hypertension, obesity, and emotional disturbances). Side effects of *other drugs* used in the management of rheumatoid arthritis include tinnitus **(Answer 1),** *from aspirin*; nausea, vomiting **(Answer 4),** headaches, and vertigo *with indomethacin* (Indocin) administration; and dermatitis ranging from erythema to exfoliative dermatitis **(Answer 2)** *with gold salts* therapy.

> **TEST-TAKING TIP**—Know the untoward effects of excessive *steroids* on the body.
> **EV, APP, 2, M/S: Meds, PhI, Pharmacological and Parenteral Therapies**

10. **(4)** Although the primary use of propantheline bromide in many clinical situations involving the gastrointestinal tract is to reduce gastric secretions and intestinal hypermotility, it is used in gallbladder disease because of its antispasmodic effects on the gallbladder and bile duct. **Answer 1** is therefore correct, but *not the best* choice. **Answers 2 and 3** are incorrect because propantheline bromide does *not* reduce bile secretions; its calming effect on gastric motility does *not* reduce the amount of chyme entering the duodenum.

> **TEST-TAKING TIP**—Look for an option that alleviates and explains a possible cause of gallbladder *pain.*
> **IMP, COM, 4, M/S: Meds, PhI, Pharmacological and Parenteral Therapies**

11. **(4)** Hydrochlorothiazide is a thiazide diuretic that promotes the excretion of water, sodium, and chloride by inhibiting the reabsorption of sodium ions in the distal ascending limb of the loop of Henle and in the distal convoluted tubule of the nephron. Natriuresis promotes the secondary loss of potassium, so this drug is classified as potassium wasting. Spironolactone is an example of an aldosterone inhibitor and is a potassium-sparing diuretic **(Answers 1, 3).** Acetazolemide (Diamox) is the most frequently employed carbonic anhydrase inhibitor **(Answer 2).**

TEST-TAKING TIP—Know the common side effects of frequently used diuretics. *Potassium* is *usually* lost (wasted). Focus on two contradictory options. You know potassium is involved; decide whether it is spared or wasted.
EV, COM, 8, M/S: Meds, PhI, Pharmacological and Parenteral Therapies

12. **(3)** Thiazide diuretics promote the excretion of sodium, chloride, bicarbonate, and potassium. However, chloride excretion tends to be proportionately greater than bicarbonate excretion, so therapy may result in hypochloremic alkalosis. Hyponatremia, *not* hypernatremia (**Answer 1**), occurs. Hypokalemia, *not* hyperkalemia (**Answer 2**), may develop, especially with brisk diuresis. Supplemental KCl therapy and/or increased dietary intake of potassium is indicated with thiazide therapy. **Answer 4** is incorrect because it says hypouricemia and hyperuricemia result, which may precipitate frank gout.

TEST-TAKING TIP—When potassium loss (*hypo*kalemia) is not a choice, think what else goes with K^+ to balance the shift (Cl^-).
AS, COM, 8, M/S: Meds, PhI, Pharmacological and Parenteral Therapies

13. **(3)** The formula for finding the correct answer is:
Dose desired/Dose on hand = x/Amount on hand.

$18/20 = x/5$
$20x = 18(5)$
$x = 18(5)/20$
$x = 4.5$ mL

TEST-TAKING TIP—The age of the client is a distractor. Know the formula; the dose on hand is 5 mL.
IMP, APP, 2, PEDS, PhI, Pharmacological and Parenteral Therapies

14. **(3)** Rifampin is the drug of choice for the prophylactic treatment of *Haemophilus influenzae* meningitis. The usual dose is 20 mg/kg/day in a single dose for 4 days. Amoxicillin/clavulanate potassium (Augmentin) (**Answer 1**), sulfisoxazole (**Answer 2**), and immune serum globulin (**Answer 4**) are *not* the drugs of choice to prevent *H. influenzae* meningitis.

TEST-TAKING TIP—Use the process of elimination—the stem says *prevent*; two options are treatment for infections, and one option has minimal effect in many situations (immune globulin). Select a broad-spectrum antibiotic for prophylaxis.
IMP, APP, 1, M/S: Meds, PhI, Pharmacological and Parenteral Therapies

15. **(4)** Pancreatin (Viokase) is an exocrine pancreatic supplement used as a digestive aid in cystic fibrosis; its primary use is to promote the absorption of fats. Pancreatin has *no effect* on the absorption of glucose (**Answer 1**), vitamin C (**Answer 2**), or sodium chloride (**Answer 3**).

TEST-TAKING TIP—Know the digestive problem (fat) with cystic fibrosis.
AN, ANL, 4, PEDS, PhI, Pharmacological and Parenteral Therapies

16. **(3)** The correct answer is found using the following formula:
Dose desired/Dose on hand = x/Amount on hand.

$0.125/0.05 = x/1$
$0.05x = 0.125(1)$
$x = 0.125(1)/0.05$
$x = 2.5$ mL

TEST-TAKING TIP—Know the formula; it works every time. Use extra care with decimal points.
IMP, APP, 6, M/S: Meds, PhI, Pharmacological and Parenteral Therapies

17. **(3)** The medication never mixes with cerebrospinal fluid, and therefore there is *no need* for the woman to lie flat for several hours after receiving this form of anesthesia (**Answer 1**). Answers 2 and 4 are incorrect because the lists are incomplete.

TEST-TAKING TIP—Choose the most complete list in this question, where **Answer 3** incorporates **Answers 2** and **4**.
AN, ANL, 5, Maternity, PhI, Pharmacological and Parenteral Therapies

18. **(1)** Hypersensitivity reactions (urticaria and hives) are common drug reactions. Photosensitization (exaggerated sunburn) in certain persons who are hypersensitive may also occur with exposure to direct or artificial sunlight during tetracycline use. Urinary retention (**Answer 2**) is a side effect of *anticholinergic* and *antihistamine* drugs. Jaundice (**Answer 3**) from drug toxicity is more common with *isoniazid* (INH), *acetaminophen*, *phenothiazines* (chlorpromazine [Thorazine]), *sulfonamides*, and *antidiabetic* drugs (e.g., tolbutamide [Orinase]). Hepatotoxicity may occur with tetracycline, but it is less common. **Answer 4**, deafness (ototoxicity), is a major side effect of the *aminoglycoside antibiotics* (e.g., gentamicin, neomycin, streptomycin, tobramycin) and *diuretics*, such as furosemide and ethacrynic acid.

TEST-TAKING TIP—This is an *expected* common side effect. Only one would be clinically acceptable, although annoying (rash).
IMP, COM, 1, M/S: Meds, PhI, Pharmacological and Parenteral Therapies

19. **(4)** This is the best choice because it *encompasses* **Answer 3**. **Answers 1** and **2** are definitely incorrect because prevention of skin reaction is to avoid sun exposure; and Cogentin decreases EPT side effects, not increases the effectiveness of phenothiazines.

TEST-TAKING TIP—When two options are correct, choose the one that covers them both.
PL, APP, 7, Psych, PhI, Pharmacological and Parenteral Therapies

20. **(1)** Blood dyscrasias often are overlooked when first symptoms of possible adverse drug effects appear in the form of a minor cold. **Answers 2, 3,** and **4** refer to extrapyramidal tract symptoms that are *not* life threatening.

TEST-TAKING TIP—Which answer is not like the others? One option is potentially life threatening (hematological system); three are not life threatening and relate to the musculoskeletal system.
AN, APP, 6, Psych, PhI, Pharmacological and Parenteral Therapies

21. **(2)** Hypertensive crisis can be precipitated by combining this drug with common cold medications and foods high in tyramine or pressor amines (e.g., yogurt, Chianti wine, cheese, cola, coffee). All other options (**Answers 1, 3,** and **4**) are incorrect because these drugs do *not* affect seizure threshold, muscle contractions, nor cause obstructive jaundice.

TEST-TAKING TIP—Application of knowledge about side effects of these two drugs and the drug classification (monoamine oxidase inhibitor) will lead you to the only correct answer.
EV, APP, 6, Psych, PhI, Pharmacological and Parenteral Therapies

22. **(4)** Kanamycin is an antibiotic that, although poorly absorbed in the GI tract, is often used as part of bowel prep before abdominal surgery. It acts as a bacteriocidal agent, thus significantly decreasing the number of intestinal flora and reducing risk of peritonitis in the postop period. Kanamycin does *not* increase peristalsis (**Answer 1**), promote passage of stool or flatus (**Answer 3**), or decrease amount of GI secretions (**Answer 2**).

    TEST-TAKING TIP—The age and diagnosis do not matter. Why would *any* client need an antibiotic preoperatively? "Mycins" such as Kana*mycin,* erythro*mycin,* strepto*mycin* are antibiotics that decrease bacterial growth.
    AN, APP, 1, PEDS, PhI, Pharmacological and Parenteral Therapies

23. **(1)** The major toxic effect of an overdose of acetaminophen (Tylenol) is liver failure; liver function should be closely monitored during the first 2 to 3 days following the ingestion of acetaminophen. Renal failure (**Answer 2**) may occur as a *late* complication of acetaminophen toxicity, as may bleeding and hemorrhage (**Answer 4**). Hyperthermia (**Answer 3**) is not a major symptom of this type of ingestion; it is more common in *salicylate* ingestion.

    TEST-TAKING TIP—Know the functions of the liver, including detoxification of substances such as medications.
    PL, APP, 1, PEDS, PhI, Pharmacological and Parenteral Therapies

24. **(1)** Acetylcysteine (Mucomyst) is the antidote for acetaminophen poisoning: it serves to protect the liver. It is usually given orally in a carbonated beverage (e.g., cola), but it can also be given via nasogastric tube. A loading dose is followed by q4h doses until a total of 18 doses have been given. KCl (**Answer 2**), aspirin (**Answer 3**), and heparin (**Answer 4**) are *not* antidotes for acetaminophen and do not serve to protect the child's liver.

    TEST-TAKING TIP—Use a process of elimination. The potential adverse effects of three of the options would likely preclude use as an antidote.
    IMP, APP, 1, PEDS, PhI, Pharmacological and Parenteral Therapies

25. **(1)** Aminophylline, a bronchodilator that acts as a smooth-muscle relaxant, is used to prevent and relieve symptoms of bronchial asthma. Anticholinergics (**Answer 2**) are used to treat muscle spasms along the GI tract. Aminophylline is neither an expectorant (**Answer 3**), which would assist in the removal of mucus from the respiratory tract, nor a mucolytic agent (**Answer 4**), which would help thin out viscid secretions.

    TEST-TAKING TIP—Know the drug classifications of frequently used medications. Remember that in asthma, bronchioles *constrict;* therefore, a broncho*dilator* is used.
    AN, APP, 6, PEDS, PhI, Pharmacological and Parenteral Therapies

26. **(1)** The formula for finding the correct answer is
    Dose desired/Dose on hand = *x*/Amount on hand.

    $100/500 = x/10$
    $500x = 100(10)$
    $x = 100(10)/500$
    $x = 2$ mL

    TEST-TAKING TIP—Know the formula and the answer is easy; the dose on hand is 10 mL.
    IMP, APP, 6, M/S: Meds, PhI, Pharmacological and Parenteral Therapies

27. **(3)** A transient side effect of IV aminophylline is an increase in heart rate; toxic effects include a prolonged increase in heart rate and abnormalities in cardiac rhythm. While receiving IV aminophylline, the client should be on a cardiac monitor, and both rate and rhythm should be closely monitored and documented by the nurse. Aminophylline may also cause a transient change in the blood pressure (**Answer 2**), but this is not as much a concern as the client's cardiac rhythm. Aminophylline should not affect level of consciousness (**Answer 1**) or temperature (**Answer 4**); thus there is no particular need for the nurse to monitor these specifically at this time.

    TEST-TAKING TIP—With two potentially correct answers, select the more encompassing choice—change in heart function will ultimately affect BP. The words "closely monitor" in the stem usually call for a *priority* answer (cardiac is usually a priority).
    PL, APP, 6, M/S: Meds, PhI, Pharmacological and Parenteral Therapies

28. **(2)** Cromolyn sodium, an uncategorized drug used as an adjunct in the treatment of asthma, is used only after the acute attack is relieved; its primary intent is prophylaxis, i.e., to prevent future attacks. Cromolyn is used in an inhaler. It is absorbed into the systemic circulation after its inhalation into the lungs. It acts on the mast cells and also inhibits the release of histamine. Theophylline (**Answer 1**), prednisone (**Answer 3**), and diphenhydramine (**Answer 4**) do *not prevent future* asthmatic attacks and have no prophylactic value.

    TEST-TAKING TIP—Look for a pattern: three of the options are used for *acute* episodes; choose the one that meets the condition of the stem (future prevention).
    AN, APP, 6, M/S: Meds, PhI, Pharmacological and Parenteral Therapies

29. **(4)** Immune serum globulin (ISG) offers the family members some protection against type A infectious hepatitis. It contains antibodies against the organism and will aid the family members in resisting this infectious disease. Amoxicillin/clavulanate potassium (Augmentin) (**Answer 1**) and sulfisoxazole (**Answer 2**) are antibiotics used for a variety of infections, but they would not prevent hepatitis. Rifampin (**Answer 3**) is used prophylactically for *Haemophilus influenzae* meningitis and to treat TB, but would not prevent hepatitis.

    TEST-TAKING TIP—Know when immune globulin may be effective (infectious hepatitis) and when it is not (*H. influenzae* meningitis). Remember that protection for hepatitis exposure is achieved through passive immunity (i.e., immune serum globulin).
    IMP, COM, 1, M/S, PhI, Pharmacological and Parenteral Therapies

30. **(3)** The nurse should give 280 mg at 10 A.M. Using the formula of 75 mg/kg/day, 75 mg (15 kg = 1125 mg per day) to be divided into 4 doses; 1125 mg divided by 4 doses = 280 mg per dose. **Answers 1, 2,** and **4** are incorrect calculations.

    TEST-TAKING TIP—Use basic math. Do not forget to divide the daily dose of 1125 mg by the total number of doses per day to get the amount to be given for a single dose at 10:00 A.M.
    IMP, ANL, 1, PEDS, PhI, Pharmacological and Parenteral Therapies

31. **(2)** In selecting the correct needle to administer an IM injection to a young child, the nurse should always look at the

child and use judgment in evaluating muscle mass and amount of subcutaneous fat. A medium-gauge needle (22 G) that is 1 inch long would be most appropriate for a young child. A $\frac{5}{8}$ inch needle (**Answer 1**) would be too small, and a $1\frac{1}{2}$ inch (18 to 20 G) needle would be too long and unnecessarily large (**Answers 3, 4**). A 23 or 25 G needle would be too thin to use on most children (**Answer 1**) and would be better suited for use with a newborn or an infant.

> **TEST-TAKING TIP**—Visualize the "average" size of a 4-year-old. *Medium* size is safe.
> **IMP, APP, 1, PEDS, PhI, Pharmacological and Parenteral Therapies**

32. **(4)** Both drugs have depressant effects; however, morphine sulfate affects rate and depth of respirations and cough reflex, which would be undesirable following chest tube insertion. *Both* drugs cause nausea and vomiting (**Answer 1**). *Morphine* sulfate is used to reduce anxiety and respiratory rate (**Answer 2**), particularly in pulmonary edema. Demerol does cause fewer smooth muscle spasms (**Answer 3**); however, that is *not the concern* in this situation, but it would be with GI surgery such as cholecystectomy.

> **TEST-TAKING TIP**—Choose "respiratory" over GI symptoms, anxiety, or muscle spasm. Know *expected* effects of opioid analgesics, and what the greatest concern is for this client situation (respiratory effectiveness).
> **PL, APP, 3, M/S: Meds, PhI, Pharmacological and Parenteral Therapies**

33. **(4)** Verapamil, a calcium channel blocker, is indicated for the management of hypertension and arrhythmia with rapid ventricular rates. Blood pressure and pulse should be taken before administration, and the medication would most likely be held or changed with persistent hypotension and bradycardia. **Answers 1, 2,** and **3** would *not* be contraindications; the medication may be given to clients with these existing conditions.

> **TEST-TAKING TIP**—To narrow the choices, focus on two contradictory options: *hyper*tension vs. *hypo*tension. Know expected therapeutic and side effects of drug classifications.
> **AN, APP, 6, M/S: Meds, PhI, Pharmacological and Parenteral Therapies**

34. **(2)** The priority is to keep the IV site open. Medications may need to be given to reverse the client's untoward reaction to the transfusion. **Answers 1, 3,** and **4** will eventually be done, but *not before* the patency of the IV is determined and maintained.

> **TEST-TAKING TIP**—Take care of the client's *safety* first, then change the equipment and do laboratory tests.
> **IMP, ANL, 6, M/S: Meds, PhI, Pharmacological and Parenteral Therapies**

35. **(2)** Metabolism and excretion of the drug are done primarily by the kidneys. In chronic renal failure, the kidneys would be unable to regulate electrolyte balance and the client would be at higher risk for the development of an electrolyte imbalance. Another classification of laxative should be used in the renal client. This laxative is *not* contraindicated for others (**Answers 1, 3,** and **4**).

> **TEST-TAKING TIP**—Use the process of elimination. Would an electrolyte-based laxative (magnesium) adversely affect one of these clients more?
> **IMP, ANL, 8, M/S: Meds, PhI, Pharmacological and Parenteral Therapies**

36. **(2)** If treatment with thyroid hormone is effective, there should be an *overall increase* in metabolic rate and a decrease in fluid retention; that is, increased blood pressure, pulse rate, pulse pressure, temperature, and rate and depth of respirations. As a result of improved renal blood flow, glomerular filtration and urine output should also increase, thus reducing the weight gain due to fluid retention. **Answers 1, 3,** and **4** are incorrect because each contains at least one outcome that is not consistent with improved status.

> **TEST-TAKING TIP**—Know the physiological effect of the thyroid on the body. ↑ Thyroid function = ↑ BP, P, T, R, pulse pressure = ↓ fluid retention.
> **EV, ANL, 3, M/S: Endocrine, PhI, Pharmacological and Parenteral Therapies**

37. **(3)** Eyedrops should be instilled into the conjunctival sac to prevent medication from hitting the sensitive cornea. The client should then be instructed to close the eye, but not squeeze shut, so that the medication can be distributed evenly over the eye. **Answers 1** and **4** are incorrect because instillation on these structures would increase corneal irritation. **Answer 2** is incorrect because drops instilled into the inner canthus are likely to run down the outer aspects of the nose or be absorbed systemically through the tear duct.

> **TEST-TAKING TIP**—The correct choice is more indirect placement of drops; the other choices are all *direct* locations.
> **IMP, APP, 2, M/S: Eye, PhI, Pharmacological and Parenteral Therapies**

38. **(2)** Diphenylhydantoin (phenytoin, Dilantin) must be injected IV slowly and in small increments to prevent vasodepression and circulatory collapse. Respiratory depression (**Answer 1**) is generally associated with *morphine sulfate*. *Adrenergic* (alpha) drugs such as norepinephrine bitartrate (Levophed) may cause vein and tissue necrosis (**Answer 3**) and have only *rarely* caused sudden malignant increases in blood pressure (**Answer 4**).

> **TEST-TAKING TIP**—Know the *expected effects* of IV Dilantin. Think circulatory.
> **IMP, APP, 2, M/S: Meds, PhI, Pharmacological and Parenteral Therapies**

39. **(1)** The most common side effects of pyridostigmine (Mestinon) and neostigmine bromide (Prostigmin) include anorexia, nausea, diarrhea, and abdominal cramps. These symptoms are due to increased gastrointestinal secretions, smooth-muscle contractions (peristalsis), and irritation of the gastric mucosa. **Answer 2** is incorrect because increased cholinergic discharge increases bladder tone and contraction, thus *facilitating* voiding. **Answers 3** and **4** are incorrect because the symptoms listed are consistent with increased adrenergic, *not* cholinergic, discharge or stimulation.

> **TEST-TAKING TIP**—Need to know expected *common outcomes*. Think GI system: nausea is a *common* side effect with many drugs. Other options are *more severe*.
> **AS, COM, 4, M/S: GI, PhI, Pharmacological and Parenteral Therapies**

40. **(3)** In order to take full advantage of the effects of anticholinesterase drugs, they should generally be scheduled 30–45 minutes before eating. **Answers 1** and **2** are not totally incorrect, in that these drugs generally act over a 3-hour period; however, *peak action* occurs *quickly,* and clients with dysphagia *need time* to eat, chew, and swallow during meals. Rushing at meals causes unnecessary fatigue. **Answer 4** may not allow *enough* time for the drug to take effect.

TEST-TAKING TIP—Clue: time frame. First, eliminate the extremes (**Answer 1, Answer 4**); look for a midpoint. Most drugs take effect within 30–45 min. What is the desired outcome? Improved swallowing of food.
IMP, COM, 3, M/S: Meds, PhI, Pharmacological and Parenteral Therapies

41. (2) Mafenide 1% (Sulfamylon) is a white antibacterial ointment applied once or twice daily. Besides causing pain on application, this medication is a carbonic anhydrase inhibitor that interferes with the kidney's ability to excrete hydrogen ions and thus may cause metabolic acidosis, *not* metabolic alkosis (**Answer 3**). Clients who are treated with mafenide 1% need to have their acid-base balance monitored by blood gas determinations. Clinical signs of metabolic acidosis are increased rate and depth of respirations. *Silver nitrate* causes black discoloration of linens, and its hypotonicity causes electrolyte imbalances (**Answers 1 and 4**). Clients treated with silver nitrate need supplemental sodium, potassium, and chloride.

TEST-TAKING TIP—Recognize expected desired and untoward *metabolic* effects. This eliminates **Answer 1**; **Answer 4** is a side effect of a different drug.
EV, COM, 1, M/S: Meds, PhI, Pharmacological and Parenteral Therapies

42. (1) The gastric distress that occurs as a side effect of these medications can be reduced by administering the drugs along with milk, soda crackers, or antacids. The nursing actions in **Answer 2** are consistent with *elimination* problems (urinary retention); those in **Answer 3** are consistent with *central nervous system* excitation (flushing, irritability); and the action in **Answer 4** is consistent with *cardiac arrhythmias* (palpitations, PVCs).

TEST-TAKING TIP—Relate the system affected (GI) to the intervention (food).
IMP, APP, 4, M/S: Meds, PhI, Pharmacological and Parenteral Therapies

Common Diagnostic Procedures, Intravenous and Oxygen Therapy, Infection Control/Isolation Precautions, and Hands-on Nursing Care

Janice McMillin and Robyn Nelson

COMMON DIAGNOSTIC PROCEDURES

I. **Noninvasive diagnostic procedures** are those procedures that provide an indirect assessment of organ size, shape, and/or function; these procedures are considered safe, are easily reproducible, require less complex equipment for recording, and generally do not require the written consent of client or guardian.

◆ **A. General nursing responsibilities:**
1. Reduce client's anxieties and provide emotional support by:
   a. Explaining purpose and procedure of test.
   b. Answering questions regarding safety of the procedure, as indicated.
   c. Remaining with client during procedure when possible.
2. Use procedures in the collection of specimens that avoid contamination and facilitate diagnosis—clean-catch urine and sputum specimens after deep breathing and coughing, for example.

B. Graphic studies of heart and brain:
1. *Electrocardiogram (ECG, also known as EKG)*—graphic record of electrical activity generated by the heart during depolarization and repolarization; *used to:* diagnose abnormal cardiac rhythms and coronary heart disease.
2. *Echocardiography* (ultrasound cardiography)—graphic record of motions produced by cardiac structures as high-frequency sound vibrations are echoed through chest wall into the heart; transesophageal echocardiography produces a clearer image, particularly in clients who are obese, barrel-chested, or with chronic obstructive pulmonary

disease (COPD); *used to:* demonstrate valvular or other structural deformities, detect pericardial effusion, diagnose tumors and cardiomegaly, or evaluate prosthetic valve function.
3. *Phonocardiogram*—graphic record of heart sounds; *used to:* keep a permanent record of client's heart sounds before and after cardiac surgery.
4. *Electroencephalogram (EEG)*—graphic record of the electrical potentials generated by the physiological activity of the brain; *used to:* detect surface lesions or tumors of the brain and presence of epilepsy.
5. *Echoencephalogram*—beam of pulsed ultrasound is passed through the head, and returning echoes are graphically recorded; *used to:* detect shifts in cerebral midline structures caused by: subdural hematomas, intracerebral hemorrhage, or tumors.

C. Roentgenological studies (x-ray)
1. *Chest*—*used to:* determine size, contour, and position of the heart; size, location, and nature of pulmonary lesions; disorders of thoracic bones or soft tissue; diaphragmatic contour and excursion; pleural thickening or effusions; and gross changes in the caliber or distribution of pulmonary vasculature.
2. *Kidney, ureter, and bladder (KUB)*—*used to:* determine size, shape, and position of kidneys, ureters, and bladder.
3. *Mammography*—examination of the breast with or without the injection of radiopaque substance into the ducts of the mammary gland; *used to:* determine the presence of tumors or cysts.
◆ *Client preparation: no* deodorant, perfume, powders, or ointment in underarm area on day of x-ray. May be uncomfortable due to pressure on the breast.

4. *Skull*—outline configuration and density of brain tissues and vascular markings, used to determine the size and location of: intracranial calcifications, tumors, abscesses, or vascular lesions.

D. **Roentgenological studies (fluoroscopy)**—require the ingestion or injection of a radiopaque substance to visualize the target organ.

◆ 1. *Additional nursing responsibilities* may include:

▶ a. Administration of *enemas or cathartics* before the procedure and a laxative after.

b. Keeping the client *NPO* 6–12 hr before examination; check with MD regarding oral medications.

c. Ascertaining client's *history of allergies* or allergic reactions (e.g., iodine, seafood).

d. Observing for *allergic* reactions to contrast medium following procedure.

e. Providing *fluid* and *food* following procedure, to counteract dehydration.

f. Observing *stool* for color and consistency until barium passes.

2. Common fluoroscopic examinations:

a. **Upper GI**—ingestion of barium sulfate or meglumine diatrizoate (Gastrografin, a white, chalky, radiopaque substance), followed by fluoroscopic and x-ray examination; *used to* determine:

(1) Patency and caliber of *esophagus;* may also detect esophageal varices.

(2) Mobility and thickness of *gastric* walls, presence of ulcer craters, filling defects due to tumors, pressures from outside the stomach, and patency of pyloric valve.

(3) Rate of passage in small bowel and presence of structural abnormalities.

b. **Lower GI**—rectal instillation of barium sulfate followed by fluoroscopic and x-ray examination; *used to:* determine contour and mobility of colon and presence of any space-occupying tumors; perform before upper GI.

◆ *Client preparation:* explain purpose; *no food after evening meal* the evening before test; *stool softeners, laxatives, enemas, and suppositories* to cleanse the bowel before the test; *NPO after midnight* before test; oral medications *not* permitted day of test. *After completion of exam:* food, *increased liquid* intake, and rest; *laxatives for at least 2 days* or until stools are normal in color and consistency.

c. *Cholecystogram* (done if gallbladder not seen with ultrasound)—ingestion of organic iodine contrast medium Telepaque (iopanoic acid), or Oragrafin (preparation of calcium or sodium salt of ipodate) followed in 12 hr by x-ray visualization; gallbladder disease is indicated with *poor* or no visualization of the bladder; accurate only if GI and liver function is intact; perform before barium enema or upper GI.

◆ *Client preparation:* explain purpose; administer large amount of *water* with contrast capsules; *low fat meal* evening *before* x-ray; *oral laxative or stool softener after meal; no food* allowed after contrast capsules; water, tea, or coffee, with *no* cream or sugar, usually allowed. *After completion of exam:* fluids, food, and rest; observe for any signs of allergy to contrast medium.

d. *Cholangiogram*—intravenous injection of a radiopaque contrast substance, followed by fluoroscopic and x-ray examination of the bile ducts; failure of the contrast medium to pass certain points in the bile duct pinpoints *obstruction.*

e. *Intravenous urography (IVU) or pyelography (IVP)*—injection of a radiopaque contrast medium, followed by fluoroscopic and x-ray films of kidneys and urinary tract; *used to:* identify lesions in kidneys and ureters and provide a rough estimate of kidney function.

f. *Cystogram*—installation of radiopaque medium through a catheter into the bladder; *used to:* visualize bladder wall and evaluate ureterovesical valves for reflux.

g. *Phlebography* (lower limb venography)—determines patency of the tibial-popliteal, superficial femoral, common femoral, and saphenous veins. A contrast medium is injected into the superficial and/or deep veins of the involved extremity, followed by x-rays, while the leg is placed in a variety of positions; *used to:* detect deep-vein thrombosis and to select a vein for use in arterial bypass grafting; localized clotting may result.

E. **Computed tomography (CT)**—an x-ray beam sweeps around the body, allowing measurement of various tissue densities; provides clear radiographic definition of structures that are not visible by other techniques, permitting earlier diagnosis and treatment and more effective and efficient follow-up. Initial scan may be followed by "contrast enhancement" using an injection of an intravenous contrast agent (iodine), followed by a repeat scan.

◆ *Client preparation:* instructions for eating before test vary. Clear liquids up to 2 hr before are usually permitted.

F. **Positron emission tomography (PET)**—A radionuclide-based imaging technique. Tracers given IV or inhalation; rarely intra-arterial. Metabolic and physiologic changes from strokes, brain tumors, epilepsy, mental illnesses such as schizophrenia and bipolar disorder, and Parkinson's disease are produced. Measures blood flow, glucose metabolism, and oxygen extraction. *Useful in:* diagnosing myocardial flow deficits and evaluating successful thrombolysis, outcomes of bypass surgery, and angioplasty (PTCA).

◆ *Client preparation:* fast for 4hr. Injection of radioactive tracers which emit signals. Must remain motionless for 45 minutes. Scanner is quiet.

G. Magnetic resonance imaging (MRI)—noninvasive, nonionic technique produces cross-sectional images by exposure to magnetic energy sources. Provides superior contrast of soft tissue, including healthy, benign, and malignant tissue, along with veins and arteries; uses no contrast medium; takes 30–90 min to complete; client must *stay still* for periods of 5–20 min at a time—equipment often very noisy.

◆ *Client preparation:* client can take food and medications except for low abdominal and pelvic studies (food/fluids withheld 4–6 hr to decrease peristalsis). *Restrictions:* clients who have metal implants, permanent pacemakers, or implanted medication pumps such as insulin, or who are pregnant or on life support systems. Clients who are obese may not be able to have full-body MRI because they may not fit in the scanner tunnel. Clients who are claustrophobic may need distraction (e.g., music) or may be referred to a facility that has an MRI chamber that is more open.

H. Multiple-gated acquisition scan (MUGA)—also known as blood pool imaging. Red blood cells are tagged with a radioactive isotope. A computer-operated camera takes sequential pictures of actual heart wall motion; *complement* to cardiac catheterization; *used to:* determine valvular effectiveness, follow progress of heart disease, diagnose cardiac aneurysms, detect coronary artery disease, determine effects of cardiovascular drug therapy. No special preparation. Painless, except for injections. Wear *gloves* if contact with client urine occurs within 24 hr after scan.

I. Ultrasound (sonogram)—scanning by ultrasound is used to diagnose disorders of the thyroid, kidney, liver, uterus, gallbladder, and fetus and the intracranial structures in the neonate. It is not useful when visualization through air or bone is required (lung studies). In some agencies the sonogram has taken the place of the oral cholecystogram in diagnosing gallbladder disease, bile duct distention, and calculi.

◆ *Client preparation* is minimal, i.e., NPO for at least 8 hr for gallbladder studies. No x-rays. Thirty-two ounces of water PO 30 min before studies of lower abdomen or uterus.

J. Pulmonary function studies:
1. *Ventilatory studies*—utilization of a spirometer to determine how well the lung is ventilating.
   a. *Vital capacity (VC)*—largest amount of air that can be expelled after maximal inspiration.

   (1) *Normally* 4000–5000 mL.

   (2) *Decreased* in restrictive lung disease.
   (3) May be normal, slightly increased, or decreased in chronic obstructive lung disease.
   b. *Forced expiratory volume (FEV)*—percentage of vital capacity that can be forcibly expired in 1, 2, or 3 sec.

   (1) *Normally* 81%–83% in 1 sec, 90%–94% in 2 sec, and 95%–97% in 3 sec.

(2) *Decreased* values indicate expiratory airway obstruction.
   c. *Maximum breathing capacity (MBC)*—maximum amount of air that can be breathed in and out in 1 min with maximal rate and depth of respiration.
   (1) Best overall measurement of ventilatory ability.
   (2) *Reduced* in restrictive and chronic obstructive lung disease.
2. *Diffusion studies*—measure the rate of exchange of gases across alveolar membrane. Carbon monoxide single-breath, rebreathing, and steady-state techniques—used because of special affinity of hemoglobin for carbon monoxide; *decreased* when fluid is present in alveoli or when alveolar membranes are thick or fibrosed.

K. Sputum studies:
1. Gross sputum evaluations—collection of sputum samples to ascertain quantity, consistency, color, and odor.
2. *Sputum smear*—sputum is smeared thinly on a slide so that it can be studied microscopically; *used to:* determine cytological changes (malignant cell) or presence of pathogenic bacteria (e.g., tubercle bacilli).
3. *Sputum culture*—sputum samples are implanted or inoculated into special media; *used to:* diagnose pulmonary infections.
4. *Gastric lavage or analysis*—insertion of a nasogastric tube into the stomach to siphon out swallowed pulmonary secretions; *used to:* detect organisms causing pulmonary infections; especially useful for detecting tubercle bacilli in children.

L. Examination of gastric contents:
1. *Gastric analysis*—aspiration of the contents of the fasting stomach for analysis of free and total acid.
   a. Gastric acidity is generally *increased* in presence of duodenal ulcer.
   b. Gastric acidity is usually *decreased* in pernicious anemia, cancer of the stomach.
2. Stool specimens—*examined for:* amount, consistency, color, character, and melena; *used to* determine presence of: urobilinogen, fat, nitrogen, parasites, and other substances.

M. Thermography—a picture of the surface temperature of the skin using infrared photography (non-ionizing radiation) detects the circulation pattern of areas in the breasts. Tumors produce more heat than normal breast tissue. Useful with large tumors, but may not detect small or deep lesions. Requires expensive equipment and is difficult to interpret accurately.

N. Doppler ultrasonography—*used to:* measure blood flow in the major veins and arteries. The transducer of the test instrument is placed on the skin, sending out bursts of ultra-high-frequency sound. The ratio of ankle to brachial systolic pressure (API ≥ 1) provides information about vascular insufficiency. Sound varies with respiration and the Valsalva maneuver. No discomfort to the client.

O. Caloric stimulation test—*used to:* evaluate the vestibular portion of the eighth cranial nerve, identify the impairment or loss of thermally induced nystagmus. Reflex eye movements (nystagmus) result in response to cold or warm irrigations of the external auditory canal if the nerve is intact. A *diminished or absent* response occurs with Meniere's or acoustic neuroma. Nausea, vomiting, or dizziness can be precipitated by the test.

P. 24-hour urine collection—a true and accurate evaluation of kidney function, primarily glomerular filtration. Substances excreted by the kidney are excreted at different rates, amounts, and times of day or night. Timed urine collection is done for *protein, creatinine, electrolytes, urinary steroids,* etc. A large container is used with or without preservative. Label with client name, type of test, and exact time test starts and ends. Not usually necessary to measure urine. Have client void, discard urine; test starts at this time. Have client void as close to the end of the 24-hr period as possible. If refrigeration is required, urine may be stored in iced container.

Q. Glucose testing—to detect disorder of glucose metabolism, such as diabetes.
1. *Fasting (FBS):* blood sample is drawn after a 12 hr fast (usually overnight). Water is allowed. If diabetes is present, value will be 126 mg/dL or greater.
2. *2 hr postprandial (PPBS):* blood is taken after a meal. For best results, client should be on a high-carbohydrate diet for 2–4 days before testing. Client fasts overnight, eats a high-carbohydrate breakfast; blood sample is drawn 2 hr after eating. Client should rest during 2 hr interval. Smoking and coffee may increase glucose level.
3. *Glucose tolerance test (GTT):* done when sugar in urine, or FBS or 2 hr PPBS is not conclusive. A timed test, usually 2 hr. high carbohydrate diet is eaten 3 days before test. Blood is drawn after overnight fast. Client drinks a very sweet glucose liquid. All of the solution must be taken. Blood and urine sample usually taken at 30 min, 1 hr, 2 hr, and sometimes 3 hr after drinking solution. Blood glucose peaks in 30–60 min, and returns to normal, usually within 3 hr.

II. Invasive diagnostic procedures—procedures that directly record the size, shape, or function of an organ and that are often complex or expensive or require utilization of highly trained personnel; these procedures may result in morbidity and occasionally death of the client and therefore require the written consent of the client or guardian.

A. General nursing responsibilities:
1. *Before procedure:* institute measures to provide for client's safety and emotional comfort.
   a. Have client sign permit for procedure.
   b. Ascertain and report any client history of allergy or allergic reactions.
   c. Explain procedure briefly, and accurately advise client of any possible sensations, such as flushing or a warm feeling, as when a contrast medium is injected.
   d. Keep client NPO 6–12 hr before procedure if anesthesia is to be used.
   e. Allow client to verbalize concerns, and note attitude toward procedure.
   f. Administer preprocedure sedative, as ordered.
   g. If procedure done at bedside:
      (1) Remain with client, offering frequent reassurance.
      (2) Assist with optional positioning of client.
      (3) Observe for indications of complications—shock, pain, or dyspnea.
2. *After procedure:* institute measures to avoid complications and promote physical and emotional comfort.
   a. Observe and record vital signs.
   b. Check injection cut-down or biopsy sites for bleeding, infection, tenderness, or thrombosis.
      (1) Report untoward reactions to physician.
      (2) Apply warm compresses to ease discomfort, as ordered.
   c. If topical anesthetic is used during procedure (e.g., gastroscopy, bronchoscopy), do *not* give food or fluid until gag reflex returns.
   d. Encourage relaxation by allowing client to discuss experience and verbalize feelings.

B. Procedures to evaluate the cardiovascular system:
1. *Angiocardiography*—intravenous injection of a radiopaque solution or contrast medium for the purpose of studying its circulation through the client's heart, lungs, and great vessels; *used to:* check the competency of heart valves, diagnose congenital septal defects, detect occlusions of coronary arteries, confirm suspected diagnoses, and study heart function and structure before cardiac surgery.
2. *Cardiac catheterization*—insertion of a radiopaque catheter into a vein to study the heart and great vessels.
   a. *Right-heart catheterization*—catheter is inserted through a cut-down in the antecubital vein into the superior vena cava, through the right atrium and ventricle, and into the pulmonary artery.
   b. *Left-heart catheterization*—catheter may be passed retrograde to the left ventricle through the brachial or femoral artery; it can be passed into the left atrium after right-heart catheterization by means of a special needle that punctures the septa; or it may be passed directly into the left ventricle by means of a posterior or anterior chest puncture.
   c. Cardiac catheterizations are *used to:*
      (1) Confirm diagnosis of heart disease and determine the extent of disease.

(2) Determine existence and extent of congenital abnormalities.

(3) Measure pressures in the heart chambers and great vessels.

(4) Obtain estimate of cardiac output.

(5) Obtain blood samples to measure oxygen content and determine presence of cardiac shunts.

◆ d. *Specific nursing interventions:*
  (1) *Preprocedure client teaching:*
    (a) Fatigue due to lying still for 3 hr or more is a common complaint.
    (b) Some fluttery sensations may be felt—occur as catheter is passed backward into the left ventricle.
    (c) Flushed, warm feeling may occur when contrast medium is injected.
  (2) *Postprocedure observations:*
    (a) Monitor ECG pattern for arrhythmias.
    (b) Check extremities for color and temperature, peripheral pulses (femoral and dorsalis pedis) for quality.

3. *Angiography (arteriography)*—injection of a contrast medium into the arteries to study the vascular tree; *used to:* determine obstructions or narrowing of peripheral arteries.

4. *Pericardiocentesis (pericardial aspiration)*—puncture of the pericardial sac is performed to remove fluid accumulating with pericardial effusion. The goal is to prevent cardiac tamponade (compression of the heart).

◆ *Nursing interventions:* monitor ECG and CVP during the procedure, have resuscitative equipment ready. Head of bed elevated to *45–60 degrees.* Maintain peripheral IV with saline or glucose. *Following the procedure:* monitor BP, CVP, and heart sounds for recurrence of tamponade (pulsus paradoxus).

C. **Procedures to evaluate the respiratory system:**

1. *Pulmonary circulation studies—used to:* determine regional distribution of pulmonary blood flow.
  a. *Lung scan*—injection of radioactive isotope into the body, followed by lung scintiscan, which produces a graphic record of gamma rays emitted by the isotope in lung tissues; *used to:* determine lung perfusion when space-occupying lesions or pulmonary emboli and infarction are suspected.
  b. *Pulmonary angiography*—x-ray visualization of the pulmonary vasculature after the injection of a radiopaque contrast medium; *used to:* evaluate pulmonary disorders (e.g., pulmonary embolism, lung tumors, aneurysms, and changes in the pulmonary vasculature due to such conditions as emphysema or congenital defects).

2. *Bronchoscopy*—introduction of a special lighted instrument (bronchoscope) into the trachea and bronchi; *used to:* inspect tracheobronchial tree for pathological changes, remove tissue for cytological

and bacteriological studies, remove foreign bodies or mucous plugs causing airway obstruction, assess functional residual capacity of diseased lung, and apply chemotherapeutic agents.

◆ a. *Prebronchoscopy nursing interventions:*
  (1) Oral hygiene.
  (2) Postural drainage is indicated.
◆ b. *Postbronchoscopy nursing interventions:*
  (1) Instruct client *not* to swallow oral secretions but to let saliva run from side of mouth.
  (2) Save expectorated sputum for laboratory analysis, and observe for frank bleeding.
  (3) NPO until gag reflex returns.
  (4) Observe for subcutaneous emphysema and dyspnea.
  (5) Apply ice collar to reduce throat discomfort.

3. *Thoracentesis*—needle puncture through the chest wall and into the pleura; *used to:* remove fluid and occasionally air from the pleural space.

◆ *Nursing interventions before* thoracentesis:
◪ a. *Position:* high-Fowler's position or sitting up on edge of bed, with feet supported on chair to facilitate accumulation of fluid in the base of the chest.
◪ b. If client is unable to sit up—turn onto *unaffected* side.
  c. Evaluate continually for signs of shock, pain, cyanosis, increased respiratory rate, and pallor.

D. **Procedures to evaluate the renal system:**

1. *Renal angiogram*—small catheter is inserted into the femoral artery and passed into the aorta or renal artery, radiopaque fluid is instilled, and serial films are taken.
  a. *Used to:* diagnose renal hypertension and pheochromocytoma and differentiate renal cysts from renal tumors.
◆ b. *Postangiogram nursing actions:* check pedal pulse for signs of decreased circulation.

2. *Cystoscopy*—visualization of bladder, urethra, and prostatic urethra by insertion of a tubular, lighted, telescopic lens (cystoscope) through the urinary meatus.
  a. *Used to:* directly inspect the bladder; collect urine from the renal pelvis; obtain biopsy specimens from bladder and urethra; remove calculi; and treat lesions in the bladder, urethra, and prostate.
◆ b. *Nursing interventions following* procedure:
  (1) Observe for urinary retention.
  (2) Warm sitz baths to relieve discomfort.

3. *Renal biopsy*—needle aspiration of tissue from the kidney for the purpose of microscopic examination.

E. **Procedures to evaluate the digestive system:**

1. *Celiac angiography, hepatoportography, and umbilical venography*—injection of a contrast medium into the portal vein or related vessel; *used to:* determine patency of vessels supplying target organ or

detect lesions in the organs that distort the vasculature.

2. *Esophagoscopy and gastroscopy*—visualization of the esophagus, the stomach, and sometimes the duodenum by means of a lighted tube inserted through the mouth.

3. *Proctoscopy*—visualization of rectum and colon by means of a lighted tube inserted through the anus.

4. *Peritoneoscopy*—direct visualization of the liver and peritoneum by means of a peritoneoscope inserted through an abdominal stab wound.

5. *Liver biopsy*—needle aspiration of tissue for the purpose of microscopic examination; *used to:* determine tissue changes, facilitate diagnosis, and provide information regarding a disease course.

◆ ◪ *Nursing interventions:* place client on *right side* and position pillow for pressure, to prevent bleeding.

6. *Paracentesis*—needle aspiration of fluid from the peritoneal cavity; *used to:* relieve excess fluid accumulation or for diagnostic studies.

◆ a. *Specific nursing interventions before paracentesis:*

(1) Have client void—to prevent possible injury to bladder during procedure.

◪ (2) *Position*—sitting up on side of bed, with feet supported by chair.

(3) Check vital signs and peripheral circulation frequently throughout procedure.

(4) Observe for signs of hypovolemic shock—may occur due to fluid shift from vascular compartment following removal of protein-rich ascitic fluid.

◆ b. *Specific nursing interventions following paracentesis:*

(1) Apply pressure to injection site and cover with sterile dressing.

(2) Measure and record amount and color of ascitic fluid; send specimens to lab for diagnostic studies.

7. *Small-bowel biopsy*—a specimen is obtained by passing a tube through the oral cavity and is microscopically examined for changes in cellular morphology.

◆ *Nursing interventions: no* food or fluids 8 hr before procedure. Obtain written consent. Remove dentures if present. Monitor vital signs before, during, and after procedure for indications of hemorrhage. Procedure takes approximately 1 hour.

F. Procedures to evaluate the reproductive system in women:

1. *Culdoscopy*—surgical procedure in which a culdoscope is inserted into the posterior vaginal cul-de-sac; *used to:* visualize: uterus, fallopian tubes, broad ligaments, and peritoneal contents.

2. *Hysterosalpingography*—x-ray examination of uterus and fallopian tubes following insertion of a radiopaque substance into the uterine cavity; *used to:* determine patency of fallopian tubes and detect pathology in uterine cavity.

3. *Breast biopsy*—needle aspiration or incisional removal of breast tissue for microscopic examina-

tion; *used to:* differentiate among benign tumors, cysts, and malignant tumors in the breast.

4. *Cervical biopsy and cauterization*—removal of cervical tissue for microscopic examination and cautery; *used to:* control bleeding or obtain additional tissue samples.

5. *Uterotubal insufflation (Rubin's test)*—injection of carbon dioxide into the cervical canal; *used to:* determine fallopian tube patency.

G. Procedures to evaluate the neuroendocrine system:

1. *Radioactive iodine uptake test (iodine[131] uptake)*—ingestion of a tracer dose of ^{131}I, followed in 24 hr by a scan of the thyroid for amount of radioactivity emitted.

a. *High* uptake indicates hyperthyroidism.

b. *Low* uptake indicates hypothyroidism.

◪ 2. *Eight-hour intravenous ACTH test*—administration of 25 units of ACTH in 500 mL of saline over an 8 hr period.

a. *Used to:* determine function of adrenal cortex.

b. 24 hr urine specimens are collected, before and after administration, for measurement of 17-ketosteroids and 17-hydroxycorticosteroids.

c. In *Addison's* disease, urinary output of steroids does *not increase* following administration of ACTH; *normally* steroid excretion *increases threefold to fivefold* following ACTH stimulation.

d. In *Cushing's* syndrome, hyperactivity of the adrenal cortex *increases* the urine output of steroids in the second urine specimen *tenfold.*

3. *Cerebral angiography*—fluoroscopic visualization of the brain vasculature after injection of a contrast medium into the carotid or vertebral arteries; *used to:* localize lesions (tumors, abscesses, intracranial hemorrhages, and occlusions) that are large enough to distort cerebrovascular blood flow.

4. *Myelogram*—through a lumbar-puncture needle, a contrast medium is injected into the subarachnoid space of the spinal column to visualize the spinal cord; *used to:* detect herniated or ruptured intervertebral disks, tumors, or cysts that compress or distort spinal cord.

◆ ◪ *Nursing interventions: elevate head of bed* with water-soluble contrast; *flat* with oil contrast; check for bladder distention with metrizamide (water soluble); vital signs every 4 hr for 24 hr.

5. *Brain scan*—intravenous injection of a radioactive substance, followed by a scan for emission of radioactivity.

a. *Increased* radioactivity at site of abnormality.

b. *Used to:* detect brain tumors, abscesses, hematomas, and arteriovenous malformations.

6. *Lumbar puncture*—puncture of the lumbar subarachnoid space of the spinal cord with a needle to withdraw samples of cerebrospinal fluid (CSF); *used to:* evaluate CSF for infections and determine presence of hemorrhage. *Not* done if increased intracranial pressure (ICP) suspected.

H. Procedures to evaluate the skeletal system. *Arthroscopy*—examination of a joint through a fiberoptic endoscope called an arthroscope. Usually done in the OR (same-day surgery) under aseptic conditions using a local anesthetic, although a general anesthetic may be used. A tourniquet is used to reduce blood flow to the area while the scope is introduced through a cannula. Saline is used as the viewing medium. Biopsy or removal of loose bodies from the joint may be done. A compression dressing (e.g., Ace bandage) is applied. Restrictions vary according to surgeon preference and nature of procedure. Weight bearing may be immediate or restricted for 24 hr. Teach client to observe for signs of infection.

DIAGNOSTIC TESTS TO EVALUATE FETAL WELL-BEING

Table 11.1.

TABLE 11.1	Diagnostic Tests to Evaluate Fetal Well-Being	
Test	**Implications of Results**	**Risks**
Nonstress Test (NST)		
Requires electronic fetal monitoring Correlates fetal movements with FHR and intact fetal CNS; 90% of gross fetal movements associated with accelerations of the FHR	*Reactive test*—indicate intact CNS. *Nonreactive test*—does not meet criteria for reactivity. May indicate fetal jeopardy.	Noninvasive procedures No known contraindications
Breast Stimulation Stress Test (BSST)		
Can be performed by stimulation of nipples until contraction occurs	Contractions can be stimulated	May be contraindicated in preterm gestation
Contraction Stress Test (CST)		
Correlates fetal heart rate response to induced uterine contractions; indicator of *uteroplacental insufficiency*	Increased doses of oxytocin are administered to stimulate uterine contractions. Interpretation: *Negative results* indicates absence of abnormal deceleration with all contractions. Reassurance that the fetus is likely to survive if labor occurs in 1 wk. *Positive results* indicate abnormal FHR decelerations with contractions. May indicate *uteroplacental insufficiency* and that the fetus is at increased risk for perinatal morbidity and death.	Invasive procedure Risk for uterine hyperstimulation and jeopardy to the fetus
Ultrasound		
Passage of high-frequency sound waves through uterus to obtain data regarding fetal growth, placental position, placental detachment, and uterine cavity; can be done abdominally or vaginally	May be *used for:* pregnancy confirmation, fetal viability, estimation of fetal age, placental location, placental abruption, detection of fetal abnormalities, identification of multiple gestation, and confirmation of fetal death.	Noninvasive procedure Inconclusive evidence of harmful effects on humans
Biophysical Profile (BPP)		
Assessment of five fetal biophysical variables: *tone, breathing movements, gross body movement, amniotic fluid volume,* and *FHR reactivity* (monitored by Nonstress Test [NST]); first four variables assessed by ultrasound; score of 2 assigned to each normal finding, and 0 to each abnormal; maximum score: 10	*Used to*: assess the fetus at risk for intrauterine compromise. Normal fetal biophysical activities indicate that the CNS is functional and the fetus is not hypoxemic. *Abnormal* findings with oligohydramnios indicate fetal jeopardy (acidosis and impending death) and necessity for **immediate** delivery. Normal: 8–10 (if amniotic fluid volume [AFV] adequate). Equivocal: 6. Abnormal: <4.	Noninvasive procedure No known contraindications

(Continued on following page)

Treatments

TABLE 11.1	Diagnostic Tests to Evaluate Fetal Well-Being *(Continued)*	
Test	**Implications of Results**	**Risks**

Amniocentesis

Invasive procedure for amniotic fluid analysis; needle placed through abdominal wall to obtain designated amount of fluid for examination; ultrasound *always precedes* this procedure; possible after 14 weeks of gestation	Amniotic fluid (fetal cells) might be analyzed for chromosomal studies to detect: aberrations, inborn errors of metabolism; determine fetal lung maturity, presence of isoimmune disease, alpha-fetoprotein (AFP) levels for determination of neural tube defects, and presence of meconium.	Complications: <1%, but risks might include: onset of contractions. infections; placental, cord, fetal, or bladder puncture Fetomaternal hemorrhage with possible Rh isoimmunization Mothers who are Rh-negative should receive RhoGAM following the procedure

Percutaneous Umbilical Blood Sampling (PUBS; also called *cordocentesis*)

Technique used to obtain pure fetal blood from the umbilical cord while the fetus is in utero; ultrasound done first to locate umbilical cord, then a needle is inserted through the maternal abdomen and into the fetal umbilical vein; done in *second and third trimesters*; a paralytic agent, such as Pavulon, may be given to prevent fetal movement during the procedure	*Indications* for fetal blood sampling: ■ Rapid fetal karyotyping. ■ Diagnosis of fetal infection. ■ Platelet disorders. ■ Fetal blood grouping. ■ Diagnosis and treatment of isoimmunization. ■ Fetal metabolic disorders. ■ Fetal blood transfusion. ■ Administration of fetal medications.	Overall fetal loss risk <2%; complication rate after PUBS: <0.5% *Complications* include: failure to obtain sample, bleeding, premature rupture of membranes, chorioamnionitis, fetal bradycardia, Rh isoimmunization (women who are Rh-negative given RhoGAM).

Chorionic Villus Sampling (CVS)

Involves obtaining a small sample of chorionic villi from edge of developing placenta between 10 and 12 weeks of gestation; can be accomplished either transcervically or transabdominally; use sterile procedure; chorionic tissue aspirated into a syringe	Because chorionic villi originate in zygote, it reflects the genetic makeup of the fetus. *Indications for CVS:* ■ Advanced maternal age (>35 yr). ■ Biochemical and molecular assays for infections. ■ Assays for metabolic disorders.	Vaginal bleeding, spontaneous abortion (SAB), rupture of membranes, limb anomalies (increased risk if done <10 weeks of gestation); intrauterine infection, Rh isoimmunization (women who are Rh-negative given RhoGAM)

NEWBORN SCREENING PROCEDURES

Table 11.2.

INTRAVENOUS THERAPY

I. Infusion systems
  A. Plastic bag:
    1. Contains no vacuum—needs no air to replace fluid as it flows from container.
    2. Medication can be added with syringe through a resealable latex port.
      a. During infusion, administration set should be completely clamped before medications are added.
      b. Prevents undiluted, and perhaps toxic, dose from entering administration set.
  B. Closed system:
    1. Requires partial vacuum—however, only filtered air enters container.

    2. Medication may be added during infusion through air vent in administration set.
  C. Administration sets:
    1. *Standard sets*—deliver 10–15 (gtt) drops/mL.
    2. *Pediatric or minidrop sets*—deliver 60 (gtt) drops/mL.
    3. *Controlled-volume sets*—permit accurate infusion of measured volumes of fluids.
      a. Particularly valuable when piggybacked into primary infusion.
      b. Solutions containing drugs can then be administered intermittently.
    4. *Y-type administration sets*—allow for simultaneous or alternate infusion of two fluids.
      a. May contain filter and pressure unit for blood transfusions.
      b. *Air embolism* significant hazard with this type of administration set.
    5. *Positive-pressure sets*—designed for rapid infusion of replacement fluids.
      a. In emergency, built-in pressure chamber increases rate of blood administration.
      b. Pump chamber *must* be filled at all times to avoid air embolism.
      c. Application of positive pressure to infusion fluids is responsibility of *physician*.

TABLE 11.2	Newborn Screening Procedures	
Test	**Implications of Results**	**◆ Nursing Priorities**
Cord blood type, group, and Coombs' test	Sample of cord blood is collected at delivery to determine newborn's *blood type* and *group* (Rh positive or negative). Coombs' test is done, especially for those whose mothers have type O or Rh-negative blood, or for neonates who are considerably jaundiced. Direct Coombs' test will determine *if antibodies* are present in the neonate's blood.	1. Review prenatal record to determine risk for ABO and Rh incompatibility. 2. Assess for jaundice. Age of the neonate in hours or days at the onset of jaundice is essential to diagnose underlying clinical causes. 3. Provide support and information to the family regarding screening procedures.
Phenylketonuria(PKU)	PKU is an autosomal recessive disease of protein synthesis in which the blood level of the amino acid phenylalanine becomes very high; the disorder results in *mental retardation*. If test is positive, retardation can be prevented through dietary control. Test is done with blood sample from neonate's heel 24–36 hr after having milk. Usually repeat screening recommended, especially if discharged early.	1. Review family history for incidence of inborn errors of metabolism. 2. Observe neonate for: lethargy, apnea, poor feeding, poor muscle tone, jaundice, enlarged tongue, diarrhea, and unusual (musty) body odor. 3. Provide support and information regarding screening procedures. Stress importance of follow-up testing.
Hypothyroidism	Mass neonatal screening for hypothyroidism is a cost-effective measure for preventing mental retardation caused by thyroid dysfunction. Sample of neonate's blood is taken for analysis (may be done with PKU analysis).	1. Review family history for thyroid dysfunction. 2. Provide support and information regarding screening procedures.
Galactosemia	Galactosemia is an autosomal recessive disease in which the inborn error of metabolism involves the body's inability to convert galactose to glucose. Surplus of galactose causes *liver* and *brain damage*. May be done with blood sample for PKU.	1. Review family history for incidence of inborn errors of metabolism. 2. Provide support and information to the family regarding screening procedures.
Sickle cell disease	Sickle cell is an autosomal recessive disorder occurring in certain ethnic groups, most commonly African-American. Other ethnic origins may include: Mediterranean, Caribbean, Arabian, East Indian, and South and Central American. Disease is marked by crescent-shaped RBCs caused by defective hemoglobin. Severe, life-threatening attacks (crises) begin in childhood (fever and abdominal pain). Blood sample is taken after birth.	1. Review family history for autosomal blood disorders, especially if member of high-risk ethnic group. 2. Provide support and information to parents regarding genetic screening. 3. Provide support and information to the family.
Tay-Sachs	Tay-Sachs disease is an autosomal recessive disease characterized by the *absence* of the enzyme hexosaminidase A (Hex-A). Especially common in people with eastern European (Ashkenazi) Jewish descent. Without Hex-A, a lipid GM_2 ganglioside accumulates abnormally in cells, especially in the nerve cells of the brain. The destructive process begins in the fetus early in pregnancy, although the disease is not clinically apparent until the child is several months old. By the time a child with TSD is 3 or 4 years old, the nervous system is badly affected. Even with the best of care, all children with classical TSD die early in childhood, usually by age 5.	1. Review family history for autosomal disorders, especially if member of high-risk ethnic group. 2. Provide information about carrier screening. 3. Provide support and information for the family

6. *Infusion pumps*—used to deliver small volumes of fluid or doses of high-potency drugs.
   a. Used primarily in neonatal, pediatric, and adult intensive care units.
   b. Have increased the safety of parenteral therapy and reduced nursing time.
D. Long-term delivery systems—centrally placed venous access catheters and ports for the administration of drugs (e.g., chemotherapy), blood and blood products, antibiotics, analgesics, antiemetics, and TPN.

Types: Hickman/Broviac, Groshong, venous access ports (VAP).
1. Inserted under strict aseptic conditions using local or general anesthesia.
2. Major concern: prevention of infection.

II. **Fluid administration**
   A. Factors influencing rate:
      1. Client's size.
      2. Client's physical condition.

3. Age of client.
4. Type of fluid.
5. Client's tolerance to fluid.
6. Client's position.

B. *Flow rates for parenteral infusions* can be computed using the following formula:

$$\frac{\text{gtt/mL of given set}}{60 \text{ min/hr}} \times \text{total volume/hr} = \text{gtt/min}$$

> **Example:** if 1000 mL is to be infused in an 8-hr (125 mL/hr) period and the administration set delivers 15 gtt/mL, the rate is 31.2 gtt/min:
> $$\frac{15}{60} \times 125 = \frac{1}{4} \times 125 = 31.2 \text{ gtt/min}$$

C. Generally the type of fluid administration set determines its rate of flow.
1. *Fluid* administration sets—approximately 15 gtt/min.
2. *Blood* administration sets—approximately 10 gtt/min.
3. *Pediatric* administration sets—approximately 60 gtt/min.
4. Always check information on the administration set box to determine the number of gtt/mL before calculating; varies with manufacturer.

D. Factors influencing flow rates:
1. *Gravity*—a change in the height of the infusion bottle will increase or decrease the rate of flow; for example, raising the bottle *higher* will *increase* the rate of flow, and vice versa.
2. *Blood clot* in needle—stopping the infusion for any reason or an increase in venous pressure may result in partial or total obstruction of needle by clot due to:
   a. *Delay* in changing infusion bottle.
   b. Blood pressure cuff on, or restraints *on* or *above* infusion needle.
   c. Client *lying on arm* in which infusion is being made.
3. Change in *needle position*—against or away from vein wall.
4. *Venous spasm*—due to cold blood or irritating solution.
5. *Plugged vent*—causes infusion to stop.

III. **Fluid and electrolyte therapy**
A. Types of therapy:
1. *Maintenance therapy*—provides water, electrolytes, glucose, vitamins, and in some instances protein to meet daily requirements.
2. *Restoration of deficits*—in addition to maintenance therapy, fluid and electrolytes are added to replace *previous* losses.
3. *Replacement therapy*—infusions to replace *current* losses in fluid and electrolytes.

B. Types of intravenous fluids (**Table 11.3**):
1. *Isotonic solutions*—fluids that approximate the osmolarity (280–300 mOsm/L) of normal blood plasma.
   a. Sodium chloride (0.9%)—normal saline.
   (1) *Indications:*
      (a) Extracellular fluid replacement when Cl^- loss is equal to or greater than Na^+ loss.
      (b) Treatment of metabolic alkalosis.
      (c) Na^+ depletion.
      (d) Initiating and terminating blood transfusions.
   (2) Possible *side effects:*
      (a) Hypernatremia.
      (b) Acidosis.
      (c) Hypokalemia.
      (d) Circulatory overload.
   b. Five percent dextrose in water (D_5W).
   (1) *Provides calories* for energy, *sparing body protein* and *preventing* ketosis resulting from fat breakdown.
      (a) 3.75 calories are provided per gram of glucose.
      (b) USP standards require use of monohydrated glucose, so only 91% is actually glucose.
      (c) D_5W yields 170.6 calories; D_5W means 5 g glucose/100 mL water.

> 50 x 3.75 = 187.5 calories/L
> 0.91 x 187.5 = 170.6 calories/L

TABLE 11.3	Commonly Used Intravenous Fluids					
IV Solution	**Na^+ (mEq/L)**	**K^+ (mEq/L)**	**Ca^{++} (mEq/L)**	**Cl^- (mEq/L)**	**Lactate (mEq/L)**	**Calories/L**
0.9% NaCl (NS)	154	0	0	154	0	0
5% Dextrose (D_5W)	0	0	0	0	0	170
5% Dextrose + 0.9% NaCl (D_5NS)	154	0	0	154	0	170
5% Dextrose + 0.45% NaCl ($D_5 \frac{1}{2}$ NS)	77	0	0	77	0	170
Lactated Ringer's solution	130	4	3	109	28	9
3% NaCl	462	0	0	462	0	0
5% NaCl	770	0	0	770	0	0
0.45% NaCl	69.3	0	0	69.3	0	0
10% Dextrose ($D_{10}W$)	0	0	0	0	0	340

(2) *Indications:*
    (a) Dehydration.
    (b) Hypernatremia.
    (c) Drug administration.
(3) Possible *side effects:*
    (a) Hypokalemia.
    (b) Osmotic diuresis—dehydration.
    (c) Transient hyperinsulinism.
    (d) Water intoxication.

c. Five percent dextrose in normal saline (D_5NS).
(1) *Prevents* ketone formation and *loss* of potassium and intracellular water.
(2) *Indications:*
    (a) Hypovolemic shock—temporary measure.
    (b) Burns.
    (c) Acute adrenocortical insufficiency.
(3) Same *side effects* as normal saline.

d. Isotonic multiple-electrolyte fluids—*used for* replacement therapy; ionic composition approximates blood plasma.
(1) Types—Plasmanate, Polysol, and lactated Ringer's.
(2) *Indicated in:* vomiting, diarrhea, excessive diuresis, and burns.
(3) Possible *side effect*—circulatory overload.
(4) Lactated Ringer's is *contraindicated* in severe metabolic acidosis and/or alkalosis and liver disease.
(5) Same *side effects* as normal saline.

2. *Hypertonic solutions*—fluids with an osmolarity much higher than 310 mOsm (+50 mOsm); increase osmotic pressure of blood plasma, thereby drawing fluid from the cells.
a. Ten percent dextrose in normal saline.
(1) Administered in large vein to dilute and prevent venous trauma.
(2) *Used for:* nutrition and to replenish Na^+ and Cl^-.
(3) Possible *side effects:*
    (a) Hypernatremia (excess Na^+).
    (b) Acidosis (excess Cl^-).
    (c) Circulatory overload.
b. Sodium chloride solutions, 3% and 5%.
(1) Slow administration essential to prevent overload (100 mL/hr).
(2) *Indicated in* water intoxication and severe sodium depletion.

3. *Hypotonic solutions*—fluids whose osmolarity is significantly less than that of blood plasma (-50 mOsm); these fluids lower plasma osmotic pressures, causing fluid to enter cells.
a. 0.45% sodium chloride—used for replacement when requirement for Na^+ use is questionable.
b. 2.5% dextrose in 0.45% saline, also 5% D in 0.2% NaCl—common rehydrating solution.

(1) *Indications:*
    (a) Fluid replacement when some Na^+ replacement is also necessary.
    (b) Encourage diuresis in clients who are dehydrated.
    (c) Evaluate kidney status before instituting electrolyte infusions.
(2) Possible *side effects:*
    (a) Hypernatremia.
    (b) Circulatory overload.
    (c) Use with *caution* in clients who are edematous with cardiac, renal, or hepatic disease.
    (d) After adequate renal function is established, appropriate electrolytes should be given to *avoid hypokalemia.*

4. *Alkalizing agents*—fluids used in the treatment of *metabolic acidosis:*
a. Ringer's:
(1) Administration—rate usually not more than 300 mL/hr.
(2) *Side effects*—observe carefully for signs of *alkalosis.*
b. Sodium bicarbonate:
(1) *Indications:*
    (a) Replace excessive loss of bicarbonate ion.
    (b) Emergency treatment of life-threatening acidosis.
(2) Administration:
    (a) Depends on client's weight, condition, and carbon dioxide level.
    (b) Usual dose is 500 mL of a 1.5% solution (89 mEq).
(3) *Side effects:*
    (a) Alkalosis.
    (b) Hypocalcemic tetany.
    (c) Rapid infusion may induce cellular acidity and death.

5. *Acidifying solutions*—fluids used in treatment of *metabolic alkalosis.*
a. Types:
(1) Normal saline (see **B. 1.** Isotonic solutions, **p. 798**).
(2) Ammonium chloride.
b. Administration—dosage depends on client's condition and serum lab values.
c. *Side effects:*
(1) Hepatic encephalopathy in presence of decreased liver function because ammonia is metabolized by liver.
(2) Toxic effects of irregular respirations, twitching, and bradycardia.
(3) *Contraindicated* with renal failure.

6. *Blood and blood products* (**Table 11.4**).
a. *Indications:*
(1) Maintenance of blood volume.
(2) Supply red blood cells to maintain oxygen-carrying capacity.

Treatments

TABLE 11.4 ● **Transfusion with Blood or Blood Products**

Treatments

Blood or Blood Product	Indications	◆ Assessment: Side Effects	◆ Nursing Care Plan/ Implementation
Whole blood	1. Acute hemorrhage 2. Hypovolemic shock	1. Hemolytic reaction 2. Fluid overload 3. Febrile reaction 4. Pyrogenic reaction 5. Allergic reaction	1. See **Unit 7, Table 7.26** (**p. 554**), for complete discussion of nursing responsibilities 2. Protocol for checking blood before transfusion is begun varies with each institution; however, at least *two* RNs must verify that the unit of blood has been crossmatched for a specific client
Red blood cells, packed	1. Acute anemia with hypoxia 2. Aplastic anemia 3. Bone marrow failure due to malignancy 4. Clients who need red blood cells but not volume	*See* Whole blood	*See* Whole blood
Red blood cells, frozen	1. *See* Red blood cells, packed 2. Clients sensitized by previous transfusions	1. Less likely to cause antigen reaction 2. Decreased possibility of transmitting hepatitis	*See* Whole blood
White blood cells (leukocytes)	Currently being used in severe leukopenia with infection (research still being done)	1. Elevated temperature 2. Graft-versus-host disease	1. Careful monitoring of temperature 2. *Must* be given as soon as collected
Platelet concentrate	1. Severe deficiency 2. Clients who have thrombocytopenia and are bleeding, with platelet counts *below* 10,000/μL.	1. Fever, chills 2. Hives 3. Development of antibodies that will destroy platelets in future transfusions *Contraindications:* 1. Idiopathic thrombocytopenic purpura 2. Disseminated intravascular coagulation (DIC)	Monitor temperature
Single-donor fresh plasma	1. Clotting deficiency or concentrates not available or deficiency not fully diagnosed 2. Shock	1. Side effects rare 2. Heart failure 3. Possible hepatitis	Use sterile, pyrogen-free filters
Plasma removed from whole blood (up to 5 days after expiration date, which is 21 days)	1. Shock due to loss of plasma 2. Burns 3. Peritoneal injury 4. Hemorrhage 5. While awaiting blood crossmatch results	*See* Single-donor fresh plasma	*See* Single-donor fresh plasma
Freeze-dried plasma	*See* Plasma removed from whole blood	*See* Single-donor fresh plasma	Must be reconstituted with sterile water before use
Single-donor fresh-frozen plasma	1. *See* Single-donor fresh plasma 2. Inherited or acquired disorders of coagulation 3. Preoperatively for hemophilia	*See* Single-donor fresh plasma	1. Notify blood bank to thaw about 30 min before administration 2. Give *immediately*
Cryoprecipitate concentrate (factor VIII—antihemophilic factor)	For hemophilia: 1. Prevention 2. Preoperatively 3. During bleeding episodes	Rare	0.55 mL of cryoprecipitate concentrate has same effect on serum level as 1600 mL of fresh-frozen plasma

(Continued on following page)

Blood or Blood Product	Indications	◆ Assessment: Side Effects	◆ Nursing Care Plan/ Implementation
Factors II, VII, IX, and X compiled	Specific deficiencies	Hepatitis	Commercially prepared
Fibrinogen (factor I)	Fibrinogen deficiency	Increased risk of hepatitis because the hepatitis virus combines with fibrinogen during fractionation	1. Reconstitute with sterile water 2. Do *not* warm fibrinogen or use hot water to reconstitute 3. Do *not* shake 4. Must be given with a filter
Albumin or salt-poor albumin	1. Shock due to hemorrhage, trauma, infection, surgery, or burns 2. Treatment of cerebral edema 3. Low serum-protein levels	None; these are heat-treated products	Commercially prepared

(3) Supply clotting factors to maintain coagulation properties.

(4) Exchange transfusion.

IV. Intravenous cancer chemotherapy

A. Usual sites: forearm, dorsum of hand, wrist, antecubital fossa.

B. Procedure:

1. Normal saline infusion usually started first, to verify vein patency, position of needle. chemotherapy "piggybacked" into IV line that is running.

2. Rate: usually 1 mL/min. Running slowly decreases nausea, vomiting, and the degree of vein damage.

3. Check vein patency every 3–5 min.

4. If more than one drug is to be infused, normal saline should be infused between drugs.

5. *Never* infuse against resistance.

6. *Stop* treatment if client reports pain at needle site. Extravasation (infiltration of toxic drugs into tissue surrounding vessel) may be present.

▶ 7. If extravasation present, begin protocol appropriate to drug administered (e.g., flushing of line with saline, applying ice or heat, local injection of site with antidote drugs, topical application of steroid creams).

8. Once treatment is completed, remove needle, apply Band-Aid, exert pressure to prevent hematoma formation.

V. Complications of IV therapy (Table 11.5).

TABLE 11.5 ⬤ **Complications of IV Therapy**			
	◆ **Assessment**		◆ **Nursing Care Plan/ Implementation**
Complication	**Subjective Data**	**Objective Data**	
Infiltration—fluid infusing into surrounding tissue rather than into vessel	Pain around needle insertion	1. Infusion rate slow 2. Swelling, hardness, coolness, blanching of tissue at site of needle 3. Blood does not return into tubing when bag/bottle lowered 4. Puffiness under surface of arm	1. Stop IV 2. Apply warm towel to area 3. Restart at another site 4. Record
Thrombophlebitis—inflammatory changes in vessel; *thromboemboli*—the development of venous clots within the inflamed vessel	Pain along the vein	Redness, swelling around affected area (red line)	1. Stop IV 2. Notify physician 3. Cold compresses or warm towel, as ordered 4. Restart in another site 5. *Rest affected limb; do not rub* 6. *See* nursing care of thrombophlebitis, **Unit 7, p. 510**
Pyrogenic reaction—contaminated equipment/solution	1. Headache 2. Backache 3. Nausea 4. Anxiety	1. ↑Temperature 2. Chills 3. Face flushed 4. Vomiting 5. ↓BP 6. Cyanosis	1. Discontinue IV 2. Vital signs 3. Send equipment for culture/analysis ⬤ 4. Antibiotic ointment, as ordered, at injection site

(Continued on following page)

Treatments

TABLE 11.5	Complications of IV Therapy *(Continued)*		
	◆ Assessment		◆ Nursing Care Plan/
Complication	**Subjective Data**	**Objective Data**	**Implementation**
			5. *Prevention:* change tubing q24–48h; meticulous sterile technique; check for precipitation, expiration dates, damage to containers, tubings, etc.; refrigerate hyperalimentation fluids; discard hyperalimentation fluids that have been at room temperature for 8–12 hr and use new bag regardless of amount left in first bag (change, to prevent infection—excellent medium for bacterial growth)
Fluid overload—excessive amount of fluid infused; infants/elderly at risk	1. Headache 2. Shortness of breath 3. Syncope 4. Dyspnea	1. ↑Pulse, venous pressure 2. Venous distention 3. Flushed skin 4. Coughing 5. ↑Respirations 6. Cyanosis, pulmonary edema 7. Shock	1. Stop IV 2. Semi-Fowler's *position* 3. Notify physician 4. Be prepared for diuretic therapy 5. *Preventive measures:* monitor flow rate and client's response to IV therapy (see **Unit 7,** Fluid volume excess, **pp. 516-517,** for subjective and objective data)
Air emboli—air in circulatory system	Loss of consciousness	1. Hypotension, cyanosis 2. Tachycardia 3. ↑Venous pressure 4. Tachypnea	1. Turn on *left* side, with head *down* 2. Administer oxygen therapy 3. **Medical emergency—call physician**
Nerve damage—improper position of limb during infusion or *tying* limb down too tight during infusion → damage to nerve	Numbness: fingers, hands	Unusual position for limb	1. Untie 2. Passive ROM exercises 3. Monitor closely for return of function 4. Record limb status
Pulmonary embolism—blood clot enters pulmonary circulation and obstructs pulmonary artery	Dyspnea	1. Orthopnea 2. Signs of circulatory and cardiac collapse	1. Slow IV to keep vein open (rate: 5–6 drops/min) 2. Notify physician 3. **Medical emergency** 4. Be prepared for lifesaving measures and anticoagulation therapy

OXYGEN THERAPY

I. **Purpose**— to relieve hypoxia and provide adequate tissue oxygenation.

II. **Clinical indications:**
   A. Any client who is likely to have significant *shunt* from:
      1. Fluid in the alveoli.
         a. Pulmonary edema.
         b. Pneumonia.
         c. Near-drowning.
         d. Chest trauma.
      2. Collapsed alveoli (atelectasis).
         a. Airway obstruction.
            (1) Any client who is unconscious.
            (2) Choking.
         b. Failure to take deep breaths.
            (1) Pain (rib fracture).
            (2) Paralysis of the respiratory muscles (spine injury).
            (3) Depression of the respiratory center (head injury, drug overdose).
         c. Collapse of an entire lung (pneumothorax).
      3. Other gases in the alveoli.
         a. Smoke inhalation.
         b. Toxic inhalations.
         c. Carbon monoxide poisoning.
      4. Respiratory arrest.
   B. Cardiac arrest.
   C. Shock.
   D. Shortness of breath.
   E. Signs of respiratory insufficiency.
   F. Breathing fewer than 10 times per minute.

G. Chest pain.

H. Stroke.

I. Anemia.

J. Fetal decelerations during labor.

III. Precautions:

A. Clients with COPD should receive oxygen at *low* flow rates (usually 1–3 L/min), to prevent inhibition of hypoxic respiratory drive.

B. *Excessive* amounts of oxygen for prolonged periods of time will cause *retrolental fibroplasia* and blindness in infants who are premature.

C. Oxygen delivered *without* humidification will result in drying and irritation of respiratory mucosa, decreased ciliary action, and thickening of respiratory secretions.

D. Oxygen supports combustion, and *fire* is a potential hazard during its administration.

1. Ground electrical equipment.

2. Prohibit smoking.

3. Institute measures to decrease static electricity.

E. *High* flow rates of oxygen delivered by ventilator or cuffed tracheostomy and endotracheal tubes can produce signs of *oxygen toxicity* in 24–48 hr:

1. Cough, sore throat, decreased vital capacity, and substernal discomfort.

2. Pulmonary manifestations due to:

a. Atelectasis.

b. Exudation of protein fluids into alveoli.

c. Damage to pulmonary capillaries.

d. Interstitial hemorrhage.

IV. Oxygen administration:

A. Oxygen is dispensed from cylinder or piped-in system.

B. Methods of delivering oxygen:

1. **Nasal prongs/cannula.**

a. Comfortable and simple, and allows client to move about in bed.

b. Delivers 25%–40% oxygen at flow rates of 4–6 L/min.

c. Difficult to keep in position unless client is alert and cooperative.

2. Jet mixing **Venturi mask.**

a. Allows for accurate delivery of prescribed concentration of oxygen.

b. Delivers 24%–50% oxygen at flow rates of 4–8 L/min.

c. Useful in long-term treatment of *COPD*.

3. **Simple O_2 face mask.**

a. Poorly tolerated—used for short periods of time; feeling of "suffocation."

b. Delivers 50%–60% oxygen at flow rates of 8–12 L/min.

c. Significant rebreathing of carbon dioxide at low oxygen flow rates.

d. Hot—may produce *pressure sores* around nose and mouth.

4. **Continuous positive airway pressure (CPAP) mask.**

a. Increases pulmonary volume; opens alveoli; may improve V/Q mismatch.

b. Used with *sleep apnea* with or without O_2 source.

5. **Nonrebreather reservoir mask.**

a. Reservoir bag has one-way valve preventing the client from exhaling back into the bag.

b. Oxygen flow rate prevents collapse of bag during inhalation.

c. Delivers 90%–95% oxygen at flow rates of 10–12 L/min.

d. Ideal for *severe hypoxia*, but client may complain of feelings of suffocation.

6. **T-tube.**

a. Provides humidification and enriched oxygen mixtures to *tracheostomy* or *endotracheal tube*.

b. Delivers up to 100% oxygen at flow rates at least twice the minute ventilation.

c. Refer to **Table 11.6** for summary of oxygen delivery equipment.

V. Intubation and mechanical ventilation:

A. *Indications:*

1. Apnea.

2. Inadequate upper airway or inability to clear secretions.

3. Worsening respiratory acidosis ($Paco_2$ >50 mm Hg) and hypoventilation.

4. Pao_2 <55 mm Hg.

5. Absent gag reflex.

6. Heavy sedation or paralysis.

7. Imminent respiratory failure (respiratory rate <8–10 breaths/min or >30–40 breaths/min).

8. Chest wall trauma.

9. Profound shock.

10. Controlled hyperventilation (e.g., increased ICP).

B. *Types of positive pressure ventilators:*

TABLE 11.6	Summary: Oxygen Delivery Equipment	
O_2	**Flow Rate Delivered**	**Percent O_2**
Nasal cannula*	1–6 L/min	24%–44%
Simple mask	6–10 L/min	35%–55%
Non-rebreather mask	6–15 L/min	50%–90%
Venti mask (Venturi)	3–15 L/min	24%–50%
Bag-valve mask (Ambu bag)	15 L/min	100% with reservoir

*Nasal cannulas should be humidified when they are used for an extended time.
From Myers, Ehren: RNotes, FA Davis, Philadelphia.

1. *Pressure cycled*—gas flows into the client until a predetermined airway pressure is reached. Tidal volume is not constant.
2. *Time cycled*—gas flows for a certain percentage of time during ventilatory cycle.
3. *Volume cycled*—most common ventilators used; tidal volume is determined, and a fixed volume is delivered with each breath.

C. *Ventilator modes:*
   1. *Controlled*—machine delivers a breath at a fixed rate regardless of client's effort or demands.
   2. *Assist-controlled*—machine senses a client's efforts to breathe and delivers a fixed tidal volume with each effort.
   3. *Intermittent mandatory ventilation (IMV)*—breaths are delivered by the machine, but the client may also breathe spontaneously without machine assistance.
   4. *Pressure support*—client breathes spontaneously and determines ventilator rate. Tidal volume determined by inflation pressure and client's lung-thorax compliance.

D. *Minute ventilation*—determined by the respiratory rate and the tidal volume. A respiratory rate of 10–15 breaths per minute is considered appropriate. Close monitoring is required to achieve desired (not necessarily normal) $Paco_2$.

E. *Positive end-expiratory pressure* (PEEP)—maintenance of positive airway pressure at the end of expiration. Applied in the form of continuous positive airway pressure (CPAP) for the client breathing spontaneously or continuous positive-pressure ventilation (CPPV) for the client receiving mechanical breaths. Applied in 3–5 cm H_2O increments. Levels >10–15 cm H_2O are associated with *cardiovascular dysfunction* and *hemodynamic* compromise.

SAFETY AND INFECTION CONTROL: GUIDELINES FOR ISOLATION PRECAUTIONS

Table 11.7.
Table 11.8.
Table 11.9.

TABLE 11.7	Guidelines for Isolation Precautions

The Hospital Infection Control Advisory Committee and the Centers for Disease Control and Prevention have concluded that some fluids, secretions, and excretions not covered under Universal Precautions (UP) represent a potential source of nosocomial and community-acquired infections. The term *Universal Precautions* has been replaced in the hospital setting by a two-tiered system of isolation: **Standard Precautions** for control of nosocomial infections; and **Transmission-based Precautions** for clients known or suspected to be infected with highly transmissible pathogens. *Standard Precautions* incorporate the major components of blood and body fluid precautions from *Universal Precautions*. *Transmission-based Precautions* may be combined for diseases that have multiple routes of transmission and are used in addition to *Standard Precautions.*

Standard Precautions

Use **Standard Precautions**, or the equivalent, for the care of all clients.

1. *Handwashing.*
   a. Wash hands **after touching:** blood, body fluids, secretions, excretions, and contaminated items, whether or not gloves are worn. Wash hands **immediately:** after gloves are removed, between client contacts, and when otherwise indicated to avoid transfer of microorganisms to other clients or environments. It may be necessary to wash hands between tasks and procedures on the same client to prevent cross-contamination of different body sites.
   b. Use a plain (non-antimicrobial) soap for routine hand washing.
   c. Use an antimicrobial agent or a waterless antiseptic agent for specific circumstances (e.g., control of outbreaks or hyperendemic infections), as defined by the infection control program (see *Contact Precautions* for additional recommendations on using antimicrobial and antiseptic agents).

2. *Gloves.* Wear gloves (clean, nonsterile gloves are adequate) **when touching:** blood, body fluids, secretions, excretions, and contaminated items. Put on clean gloves just before touching *mucous membranes* and *nonintact skin*. Change gloves between tasks and procedures on the same client after contact with material that may contain a high concentration of microorganisms. Remove gloves promptly after use, before touching noncontaminated items and environmental surfaces, and before going to another client; wash hands **immediately** to avoid transfer of microorganisms to other clients or environments.

3. *Mask, eye protection, face shield.* Wear a mask and eye protection or a face shield to protect mucous membranes of the eyes, nose, and mouth during procedures and client care activities that are likely to generate splashes or sprays of blood, body fluids, secretions, and excretions.

4. *Gown.* Wear a gown (a clean, nonsterile gown is adequate) to protect skin and to prevent soiling of clothing during procedures and client care activities that are likely to generate splashes or sprays of blood, body fluids, secretions, or excretions. Select a gown that is appropriate for the activity and amount of fluid likely to be encountered. Remove a soiled gown as promptly as possible, and wash hands to avoid transfer of microorganisms to other clients or environments.

5. *Client care equipment.* Handle used client care equipment soiled with blood, body fluids, secretions, and excretions in a manner that prevents skin and mucous membrane exposures, contamination of clothing, and transfer of microorganisms to other clients and environments. Ensure that reusable equipment is not used for the care of another client until it has been cleaned and reprocessed appropriately. Ensure that single-use items are discarded properly.

(Continued on following page)

6. *Environmental control.* Ensure that the hospital has adequate procedures for the routine care, cleaning, and disinfection of environmental surfaces, beds, bed rails, bedside equipment, and other frequently touched surfaces, and ensure that these procedures are being followed.

7. *Linen.* Handle, transport, and process used linen soiled with blood, body fluids, secretions, and excretions in a manner that prevents skin and mucous membrane exposures and contamination of clothing, and that avoids transfer of microorganisms to other clients and environments.

8. *Occupational health and blood-borne pathogens.*
   a. Take care to prevent injuries when using needles, scalpels, and sharp instruments or devices; when handling sharp instruments after procedures; when cleaning used instruments; and when disposing of used needles. *Never* recap used needles, or otherwise manipulate them using both hands, or use any other technique that involves directing the point of a needle toward any part of the body; rather, use either a one-handed "scoop" technique or a mechanical device designed for holding the needle sheath. Do *not* remove used needles from disposable syringes by hand, and do *not* bend, break, or otherwise manipulate used needles by hand. Place used disposable syringes and needles, scalpel blades, and other sharp items in appropriate puncture-resistant containers that are located as close as practical to the area in which the items were used, and place reusable syringes and needles in a puncture-resistant container for transport to the reprocessing area.
   b. Use mouthpieces, resuscitation bags, or other ventilation devices as an alternative to mouth-to-mouth resuscitation methods in areas where the need for resuscitation is predictable.

9. *Client placement.* Place a client who contaminates the environment or who does not (or cannot be expected to) assist in maintaining appropriate hygiene or environmental control in a private room. If a private room is not available, consult with infection control professionals regarding client placement or other alternatives.

Transmission-Based Precautions

Airborne Precautions

In addition to **Standard Precautions**, use *Airborne Precautions,* or the equivalent, for clients known or suspected to be infected with microorganisms transmitted by airborne droplet nuclei (small-particle residue [5 microns or smaller in size] of evaporated droplets containing microorganisms that remain suspended in the air and that can be dispersed widely by air currents within a room or over a long distance).

1. **Client placement.** Place the client in a private room that has (1) monitored negative air pressure in relation to the surrounding area, (2) 6–12 air changes per hour, and (3) appropriate discharge of air outdoors or monitored high-efficiency filtration of room air before the air is circulated to other areas in the hospital. Keep the room door closed and the client in the room. *When a private room is not available,* place the client in a room with a client who has active infection with the same microorganism, unless otherwise recommended, but with no other infection. When a private room is not available and cohorting is not desirable, consultation with infection control professionals is advised before client placement.

2. **Respiratory protection.** Wear respiratory protection when entering the room of a client with known or suspected infectious pulmonary tuberculosis. People who are susceptible should not enter the room of clients known or suspected to have *measles* (rubeola) or *varicella* (chickenpox) if other caregivers who are immune are available. If persons who are susceptible must enter the room of a client known or suspected to have measles (rubeola) or varicella, they should wear respiratory protection. Persons immune to measles (rubeola) or varicella need not wear respiratory protection.

3. **Client transport.** Limit the movement and transport of the client from the room to essential purposes only. If transport or movement is necessary, minimize client dispersal of droplet nuclei by placing a *surgical mask* on the client, if possible.

4. **Additional precautions for preventing transmission of tuberculosis.** Consult CDC "Guidelines for Preventing the Transmission of Tuberculosis in Health-Care Facilities" for additional prevention strategies.

Droplet Precautions

In addition to **Standard Precautions**, use **Droplet Precautions,** or the equivalent, for a client known or suspected to be infected with microorganisms transmitted by droplets (large-particle droplets [larger than 5 microns in size] that can be generated by the client during coughing, sneezing, talking, or the performance of procedures).

1. **Client placement.** Place the client in a private room. When a private room is not available, place the client in room with a client who has active infection with the same microorganism but with no other infection (cohorting). When a private room is not available and cohorting is not achievable, maintain spatial separation of at least 3 ft between the client who is infected and other clients and visitors. Special air handling and ventilation are not necessary, and the door may remain open.

2. **Mask.** In addition to standard precautions, wear a mask when working within 3 ft of the client. (Logistically, some hospitals may want to implement the wearing of a mask to enter the room).

3. **Client transport.** Limit the movement and transport of the client from the room to essential purposes only. If transport or movement is necessary, minimize client dispersal of droplets by masking the client, if possible.

Contact Precautions

In addition to **Standard Precautions**, use **Contact Precautions,** or the equivalent, for specified clients known or suspected to be infected or colonized with epidemiologically important microorganisms that can be transmitted by direct contact with the client (hand or skin-to-skin contact that occurs when performing client care activities that require touching the client's dry skin or indirect contact (touching) with environmental surfaces or client care items in the client's environment.

1. **Client placement.** Place the client in a private room. When a private room is not available, place the client in a room with a client who has active infection with the same microorganism but with no other infection (cohorting). When a private room is not available and cohorting is not achievable, consider the epidemiology of the microorganism and the client population when determining client placement. Consultation with infection control professionals is advised before client placement.

(Continued on following page)

| **TABLE 11.7** | **Guidelines for Isolation Precautions** *(Continued)* |

2. *Gloves and handwashing.* In addition to wearing gloves as outlined under **Standard Precautions,** wear gloves (clean, nonsterile gloves are adequate) when entering the room. During the course of providing care for a client, change gloves after having contact with infective material that may contain high concentrations of microorganisms (fecal material and wound drainage). Remove gloves before leaving the client's environment and wash hands **immediately** with an antimicrobial agent or a waterless antiseptic agent. After glove removal and hand washing, ensure that hands do *not* touch potentially contaminated environmental surfaces or items in the client's room to avoid transfer of microorganisms to other clients or environments.

3. *Gown.* In addition to wearing a gown as outlined under **Standard Precautions**, wear a gown (a clean, nonsterile gown is adequate) when entering the room if you anticipate that your clothing will have substantial contact with the client, environmental surfaces, or items in the client's room; or if the client is *incontinent* or has *diarrhea*, an *ileostomy*, a *colostomy*, or *wound drainage* not contained by a dressing. Remove the gown before leaving the client's environment. After gown removal, ensure that clothing does *not* contact potentially contaminated environmental surfaces to avoid transfer of microorganisms to other clients or environments.

4. *Client transport.* Limit the movement and transport of the client from the room to essential purposes only. If the client is transported out of the room, ensure that precautions are maintained to minimize to risk of transmission of microorganisms to other clients and contamination of environmental surfaces or equipment.

5. *Client care equipment.* When possible, dedicate the use of noncritical client care equipment to a single client (or cohort of clients infected or colonized with the pathogen requiring precautions) to avoid sharing between clients. If use of common equipment or items is unavoidable, adequately clean and disinfect them before use for another client.

Source: Centers for Disease Control and Prevention and Hospital Infection Control Practices Advisory Committee.

| **TABLE 11.8** | **Infection Control: Conditions That Need Additional Precautions** |

Clinical Syndrome or Condition	**Potential Pathogens**	**Empiric Precautions**
Diarrhea		
■ Acute diarrhea with a likely infectious cause in a client who is incontinent or is in diapers	Enteric pathogens	Contact
■ Diarrhea in an adult with a history of recent antibiotic use	*Clostridium difficile*	Contact
Meningitis	*Neisseria meningitides*	Droplet
Rash or exanthems, generalized, etiology unknown		
■ Petechial/ecchymotic with fever	*Neisseria meningitides*	Droplet
■ Vesicular	Varicella	Airborne and Contact
■ Maculopapular with coryza and fever	Rubeola (measles)	Airborne
Respiratory infections		
■ Cough/fever/upper lobe pulmonary infiltrate in a client who is *HIV-negative* or a client at *low risk* for HIV infection	*Mycobacterium tuberculosis*	Airborne
■ Cough/fever/pulmonary infiltrate in any lung location in a client who is *HIV-infected* or a client at *high risk* for HIV infection	*Mycobacterium tuberculosis*	Airborne
■ Paroxysmal or severe persistent cough during periods of *pertussis* activity	*Bordetella pertussis*	Droplet
■ Respiratory infections, particularly *bronchiolitis* and *croup*, in infants and young children	Respiratory syncytial or parainfluenza virus	Contact
Risk of multidrug-resistant microorganisms		
■ *History of infection* or colonization with multidrug-resistant organisms	Resistant bacteria	Contact
■ *Skin, wound, or urinary tract infection* in a client with a *recent* hospital or nursing home stay in a facility where multidrug-resistant organisms are prevalent	Resistant bacteria	Contact
Skin or wound infection		
■ *Abscess* or draining wound that cannot be covered	*Staphylococcus aureus,* group A streptococcus	Contact

CDC Healthcare Infection Control Practices Advisory Committee, from www.cdc.gov/ncidod/hip/ISOLAT/isopart2.htm.

TABLE 11.9	Summary: Types of Precautions and Illnesses Requiring the Precautions

Standard Precautions

Use *Standard Precautions* for the care of all clients.

Airborne Precautions

In addition to *Standard Precautions*, use *Airborne Precautions* for clients known or suspected to have serious illnesses transmitted by airborne droplet *nuclei*.
  Examples of such illnesses include:

- Measles
- Varicella (including disseminated zoster)
- Tuberculosis

Droplet Precautions

In addition to *Standard Precautions*, use *Droplet Precautions* for clients known or suspected to have serious illnesses transmitted by *large* particle droplets.
  Examples of such illnesses include:
  Invasive *Haemophilus influenzae* type b disease, including meningitis, pneumonia, epiglottitis, and sepsis
  Invasive *Neisseria meningitidis* disease, including meningitis, pneumonia, and sepsis
  Other serious bacterial respiratory infections spread by droplet transmission, including:

- Diphtheria (pharyngeal)
- Mycoplasma pneumonia
- Pertussis
- Pneumonic plague
- Streptococcal (group A) pharyngitis, pneumonia, or scarlet fever in infants and young children

Serious viral infections spread by droplet transmission, including:
- Adenovirus
- Influenza
- Mumps
- Parvovirus B19
- Rubella

Contact Precautions

In addition to *Standard Precautions*, use *Contact Precautions* for clients known or suspected to have serious illnesses easily transmitted by *direct* client contact or by contact with items in the client's environment.
Examples of such illnesses include:
Gastrointestinal, respiratory, skin, or wound infections or colonization with multidrug-resistant bacteria judged by the infection control
  program, based on current state, regional, or national recommendations, to be of special clinical and epidemiologic significance
Enteric infections with a low infectious dose or prolonged environmental survival, including:

- *Clostridium difficile*
- For clients who are in diapers or incontinent: enterohemorrhagic *Escherichia coli* O157:H7, *Shigella*, hepatitis A, or rotavirus

Respiratory syncytial virus, parainfluenza virus, or enteroviral infections in infants and young children
Skin infections that are highly contagious or that may occur on dry skin, including:
- Diphtheria (cutaneous)
- Herpes simplex virus (neonatal or mucocutaneous)
- Impetigo
- Major (noncontained) abscesses, cellulitis, or decubiti
- Pediculosis
- Scabies
- Staphylococcal furunculosis in infants and young children
- Zoster (disseminated or in the host who is immunocompromised)
- Viral/hemorrhagic *conjunctivitis*
- Viral hemorrhagic infections (*Ebola*, *Lassa*, or *Marburg*)

Adapted from Fundamentals of Isolation Precautions, CDC Healthcare Infection Control Practices Advisory Committee, from
  www.cdc.gov/ncidod/hip/ISOLAT/isopart2.htm.

Treatments

HANDS-ON NURSING CARE

◤ Positioning the Client

Table 11.10.
Figure 11.1

Commonly Used Tubes

Table 11.11.
Figure 11.2.

TABLE 11.10	◤ Positioning the Client for Specific Surgical Conditions	
Surgical Condition	**Key Points**	**Rationale**
Amputation: lower extremity	*No* pillows under stump after first 24 hr; turn client *prone* several times a day	Prevents flexion deformity of the limb
Appendicitis: ruptured	Keep in *Fowler's* position–*not* flat in bed	Keeps infection from spreading upward in the peritoneal cavity
Burns (extensive)	Usually *flat* for first 24 hr	Potential problem is hypovolemia, which will be more symptomatic in a sitting position
Cast, extremity	Keep extremity *elevated*	Prevents edema
Craniotomy	Head *elevated* with supratentorial incision; *flat* with cerebellar or brainstem incision	Reduces cerebral edema, which contributes to increased intracranial pressure
Flail chest	Position on *affected* side	Reduces the instability of the chest wall that is causing the paradoxical respiratory movements
Gastric resection	Lie down *after* meals	May be useful in preventing dumping syndrome
Hiatal hernia (*before* repair)	Head of bed *elevated* on shock blocks	Prevents esophageal irritation from gastric regurgitation
Hip prosthesis	1. Keep affected leg in *abduction* (splint or pillow between legs) 2. *Avoid* adduction and flexion of the hip 3. Use trochanter roll along outside of femur anterior joint capsule incision to keep affected leg turned slightly *inward;* no trochanter roll with posterior joint capsule incision as leg is turned slightly *outward*	If affected hip is flexed and allowed to adduct and internally rotate, the head of the femur may be displaced from the socket
Laminectomy; fusion	*Avoid* twisting motion when getting out of bed, ambulating	Prevents any shearing force on the spine
Liver biopsy	Place on *right* side, and position pillow for pressure	Prevents bleeding
Lobectomy	Do *not* put in Trendelenburg position. Position of comfort–sides, back	Pushes abdominal contents against diaphragm; may cause respiratory embarrassment
Mastectomy	1. Do *not* abduct arm first few days 2. Elevate hand and arm *higher* than shoulder if lymph glands removed	Puts tension on suture line Prevents lymphedema
Pneumonectomy	Turn *only* toward operative side for short periods; *no* extreme lateral positioning	1. Gives unaffected lung room for full expansion 2. Prevents mediastinal shift 3. In case of bleeding there will be no drainage into the unaffected bronchi
Pneumothorax	Semi-Fowler's	Gives optimal chest expansion
Radium implantation in cervix	Bedrest–usually may *elevate* head to 30 degrees	*Must* keep radium insert positioned correctly
Respiratory distress	*Orthopnea* position usually desirable	Allows for maximum expansion of lungs
Retinal detachment	1. Affected area toward bed–*complete bedrest* 2. No *sudden* movements of head 3. *Face down* if gas bubble in place	1. Gravity may help retina fall in place; prevents further tearing 2. Any sudden increase in intraocular pressure may further dislodge retina

(Continued on following page)

Surgical Condition	Key Points	Rationale
Traction		
Straight traction	Check specific orders about how much head may be elevated	Body is used as the countertraction–this must not be less than the pull of the traction
Balanced suspension	May give client more freedom to move about than in straight traction	In balanced suspension additional weights supply countertraction
Client who is unconscious	Turn on side with head slightly *lowered*–"coma" position	1. Important to let secretions drain out by gravity 2. *Must* prevent aspiration
Vascular		
Ileofemoral bypass; arterial insufficiency	1. Do *not* elevate legs 2. *Avoid* hip flexion–walk or stand, but do *not* sit	1. Arterial flow is helped by gravity 2. Flexion of the hip compresses the vessels of the extremity
Vein strippings; vein ligations	1. Keep legs *elevated* 2. Do *not* stand or sit for long periods	1. Prevents venous stasis 2. Prevents venous pooling

Jane Vincent Corbett, RN, MS, EdD, Professor Emerita, School of Nursing, University of San Francisco. Used with permission.

Treatments

POSITIONS

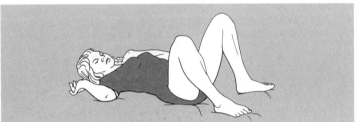

A. DORSAL RECUMBENT POSITION

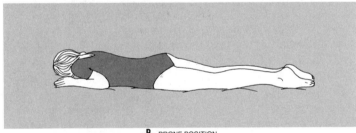

B. PRONE POSITION

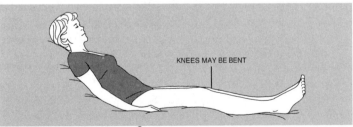

KNEES MAY BE BENT

C. FOWLER'S POSITION

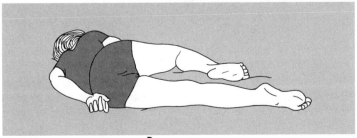

D. SIMS' POSITION

FIGURE 11.1 **Common client positions.** *(A)* **Dorsal recumbent (back-lying), legs up**—used in gynecological and obstetrical procedures such as forcep delivery or vaginal exam; **legs down**—for comfort and following spinal anesthesia. *(B)* **Prone**—may be used in clients who are unconscious to promote drainage from mouth and prevent flexion contractures. *(C)* **Fowler's**—semi-sitting; 45–60 degrees; knees may or may not be bent. Facilitates breathing and drainage. *(D)* **Sims'**—position of choice for enemas and rectal examination, prevents aspiration in clients who are unconscious, comfortable sleeping position for women who are pregnant. *(E)* **Knee-chest or genupectoral**—used for gynecological and obstetrical conditions such as impacted fetal head or transverse presentation. *(F)* **Trendelenburg**—used in abdominal surgery. **Modified Trendelenburg (torso flat and feet elevated)** preferred in shock. *(G)* **Lithotomy or dorsosacral**—used in genital tract operations and vaginal hysterectomy. *(H)* **Right lateral recumbent**—side-lying, relieves pressure on sacrum and heels.

POSITIONS

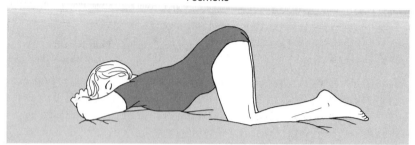

E. KNEE-CHEST OR GENUPECTORAL POSITION

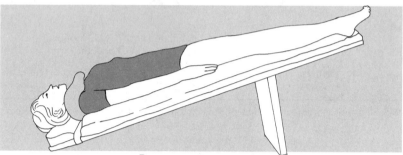

F. TRENDELENBURG POSITION

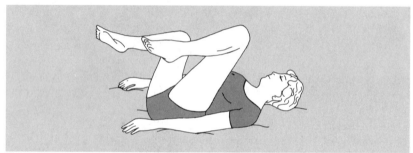

G. LITHOTOMY OR DORSOSACRAL POSITION

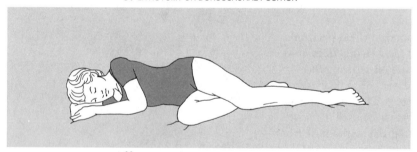

H. RIGHT LATERAL RECUMBENT POSITION

FIGURE 11.1 *(Continued)*

TABLE 11.11	Review of the Use of Common Tubes		

Tube or Apparatus	Purpose	Examples of Use	◆ Key Nursing Points
Chest tubes	1. *Anterior tube* drains mostly air from pleural space 2. *Posterior tube* drains mostly fluid from pleural space 3. Removal of fluid and air from pleural space is necessary to reestablish negative intrapleural pressure	1. *Thoracotomy* 2. *Open heart surgery* 3. *Spontaneous pneumothorax* 4. *Traumatic pneumothorax*	1. *See* Key Points for each of the three entries under Drainage system, below 2. *Sterile* technique is used when changing dressings around the tube insertions 3. Fowler's *position* to facilitate air and fluid removal 4. Cough, deep breathe qlh; splint chest; medicate for pain 5. Manage pain carefully in order *not* to depress respirations 6. Prepare for removal when there is little or no drainage, air leak disappears, or fluctuations stop in water seal; have suture set, air-occlusive dressing, and sturdy elastic tape ready; medicate for pain before removal; monitor breathing after removal (breath sounds, rate, chest pain)
Drainage system (see **Figure 11.2, p. 814**) #1: drainage compartment	Collect drainage		1. Mark level in bottle each shift to keep accurate record—*not* routinely emptied; replaced when full 2. **Never** raise container above the level of the chest; otherwise backflow will occur
#2: water-seal chamber	Water seal prevents flow of atmospheric air into pleural space; essential to prevent recollapse of the lung		1. Air bubbles from postoperative residual air *will* continue for 24–48 hr 2. *Persistent* large amounts of air bubbles in this compartment indicate an *air leak* between the alveoli and the pleural space 3. Clamp tube(s) *only* to verify a leak; replace a broken, cracked, or full drainage unit; or verify readiness of client for tube removal; not necessary to clamp when ambulating if water seal intact 4. If tube becomes disconnected, place tubing end in sterile water or saline; if dislodged from chest, seal insertion site **immediately** on expiration if possible; use *sterile air-occlusive* dressing 5. If air leak is present, clamping the tube for very long (more than 10 sec) may cause a tension pneumothorax 6. Fluctuation of the fluid level in this bottle is *expected* (when the suction is turned off) because respiration changes the pleural pressure: if there is *no fluctuation* of the fluid in the tube of this bottle (when the suction is turned off), either the lung is fully expanded or the tube is blocked by kinking or by a clot 7. Although not routinely used, milking (gently squeezing) the tubes, if ordered, will prevent blockage from clots or debris; otherwise gravity drainage is sufficient to maintain patency 8. Drainage of more than 100 mL in 1 hr should be **reported** to physician
#3: suction control—connected to wall suction	Level of the column of water (i.e., 15–20 cm) is used to control the amount of suction applied to the chest tube—if the water evaporates to only *10 cm* depth, this will be the *maximum* suction generated by the wall suction		1. Air *should continuously bubble* through this compartment when the suction is on; the bubbles are from the atmosphere—not the client; when the wall suction is turned higher, the bubbling will increase, but the increased pulling of air is from the atmosphere and *not* from the pleural space

(Continued on following page)

Treatments

TABLE 11.11	Review of the Use of Common Tubes *(Continued)*		

Tube or Apparatus	Purpose	Examples of Use	◆ Key Nursing Points
			2. Because the level of H_2O determines the maximum negative pressure that can be obtained, make sure the water does *not* evaporate—keep filling the bottle to keep the ordered level; if there is *no* bubbling of air through this container, the wall suction is *too low*
Heimlich flutter valve	1. Has a one-way valve so fluids and air can drain out of the pleural space but cannot flow back 2. Eliminates the need for water seal—no danger when tube is unclamped below the value	Same as for other chest tubes	1. Can be connected to suction if ordered 2. Sometimes can just drain into portable bag so client is more mobile
Tracheostomy tube	1. Maintains patent airway and promotes better O_2-CO_2 exchange 2. Makes removal of secretions by suctioning easier 3. Cuff on trach is necessary if need airtight fit for assisted ventilation	1. *Acute respiratory distress due to poor ventilation* 2. *Severe burns of head and neck* 3. *Laryngectomy* (trach is permanent)	1. Use oxygen *before* and *after* each suctioning 2. Humidify oxygen 3. *Sterile* technique in suctioning; clean technique at home 4. Cleanse inner cannula as needed–only leave out 5–10 min 5. Hemostat handy if outer cannula is expelled—have obturator taped to bed and another trach set handy 6. Cuff **must** be deflated periodically to prevent necrosis of mucosa, unless low-pressure cuff used
Penrose drain	Soft collapsible latex rubber drain inserted to drain serosanguineous fluid from a surgical site; usually brought out to the skin via a stab wound	*Bowel resection*	1. Expect drainage to progress from serosanguineous to more serous 2. *Sterile* technique when changing dressing—do often 3. Physician will advance tube a little each day
Nasogastric (NG) tubes			
Levin tube and small-bore feeding tubes	1. Inserted into stomach to decompress by removing gastric contents and air—prevents any buildup of gastric secretions, which are continuous 2. Used when stomach must be washed out *(lavage)* 3. Used for feedings when client is unable to swallow *(gavage)*	1. Any abdominal or other *surgery after which peristalsis is absent* for a few days 2. *Overdoses* 3. *Gastrointestinal hemorrhage* 4. *Cancer of the esophagus* 5. *Early postoperative care for client who had a laryngectomy or radical neck dissection*	1. Connect to *low* intermittent suction 2. Irrigate prn with normal saline or puffs of air 3. Clean, but *not* sterile, procedure 4. Mouth care needed 5. Report "**coffee ground**" material (digested blood) 6. For overdose, stomach is pumped out as **rapidly** as possible 7. For hemorrhage, tepid normal saline may be used to lavage 8. Critical to make sure tube still in stomach *before* beginning feeding; listen for air passing into stomach, and if possible aspirate gastric contents; small-bore tubes require placement check by x-ray 9. Follow feeding with some water to rinse out the tube 10. Clamp tube when ambulating 11. With larger-bore tubes, determine residuals and withhold feeding if large residuals obtained

(Continued on following page)

Tube or Apparatus	Purpose	Examples of Use	◆ Key Nursing Points
Salem sump	Double-lumen tube with vent to *protect gastric mucosa* from trauma of suctioning	Same as Levin tube	1. Irrigate vent (blue tubing) with air only 2. *See* Levin tube
Gastrostomy tube	1. Inserted into stomach via abdominal wall 2. May be used for decompression 3. Used *long term for feedings*	Conditions affecting *esophagus* in which it is impossible to insert a nasogastric tube	1. Principles of tube feedings same as with Levin nasogastric tube, *except* no danger that tube is in trachea 2. If permanent, tube may be replaceable
Miller-Abbott tube Cantor tube	Longer than Levin tube—has mercury or air in bags so tube can be used to *decompress the lower intestinal tract*	1. *Small-bowel obstructions* 2. *Intussusception* 3. *Volvulus*	1. Care similar to that for Levin NG tube—irrigated 2. Connected to suction, *not* sterile technique 3. Orders will be written on how to advance the tube, gently pushing tube a few inches each hour; client position may affect advancement of tube 4. X-rays determine the desired location of tube
T-tube	To *drain bile* from the common bile duct *until* edema has subsided	*Cholecystectomy* when a common duct exploration (CDE) or choledochostomy was also done	1. Bile drainage is influenced by *position* of the drainage bag 2. Clamp tube as ordered to see if bile will flow into duodenum normally
Hemovac	A type of closed-wound drainage connected to suction—used to *drain a large amount of* serosanguineous drainage from under an incision	1. *Mastectomy* 2. *Total hip procedures* 3. *Total knee procedures*	1. May compress unit, and have portable vacuum or connect to wall suction 2. Small drainage tubes may get clogged—physician may irrigate these at times
Jackson-Pratt	1. A method of *closed-wound suction* drainage—indicated when tissue displacement and tissue trauma may occur with rigid drain tubes (e.g., Hemovac) 2. *See* Hemovac	1. *Neurosurgery* 2. *Neck surgery* 3. *Mastectomy* 4. *Total knee and hip replacement* 5. *Abdominal surgery* 6. *Urological procedures*	1. Empty reservoir when full, to prevent loss of wound drainage and back-contamination 2. *See* Hemovac.
Three-way Foley	To provide avenues for *constant irrigation and constant drainage* of the urinary bladder	1. Transurethral resection (TUR) 2. *Bladder* infections	1. Watch for blocking by clots—causes bladder spasms 2. Irrigant solution often has *antibiotic* added to normal saline or sterile water 3. *Sterile* water rather than normal saline may be used for lysis of clots
Suprapubic catheter	To *drain bladder* via an opening through the abdominal wall above the pubic bone	*Suprapubic* prostatectomy	May have orders to irrigate prn or continuously
Ureteral catheter	To *drain urine* from the pelvis of one kidney, or for *splinting* ureter	1. *Cystoscopy* for diagnostic workups 2. *Ureteral surgery* 3. *Pyelotomy*	1. **Never** clamp the tube—pelvis of kidney only holds 4–8 mL 2. Use **only** 5 mL sterile normal saline if ordered to irrigate

Note: This review focuses on care of tubes, not on total client care.
Source: Jane Vincent Corbett, RN, MS, EdD, Professor Emerita, School of Nursing, University of San Francisco. Used with permission.

Treatments

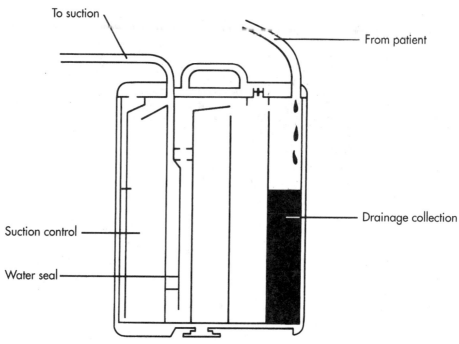

FIGURE 11.2 Chest drainage system.

Colostomy Care

Table 11.12.
Table 11.13.

Basic Prosthetic Care

Table 11.14.
Table 11.15.
Table 11.16.

Bladder Training

Table 11.17.

Bowel Training

Table 11.18.

TABLE 11.12	▶ Emptying Colostomy Appliance

Check for drainage in appliance at least twice during each shift. If drainage present (diarrhea-type stool):

Do	Do Not
1. Unclamp the bottom of bag	1. Remove appliance each time it needs emptying
2. Drain into bedpan	2. Use any materials that could irritate bowel
3. Use a squeeze-type bottle filled with warm water to rinse inside of appliance	3. Ignore client's needs
4. Clean off clamp if soiled	
5. Put a few drops of deodorant in appliance if not odorproof	
6. Fasten bottom of appliance securely (fold bag over clamp 2–3 times before closing)	
7. Check for leakage under appliance every 2–4 hr	
8. Communicate with client while attending to appliance	

TABLE 11.13 ▶ **Changing Colostomy Appliance**

Gather equipment: gloves, skin prep packet, colostomy appliance measured to fit stoma properly (if new surgical stoma, it will continue to shrink with the healing process; use stoma measuring guide), skin barrier, warm water and soap, face cloth/towel, plastic bag for disposal of old equipment. Remember that bowel is very fragile; also, working near bowel increases peristalsis, and feces and flatulence may be expelled.

Do	Do Not
1. Remove old appliance carefully, pulling from area with least drainage to area with most drainage	1. Tear appliance quickly from skin
2. Wash skin area with soap and water	2. Wash stoma with soap; put anything dry onto stoma
3. Observe skin area for potential breakdown	3. Irritate skin or stoma
4. Use packet of skin prep on the skin around the stoma; allow skin prep solution to dry on skin before applying colostomy appliance	4. Put skin prep solution onto stoma; it will cause irritation
5. Apply skin barrier you have measured and cut to size	5. Make opening too large (increases risk of leakage)
6. Put appliance on so that the bottom of the appliance is easily accessible for emptying (e.g., if client is out of bed most of the time, put the bottom facing the feet; if client is in bed most of the time, have bottom face the side); picture-frame the adhesive portion of the appliance with 1-inch tape	6. Have appliance attached so client cannot be involved in own care
7. Put a few drops of deodorant in appliance if not odor-proof	7. Use any materials that would irritate bowel
8. Use clamp to fasten bottom of appliance	8. *Avoid* conversation/eye contact
9. Talk to client (or communicate in best way possible for client) during and after procedure	9. Contaminate other incisions
10. Use good hand-washing technique	

TABLE 11.14 ▶ **Care of Dentures**

Wear gloves
If client cannot remove own dentures, grasp upper plate at the front teeth and move up and down gently to release suction
Lift the lower plate up one side at a time
Use extreme care not to damage dentures while cleaning
Use tepid, *not* hot, water to clean
Avoid soaking for long periods of time
Inspect for sharp edges
Do oral cavity assessment
Replace moistened dentures in client's mouth
Use appropriately labeled container for storage when dentures are to remain out of client's mouth

TABLE 11.15 ▶ **Caring for an Artificial Eye**

With gloved hand pull lower eyelid down over the infraorbital bone and exert pressure below the eyelid
Pressure will make the eye pop out
Handle eye prosthesis carefully
Using *aseptic* technique, cleanse socket with saline-moistened gauze, stroking from inner to outer canthus
Wash the prosthesis in warm normal saline
To reinsert, gently pull the client's lower lid down, raise the upper lid if necessary, slip the saline-moistened eye prosthesis gently into the socket, and release the lids

Treatments

TABLE 11.16 ▶ Caring for a Hearing Aid

Turn off aid when not using (open case at night to prevent draining battery)
Keep extra battery available
Wash with mild soap and warm water; use pipe cleaner to remove wax
Do *not* wear aid in shower or with ear infection
Store in same place every night and away from pets
If aid does not work: check battery insertion, on-off switch, placement (if ear-molded aid), cleanliness

TABLE 11.17 ▶ Bladder Training

1. Determine client's desire/capacity to participate in such a program.
2. Encourage client to void at certain times throughout the day (e.g., q2h then q3h, when getting up in morning, after meals, before bedtime).
3. Do *not* decrease fluid intake (would put client at risk for infection).
4. Encourage client to resist voiding when bladder is not full (use a technique such as counting while voiding and trying to increase that number to a desired level).
5. Encourage client to ask for assistance when needed, to avoid falls when attempting to get to toilet alone while unsteady on feet.
6. Respond to requests for assistance.
7. *Decrease caffeine* and *alcohol* in diet.
8. Monitor for skin breakdown in clients who are incontinent.
9. Have client practice Kegel exercises to improve tone and function of pelvic floor.
10. Refer to physical therapist who specializes in this area, if necessary.

TABLE 11.18 ▶ Bowel Training

1. Verify that the client is not impacted.
2. Determine client's desire/capacity to participate in the program.
3. Determine normal bowel habits.
4. Increase fiber and fluids in the diet.
5. Establish a routine: same time each day.
6. Give stool softener; cathartic, or suppository as ordered.
7. Offer client a hot drink before set time for defecation.
8. Provide time and privacy.
9. Encourage position that will facilitate defecation (sitting position is best, leaning forward without straining).
10. Document interventions that are successful.

Questions

Select the one answer that is best for each question, unless otherwise directed.

1. A client's laboratory values indicate hemoconcentration secondary to fluid loss. Which intravenous solution should the nurse anticipate will be ordered during initial fluid replacement therapy?
   1. 10% dextrose and saline.
   2. 5% dextrose and water with 60 mEq KCl.
   3. 5% dextrose and water only.
   4. Distilled water.
2. Before surgery, a client was instructed in the use of an incentive spirometer. The *primary* purpose of this activity is:
   1. To encourage coughing.
   2. To arouse and stimulate the client.
   3. To encourage deep breathing.
   4. To measure tidal volume and expiratory reserve volume.
3. The nurse explains to a client's family that humidification is given with oxygen administration because:
   1. Oxygen is highly permeable in water, thereby increasing gaseous diffusion.
   2. Oxygen is very drying to the mucous membranes.
   3. The partial pressures of oxygen are increased by water dilution, allowing more oxygen to reach the alveoli.
   4. Water acts as a carrier substance facilitating movement of oxygen across the respiratory membrane.
4. To correctly administer 1000 mL of 5% dextrose/water in 10 hours using a standard 15-drop administration set, the nurse would adjust the infusion rate to:
   1. 32 drops per minute.
   2. 25 drops per minute.
   3. 20 drops per minute.
   4. 15 drops per minute.

5. The nurse would conclude that a client's fasting serum-glucose levels are normal if the results are:
   1. 30–60 mg/dL of blood.
   2. 80–126 mg/dL of blood.
   3. 126–140 md/dL of blood.
   4. 140–200 mg/dL of blood.

6. A laboratory test to measure serum- and urine-glucose levels before and after ingestion of a glucose load has been ordered. The nurse knows that the test to be done is called:
   1. Fasting blood sugar.
   2. Glucose tolerance test.
   3. Postprandial blood glucose.
   4. Tolbutamide response test.

7. After a glucose tolerance test, the nurse would look for the blood-glucose levels to return to normal in about how many hours?
   1. One.
   2. Two.
   3. Three.
   4. Four.

8. The nurse knows that the most important effect of intermittent positive-pressure breathing (IPPB) is:
   1. Mobilization of bronchial secretions.
   2. Increased alveolar ventilation.
   3. Prevention of atelectasis.
   4. Decreased airway resistance.

9. Nursing preparation for an upper GI series includes:
   1. NPO for 24 hours before the procedure.
   2. Administering an enema or cathartic to enhance visualization.
   3. Discouraging the client from smoking the morning of the procedure because smoking can stimulate gastric motility.
   4. Instructing the client that the test involves insertion of a rubber gastroscopy tube.

10. Which statement by the nurse accurately describes the Miller-Abbott tube?
    1. A double-lumen tube, with one lumen leading to the inflatable balloon and the other lumen used for aspiration.
    2. A plastic or rubber tube with holes near its tip facilitating withdrawal of fluids from the stomach.
    3. A single-lumen, saline-, air-, or water-weighted tube approximately 6 feet long.
    4. A 10-foot-long rubber tube with a saline, air, or water bag at its end.

11. Fluid therapy postburn may necessitate as much as 7 liters of fluid in 24 hours for a 70 kg individual. Using a 15 gtt/mL administration set, the drops per minute that the nurse would set to deliver this volume would be:
    1. 48 gtt/min.
    2. 75 gtt/min.
    3. 60 gtt/min.
    4. 90 gtt/min.

12. Before administering oxygen therapy, the nurse would:
    1. Review client's history for indications of COPD.
    2. Observe client's respiratory pattern.
    3. Draw arterial blood gases.
    4. Auscultate bilateral breath sounds.

ANSWERS/RATIONALES/TIPS

1. **(3)** Initial fluid therapy is directed toward increasing fluid volume and urine output. **Answer 1,** being a hypertonic solution that would act to increase intracellular dehydration, is therefore *contraindicated. Once* adequate urinary output has been established, potassium salts are added (**Answer 2**) to relieve hypokalemia. The amount of added potassium chloride depends on the extent of hypokalemia. **Answer 4,** distilled water, is a hypotonic solution; that is, it does not contain any additional electrolytes. Hypotonic solutions, such as 0.45% sodium chloride, are frequently given to relieve hypertonic syndromes. However, distilled water is *never* given in fluid replacement therapy.

> **TEST-TAKING TIP**— The key word is *initial.* Use H_2O to replace fluid loss. Focus on two similar options that have 5% D/W (**Answers 2** and **3**). Eliminate the option with *KCl* (**Answer 1**) because it is added *later.*
> **AN, COM, 8, M/S: F-E, PhI, Pharmacological and Parenteral Therapies**

2. **(3)** The purpose of the incentive spirometer is to encourage deep breathing. The client is able to directly visualize progress by the number and height of balls he or she is able to raise. *After-effects* of this activity may indeed be coughing up sputum (**Answer 1**) and arousal (**Answer 2**) as the client competes with himself or herself. Incentive spirometry can be used as a rough measure of tidal volume and expiratory reserve volume (**Answer 4**) because the client breathes in deeply and exhales completely into the incentive spirometer.

> **TEST-TAKING TIP**— Key word is *primary* (or first) purpose. Clients are *first* taught to deep breathe.
> **PL, COM, 6, M/S: Resp., PhI, Reduction of Risk Potential**

3. **(2)** Humidification of oxygen is extremely important in reducing its drying effects on the mucous membranes of the bronchial tree. Humidification of oxygen is generally provided by a water nebulizer. **Answers 1, 3,** and **4** are incorrect because oxygen is *not highly permeable* in water; thus, water tends to *inhibit* rather than facilitate oxygen diffusion across the respiratory membrane. Humidification expands the volume of the inhaled gas, but by doing so it *decreases* the partial pressure of the gas in the alveoli. Normal alveolar partial pressures of oxygen are approximately 100 mm Hg, whereas the partial pressures of oxygen in the atmosphere are approximately 135 mm Hg.

> **TEST-TAKING TIP**— The question is asking why O_2 is given with humidification. Look for a simple answer. *Humidi*fication provides *moisture* because O_2 is *drying.*
> **PL, COM, 6, M/S: Resp., PhI, Reduction of Risk Potential**

4. **(2)** Maintenance of infusion rates as ordered is extremely important. In this example, the nurse can use the following equation:

$$\frac{\text{gtts/mL of given set}}{60 \text{ min/hr}} \times \text{total volume/hr} = \text{gtt/min}$$

Thus,

$$\frac{15}{60} \times 100 = \frac{1}{4} \times 100 = 25 \text{ gtt/min}$$

KEY TO CODES FOLLOWING RATIONALES:

Nursing proces: **AS,** assessment; **AN,** analysis; **PL,** plan; **IMP,** implementation; **EV,** evaluation. *Cognitive level:* **COM,** comprehension; **APP,** application; **ANL,** analysis. *Category of human function:* 1, protective; 2, sensory-perceptual; 3, comfort, rest, activity, and mobility; 4, nutrition; 5, growth and development; 6, fluid-gas transport; 7, psychosocial-cultural; 8, elimination. *Client need:* **SECE,** safe, effective care environment; **HPM,** health promotion/maintenance; **PsI,** psychosocial integrity; **PhI,** physiological integrity. (Client subneed appears after Client need code.) See appendices for full explanation.

TEST-TAKING TIP— Divide 1000 mL by 10 to determine how many mL per hour, then use this formula to calculate drops per minute.
IMP, APP, 6, M/S: Calculation, PhI, Pharmacological and Parenteral Therapies

5. **(2)** Normal fasting serum-glucose levels are 80–126 mg/dL of blood. Levels below 60 (**Answer 1**) indicate hypoglycemia; levels above 126 mg/dL (**Answers 3 and 4**) indicate hyperglycemia.

TEST-TAKING TIP— Key term is *normal.* First eliminate the extreme numbers (too low and too high). "Normal" tends to be a low-midpoint value.
IMP, COM, 4, M/S: Metab., PhI, Reduction of Risk Potential

6. **(2)** Procedurally, the client who is to receive the glucose tolerance test consumes a high carbohydrate diet for 3 days *before* the test. All drugs that may influence the test are discontinued during this period (oral contraceptives, aspirin, steroids). On the day of the test, fasting blood (**Answer 1**) and urine specimens are collected *before* the test, to provide control glucose levels. *After* ingestion of a glucose load, specimens of blood and urine are collected at hourly intervals for 3 hours. In diabetes mellitus, glucose levels are elevated. The postprandial blood glucose (**Answer 3**) is determined by giving the client an oral glucose load only. Blood-glucose levels are then evaluated in 2 hours. Usually glucose levels will return to normal during this period of time. The tolbutamide response test (**Answer 4**) may also be used to confirm diabetes. After the client fasts overnight, a baseline fasting blood sample is drawn. Intravenous tolbutamide is then given, and blood samples are drawn in 20–30 minutes. After this test the client should be given orange juice and instructed to eat breakfast.

TEST-TAKING TIP— Key phrase is *before and after;* FBS (**Answer 1**) is done only *before.* Postprandial means *after* a meal. Glucose tolerance (**Answer 2**) has *both* a "before" and an "after" component.
AN, COM, 4, M/S: Metab., PhI, Reduction of Risk Potential

7. **(3)** Within 3 hours the client's serum-glucose levels should not only have returned to normal, but some hypoglycemia should be expected. **Answers 1, 2,** and **4** are incorrect because these time frames are too soon and too long.

TEST-TAKING TIP— Eliminate the extremes (**Answers 1** and **4**). Recall that the procedure calls for *3 days* of high carbohydrate; you will make a good guess by selecting *3 hours.*
EV, COM, 4, M/S: Metab., PhI, Reduction of Risk Potential

8. **(2)** The most important effect of intermittent positive-pressure breathing (IPPB) is increased alveolar ventilation. It *also* helps mobilize secretions (**Answer 1**), decrease the occurrence of atelectasis (**Answer 3**), and decrease airway resistance (**Answer 4**) through *mechanical* bronchodilation.

TEST-TAKING TIP— When all options are correct, choose the one (alveolar ventilation) that encompasses the three other effects.
EV, COM, 6, M/S: Resp., PhI, Physiological Adaptation

9. **(3)** Clients are NPO and encouraged not to smoke or take medications the morning of an upper GI series. Clients are NPO for 6–8 hours, *not* 24 hours (**Answer 1**). Enemas and cathartics (**Answer 2**) are *not* administered before an upper GI series; however, they are given *after* the series, to aid in the elimination of the barium. The test involves an x-ray, using a barium swallow as contrast medium. Gastroscopy (**Answer 4**) is the direct visualization of the stomach.

TEST-TAKING TIP— Note the time element: *before;* this eliminates **Answer 2.** Eliminate **Answer 1** because being NPO for 24 hours is excessive. Answer 4 is the description for a different test, *not* for *UGI* series.
IMP, APP, 4, M/S: GI, PhI, Reduction of Risk Potential

10. **(1)** The Miller-Abbott tube is a double-lumen tube, with one lumen leading to the inflatable balloon and the other lumen used for aspiration of intestinal contents. **Answer 2** is an example of a *Levin* tube, used for gastric suction. **Answer 3** is an example of a *Harris* tube, and **Answer 4,** a *Cantor* tube, both used for intestinal decompression, like the Miller-Abbott.

TEST-TAKING TIP— Need to know which tubes are single vs. double lumen.
IMP, APP, 8, M/S: GI, PhI, Reduction of Risk Potential

11. **(2)** Calculating the correct rate requires computation of the hourly volume (290 mL) and the minute volume (5 mL), and then multiplying the rate, in mL/min, by the drop factor (15 gtt/mL). (The hourly and minute volumes have been rounded to the nearest whole number.) **Answers 1** and **3** are *not fast enough* to deliver this large a volume in the prescribed period. **Answer 4** is *too rapid.* A quick method of computing the drip rate is to use the first two numbers in the 24-hour fluid volume (i.e., 7000 mL in 24 hours = 70 gtt/min). This short-cut may be useful when initially starting an infusion, before mathematically calculating the rate. Use only with 15 gtt/mL factor.

TEST-TAKING TIP— Use basic IV calculation. Eliminate the extremes (**Answers 1** and **3** are too slow; **Answer 4** is too fast); select the midpoint here.
IMP, APP, 6, M/S: Calculation, PhI, Pharmacological and Parenteral Therapies

12. **(1) There is a risk to the client with COPD if the O₂** flow rate is too high. The client with COPD has a hypoxic respiratory drive. If the liter flow is above 2 L, there is a risk for respiratory depression. **Answers 2, 3,** and **4** are important nursing actions to determine the *effectiveness* of oxygen therapy.

TEST-TAKING TIP— Look for patterns in the options. Three options assess the *effectiveness* of the treatment. One validates the *appropriateness* of the order. Choose the one that is different.
AS, APP, 6, M/S: Resp., PhI, Reduction of Risk Potential

Practice Test

Sally L. Lagerquist • Janice McMillin • Robyn Nelson • Kathleen Snider

INTRODUCTION

The **Practice Test** is a *follow-up assessment* tool designed to assess areas of improvement from your initial self-assessment using the **Pre Test.** Take the **Practice Test** immediately after reading the specific *content* areas related to your individual problem areas as identified by the **Pre Test.** Determine that you are now able to meet the goal of 80% correct answers in this integrated exam.

After taking this **Practice Test,** use the units in this book again to fill in any "gaps" this test reveals in your preparation. Then take the **Final Test** to assess your readiness for NCLEX-RN®.

QUESTIONS

Select the one answer that is best for each question, unless otherwise directed.

1. For an adolescent boy, the main life-stage task is:
    1. Developing a sense of trust in others and in his environment.
    2. Finalizing his goals and plans for the future.
    3. Striving to attain independence and identity.
    4. Resolving inner conflicts and turmoil.

2. A child lying on the stretcher during admission suddenly complains of nausea and begins to vomit. The nurse should immediately:
    1. Turn the child's head to the side.
    2. Suction the child's oropharynx.
    3. Raise the head of the stretcher.
    4. Insert an NG tube.

3. The nurse can quickly assess volume depletion in a client with ulcerative colitis by:
    1. Measuring the quantity and specific gravity of the client's urine output.
    2. Taking the client's blood pressure first supine, then sitting, noting any changes.
    3. Comparing the client's present weight with weight on a previous admission.
    4. Administering the oral water test.

4. Which statement best describes the metabolic functions of the liver?
    1. Detoxification of endogenous and exogenous substances.
    2. Fluid volume control and acid-base balance.
    3. Erythrocyte and leukocyte breakdown.
    4. Concentration and storage of bile.

5. The nurse in the newborn nursery should plan any interventions with a newborn with myelomeningocele based on the knowledge that the major *short-term* complication the child is most likely to suffer is:
    1. Hydrocephalus.
    2. Meningitis.
    3. Mental retardation.
    4. Paraplegia.

6. A 32-year-old mother of three adolescents has increased her consumption of alcoholic beverages to 24 oz of 80-proof drinks per day. She gets angry with the children very quickly, cries spontaneously several times every day, and complains of headaches constantly. In planning her care, what would be considered the *least* appropriate nursing intervention?
    1. Stimulating her to work at a concrete task.
    2. Encouraging her to cry.
    3. Providing her with someone to talk to.
    4. Isolating her from stimuli.

7. The nurse explains to a client that bronchitis is characterized by:
    1. Production of mucoid sputum sometimes difficult to expectorate.
    2. Bronchoconstriction and edema of the wall of the bronchioles.
    3. Exudate in the alveoli.
    4. Increasing lung stiffness.

8. A newborn has an unrepaired myelomeningocele at the lumbosacral area. The safest position for the nurse to place the newborn in is:
    Select all that apply.
    1. Supine.
    2. Prone.
    3. Side-lying with the head slightly elevated.
    4. Side-lying.
    5. Semi-Fowler's

9. In response to a client's questions regarding the cause of glomerulonephritis, the nurse explains that acute glomerulonephritis is the result of:
    1. Acute infection of the kidney by gram-negative bacteria.
    2. An immune response of the glomerular membrane to protein of the beta-hemolytic streptococcus.
    3. Destruction of the glomerular membrane by gram-positive streptococci.
    4. Ischemia of glomerular capillary and vasa recta.

10. A client who is scheduled for repair of bilateral inguinal hernias has a history of obesity, smoker's cough, and heavy lifting following a previous inguinal hernia repair. The *most* likely cause for the herniation is:
    1. Intestinal obstruction.
    2. Failure of resected muscles in previous operations to heal properly.
    3. Chronic cough and vigorous exercise.
    4. Obesity.

11. The physician ordered Tylenol elixir for a 14-month-old with a fever of 102°F. Considering this child's developmental level and diagnosis, which would be the best approach by the nurse?
    1. Use the medicine cup and tell the child the "pretty red syrup" will taste sweet like candy.
    2. Mix the medication with 4 oz of apple juice and allow the child to drink it through a "crazy straw."
    3. Put the medication into a brightly colored plastic cup and give the child a chance to drink it.
    4. Raise the child to a sitting position, bring the medicine cup to the lips, and tell the child kindly but firmly to drink it.

12. A client has been admitted to the hospital with acute rheumatoid arthritis. The hands are painful and edematous, and there is severe pain in the left hip. The temperature is 101°F orally; pulse, 96; respirations, 22. ASA grx qid has been ordered. The nurse concludes that the client is experiencing:
    1. Increased fluid losses.
    2. Signs and symptoms of inflammation.
    3. A physiologic stress response.
    4. Side effects of salicylate therapy.

13. Which factor should the nurse identify as the most probable cause of a child's lice?
    1. The child washes the hair only once a week.
    2. The child shares the comb and brush with a friend.
    3. The child wears a hat to school every day.
    4. The child's hair is long, thick, and curly.

14. The nurse knows that the function of the gallbladder is to:
    1. Synthesize and manufacture bile.
    2. Collect, concentrate, and store bile.
    3. Collect and dilute bile.
    4. Regulate bile flow into the duodenum.

15. The most accurate description the nurse could give a colleague about a thyroid scan is that it:
    1. Assists in differentiating between primary and secondary hypothyroidism.
    2. Demonstrates increased uptake of radioactive iodine in areas of possible malignancy.
    3. Demonstrates decreased uptake of radioactive iodine in areas of possible malignancy.
    4. Measures the effect of TSH on thyroid function.

16. The nurse should review principles of care with a 12-year-old child with asthma. Which comment by the child would require additional teaching by the nurse?
    1. "I keep all my stuffed animals on my bookcase now."
    2. "I have vinyl miniblinds on the windows in my room."
    3. "I gave my cat to my best friend."
    4. "I joined the swim team at school."

17. The nurse knows that a colostomy begins functioning:
    1. Immediately.
    2. 2–3 days postoperatively.
    3. 1 wk postoperatively.
    4. 2 wk postoperatively.

18. A woman is seen in clinic complaining of amenorrhea, fatigue, urinary frequency, and morning nausea. She states that her LMP was 7 weeks ago and that her menses have been normal except for one episode following a spontaneous abortion at 8 weeks of gestation. She states she has a 5-year-old boy and 3-year-old twin girls at home. Which would accurately describe this woman if she is pregnant now?
    1. Gravida 4 para 2.
    2. Gravida 5 para 3.
    3. Gravida 4 para 3.
    4. Gravida 3 para 2.

19. The nurse knows that a decreased hematocrit occurs in chronic renal failure because:
    1. Secretion of erythropoietin factor by the diseased kidney is decreased.
    2. Chronic hypertension tends to suppress bone marrow centers.
    3. Metabolic alkalosis tends to increase red blood cell fragility.
    4. Excretion of red blood cells in the urine is increased.

20. Which laboratory studies would a routine preoperative assessment for the client having vein ligation and stripping include?
    1. VDRL, Na, K, Cl.
    2. Prothrombin time, ALT (SGOT), VDRL.
    3. UA, CBC, prothrombin time.
    4. WBC, VDRL, serum glucose.

21. A mother asks the nurse about the normal time for the onset of menstruation. The nurse would be most correct in advising her that menses usually begin at age:
    1. 11.2 years
    2. 12 years.
    3. 12.8 years.
    4. 13.5 years.

22. The *least* appropriate nursing intervention for a client experiencing alcohol withdrawal delirium would be:
    1. Reinforcing time, place, and person.
    2. Providing consistent and concrete answers to questions.
    3. Administering ordered vitamins and glucose.
    4. Applying and maintaining physical restraints.

23. Following above-the-knee amputation, a client verbalizes feelings of decreased self-worth and of being less of a person. Acceptance of the surgery is largely dependent on:
    1. What the doctor says.
    2. How the client's family is reacting.
    3. How the nursing staff reacts and responds to the client's behavior.
    4. The client's ability to grieve.

24. The nurse knows that acetonuria develops in diabetes due to:
    1. Excessive oxidation of fatty acids for energy, which increases ketones in glomerular filtrate.
    2. Osmotic diuresis, accompanying elevation in serum-glucose levels, which decreases exchange of electrolytes in renal tubules.
    3. Failure of sodium-hydrogen ion exchange mechanism in the renal tubules to secrete excess hydrogen ions.
    4. Increased volatile H^+ ions and decreased nonvolatile H^+ ions in the glomerular filtrate.

25. The nurse expects hyperkalemia on assessment to occur in chronic renal dysfunction because:
    1. As metabolic acidosis increases, the kidneys selectively secrete more H^+ than K^+ in exchange for Na^+.
    2. As edema forms, sodium diffuses into the interstitial space and is balanced by increased serum potassium.
    3. Respiratory compensation for metabolic acidosis tends to increase K^+ reabsorption by the kidneys.
    4. The nausea and vomiting that occur with metabolic acidosis tend to increase serum potassium to compensate for chloride losses.

26. A toddler is admitted to the hospital with acute bilateral otitis media, with a temperature of 103°F and tremors in arms and legs. In addition to a spinal tap to rule out bacterial meningitis, the doctor orders all the following. Which order should the nurse perform *first*?
    1. Respiratory isolation.
    2. IV 5% dextrose in 0.45 normal saline solution at 35 mL/hr.
    3. Tylenol 120 mg PO q4h.
    4. Seizure precautions.

27. After being in a community mental health day treatment center for 3 weeks, an adolescent client has become apathetic and withdrawn. The client generally sits alone and stares into space. The most appropriate nursing intervention would include:
    1. Selecting a group activity for the client to participate in.
    2. Stimulating self-growth by providing challenging activities for the client.
    3. Allowing the client to spend at least 3 hours a day in the room, for inner reflection.
    4. Encouraging staff members to sit with the client during group activities until there is voluntary socialization.

28. The nurse recognizes that the pattern of pulmonary dysfunction reflected by increased total lung capacity (TLC), functional residual capacity (FRC), and residual volume (RV) is characteristic of:
    1. Restrictive lung disease.
    2. Obstructive lung disease.
    3. Vascular lung disease.
    4. A combination of restrictive and obstructive lung disease.

29. A client has second-degree burns of the left leg and thigh. The nurse plans to help prevent contractures in the burned leg by:
    1. Maintaining abduction of the left leg, extension of the left knee, and flexion of the left ankle.
    2. Maintaining adduction of the left leg and extension of the left knee and ankle.
    3. Maintaining abduction of the left leg and flexion of the left knee and ankle.
    4. Maintaining adduction of the left leg, flexion of the left knee, and extension of the left ankle.

30. A truss is a pad of firm material that is placed over a hernial opening and held in place with a belt. When should the nurse apply a hernia truss on a client?
    1. After the client gets out of bed but before engaging in strenuous activity.
    2. After the hernia has been reduced, with the client lying down with feet elevated.
    3. At any time, whether or not the hernia has been reduced, to prevent further extrusion of the bowel.
    4. Not at all, for physicians no longer recommend the use of a truss, because athletic supporters are sufficient in preventing further herniation.

31. The doctor orders an IV to infuse at 35 mL/hr; a pediatric microdrip chamber is hanging. How many drops per minute should the nurse regulate the IV to infuse?
    1. 5–6.
    2. 7–8.
    3. 9–10.
    4. 35.

32. A client, age 25, has been scheduled for surgery to remove the lesions at the footplate of the stapes, associated with *otosclerosis*. A client who is scheduled for a *stapedectomy* should be told to expect:
    1. Tinnitus for several weeks after surgery.
    2. Rhinitis as the edema from surgery resolves.
    3. The hearing loss to continue for a while.
    4. Showering and swimming not to be permitted.

33. External fetal monitor tracings show consistent fetal decelerations of uniform shape, which begin with the contraction and return to baseline as the contraction subsides. What is the correct interpretation of these data?
    1. Acute fetal distress.
    2. Uteroplacental insufficiency.
    3. Umbilical cord compression.
    4. Physiological fetal bradycardia.

34. To correctly administer a tuberculin skin test, the nurse would inject 5 TU (tuberculin units) of PPD (purified protein derivative) of tuberculin:
    1. Intradermally.
    2. Subcutaneously.
    3. Intramuscularly.
    4. Subdermally.

35. If bile flow into the duodenum is obstructed, absorption of fat-soluble vitamins is reduced. Which complication would the nurse therefore observe?
    1. Peripheral neuritis.
    2. Scurvy.
    3. Increased bleeding tendencies.
    4. Macrocytic anemia.

36. A 20-month-old is admitted to the pediatrics unit for the third, and final, surgical procedure to correct congenital hypospadias. When admitting this toddler to the hospital, the nurse should assess all of the following. Which information will be the most important to the nursing plan of care for this toddler?
    1. The toddler's developmental level.
    2. The parents' knowledge level regarding hypospadias.
    3. The toddler's previous experience with illness and hospitalization.
    4. The parents' plans for rooming-in.

37. The nurse can increase the ventilatory efficiency of a client with COPD by positioning the client as follows:
    1. High-Fowler's.
    2. Prone.
    3. Sitting up and leaning slightly forward.
    4. Trendelenburg.

38. During the adolescent period, the *least* important task to complete is:
    1. Developing an individualized personality.
    2. Attaining adequate defense mechanisms.
    3. Establishing an ego identity.
    4. Refining and stabilizing the superego.

39. A toddler is hospitalized with laryngotracheobronchitis. When assessing the toddler, which signs and symptoms would alert the nurse that the toddler's physical condition is improving? *Select all that apply.*
    1. Progressive hoarseness.
    2. Apical pulse of 118.
    3. Increase in appetite.
    4. Pink nailbeds.

40. The preoperative nursing care plan for a client having cataract surgery includes:
    1. Keeping the client flat in bed.
    2. Applying eye patches to both eyes.
    3. Orienting the client to the environment and nursing personnel.
    4. Teaching the client eyedrop instillation.

41. Following a thyroid scan with ^{131}I for a thyroid nodule, the nurse should plan for:
    1. No special radiation precautions.
    2. Full radiation precautions to be instituted, including segregating the client in a private room.

3. Radiation precautions that are limited to urine and feces.
4. Full radiation precautions to be instituted for 8 hours (the half-life of ^{131}I).

42. A hospitalized preschooler wakes up crying at 2 A.M. and says, "I want my mommy now." The nurse should:
1. Pick the child up and rock the child for a little while.
2. Talk softly to the child while rubbing the back, but leave the child in the crib.
3. Gently but firmly tell the child to go back to sleep.
4. Call the mother and ask her to come to the hospital.

43. A 7-year-old is admitted to the burn unit in serious condition with deep partial-thickness burns over the head, face, neck, and anterior chest. On the first night in the hospital, the nurse enters the room and finds the child crying softly and moaning in pain. Recognizing the extent of the injuries, the nurse should:
1. Do nothing at this time.
2. Offer two acetaminophen (Tylenol) pills as ordered and a glass of warm milk.
3. Give an IM injection of 40 mg of meperidine HCl (Demerol) as ordered.
4. Inject 25 mg of meperidine HCl (Demerol) as ordered via central IV line.

44. The most important nursing intervention in planning care for a client with increasing symptoms of depression and alcoholism would include:
1. Referring to an alcohol rehabilitation program.
2. Identifying how the client has coped with anxiety in the past.
3. Arranging for in-patient hospitalization.
4. Requesting a prescription for an antidepressant.

45. A client who has a long-term history of smoking and a smoker's cough is scheduled for bilateral herniorrhaphy. Which preoperative nursing action will be a priority?
1. Explanation of the surgical procedure.
2. Respiratory hygiene measures and instructions in deep breathing.
3. Discussion of postoperative nursing care measures.
4. Assurance that pain medication will be available whenever needed.

46. Ascites in cirrhosis of the liver occurs because of:
1. Portal hypertension, venous dilation, and stasis.
2. Increased hepatic synthesis of albumin.
3. Decreased serum levels of aldosterone and ADH.
4. Increased blood volume causing increased blood hydrostatic pressure in the capillary bed.

47. The nurse does discharge teaching with the mother of a preschooler with epiglottitis before discharge. Which statement by the mother indicates that she has *correctly* understood the nurse's teaching?
1. "I'm so glad that my child is all better now."
2. "I will keep my child home from preschool for the rest of this month."
3. "I'm still worried that my child will get sick again when we get home."
4. "I will get a portable tank of oxygen for my child before he comes home."

48. What should the nurse recognize as an *inappropriate* method of treating *hyperthyroidism*?
1. Subtotal thyroidectomy.
2. Administration of propylthiouracil.
3. Radioiodine therapy.
4. Administration of thyroglobulin.

49. A teenager has a history of setting fires. These arson attempts may exhibit which behavior?

1. Acting out.
2. Depression.
3. Paranoia.
4. Mania.

50. After discharge following ileostomy surgery, a client calls the nurse at the hospital to report the sudden onset of abdominal cramps, vomiting, and watery discharge from the ileostomy. What should the nurse advise?
1. Call the physician if symptoms persist for 24 hours.
2. Take 30 mL of MOM (milk of magnesia).
3. NPO until vomiting stops.
4. Call the physician immediately.

51. To safely transport a client who has chest tube drainage to the x-ray department to assess the degree of lung reexpansion, the nurse would:
1. Remove the chest tubes, immediately covering the incision site with a sterile petrolatum gauze to prevent air from entering the chest.
2. Disconnect the drainage bottles from the chest tubes, covering the catheter tip with a sterile dressing to prevent contamination.
3. Send the client to x-ray with the chest tube clamped but still attached to the drainage system to prevent air from entering the chest wall if the bottles are accidentally broken.
4. Send the client to x-ray with the chest tube attached to the drainage system, taking precautions to prevent interruption in the system.

52. A toddler tries to pull the IV out, and the nurse determines that the child must be restrained to maintain the IV site. Which restraint would the nurse be most correct in applying?
1. Posey jacket.
2. Elbow.
3. Mummy.
4. Clove-hitch.

53. Which statement by the nurse correctly describes a wheeze?
1. A high-pitched musical sound produced by airflow in narrowed bronchioles.
2. A sound that is rarely considered pathological.
3. A medium-pitched sonorous sound produced by airflow in obstructed bronchi.
4. A high-pitched crowing sound produced by edema in the trachea.

54. The primary purpose of the nurse performing passive range-of-motion exercises to affected limbs of a client during acute rheumatoid arthritis is to:
1. Prevent contractures and limited range of motion.
2. Continually evaluate the client's functional abilities.
3. Assess the client's pain tolerance.
4. Evaluate the effectiveness of drug therapy.

55. The effectiveness of peritoneal dialysis will be measured by:
1. Serum potassium less than 3.5 mEq/L and serum sodium greater than 148 mEq/L.
2. Unchanged quantity and specific gravity of urine.
3. BUN less than 20 mg/dL, serum creatinine less than 1.2 mg/dL.
4. Moderately soft abdomen and dullness on percussion.

56. Which activity of daily living should the nurse recommend that a client (who has had a bilateral hernia repair) avoid after discharge?
1. Driving to and from work.
2. Walking 3 miles a day.
3. Washing and polishing the car.
4. Carrying out the garbage cans.

57. After the nurse completes preoperative teaching with a preschooler, which would be the *best* method for evaluating the effectiveness of the teaching?

1. Ask him to draw a picture of what he will look like after surgery.
2. Using puppets, ask him to show the nurse what he has learned about his surgery.
3. Tell him that this is a test and he must repeat what he has learned about his operation.
4. Suggest his parents check on their child's level of understanding and report back to the nurse.

58. The appropriate nursing action with a client experiencing expressive aphasia following a brain attack would be to:
1. Help the client and family accept this permanent disability.
2. Associate words with physical objects.
3. Wait indefinitely for the client to verbalize.
4. Tell the family that the client cannot communicate.

59. The number of first-time pregnancies in women between ages 35 and 40 years has increased by 40%. The nurse conducting a parent education class for these women, in the last trimester of pregnancy, should include discussion of:
1. Energy and stamina to meet demands of parenting.
2. Feeling troubled by pregnancy and being less adjusted during the last trimester of pregnancy.
3. The longer labor experienced by mothers who are older.
4. The greater number of labor/birth complications experienced by mothers who are older.

60. After positioning a client who has had spinal anesthesia, which initial observation should the recovery room nurse make?
1. Status of reflexes.
2. Vital signs.
3. Client's level of consciousness.
4. Integrity of airway.

61. In preparing a client for an IV cholangiogram, it is important for the nurse to ask the client if:
1. The procedure has been done before.
2. There are any known allergies, particularly to fish or other iodine-containing substances.
3. Epigastric discomfort occurs only with fatty-food ingestion.
4. There is a family history of gallstones.

62. A child is admitted to the hospital with a second attack of rheumatic fever. In doing an admission assessment on this child, which group of symptoms would the nurse most likely find?
1. Petechiae, malaise, and joint pain.
2. Chorea, anemia, and hypertension.
3. Tachycardia, erythema marginatum, and fever in late afternoon.
4. Subcutaneous nodules, dependent edema, and conjunctivitis.

63. A client is scheduled for a temporary colostomy due to severe diverticulitis. The purpose of preoperative administration of neomycin SO_4 is to:
1. Reduce the risk of postoperative wound infection.
2. Decrease bacterial count of the colon.
3. Reduce the size of a possible tumor before surgery.
4. Stimulate peristalsis and facilitate action of cleansing enemas.

64. After nebulizer treatment with isoproterenol (Isuprel), the following pulmonary function data were obtained:

	TLC	FRC	RV	VC	FEV$_1$
Before treatment	7000	5000	4200	2800	2000
After treatment	7000	4000	3000	3800	2500

The nurse would conclude that the change in lung volumes indicates:
1. Improvement.
2. Deterioration.

3. No change.
4. Data inadequate to decide.

65. Two hospitalized school-age children complain that they are "bored." The nurse should offer them:
Select all that apply.
1. A board game such as Monopoly or checkers.
2. Homework sent in from their teachers.
3. Books from the playroom.
4. An opportunity to stay up late and watch TV.

66. The nurse suspects abdominal wound dehiscence, and lifts the edges of the client's dressings. The nurse notes that the wound edges are entirely separated. What is the *next* nursing action?
1. Tell the client to remain quiet and not to cough.
2. Offer the client a warm drink to promote relaxation.
3. Position the client in a chair with the feet elevated.
4. Apply a scultetus bandage.

67. Which signs and symptoms are *least* likely to occur during peritoneal dialysis if fluid drainage is inadequate?
1. A negative balance between the amount drained and the amount instilled.
2. Confusion, lethargy, and coma.
3. Moist crackles and rhonchi.
4. Flattened neck veins in a supine position.

68. A school-age child has leukemia. Considering the diagnosis and health-teaching needs, the nurse would be most correct in advising this child to:
1. Skip brushing the teeth at this time.
2. Brush the teeth with a soft toothbrush only.
3. Brush the teeth with a firm toothbrush only.
4. Rinse the mouth with an antiseptic solution instead of brushing the teeth.

69. After an adolescent has been in a mental health day treatment center for a year and a half, the professional staff are considering discharging this client. The client asks the nurse whether other people must be told about the time spent in a mental health center. The most appropriate response the nurse could make would be:
1. "Yes, especially to all future school officials."
2. "Yes, especially to all prospective employers."
3. "No, this is an individual decision."
4. "No, there is no specific requirement."

70. A peripheral iridectomy is the surgical procedure of choice following an acute episode of closed-angle glaucoma. Which nursing measure is *inappropriate* for a client who has had an *iridectomy*?
1. Instill eyedrops to mobilize the affected pupil by alternate dilation and constriction.
2. Ambulate the client as soon as possible after the surgery.
3. Reinforce the surgical dressing as needed to prevent infection.
4. If ordered, instruct the client to massage the affected eye.

71. Which nursing action is designed to reduce ammonia intoxication in a client with bleeding esophageal varices who is jaundiced, edematous, and in a hepatic coma?
1. Active and passive range-of-motion exercises to prevent venous stasis.
2. Tap-water enemas to remove blood that may still be in the gut from the bleeding esophageal varices.
3. Administration of insulin and glucagon to reduce serum-potassium levels.
4. Holding all antibiotic medications so that the action of the intestinal bacteria on protein is enhanced.

72. Following surgery, a client with diabetes complains of nausea and appears lethargic and flushed with BP 108/78; P 100; R 24 and deep. An IV is infusing. The first nursing action should be to:

1. Call the attending physician.
2. Check the client's blood glucose.
3. Administer an antiemetic.
4. Decrease the client's IV infusion rate.

73. On admission, a preschooler is carrying a soiled and worn-looking stuffed animal. His mother states that this is his favorite toy. The most appropriate action for the nurse to take at this time is to:
    1. Offer him a choice of another stuffed animal from the hospital playroom.
    2. Place this stuffed animal somewhere in his room where he can see it but not touch it.
    3. Suggest his mother bring him a new stuffed animal.
    4. Tell him that he can keep this stuffed animal in the bed with him.

74. In monitoring the postop course of a young adult who has had surgery for a ruptured appendix, the nurse would be most correct in expecting that this client will:
    1. Have severe pain for 24 hours.
    2. Be discharged within 48 hours.
    3. Make a slow, steady recovery.
    4. Make a fairly rapid and complete recovery.

75. An adolescent may exhibit depression differently from an adult. An adolescent who is depressed is most likely to exhibit which behavior?
    1. Withdrawal.
    2. Apathy.
    3. Violence.
    4. Regression.

76. The nurse initiates ileostomy teaching with a client during the early postoperative period. The primary objective of this procedure is:
    1. To facilitate maintenance of intake and output records.
    2. To control unpleasant odors.
    3. To prevent excoriation of the skin around the stoma.
    4. To reduce the risk of postoperative wound infection.

77. Following the insertion of a catheter into the abdominal cavity, warmed dialyzing solution is allowed to run rapidly (10–20 minutes) into the abdominal cavity. The nurse warmed the solution to body temperature to prevent abdominal pain and to:
    1. Expand the molecules and increase the osmotic gradient.
    2. Increase dilation of the peritoneal vessels, thereby increasing urea clearance.
    3. Decrease the likelihood of peritonitis due to constriction of peritoneal vessels.
    4. Expedite the movement of the dialyzing solute into the abdomen.

78. Nursing actions that will facilitate medical therapy for a client with COPD include:
    1. Limiting fluid intake to prevent volume overload and right-sided heart failure.
    2. Oral and endotracheal suctioning as necessary.
    3. Instructing the client in deep breathing and coughing techniques and pursed-lip exhalations.
    4. Maintenance of bed rest and activity restrictions to reduce acidosis.

79. A client's arterial blood gases reveal: pH 7.38; Po_2 65; Pco_2 55; HCO_3 32. The nurse's interpretation of this client's blood gases is that he or she has:
    1. Uncompensated respiratory acidosis.
    2. Compensated respiratory acidosis.
    3. Uncompensated metabolic alkalosis.
    4. Compensated metabolic alkalosis.

80. Which are precautionary nursing measures to be used when caring for a client being treated with internal radioisotopes?
    1. Maintain strict client isolation, and limit professional contact with client.
    2. Limit exposure, and maximize distance between client, professional, and family.
    3. Position the client in a prone position, and restrict turning to mealtimes only.
    4. Maintain the legs in a flexed position to decrease the likelihood of dislodgement.

81. The nurse explains to a client who is diagnosed with cirrhosis that the anemia is the result of:
    1. Increased RBC fragility due to folic acid deficiencies from inadequate dietary intake.
    2. Decreased efficiency of Kupffer cells in the liver.
    3. Increased blood-ammonia levels.
    4. Decreased amino acid breakdown and synthesis.

82. The number one priority during the nurse's admission assessment of a school-age child with rheumatic fever is the child's:
    1. Weight.
    2. Apical pulse rate.
    3. Developmental level.
    4. ESR.

83. An adolescent's parents have decided that they would rather have their child placed outside of the home when discharged from the mental health day treatment center. The most appropriate intervention the nurse could make would include:
    1. Asking the parents to reassess their feelings about this decision.
    2. Suggesting that the parents discuss this decision with the entire family.
    3. Referring the parents to a social worker to assist in finding an alternative placement.
    4. Assisting the parents in finding an appropriate discharge placement.

84. The teaching plan for a client with COPD should emphasize:
    1. Smoking and alcohol restrictions.
    2. Nutrition, fluid balance, and ways to stop smoking.
    3. Vocational rehabilitation programs available in the community.
    4. Activity restrictions and pulmonary physiology.

85. Postoperative vital signs for a client with diabetes are BP 108/78; pulse 100; respirations 24 and deep. IV intake has been 2100 mL and urine output 2000 mL. The nurse recognizes that the client is experiencing:
    1. Increased ADH release in response to physiological stress of surgery.
    2. Decreased extracellular fluid (ECF) volume due to osmotic diuresis.
    3. A hypo-osmolar fluid imbalance.
    4. Circulatory overload.

86. Following bronchoscopy, what is the nurse's most important observation?
    1. Blood pressure, pulse, and temperature.
    2. Color and consistency of sputum.
    3. Function of the tenth cranial nerve.
    4. Presence of urticaria.

87. Chronic obstructive pulmonary disease can progress to respiratory failure. A client with emphysema becomes increasingly drowsy, tachypneic, and tachycardic. The nurse should first:
    1. Prepare IV aminophylline.
    2. Position the client in high-Fowler's.
    3. Give 2 liters of O_2 per nasal cannula.
    4. Administer 60% O_2 via mask.

88. A client with a history of alcohol abuse is hospitalized after an overdose of sleeping pills. The nurse should be aware that in the first 72 hours following admission to the hospital the client is most likely to exhibit:
    1. Withdrawal delirium.
    2. Suspiciousness.
    3. Mood swings.
    4. The use of coping mechanisms such as reaction formation.

89. The nurse knows that emergency procedures increase the surgical risk to the client because:
    1. The surgery is performed immediately.
    2. There is little time for psychological/physical preparation.
    3. There is decreased physiological stress.
    4. The anesthesia of choice is different for emergency surgery.

90. The nurse prepares to admit an infant with the diagnosis of Hirschsprung's disease. The nurse will expect that the infant has a strong history of:
    Select all that apply.
    1. Constipation.
    2. Abdominal distention.
    3. Anorexia
    4. Vomitus flecked with feces.
    5. Projectile vomiting

91. Care of the client on peritoneal dialysis must allow a dwell time, or equilibration period, of the dialyzing fluid, which is normally:
    1. 10–15 minutes.
    2. 20–30 minutes.
    3. 50–60 minutes.
    4. More than 1 hour.

92. A client has a smoking history of 25 years and a recent episode of 5 days of increased breathlessness. The client has a barrel chest, medium-pitched crackles, and wheezes in the right upper lobe and both lower lung lobes. The nurse observes that this client demonstrates the "increased work of breathing" during this acute period by:
    1. Increasing the rate and depth of respirations.
    2. Increasing diaphragmatic excursion.
    3. Using pursed-lip exhalations.
    4. Using accessory muscles for ventilation.

93. When administering lithium to a client with a mood disorder, what is the *least* relevant consideration?
    1. If the client's urinary output decreases significantly, diuretics should be ordered.
    2. The client must be given a complete physical examination before administering the drug.
    3. If the client experiences nausea, vomiting, and muscle weakness, the dosage may require regulating.
    4. If the client exhibits symptoms of mania during the first 10 days of receiving the drug, haloperidol (Haldol) may also be administered.

94. A client who is elderly asks about the type of anesthesia used for cataract surgery. The nurse replies that this surgery is generally performed using a:
    1. Local.
    2. General.
    3. Intravenous.
    4. Rectal.

95. Besides omission of food and fluids by mouth, other nursing considerations in the preparation of a client for IVP would include:
    1. Ingestion of contrast medium the morning of the procedure.
    2. Administration of cathartics or enemas to improve visualization of contrast medium in renal structures.

3. A low protein and low salt diet the evening before to increase hyperosmolarity of ECF.
4. Institution of an intravenous line to maintain fluid and electrolyte balance.

96. An adolescent is likely to experience several biological and psychosocial changes. Which behavior would the nurse expect to see?
    1. An increase in imaginative thinking.
    2. An increased ability to learn by rote.
    3. An increase in academic achievement.
    4. An increased ability to cope with frustration.

97. Pulmonary function data were collected on a client. The results were:

	TLC	FRC	RV	VC	FEV_1
Predicted	6000	3000	2000	4000	3000
Observed	7000	5000	4200	2800	2000

The nurse's analysis of these data reveals:
    1. Hyperinflation.
    2. Hyperventilation.
    3. Hyperpnea.
    4. Hypercapnia.

98. The nurse gives postoperative explanation to a client with diabetes that regular or crystalline insulin is used as an adjunct to NPH therapy because:
    1. There is increased tissue metabolism with surgery.
    2. Insulin production is decreased even further with the stress of surgery.
    3. Physiological and psychological stress increases serum-glucose levels via sympathetic nervous system stimulation.
    4. An increased insulin load is necessary to prevent hyperkalemia.

99. An 18-year-old with acting-out behaviors has been living in a group home for the past 2 months. The client has asked permission to visit a friend in the psychiatric hospital. The nurse should:
    1. Allow the client to visit.
    2. Assess the client's motives.
    3. Ask parents' permission.
    4. Consult with the hospital staff.

100. Signs and symptoms of postthyroidectomy respiratory obstruction vary with the degree of severity. Which early warning sign(s) and/or symptom(s) would the nurse expect with pending respiratory distress?
    Select all that apply.
    1. Hoarseness of voice.
    2. Stridor.
    3. Difficulty swallowing.
    4. Cyanosis.
    5. Choking sensation.

ANSWERS/RATIONALES/TIPS

1. **(3)** The adolescent is striving to attain a sense of independence and identity. Trust (**Answer 1**) is usually developed during infancy and matures as the individual develops. Goals and plans (**Answer 2**) are made during the adolescent period, but realistically they are rarely finalized until late adulthood. During this period, inner conflicts (**Answer 4**) are rarely resolved and are usually heightened.

TEST-TAKING TIP—Know age-appropriate psychosocial tasks.
EV, COM, 5, PEDS, PsI, Psychosocial Integrity

2. **(1)** To prevent aspiration, the first and immediate action the nurse should take is to turn the child's head to the side. All of the other actions (**Answers 2, 3,** and **4**) may also prevent aspiration, but will take considerably longer and are not immediately effective.

TEST-TAKING TIP—Patent airway is the primary concern in this question; note the use of the word *immediately*, meaning an instant action.
IMP, ANL, 8, PEDS, PhI, Reduction of Risk Potential

3. **(2)** Postural blood pressure readings are an excellent mode for assessing volume depletion. If the systolic blood pressure decreases more than 10 mm Hg and there is a concurrent increase in the pulse rate, a volume depletion problem is indicated. Urine output and specific gravity (**Answer 1**) are better measures of the adequacy of fluid volume *replacement* than of fluid volume depletion. Comparing the prior and present weight of the client (**Answer 3**) will give the nurse an estimate of the slow catabolism of body stores that occurs with ulcerative colitis. There is no *oral* water test (**Answer 4**).

TEST-TAKING TIP—Key words are "quickly" (something the nurse can do without a great deal of equipment and something that can be done easily) and "volume depletion."
AS, APP, 8, M/S: GI, PhI, Reduction of Risk Potential

4. **(1)** Liver functions are many and varied, including detoxification of chemicals (estrogen, adrenocorticoids, aldosterone, drugs, poisons, and heavy metals); synthesis of plasma proteins (albumin, fibrinogen, globulin) and several clotting factors (prothrombin, factor VII); storage of glycogen, iron, and vitamins (A, B$_{12}$, D, E, and K); gluconeogenesis (glucose from amino acids and fats); and deamination of amino acids. Fluid volume control and acid-base balance are functions of the *kidney* (**Answer 2**). Most erythrocyte and leukocyte breakdown occurs in the *spleen* (**Answer 3**). The *gallbladder* concentrates and stores bile (**Answer 4**), and the liver is involved with synthesis and secretion of bile.

TEST-TAKING TIP—The question is focusing on what is the liver supposed to do, what is the normal physiology of the liver. The key words "best describes" are asking for the most accurate and complete answer. Clue—look for a "metabolic" process.
AN, COM, 4, M/S: GI, PhI, Physiological Adaptation

5. **(2)** The major short-term complication that infants with myelomeningocele face is infection following a tear or rupture of the sac. Hydrocephalus (**Answer 1**) does occur in 90% of these cases, usually following closure of the sac, but it is thought to be part of the CNS defect rather than a complication. Likewise, paraplegia (**Answer 4**) is part of the symptom complex these clients have, rather than a complication. Mental retardation (**Answer 3**) may or may not occur, but if it does occur it is a long-term complication.

KEY TO CODES FOLLOWING RATIONALES:

Nursing process: **AS,** assessment; **AN,** analysis; **PL,** plan; **IMP,** implementation; **EV,** evaluation. *Cognitive level:* **COM,** comprehension; **APP,** application; **ANL,** analysis. *Category of human function:* **1,** protective; **2,** sensory-perceptual; **3,** comfort, rest, activity, and mobility; **4,** nutrition; **5,** growth and development; **6,** fluid-gas transport; **7,** psychosocial-cultural; **8,** elimination. *Client need:* **SECE,** safe, effective care environment; **HPM,** health promotion/maintenance; **PsI,** psychosocial integrity; **PhI,** physiological integrity. (Client subneed appears after Client need code.) See appendices for full explanation.

TEST-TAKING TIP—The question asks for a *short-term complication* rather than part of the symptoms (one that will be evident within 1 to 2 weeks).
AN, COM, 3, PEDS, SECE, Safety and Infection Control

6. **(4)** Isolation may lead to withdrawal and depression. She needs positive reinforcement and reassurance to increase her self-esteem. Isolation may also lead to an increase in her drinking and depression. Based on the symptoms she is exhibiting, involving her in simple, concrete tasks (**Answer 1**) may help her to feel useful. Crying (**Answer 2**) helps her alleviate anxiety through the physical expression of her feelings. Encouraging the verbalization of her feelings (**Answer 3**) will demonstrate that someone cares for her enough to listen, and may decrease her anxiety level.

TEST-TAKING TIP—Note key phrase: "least appropriate."
PL, ANL, 7, Psych, PsI, Psychosocial Integrity

7. **(1)** The basic pathophysiological changes associated with chronic bronchitis are hypertrophy of the mucous glands lining the bronchi and the production of increased amounts of mucus (sometimes thick and difficult to expectorate) that tend to narrow the airway and trap air distal to the mucus. Bronchoconstriction and edema of the bronchial walls (**Answer 2**) are characteristic of *asthma*. Exudate in the alveoli (**Answer 3**) and increasing lung stiffness (**Answer 4**) are consistent with *pneumonia*.

TEST-TAKING TIP—Look for inflammation ("-itis") in the bronchials.
IMP, COM, 6, M/S: Resp., PhI, Physiological Adaptation

8. **(2)** Lying on the stomach (prone) would prevent pressure from being placed on the myelomeningocele and prevent rupture of the sac. This position would also allow the nurse to assess the sac until the surgical repair can be accomplished. **Answer 1** is incorrect because lying on the back (supine) would cause pressure to be placed on the myelomeningocele and lead to rupture of the sac. This position would also prevent the nurse from assessing the sac until the surgical repair can be accomplished. **Answer 3** is incorrect because side-lying with the head slightly elevated would not provide maximum protection of the myelomeningocele and prevent rupture of the sac. This position would also present the nurse with difficulty in assessing the sac until the surgical repair can be accomplished. Slight elevation of the head might be desirable following the surgical repair of the myelomeningocele as 90% of these infants do develop hydrocephalus within 2 weeks of the surgical repair. Slight elevation of the head at that point would assist in promoting cerebral circulation until the hydrocephalus can be surgically repaired. **Answer 4** is incorrect because side-lying would not provide maximum protection of the myelomeningocele and prevent rupture of the sac. This position would also present the nurse with difficulty in assessing the sac until the surgical repair can be accomplished. **Answer 5** is incorrect because this position calls for being on the *back,* which is contraindicated.

TEST-TAKING TIP—Picture the anatomy where the problem is located and avoid on-the-back positions.
IMP, APP, 3, PEDS, SECE, Safety and Infection Control

9. **(2)** Acute glomerulonephritis is an autoimmune response to an antigen produced by beta-hemolytic streptococci. Antibodies produced to fight the antigen also react against the glomerular tissue. This causes proliferation and swelling of endothelial cells in the glomerular capillary wall and results in passage of blood cells and protein into the glomerular filtrate. Acute

glomerular nephritis is *not* the result of direct infection (**Answers 1** and **3**) or of hypoxia (**Answer 4**).

> **TEST-TAKING TIP**—The key word is "cause" of glomerulonephritis. The question is asking for an explanation of the pathophysiology of the disease. Look for a pattern—three options are *direct* infections.
> **IMP, APP, 8, M/S: Renal, PhI, Physiological Adaptation**

10. **(3)** Coughing, vigorous exercise, and straining or lifting increase intra-abdominal pressures, which tend to extrude the intestines through weakened areas of the abdominal wall. This client's history includes all of the above. Other causes of hernia include combinations of **Answers 1, 2,** and **4**; *alone* they are less likely causes.

> **TEST-TAKING TIP**—Client history identifies several risk factors/behaviors. Select the answer that is most inclusive, the one that lists more than one risk.
> **AN, APP, 8, M/S: GI, PhI, Physiological Adaptation**

11. **(4)** As a toddler, this child will probably assert autonomy by refusing to take this medication. The best approach is to be firm yet kind, and always calm. No child should be told that medicine is like candy (**Answer 1**). Medication should be mixed with no more than 1 teaspoon of any nonessential food or beverage (**Answer 2**). This toddler will probably not drink this medication (**Answer 3**), and the nurse should not offer this choice because, if the child refuses, a power struggle will follow.

> **TEST-TAKING TIP**—Look for the choice that addresses the major developmental task for toddler—autonomy.
> **IMP, APP, 5, PEDS, HPM, Health Promotion and Maintenance**

12. **(2)** Fever and increased pulse rates occur in rheumatoid arthritis due to the systemic inflammatory process of this dysfunction. If the fever is high or prolonged, increased fluid losses could occur due to insensible water loss (**Answer 1**); however, the effects on body temperature would be *secondary* to the primary inflammatory response. Though the stress response (**Answer 3**) does increase pulse rate, normally it does *not significantly* affect body temperature. **Answer 4** is incorrect because salicylates have an antipyretic effect.

> **TEST-TAKING TIP**—Look for a choice consistent with an "itis" (inflammation).
> **EV, ANL, 3, M/S: Autoimmune, PhI, Physiological Adaptation**

13. **(2)** Lice are spread by direct or indirect contact: sharing combs and brushes, sharing hats, sleeping together, etc. It is generally unrelated to frequency of hair washing (**Answer 1**), wearing a hat (**Answer 3**), or having long hair (**Answer 4**).

> **TEST-TAKING TIP**—Because lice are contagious, the best answer focuses on *prevention* of *spread* to *others*. Only one option involves *others*.
> **AS, APP, 1, PEDS, HPM, Health Promotion and Maintenance**

14. **(2)** The functions of the gallbladder are to collect, concentrate, and store bile, which is produced by the *liver, not* by the gallbladder (**Answer 1**). Bile reaches the gallbladder via the hepatic duct, which later joins the cystic duct emanating from the gallbladder to form the common bile duct. The common bile duct joins the pancreatic duct, which opens into the duodenum. Bile is not diluted (**Answer 3**). **Answer 4** is incorrect because contraction of the gallbladder and therefore flow of bile are stimulated by the hormone cholecystokinin, which is secreted by the duodenal mucosa when food enters the duodenum.

> **TEST-TAKING TIP**—This question is looking for knowledge of physiology of the gallbladder. What does the gallbladder do under normal circumstances? Be cautious of all statements in the options because some may be correct but are placed with some that are incorrect. Look at each word or phrase and decide right or wrong for each part of the option.
> **AN, COM, 4, M/S: GI, PhI, Physiological Adaptation**

15. **(3)** A thyroid scan utilizes the uptake of ^{131}I by the thyroid gland to determine the size, shape, and function of the gland. Also identified are areas of increased uptake (hot areas), indicating increased metabolic function, as in hyperthyroidism, *not* malignancy (**Answer 2**), and areas of decreased or no uptake (cold areas), which are associated with malignancy. **Answers 1** and **4** both describe the TSH stimulation test.

> **TEST-TAKING TIP**—The question is asking for the *most accurate* description of a thyroid scan. This test uses iodine uptake to identify normal and abnormal findings.
> **IMP, COM, 3, M/S: Metab., PhI, Reduction of Risk Potential**

16. **(1)** Children with asthma should have *no stuffed* animals in their rooms, because they tend to collect dust; therefore more teaching would be needed. Additional measures to "allergy proof" the room and home should include using only washable miniblinds rather than curtains (**Answer 2**) and having no pets in the home (**Answer 3**). Moderate exercise such as swimming (**Answer 4**) is recommended.

> **TEST-TAKING TIP**—The question is asking for the *incorrect* response.
> **EV, APP, 1, PEDS, HPM, Health Promotion and Maintenance**

17. **(2)** The stoma will begin to secrete mucus within 48 hours, and the proximal loop should begin to drain fecal material within 72 hours. *Ileostomies* (**Answer 1**) begin to drain immediately. **Answers 3** and **4** are incorrect because peristalsis generally returns within 48–72 hours postoperatively.

> **TEST-TAKING TIP**—Know when bowel sounds (peristalsis) return following general anesthesia.
> **EV, COM, 8, M/S: GI, PhI, Physiological Adaptation**

18. **(1)** History of three pregnancies plus current pregnancy is gravida 4. Parity refers to the number of pregnancies carried to viability, *not* the number of babies. Two pregnancies were carried past viability (para 2). This formula does not allow for indicating the number of abortions or living children. **Answers 2, 3,** and **4** are incorrect based on the definitions of gravida and parity.

> **TEST-TAKING TIP**—Be able to determine a woman's obstetric history by defining gravida and para. Use the acronym GTPAL (gravida, term, preterm, abortions, living children).
> **AN, COM, 5, Maternity, HPM, Health Promotion and Maintenance**

19. **(1)** The kidneys secrete the erythropoietin factor, which stimulates the bone marrow to produce red blood cells. In chronic kidney disease, secretion of this factor decreases as greater portions of the kidney are destroyed by the disease process. Hypertension does *not* suppress bone marrow centers (**Answer 2**), because local blood flow regulators tend to compensate over the long run by supplying tissue with adequate blood flow for metabolic purposes. Unlike metabolic acidosis, metabolic alkalosis does *not* increase RBC fragility (**Answer 3**). Frank bleeding into the urine is uncommon in chronic renal disease (**Answer 4**).

TEST-TAKING TIP—Take each option by itself and determine if it is correct or incorrect in relation to the normal or abnormal kidney function seen in chronic failure.
AN, APP, 8, M/S: Renal, PhI, Physiological Adaptation

20. (3) For clients having elective surgery, *routine* preoperative laboratory studies generally include a complete blood count, urinalysis, and prothrombin time. Some institutions also require a VDRL. The urinalysis provides information about specific gravity (indicating the ability of the kidney to concentrate and dilute urine); the presence of albumin or pus, indicating renal infection; and the presence of sugar and acetone. The CBC detects the presence of anemia, infection, allergy, and leukemia. Prothrombin time (increased) may indicate a need for preoperative vitamin K therapy. Electrolytes (**Answer 1**), enzymes such as ALT (SGOT), (**Answer 2**), and serum glucose (**Answer 4**) are ordered *only if* the client's history or physical condition warrants a more complete workup.

TEST-TAKING TIP—Key word in this question is "routine" for each client having surgery. The incorrect options all suggest an underlying medical problem, but none is discussed in the stem (e.g., VDRL).
AS, APP, 6, M/S: Preop, PhI, Reduction of Risk Potential

21. (3) The *average* age for the onset of menstruation for girls is 12.8 years of age; girls between 10.5 and 15 years *can* begin to menstruate within the normal range (**Answers 1, 2, 4**).

TEST-TAKING TIP—"Normal," "usually," and "average" are used as synonyms here. Know age-typical prepubertal and pubertal developmental norms.
IMP, COM, 3, PEDS, HPM, Health Promotion and Maintenance

22. (4) The psychological effect of being restrained can be severe. Therefore, any form of restraint should be applied as a last resort. Isolating the client from other clients during the initial adjustment period would serve to decrease stimuli and possibly prevent the need for restraints. **Answers 1, 2,** and **3** are all more appropriate interventions.

TEST-TAKING TIP—Note key phrase: "*least* appropriate."
IMP, ANL, 7, Psych, PsI, Psychosocial Integrity

23. (4) The loss of a limb is significant. The client facing the amputation must deal with self-perception, incorporate the changes in body image, and be allowed to grieve. The nurse must be sensitive to the client's stage of grieving and provide information as asked for, at a level consistent with the client's ability to comprehend. Although the attending physician (**Answer 1**), family (**Answer 2**), and nursing staff (**Answer 3**) may affect the client's perception of a situation, the work of grieving is primarily personal, with movement both forward and backward as the client progresses through the stages.

TEST-TAKING TIP—Focus on the client's needs first.
AN, ANL, 7, Psych, PsI, Psychosocial Integrity

24. (1) When excessive quantities of fatty acids are oxidized, blood buffer systems may become exhausted. Ketoacidosis develops and acetone bodies are excreted in the urine. In an emergency room situation, diabetic acidosis can be recognized not only by the increased rate and depth of respirations (Kussmaul's respirations) but also by the odor of acetone on the breath. *Neither* osmotic diuresis (**Answer 2**) *nor* failure in the sodium-hydrogen ion exchange (**Answer 3**) causes acetonuria. In the latter case, failure to excrete excess hydrogen ions would decrease urinary acids. Volatile hydrogen ions (CO_2) are excreted by the lungs; a decrease in nonvolatile hydrogen ions in the glomerular filtrate (**Answer 4**) would move the pH of the urine toward the alkaline side.

TEST-TAKING TIP—The word "acetonuria" tells you something is evident in the urine. Improper fat metabolism produces acetonuria.
AN, APP, 6, M/S: Metab., PhI, Physiological Adaptation

25. (1) Hyperkalemia tends to develop in renal dysfunction for two reasons: In the kidneys, more hydrogen ions than potassium ions are selectively secreted in exchange for sodium ions, and decreasing glomerular filtration and urine output tends to decrease the excretion of all electrolytes and waste products of metabolism. Potassium does not move out of the cell to balance sodium shifts in edema (**Answer 2**), nor does respiratory alkalosis affect potassium reabsorption in the kidneys (**Answer 3**). Nausea and vomiting (**Answer 4**) cause hypokalemia.

TEST-TAKING TIP—Know the role of potassium in the body and the pathophysiology of chronic renal failure.
AN, APP, 8, M/S: Renal, PhI, Physiological Adaptation

26. (1) In caring for a client with a potentially contagious condition such as meningitis, the first priority is protecting the nurse and other clients by observing appropriate infection control measures, in this case, respiratory isolation. All other nursing care measures would then follow in the appropriate order (**Answers 2, 3,** and **4**).

TEST-TAKING TIP—Infection control is always a priority of care.
AN, ANL, 1, PEDS, SECE, Safety and Infection Control

27. (4) The adolescent *initially* needs the staff's help in one-to-one socialization. The client *next* must be stimulated by the staff to participate in minimally demanding group activities (**Answer 1**). Allowing a minimum of 3 hours of isolated behavior (**Answer 3**) will probably increase the withdrawal. Perhaps the nurse could establish a behavior-modification program involving a trade-off of 15 minutes alone for every 45 minutes spent socializing and interacting with others. If activities are too challenging (**Answer 2**), the client may become frustrated and feel incompetent, which would lead to a decrease in self-esteem.

TEST-TAKING TIP—Note key phrase: "*most* appropriate."
PL, APP, 7, Psych, PsI, Psychosocial Integrity

28. (2) Increased lung volumes (TLC, FRC, RV) and decreased airflow—vital capacity (VC) and forced expiratory volume in 1 second (FEV_1)—are functional problems consistent with obstructive lung disease. In restrictive lung disease (**Answer 1**), volumes generally are decreased. Vascular lung disease (**Answer 3**) has no effect on ventilatory capacity but directly affects diffusion of gases; that is, pulmonary infarction decreases blood flow to the lungs, so some alveoli that are ventilated are no longer perfused. Restrictive lung disease is incorrect (**Answer 4**).

TEST-TAKING TIP—Visualize a lung with *increased* capacities: hyperinflated, trapped air (COPD).
AN, APP, 6, M/S: Resp., PhI, Physiological Adaptation

29. (1) To prevent contractures, the affected limb is kept straight (knee extension) and slightly abducted (to prevent pressure in hip joint), and the foot is supported (ankle flexion) to prevent footdrop. **Answers 2, 3,** and **4** are incorrect because all or part of each response could produce a contracture.

TEST-TAKING TIP—Key word is "contractures." Look for anything that is suggested to extend the limb or keep it straight.
PL, APP, 3, M/S: Integ., PhI, Reduction of Risk Potential

30. **(2)** A truss should be applied *before* the client gets out of bed or after the hernia has been reduced, by having the client lie down with the feet elevated in bed or in the bath. If the hernia cannot be reduced, the truss should not be applied **(Answers 1 and 3)**. Although the truss is not a cure for a hernia and its use is not as common as it once was, it is far more effective in keeping a hernia reduced than is an athletic supporter **(Answer 4)**.

> **TEST-TAKING TIP**—A truss keeps the internal organs from protruding through the herniated area. Look for the *best time.*
> **IMP, APP, 3, M/S: GI, PhI, Reduction of Risk Potential**

31. **(4)** With a pediatric microdrip chamber, the number of mL/hr = number of drops/min. Therefore, if the physician orders 35 mL/hr, the IV should infuse at 35 drops/min. Any other flow rate would be incorrect **(Answers 1, 2,** and **3).**

> **TEST-TAKING TIP**—The nurse must know how to calculate the rate of flow of IVs.
> **IMP, ANL, 1, PEDS, PhI, Pharmacological and Parenteral Therapies**

32. **(3)** Stapedectomy is the surgical procedure for the treatment of otosclerosis. Its success cannot be determined in the immediate postoperative period. The client must be told that hearing is affected for a while after surgery because of edema. Tinnitus **(Answer 1)** is a postoperative complication that must be reported, but is *not* expected. The resolution of postoperative edema **(Answer 2)** does *not* result in rhinitis. Once the ear has healed, normal activities *are* permitted, including showering and swimming **(Answer 4)**. With an upper respiratory infection, deep-sea diving and flying are usually restricted.

> **TEST-TAKING TIP**—Use a process of elimination. Ringing in the ears is *never* normal, which leaves short-term hearing impairment, given the surgery.
> **IMP, APP, 2, M/S: Ear, PhI, Reduction of Risk Potential**

33. **(4)** Early decelerations represent the normal fetal response to head compressions during contractions. **Answer 1** is incorrect because head compression does not cause fetal distress. **Answers 2** and **3** are incorrect because there are no signs of late or variable decelerations.

> **TEST-TAKING TIP**—First, decide if this is OK or not OK. Note the word "physiological," which implies an anticipated outcome. You can eliminate options with "insufficiency" and "distress," which mean there is a problem.
> **AN, ANL, 6, Maternity, PhI, Physiological Adaptation**

34. **(1)** The PPD for the tuberculin skin test is injected intradermally on the polar aspect of the forearm. If the test is correctly administered, a pale elevation similar to a mosquito bite should be apparent. **Answers 2, 3,** and **4** are not used for this test.

> **TEST-TAKING TIP**—*Correct* technique is just under the skin. Only *one* option will produce a bubble. You want to be able to see results from the administration of this injection, so you do not want to give deep injections.
> **IMP, COM, 1, M/S: Meds, PhI, Pharmacological and Parenteral Therapies**

35. **(3)** Fat-soluble vitamins, particularly vitamin K, are poorly absorbed in the absence of bile. Decreased absorption of vitamin K results in decreased levels of circulating prothrombin, thus reducing normal clotting levels. Peripheral neuritis **(Answer 1)** occurs with vitamin B_6 deficiencies, and scurvy **(Answer 2)** occurs with deficiency in vitamin C; these are *water-soluble* vitamins. Macrocytic anemia **(Answer 4)** is

consistent with a vitamin B_{12} deficiency, which may be due to lack of intrinsic factor in the stomach.

> **TEST-TAKING TIP**—Need to know fat-soluble vitamins (A, D, E, and K). Associate vitamin K with increased bleeding tendencies.
> **EV, APP, 4, M/S: Blood, PhI, Physiological Adaptation**

36. **(3)** In working with children in hospitals, the most important factor for the nurse to assess first is what that child's experience with illness and hospitalization has been thus far. This is of special importance with this child, who has previously had two hospitalizations and surgeries; the nurse needs to know if these were positive experiences for this child and how he was able to cope with them. *After* this, the nurse would continue the admitting assessment by determining the child's developmental level **(Answer 1)**, what the parents already know about hypospadias **(Answer 2)**, and whether the child's parents plan to room-in with him **(Answer 4)**.

> **TEST-TAKING TIP**—An important principle of teaching-learning is to always start with what the client already knows.
> **PL, APP, 8, PEDS, PsI, Psychosocial Integrity**

37. **(3)** The position that allows for the greatest amount of lung expansion is sitting up and leaning slightly forward. This position can be facilitated by allowing the client to rest his or her arms on a bedside table. The position that also facilitates lung expansion, but *not to the same degree*, is high-Fowler's **(Answer 1)**. Both the prone position **(Answer 2)** and the Trendelenburg position **(Answer 4)** tend to *decrease* full lung expansion due to increased pressure of abdominal contents on the diaphragm.

> **TEST-TAKING TIP**—When two options are plausible, choose the most comprehensive (two actions instead of just one).
> **IMP, APP, 6, M/S: Resp., PhI, Basic Care and Comfort**

38. **(4)** The superego may never be completely refined or stabilized. Some individuals may achieve an optimal level of functioning some time in late adulthood; however, rarely will the superego become stabilized during adolescence. As stated in **Answer 1,** the individual *does* strive to develop an independent and unique personality during adolescence. To maintain a steady state of functioning, the adolescent must learn to use defense mechanisms **(Answer 2)** in an appropriate manner. Developing a positive ego identity **(Answer 3)** is one of the major goals of adolescence.

> **TEST-TAKING TIP**—Key words: "least important" means eliminate the three options that *are* age related.
> **PL, APP, 5, Psych, HPM, Health Promotion and Maintenance**

39. **(2, 3, 4)** Answer 2 is correct because an apical pulse of 118 is normal for a toddler and would indicate a return to health. **Answer 3** is correct because as the toddler's physical condition begins to improve, so should the toddler's appetite. **Answer 4** is correct because pink nailbeds indicate a satisfactory level of oxygenation and would indicate a return to health. **Answer 1** is incorrect because progressive hoarseness, followed by aphonia (loss of speech sounds), is an ominous sign of impending airway obstruction and respiratory arrest secondary to edema and inflammation. The nurse must promptly report this to the pediatrician who will probably perform an emergency tracheostomy.

> **TEST-TAKING TIP**—Three of the responses offer options that are normal and all of them should be selected; omit selecting the one response that is abnormal.
> **EV, ANL, 6, PEDS, PhI, Physiological Adaptation**

40. (3) Even though the client will have only one eye patched after surgery, familiarization with the physical environment and with nursing personnel will decrease the occurrence of disorientation (this is especially important with elderly clients). It is not necessary to keep the client flat in bed before or after surgery (**Answer 1**). Patches (**Answer 2**) are not generally applied to both eyes. Eye-drop instillations (**Answer 4**) are part of the *postoperative* or predischarge teaching plan.

> **TEST-TAKING TIP**—The key word is "preoperative." Orienting the client to prevent injuries in the postop period is priority.
> **PL, APP, 2, M/S: Preop, SECE, Management of Care**

41. (1) Following an injection of the small dose of ^{131}I used in a thyroid scan, no radiation precautions are necessary. Full radiation precautions (**Answer 2**) are utilized for radium implants. **Answer 3** may be employed when ^{131}I therapy is utilized to control and reduce hypersecretion by the thyroid (*hyperthyroidism*). **Answer 4** is not an example of normal radiation therapy policy.

> **TEST-TAKING TIP**—There is no identification of *treatment* with radioactive substance, just a scan. Look for a pattern—three of the options are inappropriate precautions.
> **PL, APP, 3, M/S: Radiation, PhI, Reduction of Risk Potential**

42. (2) Preschoolers who are hospitalized often regress in their behavior and want "mommy," but this is obviously not practical all the time. The nurse should try to soothe the child back to sleep during the middle of the night. Calling the mother to come right in (**Answer 4**) would be inappropriate, because the family should not be called in the absence of a genuine emergency. The nurse should also not pick the child up (**Answer 1**), because preschoolers who are hospitalized frequently reject everyone except their "mommy." Simply insisting the child go back to sleep (**Answer 3**) is not enough, because the child needs some degree of comfort at this time.

> **TEST-TAKING TIP**—Look at the verbs: "pick . . . rock," "talk softly . . . rubbing back," "firmly tell," "call . . . mother." Preschoolers will regress when stressed, and respond well to verbal and physical comfort ("talk softly . . . rubbing back.")
> **IMP, APP, 7, PEDS, PsI, Psychosocial Integrity**

43. (4) The nurse should know that deep partial-thickness (second-degree) burns cause severe pain. The nurse should also know that during the first 48 to 72 hours after a serious burn, there is a very poor peripheral circulation due to hypovolemia; therefore, medications should be given via the IV route. PO (**Answer 2**) and IM (**Answer 3**) medications are generally contraindicated during this time. To do nothing (**Answer 1**) would be inappropriate, given the nature and extent of the injuries.

> **TEST-TAKING TIP**—Think impaired peripheral circulation; think IV, not IM; eliminate PO due to burns on face and neck.
> **IMP, ANL, 3, PEDS, PhI, Pharmacological and Parenteral Therapies**

44. (2) Past coping mechanisms are important in assessing the client's ability to return to a steady state of functioning. Strengths and weaknesses in the client's ability to rationally assess and cope with feelings need to be explored. Referrals may need to be made (**Answer 1**), but an initial assessment of the client needs to be completed first. Inpatient hospitalization may be needed (**Answer 3**); however, the assessment of ability to cope with the situation may assist in identifying whether hospitalization is needed. Obtaining a prescription for an antidepressant at this time (**Answer 4**) may prove to be detrimental. Even if the client does not decide to overdose, medication without psychological support is generally ineffective.

> **TEST-TAKING TIP**—Choose an assessment intervention as a most important priority (e.g., "identifying").
> **IMP, ANL, 7, Psych, PsI, Psychosocial Integrity**

45. (2) This client's smoking history and history of chronic cough necessitate directing preoperative nursing measures toward clearing the respiratory tract of excess secretions that might lead to postoperative complications. Besides oral hygiene, the following may be instituted or ordered before surgery: postural drainage, incentive spirometers, IPPB, and mucolytic agent. Because postoperative coughing is contraindicated with hernia repairs, removal of secretions is a priority, as is instruction in deep-breathing techniques. **Answers 1, 3,** and **4,** though *not top priority,* are correct and should also be included in the preoperative teaching plan.

> **TEST-TAKING TIP**—This is a *priority* question. The client is at greater risk for respiratory infection and complications.
> **AN, APP, 6, M/S: Preop, PhI, Reduction of Risk Potential**

46. (1) The portal system becomes obstructed, causing a rise in portal venous pressure and portal hypertension, venous dilation, and stasis. In cirrhosis, there is *decreased* hepatic synthesis of albumin, not increased (**Answer 2**), and *increased* levels of aldosterone, not decreased (**Answer 3**). Blood volumes are *decreased,* not increased (**Answer 4**), while total body fluid is increased due to the physiological effects of hypoproteinemia (decreased serum proteins). These factors, plus increasing obstruction of the portal vein, cause fluids, electrolytes, and serum proteins to move out of the vascular compartment and into the intestines. The abdomen provides a large potential space for the accumulation of these fluids.

> **TEST-TAKING TIP**—Know where ascites is found and how fluid is able to shift (some type of intravascular problem).
> **AN, APP, 4, M/S: GI, PhI, Physiological Adaptation**

47. (1) Although the abrupt onset and critical nature of this illness is very frightening for parents, the child is expected to make a total recovery before discharge. The parents should be aware of this very positive diagnosis. Although discharge instructions from the physician may include some rest at home, there is no need for the child to miss almost a month of school (**Answer 2**). The parents should not worry about the child getting sick again (**Answer 3**) or having oxygen in the home again (**Answer 4**); the excellent prognosis should be stressed.

> **TEST-TAKING TIP**—Eliminate the incorrect statement first. Note the use of the words "correctly understood" in this question.
> **EV, APP, 6, PEDS, HPM, Health Promotion and Maintenance**

48. (4) Thyroglobulin (Proloid) is a purified extract of pig thyroid and is used in the treatment of *hypothyroidism.* **Answers 1, 2,** and **3** *are* current methods for treating Graves' disease, or hyperthyroidism.

> **TEST-TAKING TIP**—Key word is "inappropriate," which means select the *wrong* treatment. Another key term is *hyper*thyroidism, not *hypo*thyroidism.
> **IMP, COM, 3, M/S: Endocrine, SECE, Management of Care**

49. (1) Acting out is the expression through behavior (rather than through words) of emotions that occur when the client relives or reproduces the feelings, wishes, or conflicts that are operating unconsciously. The client may be feeling frustrated, angry,

ambivalent, etc., for numerous reasons, such as conflict between self and parents, a reaction to parents' marital conflicts, sibling rivalry, or frustration due to poor self-esteem. By definition, **Answers 2, 3,** and **4** are incorrect.

> **TEST-TAKING TIP**—Review definition of *acting out.*
> **AS, APP, 7, Psych, PsI, Psychosocial Integrity**

50. **(4)** Abdominal cramps, vomiting, and watery or no discharge are signs of intestinal obstruction, a complication that requires immediate medical intervention. **Answers 1, 2,** and **3** are incorrect, not only because they can delay appropriate medical intervention but also because they increase the risk of severe fluid and electrolyte imbalance. Although obstruction of an ileostomy is a rare problem, a very small stoma or one that is contracted may need to be dilated regularly so that the little finger can be inserted easily.

> **TEST-TAKING TIP**—The key word is *"sudden."* Suspect something serious with onset of multiple symptoms. Look for a pattern—three options delay diagnosis.
> **IMP, ANL, 4, M/S: GI, PhI, Physiological Adaptation**

51. **(4)** Normal functioning of chest tubes is maintained, and the drainage system is transported below the level of the chest. Chest tubes are not removed **(Answer 1)** to facilitate transportation of the client; they are removed only after the physician is satisfied with the degree of reexpansion. Removing the chest tubes from the suction drainage system **(Answer 2)** will result in an equalization of intrapleural pressures with atmospheric pressures, thus also increasing the risk of pneumothorax. Current practice precludes the clamping of the chest tubes **(Answer 3).** It is believed that clamping increases the risk of a tension pneumothorax because air may enter the intrapleural space during inspiration but cannot escape during expiration.

> **TEST-TAKING TIP**—The reason why chest tubes are inserted is to re-expand the lung. Avoid any option that would interfere with the purpose of the chest tube. Look for the independent nursing action—nurses do *not* "remove," "disconnect," or "clamp" routinely.
> **IMP, APP, 6, M/S: Thoracic, PhI, Reduction of Risk Potential**

52. **(4)** To restrain a toddler receiving IV therapy, clove-hitch restraint to two or more limbs is most effective in maintaining the IV site. A posey jacket **(Answer 1)** would allow the toddler use of hands with which to pull at the IV. Elbow restraints **(Answer 2)** would still allow the toddler to stand and twist at the IV tubing. A mummy restraint **(Answer 3)** would be unnecessarily restrictive for a toddler.

> **TEST-TAKING TIP**—Choose the option that is effective while not restraining, by *visualizing* what these various restraints do and where they are placed.
> **IMP, APP, 1, PEDS, SECE, Safety and Infection Control**

53. **(1)** A wheeze is a high-pitched, musical chest sound produced by airflow in narrowed bronchioles. It is primarily an expiratory sound and is always, *not* rarely **(Answer 2),** considered pathological. *Rhonchi* are medium-pitched sonorous sounds **(Answer 3)** produced by airflow obstruction in larger airways. *Stridor* is a high-pitched crowing sound **(Answer 4)** on inspiration and is due to an upper-airway obstruction, such as edema, adhesions, or tracheal hypertrophy.

> **TEST-TAKING TIP**—Think "wheeze" is a "squeeze"— only one choice includes narrowing.
> **IMP, COM, 6, M/S: Resp., PhI, Physiological Adaptation**

54. **(1)** The *primary* purpose of passive range-of-motion exercises is to prevent contractures and decreased range of motion.

Secondarily, passive range-of-motion exercises assist the nurse in evaluating functional abilities **(Answer 2),** pain tolerance **(Answer 3),** and the effectiveness of drug therapy **(Answer 4).**

> **TEST-TAKING TIP**—The stem asks for a *purpose* (goal). Three of the options are nursing actions.
> **IMP, COM, 3, M/S: Ortho, PhI, Basic Care and Comfort**

55. **(3)** A BUN of less than 20 mg/dL and serum creatinine less than 1.2 mg/dL would be optimal outcome measures for this client (that is, within normal range). **Answers 1, 2,** and **4** are incorrect because a serum K^+ of less than 3.5 mEq/L would be indicative of hypokalemia and a serum Na^+ above 148 mEq/L indicates hypernatremia **(Answer 1);** quantity of urine output *should increase* to over 500 mL/24 hours **(Answer 2);** and the abdomen should be soft and tympanic to percussion; so dullness to percussion in the abdomen is consistent with *fluid excess* **(Answer 4).**

> **TEST-TAKING TIP**—The key word is "effectiveness." How well is the dialysis working? The closer to normal the values are, the more effective the treatment. Know normal lab values.
> **EV, ANL, 8, M/S: F-E, PhI, Physiological Adaptation**

56. **(4)** All straining and lifting should be avoided for at least 3 weeks to prevent undue stress on the sutures. Other less strenuous activities, such as **Answers 1, 2,** and **3,** are appropriate, though good body mechanics should be reviewed with the client.

> **TEST-TAKING TIP**—Look at all the activities and determine which one would be the most strenuous for the client.
> **PL, ANL, 3, M/S: Postop, PhI, Basic Care and Comfort**

57. **(2)** When doing preoperative teaching with preschoolers, the best method is to use puppets (doctor, nurse, hospital setup) to "act out" what the child can expect to happen. For evaluating the teaching, the nurse can then ask the child to use puppets to give a return demonstration of what was learned; this enables the nurse to clarify any misconceptions or answer any lingering questions the child might still have. Most preschoolers will not be able to *accurately* draw pictures regarding the factual information of preoperative teaching **(Answer 1),** although this might be a good way to get at feelings about the surgery or hospital. A preschooler probably has had limited experience with "tests" **(Answer 3).** The nurse should not rely on the parents to evaluate the preoperative teaching **(Answer 4),** because they are not professionals and are most likely too involved emotionally.

> **TEST-TAKING TIP**—Preschoolers respond best to *play*—therapeutic, or medical.
> **EV, ANL, 1, PEDS, PsI, Psychosocial Integrity**

58. **(2)** The client needs an opportunity to receive word images. Point to the object and clearly enunciate its name (e.g., "spoon"). Also, the client with expressive aphasia needs the chance to practice repeating words. Begin with simple words, such as *yes* and *no*, and then progress to complete phrases. Recovery from aphasia depends on the area of the brain involved and the extent of damage. There may be spontaneous recovery or improvement with speech therapy 2 years after the brain attack. To consider the impairment permanent **(Answer 1)** would be premature. **Answer 3** is incorrect because waiting may increase the client's frustration. Try to anticipate the client's needs to reduce feelings of helplessness. The nurse plays an important part in showing the family members how to communicate and in not discouraging communication **(Answer 4).**

TEST-TAKING TIP—Only one option shows "action" to improve client communication.
IMP, APP, 2, M/S: CV, PsI, Psychosocial Integrity

59. (1) The nurse needs to address the amount of energy and stamina needed to meet the demands of parenting. Older women have commented that the lack of energy and stamina came as a surprise. **Answer 2** is incorrect because older women tend to be *less troubled* by pregnancy and remain better adjusted during the last trimester. Older mothers, as a group, do *not* have longer labor (**Answer 3**), nor, with good prenatal care, do they show a greater number of labor/birth complications (**Answer 4**).

TEST-TAKING TIP—Focus on the *general expected* concerns for this age group and this trimester. You can eliminate options that focus on "troubled" feelings, "*longer* labor," "*greater* number of . . . complications."
PL, ANL, 5, Maternity, HPM, Health Promotion and Maintenance

60. (2) Clients who have had spinal anesthesia have varying degrees of hypotension due to the vasodepressor effect of the anesthetic agent on the autonomic nervous system. Reflexes (**Answer 1**) will be depressed in the lower extremities because of the anesthetic and should be checked *after* circulatory status. However, sensory impulses remain blocked longer than motor activity, so safety measures should be instituted to prevent injury from bedding, poor positioning, or sources of heat. Because the client is awake with a spinal anesthetic, level of consciousness (**Answer 3**) and airway integrity (**Answer 4**) are lower priorities than circulatory status.

TEST-TAKING TIP—Think *baseline data* in the postoperative period. You need to know what the vitals were and how they progress over time. With spinal anesthetic, circulatory problems are more likely.
AS, ANL, 1, M/S: Postop, PhI, Reduction of Risk Potential

61. (2) The contrast medium utilized in IV cholangiograms, like that used in intravenous pyelograms, contains iodine. It is important to ascertain before the test whether the client is aware of any allergy to iodine. Saltwater fish generally have a high iodine content, so it is helpful to ascertain if the client has an allergy to fish, and if so, to what kind. **Answer 1** is helpful in planning client teaching. **Answers 3** and **4** are less specific responses that provide interesting, though not essential, data.

TEST-TAKING TIP—Priority for any diagnostic study using a contrast medium is to determine if the client has an allergy to the substance being used.
AS, APP, 1, M/S: Dx Test, PhI, Reduction of Risk Potential

62. (3) The most common symptom in children with rheumatic fever is tachycardia due to cardiac involvement; in addition, these children may develop a rash, "erythema marginatum," and a characteristic fever, which spikes in the late afternoon. They do not usually have petechiae (**Answer 1**), hypertension (**Answer 2**), or conjunctivitis (**Answer 4**).

TEST-TAKING TIP—Remember that cardiac symptoms are associated with rheumatic fever; therefore, choose the option with tachycardia.
AS, COM, 6, PEDS, PhI, Physiological Adaptation

63. (2) Neomycin sulfate is used preoperatively because it is poorly absorbed in the intestinal tract and acts to decrease the bacteria count in the colon. As the result of this action, postoperative infection is reduced (**Answer 1**). Neomycin does not reduce tumor size (**Answer 3**) or directly affect peristalsis (**Answer 4**).

TEST-TAKING TIP—Timing is important *(preop)* and purpose of drug classification—antibiotic.
EV, COM, 8, M/S: Infect. Control, PhI, Pharmacological and Parenteral Therapies

64. (1) Treatment with bronchodilators such as isoproterenol will decrease bronchoconstriction, *improving* the movement of air in and out of the lungs. **Answers 2, 3,** and **4** are incorrect because these pulmonary function studies indicate that the client has been able to increase inspiratory capacity by 1000 mL (VC 2800–3800) and expiratory capacity (RV decreased, FRC decreased, and FEV_1 increased).

TEST-TAKING TIP—Know vital capacity (VC)—the amount of air in a breath.
EV, ANL, 6, M/S: Resp., PhI, Physiological Adaptation

65. (1, 3, 4) **Answer 1** is correct because school-age children are usually very competitive, and they especially enjoy the challenge of board games. This would be the most developmentally appropriate way to assist the children to relieve their boredom. **Answer 3** is correct because while reading may not be as entertaining as playing a board game, it does relieve boredom (at least on a temporary level). **Answer 4** is correct because while watching TV may not be as entertaining as playing a board game, it does relieve boredom (at least on a temporary level). **Answer 2** is incorrect because while homework is important and should receive due consideration, it will not relieve the children's boredom

TEST-TAKING TIP—Think "developmentally appropriate" and select the correct answer.
IMP, APP, 5, PEDS, HPM, Health Promotion and Maintenance

66. (1) The client should remain quiet in a low-Fowler's or horizontal position. The client should be cautioned not to cough so as not to extrude any intestines by increasing intraabdominal pressures. The physician should be notified next. Remain with the client, offer reassurance, monitor vital signs, and have others bring equipment such as IV setup, nasogastric tube, and suction equipment. The surgeon should also be notified that the client will be returning to the operating room. The client should be kept *NPO* (**Answer 2**) in low Fowler's or horizontal, not in a chair (**Answer 3**) and the dressing left in place to prevent evisceration (**Answer 4**).

TEST-TAKING TIP—This is an emergency situation. Look for the answer that will not add to the damage. Getting the client out of bed to a chair may cause the entire wound to open and all contents of the cavity to eviscerate. This new wound will need surgical correction, so client should be kept NPO.
IMP, ANL, 1, M/S: GI, PhI, Physiological Adaptation

67. (4) Flattened neck veins in a supine position are characteristic of hypovolemia. Inadequate drainage would result in fluid retention and *hypervolemia*. Indications of fluid retention include inadequate fluid drainage (**Answer 1,** greater intake than output), increased blood pressure, and signs of congestive heart failure, for example, *distended* neck veins, increased dependent edema, crackles (**Answer 3**), and decreased mentation (**Answer 2**).

TEST-TAKING TIP—The key word is "least likely"; this could also be rephrased by saying what will *not* happen. Look for fluid volume excess, *not* deficit.
EV, APP, 8, M/S: F-E, PhI, Reduction of Risk Potential

68. (2) Children with leukemia often experience bleeding gums due to thrombocytopenia; in addition, chemotherapy may

cause oral mucous membrane ulceration. Therefore, the nurse would be most correct in advising this child to use a soft toothbrush only. Using a firm toothbrush (**Answer 3**) might cause a break in the gums, leading to infection. Rinsing the mouth only (**Answer 4**) might also lead to infection, because this would not necessarily clean the gums and teeth adequately; likewise, infection might be caused by not brushing the teeth (**Answer 1**).

> **TEST-TAKING TIP**—Narrow your choices to two *contradictory* options about brushes (soft vs. hard) and choose soft, due to bleeding.
> **IMP, APP, 1, PEDS, PhI, Reduction of Risk Potential**

69. **(3)** Although there *are* several specific forms that elicit disclosure of this information, there is no law that mandates disclosure (**Answer 4**). The client has to make this decision independently. The nurse should provide therapeutic support for whatever decision. **Answers 1 and 2** are untrue statements.

> **TEST-TAKING TIP**—Note the key phrase "*most appropriate*"; it provides therapeutic support for client's decision.
> **IMP, APP, 7, Psych, PsI, Psychosocial Integrity**

70. **(3)** An iridectomy is performed in the upper segment of the iris and is covered by the upper eyelid, as normally. The excision in the iris is occluded, which decreases discomfort. Infection is less likely because bacteria are carried in the tears, by gravity, to the lower cul-de-sac. The need for a dressing is usually indicated, to decrease infection or eye movement. Because infection is *not* likely and mobilization of the eye (**Answer 1**) *is* desirable to prevent posterior synechiae (adhesion of iris to cornea or lens), no dressing is needed. **Answers 2 and 4** *are* appropriate actions. Massage of the eye, if ordered, encourages continuous flow of fluids through the surgical opening.

> **TEST-TAKING TIP**—The key word is *inappropriate*. Although dressings prevent infection, *reinforcing* the dressing would be necessary for bleeding, which is *not* indicated.
> **IMP, APP, 2, M/S: Eye, PhI, Basic Care and Comfort**

71. **(2)** Ammonia is formed in the intestines by the action of intestinal bacteria on proteins. Tap-water enemas may be given to remove protein-rich blood that has collected from bleeding esophageal varices. Because ammonia is formed during muscle contraction, active range-of-motion exercises are contraindicated (**Answer 1**). To prevent skin breakdown in a client who is jaundiced and edematous, passive exercises, turning, and frequent skin care are indicated. In an effort to reduce serum-ammonia levels, potassium levels need to be *increased,* not reduced (**Answer 3**), because potassium is necessary for cerebral metabolism of ammonia. Antibiotics that are poorly absorbed by the intestines, such as neomycin, are given, rather than withheld (**Answer 4**), to decrease the intestinal flora that manufacture ammonia.

> **TEST-TAKING TIP**—Only one option includes an intervention for a possible cause for an ammonia increase—blood.
> **IMP, APP, 8, M/S: Blood, PhI, Physiological Adaptation**

72. **(2)** Before notifying the physician (**Answer 1**), it is necessary to collect the data, blood sugar and urine sugar and acetone, on which the physician will base the insulin order. The physician should also be notified of the client's vital signs and intake and output. Generally, urinary output is depressed for about 36 hours after surgery due to increased circulating levels of ADH. Given that the client has also had insensible water loss (respirations and perspiration), the assessment data strongly indicate dehydration or hypovolemia. An antiemetic (**Answer 3**) may be administered if nausea persists *after* blood

sugar and fluid balance are rectified. The physician may order an increase in the amount and rate of intravenous fluids (contrary to **Answer 4**).

> **TEST-TAKING TIP**—The key consideration here is that the client has diabetes. During surgery the normal routine of the client with diabetes is interrupted. The first thing the nurse should do in this situation is to get baseline information, which includes glucose level for a client with diabetes. Then the nurse has accurate assessment data to report. Choose the first step of the nursing process—*assess.*
> **AN, ANL, 4 M/S: Postop, PhI, Reduction of Risk Potential**

73. **(4)** When a preschooler has a favorite "security object," be it a blanket or a doll or a stuffed animal, that child should be allowed to keep the security object, even during hospitalization. This will promote the child's sense of trust and security, thus helping to make the hospitalization a more positive experience. Offering the child another toy (**Answer 1**), putting the toy where he can see it but not touch it (**Answer 2**), or giving him a new stuffed animal (**Answer 3**) will not take the place of the child's old but well-loved original stuffed animal.

> **TEST-TAKING TIP**—Preschoolers will regress when stressed. Note that two options allow the security object to remain—one at a distance and the other *close* by.
> **IMP, APP, 7, PEDS, PsI, Psychosocial Integrity**

74. **(4)** Young adults who have had an appendectomy are expected to make a complete, rapid recovery; they should have *minimal* to moderate pain during the first 24 hours (**Answer 1**). Discharge time frame varies, not necessarily within 48 hours, or after a *slow* recovery (**Answers 2 and 3**).

> **TEST-TAKING TIP**—Consider age-appropriate expected outcome.
> **EV, APP, 8, M/S: Postop, SECE, Management of Care**

75. **(3)** Hostility and aggression are considered the underlying factors in the psychogenesis and psychodynamics of depression. The adolescent is in a stage of development in which the adolescent experiences extensive anger due to frustration. The adolescent has a greater energy level because of the increased libidinal energy available in the adolescent's system. To expend this energy, many adolescents act out their feelings of depression in violent ways rather than become withdrawn, apathetic, or regressive (**Answers 1, 2, and 4**).

> **TEST-TAKING TIP**—Choose the option that is different: violence is different from withdrawal, apathy, and regression.
> **AS, APP, 7, Psych, PsI, Psychosocial Integrity**

76. **(3)** The primary objective of stoma care is to *prevent* skin irritation and excoriation. The surrounding skin should be washed with mild soap and water, rinsed thoroughly, and patted dry. The ostomy appliance should be fitted *close to the stoma to further prevent skin irritation*. Although fecal material is measured as output (**Answer 1**), this procedure is *secondary* to control of skin damage. A tight-fitting seal on the drainage bag and a well-ventilated room will decrease odor problems (**Answer 2**). Likewise, a tight-fitting appliance will prevent contamination of the abdominal incision (**Answer 4**).

> **TEST-TAKING TIP**—The key words are "primary objective." Focus on *prevention* of skin excoriation. The gastric enzymes in the ileostomy drainage are very irritating to the tissue surrounding the stoma.
> **PL, COM, 8, M/S: GI, PhI, Reduction of Risk Potential**

77. **(2)** The dialysate is warmed to body temperature before administration to minimize discomfort and optimize clear-

ance of waste products. Warming the fluid tends to dilate the peritoneal vessels, increasing the amount of urea that passes through the membrane. It has little effect on the osmotic gradient (**Answer 1**), does not prevent peritonitis, which is secondary to infection (**Answer 3**), and does not speed infusion time (**Answer 4**), although it does make it more comfortable.

> **TEST-TAKING TIP**—The purpose of dialysis is to act as a filtration when the kidneys are unable to function correctly. Know the effect of "warming"—improves blood flow to an area.
> **PL, APP, 8, M/S: GU, PhI, Reduction of Risk Potential**

78. (3) Deep breathing, coughing, and pursed-lip exhalations are all techniques that the nurse can teach the client to improve ventilation. *Adequate* fluid intake (**Answer 1**) is essential for keeping sputum liquefied; however, very hot and very cold drinks should be avoided because they may cause bronchospasm. Clients with COPD also need to be taught to avoid exposure to infections, early signs of infection, and the need to seek medical intervention promptly should symptoms occur. **Answers 2** and **4** are not indicated in this client's therapy.

> **TEST-TAKING TIP**—Look for an option that makes the client an active participant in the care.
> **IMP, APP, 6, M/S: Resp., PhI, Physiological Adaptation**

79. (2) To read blood gases, first note the pH. In this case, pH is 7.38, which is within the normal range (7.35–7.45) but is on the acidotic side. Next, look at the Pco_2 and HCO_3 to see which one is causing the shift to acidosis. In this case the Pco_2 is 55 (acidosis) and the HCO_3 is 32 (alkalosis). Therefore, the client has compensated respiratory acidosis because the kidneys have been able to conserve enough bicarbonate to keep pH within normal range. In this case a pH below 7.35 would indicate uncompensated respiratory acidosis (**Answer 1**). If the client had uncompensated metabolic alkalosis (**Answer 3**), pH would be above 7.45. If the client had compensated metabolic alkalosis (**Answer 4**), pH would be between 7.41 and 7.45.

> **TEST-TAKING TIP**—Look at each component to determine normal, increased, or decreased. If pH is normal, it has to be *compensated*. Below 7.4 = acidosis; above 7.4 = alkalosis.
> **AN, ANL, 6, M/S: ABG, PhI, Physiological Adaptation**

80. (2) It is not necessary to isolate a client with radioactive implants (**Answer 1**), but to prevent undue exposure to radiation contacts, contact time should be brief and distance between the client and others maximized. Specific instructions as to the amount of time permitted with the client and the safe distance should be posted. **Answers 3** and **4** are incorrect because the best position for the client is supine.

> **TEST-TAKING TIP**—It is important to maintain client position so that the implant is in the correct position; but *none of these options* describes the correct position (lying flat on back). The *other important consideration* is to protect the staff and family visitor from unnecessary exposure. Clients who have radiation implants have active radiation ongoing for a number of hours. Know the concepts of *time* (as short a time of exposure to others as possible), *distance* (stay as far away as possible from the source of radiation), and *shielding* (protect with a lead barrier such as apron) when dealing with radiation therapy.
> **IMP, APP, 1, M/S: Radiation, SECE, Safety and Infection Control**

81. (1) Anemia occurs in cirrhosis due to (a) erythrocyte destruction in the engorged spleen, (b) gastrointestinal blood losses, and (c) folic acid deficiencies from inadequate dietary intake. Kupffer cells (**Answer 2**) line the venous sinusoids in the liver and are primarily macrophagic. **Answers 3** and **4** are incorrect because decreased amino acid breakdown and synthesis result in increasing serum-ammonia levels, which may further inhibit dietary intake.

> **TEST-TAKING TIP**—Use process of elimination and a clue from the stem—anemia; look for low RBCs.
> **AN, COM, 6, M/S: GI, PhI, Physiological Adaptation**

82. (2) Carditis is the only manifestation of rheumatic fever that can lead to permanent damage; the best way to evaluate a child for the presence of carditis is to monitor the apical pulse at least q4h. Growth and development (**Answers 1** and **3**) and ESR (**Answer 4**) deserve *secondary* consideration after checking the apical pulse.

> **TEST-TAKING TIP**—When performing an assessment, *priority* always implies either heart or lungs.
> **AN, ANL, 1, PEDS, PhI, Reduction of Risk Potential**

83. (2) Although the adolescent's parents may perceive this as a parental decision, it is important for the entire family to be included in the decision-making process because the entire family system will be affected by this change. Asking the parents to reassess their feelings (**Answer 1**) may help them evaluate the situation, but it avoids facing the issue as a family decision. A referral may be appropriate (**Answers 3** and **4**); however, all parties involved in the decision must be listened to before making a referral or searching for an alternative placement.

> **TEST-TAKING TIP**—Key phrase: "*most* appropriate." It is most appropriate to involve the family system in decision making related to an adolescent.
> **IMP, ANL, 7, Psych, PsI, Psychosocial Integrity**

84. (2) Although it is not possible to make a client stop smoking, the client should be presented with information about methods used by other people who were successful in stopping. Although most people are aware of the deleterious effects of smoking, clients need to be reminded of the relationship between smoking and their present condition. Fluid intake and nutrition should be discussed and adapted to individual needs. Clients should be able to identify drugs, giving the name, correct dosage, timing, and potential side effects. Alcohol in moderation is not restricted (**Answer 1**). Vocational rehabilitation should be present as an option but *not* emphasized (**Answer 3**). Activities should be *encouraged* to tolerance (**Answer 4**).

> **TEST-TAKING TIP**—Look for the option that is broadest and encompasses the most areas for teaching.
> **IMP, APP, 6, M/S: Resp., PhI, Physiological Adaptation**

85. (2) The client's vital signs and urine output reflect a decrease in extracellular volume secondary to osmotic diuresis. Increased ADH release *decreases* urinary output (**Answer 1**). A hypo-osmolar fluid imbalance is one in which there is more water than solute in the extracellular fluid compartment (**Answer 3**). Like circulatory overload (**Answer 4**), symptoms of a hypo-osmolar imbalance include: widened pulse pressure, increased blood pressure, distended neck veins, and respiratory crackles.

> **TEST-TAKING TIP**—Blood pressure is low and pulse is fast in fluid volume deficit.
> **AN, ANL, 6, M/S: F-E, PhI, Physiological Adaptation**

86. **(2)** After bronchoscopy the client generally produces a large amount of sputum that must be observed carefully for signs of hemorrhage, particularly if a biopsy specimen has been taken during the procedure. Although the sputum is generally blood streaked, any pronounced bleeding should be reported immediately. Patency of the airway is the *first priority*. **Answers 1** and **3** are also observations made after a bronchoscopy. Vital signs are observed until stable, and food and fluids are withheld until the gag reflex returns. **Answer 4,** urticaria, does not occur following bronchoscopy, though it may after a bronchogram if the client reacts to the iodine-based dye.

> **TEST-TAKING TIP**—Think of the organ just examined and look for any signs and symptoms that identify a problem in that organ or system. Priority—assessment of system affected by procedure (e.g., patency of airway).
> **AS, APP, 6, M/S: Dx Test, PhI, Reduction of Risk Potential**

87. **(2)** Position the client who is conscious to sit upright in a supported, forward-leaning position (high-Fowler's, orthopneic) to improve ventilation and oxygenation. A calm and reassuring approach will decrease hyperactivity of the client and oxygen need. Acute respiratory failure is a medical emergency. Aminophylline (**Answer 1**) is indicated to combat bronchospasm, but it is *not an independent nursing* action. Low-flow oxygen (2 L) is also administered to the client in respiratory failure; however, nasal cannulas (**Answer 3**) do not provide predictable O_2 concentrations. A Venturi mask would be more appropriate. **Answer 4** is incorrect because the higher concentration of O_2 (60%) may lead to respiratory depression unless the client is maintained on controlled mechanical ventilation.

> **TEST-TAKING TIP**—Focus on the client first, then the equipment.
> **AN, ANL, 6, M/S: Resp., PhI, Physiological Adaptation**

88. **(1)** Individuals who have used alcohol habitually over an extended time period usually exhibit symptoms of withdrawal delirium when the alcohol intake is severely decreased or curtailed. **Answers 2, 3,** and **4** are less likely reactions.

> **TEST-TAKING TIP**—Note the phrase "most likely to exhibit" and review signs and symptoms of alcohol withdrawal.
> **AS, ANL, 7, Psych, PsI, Psychosocial Integrity**

89. **(2)** Few surgeries warrant immediate treatment (**Answer 1**); however, the urgency of the situation does decrease preparation time. Consequently, the client's physiologic stress will increase, not decrease (**Answer 3**), placing greater demands on metabolic functions and increasing the risk of complications. Emergency surgery does not compromise the use of general anesthesia (**Answer 4**). It is imperative to ascertain before an emergency surgery the time, type, and amount of the last oral intake, as gastric lavage or suctioning may be necessary to prevent aspiration during the surgery. Generally clients are NPO 12 hours before surgery.

> **TEST-TAKING TIP**—When more than one answer looks good look for an answer that is broad and includes another option.
> **AN, APP, 1, M/S: Preop, PhI, Physiological Adaptation**

90. **(1)** The classic sign of Hirschsprung's disease is obstinate constipation that persists despite all efforts of treatment. Normally, when a stool bolus enters the rectum, the internal sphincter relaxes, and the stool is evacuated. In Hirschsprung's disease, the absence of ganglion cells in the affected bowel results in a lack of enteric nervous system stimulation, which decreases the ability of the internal sphincter to relax and obstinate constipation occurs. **Answers 2, 3,** and **4** are incorrect because while other symptoms, such as abdominal distention, anorexia, and vomitus flecked with feces, may be present, they are not generally considered *specific* to Hirschsprung's disease. Symptoms such as abdominal distention, anorexia, and vomitus flecked with feces are *general* symptoms that could be associated with a variety of gastrointestinal disorders. **Answer 5** is incorrect because projectile vomiting is seen most commonly with pyloric stenosis.

> **TEST-TAKING TIP**—Note the use of the word *strong* in the stem of the question; then respond with the answer that is most *specific* for Hirschsprung's disease.
> **AS, APP, 8, PEDS, PhI, Physiological Adaptation**

91. **(2)** Generally, the dwell time of the dialysate is 20–30 minutes, occasionally longer. The dwell time as well as the instillation and outflow times are prescribed by the physician according to the client's needs. Ten to 15 minutes (**Answer 1**) is too short a time to allow for diffusion of waste products. Equilibrium between dialysate and body fluids occurs in 15–30 minutes. Longer times (**Answers 3** and **4**) are not necessary.

> **TEST-TAKING TIP**—Think about what is happening in the procedure and determine how long it would take to be effective.
> **IMP, COM, 1, M/S: Renal, PhI, Physiological Adaptation**

92. **(4)** Indications of respiratory distress and the increased work of breathing in this client are characterized by the use of the accessory muscles of respiration, the sternocleidomastoid and trapezius muscles. Using these muscles enables the client to *increase the size* of the thorax, thus allowing air to move in. Clients with chronic bronchitis and air trapping generally are *not* able to increase the depth of breathing (**Answer 1**) by increasing diaphragmatic excursion (**Answer 2**). Some clients may be using pursed-lip exhalations (**Answer 3**), but these help maintain open airways for the expulsion of gases.

> **TEST-TAKING TIP**—Visualize the client. If the client was "working" to take in a breath, what would you see?
> **AS, APP, 6, M/S: Resp., PhI, Physiological Adaptation**

93. **(1)** Lithium is excreted through the kidneys. Consequently, the kidneys must function adequately to avoid lithium toxicity. Diuretics should *not* be given concurrently with lithium because they may potentiate sodium and fluid depletion, which may lead to lithium toxicity. Haloperidol (Haldol) (**Answer 4**) is a major tranquilizer that is sometimes administered simultaneously with lithium during the first week to 10 days to control manic symptoms. Nausea, vomiting, and muscle weakness (**Answer 3**) are all possible side effects of lithium. They indicate a need for close observation and regulation of the drug if they disrupt the person's level of functioning. Every client should be screened before the administration of any medication (**Answer 2**). However, because lithium is a drug that is taken over a long period of time, blood levels must be consistently regulated and physical examinations routinely scheduled (every 3 months initially; then every 6 months once the client appears to be regulated).

> **TEST-TAKING TIP**—Note the phrase "least relevant" and turn this into a "true or false" question. Know that lithium is a salt depleter; therefore, diuretics should *not* be given.
> **EV, ANL, 7, Psych, PhI, Pharmacological Therapy**

94. **(1)** Local anesthesia is used in cataract surgery, not only because this surgery is a short procedure but also because

most clients are elderly, with one chronic disease or more, which may be exacerbated by general anesthesia (**Answer 2**). Intravenous anesthesia (**Answer 3**) with thiopental sodium (Pentothal) is most frequently used when unconsciousness is desirable for short procedures or when an anesthetic induction is desired for general anesthesia. Rectal anesthesia (**Answer 4**), though rarely used today, has been employed to induce short-term anesthesia in children.

> **TEST-TAKING TIP**—The procedure is fast, and the eye is easily anesthetized. Most clients are elderly, and are high risk with general anesthesia.
> **IMP, COM, 2, M/S: Eye, PhI, Reduction of Risk Potential**

95. (2) The evening before an intravenous pyelogram (IVP), the client is administered oral cathartics or enemas to clean the bowel of fecal material and flatus, thereby improving visualization of the kidneys and ureters. The radiopaque dye used in this procedure is injected by a physician in the radiology department, not by the nurse before the procedure (**Answer 1**). **Answer 3** is *not* part of IVP preparation. If the client is having difficulty maintaining fluid volume balance, an intravenous infusion *may* be initiated to prevent dehydration, but it is not standard (**Answer 4**).

> **TEST-TAKING TIP**—If the intestine was not empty, would visualization of the kidney be accurate?
> **PL, APP, 8, M/S: Dx Test, PhI, Reduction of Risk Potential**

96. (1) Adolescents are preoccupied with their changing bodies, their relationships, and their fantasies. Although they have difficulty with rote learning (**Answer 2**), they have an increased potential for imaginative thinking. During this period they are less able to concentrate on their academic work (**Answer 3**), which leads to increased feelings of frustration that are usually *not* accompanied by an increased ability to cope (**Answer 4**).

> **TEST-TAKING TIP**—Know age-appropriate behavior.
> **EV, APP, 5, PEDS, PsI, Psychosocial Integrity**

97. (1) The observed total lung capacity (TLC), functional residual capacity (FRC), and residual volume (RV) are all increased over expected values. These values indicate that the client is hyperinflated, a common phenomenon with air obstruction and air trapping. Hyperventilation is characterized by an increase in P_{O_2} and pH (**Answer 2**). Hyperpnea is simply an increase in respiratory rate (**Answer 3**). Hypercapnia is identified when P_{CO_2} is elevated (**Answer 4**).

> **TEST-TAKING TIP**—Look at the *total* capacity (TLC). Visualize a balloon—hyperinflated.
> **AN, ANL, 6, M/S: Resp., PhI, Physiological Adaptation**

98. (3) Glycogenolysis and therefore serum-glucose levels are increased due to the stresses of surgery. To control blood-glucose levels and prevent ketoacidosis, *secondary* to increased tissue metabolism (**Answer 1**), regular insulin is given in doses adjusted according to the results of urine tests (rainbow or sliding scale). Regular insulin may be given alone until results of urine tests for glucosuria and ketonuria stabilize or as a supplement along with an intermediate-acting insulin such as NPH. **Answer 2**, decreased insulin production, results from the extent of the client's *dysfunction*, *not* the stress of surgery. Insulin does facilitate the movement of potassium across the cellular membrane, thus preventing hyperkalemia (**Answer 4**) but this is *not* the *best* answer.

> **TEST-TAKING TIP**—Think of the stress reaction and its effects on the body. Increased stress leads to increased glucose level.
> **AN, COM, 4, M/S: Postop, PhI, Pharmacological and Parenteral Therapies**

99. (2) The 18-year-old may have valid reasons for wanting to visit a friend, but allowing the client to visit without assessing motives (**Answer 1**) may prove detrimental to the client, to the friend, and to the staff. The parents (**Answer 3**) essentially relinquished their decision-making authority by allowing their child to live in the group home. The hospital staff would have to be consulted before the visit, regardless of the client's motive. However, **Answer 4** is too vague, in that it does not specify what issues would be covered in the consultation.

> **TEST-TAKING TIP**—Key word: "assess," the first step of the nursing process.
> **IMP, ANL, 7, Psych, PsI, Psychosocial Integrity**

100. (3, 5) **Answer 3** is correct because in early respiratory obstruction, the client generally complains of difficulty swallowing and a feeling of fullness or a choking sensation. Difficulty swallowing without the complaint of fullness or choking may be due to tracheal irritation from the surgery. **Answer 5** is correct because choking, a feeling of fullness combined with difficulty swallowing, would be early indications of a potential airway obstruction. **Answer 1** is incorrect because hoarseness is *common* following thyroidectomy and is secondary to edema of the larynx. **Answer 2** is incorrect because it would be a *late* sign of airway obstruction and respiratory distress. **Answer 4** is incorrect because cyanosis would be a *late* sign of respiratory obstruction.

> **TEST-TAKING TIP**—Differentiate *early* signs from *late* signs.
> **AS, ANL, 6, M/S: Resp., PhI, Physiological Adaptation**

Final Test

Sally L. Lagerquist • Janice McMillin • Robyn Nelson • Kathleen Snider

WHAT IS THE FINAL TEST?

The **Final Test** is a multiple-choice exam with 4, 5, or 6 options designed to assess your baseline nursing knowledge and evaluate your ability to apply that knowledge to various clinical situations and to items presented in a simulated NCLEX-RN® exam. Self-analysis of your scores will help you prioritize what to study by identifying your individual problem areas.

Written to reflect the content framework and the purpose of the NCLEX-RN® Test Plan (to measure a candidate's ability to practice safely and effectively as a Registered Nurse in an entry-level position), the **Final Test** can be used as preparation and review for the licensure examination. It can also be used for review by *nurses returning to active practice* and by **international nurses** who are *graduates of nursing schools* outside of the United States and are preparing for qualifying examinations.

Each question on the **Final Test** was field tested in a pilot test given to NCLEX-RN® candidates representing a wide geographic distribution, as well as various types of nursing programs.

Selection of Content and Distribution of the Questions

The **Final Test** is composed of 100 content-integrated, multiple-choice questions, most with four options. *One of the answers is most complete and therefore the best choice.* The other three answers (distractors) are not always wrong but are usually not as complete or as important as the best answer. In addition, five alternate item format questions have been added to this test, where you will be asked to *select all that apply* from 5–6 options.

Using a nursing process framework, the questions on the **Final Test** reflect nursing situations that involve different clinical areas and diagnoses. As on the NCLEX-RN®, the number of questions for each content area varies. The percentage distribution of items in this test related to client

needs follows the NCLEX-RN® blueprint (see **Table 1.1** in **Unit 1,** Orientation, for percentages).

Based on the blueprint for the *Test Plan for The National Council Licensure Examination* (NCLEX-RN®) published by the National Council of State Boards of Nursing, Inc., the **Final Test** assesses your knowledge, skills, and abilities in the five phases of the *nursing process:* Assessment (AS), Analysis (AN), Plan (PL), Implementation (IMP), and Evaluation (EV), and **four** broad areas of *client needs:* Safe, Effective Care Environment (SECE), Physiological Integrity (PhI), Psychosocial Integrity (PsI), and Health Promotion and Maintenance (HPM); and six *client subneeds,* including eight detailed areas of *human functions* (Protective; Sensory-Perceptual; Comfort, Rest, Activity and Mobility; Nutrition; Growth and Development; Fluid-Gas Transport; Psychosocial-Cultural; Elimination). Each question in the **Final Test** has been classified according to the above categories, and according to clinical area.

Timing

Allow about 1 minute per question. Time yourself and plan to complete the 100-question test in no more than 1 hour and 40 minutes. Simulate test-taking conditions by having uninterrupted time of 1 hour and 40 minutes, or divide the exam into two sessions of 50 questions for 50 minutes for each session.

Test Results

When you check your answers, keep track not only of how many are incorrect, but also how many are incorrect in *each category* of nursing process, client needs, and human functions.

Suggestions for Further Study

You can use your test results, in combination with the following appendices, to assess your NCLEX-RN® strengths and weaknesses.

I. When you have problems with **types** of questions · Refer to Appendix:

    A. **Nursing process**
       1. Definitions/Descriptions · F
       2. Index to nursing process *questions* · G

II. When you have problems with **content/subject areas** · Refer to Appendix:

    A. **Client needs** (4 broad categories and 6 client subneeds)
       1. Definitions/Descriptions · B
       2. Index to *content* · C
       3. Index to *practice questions that cover these content areas* · D, E

    B. **Human functions** (8 specific concepts and detailed areas)
       1. Definitions/Descriptions · H
       2. Index to *content* · I
       3. Index to *practice questions that cover these content areas* · J

You now have an individualized evaluation with which to develop your plan for *what* you need to study and *where* to find the material for further study. Our good wishes for your success!

QUESTIONS

Select the one answer that is best for each question, unless otherwise directed.

1. In assessing a woman's reasons for suspecting she may be 3 months pregnant, the most relevant question for the nurse to ask would be:
   1. "Are you currently taking oral contraceptives?"
   2. "When was your last menstrual period?"
   3. "How much weight have you gained?"
   4. "Have you been pregnant before?"

2. Postoperative orders include "IV of D5 $\frac{1}{4}$ NS at 75 mL per hour." At 7:00 P.M., a new 1000 mL bag of fluid is hung. If the IV infuses at the prescribed rate, how much fluid should be left in the bag at 7:00 A.M.?
   1. 100 mL.
   2. 900 mL.
   3. Nothing should be left; bag should be empty.
   4. Not enough information is given to determine this.

3. As a client with a cardiac condition gets up to use the commode, he turns ashen and is diaphoretic. Vital signs are as follows: BP 128/60; pulse 42; respirations 24. EKG shows patterns of complete heart block. The nurse knows that the client's signs and symptoms are related to:
   1. Inability of heart to increase its rate during exertion.
   2. Insufficient blood flow to the coronary arteries.
   3. Increased stroke volume.
   4. Inability of the circulatory reflexes to increase venous return.

4. Preoperative teaching includes deep breathing and coughing. What is the *least* desired outcome of the teaching plan? The client:
   1. States the rationale for repeating these exercises every 1–2 hours postoperatively.
   2. Demonstrates coughing technique.

3. Inhales through both nose and mouth and raises abdomen with each respiration.
   4. States the need to repeat exercises until feeling light-headed.

5. If the first day of a pregnant woman's last menstrual period (LMP) was July 10, what is her baby's expected date of delivery (EDD)?
   1. April 17.
   2. May 30.
   3. March 14.
   4. June 1.

6. At 7:00 A.M., the night nurse hangs a new 500 mL bag of D5 $\frac{1}{2}$ NS and adjusts the flow rate to 35 mL/hr per MD order. If the IV infuses at the proper rate, how much fluid should be left in the bag when the day nurse makes rounds at 11:30 A.M., halfway through the shift?
   1. 160 mL.
   2. 250 mL.
   3. 340 mL.
   4. Unable to determine.

7. The nurse should know that the majority of amputations are attributed to:
   1. Chemical burns.
   2. Diabetic ulcers.
   3. Arteriosclerosis obliterans.
   4. Bone tumors.

8. An 18-year-old is admitted to the hospital with a compound fracture of the left tibia and patella following a minibike accident. The fractures are repaired surgically, and a long leg cast is applied. During the first night in the hospital, the client complains of severe pain in the left leg. At this time, it would be most appropriate for the nurse to:
   1. Obtain more information about the characteristics of the pain.
   2. Give the client a dose of "Demerol 50 mg IM prn q4–6h" as ordered.
   3. Reassure the client that the pain will diminish in a few days.
   4. Distract the client by turning on the television.

9. When caring for a child who has received a diazepam (Valium) "IV push" × 2 during a procedure, which vital sign should the nurse evaluate *first*?
   1. Temperature.
   2. Pulse.
   3. Respirations.
   4. Blood pressure.

10. An infant weighs 3500 g. The recommended dose for oral ampicillin is 50–100 mg/kg/24 hrs divided q 6 hrs. What is the maximum daily dose that the nurse can safely administer? *Fill in the blank.*
    —————mg

11. The nurse has established the unresponsiveness of a client. After the airway is opened, the next nursing action would be to:
    1. Look, listen, and feel for breathing.
    2. Pinch the client's nostrils and give two full breaths.
    3. Check the client's carotid pulse for 5–10 seconds.
    4. Finger sweep the client's mouth for any foreign object.

12. A client is to be discharged on a 2 g sodium diet. The nurse would know that the client understands the dietary limitations if he or she selected:
    1. Filet of sole, tossed salad with lemon juice, coffee.
    2. Chow mein, fried rice, tea.
    3. Canned tomato soup, unsalted crackers, skim milk.
    4. Two hot dogs with mustard, macaroni salad, ginger ale.

13. Which recreational activity will most likely be restricted for an adult following recovery from pacemaker insertion?
    1. Swimming.
    2. Fashioning lamps from driftwood and metal.
    3. Operating ham radio.
    4. Playing golf.

14. After determining that a client is pulseless, the nurse would begin adult one-person CPR at a minimum compression rate of:
    1. 60 compressions per minute.
    2. 80 compressions per minute.
    3. 90 compressions per minute.
    4. 100 compressions per minute.

15. With which risk factor does sudden infant death syndrome (SIDS) occur most frequently?
    1. Hispanic.
    2. Low birth weight.
    3. Midrange socioeconomic status.
    4. Breastfeeding.

16. After a client returns from surgery following craniotomy, the nurse knows that the optimum positioning of a client after neurosurgery, unless otherwise indicated, would be:
    1. Flat on back.
    2. Head elevated 30 degrees.
    3. Head elevated 45 degrees.
    4. Head elevated 90 degrees.

17. On turning a client who has had a right modified mastectomy to her left side, the nurse notes a moderately large amount of serosanguineous drainage on the bedsheets. The nurse should:
    1. Remove the dressing to ascertain the origin of the bleeding.
    2. Milk the Hemovac tubing, using a downward motion.
    3. Note vital signs, reinforce the dressing, and notify the surgeon immediately.
    4. Recognize that this is a frequent occurrence with this type of surgery.

18. A couple who are expecting a baby is informed that a cesarean will be performed immediately. The couple inquires whether the mother must be put to sleep. The most appropriate nursing response would be to:
    1. Refer the couple to the anesthesiologist.
    2. Ask the attending physician to explain the procedure to the couple.
    3. Tell the couple that she probably will receive general anesthesia.
    4. Inform the couple that most women who have a cesarean birth receive spinal anesthesia.

19. What should the nurse see in the vomitus that is characteristic of infants with pyloric stenosis?
    1. Stomach contents only.
    2. Stomach contents plus bile.
    3. Stomach contents streaked with blood.
    4. Stomach contents with flecks of feces.

20. Which system should the nurse monitor carefully for possible toxic effects of EDTA?
    1. Neurological.
    2. Renal.
    3. Cardiovascular.
    4. Hematological.

21. The nurse knows that a modified radical mastectomy involves removal of:
    1. The breast only.
    2. The breast and axillary nodes.

3. The breast, pectoralis major muscle, and axillary lymph nodes.
4. The breast, underlying chest muscle, axillary lymph nodes, and internal mammary lymph nodes.

22. A child admitted to rule out intussusception is scheduled for a barium enema. The nurse should teach the child's parents that the major purpose of this procedure is to:
    1. Confirm the diagnosis.
    2. Reduce the telescoping.
    3. Ease the passage of stool.
    4. Provide symptomatic relief.

23. At 2:30 A.M., the nurse hangs a 1000 mL bottle of IV fluid. If the IV infuses at 110 mL per hour as ordered, how much fluid should infuse by 6:00 A.M.?
    1. 385 mL.
    2. 500 mL.
    3. 615 mL.
    4. 740 mL.

24. On the third day of hospitalization following an anterior MI, a client becomes increasingly restless. Pulse rate has increased to 126 beats per minute. The first nursing action is to:
    1. Do a partial physical assessment, which includes vital signs, pulmonary auscultation, and cognitive functions.
    2. Ask if the client is upset, because depression is common on the third day of hospitalization.
    3. Readminister oxygen per nasal catheter (prongs or tongs) at 6 liters, because restlessness is an early sign of cerebral hypoxia.
    4. Decrease the rate of intravenous infusion to prevent fluid volume overload.

25. While observing a client throughout a blood transfusion, the nurse should be alert to which possible sign of a hemolytic reaction?
    1. Urticaria.
    2. Polyuria.
    3. Flank pain.
    4. Hypothermia.

26. In considering the equipment for Bryant's traction, the nurse should expect to see:
    1. A Kirschner wire in the fractured femur.
    2. A Steinmann pin in the fractured femur.
    3. Adhesive material taped to the skin of both legs.
    4. Adhesive material taped to the skin of the fractured leg only.

27. The nurse has discussed important aspects of breastfeeding with a new mother. To evaluate the effects of the teaching, the nurse asks her to put it in her own words. Which response indicates a need for further teaching?
    1. "Rest and relaxation are essential."
    2. "An adequate diet is important."
    3. "Large breasts produce more milk."
    4. "Birth control is necessary throughout breastfeeding if I don't want to become pregnant."

28. In discussing what clothes a toddler with eczema should wear, both in the hospital and at home, the nurse would be most correct in teaching the mother that this child should wear only:
    1. Cotton.
    2. Linen.
    3. Natural wool.
    4. Polyester blend.

29. A client with a left leg fracture is to be taught the three-point gait before discharge. Which instruction should the nurse give to this client?

1. "Advance your right crutch, swing the left foot forward, advance the left crutch, and then bring the right foot forward."
2. "Move your right crutch and left foot forward together, and then swing the right foot and left crutch in one movement."
3. "While partially bearing weight on your left leg, advance both crutches and then bring your right leg forward."
4. "Using one movement, advance your left foot and both crutches and then bring your right leg forward."

30. Immediately after general anesthesia, a client has an airway in place and is in a supine position. To prevent airway obstruction, the nurse should:
    1. Leave the airway tube in and turn the client's head to the side.
    2. Maintain the client's present position.
    3. Remove the airway tube and turn the client's head to the side.
    4. Remove the airway tube and maintain the client's prone position.

31. A woman who had rheumatic fever in early childhood is admitted to labor and delivery in active labor at 38 weeks' gestation. When planning her care, which nursing intervention(s) would be appropriate for this client?
    Select all that apply.
    1. Preparing a fluid bolus of lactated Ringer's solution to ensure good hydration.
    2. Closely monitoring maternal heart rate during labor.
    3. Encouraging valsalva pushing during the second stage of labor.
    4. Encouraging client to rest on her side during labor.
    5. Preparing client for a labor epidural to decrease pain.

32. A client with a history of substance abuse asks the nurse not to tell anyone about the client smoking a marijuana joint in the hospital room, and the client promises to never do it again. The nurse should realize that this client is *mostly*:
    1. Being sincere and wanting to change.
    2. Seeking attention.
    3. Being manipulative.
    4. Trying to avoid punishment.

33. The proper method of suctioning a tracheostomy tube includes:
    1. Suctioning only while inserting the catheter.
    2. Suctioning only while withdrawing the catheter.
    3. Suctioning during both insertion and withdrawal of the catheter.
    4. Suctioning on insertion only if secretions are copious.

34. To help a preschooler cope most effectively with repeated painful injections of EDTA, the nurse should:
    1. Teach the mother the importance of bringing favorite toys.
    2. Encourage the child to spend most of the day in the playroom, engaged in free play.
    3. Offer the opportunity for therapeutic play.
    4. Allow play with other preschool children as much as the child wants.

35. Which arm position will best facilitate venous return on the operative side of a client who has had a modified mastectomy, and reduce the occurrence of lymphedema?
    1. Semi-Fowler's position with the elbow flexed and the arm across the chest.
    2. Low-Fowler's position with the arm elevated so that the hand and elbow are slightly higher than the shoulder.
    3. High-Fowler's position with the elbow flexed and the right hand positioned next to the head.
    4. Adduction of the shoulder, extension of the elbow, and flexion of the wrist.

36. The most important aspect of treatment for a client who is a substance abuser is:
    1. Teaching the client about the hazards of taking drugs.
    2. Informing the client that using drugs is illegal.
    3. Encouraging the client to want to change behavior.
    4. Assisting the client to develop alternative coping mechanisms.

37. Two hours after a child returns to the unit following cardiac catheterization, the dressing is soaked with bright-red blood. The nurse first reinforces the dressing. What should the nurse do next?
    1. Check vital signs.
    2. Increase the flow rate of the IV.
    3. Place the child in reverse Trendelenburg position.
    4. Notify the cardiologist.

38. A client is awaiting the insertion of a permanent pacemaker because of complete heart block. The nurse knows that isoproterenol hydrochloride (Isuprel) is used for this client because of which effect?
    1. Beta-mimetic.
    2. Cardiac glycoside.
    3. Anticholinergic.
    4. Beta-blocker.

39. A client has had an above-the-knee amputation on the left side. While being repositioned onto the abdomen, the client cannot turn because the "left foot is causing too much pain." The first response by the nurse should be:
    1. To insist that the client lie on the abdomen.
    2. To ignore the comment and state that the nurse will return later.
    3. To discuss the principle of phantom pain after amputation.
    4. To offer some form of pain control.

40. During a predischarge teaching session for a client who has had a permanent pacemaker inserted, the client's wife states, "Don't worry, I'll be sure that he obeys the doctor's orders to the letter." The nurse's best response would be:
    1. "I can see that with your help, he should do just fine."
    2. "Are you worried?"
    3. "I'm not worried. You both have a lot of common sense."
    4. "This has been a difficult period for both of you. Can you foresee any problems with these instructions?"

41. Upon return from the OR at 11:30 A.M., a client has 425 mL left in an IV bag of 5% dextrose and $\frac{1}{2}$ NS. The postop MD orders include "IV to infuse at 320 mL every 8 hours." When should the nurse anticipate having to change the IV bag?
    1. 3:00 P.M.
    2. 6:00 P.M.
    3. 9:00 P.M.
    4. 12:00 midnight.

42. Before entering a client's room, the nurse should wash her or his hands for a minimum of:
    1. 10 seconds.
    2. 30 seconds.
    3. 45 seconds.
    4. 60 seconds.

43. The preoperative medications ordered by the anesthesiologist are morphine sulfate, 15 mg, and atropine SO_4, 0.4 mg, subcutaneously. The nurse can expect to give these drugs:
    1. Right before the client leaves for surgery.
    2. 45–60 minutes before anesthetic induction.
    3. 20–30 minutes before anesthetic induction.
    4. 10–15 minutes before anesthetic induction.

44. The nurse knows that a person who is on a bland diet may *lack* which essential nutrient?

1. Vitamin C.
2. Carbohydrates.
3. Protein.
4. Vitamin A.

45. When assessing a client who has been abusing amphetamines, which symptom would the nurse expect to see?
    1. Bradycardia.
    2. Increased irritability.
    3. Hypotension.
    4. Constipation.

46. Which action is *least* likely to be within the role and legal responsibilities of the nurse who is assisting with an amniocentesis?
    1. Informing the woman about the risks involved in amniocentesis.
    2. Explaining/reinforcing how the procedure will be done.
    3. Monitoring the fetal heart rate.
    4. Observing the woman for signs of bleeding or contractions after the procedure is completed.

47. Two weeks after a cast is applied, a foul odor is detected at the lower end of the cast. A window is made in the cast over the infected area and an antibiotic is prescribed. After 3 days on antibiotic therapy, which effect would be most indicative of a therapeutic response?
    1. White blood cell count is 7900/mm^3.
    2. Temperature is 99.4°F.
    3. No complaints of pain.
    4. Appetite is fairly good.

48. Which drugs may the nurse administer to prevent pseudoparkinsonism?
    Select all that apply.
    1. Trihexyphenidyl HCL (Artane).
    2. Diphenhydramine (Benadryl).
    3. Chlorpromazine HCL (Thorazine).
    4. Benztropine (Cogentin).
    5. Trifluoperazine HCL (Stelazine).
    6. Risperidone (Risperdal).

49. What will the nurse encourage a client, who has had a modified right mastectomy, to do which is appropriate as *initial* therapy 24 hours after surgery?
    1. Self-feeding and hair combing.
    2. Passive/active flexion and extension of the elbow and pronation and supination of the wrist.
    3. Abduction and external rotation of the right shoulder.
    4. Early ambulation and active extension and flexion of the elbow.

50. The doctor orders Burow's solution soaks for a toddler with eczema. In order to gain the toddler's cooperation with this treatment, the nurse should tell the toddler:
    1. "Let's do this real fast and then you can see mommy and daddy."
    2. "You don't want to have to stay here forever, do you? Let's make you all better now!"
    3. "This medicine will help you get better so you can go home. Help me pour some on your arms."
    4. "This is magic medicine that will make all your boo-boos go away. Don't you want to chase away those boo-boos?"

51. While preparing a client's preoperative medication, the nurse notes that the atropine SO$_4$ on hand is in a strength of 0.6 mg/mL. The prescribed dosage is 0.4 mg. The correct amount of atropine to administer is:
    1. 1.5 mL.
    2. 1 mL.
    3. 10 minims.
    4. 8 minims.

52. The rationale for using humidified oxygen with tracheal tubes is that:
    1. It is a traditional procedure.
    2. It is a means of providing fluid intake.
    3. It decreases insensible water loss.
    4. The natural humidifying pathway has been bypassed.

53. Parents of a 6-month-old infant bring the infant in for a physical examination; all immunizations are up-to-date. This infant should receive three of the following immunizations at this time; which immunization should not be given?
    1. Hepatitis B.
    2. Diphtheria, tetanus, and pertussis (DTaP).
    3. *H. influenzae* type b.
    4. Measles, mumps, rubella.

54. An IV rate is to be regulated to keep vein open (KVO). The nurse knows that the longest possible time that a single 1000 mL bottle or bag can infuse safely is:
    1. 24 hours.
    2. 5 hours.
    3. 18 hours.
    4. 12 hours.

55. The nurse should know that the best position to check an adolescent for scoliosis is:
    1. Standing up straight.
    2. Lying flat on the stomach.
    3. Standing and bending 90 degrees at the waist.
    4. Sitting in a straight-back chair.

56. A unit of blood is ordered for a client when the BP drops to 90/60. What is the most important safeguard before administering blood?
    1. Refrigerate unit of blood until immediately before giving.
    2. Agitate the blood so it is well mixed.
    3. Carefully check labeled blood against client's wristband.
    4. Infuse the blood through a blood warmer.

57. Potassium chloride is to be added to an infant's intravenous fluids. Before adding this electrolyte, the nurse should determine that:
    1. The infant has voided recently.
    2. Moro reflex is present.
    3. Respiratory rate is between 25 and 40.
    4. Mucous membranes are moist.

58. When a client is admitted to the unit following an appendectomy, the *first* action the nurse should take is to:
    1. Attach nasogastric tube to suction.
    2. Calculate the IV flow rate and adjust the drip.
    3. Monitor vital signs.
    4. Check client's ID band.

59. The nurse planning to administer a unit of blood to a child should know that after it is removed from the refrigerator, the blood should be transfused within:
    1. Six hours.
    2. Two hours.
    3. Four hours.
    4. One hour.

60. In observing women in the latent phase of the first stage of labor, which behavior would the nurse expect to see?
    1. Tendency to hyperventilate.
    2. Euphoria, excitement, and talkativeness.
    3. Fairly quiet and introverted behavior.
    4. Irritability and crying.

61. What would the nurse expect to find when doing an assessment of a person who has a history of substance abuse:
    1. An individual who is very assertive.
    2. An individual who is very dependent.

3. An individual who is very mature.

4. An individual who is very aggressive.

62. A client has had a permanent pacemaker inserted, with the pacing catheter introduced into the right external jugular vein and positioned in the right ventricle. Which nursing care activity is the nurse's first priority in the *early* postimplantation period?
    1. Restricting activity to prevent pacing catheter displacement.
    2. Monitoring the EKG continually, noting rhythm, rate, appearance, and amplitude of pacing spike.
    3. Implementing passive range-of-motion exercise to the right arm to prevent "frozen shoulder."
    4. Maintaining sterile dressings over the operative site to prevent infection.

63. A client takes secobarbital (Seconal) whenever feeling "too stressed," such as whenever there is an exam or whenever the client feels too pressured, which happens at least four or five times a week. The nurse should be aware that large doses of secobarbital can cause:
    1. Tachycardia.
    2. Hypertension.
    3. Assaultive behavior.
    4. Increased respirations.

64. The nursing assistant caring for a child in Bryant's traction reports that the child's buttocks are resting on the mattress. The nurse would be most correct in telling the nursing assistant that:
    1. This is where the buttocks should be.
    2. The buttocks should be slightly off the mattress.
    3. This is the responsibility of the nurse.
    4. The child will need special skin care to avoid pressure areas or breakdown.

65. Which nursing intervention for a client with a Hemovac is *inappropriate*?
    1. Observing and recording the amount and color of the drainage.
    2. Maintaining suction by emptying and recompressing the apparatus regularly.
    3. Increasing suction by attaching the Hemovac to wall suction as the drainage increases.
    4. Preventing traction on the drainage tubes by repositioning the Hemovac each time the client is repositioned.

66. The nurse would interpret a client's central venous pressure (CVP) as normal if the pressure were:
    1. 4–10 cm H_2O.
    2. 20–30 mm Hg.
    3. 10–20 cm H_2O.
    4. 7–14 mm Hg.

67. The nurse recognizes dyspnea as:
    1. Increased awareness of respiratory effort.
    2. Decreased alveolar ventilation.
    3. Increased rate and depth of respiration.
    4. Decreased oxygen saturation of venous blood.

68. A client asks what type of anesthesia is usually used during vein-stripping. The nurse tells the client to expect:
    1. Local.
    2. Topical.
    3. Regional.
    4. General.

69. In reviewing an infant's admission history, the nurse should anticipate that intussusception most typically presents with which of the following assessment findings?
    Select all that apply.
    1. Inconsolable crying.
    2. Crampy abdominal pain.

3. Drawing up of knees to the chest.

4. Bloody stools.

5. "Currant jelly" stools.

6. Non-bile stained emesis.

70. The nurse finds a marijuana joint under an adolescent client's pillow. After being confronted, the client promises not to smoke marijuana again if the nurse will not report the incident. The nurse fears that the client is being manipulative. The *most* therapeutic nursing intervention when working with clients who are manipulative is to:
    1. Make decisions for them.
    2. Reinforce use of alternative behaviors.
    3. Set rigid limits.
    4. Confront them in front of others.

71. A client with a history of many years of smoking and a smoker's cough is scheduled for bilateral herniorrhaphy. Which type of surgical anesthesia may be most appropriate for this situation?
    1. General.
    2. Intravenous.
    3. Spinal.
    4. Local infiltration.

72. Pulmonary function testing on a client with a long history of smoking revealed a vital capacity within normal limits but a reduced forced expiratory volume (FEV_1).
    The nurse explains to the family that this means that the client:
    1. Has difficulty moving air in and out of the lungs.
    2. May have some airway obstruction.
    3. Has weakened expiratory muscles of respirations.
    4. May have some areas of atelectasis in the lungs.

73. New parents of an infant with a cleft lip and palate are experiencing a reactive depression in response to the birth of their infant, who is in the high-risk newborn nursery. The primary difference between a reactive (situational) depression and major depressive disorder—melancholic type (endogenous depression) is that in a reactive depression:
    1. There is substantial weight loss, usually over 10 pounds.
    2. The individual does not respond to environmental stimuli.
    3. The individual generally feels worse as the day progresses.
    4. The precipitating event is usually difficult to identify.

74. A client has a long leg cast due to a fractured right tibia and fibula. Which is an appropriate exercise for this client to prevent complications of immobility?
    1. Quadriceps setting.
    2. Extension of the right knee.
    3. Passive range of motion of the hip.
    4. Flexion of the right knee.

75. A toddler who fractured the right femur in a car accident is placed in Bryant's traction and admitted to the hospital. During the first night in the hospital, the toddler lies still in the crib, sucks a thumb, and occasionally sobs quietly in a monotone voice. The nurse should interpret these behaviors to mean that the toddler:
    1. Wants the mother.
    2. Might prefer to sleep in a bed.
    3. Probably does not sleep through the night at home.
    4. May be experiencing painful muscle spasms due to the fracture.

76. The parents of an infant born with a cleft lip and palate express concern about caring for their baby. They are especially worried about paying excessive hospital bills because insurance has set limits. The most appropriate nursing action would be to:

1. Refer the couple to a social worker.
2. Validate the couple's perceived needs.
3. Discuss alternatives with the couple.
4. Implement health teaching regarding the physical care of the baby.

77. The nurse concludes that an intradermal TB test result is positive if the following is present:
    1. An induration of 10 mm or more.
    2. An induration of 10 cm or more.
    3. An induration of 5–9 mm.
    4. A hivelike vesicle.

78. What side effects would a client demonstrate if he or she received hyperalimentation solution at too rapid an infusion rate?
    1. Cellular dehydration and potassium depletion.
    2. Circulatory overload and hypoglycemia.
    3. Hypoglycemia and hypovolemia.
    4. Potassium excess and congestive heart failure.

79. When teaching families about cleft lip and palate, the nurse would need to be aware that:
    1. Cleft lip occurs most frequently in girls.
    2. Cleft palate occurs most frequently in boys.
    3. Cleft lip and palate almost always occur simultaneously.
    4. Cleft lip and palate are both influenced by hereditary factors.

80. A 3-month-old infant brought unconscious to the emergency department (ED) by the parents was pronounced dead. The mother becomes hysterical, crying uncontrollably. The father asks the nurse to "do something." The most appropriate nursing action would be:
    1. Providing the parents with privacy.
    2. Obtaining an order for a tranquilizer.
    3. Sitting quietly with the couple.
    4. Asking the mother to calm down.

81. A woman is in preterm labor and is bleeding. She requests a sip of water after being in labor for 2 hours in the hospital. The most appropriate nursing action would be:
    1. Checking the physician's orders.
    2. Giving her a small sip of water.
    3. Offering her ice chips.
    4. Telling her she cannot have fluids at this time.

82. A mother states that the pediatrician told her that her infant has numerous allergies, including milk allergies. Which formula should the nurse offer?
    1. Lofenalac.
    2. Enfamil.
    3. Similac with iron.
    4. Isomil.

83. What information would receive the *least* emphasis in the nurse's predischarge education plan for a client who has had a permanent pacemaker inserted?
    1. Rationale for pacemaker implantation.
    2. Pacemaker function and signs indicating malfunction.
    3. Therapeutic program, including medication, diet, activity schedule, and safety precautions.
    4. Necessity for periodic follow-up visits to physician.

84. The nurse needs to know that SIDS usually occurs:
    1. Within 2–4 weeks after birth.
    2. Between 2 and 4 months after birth.
    3. More than 6 months after birth.
    4. Between 6 and 9 months after birth.

85. The nurse must recognize the side effects of morphine and atropine administration given preoperatively, which include:

1. Bradycardia, anorexia, and decreased urine output.
2. Hypertension, nausea, vomiting, tachycardia.
3. Hypotension, cotton mouth, nausea, and vomiting.
4. Dryness, cotton mouth, constricted pupils, and bradycardia.

86. The MD orders an IV of D_5W at 40 mL/hr. A 500 mL bag, with a pediatric microdrip chamber, is hung at 11:00 A.M. At 3:15 P.M., the nurse notes that the bag has 100 mL left. What should be the nurse's initial action?
    1. Readjust the flow rate to 40 microdrops per minute.
    2. Hang a new 500 mL bag of fluid.
    3. Maintain the flow rate at 20 microdrops per minute until the IV is back on schedule.
    4. Notify the physician.

87. The nurse would expect to find drug abuse *least* prevalent in:
    1. An upper socioeconomic family.
    2. An elderly individual.
    3. A lower socioeconomic family.
    4. An adolescent.

88. The nurse must assess past medical history and use of medications for any surgical candidate. Which drugs can negatively interfere with anesthesia or contribute to postoperative complications?
    1. Anticoagulants and antihypertensives.
    2. Anticoagulants and insulin.
    3. Digoxin and thiazide diuretics.
    4. Vitamins and mineral replacements.

89. To assess accurately a client's functional and vocational rehabilitation potential with myasthenia gravis, the nurse must *first* ascertain:
    1. The degree of physical and emotional stress in the client's present occupation.
    2. The activities of daily living that cause the greatest degree of muscle weakness and fatigue.
    3. The client's understanding of and attitude toward myasthenia gravis, as well as the ability to cope with activity restrictions.
    4. Whether or not the client's current occupation allows opportunities to sit down and rest when necessary.

90. In providing postoperative nursing care for the infant after a cleft lip repair, the nurse should:
    1. Place the infant in a prone position to facilitate drainage.
    2. Avoid moving the infant too much in order to keep from dislodging the Logan bar.
    3. Cleanse the suture area frequently to prevent scarring.
    4. Encourage the infant to cry to promote adequate lung aeration.

91. A client has multiple fractures of both legs; treatment includes bed rest with skeletal traction. The nursing intervention that would be *most* effective in prevention of footdrop would be use of:
    1. A bed cradle.
    2. A footboard.
    3. Passive range of motion every shift.
    4. A trochanter roll.

92. The physician recommends an inpatient, short-term drug treatment program for an 11-year-old with a substance abuse problem. The adolescent's father becomes very hostile and states, "My child is no addict and isn't going to be put away in any crazy house." To assess the father's reaction to the physician's recommendation, the nurse should realize that the father is:
    1. Expressing anger about the accurate diagnosis.
    2. Denying that his child is a drug abuser.
    3. Projecting the blame elsewhere.
    4. Looking for another, better solution.

93. A hospitalized toddler's mother comes in to visit. The toddler clings to the nurse who is bathing the toddler and refuses to look at the mother. The nurse recognizes that this behavior is characteristic of what phase of separation anxiety? *Select all that apply.*
    1. Anaclitic depression.
    2. Protest.
    3. Despair.
    4. Denial.
    5. Stranger fear.

94. Which nursing action is inappropriate in the preparation of a client for *oral* cholecystography?
    1. Administering a fat-free diet the evening before the test.
    2. Administering Telepaque (iopanoic acid) tablets in 5-minute intervals 1 hour after supper.
    3. Administering at least 6 oz of water with each Telepaque (iopanoic acid) tablet.
    4. Allowing the client, after ingesting the tablets, to drink water until midnight, then NPO.

95. A preoperative *nursing priority* for a client having a tracheostomy is:
    1. Establishing postoperative communication.
    2. Drawing blood for serum-electrolyte and blood gas determinations.
    3. Inserting a Foley catheter and attaching it to dependent drainage.
    4. Doing a surgical prep of the neck and upper chest wall.

96. The husband of a woman having a modified radical mastectomy has arrived early to be with his wife before surgery. After his wife leaves for the operating room, the nurse would *initially:*
    1. Tell him to go on to work and come back in the early evening, when his wife is likely to be more responsive.
    2. Explain that, following surgery, his wife will be taken to the recovery room, but the surgeon will contact him when the procedure is over.
    3. Get him a cup of coffee and tell him to make himself comfortable, because it will be some time before his wife returns to her room.
    4. Encourage him to express his feelings and concerns so as to plan for postoperative family teaching.

97. The nurse explains to a client that the purpose of intermittent positive-pressure breathing (IPPB) with normal saline is to maintain patent airways and to mobilize secretions. To accomplish this, IPPB exerts:
    1. Positive pressures on inspiration.
    2. Negative pressures on inspiration.
    3. Positive pressures on expiration.
    4. Negative pressures on expiration.

98. The drainage period during peritoneal dialysis generally takes 20 minutes, though this may vary from client to client. If fluid is not draining properly, the nurse can facilitate return by:
    1. Turning the client to a prone position.
    2. Manipulating the indwelling catheter.
    3. Elevating the head of the bed, thereby increasing intraabdominal pressures.
    4. Elevating the foot of the bed, thereby increasing abdominal pressures and gravity flow.

99. The nurse working with a family who experienced SIDS (sudden infant death syndrome) should:
    1. Be knowledgeable about various theories of psychotherapy.
    2. Have extensive experience working with clients who are dying.
    3. Be able to identify personal feelings about death.
    4. Be able to suppress personal feelings about death.

100. When teaching the parents about the care of their infant with a cleft lip and palate, the nurse should inform them that:
    1. It is important to use a nipple with large holes to make sucking easier.
    2. The infant will have difficulty feeding because the infant cannot create a vacuum in the mouth.
    3. The infant should be given small amounts of formula while being maintained in a supine position to facilitate feeding.
    4. It is important to isolate the infant from others to prevent possible infection.

ANSWERS/RATIONALES/TIPS

1. **(2)** The date of the woman's last period is the most relevant question to ask in performing the initial assessment because it will assist the nurse in making a preliminary determination of possible pregnancy. **Answer 1** is incorrect because whether the woman is presently taking oral contraceptives may be relevant, it would be more pertinent to assess what *general* type of birth control the couple may be using and if they have been using it effectively. **Answers 3** and **4** are incorrect because whether she has been pregnant before and how much weight she has gained are both relevant to performing the assessment, it is *not* essential to determine *whether* she is pregnant at the present time.

> **TEST-TAKING TIP**—Choose the answer that meets the condition of the stem: to find out *if* she is pregnant *now*. Review presumptive, probable, and positive signs of pregnancy.
> **AS, APP, 5, Maternity, HPM, Health Promotion and Maintenance**

2. **(1)** If the IV infuses at the prescribed rate of 75 mL per hour from 7:00 P.M. to 7:00 A.M., or 12 hours, 75 mL x 12 hours = 900 mL infused. If a 1000 mL bag were hung and 900 mL infused, 1,000 − 900 = 100 mL *left* in the bag. **Answers 2** and **3** are incorrect calculations. **Answer 4** is incorrect because there *is* enough information to determine this.

> **TEST-TAKING TIP**—Looks more difficult than it is. Just multiply and subtract.
> **EV, APP, 6, M/S: Calculation, PhI, Pharmacological and Parenteral Therapies**

3. **(1)** The inherent rate of ventricular excitable tissue is between 20 and 40 and does not increase significantly with exertion in complete heart block. **Answers 2** and **3** are incorrect because this phenomenon results in decreased cardiac output despite increased diastolic filling time, coronary artery blood flow, and stroke volume with each ventricular contraction. **Answer 4** is incorrect because the decreased cardiac output results in stimulation of circulatory reflexes to increase venous return, which produces peripheral vasoconstriction, the cause of the client's pallor and diaphoresis.

KEY TO CODES FOLLOWING RATIONALES:

Nursing process: **AS,** assessment; **AN,** analysis; **PL,** plan; **IMP,** implementation; **EV,** evaluation. *Cognitive level:* **COM,** comprehension; **APP,** application; **ANL,** analysis. *Category of human function:* **1,** protective; **2,** sensory-perceptual; **3,** comfort, rest, activity, and mobility; **4,** nutrition; **5,** growth and development; **6,** fluid-gas transport; **7,** psychosocial-cultural; **8,** elimination. *Client need:* **SECE,** safe, effective care environment; **HPM,** health promotion/maintenance; **PsI,** psychosocial integrity; **PhI,** physiological integrity. (Client subneed appears after Client need code.) See appendices for full explanation.

💡 **TEST-TAKING TIP**—Look for a similar idea in stem and in answer—"heart block" and "blocked rate increase."
AN, ANL, 6, M/S: Cardiac, PhI, Physiological Adaptation

4. **(4)** To repeat the breathing exercises until the client is light-headed is inappropriate. It indicates hyperventilation, which may lead to tetany due to loss of volatile hydrogen ions. Clients *should,* however, be able to supply a rationale for deep breathing and coughing techniques (**Answer 1**), as well as demonstrate them correctly (**Answer 2**). Answer 3 is also a desirable outcome.

TEST-TAKING TIP—*Least* desired outcome will be low priority or undesirable
EV, APP, 3, M/S: Preop, PhI, Basic Care and Comfort

5. **(1)** According to Nägele's rule (LMP − 3 months + 7 days), the calculations would be: 7/10 − 3 months = 4/10 + 7 days = 4/17. Nägele's rule assumes that the woman has a 28-day cycle and that pregnancy occurred on the fourteenth day. If the woman's cycle is longer or shorter than 28 days, appropriate adjustments must be made. Only about 4%–5% of women give birth on the EDD plus or minus 7 days. **Answers 2, 3,** and **4** are incorrect calculations.

TEST-TAKING TIP—Use Nägele's rule. A simple method is to count 9 months from the LMP, +7 days.
AN, COM, 5, Maternity, HPM, Health Promotion and Maintenance

6. **(3)** If the IV infusion was at the prescribed rate of 35 mL/hr for 4.5 hours, from 7:00 A.M. to 11:30 A.M., 35 mL x 4.5 hours = 157.5 mL absorbed. If 500 mL was hung at 7:00 A.M., and approximately 160 mL was infused, 500–160 = 340 mL left in the bag at 11:30 A.M. **Answers 1** and **2** are incorrect calculations. **Answer 4** is incorrect because amount of fluid left *is* determinable.

TEST-TAKING TIP—Use basic math, not a formula.
EV, APP, 6, M/S: Calculation, PhI, Pharmacological and Parenteral Therapies

7. **(3)** Although some complete or partial amputations may result from trauma (**Answer 1**), the majority are necessitated by arteriosclerosis obliterans. **Answer 2** is incorrect because long-standing complications of diabetes mellitus are peripheral vascular insufficiency and infections, which in turn may increase the likelihood of amputation. **Answer 4** is incorrect because bone tumors, particularly of the knee, necessitate amputation *less often* than arteriosclerosis obliterans.

TEST-TAKING TIP—Think broad and most encompassing.
AN, COM, 3, M/S: Vascular, PhI, Physiological Adaptation

8. **(1)** Initially, the nurse must obtain more information about the client's pain before giving medication. **Answer 2** is incorrect because if the pain were due to compression of the leg by a cast that is too tight, medicating the client could result in serious neurovascular complications. **Answers 3** and **4** are incorrect because offering reassurance or distraction is not appropriate at this time, or a sufficient nursing intervention.

TEST-TAKING TIP—Assessment is always the first step of the nursing process.
IMP, ANL, 3, M/S: Ortho, PhI, Physiological Adaptation

9. **(3)** Diazepam is a CNS depressant, and in children and elderly adults, it may depress the respiratory center. Thus, when the client returns to the unit, the nurse should first evaluate respirations. **Answers 1, 2,** and **4** are incorrect. *After* determining that the client is breathing adequately, the nurse can then evaluate the temperature, pulse, and blood pressure.

TEST-TAKING TIP—Patent airway and respirations are always the priority of care.
EV, ANL, 1, PEDS, PhI, Pharmacological and Parenteral Therapies

10. **350 mg** 3500 gm = 3.5 kg (7.7 lb). The minimum recommended dose of ampicillin is 50 mg per kg per 24 hrs or 175 mg in 24 hrs. The maximum recommended dose of ampicillin is 100 mg per kg per 24 hr or 350 mg in 24 hr.

TEST-TAKING TIP—Know how to convert gm to kg (divide gm by 1000) before proceeding on to the actual mathematical calculation.
IMP, APP, 1, PEDS, PhI, Pharmacological and Parenteral Therapies

11. **(1)** After opening the airway by head tilt and chin lift, the nurse must look, listen, and feel for any movement of air. Often opening the airway may be all that is needed. Giving two breaths (**Answer 2**) is done *after* establishing breathlessness, *followed by* checking the pulse (**Answer 3**). Finger sweeps (**Answer 4**) are only done if ventilation is *unsuccessful* and back blows have been done.

TEST-TAKING TIP—Remember the ABCs of CPR.
IMP, APP, 1, M/S: CPR, PhI, Physiological Adaptation

12. **(1)** Fresh fish with scales would be permitted on a mildly restricted (2 g) to an extremely restricted (200 mg) sodium diet. Only shellfish are restricted. **Answers 2, 3,** and **4** are incorrect because foods to be avoided on a sodium-restricted diet include ethnic foods, particularly Chinese, which usually has soy sauce as an additive; commercially-prepared soups, such as canned tomato soup; and hot dogs, which are a commercially-prepared meat.

TEST-TAKING TIP—Look for similarities in answers. Only one choice is fresh-cooked with no additives.
EV, APP, 4, M/S: Diet, PhI, Basic Care and Comfort

13. **(3)** Clients with permanent pacemakers are cautioned to avoid all sources of high electronic output because they may cause pacemaker malfunction. Other sources of high electronic output include older, noninsulated microwave ovens, running car engines, and dental drills. **Answers 1** and **4** are incorrect because activities such as swimming and golf *can* be resumed usually after 5 weeks. **Answer 2** is incorrect because creative hobbies such as fashioning lamps *are* indicated *as long as* precautions are taken to avoid electrical shocks.

TEST-TAKING TIP—Look for a restricted or potentially "risky" activity.
IMP, APP, 1, M/S: Hazard, SECE, Safety and Infection Control

14. **(2)** One-person or two-person CPR for adults is done at a minimum rate of 80 compressions per minute (up to a rate of 100). Sixty compressions per minute (**Answer 1**) is no longer considered adequate in CPR. **Answers 3** and **4** are both within the range of acceptable rates; however, the question asks for the *minimum* rate.

TEST-TAKING TIP— Look for current minimum rate (know 80).
IMP, COM, 6, M/S: CPR, PhI, Physiological Adaptation

15. **(2)** SIDS occurs most frequently in low birthweight, preterm infants, and in the lower, not middle (**Answer 3**), socioeconomic groups. **Answer 1** is incorrect because SIDS occurs most frequently in blacks and Native Americans, not Hispanics. **Answer 4** is incorrect because SIDS has a lower incidence in infants who are breastfed.

TEST-TAKING TIP—Review risk factors; when in doubt, choose an objective risk factor.
AS, APP, 5, PEDS, HPM, Health Promotion and Maintenance

16. **(2)** Elevation of 20–30 degrees is the optimum position to reduce intracranial pressure, aid venous drainage from the brain, and facilitate respiration. **Answer 1** is incorrect because flat on the back may increase the chance of aspiration. A lateral or semiprone position may be indicated in the early postoperative period if there are no signs of cerebral edema. **Answers 3** and **4** are incorrect because they may increase the amount of hip flexion and can contribute to an increase in intracranial pressure.

TEST-TAKING TIP—Picture the client position. *Optimum* is key to head *and* limb positioning.
PL, COM, 2, M/S: Neuro, PhI, Reduction of Risk Potential

17. **(3)** Pressure dressings are **never** removed (**Answer 1**), but if saturated, they should be reinforced with sterile dressings. The possibility of hemorrhage is ever-present, and signs of increased bleeding should be immediately reported to the surgeon. This is not a normal occurrence. Vital signs and Hemovac drainage and function should also be assessed. **Answer 2** is incorrect because Hemovacs may be irrigated, but generally they are not milked. **Answer 4** is incorrect because this is *not a normal occurrence*.

TEST-TAKING TIP—Gather data to interpret finding. Assess!
IMP, APP, 6, M/S: Wound Care, PhI, Reduction of Risk Potential

18. **(2)** This response allows the couple to become informed without infringing on the physician's role. The physician can then decide either to inform the couple of the procedure to be used or to have the anesthesiologist inform them. **Answer 1** is incorrect because time is limited and the physician may decide to inform the couple himself or herself. **Answers 3** and **4** are incorrect because it is not the nurse's role to discuss anesthesia of choice.

TEST-TAKING TIP—Choose the appropriate nursing role rather than the MD's role when it deals with explaining emergency procedures.
IMP, APP, 7, Maternity, SECE, Management of Care

19. **(1)** In pyloric stenosis, the pyloric sphincter at the distal end of the stomach is thickened, or stenotic. This sphincter blocks the flow of formula into the small intestine, causing vomiting; it also blocks the flow of bile back into the stomach. Thus, the infant with pyloric stenosis characteristically vomits only stomach contents, not bile (**Answer 2**), blood (**Answer 3**), or feces (**Answer 4**).

TEST-TAKING TIP—The correct choice is the one that is different ("only"). All of the other choices contain another element that does not relate to correct anatomy and pathophysiology.
AS, ANL, 8, PEDS, PhI, Basic Care and Comfort

20. **(2)** EDTA and BAL work by binding to the heavy metal lead and promoting its excretion via the kidneys. Renal toxicity may occur as a result. The nurse should force fluids and monitor kidney function carefully. The other choices are incorrect because calcium disodium edetate (EDTA) and dimercaprol (BAL) do *not* adversely affect the neurological system (**Answer 1**), the cardiovascular system (**Answer 3**), or the hematological system (**Answer 4**).

TEST-TAKING TIP—Determine where the drug is excreted; omit neurological, cardiovascular, and hematological systems.
EV, APP, 8, PEDS, PhI, Pharmacological and Parenteral Therapies

21. **(2)** Modified radical mastectomy consists of removal of the breast and all or selected lymph nodes with preservation of the pectoralis major muscle. The other choices are incorrect because they are examples of a simple mastectomy (**Answer 1**), classic radical mastectomy (**Answer 3**), and supraradical mastectomy (**Answer 4**).

TEST-TAKING TIP—The key word is *modified*, something less than radical but more than simple.
AS, COM, 1, M/S: Cancer, PhI, Physiological Adaptation

22. **(1)** The definitive diagnosis of intussusception is based on a barium enema, which clearly demonstrates the telescoping of the bowel wall, which blocks the flow of the barium. **Answer 2** is incorrect because although a secondary effect may be a nonsurgical reduction of the telescoping (which may occur due to hydrostatic pressure), this is uncertain and is not the main reason the procedure is performed. **Answers 3** and **4** are incorrect because a barium enema is not administered to ease the passage of stool or provide symptomatic relief.

TEST-TAKING TIP—Barium enema is a diagnostic procedure; therefore, the answer involves "diagnosis."
IMP, APP, 8, PEDS, PhI, Reduction of Risk Potential

23. **(1)** If the IV infuses at the proper rate, 110 mL per hour, from 2:30 A.M. to 6:00 A.M., 110 mL x 3.5 hours = 385 mL infused. **Answers 2, 3,** and **4** are incorrect calculations.

TEST-TAKING TIP—Basic math, not a formula.
EV, APP, 6, M/S: Calculation, PhI, Pharmacological and Parenteral Therapies

24. **(1)** An early indication of cardiac decompensation is tachycardia. Therefore, the client's vital signs, mentation, and pulmonary status should be assessed to rule out this complication of myocardial infarction. Other causes of tachycardia are hypovolemia, anxiety, and pain. Assessment of pain and emotional status can be determined during cognitive assessment. **Answers 2, 3,** and **4** are incorrect because actions such as encouraging verbalization of feelings, administering oxygen, and decreasing the rate of intravenous infusion will be determined by the nurse's assessment of vital signs.

TEST-TAKING TIP—Choose the first step of the nursing process: *assess*.
IMP, ANL, 6, M/S: Cardiac, PhI, Physiological Adaptation

25. **(3)** Signs and symptoms of a hemolytic reaction usually include: chills, shaking, fever, red (or black) urine, headache, and flank pain. **Answer 1** is incorrect because urticaria is not a common sign in a hemolytic reaction, although it is common with an allergic reaction. **Answers 2** and **4** are incorrect because neither polyuria nor hypothermia is a common sign in a hemolytic reaction.

TEST-TAKING TIP—Recognize possible complications (kidney with hemolysis).
AS, COM, 6, M/S: Blood, PhI, Pharmacological and Parenteral Therapies

26. **(3)** Bryant's traction is a form of skin traction used in infants and toddlers with fractured femurs; when applied correctly, adhesive material should be taped to the skin of both legs. **Answers 1** and **2** are incorrect because skeletal traction in the form of a Kirschner wire or Steinmann pin is not used in

Bryant's traction. **Answer 4** is incorrect because adhesive material should be taped to the skin of both legs, *not* one leg.

> **TEST-TAKING TIP**—Choose the option that is different: three options have *one* leg; one option involves *both* legs. Bryant's traction is always applied bilaterally.
> **AS, APP, 3, PEDS, PhI, Basic Care and Comfort**

27. **(3)** Breast size is not as important as the amount of glandular tissue, because it is not the adipose tissue but the secreting tissues of the mammary glands that produce the milk. **Answers 1 and 2** are incorrect responses because adequate diet and rest *are* essential to promoting lactation. **Answer 4** is incorrect because she may ovulate and could become pregnant while lactating.

> **TEST-TAKING TIP**—When a question asks for the "need for further teaching," choose the *incorrect* answer; in this case eliminate the one that is a myth.
> **EV, APP, 4, Maternity, HPM, Health Promotion and Maintenance**

28. **(1)** To prevent exacerbating the eczema, it is generally recommended that the child wear pure, natural cotton clothing only. **Answers 2, 3, and 4** are incorrect because linen, wool, and polyester blends are more likely to cause the eczema to be worse.

> **TEST-TAKING TIP**—Because of the allergic nature of eczema, any food or clothing should be hypoallergenic.
> **IMP, APP, 1, PEDS, PhI, Basic Care and Comfort**

29. **(4)** In the three-point gait, both crutches and the affected "bad" leg and foot are moved together, with the unaffected "good" leg and foot following. **Answers 1 and 2** are incorrect because the crutches are both moved simultaneously, not independently. **Answer 3** is incorrect because the client should not bear any weight on the fractured leg when using the three-point gait.

> **TEST-TAKING TIP**—Visualize each answer. Which one avoids weight bearing?
> **IMP, APP, 3, M/S: Ortho, PhI, Basic Care and Comfort**

30. **(1)** The airway tube should remain in place and the client's head should be turned to the side to prevent obstruction of the airway by the tongue and to allow secretions to drain from the mouth. **Answer 2** is incorrect because the head is not turned to the side. **Answers 3 and 4** are incorrect because the airway tube should **never** be removed until the client is alert enough to begin attempting to eject it. Leaving the airway tube in after this point may cause vomiting due to stimulation of the gag reflex.

> **TEST-TAKING TIP**—Think client safety as a priority.
> **IMP, APP, 6, M/S: Postop, PhI, Reduction of Risk Potential**

31. **(2, 4, 5)** **Answer 2** is correct because an increased heart rate may be an early sign of cardiac decompensation. **Answer 4** is correct because rest on either side reduces stress on the heart. **Answer 5** is correct because a labor epidural decreases pain and the decreased cardiac stress that is increased by the physiological response to pain. The epidural also decreases the rapid cardiac output immediately following birth. **Answer 1** is incorrect because this client has cardiac disease, and a fluid bolus may lead to a fluid overload and cardiac decompensation. **Answer 3** is incorrect because valsalva pushing causes too much stress in a client with cardiac disease.

> **TEST-TAKING TIP**—The question asks for appropriate actions for a client with cardiac disease. Three options are actions that *decrease* cardiac output (**Answers 2, 4, and 5**);

two options *increase* cardiac load and are inappropriate (**Answers 1 and 3**).
> **PL, ANL, 6, Maternity, PhI, Reduction of Risk Potential**

32. **(3)** Attempting to control the situation and do as the client pleases is most likely the client's primary goal, in light of the history of drug abuse. Bending the rules for a severe violation of hospital policy, the treatment, and the law is not justified. For **Answer 1** to be correct, the nurse would need further evidence of the client's desire to change, such as overt, consistent changes in the client's pattern of behavior and open verbalization of feelings. **Answers 2 and 4** are incorrect because they are aspects of manipulation.

> **TEST-TAKING TIP**—Choose the broad concept (manipulation), which *covers* attention-seeking and avoidance.
> **AN, ANL, 7, Psych. PsI, Psychosocial Integrity**

33. **(2)** Suction is applied only after the catheter is in place and ready for withdrawal. Applying suction intermittently and rotating the suction catheter assist in reducing the negative pressure effects of suctioning. Suctioning should be limited to periods of 10 to 15 seconds. **Answers 1, 3, and 4** are incorrect because of the negative effects these actions would have on client aeration.

> **TEST-TAKING TIP**—Look for one proper and safe technique; eliminate three choices that include during "insertion."
> **IMP, APP, 6, M/S: Resp., PhI, Reduction of Risk Potential**

34. **(3)** The most effective intervention to help preschoolers cope with painful experiences during hospitalization is to offer the opportunity for therapeutic play with puppets or dolls and medical equipment. This type of play experience allows the child to "act out" frustrations and anger in a safe, controlled manner, enabling the child to work through feelings about a difficult experience. **Answers 1, 2, and 4** are incorrect because playing with toys, engaging in free play, and playing with other children are not as effective as offering an opportunity for therapeutic play.

> **TEST-TAKING TIP**—*Therapeutic* release of feelings (pain) is accomplished best via *therapeutic* (medical) play.
> **IMP, APP, 5, PEDS, PsI, Psychosocial Integrity**

35. **(2)** Low-Fowler's to semi-Fowler's position with the arm elevated on pillows so that the wrist and elbow are slightly higher than the shoulder best facilitates venous return, reducing the occurrence of edema. Some physicians may order that the client be positioned so that the hand is raised above the head. **Answers 1, 3, and 4** are incorrect because venous return is not enhanced, or muscle contractures may possibly develop.

> **TEST-TAKING TIP**—Visualize the position of the arm.
> **IMP, APP, 6, M/S: Postop, PhI, Basic Care and Comfort**

36. **(3)** The treatment of drug abuse is only effective if the client is motivated to make changes in style and pattern of living. Although the hazards of drugs (**Answer 1**), the fact that using drugs is illegal (**Answer 2**), and developing alternative coping mechanisms (**Answer 4**) are all significant components to be incorporated in health teaching, the client must first be motivated to learn.

> **TEST-TAKING TIP**—Key phrase is "most important aspect of treatment"; in this question, "motivation" precedes other choices.
> **PL, ANL, 7, Psych, PsI, Psychosocial Integrity**

37. **(1)** After marking the original dressing (to indicate the extent of the bleeding) and reinforcing the dressing (to prevent infection), the nurse should check the vital signs to determine

if the bleeding episode has had any effect on the child's physiological status. **Answer 2** is incorrect because in general the nurse should never change the flow rate of the IV without a physician's order. **Answers 3** and **4** are incorrect because *after* checking vital signs, depending on the status of the bleeding and the vital signs, the nurse might change the client's position and notify the cardiologist.

> **TEST-TAKING TIP**—Look at the verbs; select a verb that assesses ("*check*" before "increase," "place," or "notify"). Assessment is the first step of the nursing process.
> **IMP, ANL, 6, PEDS, PhI, Physiological Adaptation**

38. **(1)** Isoproterenol is categorized as a beta-mimetic, in that its action simulates beta-adrenergic discharge. Actions include: increased strength of cardiac contraction, increased heart rate, and decreased venous pooling, which increases venous return. An additional effect of isoproterenol is increased myocardial consumption resulting from increased rate and contractility. Isoproterenol is not a cardiac glycoside (**Answer 2**) like *digoxin,* an anticholinergic (**Answer 3**) like *atropine,* or a beta-blocker (**Answer 4**) like *propanolol.*

> **TEST-TAKING TIP**—Recognize expected drug effects.
> **PL, COM, 6, M/S: Meds, PhI, Pharmacological and Parenteral Therapies**

39. **(3)** Phantom limb pain or sensation is an unpleasant complication that sometimes follows amputation. This phenomenon is not completely understood but is believed to result from afferent nerve fibers (sensory) severed during surgery. The pain in the limb may be identical to that perceived by the client before surgery. The client needs to be aware of the nature of this discomfort. Sometimes the sensation will disappear if the client looks at the stump and recalls that the limb has been amputated. In cases where discomfort persists, alcohol may be injected into the nerve endings for temporary relief, the nerve endings may be removed, or on rare occasions reamputation may be required. **Answers 1** and **2** are incorrect because they negate the client's perceptions of discomfort and avoid the issue. **Answer 4** is incorrect because an explanation of the phenomenon and other palliative measures should *precede* the administration of a narcotic.

> **TEST-TAKING TIP**—*First* response: address the client's comment.
> **IMP, ANL, 2, M/S: Ortho, PhI, Basic Care and Comfort**

40. **(4)** Conflicts concerning discharge instructions following myocardial infarction and pacemaker insertion are common. When the nurse prepares a client for discharge, it is important to recognize that both client and spouse may have several fears they have not verbalized. Allow time for and encourage verbalization of feelings. Likewise, be sure that discharge instructions are feasible for the individual's life-style; if they are not, work out a plan of modification with the client, family, and physician. Referral to a community health nurse or local cardiac rehabilitation support group may also facilitate the rehabilitation. **Answers 1, 2,** and **3** are incorrect because they cut off the client's and spouse's range of response and may therefore preclude obtaining pertinent data.

> **TEST-TAKING TIP**—Look for the broadest response.
> **IMP, ANL, 7, M/S: Cardiac, PsI, Psychosocial Integrity**

41. **(3)** Per MD order, the IV should infuse at 320 mL every 8 hours, or 40 mL per hour. Thus, if there is 425 mL left in the IV and it runs at 40 mL per hour, the present bag should last 10 hours, or from 11:30 A.M. to 9:30 P.M. The nurse should plan to change the bag at 9:00 P.M., before it runs out completely. **Answers 1** and **2** are incorrect because changing it earlier would waste IV fluid, which is costly. **Answer 4** is incorrect because changing it later would mean the IV would run out completely, which may result in an embolism or a clogged IV line.

> **TEST-TAKING TIP**—Basic math, no formula required.
> **IMP, APP, 6, M/S: Calculation, PhI, Pharmacological and Parenteral Therapies**

42. **(1)** To be sure a typical antimicrobial will have the desired effect, it must be in contact with the skin for a minimum of 10 seconds. **Answers 2, 3,** and **4** are incorrect because durations longer than 10 seconds are not necessary.

> 💡 **TEST-TAKING TIP**—The minimum duration of time for proper handwashing is approximately equal to the amount of time it takes to sing "Happy Birthday" (about 10 seconds)!
> **IMP, COM, 1, M/S: Infect. Control, SECE, Safety and Infection Control**

43. **(2)** To reduce anxiety and ensure ease of induction, a preoperative medication should be administered 45–60 minutes before anesthesia. Side rails should be raised after administration of medication, because the client will begin to feel drowsy and light-headed. **Answers 1, 3,** and **4** are incorrect because giving medication less than 45–60 minutes before induction of anesthesia would not allow sufficient time for the medication to reach its peak effect.

> **TEST-TAKING TIP**—Correct answer is broadest and most optimal for desired outcome.
> **PL, COM, 1, M/S: Preop, PhI, Pharmacological and Parenteral Therapies**

44. **(1)** The client should be given diluted orange juice to ensure an adequate supply of ascorbic acid (vitamin C). **Answers 2, 3,** and **4** are incorrect because carbohydrates, protein, and vitamin A can be easily obtained by ensuring a variety of foods in the bland diet.

> **TEST-TAKING TIP**—Choose the option that would potentially increase acid (ascorbic *acid*).
> **EV, COM, 4, M/S: Diet, PhI, Basic Care and Comfort**

45. **(2)** Although in moderation these drugs produce feelings of well-being and alertness, an overdose of amphetamines causes an increase in tension and irritability. **Answers 1** and **3** are incorrect because an increase in the heart rate and blood flow is exhibited (these drugs stimulate the release of norepinephrine). **Answer 4** is incorrect because diarrhea, *not* constipation, is a common side effect.

> **TEST-TAKING TIP**—Review signs and symptoms of amphetamine abuse.
> **EV, COM, 7, Psych, PhI, Pharmacological and Parenteral Therapies**

46. **(1)** Obtaining consent and informing the woman about the risks involved are legally the *physician's* role. The nurse's role is to reinforce the physician's teaching and to confirm that the information has been given to the woman. **Answer 2** is an incorrect response because it *is* an appropriate nursing action to reinforce the physician's teaching and to confirm that the information has been given to the woman. **Answers 3** and **4** are incorrect because monitoring the fetal heart rate and observing for bleeding *are* both appropriate nursing actions.

> **TEST-TAKING TIP**—When asked to choose the *least* likely, choose an *incorrect* answer. Review the nurse's legal responsibilities regarding informed consent for procedures.
> **PL, APP, 7, Maternity, SECE, Management of Care**

47. **(1)** The most objective measure of the effectiveness of an antibiotic is a return of the white blood cell count to normal. **Answer 2** is incorrect because a low-grade temperature may indicate a lingering infection. **Answers 3** and **4** are incorrect because no pain and a good appetite are both good clinical indicators, but not as objective or as clearly measurable as the white blood cell count.

> **TEST-TAKING TIP**—Key term is "*most indicative*" of a therapeutic response (*no infection*).
> EV, ANL, 1, M/S: Infect. Control, PhI, Pharmacological and Parenteral Therapies

48. **(1, 2, 4)** Answers 1, 2, and 4 are correct because these medications are used to treat pseudoparkinsonism or EPS. **Answer 3** is incorrect because this medication is used to treat psychotic symptoms and is a *cause* of pseudoparkinsonism. **Answer 5** is incorrect because this medication is used to treat psychotic symptoms and is a *cause* of pseudoparkinsonism. **Answer 6** is incorrect because this medication is used to treat psychotic symptoms and is a *cause* of pseudoparkinsonism.

> **TEST-TAKING TIP**—Know the drug categories to help you choose the correct responses.
> IMP, APP, 7, Psych, PhI, Pharmacological/Parenteral Therapies

49. **(2)** The earliest exercises initiated are passive range of motion of the elbow, wrist, and hand; these exercises are begun on the first postoperative day. As the client is able, she is encouraged to put those joints through active range of motion. These exercises assist in maintaining function and in reducing lymphedema. Progression to other exercises, such as hair combing and wall reaching, is dependent on wound healing, grafts, presence of drainage tubes, and the client's tolerance. **Answers 1, 3,** and **4** are incorrect responses because they are implemented *after* a modified mastectomy; they are not appropriate as *initial* therapy.

> **TEST-TAKING TIP**—When all are correct answers, consider the time period and client limitations in the early postoperative period.
> PL, APP, 3, M/S: Postop, PhI, Basic Care and Comfort

50. **(3)** To best gain the cooperation of a toddler, the nurse should help her or him focus on how the treatment will help the toddler go home; the nurse should also use distraction. **Answers 1, 2,** and **4** are incorrect because the nurse should never bribe, threaten, or lie to the child.

> **TEST-TAKING TIP**—Choose the one option that is *not* manipulative, frightening, or fantasy.
> IMP, APP, 5, PEDS, PsI, Psychosocial Integrity

51. **(3)** Correct medication administration is extremely important. When the medication order is of a different strength from the supplies at hand, using the following formula will be helpful in determining the correct dose:

$$\frac{\text{Desired}}{\text{Available}} \times \frac{\text{Quantity}}{\text{on hand}} = \frac{0.4}{0.6} \times \frac{15 \text{ minims}}{1}$$

$$= \frac{2}{3} \times \frac{15}{1}$$

$$= \frac{30}{3}$$

$$= 10 \text{ minims}$$

Answers 1, 2, and **4** are inaccurate calculations.

> **TEST-TAKING TIP**—Know the correct *ratio* formula.
> IMP, APP, 1, M/S: Calculation, PhI, Pharmacological and Parenteral Therapies

52. **(4)** The natural pathway of humidification, the upper respiratory tract, has been bypassed. Therefore, to prevent drying out of the mucous membranes of the bronchi, as well as crusting of secretions, humidification by nebulization is provided. **Answer 1** is incorrect because although supplying humidification during oxygen therapy has become standard, it is not a rationale for its use. **Answers 2** and **3** are incorrect because they are not specific to this question, though probably true to some extent.

> **TEST-TAKING TIP**—Identify the key concept—humidification.
> AN, APP, 6, M/S: Resp., PhI, Reduction of Risk Potential

53. **(4)** Measles, mumps, and rubella are first given at 12–15 months, and repeated at either 4–6 years or 11–12 years. Hepatitis B (**Answer 1**), DTaP (**Answer 2**), and *H. influenzae* type b (**Answer 3**) *should* all be given at 6 months.

> **TEST-TAKING TIP**—Knowing immunization schedule is the only way to select this answer. Note that the question asks which is *not* given.
> IMP, APP, 1, PEDS, HPM, Health Promotion and Maintenance

54. **(1)** The likelihood of product contamination after opening the bottle or bag increases over time, but the bottle or bag can hang safely for a maximum of 24 hours. Bottles or bags used for intermittent IV medications should be timed and dated, and not left hanging at the bedside for over 24 hours. The use of the heparin lock has decreased the need for KVO IVs, and medications are administered with 50 mL or 100 mL single-use solution bags. **Answers 2, 3,** and **4** are incorrect because the times are all too soon and would unnecessarily increase the cost of hospitalization.

> **TEST-TAKING TIP**—The best answer includes all the other choices.
> EV, COM, 1, M/S: Hazard, PhI, Pharmacological and Parenteral Therapies

55. **(3)** To effectively screen for the S-shaped lateral curvature of scoliosis, the nurse should ask the adolescent to stand and bend over 90 degrees at the waist. The nurse should look for unevenness of the shoulders or hips, or any curves or humps, which require further follow-up and evaluation. **Answers 1, 2,** and **4** are incorrect because no other position is recommended.

> **TEST-TAKING TIP**—Select the position that is not like the others; three describe a straight or flat position, only one involves bending.
> AS, APP, 3, PEDS, HPM, Health Promotion and Maintenance

56. **(3)** Some of the most serious reactions occurring with blood transfusions are the result of human error. To reduce human error, it is essential for two nurses to verify that the client's name and hospital number on the blood bag correspond exactly to that on the wristband. **Answers 1, 2,** and **4** are incorrect because although they are proper safeguards, they are not the *first* priority.

> **TEST-TAKING TIP**—Only one choice deals with direct client safety.
> IMP, COM, 1, M/S: Blood, PhI, Pharmacological and Parenteral Therapies

Final Test

57. (1) Before adding potassium chloride to any IV line, the nurse must check that the client's kidneys are functioning to avoid potassium overload and hyperkalemia. **Answers 2, 3, and 4** are incorrect because it is not necessary to check reflexes, respiratory rate, or mucous membranes before adding potassium to the IV line.

> 💡 **TEST-TAKING TIP**—Remember: "no pee = no potassium."
>
> **AN, ANL, 8, PEDS, PhI, Pharmacological and Parenteral Therapies**

58. (4) When a nurse is admitting a new client to the unit, the first action the nurse should take is to correctly identify the client. If the client is fully awake and alert, the nurse can ask the client for his or her name; if the client is newly postop, still under the influence of anesthesia and medication, the nurse should first check the ID band. After identifying the client, the nurse could *then* proceed to monitor vital signs **(Answer 3)**, check the IV **(Answer 2)**, and attach the Salem sump tube to suction **(Answer 1)**.

> 💡 **TEST-TAKING TIP**—Focus on the client, then the procedures with priority questions. Order of priority starts with a KIS (keep it simple) option (i.e., identify the *client*).
>
> **IMP, APP, 1, M/S: Mgmt., SECE, Management of Care**

59. (3) Refrigerating blood assists in delaying the growth of bacteria. The blood must be administered within 4 hours, not 6 hours **(Answer 1)**, but not within 1 and 2 hours because it would be so rapid that the client may experience overload **(Answers 2 and 4)**.

> **TEST-TAKING TIP**—Eliminate the "extremes" first (too short, too long time periods).
>
> **IMP, COM, 6, PEDS, PhI, Pharmacological and Parenteral Therapies**

60. (2) Euphoria, excitement, and talkativeness are all seen *initially,* when the woman is fairly energetic and anxious to have labor begin. **Answer 1** is incorrect because a tendency to hyperventilate usually occurs during the *midactive* phase. Introverted behavior **(Answer 3)** and irritability or crying **(Answer 4)** usually occur in the *transitional* or deceleration period of the active phase of the first stage.

> 💡 **TEST-TAKING TIP**—The key is a *time* element. *First* stage, *first* euphoria. Review phases and stages of labor and a woman's expected responses.
>
> **EV, APP, 5, Maternity, PsI, Psychosocial Integrity**

61. (2) People who abuse drugs tend to be excessively dependent and passive, become easily frustrated, and cannot cope with anxiety. **Answers 1, 3, and 4** are incorrect because individuals who are assertive, mature, or aggressive are generally able to externalize their feelings and fears or to cope effectively with stress.

> **TEST-TAKING TIP**—Choose the option that is different (*dependent* vs. outgoing).
>
> **AS, APP, 7, Psych, PsI, Psychosocial Integrity**

62. (1) Each of these activities (restricting activity, monitoring EKG, implementing passive range of motion, maintaining sterile dressings) is a priority in the early postinsertion period. However, because a transvenous approach was used with this client, it is essential that activities be restricted for the first few days to reduce the risk of catheter dislodgement. To monitor for this complication, periodic comparisons of the client's current rhythm strip should be made with the tracing taken at the time of insertion. Changes in either the pacemaker artifact or pacemaker-initiated QRS indicate a change in position. Although this may not always be significant, it becomes so if the pacemaker fails to capture, causing a decrease in heart rate and cardiac output. **Answers 2, 3, and 4** are incorrect because *restricting activity* is the nurse's *first priority.*

> **TEST-TAKING TIP**—When all answers are correct, look for the most important at that point.
>
> **PL, APP, 1, M/S: Cardiac, PhI, Reduction of Risk Potential**

63. (3) With large dosages of secobarbital there may be an increase in anger or a deep sleep, depending on the individual's reaction. Secobarbital, a barbiturate, causes a depression of the CNS, so its effects usually include bradycardia (*not* tachycardia, **Answer 1**), hypotension (*not* hypertension, **Answer 2**), and depressed respiration (*not* increased respirations, **Answer 4**).

> **TEST-TAKING TIP**—Look at the pattern of responses and choose the one that is different (in this case, the psychosocial answer).
>
> **EV, APP, 7, M/S: Meds, PhI, Pharmacological and Parenteral Therapies**

64. (2) In Bryant's traction, the hips and buttocks should be raised slightly (1 inch) *above* the mattress, *not* resting on the mattress **(Answer 1)**, for the traction to be effective. **Answer 3** is incorrect because although the nurse is ultimately responsible, the nursing assistant should be commended for having brought this concern to the nurse's attention. **Answer 4** is incorrect because although it is true that this child will need special skin care due to prolonged immobility, the nurse should first take measures to correct the problem with the traction.

> **TEST-TAKING TIP**—Visualize Bryant's traction. It is applied to the legs, which are *flexed* at a 90-degree angle at the hips. The child's trunk (buttocks are raised slightly off the bed). This provides the needed countertraction. Remember that weights and pulleys must hang free and clear for traction to be most effective.
>
> **IMP, APP, 3, PEDS, PhI, Basic Care and Comfort**

65. (3) The Hemovac is a portable suction system that provides low negative pressure (30–45 mm Hg) to gently remove excess fluid and debris from the wound. It does not require attachment to any other suction system. **Answers 1, 2, and 4** are incorrect because they *are* standard and appropriate nursing measures.

> **TEST-TAKING TIP**—Look for an *incorrect* nursing action.
>
> **IMP, APP, 1, M/S: Wound Care, PhI, Reduction of Risk Potential**

66. (1) Central venous pressures of 4–10 cm H_2O are normal. Some clinicians consider up to 15 cm H_2O to be normal, but pressures over 15 cm H_2O **(Answer 3)** clearly indicate hypervolemia or heart failure. **Answers 2 and 4** are incorrect because CVP is measured by water, not mercury.

> **TEST-TAKING TIP**—Know normal ranges to interpret changes.
>
> **EV, COM, 6, M/S: Cardiac, PhI, Physiological Adaptation**

67. (1) *Dyspnea* is a term that describes the client's subjective awareness of increased respiratory effort. The increased work of breathing may indeed be *related* to alveolar hypoventilation **(Answer 2)**, which *results* in an increased rate and depth of respiration **(Answer 3)**. Oxygen saturation **(Answer 4)** shows whether the *circulation* is normal or tissue demands have changed.

> **TEST-TAKING TIP**—Look for the option that is broad: dyspnea is *subjective* data. The other options have components of *objective* data.
>
> **AN, COM, 6, M/S: Resp., PhI, Physiological Adaptation**

68. **(4)** Vein-stripping is a painful and tiresome procedure and, for the client's comfort, is almost always done under general anesthesia. **Answer 1** is incorrect because local anesthesia is limited to small areas such as with laceration repair. Topical anesthesia (**Answer 2**) only decreases pain sensation in mucous membranes, and because the incisions for vein-stripping are made in the groin as well as the ankle, regional anesthesia (**Answer 3**) would be impractical. Vein-stripping could also be done using spinal anesthesia.

> **TEST-TAKING TIP**—The best option is the one that would provide most comfort for length of the surgical procedure.
> **IMP, COM, 6, M/S: Vascular, PhI, Basic Care and Comfort**

69. **(1, 2, 3, 4, 5)** Answers 1, 2, 3, 4 and **5** are correct because intussusception occurs when a proximal segment of the bowel telescopes into a more distal segment, pulling the mesentery with it. The mysentery is compressed and angled, resulting in lymphatic and venous obstruction. As the edema from the obstruction increases, pressure within the area of intussusception increases. When the pressure equals the arterial pressure, arterial blood flow stops, resulting in ischemia and the pouring of mucus into the intestine. Venous engorgement also leads to leaking of blood and mucus into the intestinal lumen. This results in the paroxysmal (crampy) abdominal pain and bloody or "currant jelly" stools associated with intussusception. Due to the abdominal pain, the child also exhibits inconsolable crying and drawing up of knees to the chest during the cramping episode.

Answer 6 is incorrect because intussusception occurs most commonly at the ileocecal valve where the ileum (small intestine) invaginates into the cecum (large intestine). The common bile duct, which allows for the passage of both bile and pancreatic secretions, empties into the duodenum (small intestine) at the ampulla of Vater. As the intussusception (a form of obstruction) occurs below the ampulla of Vater, the emesis would be bile stained.

> **TEST-TAKING TIP**—Know how pathophysiology contributes to the classic signs and symptoms of a disease.
> **AS, APP, 3, PEDS, PhI, Physiological Adaptation**

70. **(2)** Many times, clients who are manipulative are not aware of any other mechanisms for fulfilling their needs. Teaching them to identify manipulative behaviors may help them to avoid being manipulative and to eventually adopt more appropriate means for meeting their needs. The clients should be *involved* in the decision-making process (**Answer 1**). Limits must be *realistically* established (**Answer 3**). Public confrontation (**Answer 4**) may only exacerbate the power struggle.

> **TEST-TAKING TIP**—Therapeutic nursing process calls for supportive care (e.g., reinforce), *not* a dominant, controlling approach (e.g., rigid, confronting).
> **PL, APP, 7, Psych, PsI, Psychosocial Integrity**

71. **(3)** Because the client has a history of chronic cough, and because hernias can be repaired with spinal anesthesia, this approach may have the least amount of risk for postoperative complications. General anesthesia (**Answer 1**) has the greatest risk for respiratory complications after surgery. Intravenous (**Answer 2**) and local infiltration (**Answer 4**) would not supply the depth of anesthesia needed to complete the repair.

> **TEST-TAKING TIP**—Look for the anesthesia that will be safest for a client who is high-risk.
> **PL, COM, 1, M/S: Meds, PhI, Reduction of Risk Potential**

72. **(2)** Timed forced expiratory volume measures the functional ability of an individual to remove air from his or her lungs. Reduction in FEV_1 is usually due to airway obstruction from excess mucus. Vital capacity measures the individual's ability to move a volume of air in and out of the lungs (**Answer 1**). Though inadequate innervation of the intercostals (**Answer 3**) would also reduce the FEV_1, there is nothing in this case to indicate that this client has neuromuscular problems. Atelectasis (**Answer 4**) is determined by x-ray, clinical symptomatology, and blood gases.

> **TEST-TAKING TIP**—Distinguish between the normal and the abnormal findings. Normal vital capacity means no difficulty in moving air in and out of the lungs. Reduced forced expiratory volume means something is interfering with expiratory phase of respiration; air is trapped (possible COPD).
> **IMP, ANL, 6, M/S: Dx Test, PhI, Physiological Adaptation**

73. **(3)** This diurnal variation is characteristic of a *reactive* (situational) depression. The individuals experiencing a melancholic type depression usually feel worse in the morning but better as the day progresses. In reactive depression there is usually a weight loss of *less* than 10 pounds (**Answer 1**). The individuals usually do respond to environmental stimuli (**Answer 2**). The precipitating event is usually an *identifiable* stressor, such as the birth of an unhealthy baby (**Answer 4**).

> **TEST-TAKING TIP**—Knowing the difference between reactive depression (situational) and melancholia will point to the correct answer. You can also eliminate **Answers 2** and **4** because of similarity of terms, such as "reactive" (situational); you *would* expect a response (reaction) to environment and external stressors (events).
> **AN, COM, 7, Psych, PsI, Psychosocial Integrity**

74. **(1)** Quadriceps-setting exercise is an appropriate activity to prevent complications of immobility. Range-of-motion exercises for joints not enclosed in the cast are encouraged. The primary purpose of the cast is to immobilize those joints above and below the fracture site; therefore extension (**Answer 2**) and flexion (**Answer 4**) of the knees are inappropriate. **Answer 3** is not correct because passive range of motion is *not as effective as active* range of motion in the prevention of complications of immobility.

> **TEST-TAKING TIP**—Visualize the cast; joints above and below the fracture site will be enclosed in the cast. That eliminates any activity for the ankle and knee. Prevention of complications from immobility is best accomplished with active range of motion rather than passive. The best answer would be quadriceps setting. Prevent atrophy while in the cast.
> **PL, APP, 3, M/S: Ortho, PhI, Reduction of Risk Potential**

75. **(1)** Toddlers will most likely experience separation anxiety when separated from parents. In the "despair" phase, the child appears to be mourning the apparent loss of the parent, as evidenced by nonverbal behavior cues such as monotone crying, regressive behavior (thumb sucking), and sleep disturbances. If this child were experiencing muscle spasms due to her fracture (**Answer 4**), she would most likely cry out in severe pain intermittently. The other explanations for her behavior (**Answers 2** and **3**) do not take her developmental level into account.

> **TEST-TAKING TIP**—Know age-typical (toddler) behavior in relation to the concept of separation anxiety.
> **AN, ANL, 5, PEDS, PsI, Psychosocial Integrity**

76. **(2)** It is important to assess and validate the parents' perceived needs in order to plan care effectively. The parents may need a social worker as well as a community health nurse, speech pathologist, audiologist, etc. Therefore it is essential to first make an accurate and continual assessment

of the family's needs before referral (**Answer 1**). Alternatives (**Answer 3**) may be more appropriately identified *after* performing a total assessment. Health teaching (**Answer 4**) is necessary, but it must be based on an assessment and validation of the family's needs as well as of their level of readiness.

> **TEST-TAKING TIP**—Assessment ("validate") comes before referral (**Answer 1**), discussing alternatives (**Answer 3**), or doing health teaching (**Answer 4**).
> **PL, APP, 7, Psych, PsI, Psychosocial Integrity**

77. (**1**) An induration of 10 mm or more (not cm, as in **Answer 2**) is considered a positive reaction. The skin is generally reddened. Indurations of 5 to 9 mm (**Answer 3**) are considered *doubtful* reactions. Individuals with doubtful reactions should be retested, unless they have had a known contact with persons with tuberculosis. Indurations of less than 5 mm are considered *negative* reactions. The reaction is *not* hivelike (**Answer 4**).

> **TEST-TAKING TIP**—Visualize the size of each of the options given. Watch the unit of measure (mm versus cm).
> **EV, COM, 1, M/S: Infect. Control, SECE, Safety and Infection Control**

78. (**1**) The primary effect of rapid infusion of hyperalimentation solutions is cellular dehydration due to osmosis of water from the cell in response to vascular hyperosmolarity. Occasionally circulatory overload (**Answer 2**) does occur, but with hyperglycemia. When infusion rates are rapid, supplementary insulin should be administered to prevent the effects of hyperglycemia. Hypoglycemia (**Answer 3**) may occur if the infusion rate is suddenly decreased because the body generally adapts to hyperosmolar solutions by increasing insulin release from the pancreas. However, *hypervolemia*, not hypovolemia, generally occurs. Potassium *depletion*, not excess (**Answer 4**), also results.

> **TEST-TAKING TIP**—Know the concepts of osmosis and diffusion as they relate to a hypertonic solution, *high* in glucose.
> **EV, ANL, 6, M/S: F-E, PhI, Pharmacological and Parenteral Therapies**

79. (**4**) The exact cause of the failure of the embryonic structures of the face to form a union is unclear. However, there is a significant familial pattern, and a hereditary factor is involved. Cleft palate is seen more frequently in girls, whereas cleft lip is seen more frequently in boys (**Answers 1** and **2**). Although cleft lip and palate sometimes do occur together (**Answer 3**), in many cases they occur independently.

> **TEST-TAKING TIP**—Choose the more general "heredity" response than gender-specific responses (**Answers 1** and **2**); eliminate the option with "always" in the stem.
> **AN, ANL, 5, PEDS, HPM, Health Promotion and Maintenance**

80. (**3**) It is essential that the nurse be readily available to provide physiological, sociological, and psychological support when needed. The father has requested assistance; therefore, although privacy (**Answer 1**) is important, remaining with the couple to provide support and guidance is paramount. **Answer 2** may be appropriate if sitting with the couple does not decrease the mother's anxiety. **Answer 4** will probably be ineffective. Furthermore, she may need to feel that it is OK to express her feelings, and the nurse should encourage her to be as open as possible.

> **TEST-TAKING TIP**—In crisis intervention, *support* (sitting quietly) is a first priority.
> **PL, ANL, 7, Psych, PsI, Psychosocial Integrity**

81. (**1**) Fluid orders vary among hospitals, physicians, and childbirth methods. Because the woman is in preterm labor and is bleeding, the orders will probably maintain her NPO with an IV. **Answers 2** and **3** are incorrect because giving her a small sip of water or ice chips may be contraindicated at this time. **Answer 4** is incorrect because the physician may allow sips of water or ice chips.

> **TEST-TAKING TIP**—Look at the verbs: "check" with the MD, "give," "offer," "tell… cannot have." Two options *give* the water; one option *withholds* it. The best answer is to *check* with the MD because this is a complicated labor.
> **IMP, ANL, 6, Maternity, PhI, Reduction of Risk Potential**

82. (**4**) Infants or children with milk allergies should be offered a lactose-free formula such as Isomil. **Answers 1, 2,** and **3** are incorrect because these formulas are lactose-based and are contraindicated for infants or children with milk allergies.

> **TEST-TAKING TIP**—Know which formulas are lactose free: Isomil, Prosobee, and Nutramigen.
> **IMP, COM, 4, PEDS, PhI, Basic Care and Comfort**

83. (**1**) The rationale for pacemaker implantation is presented in the preinsertion period and is reinforced in the postinsertion period and therefore receives the least emphasis in the predischarge plan. **Answers 2, 3,** and **4** are incorrect: they *are* essential components of a predischarge teaching plan, because the client must focus on management of the pacemaker, and they all receive great emphasis.

> **TEST-TAKING TIP**—Look for a pattern. The *least* emphasis would be on a preinsertion education topic.
> **PL, APP, 6, M/S: Cardiac, HPM, Health Promotion and Maintenance**

84. (**2**) SIDS usually occurs within the first year of life. The peak time appears to be between 2 and 4 months after birth. **Answer 1** is incorrect because SIDS rarely occurs within 2–4 *weeks* after birth. **Answers 3** and **4** are incorrect because SIDS is comparatively unusual *after* 6 months of age; 95% of all cases occur by 6 months of age.

> **TEST-TAKING TIP**—Answers 3 and 4 are virtually the same; therefore, neither choice is the correct answer.
> **AS, COM, 5, PEDS, HPM, Health Promotion and Maintenance**

85. (**3**) Morphine sulfate acts not only to reduce pain and anxiety by blocking the activity of the reticular substance in the brainstem, but also to relax vascular smooth muscle, thereby decreasing blood pressure. Nausea and vomiting are common adverse side effects of this medication. Atropine is an anticholinergic whose drying effects tend to cause the client to complain that the mouth feels like cotton. **Answers 1** and **4** are incorrect because atropine also blocks vagal effects on the heart, increasing pulse rate, *not* decreasing it. **Answer 2** is incorrect because blood pressure is decreased, *not* increased.

> **TEST-TAKING TIP**—Look for side effects that relate to the drug action: vasodilation (morphine) and decreased secretions (atropine)
> **EV, COM, 1, M/S: Meds, PhI, Pharmacological and Parenteral Therapies**

86. (**1**) If the IV infused at the correct rate of 40 mL/hr from 11:00 A.M. to 3:15 P.M., the client should have received 170 mL of IV fluid; because the client has received twice the prescribed amount, the nurse should *first* correct the rate, *then* notify the physician (**Answer 4**). (The nurse should also check at this time to see if the IV line is being affected by the position of the limb.) If, after contacting the physician, a new rate is ordered, only then would the nurse adjust the rate to a level lower than

originally prescribed (**Answer 3**). **Answer 2** is incorrect because there is no reason to hang a new bag at this time.

> **TEST-TAKING TIP**—First, decide whether this is OK or *not* OK. Next, choose a corrective action *before* calling the MD. Look for a choice that *first* addresses the client's safety.
> **IMP, ANL, 6, M/S: F-E, PhI, Pharmacological and Parenteral Therapies**

87. (2) Although drug abuse may be found at every age level, the elderly seem least likely to abuse substances in general. This is probably due to generational differences in cultural norms and morals. (It was thought that one was "weak" or "sick" to rely on drugs to escape problems.) However, many times the elderly specifically use alcohol as an escape mechanism. **Answers 1** and **3** are incorrect because drug abuse is found among all socioeconomic classes. **Answer 4** is incorrect because many adolescents use drugs to escape reality, cope with stress, identify with their peers, etc. The reasons for abuse vary from individual to individual, depending on their particular needs.

> **TEST-TAKING TIP**—Note key phrase: "*least* prevalent."
> **AN, APP, 7, Psych, PsI, Psychosocial Integrity**

88. (1) Anticoagulants increase bleeding time and tendency to hemorrhage. Antihypertensives such as reserpine, hydralazine, and methyldopa potentiate the hypotensive effects of anesthetic agents, thereby creating problems with maintenance of blood pressure. Thiazide diuretics may induce potassium depletion and lead to respiratory depression during anesthesia. **Answers 2, 3,** and **4** are incorrect because neither insulin, digoxin, nor vitamins and minerals potentiate the central nervous system depression due to anesthesia.

> **TEST-TAKING TIP**—Review the options as to potential risk in the postoperative phase. If a part of the option is wrong, the option is wrong even if it contains some part that is correct. Once you have eliminated those components that have something wrong in them, there is usually only one correct answer left. Use the process of elimination.
> **EV, COM, 1, M/S: Meds, PhI, Reduction of Risk Potential**

89. (3) Before assessing and planning any rehabilitation program, the nurse must *first* assess the client's and the family's understanding of and attitudes toward myasthenia, as well as their emotional response and coping abilities. *Before* ascertaining any further information about job stresses (**Answers 1** and **4**) or lifestyle (**Answer 2**), any unusual fears, misconceptions, or problems relating to the client's condition need to be identified and dealt with. It may be necessary to utilize the skills of a psychiatric nurse specialist, health psychologist, or psychiatrist to evaluate the situation and assist in planning interventions.

> **TEST-TAKING TIP**—The question is asking for priority (i.e., *first*).
> **AS, ANL, 3, M/S: NM, PsI, Psychosocial Integrity**

90. (3) The prevention of scarring is essential. All crusts should be cleaned away as gently as possible, and the area should be cleansed frequently to prevent infection. The infant should be placed on the back or side and minimally restrained to prevent him or her from turning onto the face. The side position is preferred in order to prevent the aspiration of mucus or the regurgitation of milk (**Answer 1**). The infant needs to be repositioned frequently to lessen the danger of hypostatic pneumonia (**Answer 2**). Crying should be minimized as much as possible to avoid unnecessary strain on the suture line (**Answer 4**).

> **TEST-TAKING TIP**—Visualize the surgical site anatomically and eliminate **Answer 1** (needs to be face up) and

Answer 4 (what happens to suture line when crying?). Choose the option that *prevents* (**Answer 3**).
> **IMP, ANL, 1, PEDS, PhI, Reduction of Risk Potential**

91. (2) Keeping the foot in the correct anatomical position is the *best* method of preventing footdrop, and a footboard is best when the client is in traction. A bed cradle (**Answer 1**) is effective in keeping pressure off the legs and feet. Passive range of motion (**Answer 3**) is most effective in preventing contractures. A trochanter roll (**Answer 4**) is most effective in preventing external rotation of the hip.

> **TEST-TAKING TIP**—Visualize the traction; it has ropes and pulleys and weights. This eliminates the bed cradle. A trochanter roll is used to prevent external rotation, not footdrop. The key phrase is "most effective." Something that is continuous rather than three times a day would be best. Look for clues in the stem—*foot*drop… *foot* board.
> **IMP, COM, 3, M/S: Ortho, PhI, Basic Care and Comfort**

92. (2) He is attempting to cope with his anxiety by denying reality. He may also be angry (**Answer 1**), but his behavior and verbalization indicate denial. It is through the use of denial that he is displacing the blame (**Answer 3**), so denial is the more appropriate answer. He is unable to think clearly enough to seek any type of intervention (**Answer 4**); he is reacting rather than problem solving.

> **TEST-TAKING TIP**—Denial is the most common coping mechanism. One manifestation of denial can be anger, but denial is the more inclusive answer. Eliminate **Answers 3** and **4** because they are not related to the stem.
> **AN, ANL, 7, Psych, PsI, Psychosocial Integrity**

93. (4) During the phase of denial (also known as detachment), the child covers up painful feelings toward the mother and turns instead to others, such as the nurse. The nurse should explain to the toddler's mother that the toddler is not trying to make the mother jealous and that the toddler shoud not be scolded or disciplined for turning away from the mother. This behavior can usually be modified by increased visitation of the toddler by the mother and a quick return home to reestablish the toddler's routines.

Answer 1 is incorrect because the major stress from middle infancy throughout the preschool years, especially for children ages 16–30 months, is separation anxiety, also called anaclitic depression. This term describes three distinct phases (protest, despair, denial) as opposed to the specific phase of separation anxiety, which the toddler is demonstrating. Separation anxiety is usually manifested during illness and hospitalization because of the child's limited number of coping mechanisms when confronted with a change from the usual state of health and routine.

Answer 2 is incorrect because during the phase of protest, the child cries loudly, screams for the parent, refuses the attention of anyone else, and is inconsolable.

Answer 3 is incorrect because during the phase of despair, the crying stops. The child is much less active, is disinterested in play or food, and withdraws from others.

Answer 5 is incorrect because this is a normal stage of social development and is not related to the process of hospitalization. As infants demonstrate attachment to one person (usually the mother), they correspondingly exhibit less friendliness to others. From ages 6–8 months, fear of strangers becomes prominent and is related to the infant's ability to discriminate between familiar and nonfamiliar people.

> **TEST-TAKING TIP**—Know the manifestations and stages of separation anxiety versus age-appropriate stranger fear.
> **AN, APP, 7, PEDS, PsI, Psychosocial Integrity**

Final Test

94. **(3)** Drinking 6 oz with each pill is too much! Iopanoic acid (Telepaque) tablets are administered *1 hour after* eating a *fat free meal* (**Answers 1 and 2**), one at a time and in *5-minute* intervals, with a *minimal* amount of water (usually 8 oz) to swallow *all* the tablets. Water *is* allowed until bedtime (**Answer 4**), but food is withheld to allow as much dye as possible to concentrate in the gallbladder. The next morning an initial x-ray is taken, after which the client is given a fatty meal, and several more pictures are taken to observe the functioning of the gallbladder.

> **TEST-TAKING TIP**—The key word is "inappropriate" or what would you *not* do for this client. Look for the wrong answer, not the correct one, when it asks for what is "inappropriate."
> **PL, APP, 4, M/S: Dx Test, PhI, Reduction of Risk Potential**

95. **(1)** Since tracheostomy inhibits the client from talking, it is essential to establish a mode of postoperative communication so that the client can express needs. The mode chosen should be communicated to the rest of the staff so that the approach to the client is consistent. Blood work (**Answer 2**) may or may not be ordered before tracheostomy, though blood gas analysis is frequently ordered to establish baseline data in order to evaluate the effectiveness of the intervention. Inserting a Foley catheter (**Answer 3**) is not a priority *unless* urinary output has decreased. A standard surgical prep (**Answer 4**), cleansing and shaving the operative area, is not done before tracheostomy. However, the physician does cleanse the area with an antiseptic before performing the tracheostomy.

> **TEST-TAKING TIP**—Do something for the client directly, then take care of procedures.
> **AN, APP, 7, M/S: Preop, PsI, Psychosocial Integrity**

96. **(2)** After the client has left for surgery, family members should be told the approximate time the client will be in surgery and that from there the client will go to the recovery room until awake and all vital signs are stable. Clarify that delays may occur and that the induction of, as well as the emergence from, anesthesia takes time. **Answers 1 and 3** are incorrect because family members should be allowed to decide whether they will stay or go and come back later. If family members decide to wait, direct them to a waiting area where they can be comfortable. Assure them that you will direct the surgeon to them after the surgery is finished. **Answer 4** is not an initial action. The nurse does answer any questions and concerns the family members may have, being as supportive as possible.

> **TEST-TAKING TIP**—Look at the action words carefully: "*tell* him," "*explain* that," "*get* him," or "*encourage* him." Best answer is to *encourage* him.
> **IMP, APP, 7, Psych, PsI, Psychosocial Integrity**

97. **(1)** IPPB facilitates the flow of air deep into the lungs by exerting pressures greater than atmospheric pressure (positive pressure) on inspiration. The client needs to learn to take slow, controlled inspirations to prevent hyperventilation. **Answers 2, 3,** and **4** are incorrect because negative inspiratory pressures are consistent with CPAP or PEEP ventilatory systems, and pressures normally become more negative as the client exhales.

> **TEST-TAKING TIP**—Key term in this question is "positive pressure." This eliminates two options immediately. To improve respiratory hygiene, you attempt to get more air in during inspiration.
> **AN, COM, 6, M/S: Resp., PhI, Physiological Adaptation**

98. **(3)** The cumulative inflow and outflow records should show an outflow equal to or in excess of the amount instilled. The amount of excess outflow allowed is also determined by the physician; this rarely exceeds 200 mL per cycle. Occasionally, drainage is less then expected. Nursing measures to enhance outflow include turning the client from side to side, elevating the *head* of the bed (increases intraabdominal pressures), and/or gently massaging the abdomen. If the problem continues, notify the physician before initiating another cycle; the *physician* may attempt to clear the catheter by rotation or by probing it for fibrin clots (**Answer 2**). **Answers 1** and **4** will not improve flow.

> **TEST-TAKING TIP**—Visualize where the catheter is placed and what would facilitate the return of fluid. By elevating the head of the bed, intra-abdominal pressure is increased; this in turn helps to force the fluid out through the catheter.
> **IMP, APP, 6, M/S: F-E, PhI, Reduction of Risk Potential**

99. **(3)** It is important for all health team members to be in touch with their feelings about death and dying in order to help the family work through *their* feelings. **Answers 1** and **2** may help the nurse teach the family to express their feelings, but **Answer 3** is still primary. **Answer 4** is inappropriate because suppression may lead to avoidance and to the ineffective resolution of feelings.

> **TEST-TAKING TIP**—Ask yourself, is it knowledge and experience that is primary? Or is it "feelings"? "Feelings" are primary. Then ask, is it suppression or identification of feelings? Being in touch with your own feelings is a primary nursing concept.
> **PL, ANL, 7, Psych, PsI, Psychosocial Integrity**

100. **(2)** The nurse must meet the parents at their level of readiness while at the same time providing them with enough information to allow them to care adequately for the infant. Sucking needs to be *avoided* in an infant with a cleft palate because of the possibility of aspiration and because the infant will not be allowed to suck postoperatively (**Answer 1**). A special nipple or feeder is helpful, such as Lamb's nipple or Brecht feeder. The infant should be fed in an *upright* position to decrease the likelihood of aspiration (**Answer 3**). The infant needs to be isolated *only* from those individuals with *infectious* diseases such as colds or chickenpox (**Answer 4**). The infant should be treated as normally as possible to stimulate growth and development.

> **TEST-TAKING TIP**—Eliminate three of the options (too specific *and* incorrect); instead, select the most *general* response ("difficulty feeding").
> **IMP, APP, 4, PEDS, PhI, Basic Care and Comfort**

Laboratory Values

This chart gives a quick overview of what is normal and the conditions that result in high or low values.

Test	Normal Values	Possible Significance	
		Increases	Decreases
Hematology			
Aspartate aminotransferase (AST)—formerly called serum glutamic oxaloacetic transaminase (SGOT)	*Men:* 10–40 U/L *Women:* 9–25 U/L	Myocardial infarction, cardiac surgery, hepatitis, cirrhosis, trauma, severe burns, progressive muscular dystrophy, infectious mononucleosis, acute renal failure, Reye syndrome, HELLP syndrome	Uremia, chronic dialysis, ketoacidosis
Bleeding time—indication of hemostatic efficiency	1–9 min	Hemorrhagic purpura, acute leukemia, aplastic anemia, DIC, oral anticoagulant therapy, Reye syndrome	
Hematocrit—volume of packed red blood cells/100 mL of blood	*Men:* 45% (40%–50%) *Women:* 40% (38%–47%)	Dehydration, polycythemia, congenital heart disease	Anemia, hemorrhage, leukemia, dietary deficiencies
Hemoglobin—oxygen-combining protein	*Men:* 13.5–18 g/dL *Women:* 12–16 g/dL	Same as for Hematocrit	Same as for Hematocrit
Activated partial thromboplastin time (aPTT)— tests coagulation mechanism; stage I deficiencies	*aPTT:* 25–41	Deficiency of factors VIII, IX, X, XI, XII; anticoagulant therapy	Extensive cancer, DIC
Platelets—thrombocytes	150,000–400,000/mm³	Polycythemia vera, postsplenectomy, anemia, Kawasaki disease	Leukemia, aplastic anemia, cirrhosis, multiple myeloma, chemotherapy, HELLP syndrome
Prothrombin time—tests extrinsic clotting; stages II and III	10–13 sec	Anticoagulant therapy, DIC, hepatic disease, malabsorption, Reye syndrome	Digitalis therapy, diuretic reaction, vitamin K therapy
Red blood cell count—number of circulating erythrocytes in 1 μL of whole blood	*Men:* 4.5–6.2 million/μL *Women:* 4.2–5.4 million/μL	Polycythemia vera, anoxia, dehydration	Leukemia, hemorrhage, anemias, Hodgkin's
Sedimentation rate—speed at which red blood cells settle in uncoagulated blood	*Men:* 0–15 mm/hr *Women:* 0–20 mm/hr	Acute bacterial infection, cancer, infectious disease, numerous inflammatory states, rheumatic fever, Kawasaki disease	Polycythemia vera, sickle cell anemia
White blood cell count—number of leukocytes in 1 μL	4.5–11 × 10³/μL	Leukemia, bacterial infection, severe sepsis, Kawasaki disease	Viral infection, overwhelming bacterial infection, lupus erythematosus, antineoplastic chemotherapy, bone marrow depression

(Continued on following page)

Test	Normal Values	Possible Significance	
		Increases	Decreases
White blood cell differential—enumeration of individual leukocyte distribution			
Neutrophils	56% mean cell count 1800–7800/µL	Bacterial infection, tumor, inflammation, stress, drug reaction, trauma, metabolic disorders	Acute viral infection, anorexia nervosa, radiation therapy, drug induced, alcoholic ingestion
Eosinophils	2.7% cell count 0–450/µL	Allergic disorder, parasitic infestation, eosinophilic leukemia	Acute or chronic stress; excess ACTH, cortisone, or epinephrine; endocrine disorder
Basophils	25–100/µL, or 0–1% cell count 0–200/µL	Myeloproliferative disease, leukemia	Anaphylactic reaction, hyperthyroidism, radiation therapy, infections, ovulation, pregnancy, aging
Lymphocytes	20%–40% cell count 1000–4800/µL	Chronic lymphocytic leukemia, infectious mononucleosis, chronic bacterial infection, viral infection	Leukemia, systemic lupus erythematosus, immune deficiency disorders
Blood Chemistry			
Alkaline phosphatase (ALP)	32–92 U/L	Hyperparathyroidism, Paget's disease, cancer with bone metastasis, obstructive jaundice, cirrhosis, hepatitis A, rickets	Malnutrition, scurvy, celiac disease, chronic nephritis, hypothyroidism, cystic fibrosis
Amylase	80–180 IU/L	Acute pancreatitis, mumps, duodenal ulcer, pancreatic cancer, perforated bowel, renal failure	Advanced chronic pancreatitis, chronic alcoholism
Bilirubin, serum	*Direct:* 0.0–0.4 mg/dL *Indirect:* 0.2–0.8 mg/dL *Total:* 0.3–1.0 mg/dL	Massive hemolysis, low-grade hemolytic disease, cirrhosis, obstructive liver disease, hepatitis, biliary obstruction, neonatal (physiological) jaundice	
B-type natriuretic peptide	NON-CHF *Men:* 10 pg/mL (picogram) *Women:* 17 pg/mL CHF *Men:* 146–928 pg/mL *Women:* 149–858 pg/mL	Heart failure	
Calcium, serum	8.2–10.2 mg/dL	Hyperparathyroidism, multiple myeloma, bone metastasis, bone fracture, thiazide-diuretic reaction, milk-alkali syndrome	Hypoparathyroidism, renal failure, pregnancy, massive transfusion
Carbon dioxide	22–30 mEq/L	Emphysema, salicylate toxicity, vomiting	Starvation, diarrhea
Chloride, serum	98–107 mEq/L	Hyperventilation, diabetes insipidus, uremia, cystic fibrosis	Heart failure, pyloric obstruction, hypoventilation, vomiting, chronic respiratory acidosis
Creatine, serum	*Men:* 0.7–1.3 mg/dL *Women:* 0.5–1.0 mg/dL	Chronic glomerulonephritis, nephritis, heart failure, muscle disease	Debilitation, long-term corticosteroid therapy
Creatine kinase (CK) (creatine phosphokinase [CPK])	*Men:* 17–148 IU/L *Women:* 10–79 IU/L	Acute myocardial infarction, acute stroke, convulsions, surgery, muscular dystrophy, hypokalemia	Addison's disease
Isoenzymes			

(Continued on following page)

Test	Normal Values	Possible Significance	
		Increases	Decreases
CPK-MM/CK-MM	100%	Muscular dystrophy, delirium tremens, surgery, hypokalemia, crush injuries, hypothyroidism	
CPK/MB/CK-MB	0.6% of total CPK	Acute myocardial infarction, cardiac defibrillation, myocarditis, cardiac ischemia	
CPK-BB/CK-BB	0%	Pulmonary infarction, brain surgery, stroke, pulmonary embolism, seizures, intestinal ischemia	
Fibrinogen, serum	0.2–0.4 g/100 dL or 200–400 mg/dL	Pneumonia, acute infection, nephrosis, rheumatoid arthritis	Cirrhosis, toxic liver necrosis, anemia, obstetric complications, DIC, advanced carcinoma
Glucose (fasting)	60–110 mg/100 mL (serum)	Acute stress, Cushing's syndrome, hyperthyroidism, acute or chronic pancreatitis, diabetes mellitus, hyperglycemia	Addison's disease, liver disease, reactive hypoglycemia, pituitary hypofunction
Glycosylated hemoglobin (HbA_{1c})	4.0%–7.0%	Newly diagnosed or poorly controlled diabetes mellitus	Iron deficiency anemia, chronic blood loss
Iron-binding capacity (total)	218–385 g/dL	Lead poisoning, hepatic necrosis	
Lactic dehydrogenase (LDH)	60–120 U/mL (Wacker Scale) 150–450 U/mL (Wroblewski)	Myocardial infarction, pernicious anemia, chronic viral hepatitis, pneumonia, pulmonary emboli, stroke, renal tissue destruction, leukemia, non-Hodgkin's lymphoma, shock, trauma, Reye syndrome	
LDH-1	17%–27%		
LDH-2	27%–37%		
LDH-3	18%–25%		
LDH-4	3%–8%		
LDH-5	6%–16%		
Lipids:			
Cholesterol (total serum)	<200 mg/dL	Hypercholesterolemia, hyperlipidemia, myocardial infarction, uncontrolled diabetes mellitus, high cholesterol diet, hypothyroidism, atherosclerosis, stress, familial biliary obstruction, nephrotic syndrome	Malnutrition, cholesterol-lowering medication, anemia, liver disease, hyperthyroidism
Low-density lipoprotein (LDL)	<130 mg/dL		
High-density lipoprotein (HDL)	35–75 mg/dL		
Triglycerides	40–150 mg/100 mL		
Phosphorus, inorganic serum	3.0–4.5 mg/dL	Chronic glomerular disease, hypoparathyroidism, milk-alkali syndrome, sarcoidosis	Hyperparathyroidism, rickets, osteomalacia, renal tubular necrosis, malabsorption syndrome, vitamin D deficiency
Potassium, serum	3.5–5.0 mEq/L	Diabetic ketosis, renal failure, Addison's disease, excessive intake, APSGN	Thiazide diuretics, Cushing's syndrome, cirrhosis with ascites, hyperaldosteronism, steroid therapy, malignant hypertension, poor dietary habits, chronic diarrhea, diaphoresis, renal tubular necrosis, malabsorption syndrome, vomiting
Protein, serum (albumin/globulin)	*Total:* 6.4–8.3 g/dL *Albumin:* 3.5–5.0 g/dL *Globulin:* 2.8–4.4 g/dL	Dehydration, multiple myeloma, APSGN	Chronic liver disease, myeloproliferative disease, burns, nephrotic syndrome, Hirschsprung's disease

(Continued on following page)

Appendix A

Test	Normal Values	Possible Significance	
		Increases	Decreases
Serum glutamic-oxaloacetic transaminase (SGOT)—see AST			
Sodium, serum	136–145 mEq/L	Increased intake, either orally or IV; Cushing's syndrome, excessive sweating, diabetes insipidus, cystic fibrosis	Addison's disease, sodium-losing nephropathy, vomiting, diarrhea, fistulas, tube drainage, burns, renal insufficiency with acidosis, starvation with acidosis, paracentesis, thoracentesis, ascites, heart failure, SIADH
T$_3$ uptake	24%–34%	Hyperthyroidism, thyroxine-binding globulin (TBG) deficiency	Hypothyroidism, pregnancy, TBG excess
Thyroxine	5–12 μg/dL	Hyperthyroidism, pregnancy	Hypothyroidism, renal failure
Troponin 1	0–0.5 ng/ml	Acute myocardial infarction	
Urea nitrogen, serum (BUN)	5–20 mg/dL	Acute or chronic renal failure, heart failure, obstructive uropathy, dehydration, HELLP syndrome	Cirrhosis, malnutrition
Uric acid, serum	*Men:* 4.5–8 mg/dL *Women:* 2.5–6.2 mg/dL	Gout, chronic renal failure, starvation, diuretic therapy	
Blood Gases			
Bicarbonate (HCO$_3$)	21–28 mEq/L	Metabolic alkalosis	Metabolic acidosis
Carbon dioxide pressure (Pco$_2$), whole blood, arterial	35–45 mm Hg	Primary respiratory acidosis, loss of H$^+$ through nasogastric suctioning or vomiting	Primary respiratory alkalosis
Oxygen pressure (Po$_2$), whole blood, arterial	80–100 mm Hg	Oxygen administration in the absence of severe lung disease	Chronic obstructive lung disease, severe pneumonia, pulmonary embolism, pulmonary edema, respiratory muscle disease
pH, serum	7.35–7.45	Metabolic alkalosis–alkali ingestion, respiratory alkalosis–hyperventilation	Metabolic acidosis–ketoacidosis, shock, respiratory acidosis–alveolar hypoventilation
Immunodiagnostic Studies			
Carcinoembryonic antigen	<2.5 ng/mL	*Cancer* of: colon, lung, metastatic breast, pancreas, stomach, prostate, ovary, bladder, limbs; also neuroblastoma, leukemias, osteogenic carcinoma; *non-cancer* conditions such as: hepatic cirrhosis, uremia, pancreatitis, colorectal, polyposis, peptic ulcer disease, ulcerative colitis, regional enteritis	
Urinalysis			
pH	4.5–7.8	Metabolic alkalosis	Metabolic acidosis
Specific gravity	1.003–1.029	Dehydration, pituitary tumor, hypotension, APSGN	Distal renal tubular disease, polycystic kidney disease, diabetes insipidus, overhydration
Glucose	Negative	Diabetes mellitus	
Protein	Negative	Nephrosis, glomerulonephritis, lupus erythematosus, preeclampsia	
Casts	0–0.4 hyaline casts per LPF	Nephrosis, glomerulonephritis, lupus erythematosus, infection	

(Continued on following page)

Test	Normal Values	Possible Significance	
		Increases	**Decreases**
Red blood cells	Negative	Renal calculi, hemorrhagic cystitis, tumors of the kidney, APSGN	
White blood cells	Negative	Inflammation of the kidneys, ureters, or bladder	
Color	Normal yellow, clear	*Abnormal: red to reddish brown*—hematuria; *brown to brownish gray*—bilirubinuria or urobilinuria; *tea colored*—possible obstructive jaundice	*Almost colorless:* chronic kidney disease, diabetes insipidus, diabetes mellitus
Sodium	40–220 mEq/L/24 hr	Salt-wasting renal disease, SIADH, dehydration	Heart failure, primary aldosteronism
Chloride	110–250 mEq/24 hr	Chronic obstructive lung disease, dehydration, salicylate toxicity	Gastric suction, heart failure, emphysema
Potassium	25–125 mEq/L/24 hr	Diuretic therapy	Renal failure
Creatinine clearance	90–139 mL/min		Renal disease
Hydroxycorticosteroids	2–10 mg/24 hr	Cushing's disease	Addison's disease
17-Ketosteroids	*Men:* 4.5–12 mg/24 hr *Women:* 2.5–10 mg/24 hr	Hirsutism, adrenal hyperplasia	Thyrotoxicosis, Addison's disease
Catecholamines (VMA)	*Epinephrine:* <20 μg/24 hr *Norepinephrine:* <100 μg/24 hr	Pheochromocytoma, severe anxiety, numerous medications	
Urine Test			
Schilling test	Excretion of 8%–40% or more of test dose should appear in urine		Gastrointestinal malabsorption, pernicious anemia

NCLEX-RN® Test Plan:
Four General Client Needs and Six Client Subneeds:
Definitions/Descriptions*

The latest NCLEX-RN® test plan follows the categories of client needs and client subneeds described below.

A. Safe, Effective Care Environment

See also **Appendix H**, Eight Detailed Areas of Human Functions Definitions/Descriptions—*Protective Functions.*

The nurse meets client needs for a safe and effective care environment by providing and directing nursing care that protects clients, family/significant others, and other health-care personnel and promotes achievement of the following client needs and subneeds:

1. **Management of care**—providing coordinating, supervising, and collaborating with all other multidisciplinary health-care team members to provide integrated cost-effective client care, including activities related to ethical and legal issues.
2. **Safety and infection control**—protecting clients, family and significant others, and health-care personnel from health and environmental hazards.

Knowledge, Skills, and Abilities

To meet client needs for a safe, effective care environment, the nurse should possess knowledge, skills, and abilities that include but are not limited to the following areas:

1. *Management of care*
   - Accountability
   - Advance Directives
   - Advocacy
   - Case Management
   - Client Rights
   - Collaboration with Multidisciplinary Team
   - Concepts of Management
   - Confidentiality
   - Consultation
   - Continuity of Care
   - Continuous Quality Improvement
   - Delegation
   - Establishing Priorities
   - Ethical Practice
   - Group Dynamics
   - Informed Consent
   - Legal Rights and Responsibilities
   - Organ Donation
   - Performance Improvement (Quality Assurance)
   - Referrals
   - Resource Management
   - Staff Education
   - Supervision
2. *Safety and infection control*
   - Accident Prevention
   - Disaster Planning: Environmental and Personal Safety
   - Emergency Response Plan
   - Error Prevention
   - Handling Hazardous and Infectious Materials
   - Home Safety
   - Injury Prevention
   - Medical and Surgical Asepsis
   - Reporting of Incident/Event/Irregular Occurrence/Variance
   - Safe Use of Special Equipment
   - Security Plan
   - Standard (Universal)/Transmission-Based/Other Precautions
   - Use of Restraints/Safety Devices

---

*Adapted from National Council of State Boards of Nursing: NCLEX-RN® Test Plan. National Council of State Boards, Chicago, 2004.

B. Health Promotion and Maintenance

See also **Appendix H**, Eight Detailed Areas of Human Functions Definitions/Descriptions—*Growth and Development, Nutrition.*

The nurse meets client needs for health promotion and maintenance throughout the life span by providing and directing nursing care of the client and family/significant others that incorporates the knowledge of expected growth and development principles, prevention and/or early detection of health problems, and strategies to achieve optimum health.

Growth and development throughout the life span—assisting clients and significant others through normal and expected stages of *growth and development,* from conception through advanced old age (includes routine newborn care and normal prepartum, intrapartum, and postpartum care).

Prevention and early detection of disease—managing and providing for clients and significant others in need of prevention and/or early detection of health problems and strategies to achieve optimal health; assisting clients to recognize alterations in health and to develop health practices that promote and support wellness.

Knowledge, Skills, and Abilities

To meet client needs of health promotion and maintenance, the nurse should possess knowledge, skills, and abilities that include but are not limited to the following areas:

Growth and development throughout the life span
- Aging Process
- Ante/Intra/Postpartum and Newborn Care; Birthing and Parenting
- Developmental Stages and Transitions
- *Expected* Body Image Changes
- Family Planning
- Family Systems
- Human Sexuality; Reproduction

Prevention and early detection of disease
- Community Resources
- Disease Prevention
- Health and Wellness
- Health Promotion Programs
- Health Screening
- High-Risk Behaviors
- Immunizations: Principles of Immunity
- Lifestyle Choices
- Principles of Teaching and Learning
- Self-Care
- Techniques of Physical Assessment

C. Psychosocial Integrity

See also **Appendix H**, Eight Detailed Areas of Human Functions Definitions/Descriptions—*Psychosocial-Cultural Functions.*

The nurse meets client needs for psychosocial integrity in stress- and crisis-related situations throughout the life span by providing and directing nursing care that promotes and supports the emotional, mental, and social well-being of the client and family/significant others experiencing stressful events, as well as of clients with *acute or chronic mental illness* and maladaptive behaviors.

The nurse promotes client's ability to cope, adapt, and problem-solve situations related to illness or stressful events; provides assistance to clients and families or significant others to promote client self-care; and supports families or significant others in order to enhance the overall management of client care, including self-care–related teaching provided in any care delivery environment.

Knowledge, Skills, and Abilities

To meet client needs for psychosocial integrity, the nurse should possess knowledge, skills, and abilities that include but are not limited to the following areas:

Coping and adaptation
- Coping Mechanisms
- Cultural Diversity
- Grief and Loss
- Mental Health Concepts
- Religious and Spiritual Influences on Health
- Sensory/Perceptual Alterations
- Situational Role Changes
- Stress Management
- Support Systems
- Therapeutic Communication, Counseling Techniques
- *Unexpected* Body Image Changes

Psychosocial adaptation
- Abuse/Neglect: Child, Domestic Violence, Elder, Sexual
- Behavioral Interventions
- Chemical Dependency
- Crisis Intervention
- End-of-Life
- Family Dynamics
- Psychopathology; Psychodynamics of Behavior
- Therapeutic Environment
- Treatment Modalities

D. Physiological Integrity

See also **Appendix H**, Eight Detailed Areas of Human Functions Definitions/Descriptions—*Sensory-Perceptual; Comfort, Rest, Activity, and Mobility; Nutrition; Fluid-Gas Transport; Elimination.*

The nurse meets the physiological integrity needs of clients with potentially life-threatening or chronically recurring physiological conditions, and of clients at risk for the development of complications or untoward effects of treatments or management modalities by providing and directing nursing care that promotes achievement of the following client needs:

3. **Basic care and comfort**—providing comfort and assistance in the performance of *activities of daily living,* including those that have been modified because of health deviations; providing assistance to clients and families

or significant others to promote client self-care; supporting families or significant others in order to enhance the overall management of client care, including self-care–related teaching provided in any care delivery environment.

4. **Pharmacological and parenteral therapies** —managing and providing care related to the administration of *medications and parenteral therapies*.

5. **Reduction of risk potential** —reducing the likelihood that clients will develop *complications* or health problems related to *existing conditions, treatments, or procedures*. Also included are those activities that involve monitoring changes in status and preparing or caring for clients undergoing diagnostic procedures and invasive therapies.

6. **Physiological adaptation** —managing and providing care for clients with *acute, chronic, or life-threatening* physical health conditions.

Knowledge, Skills, and Abilities

To meet client needs for physiological integrity, the nurse should possess knowledge, skills, and abilities that include but are not limited to the following areas:

3. *Basic care and comfort*
   - Alternative and Complementary Therapies
   - Assistive Devices
   - Elimination
   - Mobility/Effects of Immobility
   - Nonpharmacological Comfort Interventions
   - Nutritional Therapies and Oral Hydration
   - Palliative/Comfort Care
   - Personal Hygiene: teeth, hearing aids
   - Rest and Sleep; Activities of Daily Living

4. *Pharmacological and parenteral therapies*
   - Adverse Effects/Contraindications and Side Effects
   - Blood and Blood Products
   - Central Venous Access Devices
   - Chemotherapy
   - Dosage Calculations
   - Expected Outcomes/Effects
   - Intravenous Therapy
   - Medication Administration
   - Parenteral Fluids
   - Pharmacological Agents/Actions

   - Pharmacological Interactions
   - Pharmacological Pain Management
   - Total Parenteral Nutrition

5. *Reduction of risk potential*
   - Diagnostic Tests
   - Lab Values
   - Monitoring Conscious Sedation
   - **Potential** for Alterations in Body Systems
   - **Potential** for Complications of Diagnostic Tests/Procedures/Treatments
   - **Potential** for Complications from Surgical Procedures and Health Alterations
   - Skin and Wound Care
   - System-Specific Assessments
   - Therapeutic Procedures
   - Use of Special Equipment
   - Vital Signs

6. *Physiological adaptation*
   - Alterations in Body Systems
   - Fluid and Electrolyte Imbalances
   - Hemodynamics
   - Illness Management
   - Infectious Diseases
   - Medical Emergencies
   - Pathophysiology
   - Radiation Therapy
   - Respiratory Care
   - Unexpected Response to Therapies

The practice questions in this book (end-of-unit questions, **Pre Test, Practice Test,** and **Final Test**) are coded as to the client need being tested; the codes are found following the answer/rationale for each question. *Key to client need codes:*

SECE	Safe, Effective Care Environment
HPM	Health Promotion and Maintenance
PsI	Psychosocial Integrity
PhI	Physiological Integrity

For an index to *questions* relating to each general client need, see **Appendix D.**

For page references for specific *topics (content, theory) to review* relating to each client subneed, see **Appendix C.**

Index: Content Related to NCLEX-RN® Test Plan: Four General Client Needs and Six Client Subneeds (with Detailed Knowledge, Skills, and Abilities)

The following outline of content (nursing knowledge, skills, and abilities) is organized in terms of **four categories of client need:** *Safe, Effective Care Environment* (SECE), *Health Promotion/Maintenance* (HPM), *Psychosocial Integrity* (PsI), and *Physiological Integrity* (PhI). Included in the outline of topics are **six** numbered **client subneeds** and corresponding task statements. These items are derived from a study of nursing tasks and are *used in the development of the NCLEX-RN® test plan.*

Students who have taken and evaluated their performance on the **Pre Test, Practice Test,** or **Final Test** in this book will find this outline a useful guide for a concentrated review of specific problem topics. **Repeat NCLEX-RN® test takers** will also find this outline to be a useful guide for review of their problem areas. Refer to the pages listed in the right column for review of content in a particular topic.

The shaded areas and **bold-faced** topics and *italics* for subtopics are directly linked to the **official NCLEX-RN® Test Plan.**

A. SAFE, EFFECTIVE CARE ENVIRONMENT (SECE)

	Pages
1. Management of care: 13–19 %	
a. Advance directives	125
b. Advocacy	126, 265
c. Case management	119, 135, 265
d. Client rights	125
e. Collaboration with multidisciplinary team, **consultation, and referral**	170, 218, 232, 265, 322, 328, 331, 400, 401, 402, 410, 411, 412, 428, 436, 437, 443, 446, 493, 494, 495, 500, 502-503, 545, 595, 596, 599, 602, 608, 609, 629, 635, 636, 647-650, 663
f. Concepts of management	119
g. Confidentiality	127, 128-130
h. Continuity of care	135, 265
i. *Delegation*	116, 119, 265
j. Establishing **priorities**	115, 120
k. **Ethical** practice	125-126, 131-132
l. Informed consent	126, 128, 133
m. **Legal** principles, rights and responsibilities (incorporated into client care)	126-133
n. **Performance improvement** (quality assurance)	119, 265
o. Organ donation	128, 265, 590
p. Resource management	119, 265
q. Supervision	119, 265
2. Safety and infection control: 8–14 %	
a. *Accident prevention*	
(1) Safety (by ages)	231, 271, 272, 273, 275, 277, 278, 279
(2) Assess *safety in home* environment	272, 273, 309, 703
(3) Safety needs of clients with perceptual disorders (e.g., Meniere's)	597, 600, 602, 606, 607, 610
b. **Disaster planning**	120, 265
c. **Emergency response plan**	120-121

(Continued on following page)

(Continued on following page)

Integrated Concepts and Processes

The following concepts and processes are basic to nursing practice. They are integrated throughout the four major categories of *client needs:*

For an index to *questions* relating to each client need, see **Appendixes D** and **E.**

Index: Questions Related to Four General Client Needs

Use this index to locate *practice questions* throughout the book in each of the *four general categories of client needs* that are tested on NCLEX-RN®.

FOUR CATEGORIES OF CLIENT NEEDS

Unit	Safe, Effective Care Environment (SECE) Question No.	Health Promotion and Maintenance (HPM) Question No.	Psychosocial Integrity (PsI) Question No.	Physiological Integrity (PhI) Question No.
Unit 1: Orientation and Pre Test (Q/A:1–100)	1, 10, 20, 30, 40, 50, 51, 59, 60, 64, 70, 75, 80, 87, 89, 90, 97, 100	2, 4, 7, 12, 13, 15, 16, 17, 26, 28, 31, 32, 35, 36, 45, 46, 58, 68, 71, 79, 81	29, 76	3, 5, 6, 8, 9, 11, 14, 18, 19, 21, 22, 23, 24, 25, 27, 33, 34, 37, 38, 39, 41, 42, 43, 44, 47, 48, 49, 52, 53, 54, 55, 56, 57, 61, 62, 63, 65, 66, 67, 69, 72, 73, 74, 77, 78, 82, 83, 84, 85, 86, 88, 91, 92, 93, 94, 95, 96, 98, 99
(Q/A: 101–200)	101, 104, 109, 113, 114, 115, 119, 121, 123, 128, 131, 132, 134, 136, 137, 138, 144, 154, 168, 171, 181, 185, 186, 194	106, 107, 110, 111, 112, 120, 125, 127, 129, ,130, 140, 142, 150, 152, 160, 161, 162, 170, 176, 180, 190, 200	116, 117, 122, 146, 147, 159	102, 103, 105, 108, 118, 124, 126, 133, 135, 139, 141, 143, 145, 148, 149, 151, 153, 155, 156, 157, 158, 163, 164, 165, 166, 167, 169, 172, 173, 174, 175, 177, 178, 179, 182, 183, 184, 187, 188, 189, 191, 192, 193, 195, 196, 197, 198, 199
(Q/A: 201–300)	203, 204, 206, 207, 209, 211, 222, 253, 261, 268, 283, 298, 299	212, ,234, 235, 240, 241, 247, 249, 252, 258, 259, 264, 271, 282	210, 213, 215, 216, 217, 218, 220, 221, 224, 225, 226, 229, 230, 231, 232, 239, 240, 244, 250, 260, 270, 272, 280, 290, 294, 300	201, 202, 205, 208, 214, 219, 223, 227, 228, 233, 236, 237, 238, 242, 243, 245, 246, 248, 251, 254, 255, 256, 257, 262, 263, 265, 266, 267, 269, 273, 274, 275, 276, 277, 278, 279, 281, 284, 285, 286, 287, 288, 289, 291, 292, 293, 295, 296, 297
(Q/A: 301–400)	305, 313, 326, 334, 337, 338, 356, 373	303, 304, 318, 322, 325, 327, 329, 333, 336, 344, 345, 347, 349, 352, 353, 357, 363, 364, 367, 371, 376, 381, 383, 396, 397, 399	310, 328, 387	301, 302, 306, 307, 308, 309, 311, 312, 314, 315, 316, 317, 319, 320, 321, 323, 324, 330, 331, 332, 335, 339, 340, 341, 342, 343, 346, 348, 350, 351, 354, 355, 358, 359, 360, 361, 362, 365, 366, 368, 369, 370, 372, 374, 375, 377, 378, 379, 380, 382, 384, 385, 386, 388, 389, 390, 391, 392, 393, 394, 395, 398, 400
(Q/A: 401–500)	408, 418, 419, 426, 427, 428, 431, 432, 436, 437, 438, 445, 446, 447, 457, 462, 467, 471, 472, 496	403, 406, 409, 414, 429, 435, 442, 453, 465, 466, 484, 486, 487, 492	434, 478, 479, 494, 497	401, 402, 404, 405, 407, 410, 411, 412, 413, 415, 416, 417, 420, 421, 422, 423, 424, 425, 430, 433, 439, 440, 441, 443, 444, 448, 449, 450, 451, 452, 454, 455, 456, 458, 459, 460, 461, 463, 464, 468, 469, 470, 473, 474, 475, 476, 477, 480, 481, 482, 483, 485, 488, 489, 490, 491, 493, 495, 498, 499, 500

(Continued on following page)

FOUR CATEGORIES OF CLIENT NEEDS

Unit	Safe, Effective Care Environment (SECE) Question No.	Health Promotion and Maintenance (HPM) Question No.	Psychosocial Integrity (PsI) Question No.	Physiological Integrity (PhI) Question No.
Unit 3: Management of Care, Cultural Diversity, Ethical and Legal Aspects, and Nursing Trends (Q/A: 1–28)	1, 2, 3, 4, 5, 6, 7, 8, 9, 10, 11, 12, 13, 14, 15, 16, 17, 18, 19, 20, 21, 22, 23, 24, 25, 26, 27, 28			
Unit 4: Nursing Care of the Child-bearing Family (Q/A: 1–100)	11, 20, 23, 24, 25, 36, 45, 46, 48, 50, 52, 59, 78, 79	1, 3, 4, 10, 12, 13, 16, 18, 19, 27, 32, 33, 34, 35, 39, 40, 41, 42, 43, 47, 49, 54, 63, 64, 65, 66, 70, 74, 77, 81, 94, 95, 96, 97, 98	17, 28, 30, 31, 56, 67, 76, 99	2, 5, 6, 7, 8, 9, 14, 15, 21, 22, 26, 29, 37, 38, 44, 51, 53, 55, 57, 58, 60, 61, 62, 68, 69, 71, 72, 73, 75, 80, 82, 83, 84, 85, 86, 87, 88, 89, 90, 91, 92, 93, 100
Unit 5: Nursing Care of Children and Families (Q/A:1–100)	15, 26, 30, 31, 44, 51, 79, 80, 85 86, 89, 91, 92, 94, 97, 98, 99, 100	3, 10, 11, 17, 18, 25, 27, 29, 32, 37, 41, 45, 46, 50, 53, 57, 58, 59, 62, 68, 72, 74, 75, 76, 82, 83, 84, 88	12, 14, 43, 54, 61, 64, 87	1, 4, 5, 6, 7, 8, 9, 13, 16, 19, 20, 21, 22, 23, 24, 28, 33, 34, 35, 36, 38, 39, 40, 42, 47, 48, 49, 52, 55, 56, 60, 63, 65, 66, 67, 69, 70, 71, 73, 77, 78, 81, 90, 93, 95, 96
Unit 6: Nursing Care of Behavioral and Emotional Problems Throughout the Life Span (Q/A: 1–100)	11, 20, 29, 37, 64, 92, 97, 98, 99, 100	16, 18, 50, 56, 75, 79, 87	2, 3, 5, 6, 7, 8, 9, 12, 13, 14, 15, 17, 19, 21, 23, 24, 25, 26, 27, 28, 30, 31, 32, 33, 34, 36, 38, 39, 40, 41, 42, 43, 44, 46, 47, 48, 49, 51, 52, 53, 54, 55, 57, 59, 60, 61, 62, 66, 67, 68, 69, 72, 73, 74, 76, 77, 78, 80, 81, 82, 83, 84, 85, 86, 89, 90, 93, 94, 95, 96	1, 4, 10, 22, 35, 45, 58, 63, 65, 70, 71, 88, 91
Unit 7: Nursing Care of the Acutely Ill and the Chronically Ill Adult (Q/A: 1–100)	1, 46, 49, 55, 95		5, 19, 21, 22, 23, 40	2, 3, 4, 6, 7, 8, 9, 10, 11, 12, 13, 14, 15, 16, 17, 18, 20, 24, 25, 26, 27, 28, 29, 30, 31, 32, 33, 34, 35, 36, 37, 38, 39, 41, 42, 43, 44, 45, 47, 48, 50, 51, 52, 53, 54, 56, 57, 58, 59, 60, 61, 62, 63, 64, 65, 66, 67, 68, 69, 70, 71, 72, 73, 74, 75, 76, 77, 78, 79, 80, 81, 82, 83, 84, 85, 86, 87, 88, 89, 90, 91, 92, 93, 94, 96, 97, 98, 99, 100
Unit 8: The Older Adult (Q/A: 1–14)	1, 11	2, 4, 6, 7, 9, 13		3, 5, 8, 10, 12, 14
Unit 9: Review of Nutrition (Q/A: 1–6)				1, 2, 3, 4, 5, 6
Unit 10: Review of Pharmacology (Q/A: 1–42)				1, 2, 3, 4, 5, 6, 7, 8, 9, 10, 11, 12, 13, 14, 15, 16, 17, 18, 19, 20, 21, 22, 23, 24, 25, 26, 27, 28, 29, 30, 31, 32, 33, 34, 35, 36, 37, 38, 39, 40, 41, 42
Unit 11: Common Diagnostic Procedures, Intravenous and Oxygen Therapy, Infection Control/Isolation Precautions, and Hands-on Nursing Care (Q/A:1–12)				1, 2, 3, 4, 5, 6, 7, 8, 9, 10, 11, 12

(Continued on following page)

FOUR CATEGORIES OF CLIENT NEEDS

Unit	Safe, Effective Care Environment (SECE) Question No.	Health Promotion and Maintenance (HPM) Question No.	Psychosocial Integrity (PsI) Question No.	Physiological Integrity (PhI) Question No.
Unit 12: Practice Test (Q/A: 1–100)	5, 8, 26, 40, 48, 52, 74, 80	11, 13, 16, 18, 21, 38, 47, 59, 65	1, 6, 22, 23, 27, 36, 42, 44, 49, 57, 58, 69, 73, 75, 83, 88, 96, 99	2, 3, 4, 7, 9, 10, 12, 14, 15, 17, 19, 20, 24, 25, 28, 29, 30, 31, 32, 33, 34, 35, 37, 39, 41, 43, 45, 46, 50, 51, 53, 54, 55, 56, 60, 61, 62, 63, 64, 66, 67, 68, 70, 71, 72, 76, 77, 78, 79, 81, 82, 84, 85, 86, 87, 89, 90, 91, 92, 93, 94, 95, 97, 98, 100
Unit 13: Final Test (Q/A: 1–100)	13, 18, 42, 46, 58, 77	1, 5, 15, 27, 53, 55, 79, 83, 84	32, 34, 36, 40, 50, 60, 61, 70, 73, 75, 76, 80, 87, 89, 92, 93, 95, 96, 99	2, 3, 4, 6, 7, 8, 9, 10, 11, 12, 14, 16, 17, 19, 20, 21, 22, 23, 24, 25, 26, 28, 29, 30, 31, 33, 35, 37, 38, 39, 41, 43, 44, 45, 47, 48, 49, 51, 52, 54, 56, 57, 59, 62, 63, 64, 65, 66, 67, 68, 69, 71, 72, 74, 78, 81, 82, 85, 86, 88, 90, 91, 94, 97, 98, 100

For an index to *topics* (i.e., content, theory) relating to each client need, see **Appendix C**.

Index: Questions Related to Six Client Subneeds

Use this index to locate *practice questions* throughout the book in each of the *six client subneeds* that are tested on NCLEX-RN®. For an index to locate practice questions in the *four general categories* of client needs, see **Appendix D.**

SIX CLIENT SUBNEEDS

Unit	1. Management of Care — Question No.	2. Safety and Infection Control — Question No.	3. Basic Care and Comfort — Question No.	4. Pharmacological and Parenteral Therapies — Question No.	5. Reduction of Risk Potential — Question No.	6. Physiological Adaptation — Question No.
Unit 1: Orientation and Pre Test (Q/A:1–100)	10, 20, 30, 40, 50, 59, 64, 87, 89, 97	1, 51, 60, 70, 75, 80, 90, 100	3, 25, 38, 47, 62, 73, 74, 82, 84, 94, 99	11, 21, 23, 37, 48, 86, 91, 93, 95, 96, 98	5, 6, 8, 14, 19, 22, 33, 34, 42, 44, 49, 52, 53, 54, 57, 63, 65, 66, 77, 78, 83, 88, 92	9, 18, 24, 27, 41, 43, 55, 56, 61, 67, 69, 72, 85
(Q/A: 101–200)	101, 104, 109, 113, 119, 121, 123, 128, 131, 132, 134, 136, 137, 138, 144, 168, 186, 194	114, 115, 154, 171, 181, 185	103, 124, 135, 149, 153, 155, 156, 164, 165, 167, 169, 179, 193, 195, 197	108, 141, 145, 148, 151, 166, 177, 184, 191, 196, 198	105, 118, 126, 139, 157, 158, 163, 172, 173, 174, 175, 178, 182, 187, 188, 189, 192	102, 133, 143, 183, 199
(Q/A: 201–300)	253, 268, 283, 299	203, 204, 206, 207, 209, 211, 222, 261, 298	201, 227, 233, 236, 237, 242, 246, 263, 265, 284, 297	208, 238, 243, 245, 248, 286, 287, 288, 289, 291, 295	202, 205, 214, 223, 228, 251, 254, 255, 257, 266, 267, 269, 273, 274, 276, 277, 279, 281, 285	219, 256, 262, 275, 278, 292, 293, 296
(Q/A: 301–400)	305, 313, 334, 337, 338, 356, 373	326	319, 320, 330, 331, 332, 335, 340, 350, 378, 388	301, 302, 306, 341, 342, 348, 355, 360, 362, 369, 370, 372, 374, 379, 380, 390, 393, 400	308, 309, 321, 324, 343, 358, 359, 365, 366, 368, 375, 384, 386, 389, 392, 394	307, 311, 312, 314, 316, 317, 323, 339, 345, 351, 354, 361, 377, 382, 385, 391, 395, 398
(Q/A: 401–500)	428, 431, 438, 445, 446, 462	408, 418, 419, 426, 427, 432, 436, 437, 447, 467, 471, 472, 496	423, 424, 443, 448, 449, 457, 475, 476, 485, 491, 493	401, 411, 420, 444, 468, 469, 482, 489, 495, 499	402, 404, 405, 410, 415, 417, 422, 425, 430, 433, 440, 441, 450, 455, 456, 461, 464, 473, 474, 498	407, 412, 413, 416, 421, 439, 451, 452, 454, 458, 459, 460, 463, 470, 477, 480, 481, 483, 488, 497, 500
Unit 3: Management of Care, Cultural Diversity, Ethical and Legal Aspects, and Nursing Trends (Q/A:1–28)	1, 2, 3, 4, 5, 6, 8, 9, 10, 11, 12, 13, 15, 16, 17, 18, 19, 21, 22, 23, 24, 25, 26, 27, 28	7, 14, 20				
Unit 4: Nursing Care of the Childbearing Family (Q/A:1–100)	20, 23, 24, 50, 52	11, 25, 36, 45, 46, 48, 59, 78, 79	6, 14, 57, 60, 62, 100	9, 21, 44, 51, 55	5, 7, 8, 15, 22, 29, 37, 38, 53, 58, 68, 71, 72, 73, 75, 80, 83, 85, 86, 87, 88, 90, 91, 92, 93	2, 26, 61, 69, 82, 84, 89
Unit 5: Nursing Care of Children and Families (Q/A:1–100)	15, 51, 85, 86, 91, 92, 94, 97, 98, 99, 100	26, 30, 31, 44, 79, 80, 89	1, 4, 19, 20, 23, 48, 70, 71, 96	7, 16, 22, 34, 38, 39, 52, 67, 69, 73, 77, 78, 81, 93	6, 13, 21, 33, 35, 36, 55, 56, 60, 63, 65, 66, 95	5, 9, 24, 28, 40, 42, 47, 90
Unit 6: Nursing Care of Behavioral and Emotional Problems Throughout the Life Span (Q/A:1–100)	20, 29, 64, 97, 98, 100	11, 37, 92, 99	4, 35, 58	70, 91	22, 63	1, 10, 45, 65, 71

(Continued on following page)

SIX CLIENT SUBNEEDS

Unit	1. Management of Care Question No.	2. Safety and Infection Control Question No.	3. Basic Care and Comfort Question No.	4. Pharmacological and Parenteral Therapies Question No.	5. Reduction of Risk Potential Question No.	6. Physiological Adaptation Question No.
Unit 7: Nursing Care of the Acutely Ill and the Chronically Ill Adult (Q/A:1–100)	1, 46	49, 55, 95	7, 15, 20, 25, 27, 29, 31, 48, 59, 71, 76, 88, 90	10, 16, 32, 38, 53, 63, 66, 70, 77, 79	3, 9, 11, 18, 24, 43, 44, 47, 56, 57, 61, 67, 69, 72, 73, 74, 78, 80, 81, 83, 84, 86, 87, 91, 93, 100	2, 4, 6, 8, 12, 13, 14, 17, 26, 28, 30, 33, 34, 35, 36, 37, 39, 41, 42, 45, 50, 51, 52, 54, 58, 60, 62, 64, 65, 68, 75, 82, 85, 89, 92, 94, 96, 97, 98, 99
Unit 8: The Older Adult (Q/A:1–14)	1	11	3, 5, 8, 14		10, 12	
Unit 9: Review of Nutrition (Q/A:1–6)			1, 2, 3, 6		4, 5	
Unit 10: Review of Pharmacology (Q/A:1–42)				1, 2, 3, 4, 5, 6, 7, 8, 9, 10, 11, 12, 13, 14, 15, 16, 17, 18, 19, 20, 21, 22, 23, 24, 25, 26, 27, 28, 29, 30, 31, 32, 33, 34, 35, 36, 37, 38, 39, 40, 41, 42		
Unit 11: Common Diagnostic Procedures, Intravenous and Oxygen Therapy, Infection Control/Isolation Precautions, and Hands-on Nursing Care (Q/A:1–12)				1, 4, 11	2, 3, 5, 6, 7, 9, 10, 12	8
Unit 12: Practice Test (Q/A:1–100)	40, 48, 74	5, 8, 26, 52, 80	37, 54, 56, 70	31, 34, 43, 63, 93, 98	2, 3, 15, 20, 29, 30, 32, 41, 45, 51, 60, 61, 67, 68, 72, 76, 77, 82, 86, 94, 95	4, 7, 9, 10, 12, 14, 17, 19, 24, 25, 28, 33, 35, 39, 46, 50, 53, 55, 62, 64, 66, 71, 78, 79, 81, 84, 85, 87, 89, 90, 91, 92, 97, 100
Unit 13: Final Test (Q/A:1–100)	18, 46, 58	13, 42, 77	4, 12, 19, 26, 28, 29, 35, 44, 49, 64, 68, 82, 91, 100	2, 6, 9, 10, 20, 23, 25, 38, 41, 43, 45, 47, 48, 51, 54, 56, 57, 59, 63, 78, 85, 86	16, 17, 22, 30, 31, 33, 52, 62, 65, 71, 74, 81, 88, 90, 94, 98	3, 7, 8, 11, 14, 21, 24, 37, 66, 67, 69, 72, 97

For an index to *questions* throughout this book relating especially to Health Promotion and Maintenance and Psychosocial Integrity (as well as the other 2 general client needs) see Appendix D.

For an index to *topics* (i.e. content, theory) relating to each client subneed, see Appendix C.

NCLEX-RN® Test Plan:
◆ Nursing Process Definitions/Descriptions

The phases of the nursing process include:

I. Assessment: establishing a database.

A. *Gather objective and subjective information relative to the client:*
- Collect information from the client, significant others, and health-care team members; current and prior health records; and other pertinent resources.
- Use assessment skills appropriate to client's condition.
- Recognize *symptoms* and significant findings.
- Determine client's ability to assume care of daily health needs.
- Determine health-care team member's ability to provide care.
- Assess environment of client.
- Identify own or staff reactions to client, significant others, and health-care team members.

B. *Confirm data:*
- Verify observation or perception by obtaining additional information.
- Question prescriptions and decisions by other health-care team members when indicated.
- Observe condition of client directly when indicated.
- Validate that an appropriate client assessment has been made.

C. *Communicate information gained in assessment:*
- Document assessment findings thoroughly and accurately.
- Report assessment findings to relevant members of the health-care team.

II. Analysis: identifying actual or potential health-care needs and problems based on assessment.

A. *Interpret data:*
- Validate data.
- Organize related data.
- Determine *need for additional* data.
- Determine client's unique needs or problems.

B. *Formulate client's nursing diagnoses:*
- Determine significant relationship between data and client needs or problems.
- Use *standard taxonomy* for formulating nursing diagnoses.

C. *Communicate results of analysis:*
- *Document client's nursing diagnoses.*
- Report results of analysis to relevant members of the health-care team.

III. Planning: setting goals for meeting client's needs and designing strategies to achieve these goals.

A. *Prioritize nursing diagnoses:*
- Involve client, significant others, and health-care team members when establishing nursing diagnoses.
- Establish priorities among nursing diagnoses.
- Anticipate needs and problems on the basis of established priorities.

B. *Determine goals of care*
- Involve client, significant others, and health-care team members in setting goals.
- Establish *priorities among goals.*
- Anticipate needs or problems on the basis of established priorities.

C. *Formulate outcome criteria for goals of care:*
- Involve client, significant others, and health-care team members in formulating outcome criteria for goals of care.
- Establish *priorities among outcome criteria* for goals of care.
- Anticipate needs or problems on the basis of established priorities.

D. *Develop plan of care and modify as necessary:*
- Involve the client, significant others, and health-care team members in designing strategies.
- Individualize the plan of care based on such information as *age, gender, culture, ethnicity, and religion.*
- Plan for client's safety, comfort, and maintenance of optimal functioning.

- Select nursing interventions for delivery of client's care.
- Select *appropriate teaching* approaches.

E. *Collaborate with other health-care team members when planning delivery of client's care:*
- Identify health or social resources available to the client and significant others.
- Select appropriate health-care team members when planning assignments.
- Coordinate care provided by health-care team members.

F. *Communicate plan of care:*
- Document plan of care thoroughly and accurately.
- Report plan of care to relevant members of the health-care team.
- Review plan of care with client.

IV. Implementation: initiating and completing actions necessary to accomplish the defined goals.

A. *Organize and manage client's care:*
- Implement a plan of care.
- Arrange for a client-care conference.

B. *Counsel and teach client, significant others, and health-care team members:*
- Assist client, significant others, and health-care team members to recognize and manage stress.
- Facilitate client relationships with significant others and health-care team members.
- *Teach* correct principles, procedures, and techniques for maintenance and promotion of health.
- Provide client with health status information.
- Refer client, significant others, and health-care team members to appropriate *resources.*

C. *Provide care to achieve established goals of care:*
- Use safe and appropriate techniques when administering client care.
- Use precautionary and *preventive* interventions in providing care to client.
- *Prepare client for surgery,* delivery, or other procedures.
- Institute *interventions* to compensate for *adverse* responses.
- Initiate *lifesaving interventions* for emergency situations.
- Provide an environment conducive to attainment of goals of care.
- Adjust care in accord with client's expressed or implied needs, problems, and preferences.
- Stimulate and motivate client to achieve self-care and independence.
- Encourage client to follow a treatment regimen.
- Assist client to maintain optimal functioning.

D. *Supervise and coordinate the delivery of client's care provided by nursing personnel:*
- Delegate nursing interventions to appropriate nursing personnel.

- Monitor and follow up on delegated interventions.
- Manage health-care team members' reactions to factors influencing therapeutic relationships with clients.

E. *Communicate nursing interventions:*
- Record actual client responses, nursing interventions, and other information relevant to implementation of care.
- Provide complete, accurate reports on assigned client(s) to relevant members of the health-care team.

V. Evaluation: determining the extent to which goals have been achieved and interventions have been successful.

A. *Compare actual outcomes with expected outcomes of care:*
- Evaluate responses (expected and unexpected) in order to determine the degree of success of nursing interventions.
- Determine impact of therapeutic interventions on the client and significant others.
- Determine need for modifying the plan of care.
- Identify factors that may interfere with the client's ability to implement the plan of care.

B. *Evaluate the client's ability to implement self-care:*
- Verify that tests *or measurements are performed correctly* by the client and other caregivers.
- Ascertain client's and others' understanding of information given.

C. *Evaluate health-care team members' ability to implement client care:*
- Determine impact of teaching on health-care team members.
- Identify factors that might alter health-care team members' response to teaching.

D. *Communicate evaluation findings:*
- Document client's response to therapy, care, and teaching.
- Report client's response to therapy, care and teaching to relevant members of the health-care team.
- Report and document others' responses to teaching.
- Document other caregivers' responses to teaching.

The practice questions in this book (end-of-unit questions, **Pre Test, Practice Test,** and **Final Test**) are coded as to the phase of the nursing process being tested; the codes are found following the answer/rationale for each question. *Key to nursing process codes:*

◆	AS	Assessment
◆	AN	Analysis
◆	PL	Planning
◆	IMP	Implementation
◆	EV	Evaluation

For an index to questions relating to each phase of the nursing process, see **Appendix G.**

Index: Questions Related to
◆ Nursing Process

Use this index to locate *practice questions* throughout the book in each of the five phases of the *nursing process.*

FIVE PHASES OF THE NURSING PROCESS AND THEIR CODES

Unit	Assessment (AS) Question No.	Analysis (AN) Question No.	Plan (PL) Question No.	Implementation (IMP) Question No.	Evaluation (EV) Question No.
Unit 1: Orientation and Pre Test (Q/A: 1–100)	10, 12, 26, 27, 30, 51, 56, 59, 70, 77, 87, 99	2, 5, 15, 19, 22, 24, 31, 32, 39, 61, 63, 68, 71, 79, 80	8, 13, 14, 16, 45, 46, 50, 60, 65, 75, 78, 85, 90, 92, 93	1, 4, 6, 7, 9, 11, 17, 20, 21, 33, 34, 35, 37, 38, 40, 41, 42, 44, 47, 48, 49, 52, 54, 55, 57, 58, 62, 67, 69, 72, 73, 74, 76, 81, 82, 83, 86, 89, 91, 95, 96, 100	3, 18, 23, 25, 28, 29, 36, 43, 53, 64, 66, 84, 88, 94, 97, 98
(Q/A: 101–200)	106, 107, 110, 118, 124, 125, 150, 170, 175, 179, 180, 186, 199	102, 113, 114, 126, 130, 132, 133, 142, 154, 157, 168, 169, 176, 188	108, 116, 137, 138, 141, 145, 151, 153, 156, 161, 163, 164, 174, 177, 181, 185, 192, 195, 197	103, 104, 105, 111, 112, 117, 119, 120, 121, 122, 123, 127, 128, 129, 131, 134, 135, 136, 139, 140, 146, 147, 148, 152, 155, 158, 159, 160, 162, 165, 166, 167, 171, 172, 173, 178, 184, 187, 189, 190, 193, 194, 196, 198, 200	101, 109, 115, 143, 144, 149, 182, 183, 191
(Q/A: 201–300)	207, 210, 220, 224, 226, 229, 249, 252, 259, 260, 266, 271, 272, 277, 280, 290	202, 204, 209, 212, 216, 218, 219, 222, 225, 228, 232, 234, 239, 240, 241, 246, 247, 254, 255, 258, 268, 275, 276, 278, 282, 294, 296	244, 251, 270, 285, 287, 288, 289, 291	201, 203, 205, 206, 208, 211, 213, 214, 215, 217, 221, 223, 230, 231, 233, 235, 236, 237, 238, 242, 243, 245, 248, 256, 257, 261, 263, 265, 267, 279, 281, 284, 286, 292, 295, 297, 298, 299, 300	227, 250, 253, 262, 264, 269, 273, 274, 283, 293
(Q/A: 301–400)	307, 310, 311, 312, 314, 323, 328, 350, 352, 357, 358, 378, 379, 382, 386, 389, 390, 392, 393	313, 318, 325, 327, 329, 331, 332, 333, 334, 336, 337, 338, 345, 353, 363, 365, 371, 376, 377, 381, 383, 384, 391, 394, 398, 399	321, 341, 349, 351, 354, 355, 359, 361, 369, 372, 374, 380, 385	301, 302, 303, 304, 306, 308, 309, 315, 316, 317, 319, 320, 322, 326, 330, 335, 339, 343, 344, 346, 347, 348, 360, 362, 364, 366, 367, 368, 375, 387, 388, 395, 396, 397, 400	305, 324, 340, 342, 356, 370, 373
(Q/A: 401–500)	405, 406, 407, 412, 420, 425, 428, 429, 430, 460, 461, 464, 465, 471, 477, 485, 488, 496, 500	401, 409, 410, 427, 431, 432, 442, 447, 450, 451, 452, 458, 459, 463, 467, 469, 473, 483, 486, 494	402, 403, 413, 421, 441, 474, 480, 487, 489, 493	404, 408, 411, 414, 415, 416, 419, 420, 426, 433, 434, 435, 436, 437, 440, 443, 449, 453, 454, 455, 462, 466, 468, 472, 475, 476, 478, 479, 481, 482, 484, 490, 491, 492, 495, 497, 498	417, 418, 422, 424, 438, 439, 444, 445, 446, 448, 456, 457, 470, 499
Unit 3: Management of Care, Cultural Diversity, Ethical and Legal Aspects, and Nursing Trends (Q/A: 1–28)		11, 12, 17, 18, 19, 20	5	1, 2, 3, 4, 8, 13, 14, 26, 28	6, 7, 9, 10, 15, 16, 21, 27
Unit 4: Nursing Care of the Childbearing Family (Q/A: 1–100)	1, 2, 10, 13, 15, 29, 38, 41, 82, 85, 86, 92, 96, 99	3, 4, 5, 7, 8, 12, 14, 18, 22, 33, 34, 37, 40, 42, 44, 55, 58, 59, 61, 63, 64, 68, 69, 70, 74, 75, 77, 81, 83, 84, 89, 95, 97	11, 35, 52, 66, 87, 88, 98	6, 9, 17, 19, 20, 21, 23, 24, 25, 27, 28, 30, 31, 36, 39, 45, 46, 48, 49, 50, 51, 53, 54, 56, 57, 62, 65, 67, 71, 72, 73, 76, 78, 79, 80, 90, 93, 94, 100	16, 26, 32, 43, 47, 60, 91

(Continued on following page)

FIVE PHASES OF THE NURSING PROCESS AND THEIR CODES

Unit	Assessment (AS) Question No.	Analysis (AN) Question No.	Plan (PL) Question No.	Implementation (IMP) Question No.	Evaluation (EV) Question No.
Unit 5: Nursing Care of Children and Families (Q/A: 1–100)	5, 59, 62, 72, 73, 88	4, 6, 7, 8, 10, 21, 24, 26, 29, 31, 44, 45, 46, 47, 49, 58, 68, 71, 74, 78, 81, 85, 86, 87, 95	30, 34, 40, 77, 100	1, 2, 3, 9, 11, 12, 13, 15, 17, 19, 20, 22, 23, 27, 28, 32, 35, 38, 39, 41, 43, 48, 50, 52, 53, 54, 55, 56, 57	14, 16, 18, 25, 33, 36, 37, 42, 51, 67, 83, 89, 91, 93, 94, 99
Unit 6: Nursing Care of Behavioral and Emotional Problems Throughout the Life Span (Q/A: 1–100)	3, 7, 28, 43, 65, 71, 85, 88, 89, 90	8, 9, 16, 21, 23, 26, 27, 30, 34, 35, 39, 40, 41, 42, 44, 45, 47, 49, 50, 51, 63, 66, 67, 69, 73, 74, 75, 76, 77, 84, 87, 93, 94, 95, 96, 97, 98	1, 10, 14, 17, 22, 25, 32, 37, 46, 56, 57, 68, 78, 80, 100	2, 4, 5, 6, 11, 12, 13, 18, 19, 20, 24, 29, 33, 36, 38, 48, 52, 53, 54, 55, 59, 61, 64, 81, 82, 83, 92, 99	15, 31, 58, 60, 62, 70, 72, 79, 86, 91
Unit 7: Nursing Care of the Acutely Ill and the Chronically Ill Adult (Q/A: 1–100)	3, 6, 16, 18, 23, 30, 38, 42, 50, 58, 61, 62, 93, 97, 98	4, 5, 8, 9, 11, 12, 13, 14, 17, 26, 28, 33, 36, 37, 39, 40, 46, 52, 54, 63, 65, 68, 69, 73, 74, 77, 82, 86, 88, 89, 94, 99	2, 7, 10, 31, 47, 51, 55, 56, 76, 80, 84, 92, 100	1, 19, 20, 21, 22, 24, 25, 27, 29, 32, 48, 49, 57, 59, 64, 66, 67, 70, 71, 72, 78, 79, 81, 83, 85, 87, 90, 91, 95, 96	15, 34, 35, 41, 43, 44, 45, 53, 60, 75
Unit 8: The Older Adult (Q/A: 1–14)	1, 3, 4, 7, 9, 12, 13	10, 11		2, 5, 6, 8, 14	
Unit 9: Review of Nutrition (Q/A: 1–6)			2, 4, 6	1, 3, 5	
Unit 10: Review of Pharmacology (Q/A: 1–42)	1, 12, 39	8, 15, 17, 20, 22, 25, 28, 33	5, 7, 19, 23, 27, 32	2, 3, 6, 10, 13, 14, 16, 18, 24, 26, 29, 30, 31, 34, 35, 37, 38, 40, 42	4, 9, 11, 21, 36, 41
Unit 11: Common Diagnostic Procedures, Intravenous and Oxygen Therapy, Infection Control/Isolation Precautions, and Hands-on Nursing Care (Q/A: 1–12)	12	1, 6	2, 3	4, 5, 9, 10, 11	7, 8
Unit 12: Practice Test (Q/A: 1–100)	3, 13, 20, 49, 60, 61, 62, 75, 86, 88, 90, 92, 100	4, 5, 10, 14, 18, 19, 23, 24, 25, 26, 28, 33, 45, 46, 72, 79, 81, 82, 85, 87, 89, 97, 98	6, 27, 29, 36, 38, 40, 41, 56, 59, 76, 77, 95	2, 7, 8, 9, 11, 15, 21, 22, 30, 31, 32, 34, 37, 42, 43, 44, 48, 50, 51, 52, 53, 54, 58, 65, 66, 68, 69, 70, 71, 73, 78, 80, 83, 84, 91, 94, 99	1, 12, 16, 17, 35, 39, 47, 55, 57, 63, 64, 67, 74, 93, 96
Unit 13: Final Test (Q/A: 1–100)	1, 15, 19, 21, 25, 26, 55, 61, 69, 84, 89	3, 5, 7, 32, 52, 57, 67, 73, 75, 79, 87, 92, 93, 95, 97	16, 31, 36, 38, 43, 46, 49, 62, 70, 71, 74, 76, 80, 83, 94, 99	8, 10, 11, 13, 14, 17, 18, 22, 24, 28, 29, 30, 33, 34, 35, 37, 39, 40, 41, 42, 48, 50, 51, 53, 56, 58, 59, 64, 65, 68, 72, 81, 82, 86, 90, 91, 96, 98, 100	2, 4, 6, 9, 12, 20, 23, 27, 44, 45, 47, 54, 60, 63, 66, 77, 78, 85, 88

Appendix G

885

Eight Detailed Areas of Human Functions: Definitions/Descriptions

The following eight detailed areas are incorporated under specific client needs (see Appendix B). These functions are *detailed* areas of eight selected topics included under four client needs and six client subneeds (i.e., they provide a **further breakdown of the most important concepts to master** related to client needs).

1. **Protective Functions (Safety and Infection Control)**

   Client's ability to maintain defenses and prevent physical and chemical *trauma, injury, infection,* and threats to health status. Examples: *communicable* diseases (including sexually transmitted disease), *immunity, physical trauma* and *abuse,* asepsis, *safety hazards, poisoning,* skin disorders, and preoperative care and postoperative complications.

2. **Sensory-Perceptual Functions (Physiological Adaptation)**

   Client's ability to perceive, interpret, and respond to sensory and cognitive stimuli. Examples: *auditory, visual,* and verbal impairments, sensory *deprivation,* sensory *overload, aphasia, brain tumors, laryngectomy, dementia, body image, reality orientation,* learning disabilities, and *seizure* disorders.

3. **Comfort, Rest, Activity, and Mobility Functions (Basic Care and Comfort)**

   Client's ability to maintain mobility, desirable level of activity, and adequate sleep, rest, and comfort. Examples: joint impairment, body alignment, *pain, sleep* disturbances, *activities of daily living, neuromuscular* impairment, *musculoskeletal* impairment, and *endocrine* disorders that affect activity.

4. **Nutrition (Basic Care and Comfort)**

   Client's ability to maintain the intake and processing of essential nutrients. Examples: *normal* nutrition, diet in *pregnancy* and *lactation, obesity,* conditions such as *diabetes, gastric* disorders, and *metabolic* disorders that affect primarily the nutritional status.

5. **Growth and Development (Health Promotion and Maintenance)**

   Client's ability to maintain maturational processes throughout the life span. Examples: *childbearing, child rearing,* conditions that interfere with the maturation process, maturational crises, changes in *aging, psychosocial development,* sterility, and conditions of the *reproductive system.*

6. **Fluid-Gas Transport Functions (Physiological Adaptation)**

   Client's ability to maintain fluid-gas transport. Examples: *fluid volume deficit and overload, cardiopulmonary* diseases, *acid-base balance,* cardiopulmonary resuscitation, *anemias, hemorrhagic* disorders, leukemias, and *infectious pulmonary* diseases.

7. **Psychosocial-Cultural Functions (Psychosocial Integrity)**

   Client's ability to function in intrapersonal, interpersonal, intergroup, and sociocultural relationships. Examples: *grieving, death and dying, psychopathology, self-concept,* therapeutic *communication, group* dynamics, *ethical-legal* aspects, *community resources, spiritual* needs, situational *crises,* and *substance abuse.*

8. **Elimination Functions (Physiological Adaptation)**

   Client's ability to maintain functions related to relieving the body of waste products. Examples: conditions of the *gastrointestinal* system, such as vomiting, diarrhea, constipation, ulcers, neoplasms, colostomy, and hernia; conditions of the *urinary* system, such as kidney stones, transplants, renal failure, and prostatic hyperplasia.

The practice questions in this book (end-of-unit questions, **Pre Test, Practice Test,** and **Final Test**) are coded as to the category of human function being tested; the codes are found following the answer/rationale for each question. *Key to category of human function codes:*

1. Protective
2. Sensory-Perceptual
3. Comfort, Rest, Activity, and Mobility
4. Nutrition
5. Growth and Development
6. Fluid-Gas Transport
7. Psychosocial-Cultural
8. Elimination

For an index to *questions* relating to each human function, see **Appendix J.**

For page references of specific *topics to review* relating to each human function, see **Appendix I.**

Index: Content Related to Eight Detailed Areas of Human Functions

These eight detailed areas of human functions/concepts provide detailed examples of *content* areas incorporated under the six client *subneeds* of the four *general* areas of client needs on which the NCLEX-RN® test plan is based.

How to use this index: If, for example, after you take the tests in this book, you notice that you are mostly missing questions under VI (6) *Fluid-Gas Transport Functions,* this means that you have identified your *specific* problem area under the general client need of **Physiological Integrity,** subneed 6, *Physiological Adaptation.* In other words, **Appendix I** will lead you to the pages in this book that cover the specific problem area that you identified for extra focus in your exam prep.

To summarize, this is a diagram of how these various categories relate to each other:

First, there are the: | 4 general **Client Needs**

This breaks down into: | 6 categories of **Client Subneeds**

Finally, these are detailed areas to master: | 8 detailed areas (concepts of *human function*) under Client Subneeds

For an index to *questions* relating to each category of human function, see **Appendix J.**

Index: Questions Related to Eight Detailed Areas of Human Functions

This index lists *practice questions* for you to use in reviewing the eight detailed areas of *human functions* (that are detailed examples of what is covered by the four general client needs and six client subneeds).

EIGHT CATEGORIES OF HUMAN FUNCTIONS

Unit	Protective Functions (1) Question No.	Sensory-Perceptual Functions (2) Question No.	Comfort, Rest, Activity, and Mobility Functions (3) Question No.	Nutrition (4) Question No.	Growth and Development (5) Question No.	Fluid-Gas Transport Functions (6) Question No.	Psychosocial-Cultural Functions (7) Question No.	Elimination Functions (8) Question No.
Unit 1: Orientation and Pre Test (Q/A: 1–100)	1, 2, 8, 11, 14, 21, 23, 24, 28, 30, 34, 45, 46, 51, 56, 58, 60, 64, 68, 75, 80, 86, 87, 88, 90, 91, 93, 95, 97, 100	41, 65, 70, 79	3, 17, 57, 66, 73, 74, 77, 82, 99	9, 25, 36, 47, 62, 63, 69, 72, 81, 83, 94, 98	7, 12, 13, 16, 26, 31, 35, 48, 61, 67, 71, 76	4, 6, 15, 18, 22, 27, 32, 33, 37, 38, 39, 42, 43, 44, 53, 55, 85, 92, 96	10, 19, 20, 29, 40, 50, 59, 89	5, 49, 52, 54, 78, 84
(Q/A: 101–200)	101, 104, 105, 108, 113, 114, 115, 118, 119, 123, 131, 137, 145, 148, 152, 154, 161, 168, 171, 177, 185, 186, 187, 189, 191, 192, 194	107, 170, 179	102, 103, 117, 153, 169, 178, 181, 184, 188	124, 129, 135, 149, 158, 163, 165, 167, 193	106, 110, 120, 122, 125, 127, 130, 140, 141, 142, 147, 150, 160, 176, 180, 190, 196, 199, 200	109, 155, 156, 157, 162, 166, 182, 183, 198	111, 112, 116, 121, 126, 128, 132, 134, 136, 138, 139, 144, 146, 159	133, 143, 151, 164, 172, 173, 174, 175, 195, 197
(Q/A: 201–300)	203, 204, 206, 207, 209, 211, 218, 222, 223, 229, 243, 257, 261, 267, 268, 272, 274, 276, 277, 278, 279, 282, 283, 285, 286, 289, 291, 299	215, 217, 245, 260, 266, 298	201, 227, 244, 246, 265, 270, 287, 288, 292, 297	219, 228, 234, 236, 237, 238, 242, 263, 284	202, 205, 212, 235, 241, 247, 259, 264	208, 214, 233, 262, 269, 271, 273, 275, 281, 295, 296	210, 213, 216, 220, 224, 225, 226, 230, 231, 232, 239, 240, 280, 290, 294, 300	221, 258, 293
(Q/A: 301–400)	305, 307, 312, 313, 321, 325, 326, 335, 337, 338, 356, 357, 363	328, 385, 386	310, 318, 320, 331, 332, 339, 358, 359, 362, 390	301, 330, 340, 341, 355, 368, 388, 398	303, 304, 322, 327, 333, 336, 353, 364, 367, 371, 373, 381, 383, 396, 397	302, 306, 308, 311, 314, 315, 316, 317, 319, 323, 324, 334, 343, 352, 354, 365, 366, 369, 372, 374, 382, 384, 389, 391, 392, 393, 394, 395, 399	360, 370, 387, 400	329, 342, 361
(Q/A: 401–500)	401, 402, 408, 411, 418, 419, 422, 426, 427, 432, 436, 437, 445, 447, 455, 456, 458, 462, 465, 467, 470, 472	425, 431, 481, 483, 492, 495	420, 423, 428, 438, 471, 482, 489, 493, 496	435, 443, 448, 457, 460, 475, 476, 480, 484, 500	403, 406, 429, 449, 453, 461, 466, 468, 469, 473, 474, 477, 478, 479, 486, 498	407, 409, 412, 413, 414, 415, 416, 417, 421, 433, 439, 441, 444, 446, 451, 452, 454, 459, 463, 464, 499	410, 430, 434, 440, 450, 490, 494, 497	404, 405, 424, 442, 485, 487, 488, 491
Unit 3: Management of Care, Cultural Diversity, Ethical and Legal Aspects, and Nursing Trends (Q/A: 1–28)	1, 2, 4, 14, 16, 17, 20						3, 5, 6, 7, 8, 9, 10, 11, 12, 13, 15, 18, 19, 21, 22, 23, 24, 25, 26, 27, 28	

(Continued on following page)

EIGHT CATEGORIES OF HUMAN FUNCTIONS

Unit	Protective Functions (1) Question No.	Sensory-Perceptual Functions (2) Question No.	Comfort, Rest, Activity, and Mobility Functions (3) Question No.	Nutrition (4) Question No.	Growth and Development (5) Question No.	Fluid-Gas Transport Functions (6) Question No.	Psychosocial-Cultural Functions (7) Question No.	Elimination Functions (8) Question No.
Unit 4: Nursing Care of the Childbearing Family (Q/A: 1–100)	5, 9, 15, 21, 22, 23, 25, 36, 42, 43, 45, 46, 47, 48, 51, 53, 55, 56, 59, 71, 77, 78, 79, 89, 91, 92		66, 70, 88, 98, 100	6, 14, 57, 62, 65, 72, 73, 75, 81	1, 2, 3, 4, 10, 13, 16, 17, 18, 19, 24, 27, 32, 34, 35, 38, 39, 40, 41, 49, 50, 54, 60, 64, 68, 74, 94, 95, 96, 97	8, 11, 12, 26, 37, 44, 52, 58, 61, 63, 69, 80, 82, 83, 84, 85, 86, 87, 93	7, 20, 28, 30, 31, 33, 67, 99	29
Unit 5: Nursing Care of Children and Families (Q/A: 1–100)	1, 3, 6, 7, 13, 22, 26, 30, 31, 40, 41, 48, 52, 57, 58, 64, 79, 81, 85, 86, 89, 92, 94, 100	2, 62, 74	43, 60, 68, 75	9, 19, 24, 39, 42, 63, 82, 93, 96	11, 12, 17, 27, 32, 45, 49, 59, 83, 84, 87, 88, 99	4, 5, 10, 16, 18, 20, 23, 25, 28, 34, 35, 36, 38, 46, 47, 50, 51, 53, 55, 56, 65, 66, 69, 72, 73, 76, 77, 78, 80, 90, 95, 97	2, 8, 14, 29, 54, 98	15, 33, 37, 44, 61, 67, 70, 71, 91
Unit 6: Nursing Care of Behavioral and Emotional Problems Throughout the Life Span (Q/A: 1–100)	11, 24, 92, 97, 98, 99	2, 3, 5, 9, 12, 17, 22, 28, 32, 35, 45	71, 81, 82	4, 94	16, 21, 53, 75, 89	1, 37	6, 7, 8, 10, 13, 14, 15, 18, 19, 20, 23, 25, 26, 27, 29, 30, 31, 33, 34, 36, 38, 39, 40, 41, 42, 43, 44, 46, 47, 48, 49, 50, 51, 52, 54, 55, 56, 57, 58, 59, 60, 61, 62, 63, 64, 65, 66, 67, 68, 69, 70, 72, 73, 74, 76, 77, 78, 79, 80, 83, 84, 85, 86, 87, 88, 90, 91, 93, 95, 96, 100	
Unit 7: Nursing Care of the Acutely Ill and the Chronically Ill Adult (Q/A: 1–100)	20, 84, 96, 99	2, 26, 29, 33, 38, 52, 67, 79, 80, 87, 95	13, 25, 31, 32, 37, 42, 46, 47, 53, 59, 71, 73, 83, 90	1, 7, 9, 12, 17, 30, 35, 45, 57, 63, 74, 76, 88		3, 6, 8, 10, 11, 14, 16, 18, 28, 34, 39, 41, 43, 44, 48, 50, 51, 54, 55, 56, 58, 61, 62, 64, 65, 66, 68, 69, 70, 72, 78, 81, 86, 91, 92, 93, 94, 97, 98, 100	5, 19, 21, 22, 23, 40, 75	4, 15, 24, 27, 36, 49, 60, 77, 82, 85, 89
Unit 8: The Older Adult (Q/A: 1–14)	3, 10, 11	4, 5, 13	6, 8, 9, 12, 14		1, 2, 7			
Unit 9: Review of Nutrition (Q/A: 1–6)				1, 2, 3, 4, 5, 6				

(Continued on following page)

 Appendix J

EIGHT CATEGORIES OF HUMAN FUNCTIONS

Unit	Protective Functions (1) Question No.	Sensory-Perceptual Functions (2) Question No.	Comfort, Rest, Activity, and Mobility Functions (3) Question No.	Nutrition (4) Question No.	Growth and Development (5) Question No.	Fluid-Gas Transport Functions (6) Question No.	Psychosocial-Cultural Functions (7) Question No.	Elimination Functions (8) Question No.
Unit 10: Review of Pharmacology (Q/A: 1–42)	14, 18, 22, 23, 24, 29, 30, 31, 41	9, 13, 37, 38	1, 2, 8, 32, 36, 40	5, 7, 10, 15, 39, 42	17	3, 6, 16, 20, 21, 25, 26, 27, 28, 33, 34	19	4, 11, 12, 35
Unit 11: Common Diagnostic Procedures, Intravenous and Oxygen Therapy, Infection Control/Isolation Precautions, and Hands-on Nursing Care (Q/A: 1–12)				5, 6, 7, 9		2, 3, 4, 8, 11, 12		1, 10
Unit 12: Practice Test (Q/A: 1–100)	13, 16, 26, 31, 34, 52, 57, 60, 61, 66, 68, 80, 82, 89, 91	32, 40, 58, 70, 94	5, 8, 12, 15, 21, 29, 30, 41, 43, 48, 54, 56	4, 14, 35, 46, 50, 72, 98	1, 11, 18, 38, 59, 65, 96	7, 20, 24, 28, 33, 37, 39, 45, 47, 51, 53, 62, 64, 78, 79, 81, 84, 85, 86, 87, 92, 97, 100	6, 22, 23, 27, 42, 44, 49, 69, 73, 75, 83, 88, 93, 99	2, 3, 9, 10, 17, 19, 25, 36, 55, 63, 67, 71, 74, 76, 77, 90, 95
Unit 13: Final Test (Q/A: 1–100)	9, 10, 11, 13, 21, 28, 42, 43, 47, 51, 53, 54, 56, 58, 62, 65, 71, 77, 85, 88, 90	16, 39	4, 7, 8, 26, 29, 48, 49, 55, 64, 69, 74, 89, 91	12, 27, 44, 82, 94, 100	1, 5, 15, 34, 50, 60, 75, 79, 84	2, 3, 6, 14, 17, 23, 24, 25, 30, 31, 33, 35, 37, 38, 41, 52, 59, 66, 67, 68, 72, 78, 81, 83, 86, 97, 98	18, 32, 36, 40, 45, 46, 48, 61, 63, 70, 73, 76, 80, 87, 92, 93, 95, 96, 99	19, 20, 22, 57

For an index to *content* (theory) related to each of the above, see **Appendix I.**

Reduction of Risk Potential: Index to Diagnostic Procedures/Tests

This is an important area to review because it is a **subcategory** of the NCLEX-RN® Test Plan that is often tested. Refer also to **Unit 11.** These tests below are listed in chronological order by unit.

Common Acronyms and Abbreviations

This list provides a review of what you need to know about acronyms and abbreviations used in charting, verbal directives, and study guides.

a	Before (*ante*)
AAA	Abdominal aortic aneurysm
Ab	Antibody; Abortion
Abd	Abdomen; Abdominal
ABG	Arterial blood gas
ac	Before meals (*ante cibum*)
ACE	Angiotensin-converting enzyme
ACTH	Adrenocorticotropic hormone
ADH	Antidiuretic hormone
ADHD	Attention deficit-hyperactivity disorder
ad lib	As much as desired (*ad libitum*)
ADLs	Activities of daily living
AED	Automatic external defibrillator
AFB	Acid-fast bacillus
Afib	Atrial fibrillation
Aflutter	Atrial flutter
AFP	Alpha-fetoprotein
AG	Antigen
AGA	Average for gestational age
AGE	Acute gastroenteritis
AHF	Antihemophilic factor
AIDS	Acquired immunodeficiency syndrome
AK (or AKA)	Above-the-knee (amputation)
ALL	Acute lymphocytic (lymphoblastic) leukemia
ALS	Amyotrophic lateral sclerosis
AMA	Against medical advice
AML	Acute myelogenous leukemia
Amp	Ampule
ANP	Adult Nurse Practitioner
ANS	Autonomic nervous system
A&O $\times$ 3	Alert, oriented to person, place, time
AP	Anteroposterior; Alkaline phosphatase
aPPT	Activated partial thromboplastin time
APSGN	Acute poststreptococcal glomerulonephritis
ARC	AIDS-related complex
ARDS	Adult respiratory distress syndrome
ARF	Acute renal failure
ARMD	Age-related macular degeneration
AROM	Artificial rupture of membranes
ASA	Acetylsalicylic acid (aspirin)
ASAP	As soon as possible
ASD	Atrial septal defect
AST	Aspartate aminotransferase
AV	Atrioventricular; Arteriovenous; Aortic valve
AVB	Atrioventricular block
AVM	Arteriovenous malformation
AVR	Aortic valve repair
BAC	Blood alcohol concentration
BBT	Basal body temperature
BCLS	Basic cardiac life support
bid	Twice daily (*bis in die*)
BK (or BKA)	Below-the-knee (amputation)
BM	Bowel movement; Bone marrow
BMA	Bone marrow aspiration
BMI	Body mass index
BMR	Basal metabolic rate
BMT	Bone marrow transplant
BOM	Bilateral otitis media
BP	Blood pressure
BPD	Bronchopulmonary dysplasia
BPH	Benign prostatic hyperplasia
bpm	Beats per minute
BPP	Biophysical profile
BRP	Bathroom privileges
BSE	Breast self-examination
BUN	Blood urea nitrogen
c̄	With (*cum*)
CA	Carcinoma; Cancer
CABG	Coronary artery bypass graft operation ($\times$1, 2, 3, 4 number of grafts)
CAD	Coronary artery disease
CBC	Complete blood count
CC	Chief complaint
cc	Cubic centimeter
CCU	Cardiac (intensive) care unit
CD	Communicable disease
CDC	Centers for Disease Control and Prevention
CF	Cystic fibrosis

CHD	Congenital heart disease; Coronary heart disease
CHF	Congestive heart failure
CICU	Cardiac intensive care unit
CMV	Cytomegalovirus
CNS	Central nervous system; Coagulase-negative *Staphylococcus*; Clinical nurse specialist
C/O	Complains of
COA	Coarctation of aorta
COPD	Chronic obstructive pulmonary disease
CP	Cerebral palsy
CPD	Cephalopelvic disproportion
CPK	Creatine phosphokinase (now creatine kinase [CK])
CPR	Cardiopulmonary resuscitation
CRF	Chronic renal failure; Cardiac risk factors
CRP	C-reactive protein
C&S	Culture and sensitivity
CSF	Cerebrospinal fluid
CSM	Circulation, sensory, and motor
CST	Contraction stress test
CT	Computerized tomography
CV	Cardiovascular
CVA	Cerebrovascular accident (now called brain attack); Costovertebral angle
CVP	Central venous pressure
Δ	Change (Greek letter delta)
D/C	Discharge; Discontinue
D&C	Dilation and curettage
D&D	Dehydration and diarrhea
DDH	Developmental dysplasia of the hip
D&E	Dilation and evacuation
DI	Diabetes insipidus
DIC	Disseminated intravascular coagulation
Dig	Digitalis
DJD	Degenerative joint disease
DKA	Diabetic ketoacidosis
DM	Diabetes mellitus
DMD	Duchenne's muscular dystrophy
DNR	Do not resuscitate
DOA	Dead on arrival
DOB	Date of birth
DOE	Dyspnea on exertion
DPT	Diphtheria, pertussis, and tetanus
DRG	Diagnosis-related group
DRI	Dietary reference intakes
DTR	Deep-tendon reflex
DTs	Delirium tremens
DVT	Deep vein thrombosis
D_5W/D5W	5% dextrose in water
Dx	Diagnosis
ECF	Extended care facility; Extracellular fluid
ECG	Electrocardiogram (purist's version)
Echo	Echocardiogram
ECMO	Extracorporeal membrane oxygenation
ECT	Electroconvulsive therapy (see EST)
ED	Emergency department (commonly called *emergency room*); Erectile dysfunction
EDD	Estimated date of delivery
EEG	Electroencephalogram
EENT	Eye, ear, nose, and throat
EFM	Electronic fetal monitoring
EKG	Electrocardiogram (common version)
EMG	Electromyogram
EMS	Emergency medical service
EMT	Emergency medical technician
ENT	Ear, nose, and throat
EPS	Extrapyramidal symptoms
ER	Emergency room
ESR	Erythrocyte sedimentation rate
EST	Electroshock therapy
ETOH	Alcohol (ethanol)
FAS	Fetal alcohol syndrome
FBS	Fasting blood sugar
FEV_1	Forced expiratory volume in 1 second
FHR	Fetal heart rate
FHT	Fetal heart tones
FNP	Family nurse practitioner
FRC	Functional residual capacity
FSH	Follicle-stimulating hormone
FTT	Failure to thrive
FUO	Fever of unknown origin
FVC	Forced vital capacity
Fx	Fracture
g	Gram
G	Gravida
GABS	Group A beta-hemolytic streptococcus
GB	Gallbladder
GBS	Group B streptococcus
GBS	Guillain-Barré syndrome
GC	Gonococcus; Gonorrhea
GCS	Glasgow coma scale
G&D	Growth and development
GDM	Gestational diabetes mellitus
GER	Gastroesophageal reflux
GI	Gastrointestinal
gm	Gram
gr	Grain
GTT	Glucose tolerance test
gtt(s)	Drop(s) (*guttae*)
GU	Genitourinary
GYN	Gynecological
HAV	Hepatitis A virus
HBGM	Home blood glucose monitoring
HBV	Hepatitis B virus
HCG	Human chorionic gonadotropin
Hct	Hematocrit
HCV	Hepatitis C virus
HDL	High-density lipoprotein
HEENT	Head, eyes, ears, nose, throat
Hgb	Hemoglobin
$HgbA_{1c}$	Glycosylated hemoglobin

HIB	*Haemophilus influenzae* type B		MD	Muscular dystrophy
HIV	Human immunodeficiency virus		MDI	Metered-dose inhaler
HMO	Health maintenance organization		Med	Medication
HOB	Head of bed		mEq	Milliequivalent
HPL	Human placental lactogen		MI	Myocardial infarction
HPS	Hypertrophic pyloric stenosis		mL	Milliliter
HPV	Human papilloma virus		MMR	Measles, mumps, rubella
HR	Heart rate		MOM	Milk of magnesia
HRT	Hormone replacement therapy		Mono	Mononucleosis
hs	Bedtime *(hora somni)*		MR	Mitral regurgitation; Mental retardation
HSP	Henoch-Schönlein purpura		MRI	Magnetic resonance imaging
HSV	Herpes simplex virus		MRSA	Methicillin-resistant *Staphylococcus aureus*
HTN	Hypertension			
Hx	History		MS	Mental status; Mitral stenosis; Multiple sclerosis; Morphine sulfate
ICP	Intracranial pressure		MVR	Mitral valve repair/replacement
ICU	Intensive care unit			
I&D	Incision and drainage		NA	Not applicable
IDDM	Insulin-dependent diabetes mellitus		NEC	Necrotizing enterocolitis
Ig	Immunoglobulin		NG	Nasogastric
IM	Intramuscular		NICU	Neonatal intensive care unit
INH	Isoniazid		NIDDM	Non–insulin-dependent diabetes mellitus
I/O, I&O	Intake and output		NL	Normal
IPPB	Intermittent positive-pressure breathing		NM	Neuromuscular
IQ	Intelligence quotient		NOC	Night (nocturnal)
IUD	Intrauterine device		NPH	Neutral protamine Hagedorn (intermediate-acting insulin)
IUFD	Intrauterine fetal death		NPO	Nothing by mouth *(nil per os)*
IV	Intravenous		NS	Normal saline
IVC	Inferior vena cava		NSAID	Nonsteroidal antiinflammatory drug
IVP	Intravenous pyelogram; Intravenous push		NSR	Normal sinus rhythm
IVH	Intraventricular hemorrhage		NST	Nonstress test
			NTG	Nitroglycerin
JCAHO	Joint Commission on Accreditation of Healthcare Organizations		N/V	Nausea, vomiting
			NVD	Nausea, vomiting, diarrhea
JRA	Juvenile rheumatoid arthritis			
			O_2	Oxygen
KD	Kawasaki disease		OB	Obstetrics
KUB	Kidneys, ureters, bladder (flat/upright abdominal x-ray)		OD	Right eye *(oculus dexter);* Overdose
			OFTT	Organic failure to thrive
			OM	Otitis media
L&B	Laryngoscopy and bronchoscopy		OOB	Out of bed; out of breath
L-C-P, LCPD	Legg-Calvé-Perthes disease		O&P	Ova and parasites
LDL	Low-density lipoprotein		OR	Operating room
LFTs	Liver function tests		OS	Left eye *(oculus sinister)*
LGA	Large for gestational age		OT	Occupational therapy
LGI	Lower gastrointestinal		OTC	Over-the-counter
LLL	Left lower (lung) lobe		OU	Both eyes *(oculo utro)*
LLQ	Left lower quadrant			
LMP	Last menstrual period		P	Para; Pulse
LOC	Loss of consciousness; Level of consciousness		p	Post (after)
LPN	Licensed practical nurse		PA	Posteroanterior; Physician's assistant; Pulmonary artery
LTB	Laryngotracheobronchitis		PAC	Premature atrial contraction
LTE	Life-threatening event		PACU	Postanesthesia care unit
LUL	Left upper (lung) lobe		PAF	Paroxysmal atrial fibrillation
LUQ	Left upper quadrant		P_{AO_2}	Alveolar oxygen pressure
			Pa_{O_2}	Arterial partial pressure of oxygen
MAOI	Monoamine oxidase inhibitor		PAS	Para-aminosalicylic acid
MAP	Mean arterial pressure		PAT	Paroxysmal atrial tachycardia
MCL	Midclavicular line			

pc	After meals (*post cibum*)	ROP	Retinopathy of prematurity
PCA	Patient-controlled analgesia (pump); Patient care assistant	ROS	Review of systems
		RR	Respiratory rate
PCP	*Pneumocystis carinii* pneumonia; Phencyclidine	RSV	Respiratory syncytial virus
		RT	Respiratory therapy
PDA	Patent ductus arteriosus	R/T	Related to
PE	Pulmonary embolus; Pulmonary edema	RUL	Right upper (lung) lobe
PEEP	Positive end-expiratory pressure	RUQ	Right upper quadrant
PERRL(A)	Pupils equally round and reactive to light (and accommodation)	Rx	Prescription/Therapy/Treatment
PFTs	Pulmonary function tests	s	Without (*sine*)
PICU	Pediatric intensive care unit	S_1	First heart sound
PID	Pelvic inflammatory disease	S_2	Second heart sound
PIH	Pregnancy-induced hypertension	S_3	Third heart sound
PKU	Phenylketonuria	S_4	Fourth heart sound
PMI	Point of maximum impulse	SAB	Spontaneous abortion
PMS	Premenstrual syndrome	Sao_2	Arterial blood-oxygen saturation
PND	Paroxysmal nocturnal dyspnea	SBE	Subacute bacterial endocarditis
PNP	Pediatric nurse practitioner	SC	Subcutaneously
PO	By mouth (*per os*)	SCA	Sickle cell anemia
PPD	Purified protein derivative (TB skin test); Percussion and postural drainage	SGA	Small for gestational age
		SIADH	Syndrome of inappropriate antidiuretic hormone
PPHN	Persistent pulmonary hypertension of the newborn	SICU	Surgical intensive care unit
		SIDS	Sudden infant death syndrome
PPO	Preferred provider organization	SL	Sublingually
PQRST	Provoke-quality-radiation-severity-time	SLE	Systemic lupus erythematosus
prn	When necessary (*pro re nata*)	SNF	Skilled nursing facility
PSA	Prostate-specific antigen	SOB	Short(ness) of breath
Pt	Patient	SQ	Subcutaneously
PT	Prothrombin time; Physical therapy	SR	Sinus rhythm
PTA	Prior to admission	SROM	Spontaneous rupture of membranes
PTCA	Percutaneous transluminal coronary angioplasty	S/Sx	Signs, symptoms
		Stat	Immediately (*statim*)
PTL	Preterm labor	STD	Sexually transmitted disease
PTSD	Post-traumatic stress disorder	SVG	Spontaneous vaginal delivery
PTT	Partial thromboplastin time	Sx	Symptoms
PUD	Peptic ulcer disease		
PVC	Premature ventricular contraction	T	Temperature
		TAB	Therapeutic abortion
q	Each, every (*quaque*)	TAR	Total all routes (intake)
qd	Each day (*quaque die*)	T&A	Tonsillectomy and adenoidectomy
qh	Every hour	TB	Tuberculosis
qhs	Every night before sleep (*quaque hora somni*)	TCA	Tricyclic antidepressant
		TEF	Tracheoesophageal fistula
qid	Four times a day (*quarter in die*)	TENS	Transcutaneous electrical nerve stimulation
qod	Every other day		
		TGV	Transposition of great vessels
R	Respirations	TIA	Transient ischemic attack
RA	Rheumatoid arthritis; Right atrium	TID	Three times a day (*ter in die*)
RAD	Reactive airway	TKO	To keep open
RBC	Red blood cell	TLC	Total lung capacity; Tender loving care; Therapeutic lifestyle change
RDA	Recommended daily/dietary allowances		
RDS	Respiratory distress syndrome	TOF	Tetralogy of Fallot
RHD	Rheumatic heart disease	TOLAC	Trial of labor after cesarean section
RLL	Right lower (lung) lobe	TORCH	Toxoplasmosis, other (hepatitis B, syphilis), rubella, cytomegalovirus, herpes simplex 2
RLQ	Right lower quadrant		
RML	Right middle (lung) lobe		
R/O	Rule out		
ROM	Range of motion; Rupture of membranes	TPA	Tissue plasminogen activator

TPN	Total parenteral nutrition		UV	Ultraviolet
TPR	Temperature, pulse, respirations			
TSE	Testicular self-examination		VBAC	Vaginal birth after cesarean
TSH	Thyroid-stimulating hormone		VC	Vital capacity
TSS	Toxic shock syndrome		VCUG	Voiding cystourethrography
TURP	Transurethral resection of prostate		VD	Venereal disease
TV	Total volume; Tidal volume		VF, Vfib	Ventricular fibrillation
TVH	Total vaginal hysterectomy		VS	Vital signs
Tx	Treatment		VSD	Ventricular septal defect
			VZV	Varicella-zoster virus
UA	Urinalysis			
UAP	Unlicensed assistive personnel		w/	With
UDAB	Urine drugs of abuse		WBC	White blood cell; White blood (cell) count
UGI	Upper gastrointestinal		WHO	World Health Organization
UQ	Upper quadrant		WIC	Women, infants, and children
URI	Upper respiratory infection		WNL	Within normal limits
UTI	Urinary tract infection		w/o	Without

Quick Guide to Common Clinical Signs

Many clinical signs have been named for the physicians who first described them, or the phenomena they resemble. Following is a list of 34 *of the most common clinical signs* for use as a quick reference as you review.

Babinski reflex Dorsiflexion of the big toe after stimulation of the lateral sole. It is a normal reflex in infants under the age of 6 months, but indicates a *lesion of the pyramidal (corticospinal) tract* in older individuals.

Barlow test *Developmental hip dysplasia* is present if femoral head moves in and out of the back of the acetabulum while exerting pressure from the front.

Blumberg's sign Transient pain in the abdomen after approximated fingers pressed gently into abdominal wall are suddenly withdrawn—rebound tenderness; associated with *peritoneal inflammation.*

Braxton-Hicks contractions Irregular painless uterine contractions.

Brudzinski's sign Flexion of the hip and knee induced by flexion of the neck; associated with *meningeal irritation.*

Brushfield's spots Speckling of iris associated with *Down syndrome.*

Chadwick's sign Cyanosis of vaginal and cervical mucosa; associated with *pregnancy.*

Cheyne-Stokes respiration Rhythmic cycles of deep and shallow respiration, often with apneic periods; associated with *central nervous system respiratory center dysfunction.*

Chvostek's sign Facial muscle spasm induced by tapping on the facial nerve branches; associated with *hypocalcemia.*

Coopernail's sign Ecchymoses on the perineum, scrotum, or labia; associated with *fracture of the pelvis.*

Cullen's sign Bluish discoloration of the umbilicus; associated with *acute pancreatitis* or *hemoperitoneum,* especially *rupture of fallopian tube* in ectopic pregnancy.

Doll's-eyes sign Dissociation between the movements of the head and eyes: as the head is raised the eyes are lowered, and as the head is lowered the eyes are raised; associated with *global-diffuse disorders of the cerebrum.* By contrast, in the evaluation of newborns (whose nervous systems are immature), the irises normally remain in midline despite the rotation of the head.

Fluid wave Transmission across the abdomen of a wave induced by snapping the abdomen; associated with *ascites.*

Goldstein's sign Wide distance between the great toe and the adjoining toe; associated with *cretinism* and *trisomy 21.*

Harlequin sign In the newborn infant, reddening of the lower half of the laterally recumbent body and blanching of the upper half, due to a *temporary vasomotor disturbance.*

Hegar's sign Softening of the fundus of the uterus; associated with the *first trimester of pregnancy.*

Homans' sign Pain behind the knee, induced by dorsiflexion of the foot; associated with peripheral vascular disease, especially *venous thrombosis* in the calf (*not* a diagnostic test itself).

Kehr's sign Severe pain in the left upper quadrant, radiating to the top of the shoulder; associated with *splenic rupture.*

Kernig's sign Inability to extend leg when sitting or lying with the thigh flexed on the abdomen; associated with *meningeal irritation.*

Knie's sign Unequal dilation of the pupils; associated with *Graves' disease.*

Kussmaul's respiration Paroxysmal air hunger; associated with acidosis, especially *diabetic ketoacidosis.*

Lasègue's sign Straight leg raising with hip flexed and knee extended will elicit sciatic pain associated with *herniated lumbar disk.*

Lhermitte's sign Sudden electric shock–like sensation along spine on flexion of the head caused by *trauma* to the cervical spine, *multiple sclerosis, cervical cord tumor,* or *spondylosis.*

McBurney's sign Tenderness at McBurney's point (located two-thirds of the distance from the umbilicus to the anterior-superior iliac spine); associated with *appendicitis.*

Murphy's sign Pain on taking a deep breath when pressure is applied over location of the gallbladder; a sign of *gallbladder disease.*

Ortolani's maneuver Manual procedure performed to rule out the possibility of congenital hip dysplasia. A "click" sound sometimes is heard if *hip dysplasia* is present; on assessment, head of femur can be felt (or heard as a click) as it slips forward in the acetabulum and slips back when pressure is released and legs are returned to their original position.

Osler's sign Small painful erythematous swellings in the skin of the hands and feet; associated with bacterial endocarditis.

Psoas sign Pain induced by hyperextension of the right thigh while lying on the left side; associated with *appendicitis.*

Setting-sun sign Downward deviation of the eyes so that each iris appears to "set" beneath the lower lid, with white sclera exposed between it and the upper lid; associated with *increased intracranial pressure* or irritation of the *brainstem;* also seen in *hydrocephalus.* Seen occasionally for brief periods in normal infants.

Simian crease Transverse palmar or plantar crease; associated with *Down syndrome.*

Tinel's sign Tingling sensation felt from light percussion on the radial side of the palmaris longus tendon; associated with *carpal tunnel syndrome.*

Trendelenburg's sign When child bears weight on affected hip, pelvis tilts downward on the unaffected side instead of upward, as it should; associated with *developmental hip dysplasia.*

Trousseau's sign Carpopedal spasm develops when BP cuff is inflated above systolic pressure for 3 minutes; associated with *hypocalcemia.*

Williamson's sign Markedly diminished blood pressure in the leg as compared with that in the arm on the same side; associated with *pneumothorax* and *pleural effusions.*

Memory Aids

Acid-base—"RAMS" (*Respiratory Alternate, Metabolic Same*)

	Respiratory (alternate)		Metabolic(same)	
Acidosis	$\downarrow$pH	$\uparrow$P$_{CO_2}$	$\downarrow$pH	$\downarrow$HCO$_3$
Alkalosis	$\uparrow$pH	$\downarrow$P$_{CO_2}$	$\uparrow$pH	$\uparrow$HCO$_3$

Alcohol withdrawal: clinical features—"HITS"[a]

Hallucinations (visual, tactile)
Increased vital signs and insomnia
Tremens → delirium tremens (potentially lethal)
Shakes/Sweats/Seizures/Stomach pains (nausea, vomiting)

Angina: precipitating factors—"three E's"

Eating
Emotion
Exertion (Exercise)

Anorexia nervosa: clinical features—"A²NOREXI²C"[a]

Adolescent women/Amenorrhea
NGT alimentation (most severe cases)
Obsession with losing weight/becoming fat though underweight
Refusal to eat (≥5% die)
Electrolyte abnormalities (e.g., $\downarrow$K$^+$, cardiac arrhythmia)/$\uparrow$eXercise
Intelligence often above average/Induced vomiting
Cathartic use (and diuretic abuse)

Appendicitis: assessment—"PAINS"

Pain (RLQ)
Anorexia
Increased temperature, WBC (15,000–20,000)
Nausea
Signs (McBurney's, Psoas)

Arterial occlusion: symptoms—"six P's"

Pain
Pale
Pulseless
Paresthesia
Poikilothermic
Paralysis

Blood glucose *(rhyme)*

Symptom	Implication
Cold and **clammy** . . .	give hard **candy**
Hot and **dry** . . .	glucose is **high**

Blood vessels in umbilical cord—"AVA"

Artery
Vein
Artery

Cancer: focus of patient care—"CANCER"

Chemotherapy
Assess body image disturbance (related to alopecia)
Nutritional needs when N/V present
Comfort from pain
Effective response to Tx? (Evaluate)
Rest (for patient and family)

Cholecystitis: risk factors—"five F's"

Female
Fat
Forty
Fertile
Fair

Cleft lip: nursing care plan (postoperative)—"CLEFT² LIP"

Crying, minimize
Logan bow
Elbow restraints
Feed with Brecht feeder
Teach feeding techniques; two months of age (average age at repair)
Liquid (sterile water), rinse after feeding
Impaired feeding (no sucking)
Position—*never* on abdomen

Cognitive disorders: assessment of difficulties—"JOCAM"

Judgment
Orientation
Confabulation
Affect
Memory

---

[a]Modified from Rogers, PT: The Medical Student's Guide to Top Board Scores. Little, Brown, Boston (out of print).

Coma: causes—"A^2-E^3-I-O-U T^2IPS^2"[b]

Alcohol, acidosis (hyperglycemic coma)

Epilepsy (also electrolyte abnormality, endocrine problem)

Insulin (hypoglycemic shock)

Overdose (or poisoning)

Uremia and other renal problems

Trauma; temperature abnormalities (hypothermia, heat stroke)

Infection (e.g., meningitis)

Psychogenic ("hysterical coma")

Stroke or space-occupying lesions in the cranium

Complication of severe preeclampsia—"HELLP" *syndrome*

Hemolysis

Elevated Liver enzymes

Low Platelet count

Cushing's syndrome: symptoms—*"three S's"*

Sugar (hyperglycemia)

Salt (hypernatremia)

Sex (excess androgens)

Diabetes: signs and symptoms—*"three P's," "three poly's"*

Polydipsia (very thirsty)

Polyphagia (very hungry)

Polyuria (urinary frequency)

Diet: low cholesterol—*avoid the three C's:*

Cake

Cookies

Cream (dairy, e.g., milk, ice cream)

Dystocia: etiology—*"three P's"*

Power

Passageway

Passenger

Dystocia: general aspects (maternal)—*"three P's"*

Psych

Placenta

Position

Episiotomy assessment—*"REEDA"*

Redness

Edema

Ecchymosis

Discharge

Approximation of skin

Eye medications

Mydriatic = dilated pupils

Miotic = tiny (constricted) pupils

Hypertension: complications—*"four C's"*

CAD (coronary artery disease)

CHF (congestive heart failure)

CRF (chronic renal failure)

CVA (cardiovascular accident; now called brain attack or stroke)

Hypertension: nursing care plan—*"I TIRED"*

Intake and output (urine)

Take blood pressure

Ischemia attack, transient (watch for TIAs)

Respiration, pulse

Electrolytes

Daily weight

Hypoglycemia: signs and symptoms—*"DIRE"*

Diaphoresis

Increased pulse

Restless

Extra hungry

Infections during pregnancy—*"TORCH"*

Toxoplasmosis

Other (hepatitis B, syphilis, group B beta strep)

Rubella

Cytomegalovirus

Herpes simplex virus

IUD: potential problems with use—*"PAINS"*[c]

Period (menstrual: late, spotting, bleeding)

Abdominal pain, dyspareunia

Infection (abnormal vaginal discharge)

Not feeling well, fever or chills

String missing

Manipulation: nursing plan—promote the *"three C's"*

Cooperation

Compromise

Collaboration

Medication administration—*"six rights"*

RIGHT medication

RIGHT dosage

RIGHT route

RIGHT time

RIGHT client

RIGHT technique

Melanoma characteristics—*"ABCD"*

Asymmetry

Border

Color

Diameter

Mental retardation: nursing care plan—*"three R's"*

Regularity (provide routine and structure)

Reward (positive reinforcement)

Redundancy (repeat)

Myocardial infarction: treatment—*"M^2ONA"*

MONA greets every M.I:

Monitor/morphine

Oxygen

---

[b]Adapted from Caroline, NL: Emergency Care in the Streets, ed 5. Little, Brown, Boston (out of print)

[c]From Hatcher, RA, et al: Contraceptive Technology. ed 16. Irving, New York.

Nitroglycerin
Aspirin

Newborn assessment components—*"APGAR"*
Appearance
Pulse
Grimace
Activity
Respiratory effort

Obstetric (maternity) history—*"GTPAL"*
Gravida
Term
Preterm
Abortions (SAB, TAB)
Living children

Oral contraceptives: signs of potential problems—*"ACHES"*[c]
Abdominal pain (possible liver or gallbladder problem)
Chest pain or shortness of breath (possible pulmonary embolus)
Headache (possible hypertension, brain attack)
Eye problems (possible hypertension or vascular accident)
Severe leg pain (possible thromboembolic process)

Pain: assessment—*"PQRST"*
What	Provokes the pain?
What is the	Quality of the pain?
Does the pain	Radiate?
What is the	Severity of the pain?
What is the	Timing of the pain?

Pain: management—*"ABCs"*
Ask about the pain
Believe when clients say they have pain
Choices—let clients know their choices
Deliver what you can, when you said you would
Empower/Enable clients' control over pain

Postoperative complications: order—*"four W's"*
Wind (pulmonary)
Wound
Water (urinary tract infection)
Walk (thrombophlebitis)

Preterm infant: anticipated problems—*"TRIES"*
Temperature regulation (poor)
Resistance to infections (poor)
Immature liver
Elimination problems (necrotizing enterocolitis [NEC])
Sensory-perceptual functions (retinopathy of prematurity [ROP])

Psychotropic medications: common antidepressives (tricyclics)—*"VENT"*
Vivactil
Elavil
Norpramin
Tofranil

Schizophrenia: primary symptoms—*"four A's"*
Affect
Ambivalence
Associative looseness
Autism

Sprain: nursing care plan—*"RICE"*
Rest
Ice
Compression
Elevation

Stool assessment—*"ACCT"*
Amount
Color
Consistency
Timing

Tracheoesophageal fistula: assessment—*"three C's"*
Coughing
Choking
Cyanosis

Traction: nursing care plan—*"TRACTION"*
Trapeze bar overhead to raise and lower upper body
Requires free-hanging weights; body alignment
Analgesia for pain, prn
Circulation (check color and pulse)
Temperature (check extremity)
Infection prevention
Output (monitor)
Nutrition (alteration related to immobility)

Transient ischemic attacks: assessment—*"three T's"*
Temporary unilateral visual impairment
Transient paralysis (one-sided)
Tinnitus = vertigo

Trauma care: complications—*"T²RAUMA"*
Thromboembolism; Tissue perfusion, altered
Respiration, altered
Anxiety related to pain and prognosis
Urinary elimination, altered
Mobility impaired
Alterations in sensory-perceptual functions and skin integrity (infections)

Wernicke-Korsakoff syndrome (alcohol-associated neurological disorder)—*"COAT RACK"*[d]
Wernicke's encephalopathy (acute phase): clinical features:
Confusion
Ophthalmoplegia
Ataxia
Thiamine is an important aspect of Tx

Korsakoff's psychosis (chronic phase): characteristic findings:
Retrograde amnesia (↓recall of some old memories)
Anterograde amnesia (↓ability to form new memories)
Confabulation
Korsakoff's psychosis

---

[d]Adapted from Rogers, PT: The Medical Student's Guide to Top Board Scores. Little, Brown, Boston, (out of print).

Directory of State Boards of Nursing

Alabama Board of Nursing
770 Washington Avenue
RSA Plaza, Ste 250
Montgomery, AL 36130-3900
Phone: (334) 242-4060
www.abn.state.al.us/

Alaska Board of Nursing
550 West Seventh Ave., Suite 1500
Anchorage, AK 99501-3567
(907) 269-8161
www.dced.state.ak.us/occ/pnur.htm

American Samoa Health Services
Regulatory Board
LBJ Tropical Medical Center
Pago Pago, AS 96799
(684) 633-1222

Arizona State Board of Nursing
1651 E. Morten Ave., Suite 210
Phoenix, AZ 85020
(602) 331-8111
www.azboardofnursing.org/

Arkansas State Board of Nursing
University Tower Building
1123 S. University, Suite 800
Little Rock, AR 72204-1619
(501) 686-2700
www.state.ar.us/nurse

California Board of Registered Nursing
400 R St., Ste. 4030
Sacramento, CA 95814-6239
(916) 322-3350
www.rn.ca.gov/

**California Board of Vocational Nursing and
Psychiatric Technicians**
2535 Capitol Oaks Drive, Suite 205
Sacramento, CA 95833
(916) 263-7800
www.bvnpt.ca.gov/

Colorado Board of Nursing
1560 Broadway, Suite 880
Denver, CO 80202
(303) 894-2430
www.dora.state.co.us/nursing/

Connecticut Board of Examiners for Nursing
Dept. of Public Health
410 Capitol Ave., MS# 13PHO
P.O. Box 340308
Hartford, CT 06134-0328
(860) 509-7624
www.state.ct.us/dph/

Delaware Board of Nursing
861 Silver Lake Blvd.
Cannon Building, Suite 203
Dover, DE 19904
(302) 739-4522
www.professionallicensing.state.de.us/boards/nursing/index
.shtml

District of Columbia Board of Nursing
Department of Health
825 N. Capitol St., NE, 2nd Floor
Room 2224
Washington, DC 20002
(202) 442-4778
www.dchealth.dc.gov

Florida Board of Nursing
4052 Bald Cypress Way, BIN C02 (mailing address)
4042 Bald Cypress Way, Rm 120 (physical address)
Tallahassee, FL 32399-3252
(850) 245-4125
www.doh.state.fl.us/mqa/

Georgia Board of Nursing
237 Coliseum Drive
Macon, GA 31217-3858
(478) 207-1640
www.sos.state.ga.us/plb/rn

Georgia State Board of Licensed Practical Nurses
237 Coliseum Drive
Macon, GA 31217-3858
(478) 207-1300
www.sos.state.ga.us/plb/lpn

Guam Board of Nurse Examiners
P.O. Box 2816
Hagatna, Guam 96932
(671) 735-7406; (671) 725–7411
(671) 725-7411

Hawaii Board of Nursing
King Kalakaua Building
335 Merchant St., 3rd Floor
Honolulu, HI 96813
(808) 586-3000
www.state.hi.us/dcca/pvl/areas_nurse.html

Idaho Board of Nursing
280 N. 8th St., Suite 210
P.O. Box 83720
Boise, ID 83720
(208) 334-3110
www.state.id.us/ibn/ibnhome.htm

Illinois Department of Professional Regulation
Chicago Office
James R. Thompson Center
100 West Randolph, Suite 9-300
Chicago, IL 60601
(312) 814-2715
Springfield Office
320 W. Washington St., 3rd Floor
Springfield, IL 62786
(217) 782-8556
www.dpr.state.il.us/

Indiana State Board of Nursing
Health Professions Bureau
402 W. Washington St., Room W066
Indianapolis, IN 46204
(317) 234-2043
www.state.in.us/hpb/boards/isbn/

Iowa Board of Nursing
RiverPoint Business Park
400 S.W. 8th St., Suite B
Des Moines, IA 50309-4685
(515) 281-3255
www.state.ia.us/government/nursing/

Kansas State Board of Nursing
Landon State Office Building
900 S.W. Jackson, Suite 1051
Topeka, KS 66612
(785) 296-4929
www.ksbn.org

Kentucky Board of Nursing
312 Whittington Parkway, Suite 300
Louisville, KY 40222
(502) 329-7000
www.kbn.ky.gov/

Louisiana State Board of Nursing
3510 N. Causeway Boulevard, Suite 501
Metairie, LA 70002
(504) 838-5332
www.lsbn.state.la.us/

Louisiana State Board of Practical Nurse Examiners
3421 N. Causeway Boulevard, Suite 505
Metairie, LA 70002
(504) 838-5791
www.lsbpne.com/

Maine State Board of Nursing
158 State House Station
Augusta, ME 04333
(207) 287-1133
www.maine.gov/boardofnursing/

Maryland Board of Nursing
4140 Patterson Ave.
Baltimore, MD 21215
(410) 585-1900
www.mbon.org

Massachusetts Board of Registration in Nursing
Commonwealth of Massachusetts
239 Causeway St.
Boston, MA 02114
(617) 727-9961
www.state.ma.us/reg/boards/rn/

Michigan CIS/Bureau of Health Professions
Ottawa Towers North
611 W. Ottawa, 1st Floor
Lansing, MI 48933
(517) 335-0918
www.michigan.gov/healthlicense

Minnesota Board of Nursing
2829 University Ave. SE, Suite 500
Minneapolis, MN 55414
(612) 617-2270
www.nursingboard.state.mn.us/

Mississippi Board of Nursing
1935 Lakeland Drive, Suite B
Jackson, MS 39216-5014
(601) 987-4188
www.msbn.state.ms.us/

Missouri State Board of Nursing
3605 Missouri Boulevard
P.O. Box 656
Jefferson City, MO 65102-0656
(573) 751-0681
www.ecodev.state.mo.us/pr/nursing/

Montana State Board of Nursing
301 South Park
PO Box 200513
Helena, MT 59620-0513
(406) 841-2340
www.discoveringmontana.com/dli/bsd/license/bsd_boards/
nur_board/board_page.htm

Nebraska Health and Human Services System
Dept. of Regulation & Licensure, Nursing Section
301 Centennial Mall South
Lincoln, NE 68509-4986
(402) 471-4376
www.hhs.state.ne.us/crl/nursing/nursingindex.htm

Nevada State Board of Nursing
Administration, Discipline & Investigations
5011 Meadowood Mall #201
Reno, NV 89502-6547
(775) 688-2620
www.nursingboard.state.nv.us/

Nevada State Board of Nursing
Licensure and Certification
2500 West Sahara Ave., Suite 207
Las Vegas, Nevada 89102-4293
(702) 486-5800
FAX: (702) 486-5803
www.nursingboard.state.nv.us/

New Hampshire Board of Nursing
21 South First St., Ste. 16
Concord, NH 03301-2431
(603) 271-2323
www.state.nh.us/nursing/

New Jersey Board of Nursing
P.O. Box 45010
124 Halsey St., 6th Floor
Newark, NJ 07101
(973) 504-6586
www.state.nj.us/lps/ca/medical.htm

New Mexico Board of Nursing
6301, Indian School Road NE, Suite 710
Albuquerque, NM 87110-8188
(505) 841-8340
www.state.nm.us/clients/nursing

New York State Board of Nursing
Education Building
89 Washington Ave.
2nd Floor West Wing
Albany, NY 12234
(518) 474-3817 Ext. 120
www.nysed.gov/prof/nurse.htm

North Carolina Board of Nursing
3724 National Drive, Suite 201
Raleigh, NC 27612
(919) 782-3211
www.ncbon.com/

North Dakota Board of Nursing
919 South 7th St., Suite 504
Bismarck, ND 58504
(701) 328-9777
www.ndbon.org/

Northern Mariana Islands—Commonwealth
Board of Nurse Examiners
P.O. Box 501458
Saipan, MP 96950
(670) 664-4812

Ohio Board of Nursing
17 South High St., Suite 400
Columbus, OH 43215-3413
(614) 466-3947
www.nursing.ohio.gov

Oklahoma Board of Nursing
2915 N. Classen Boulevard, Suite 524
Oklahoma City, OK 73106
(405) 962-1800
www.youroklahoma.com/nursing

Oregon State Board of Nursing
800 NE Oregon St., Box 25
Suite 465
Portland, OR 97232
(503) 731-4745
www.osbn.state.or.us/

Pennsylvania State Board of Nursing
P.O. Box 2649
Harrisburg, PA 17105-2649
(717) 783-7142
www.dos.state.pa.us/bpoa/cwp/view.asp?a=1104&q=
432869

Puerto Rico—Commonwealth of Puerto Rico
Board of Nurse Examiners
800 Roberto H. Todd Avenue
Room 202, Stop 18
Santurce, PR 00908
(787) 725-7506

Appendix O

Rhode Island Board of Nurse Registration and Nursing Education
105 Cannon Building
Three Capitol Hill
Providence, RI 02908
(401) 222-5700
www.healthri.org/hsr/professions/nurses.htm

South Carolina State Board of Nursing
110 Centerview Drive, Suite 202
Columbia, SC 29210
(803) 896-4550
www.llr.state.sc.us/pol/nursing

South Dakota Board of Nursing
4305 South Louise Ave., Suite 201
Sioux Falls, SD 57106-3115
(605) 362-2760
www.state.sd.us/dcr/nursing/

Tennessee State Board of Nursing
425 Fifth Ave. North
Cordell Hull Building, 1st Floor
Nashville, TN 37247
(615) 532-5166
www.tennessee.gov/health

Texas Board of Nurse Examiners
333 Guadalupe, Suite 3-460
Austin, TX 78701
(512) 305-7400
www.bne.state.tx.us/

Texas Board of Vocational Nurse Examiners
William P. Hobby Building, Tower 3
333 Guadalupe Street, Suite 3-400
Austin, TX 78701
(512) 305-8100
www.bvne.state.tx.us/

Utah State Board of Nursing
Heber M. Wells Building, 4th Floor
160 East 300 South
Salt Lake City, UT 84111
(801) 530-6628
www.commerce.state.ut.us/

Vermont State Board of Nursing
81 River St.
Heritage Building

Montpelier, VT 05609-1106
(802) 828-2396
www.vtprofessionals.org/opr1/nurses/

Virgin Islands Board of Nurse Licensure
Veterans Drive Station
St. Thomas, VI 00803
(340) 776-7397

Virginia Board of Nursing
6603 West Broad St., 5th Floor
Richmond, VA 23230-1712
(804) 662-9909
www.dhp.state.va.us/

Washington State Nursing Care Quality Assurance Commission
Department of Health HPQA #6
310 Israel Road SE
Tumwater, WA 98501-7864
(360) 236-4700
wws2.wa.gov/doh/hpqa-licensing/HPS6/Nursing/default.htm

West Virginia Board of Examiners for Registered Professional Nurses
101 Dee Drive
Charleston, WV 25311
(304) 558-3596
www.wvrnboard.com

West Virginia State Board of Examiners for Licensed Practical Nurses
101 Dee Drive
Charleston, WV 25311
(304) 558-3572
www.lpnboard.state.wv.us/

Wisconsin Department of Regulation and Licensing
1400 E. Washington Ave., RM 173
Madison, WI 53708
(608) 266-0145
www.drl.state.wi.us/

Wyoming State Board of Nursing
2020 Carey Ave., Suite 110
Cheyenne, WY 82001
(307) 777-7601
nursing.state.wy.us/

APPENDIX P

Complementary and Alternative Therapies

Complementary and alternative therapies can be integrated into the treatment plan for many conditions, including the following.

Condition	Complementary/Alternative Therapies
Anxiety (see also **Unit 10, Table 10.11**)	*Herbals:* St. John's wort Tea: chamomile, peppermint Valerian *Diet/Nutrition:* *Eliminate:* caffeine, alcohol, tobacco, sugar *Lifestyle:* Exercise *Mind-Body Interventions:* Biofeedback Cognitive behavioral therapy Deep breathing Group therapy Meditation Relaxation response *Bioelectromagnetic Therapies:* Energy healing *Alternative Systems of Care:* Acupuncture *Hands-on Healing Techniques:* Massage
Arthritis	*Herbals:* Ginger concentrate Topical: capsaicin *Diet/Nutrition:* Weight Loss Vitamins C and E *Lifestyle:* Exercise *Mind-Body Interventions:* Cognitive-behavioral therapy; biofeedback Tai chi, qi gong, yoga *Pharmacological and Biological Treatments:* Glucosamine sulfate SAMe *Bioelectromagnetic Therapies:* Static magnet therapy *Alternative Systems of Care:* Acupuncture, acupressure Ayurveda Traditional Chinese medicine

(Continued on following page)

Appendix P

Condition	Complementary/Alternative Therapies
Arthritis (cont'd)	*Hands-on Healing Techniques:* Physical therapy

Asthma	*Herbals:*
	    Grape-seed extract
	    Guaifenesin
	Diet/Nutrition:
	    Have: omega-3 fatty acids; onions, garlic; vitamins C, E; zinc
	    Avoid: milk, egg, wheat, sulfites, aspirin
	    Reduce: sodium intake
	Mind-Body Interventions:
	    Biofeedback
	    Yoga breathing techniques
	Alternative Systems:
	    Acupuncture
	    Ayurvedic
	    Chinese herbals
	Hands-on Healing Techniques:
	    Massage

Coronary artery disease	*Diet/Nutrition:*
	    Eliminate: tobacco, caffeine, alcohol
	    Low fat, vegetarian
	    Vitamins C, E, B_6, B_{12}, folic acid
	Lifestyle:
	    Dr. Dean Ornish program
	Mind-Body Interventions:
	    Relaxation and stress management
	    Guided imagery
	    Treat for depression (anger/hostility management)

Depression (see also **Unit 10, Table 10.11**)	*Herbals:*
	    St. John's wort
	Diet/Nutrition:
	    Folic acid, vitamins B_{12} and C, thiamine, niacin
	Lifestyle:
	    Exercise, relaxation, stress reduction
	Mind-Body Interventions:
	    Biofeedback
	    Cognitive behavioral therapy
	    Meditation
	    Spiritual approaches
	    Tai chi, qi gong
	Bioelectromagnetic Therapies:
	    Light therapy (for S.A.D.)
	Alternative Systems of Care:
	    Acupuncture
	Hands-on Healing Techniques:
	    Massage

Diabetes	*Herbals:*
	    Garlic
	    Green tea
	    Fenugreek
	Diet and Nutrition/Lifestyle:
	    Regular exercise
	    Weight loss
	    Diet; high fiber; low simple sugars and fats; potassium; Ornish diet
	        Onion, cold water fish
	    Alpha-lipoic acid
	    Biotin
	    Chromium
	    Flaxseed oil
	    Vitamins C, B_3, B_6, B_{12}, E

Appendix P

(Continued on following page)

Condition	Complementary/Alternative Therapies
Gastroesophageal reflux disease	*Herbals:* 　　Licorice 　　Raspberry tea 　　Caraway *Diet and Nutrition/Lifestyle:* 　　Weight loss 　　Small meals 　　Don't lie down for 2 hr pc 　　Elevate HOB 6 in. 　　*Avoid:* onions, spicy foods, peppermint, caffeine, alcohol (although white wine 　　　may ↑ gastric emptying)
Other gastrointestinal problems 　Constipation 　Diarrhea (antibiotic-induced) 　Indigestion 　Peptic ulcer	 *Herbals:* 　　Aloe, cascara, senna *Diet:* 　　Yogurt *Herbals:* 　　Peppermint oil *Herbals:* 　　Licorice (may cause sodium concentration and counteract antihypertensive meds)
Migraine headache	*Herbals:* 　　Feverfew (**caution:** ↑ risk of post-op bleeding and stomach upset if also on NSAIDs) 　　Ginger (dried) *Diet and Nutrition/Lifestyle:* 　　Vitamin B_2 (riboflavin) 　　*Avoid:* chocolate, cheese, beer, red wine, dairy, wheat *Mind-Body Interventions:* 　　Relaxation therapy 　　Biofeedback 　　Guided imagery 　　Meditation 　　Stress management 　　Tai chi, yoga
Hypercholesterolemia	*Herbals:* 　　Garlic cloves 　　Chinese red yeast rice *Diet and Nutrition/Lifestyle:* 　　Exercise, weight loss 　　Fruits/vegetables: 5–7 servings/daily (for bioflavonoids and beta carotene) 　　Fiber 　　Mediterranean diet 　　Vegetarian diet 　　Soy protein 　　Very low fat (Ornish diet) *Mind-Body Interventions:* 　　Modifying type A behavior: 　　↓: stress, hostility, time urgency, competitiveness 　　↑: sleep pattern 　　Relaxation therapy *Alternative Systems of Care:* 　　Ayurveda 　　Traditional Chinese medicine
Hypertension	*Herbals:* 　　Garlic, ginseng dried root, hawthorn *Diet and Nutrition/Lifestyle:* 　　DASH diet; fiber, potassium, low sodium; reduce caffeine 　　Weight loss 　　Aerobic exercise 　　Quit smoking 　　CoQ10 　　Alcohol intake <3 drinks/day

Appendix P

(Continued on following page)

Condition	Complementary/Alternative Therapies
Hypertension (cont'd)	Calcium, magnesium Reduce sugar intake Check for heavy metals, such as lead *Mind-Body Interventions:* 　Anger prevention/management 　Guided imagery 　Music therapy 　Tai chi, yoga *Alternative Systems of Care:* 　Ayurveda 　Traditional Chinese medicine
Irritable bowel syndrome	*Herbals:* 　Peppermint 　Chamomile tea, fennel tea, raspberry tea 　Sage 　Garlic 　Lemon balm *Diet and Nutrition/Lifestyle:* 　Charcoal (for excess gas) 　Fiber 　Food allergy: identify/eliminate most common (dairy, grain) 　Lactase (if lactose intolerance) 　Lactobacillus acidophilus 　Reduce refined sugar in diet *Mind-Body Interventions:* 　Cognitive behavioral therapy 　Treat depression; psychotherapy 　Exercise 　Progressive muscle relaxation 　Biofeedback 　Stress management *Alternative Systems of Care:* 　Acupuncture 　Ayurveda 　Traditional Chinese medicinal herbals
Musculoskeletal problems	*Herbals:* 　Arnica ointment/gel (topical) 　Tiger balm (topical) 　Salicylate ointment 　Aloe gel 　Curcumin (antiinflammatory) 　Lavender 　Camphor *Diet and Nutrition/Lifestyle:* 　Regular exercise 　Stretching, conditioning; warm-up exercises 　Bioflavonoids: citrus 　Calcium (bone, muscle injury) 　Magnesium (muscle spasm, injury) 　Vitamin C (connective tissue and muscle damage) 　Vitamin E (muscle damage); topical for scars 　Bursitis: Vitamin B_{12} 　Fibromyalgia: vitamin B_1, magnesium, vitamin E *Mind-Body Interventions:* 　Guided imagery 　Tai chi, yoga, qi gong 　Music therapy *Alternative Systems of Care:* 　Acupuncture, acupressure 　Cupping; massage, oil
Upper respiratory infections	*Herbals:* 　Echinacea (dried root or tea) (**Caution:** may interfere with immunosuppressant meds) 　Garlic cloves

(Continued on following page)

Condition	Complementary/Alternative Therapies
Upper respiratory infections (cont'd)	Horseradish
	Slippery elm tea
	Diet and Nutrition/Lifestyle:
	Avoid exhausting exercise; bedrest
	Drink large amounts of fluids
	Gargle: salt water and vinegar
	Hot water with lemon juice and honey
	Mind-Body Interventions:
	Social support
	Stress management
	Alternative Systems of Care:
	Ayurveda
	Acupuncture
	Cupping
	Traditional Chinese medicine
	Hands-on Healing Techniques:
	Percussion
Urinary tract infections	*Diet/Nutrition*
	Large amounts of low sugar juices, water (2 L/day)
	Cranberry juice
	Blueberry juice
	Lifestyle:
	Urinate after intercourse (women)

Source: Adapted from Sierpina, VS: Integrative Health Care: Complementary and Alternative Therapies for the Whole Person, FA Davis, Philadelphia, 2000.

Appendix P

Note: Page number followed by the letter f refer to figures; those followed by the letter t refer to tables.

Human immunodeficiency virus (HIV) infection.
  Lyme disease, 543–544
  neonatal, 234–235
  resistance to, in preterm infant, 238
  total parenteral nutrition causing, 573t
Infection control
  for infant, child, and adolescent, 265, 274t
  in congenital heart disease and, 285
  in cystic fibrosis, 290
  in leukemia, 285
  in sickle cell anemia, 287
Infertility, 148, 149f
Infestation
  lice, 315
  pinworms, 315
Inflammatory bowel disease, 582. *See also* Crohn's disease; Ulcerative colitis.
Influenza, avian, 546t
Influenza vaccine, 300t
  for adults, 478t
Informed consent, 133
Infusion systems, 805–806
Ingestion, accidental, in childhood, 315–318
Inhalational anesthesia, stages of, 552
Inhalational anthrax, 547t
Injury. *See specific injury, e.g.,* Fractures; *under anatomy.*
Injury prevention
  in cerebral palsy, 331
  in hemophilia, 289
  in leukemia, 285
Insanity, definition of, 457
Insomnia
  in older adults, 381
  in pregnancy, 156t
Insulin, 761t–762t
  for diabetes in pregnancy, 167, 168
  for diabetes mellitus, 574–575
Integumentary system. *See* Skin *entries.*
Intellectual immobility, 613
Intelligence quotient, in Down syndrome, 279
Interferon(s), 779t
Intermittent peritoneal dialysis, 590t, 591
Internal radiation
  sealed, 659–660
    nursing precautions for, 660
  unsealed, 660
International Council of Nurses (ICN), 135
Interstitial cell-stimulating hormone, 142
Intervertebral disk, herniation of, 634
Interviewing
  purpose and goals of, 417
  verbal interactions in, principles of, 417
Intestinal obstruction, 583
  postoperative, 557t
Intracranial pressure, increased, 605
  signs of, 332–333
Intrafamily relationships, pregnancy and, 158
Intramuscular medications, administration of, in infants and children, 739
Intraoperative preparation
  anesthesia in, 551–552
  hypothermia in, 552
Intrapartal period, 186–210
Intrapartum period. *See also* Labor.
  clinical pathway in, 210t–212t
  complications in, 202t–210t
Intrapersonal/interpersonal theory, 119
Intrauterine device, 145t–146t
  potential problems of, 144

Intravenous agents, in anesthesia, 552
Intravenous conscious sedation, 551
Intravenous therapy, 796–801
  complications of, 801t–802t
  fluids and electrolytes in, 798t, 798–799, 801, 800t–801t
  fluids in, 797–798, 798t
  for cancer, 801
  infusion systems in, 796–797
Intravenous urography, 790
Intraventricular hemorrhage, in neonate, 239–240
Intussusception, 325–326
Invasion of privacy, legal aspects of, 127
Involuntary admission, to psychiatric care, 132, 133f
Iodine
  deficiency of, 559t
  radioactive, 659
Ipecac syrup, 768t
Iron
  deficiency of, 559t
  during pregnancy, 714t
  foods high in, 726
Iron deficiency anemia, 511–512
Irreducible hernia, 579
Irresistible impulse test, 132
Irrigation, colostomy, 585t
Ischemic stroke, 606
Isolation precautions, guidelines for, 804t–806t
Isoniazid, 769t
  for tuberculosis, 528
Isoproterenol, 742t
Isosorbide, 745t
Isotonic solutions, intravenous, 798–799
Italians, food patterns of, 716t

J

J pouch, 582–583
Jacksonian march, 606
Jackson-Pratt apparatus, 813t
Jarisch-Herxheimer reaction, 544
Jaundice, physiologic, 231
Jews, Orthodox, religious considerations in meal planning for, 721
Joint degeneration, in hemophilia, prevention of, 289
Juvenile rheumatoid arthritis, 330t

K

Kaolin with pectin, 749t
Kava, 779t
Kawasaki's disease, 310–312
Kegel exercises, 594
Kehr's sign, 176
Kernicterus, 243
Ketoacidosis, vs. hypoglycemia, in diabetes mellitus, 575t
Ketoconazole, 750t
Ketorolac, 744t
Kidney(s). *See also* Renal *entries.*
  cancer of, 672t
  effect of preeclampsia/eclampsia on, 181
Knee replacement, total, 632
Kock pouch, 594
Koplik spots, in measles, 303f
Korsakoff's syndrome (alcohol amnestic syndrome), 407

L

Labia majora, 141
Labia minora, 141
Labile, definition of, 456

Labor
  analgesic and anesthetic drugs for, 741t
  biologic foundations of, 186–191
  Braxton-Hicks contractions in, 186
  cesarean birth and, 201–202
    vaginal birth after, 202
  clinical pathway in, 210–212
  complications of, 202–210
  danger signs during, summary of, 210
  degree of descent in, 190–191
  dysfunctional (dystocia), 203
    hypertonic, 206–207
    hypotonic, 207
  episiotomy in, 200
  false vs. true, 188t
  fetal head in, 188, 188f
  fetal heart tones in, 189–190
  fetal jeopardy during, 208–209
  fetal lie in, 188
  fetal loss during, grief and, 205–206
  fetal presentation in, 188–189, 189f
  forceps-assisted birth and, 200–201
  induction of, 198–200
    criteria for, 199
    indications for, 198–199
    methods of, 199
  Leopold's maneuvers in, 189
  lightening in, 186
  mechanism of, cardinal movements in, 190, 190f
  participatory childbirth techniques in, 191
  pelvic structure and configuration in, 187–188
  premonitory signs of, 186
  preterm, 203–205
  prolapsed umbilical cord during, 209
  psychoprophylaxis in, Lamaze method of, 191
  stage(s) of, 187
    first
      amniotic fluid in, 191
      antepartal history and, 191, 193
      contractions during, 191
      nursing actions during, 191, 192f, 193–194
      phases in, 186t–187t
    second, nursing actions during, 193–194
    third, nursing actions during, 194
    fourth
      location and tone of fundus in, 194
      nursing actions during, 194–196
      vaginal flow during, 194
      vital signs during, 194
  suppression of, contraindications to, 204
  uterine contractions during, 187
  uterine rupture during, 207–208
  vacuum extraction birth and, 201
  warning signs during, 191
Laboratory values, neonatal, 228t
Laceration, brain, 602
Lactation, 216–217
  nutrition during, 713
Lactogen, human placental, in pregnancy, 154t
Lactose-free diet, 724
Lamaze method, of psychoprophylaxis, 191
Laminectomy, 634, 639
Language, cultural aspects of, 121
Lansoprazole, 762t
Large for gestational age, 237
Large-cell carcinoma, of lung, 661

Soon you'll graduate and pass your test. Prepare for what comes next.

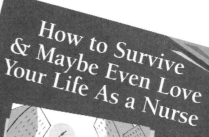

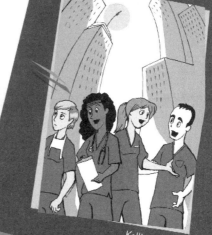

How to Survive
& Maybe Even Love
Your Life As a Nurse

Kelli S. Dunham
Staci J. Smith

How to Survive & Maybe Even Love Your Life As a Nurse

Kelli S. Dunham, RN, BSN
Drexel University, Philadelphia, PA

Staci J. Smith, RN-C
Graduate Hospital, Philadelphia, PA

ISBN 0-8036-1158-7. 2005. 212 pages.

Kelli Dunham has helped thousands learn *How to Survive and Maybe Even Love Nursing School.* Now she and fellow RN Staci Smith, a 20-year nursing veteran, share their knowledge along with that of hundreds of working RNs who love what they do.

How to Survive and Maybe Even Love Your Life as a Nurse is a light-hearted, fresh, and easy-to-read guide that will take you from graduation through your first nursing job and into a successful, fulfilling career. With a healthy dose of comic relief, this life-saving book serves as your mentor and cheerleader, guiding and supporting you through both the challenging and rewarding times ahead. Loaded with solid, specific, practical advice and tools to reduce anxiety, *How to Survive and Maybe Even Love Your Life as a Nurse* is fun to read and definitely worth reading!

- Your job search and evaluating job offers
- Handling difficult patients, co-workers, supervisors, and situations
- Diversity in the workplace
- Managing your finances and your time
- Burnout and coping with stress

Plus you'll find comprehensive lists of resources and real life anecdotes!